D0083520

Berry & Kohn's

Operating Room Technique

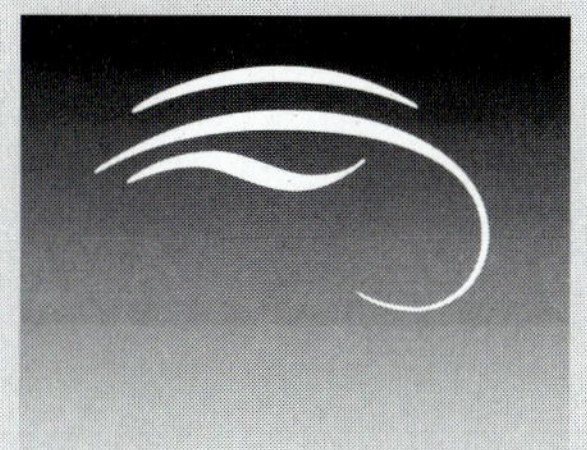

EIGHTH EDITION

Berry & Kohn's Operating Room Technique

Lucy Jo Atkinson, RN, BSN, MS

Consultant in Operating Room Practice
Formerly Director of Educational Services, Ethicon, Inc.
Assistant Director of Nursing for Operating Rooms and Recovery Room
Cedars of Lebanon Hospital, Los Angeles, California

Nancymarie Howard Fortunato, RN, BSN, BA, MEd, RNFA, CNOR

Perioperative Nursing, Cleveland Clinic Foundation, Cleveland, Ohio
Perioperative Program Developer and Educator, Lakeland Community College, Mentor, Ohio
RNFA Program Developer and Educator, Educational Services for Professionals, Ashtabula, Ohio
Consultant for Medical Research and Program Design, Delphi, LTD Professional Services, Wickliffe, Ohio
Captain, United States Army Nurse Corps, Reserve Component
Perioperative Nursing Education, 256th Combat Support Hospital/HUS, Parma, Ohio

with 354 illustrations

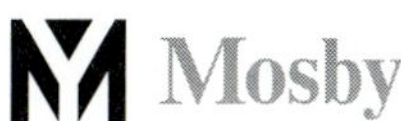

St. Louis Baltimore Boston Carlsbad Chicago Naples New York Philadelphia Portland
London Madrid Mexico City Singapore Sydney Tokyo Toronto Wiesbaden

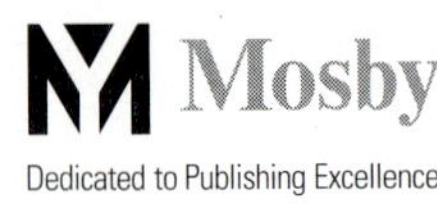

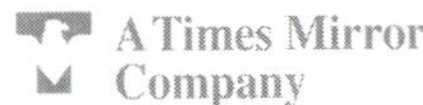

Publisher: Nancy L. Coon
Editor: Michael S. Ledbetter
Editorial Assistant: Julie Council
Project Manager: Linda McKinley
Production Editor: Rich Barber
Manufacturing Supervisor: Linda Ierardi
Editing and Production: Top Graphics
Designer: Elizabeth Fett

EIGHTH EDITION

A Note to the Reader
The author and publisher have made every attempt to check dosages and nursing content for accuracy. Because the science of pharmacology is continually advancing, our knowledge base continues to expand. Therefore we recommend that the reader always check product information for changes in dosage or administration before administering any medication. This is particularly important with new or rarely used drugs.

Printed in the United States of America
Composition by Top Graphics
Printing/binding by Maple-Vail Book Manufacturing Group

Mosby–Year Book, Inc.
11830 Westline Industrial Drive
St. Louis, Missouri 63146

Library of Congress Cataloging-in-Publication Data

Atkinson, Lucy Jo.
Berry & Kohn's operating room technique. — 8th ed. / Lucy Jo Atkinson, Nancymarie Howard Fortunato.
p. cm.
ISBN 0-8151-0103-1
1. Operating room nursing. I. Fortunato, Nancymarie Howard. II. Berry, Edna Cornelia. III. Kohn, Mary Louise. IV. Title.
[DNLM: 1. Operating Room Nursing. 2. Operating Room Technicians. WY 162 A876b 1996]
RD32.3.B4 1996
617'.91—dc20
DNLM/DLC
for Library of Congress 95-41189
CIP

96 97 98 99 00 / 9 8 7 6 5 4 3 2 1

DEDICATED TO

Mary Louise Kohn
whose teachings brought forth this text, with love for perioperative caregivers.
She taught that the patient is the reason for our existence.
Her selflessness is an inspiration.

A N D

To the memory of
Edna Cornelia Berry
whose devotion to teaching was surpassed only by her devotion
to the care of surgical patients in the operating room.

CONSULTANTS

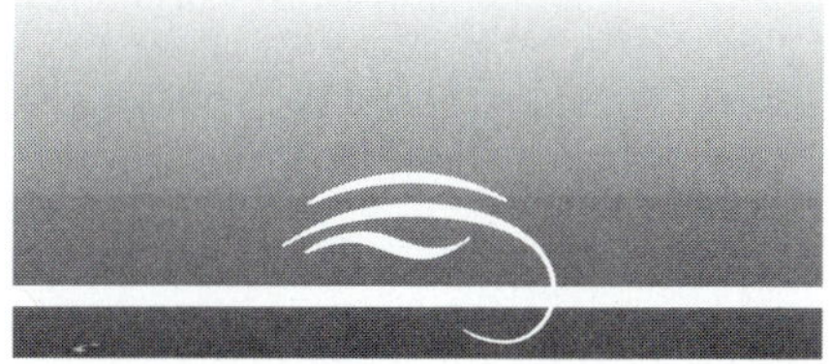

Ruth Bakst, RN, CNOR
Perioperative Educator, St. Luke's Medical Center, Cleveland, Ohio; Registered Nurse-Midwife, Capetown, South Africa

Patricia A. Chapek, RN, BA, CNOR
Perioperative Nursing, Cardiac Department, Cleveland Clinic Foundation, Cleveland, Ohio

Mary Gilley, RN, MS, CNOR
Nurse Clinician, Washington University Medical Center, St. Louis, Missouri

Judith C. Greig, RN, MSN
Nursing Program Director, Lakeland Community College, Mentor, Ohio

Katrina E. Hegedus, RN, BSN, CNOR
Perioperative Nurse Manager, MetroHealth Medical Center, Cleveland, Ohio

Sherrie Holliman, RN, CNOR
Director, Surgical Technology, Thomas Technical Institute, Thomasville, Georgia

H. Patricia P. Kapsar, RN, MBA
Director of Nursing, Bethesda General Hospital; Instructor, Continuing Education, St. Louis Community College, St. Louis, Missouri

Maryann Mawhinney, RN, BSN, CNOR
Perioperative Nursing, Holy Spirit Hospital, Camp Hill, Pennsylvania

Susan M. McCullough, RN, BSN, CNOR
Perioperative Nursing, Eye Institute, Cleveland Clinic Foundation, Cleveland, Ohio

Michelle R. Pamer, RN, RNFA, CNOR
Vitreo Retinal Consultants, Canton, Ohio

Martin A. Phillips III, RN, BSN, CNOR
Director of Perioperative Services, Marymount Hospital, Garfield Heights, Ohio; Captain, United States Army Nurse Corps; Reserve Component, Head Nurse–OR/HUS, 256th Combat Support Hospital, Parma, Ohio

M. Jane Rua, RN, BSN, JD
Attorney at Law, Jeffries, Kube, Forrest, and Monteleone Co., LPA, Cleveland, Ohio

Mary Senna, RN
Westfield Orthopaedic Group, Westfield, New Jersey

Patricia Seymour, RN, MS
Administrator, Educational Services for Professionals; Nursing Educator, Kent State University, Ashtabula, Ohio

Joanne Stolla, RN, RNFA, CNOR, CRNO
Vitreo Retinal Consultants, Canton, Ohio

Mae L. Wykle, RN, PhD, FAAN
Associate Dean for Community Affairs; Professor of Nursing and Director of Center on Aging and Health, Frances Payne Bolton School of Nursing, Case Western Reserve University, Cleveland, Ohio

Student perioperative nurses from Lakeland Community College and RNFA interns from Educational Services for Professionals reviewed each new table and box for this edition.

PREFACE

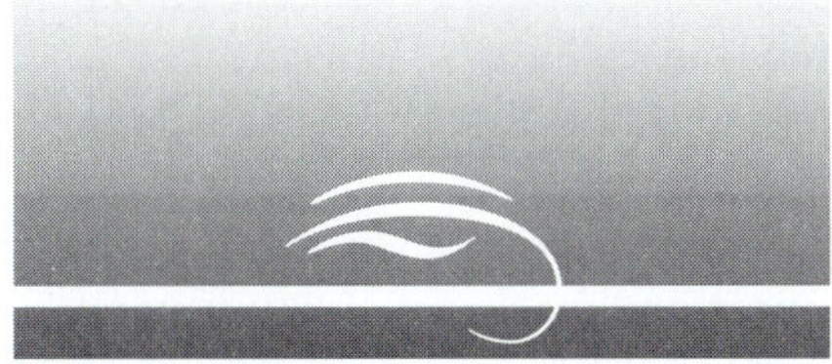

This time-honored text has its roots in the operating room (OR) orientation manual created by Mary Louise Kohn in the late 1940s, while she was working as an OR educator at University Hospitals of Cleveland, Ohio. Her impeccable notes were a source of interest to many OR supervisors and educators, who wanted to standardize their teaching techniques in accordance with Mary Louise's orientation tool. Many observers requested copies of her writings. Eventually, the cost of providing copies became prohibitive. At the suggestion of her superiors in 1951, Mary Louise decided to assemble her material into manuscript style for publication. She spent countless hours writing and revising material until the birth of her daughter. Her dedication to her family led her to seek assistance for this project from Edna Cornelia Berry, who became her willing partner and coauthor throughout the first four editions.

The first edition of *Introduction to Operating Room Technique* by Edna Cornelia Berry and Mary Louise Kohn was published in 1955. Its goals were:

- To explain the principles of sterile and aseptic technique
- To stress the necessity for their application in all surgical procedures
- To provide insight into the physiologic and psychologic impact of surgical intervention on each patient as a unique individual

Every new edition of this classic text has addressed changing needs and evolving technologies, while maintaining the fundamental focus that still remains valid after 40 years, the care of the surgical patient.

Berry and Kohn's Operating Room Technique is designed to meet the needs of educators, learners, and practicing perioperative caregivers. Knowing the "why" of patient care is as important as knowing the "how." A strong emphasis is placed on understanding the rationale behind each patient care activity.

FEATURES

The following features have made *Berry and Kohn's Operating Room Technique* the perioperative text of choice for more than 40 years.

- Focus on the physiologic, psychologic, and spiritual considerations of perioperative patients to provide guidelines and standards for planning and implementing comprehensive individualized care.
- In-depth discussion of patients with special needs related to age or health status considerations with an emphasis on the development of a plan of care tailored to the unique care parameters of these patients.
- Discussion of perioperative patient care for both inpatient and ambulatory procedures to highlight considerations based on the setting as well as the surgical procedure.
- Encouragement of the caregiver to identify and examine personal and professional development issues that influence the manner in which care is rendered.
- Emphasis on teamwork among perioperative caregivers to encourage cooperation in attaining positive patient care outcomes.
- Building of knowledge in a logical sequence from fundamental concepts to implementation during surgical intervention to enable readers to apply theory to practice.
- Presentation of content in a concise, readily accessible modified outline format to enhance reader comprehension and facilitate retrieval of specific information. This is supplemented with an extensive bibliography and cross-referenced index.
- Comprehensive coverage of a broad range of essential topics to provide a thorough understanding of fundamental principles and tech-

niques and an understanding of their applications in various surgical procedures.

NEW TO THIS EDITION

This edition was reviewed, updated, and reorganized into 11 sections with the content synthesized in manageable segments. Educators and learners will find the arrangement user friendly in the classroom setting. The logical and sequential order of the subject matter will enable perioperative caregivers of all educational backgrounds to review and sharpen their knowledge and skill levels. The carefully planned tables, boxes, and figures will further clarify the textual content.

Noteworthy features include the following:

- A new chapter on Postoperative Patient Care provides the reader with an understanding of the recovery process.
- A new chapter on Perioperative Geriatrics discusses the unique needs of older adults, a diverse and growing population.
- Anesthesia coverage has been divided into two chapters—(1) General Anesthesia: Techniques and Agents and (2) Local and Regional Anesthesia.
- Over 200 new illustrations have been added to enhance the visual detail of basic principles and surgical technique.
- New boxes and tables serve to clarify and highlight information critical to perioperative practice.
- The most up-to-date AORN Standards and Recommended Practices and modern terminology have been incorporated to reflect today's perioperative practice.

ORGANIZATION

Section One is dedicated to the learner and the educator. The correlation of theory and practice is integral to the success of patient care in the perioperative environment. Professional and personal attributes of the caregiver are examined, with an emphasis on objectivity in the development of the plan of care.

Section Two delineates team members' roles, both as direct and indirect caregivers. Nonphysician first assistants are discussed.

Section Three develops, in depth, a plan of care with the patient viewed as a unique individual. A new segment on the pregnant surgical patient is featured.

Section Four examines the perioperative environment, occupational hazards, and safety issues.

Section Five delineates aseptic and sterile techniques in fundamental aspects, such as attire, scrubbing, gowning and gloving, sterilization, and disinfection. Processing instrumentation and the safe use of specialized surgical equipment are presented. New illustrations reflect current attire with an emphasis on universal precautions.

Section Six discusses preoperative patient care and includes the family/significant other in the plan of care.

Section Seven covers anesthesia methods and physiologic patient monitoring and related complications.

Section Eight describes intraoperative patient care, including positioning, prepping, and draping. Interactive roles of the circulator and the scrub person are specified. Hemostasis, blood replacement, and intraoperative wound care considerations are discussed in detail. New illustrations reinforce the discussions.

Section Nine presents postoperative patient care, wound infection, and postoperative care of the physical environment. The postanesthesia care unit is explained. Death of a patient is discussed, and the importance of legal evidence is stressed.

Section Ten covers surgical specialties, including diagnostics, presented as individual chapters throughout this section. New illustrations help to clarify procedures.

Section Eleven divides multidisciplinary patient care into categories including ambulatory surgery, pediatrics, geriatrics, organ procurement and transplantation, and surgical oncology.

ANCILLARIES

Perioperative Learner's Resource Manual (Book Code 27886; ISBN 0-8151-0827-3)

This companion resource manual enhances the learner's comprehension and provides exercises for using newly gained knowledge. The manual follows the content of the main text chapter by chapter. It is an excellent tool for reviewing for examinations and applying new information to written course work. Suggested learning activities and additional references are included.

Perioperative Educator's Resource Manual (Book Code 27885; ISBN 0-8151-0826-5)

The educator's resource manual parallels the learner's resource manual but contains additional classroom material, answer keys, and critical thinking exercises to aid in the education process.

Lucy Jo Atkinson
Nancymarie Fortunato

ACKNOWLEDGMENTS

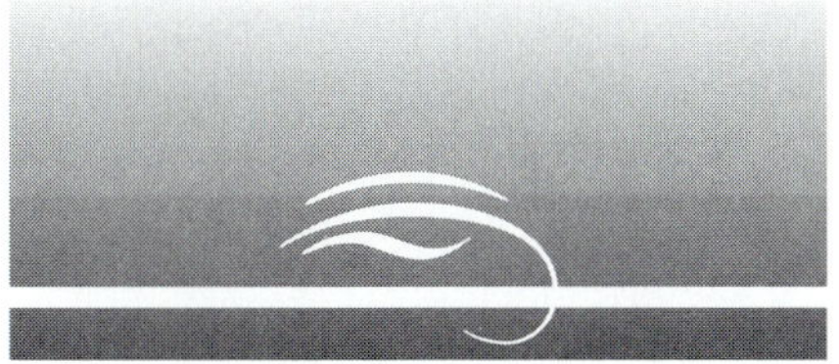

To Nancy Lynam-Davis, MSLS, AHIP, medical librarian at Meridia Hillcrest Hospital, Mayfield Heights, Ohio

To the officers and membership of the Greater Cleveland Chapter of AORN, #3608, for serving as a sounding board for the structural reorganization of this edition

To librarians and library assistants at Cleveland Clinic Foundation, Cleveland, Ohio

To family, friends, and colleagues, who extended endless patience and perseverance during the preparation of this manuscript

To surgeons and anesthesiologists, who were supportive and informative throughout this project

With deep appreciation to Michael Ledbetter, Teri Merchant, and Julie Council, for their guidance and patience in helping make this eighth edition a reality

A special thanks to kind and loving mentors, who believed in miracles and offered encouragement

and especially to

Mary Louise Kohn, who has entrusted her labor of love to our care

CONTENTS

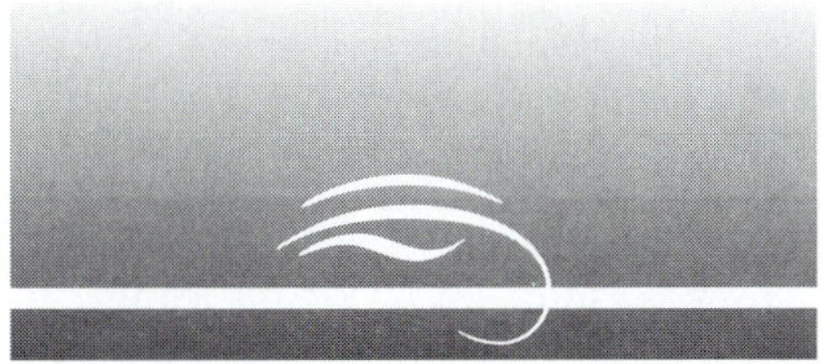

SECTION ONE

Correlation of Theory and Practice

SECTION TWO

The Perioperative Health Care Team

SECTION THREE

The Patient as a Unique Individual

SECTION FOUR

The Surgical Environment

SECTION FIVE

Surgical Asepsis, Instrumentation, and Equipment

SECTION SIX

Preoperative Patient Care

SECTION SEVEN

Anesthesia Concepts and Considerations

SECTION EIGHT

Intraoperative Patient Care

SECTION NINE

Postoperative Care of the Patient and Environment

SECTION TEN

Surgical Specialties

SECTION ELEVEN

Multidisciplinary Perioperative Considerations

SECTION ONE

Correlation of Theory and Practice

CHAPTER 1

Introduction for the Learner

MODERN SURGERY

Health is a personal and economic asset. Needs are altered in proportion to an individual's ability to function normally. *Optimal health* has been defined as the best an individual can feel and function in the particular circumstances or with a disease process. *Disease* is a failure of the adaptive mechanisms to adequately counteract stimuli or stresses, resulting in disturbance in function or structure of any part, organ, or system of the body. *Illness* is often a composite of many reactions or diseases.

Surgical intervention, one step in the total process of restoring or maintaining health, offers hope to those of all ages with conditions that can be treated surgically. The number of surgical procedures performed and anesthetics administered increase annually. This is related to health consciousness of the population, incidence of trauma and congenital abnormalities, increasing number of aged persons with degenerative diseases, developments in biotechnology, and the rapid progress in all facets of medicine. Many former contraindications to surgery have been eliminated. Because of better diagnostic and supportive services and drug therapies, many persons are now considered candidates for surgery.

Surgery designates the branch of medicine that encompasses preoperative preparation, intraoperative judgment and management, and postoperative care of patients. Surgery as a discipline is total care of illness with an extra modality of treatment, the *surgical procedure.* The purpose of a surgical procedure, either invasive or noninvasive, is to correct deformities or defects, repair injuries, alter form or structure, diagnose and cure disease processes, relieve suffering, or prolong life. At the time of the surgical procedure, pathologic conditions are documented and treated. Surgical intervention encompasses more than technical performance of an operative procedure. In fact, the surgical procedure may constitute a minor part of the total therapy for surgical patients. A surgical procedure may be an *invasive* incision into body tissues or entrance into a body cavity or a *noninvasive* manipulation of a body structure. Surgery is both a science and an art.

Surgical science has progressed during the twentieth century far beyond what was envisioned centuries ago. Surgery was not a medical discipline until the time of the Greek physician Galen (130-200 AD). However, it remained primitive and without a scientific base for the next 1200 years. Surgery did not truly progress as a science until the age of technology in this century. Reliable diagnostic techniques and equipment enable physicians to measure precisely the effects of illness and injury and to diagnose and predict surgical outcomes. Surgeons and nurses consult with equipment manufacturers to develop and perfect instrumentation. Knowledge and management of the surgical patient's nutrition and physiologic condition combined with the precise skills of the surgeon enhance the effectiveness and safety of surgical care. Advances in the development of safe anesthetics also have contributed to favorable surgical outcomes. Specialization in all areas of medicine and nursing brings to patient care a vast array of services for helping to determine what is wrong, what needs to be done, and how best to do it. Some of the greatest gains have been in methods for preparing patients for the surgical procedure and caring for them postoperatively in the rehabilitation period. These methods are based on the premise that each patient is unique and requires individualized care.

The art of surgery encompasses the entire surgical team's attitude, which should be one of concern, compassion, and empathy for the patient. Dedication to the safety and welfare of the patient should be manifested by applying scientific knowledge and professional skills. Although surgery can alter the course of a disease process, side effects and potential complications present hazards. Mortality is higher following surgical intervention than after other types of medical management. This is why surgery is the most dramatic branch of medicine, and the one most feared by patients.

DEFINITION OF TERMS

This introductory chapter establishes the framework for an in-depth study of surgical technology and surgical patient care. Terms commonly used throughout the text need to be understood as the basis for learning about and participating in the science and art of surgery (Box 1-1).

REASON FOR SURGICAL INTERVENTION

Patients submit to surgical intervention for a variety of reasons, including:

1. To preserve life (e.g., relief of intestinal obstruction or decompression of a skull fracture)
2. To maintain dynamic bodily equilibrium (e.g., removal of a diseased kidney)
3. To undergo diagnostic procedures (e.g., breast biopsy, bronchoscopy)

BOX 1-1

Glossary of Terms Pertinent to Surgical Patient Care

behavior Actions or conduct indicative of a mental state or predisposition that is influenced by emotions, feelings, beliefs, values, morals, and ethics.

cognition Process of knowing or perceiving, such as learning scientific principles and observing their application.

competency Creative application of knowledge, skills, and interpersonal abilities in fulfilling functions to provide individualized patient care.

disease Failure of the adaptive mechanisms to counteract stimuli or stresses adequately, resulting in disturbance in function or structure of any part, organ, or system of the body.

health, optimal Best an individual can feel and function in the particular circumstance or with a disease process.

illness Composite of many reactions or diseases.

knowledge Organized body of factual information.

learning style Methods used by the learner to understand new information. These may be visual, auditory, tactile, or performance-oriented behaviors.

objectives Written in behavioral terms, statements that determine expected outcomes of a behavior or process.

operation Invasive modality of treatment (i.e., incision into body tissues for purpose of repair or removal, or entrance into a body cavity). Reference is made throughout this text to *surgical procedure*.

perioperative Total surgical experience that encompasses preoperative, intraoperative, and postoperative phases of surgical patient's care.

profession Highly specialized discipline that systematically combines and coordinates unique knowledge, skills, and behavioral attributes.

psychomotor Pertaining to physical demonstration of mental processes (i.e., applying cognitive learning).

skill Application of knowledge into observable, measurable, and quantifiable performance.

standard Usually a written document sanctioned by an authoritative body that directs or guides interventions to achieve objectives.

surgery Branch of medicine that encompasses preoperative, intraoperative, and postoperative care of patients. The work of a surgeon is both a science and an art.

surgical conscience Awareness, which develops from a knowledge base, of the importance of strict adherence to principles of aseptic and sterile techniques.

surgical intervention Therapeutic process to restore or maintain health (i.e., the ability to function).

surgical procedure Invasive incision into body tissues or a minimally invasive entrance into a body cavity for either therapeutic or diagnostic purpose during which protective reflexes or self-care abilities are potentially compromised.

team Group of two or more persons who recognize common objectives and coordinate their efforts to achieve them. The health care team includes all personnel relating to the patient directly or indirectly.

4. To prevent infection and to promote healing (e.g., burn debridement)
5. To obtain comfort (e.g., relief of chronic, persistent pain)
6. To ensure the ability to earn a living (e.g., elective herniorrhaphy)
7. To restore or reconstruct a part of the body that is congenitally malformed or damaged by trauma or disease (e.g., cleft palate, hip reconstruction)
8. To alter cosmetic appearance (e.g., facelift)

Not all surgical procedures are performed in hospitals. Many are performed in surgeons' offices or in independent, nonhospital-based, freestanding surgical facilities if they are not complex enough to require hospitalization. Not all patients undergoing surgical intervention in a hospital-contained operating room (OR) unit are admitted to the hospital. Surgeons view postoperative activity as beneficial rather than hazardous for surgical patients. Consequently, a surgical procedure on an ambulatory care or an outpatient basis is feasible and safe for carefully selected patients. Ambulatory surgery is discussed in Chapter 41. Although reference will be made throughout this text to the *hospital*, the practices and procedures described are applicable in all surgical care settings, including diagnostic and therapeutic environments and facilities.

The types of procedures performed in a hospital or other health care facility vary according to the expertise of the surgeons on the staff, the community in which the facility is located, and the equipment available. The daily schedule of surgical procedures is as variable as the type of facility and the types of surgical procedures performed. Regardless of the circumstances that bring patients to the OR, the intraoperative phase of care becomes an integral part of nursing service, filling a need that cannot be met by the individual patient or his or her family. Nursing care of patients undergoing surgical intervention as the therapeutic modality of choice is carried out at two levels: professional and technical. The purpose of this text is to provide a basis for learning professional and technical issues that make the surgical patient unique in all aspects of nursing care.

LEARNER

The beginning learner in the OR may be either a medical, nursing, or surgical technology student enrolled in a formalized educational program. Medical students have a surgical rotation that includes participation in operative procedures. They should learn some of the basic principles of surgical technology to ensure the safety and welfare of patients.

Some schools of nursing offer a course in perioperative nursing either in the core curriculum or as a student elective. However, education for first-level entry into professional practice prepares nurses to be generalists. After graduation from any program, the nurse needs further preparation in the clinical area of specialization. This may take place in a postbasic/postgraduate perioperative nursing course offered by a community college or a hospital. The purpose of a formalized postgraduate program is to meet the nurse's needs for theoretical and technical knowledge and to provide supervised clinical experience. This may be offered through a well-planned and well-taught on-the-job inservice educational program, plus self-study, or through an internship program sponsored by a hospital. Participants in these programs may be registered nurses (RNs) or licensed practical/vocational nurses (LPNs/LVNs) who have recently graduated, desire a change in clinical practice setting, or are reentering the profession.

Because of the rapidly advancing technology creating the need for specialized competencies, all practicing surgeons, operating room nurses, and surgical technologists should continuously learn new procedures and technologies. An experienced nurse or surgical technologist new to a particular practice setting should learn the specific performance expectations of that institution. All personnel should go through an orientation process to introduce them to the philosophy, goals, policies, procedures, role expectations, and physical facilities. All learners in the OR environment are adults. Therefore, regardless of level of learning, advanced or beginning, the general characteristics of the adult learner apply.

1. As a person matures, time perspective changes from one of postponed application of knowledge to immediacy of application. Accordingly, learning shifts from a subject-centered orientation to a problem-solving approach. Adults will learn what they need to know to solve problems (i.e., to function effectively).
2. An ego involvement, with a positive goal-oriented self-concept, moves an adult from a dependent personality toward that of a self-directed individual, who wants to be responsible for his or her own behavior. Learning is performance based.
3. The readiness to learn becomes oriented to the need to increase developmental skills. Adults with a high level of self-esteem are responsive to learning. Learning is enhanced in an environment that does not threaten self-concept and self-esteem. It is a normal adult activity.
4. As experience accumulates, the resources for learning enhance individual participation and involvement in the learning process (i.e., practical application of developing skills through an expanded knowledge base). Immediate feedback helps focus on objectives and accomplishments. The adult learner enjoys participation in the planning, implementation, and evaluation of learning.

5. Motivation for learning new behaviors intensifies through achievement of learning objectives. The subjective feelings of successful learning promote the desire to learn more.
6. The fear of failure to learn will decrease the adult learner's desire to be a risk taker as an independent decision maker. Although not a function of the beginning learner, major decision making is a function of practicing health care providers. As knowledge and confidence increase, so does the ability to make decisions. In the learning environment, the learner needs to be supported for honest mistakes made during the learning process. Evaluation of learning attainment should be an ongoing process to assist the learner in gaining the knowledge and skill necessary for decision making.

Not everyone learns at the same speed or assimilates information in the same manner. Theoretical knowledge or a skill learned quickly by one learner may be difficult for another. Learning styles vary among individuals. Influencing factors include:

1. Intelligence/intellect
2. Cultural background
3. Educational background
4. Motivation to learn
5. Personality characteristics
6. Psychologic strengths or deficiencies
7. Social skills, including communication skills
8. Manual dexterity
9. Physical senses
10. Perceptual preferences and sensory partiality (e.g., visual vs. auditory)
11. Environment

Each hospital has a learner/beginner level of work more or less defined. In most hospitals, beginning learners are not used to fill staff positions. Learners actually help prepare for, assist during, and clean up following surgical procedures. Novices will not be expected to assume responsibilities for which they are not fully prepared. Only through continued study and experience can individuals qualify as team members during the most complex surgical procedures.

The learner is usually taught the scrub role functions at the operating table early in the OR experience. These functions are discussed in detail in Chapter 20 and throughout this text. At first, an experienced instructor, preceptor, or other staff member scrubs with the new person, gradually permitting the learner to take over more of the work in the sterile field until the learner is able to function without help. The types of surgical procedures to which the novice may be assigned vary from hospital to hospital, depending on many factors peculiar to each. However, rarely does the beginning learner scrub on surgical procedures of the heart, lung, hip, or brain.

Since one of the objectives of learning is to gain a thorough knowledge of sterile technique, repetition of the scrub functions serves a valuable purpose by impressing it indelibly in the mind of the learner. It is better to learn the fundamentals thoroughly than to try to observe many complicated surgical procedures and retain little. Knowing how to do a procedure is not enough. All OR procedures should be practiced. Greater satisfaction is sensed as skill is gained. To make the experience as profitable as possible, the learner should assist in circulating duties in addition to performing scrub functions. This necessitates constant supervision and help from the instructor or another experienced staff member. Contribution to the accomplishment of the work of the entire team becomes real and is a necessary part of the learning process.

The learner is not the only one who benefits from this learning process. The OR team gains from each learner contact. The surgeons actively participate in the learning experience by acquainting the learner with patients' situations, by explaining why surgical procedures are being performed, and by answering questions.

CLINICAL INSTRUCTOR

Experience in the OR clinical setting should be planned and supervised. Learning objectives should be established and evaluated. A designated resource person, either a faculty member or nursing staff member employed by the hospital, is available to instruct and assist the learner in competently applying newly acquired knowledge and skills. The term *instructor* will be used throughout this text to refer to the resource person responsible for planning, implementing, and evaluating the learner's experiences in the classroom, self-study laboratory, and clinical OR setting. The instructor who is a faculty member employed by a teaching institution may not be a member of the hospital staff. Hospitals offering the clinical setting for educational programs have their own policies and procedures that should be adapted and adhered to by both the instructor and the learner. During clinical experience, the instructor supervises learner activities.

The instructor should consider the impact on the learner seeing the OR for the first time. The room can appear large and overwhelming to a learner who has not seen one before. A tour of the facility before actually beginning the program can help decrease the learner's anxiety. Personal or subjective traits such as emotional stability, social skills, and psychologic characteristics should continually be assessed by the instructor. An ill-tempered, easily angered learner can be very difficult to deal with as a future team member. The learner who does not have assertive skills in dealing with a stressful event also cannot function effectively. Subjective responses should be monitored and should remain on a professional level for the team to function efficiently. Learning is more effective when the instructor takes the learning style and its influence into consideration when developing a program of instruction.

The instructor objectively assesses the learner's skills and knowledge. When deficiencies are identified, the learner should be provided with the appropriate learning experiences to enable the attainment of his or her highest potential. The learner takes an active role in the teaching/learning process. By identifying learner needs, behavioral objectives are determined; then effective and organized educational experiences can be developed. The instructor and the learner should establish behavioral objectives within the guidelines of the anticipated future scope of practice. Evaluation of the learner's progress is measured by how successfully the learner has met the behavioral objectives.

The instructor should use a variety of approaches with learners to enable them to achieve the identified behavioral objectives. Skill in questioning and encouragement in making discoveries and correlations allow the learner to use critical thinking as a learning tool. A structured curriculum employs written guidelines and relevant assignments for feedback to ensure that learning has taken place. Learner conferences should be held on a regular basis to discuss procedures and problems. Positive reinforcement helps the learner build confidence and competence. The instructor should not punish a learner for making honest errors during supervised learning. Degradation and damage to self-esteem are barriers that will not facilitate learning. The learner should not be put in a position to perform any function for which he or she has not had adequate training or guided practice.

The organization of the material to be taught and the experiences to be assigned are further enhanced by the way the program is presented. The elements of effective instruction may be summarized as follows:

1. Set clear and concise behavioral objectives that are measurable in performance terminology descriptive of knowledge, comprehension, application, analysis, understanding, and evaluation.
2. Establish a learning environment that is controlled by the instructor.
3. Provide stimulus variation in presenting material. Videotapes and photographs can be alternated with lecture and hands-on practice. The opportunity to handle instruments and supplies in a classroom is less threatening than handling them in the OR for the first time.
4. Encourage the exchange of questions as an assessment tool. Many times learners will ask exactly what they need to know. The instructor can determine areas of knowledge deficit.
5. Reinforce learning. After a skill has been taught, provide guided practice in the clinical laboratory before actually performing the task in the OR. Provide positive support for desired behaviors. Self-assessment and performance assessment provide feedback about the learner's progress.
6. Provide a summary of the day's accomplishments. Review of the activities helps reinforce the learning process by allowing the learner to associate the events of his or her experience with newly acquired knowledge.

The instructor should work closely with the OR nurse manager. Classroom hours and clinical experience assignments are worked out together. The manager offers suggestions and constructive criticism for the benefit of the learner. The instructor offers suggestions for the experiences of the learner. The manager is aware of the program planned for the learner. An effort is made to confer and to coordinate any changes in the program. This fosters a friendly and cooperative relationship. The manager is advised of each learner's progress. The instructor maintains a list of procedures for each surgical service on which learners have scrubbed or circulated. This enables the nurse manager to identify experience needed by each learner when making out assignments.

The instructor should also acquaint the entire OR staff with the proposed learning experiences. All staff members should assist in teaching the learners within the guidelines of the structured learning experience. Everyone should be familiar with the level of the learners, the learning objectives, and the roles that staff members will be expected to assume with respect to teaching.

The instructor should determine in what areas the learner is knowledgeable and in what areas additional experience is needed. A competency-based skills inventory checklist can assist in identifying learning needs (Box 1-2). This involves rating the actual skills and knowledge of the learner against a standardized listing of the skills and knowledge required for optimum performance. This framework provides a means for the learner to identify his or her own learning needs and to request new learning experiences.

The instructor provides a checklist of work assignments for the learners. Learners check off their assignments as they observe or complete them. New assignments are made each day from this list, according to the experience needs of each learner. Learners should avail themselves of every opportunity to learn by observation and practice to enhance their competency.

BOX 1-2

Learner Skills Checklist

This is an abbreviated sample of psychomotor skills (elaborated further in Chapter 20) that a learner must master to perform scrub role.

S = Satisfactory U = Unsatisfactory	S	U	Comments
Wears OR attire properly			
Housekeeping duties: Before first operation of day			
Between operations			
Sterile supplies: Check integrity of package			
Check sterility indicator			
Opening: Muslin wrappers			
Paper wrappers			
Sealed packages			
Sutures			
Packs			
Scrubs per procedure			
Gowns correctly			
Gloves: Closed method			
Open method			
Assist surgeon			
Sterile set-up: Drape tables			
Cover Mayo stand			
Counts: Sponges			
Sharps			
Instruments			
Arrangement of instruments			
Knife blades on handles			
Suture preparation			

LEARNING RESOURCES

Some learning of OR technique can take place in a classroom setting or a self-study laboratory. Lecture and demonstration may be given to learners who then practice the procedure, which, in turn, is followed by the instructor's evaluation of their performance. Books, journals, films, slides, photographs, and other audiovisual materials may supplement the lecture approach. Live closed-circuit television and interactive telecommunication systems permit instructors and learners to communicate from remote locations. Many audiovisual materials, such as videodiscs and audiotapes, computer-assisted instruction (CAI), and computer-assisted interactive video instruction (CAIVI) are self-contained units for self-study. A bibliography in a text such as this provides reference leads to add to and broaden the learner's theoretical knowledge. The volume of literature is almost without limit. Each instructor plans classes or self-study units according to available materials and learner needs. Selection of appropriate instructional methods will depend on availability of time, facilities, and equipment and on class size, learner capabilities, subject matter, and objectives. Review of a videotape of a learner's performance in a laboratory setting can be a useful tool, for example, to help the learner self-critique and to assist the instructor in providing feedback. The following are useful resources for acquiring and reinforcing knowledge:

1. *Library and literature file.* Books and current periodicals are available for learner reference in the department library. These may be found in the manager's office, the nursing staff lounge, or the classroom or conference room if there is one within the OR suite. In addition to books and periodicals, educational literature is available from surgical supply and instrument manufacturers. The literature that accompanies new equipment is of inestimable value to all the staff and to learners. This is filed and kept available as part of the inservice educational program.
2. *Computer database information systems.* Several networks are available to research topics of interest for self-study or to supplement classroom presentations.
   a. *Cumulative Index to Nursing and Allied Health Literature (CINAHL)* is the most widely used index for nursing and allied health. In addition to the printed version, the on-line computer version is available through the database vendors DIALOG, BRS, and Data-Star. The database includes indexing by subject headings from virtually all English-language nursing journals and allied health literature from January 1983, with bimonthly updates. CINAHL also indexes pertinent articles from the medical literature and lists nursing and allied health books.
   b. *NurseSearch* is a computer retrieval system from 60 nursing journals by subject or author. Software and data on floppy disks can be used with all IBM-compatible personal computers.
   c. *Medical Literature Analysis and Retrieval System On-Line (MEDLINE)* is a computer-based reference system available at most libraries in institutions and government agencies in the United States and Canada. More than 3000 biomedical journals, including nursing journals, are referenced. The file contains references dating from 1966 at the National Library of Medicine.
   d. *Audiovisual On-Line (AVLINE)* is a database of references to audiovisual aids in the health sciences. Established by the National Library of Medicine, AVLINE is available through the same networks as MEDLINE.
   e. *CARL* is a computer access system to books and journals published by the Association of Operating Room Nurses, Inc. Personal computers and modems or a library's interfacing system can access these references.
   f. *Educational Technology Network (E.T. NET)* is an electronic conferencing system to share and exchange information about existing interactive instructional materials, hardware, and all types of software. The system is accessible via Internet, SprintNet, and DATA PAC.
3. *Videotape library.* The Hospital Satellite Network (HSN) is a telecommunication service provided to hospitals. Subscribers can view videotape programs transmitted by satellite. *Video Journal* provides a new videotape program to subscribers every 2 months. These are but two of several sources of audiovisual programs available for purchase or rental. Many sales representatives from equipment and instrumentation manufacturers offer free educational videotapes.

BEHAVIORAL OBJECTIVES

The surgical procedure itself is the focal point of the perioperative experience for the patient. Management of this critical act requires an educated team whose members understand the dynamics of the problems presented and the methods to solve them. Each team member is responsible for maintaining the knowledge and skills necessary for safe and efficient performance. The learner, as he or she progresses through the learning process, should accomplish a baseline level of knowledge and assume responsibility for progressing along a continuum to develop advanced skills.

Behavioral objectives should be written in behavioral terms and based on standards of expected performance and accepted standards of patient care. Therefore the concepts to be learned and the objectives to be met for all beginning learners of OR technology should include the following as a basis on which to build their practice. Each behavioral objective is measurable and can be evaluated by performance standards.

1. To demonstrate ability to apply the principles of sterilization, disinfection, and aseptic and sterile techniques in preparation and use of all supplies and equipment under all conditions and circumstances imperative to prevent the potential eventuality of an environmentally acquired infection.
2. To increase and clarify knowledge of anatomy and physiology in normal structure and function and of pathophysiology altered by disease

processes. This knowledge will be demonstrated by the ability to position patients on the operating table correctly and to select appropriate instrumentation, equipment, and supplies.

3. To comprehend the interrelationships between physiologic, ethnocultural, and psychosocial factors that affect patients' and their families' adaptation to the risk factors and outcomes of surgical intervention.
4. To identify the procedures necessary to prepare each patient as an individual for the intended surgical procedure.
5. To demonstrate an understanding of the surgical procedures by anticipating the needs of OR team members and by organizing work efficiently in the best interests of patients' safety and welfare.
6. To understand actions and uses of anesthetic agents, fluids, and electrolytes and patients' responses to them by having appropriate supplies available in the event of adverse reactions.
7. To understand the principles of wound management and healing and to prevent inadvertent trauma during surgical intervention.
8. To identify the potential environmental dangers to the patient through an understanding of the function and care of surgical instruments, supplies, and equipment.
9. To identify the members of the OR team and the legal responsibility of each for the care of the conscious or the unconscious patient as a basis for maintaining continuity of patient care.
10. To participate in making decisions that demonstrate willingness to collaborate with members of the OR team to ensure positive patient outcomes.
11. To function as a team member by showing consideration for and cooperation with others within the OR and by communicating with the interdependent departments of the hospital that work together for the well-being of the patient.
12. To develop flexibility, adaptability, manual dexterity, and self-reliance as a team member by acquiring a working knowledge of all aspects of the OR environment and the functions of all personnel.
13. To develop self-control and the ability to manage personal anxiety by learning basic techniques that enable the correct responses to emergency or stressful situations and to normal circumstances.
14. To identify factors that create stress among the members of the OR team as a basis for evaluating and modifying own behavior to enhance personal participation in the team effort on behalf of the patient.
15. To exert a conscientious effort to carry out all duties accurately and with integrity, in compliance with hospital policies and recognized standards of practice, and thus to develop pride in performance consistent with personal, professional, and vocational ethical and moral values.
16. To help control patient and hospital costs through the correct, safe, and economical use of supplies and equipment and personal efficiency in time and motion.

APPLICATION OF THEORY TO PRACTICE

Learning is a process of discovery and mastery of skills. Performance-based learning to function competently in an environment such as the OR should take place on three levels: cognitive, psychomotor, and affective (Figure 1-1). The learner should understand the scientific principles (cognitive learning) underlying the technical skills (psychomotor learning) and appreciate the necessity for adhering to these principles (affective learning). In simpler terms, the learner should know why to do what (cognitive), how (psychomotor), when, where, and by whom (affective).

Reading the literature, using audiovisual teaching aids, and attending lectures are only part of providing adequate preparation for clinical practice. Skills are gained by active participation. Practice will give the learner an opportunity to apply his or her knowledge of the basic sciences. Theory becomes meaningful and of value only when it is put to practical use. Some learning will be accomplished through observation, but skills will be learned through actual hands-on experience in applying the theory learned in the classroom or self-study laboratory.

In the OR the learner will see living anatomy; its alteration by congenital deformities, disease, or injury; and its restoration or reconstruction. Experience in the OR enables the learner to be a more understanding, observant, and efficient person. In close teamwork with surgeons and anesthesiologists, the nurse and the surgical technologist participate in vital resuscitative measures and learn to care for anesthetized, unconscious, and/or critically ill patients. Learning to function in life-threatening situations is critical to the patient's welfare. In addition, the learner discovers that emergencies such as cardiac arrest are more easily prevented than treated. He or she gains valuable experience applicable to any nursing situation by learning:

1. To fully realize what surgical intervention in all its aspects means to a patient. The learner will understand the *whys* of postoperative pain, complications, and care.
2. To realize the importance of optimal physical and emotional preoperative preparation for all patients and the need for constant patient observation intraoperatively.

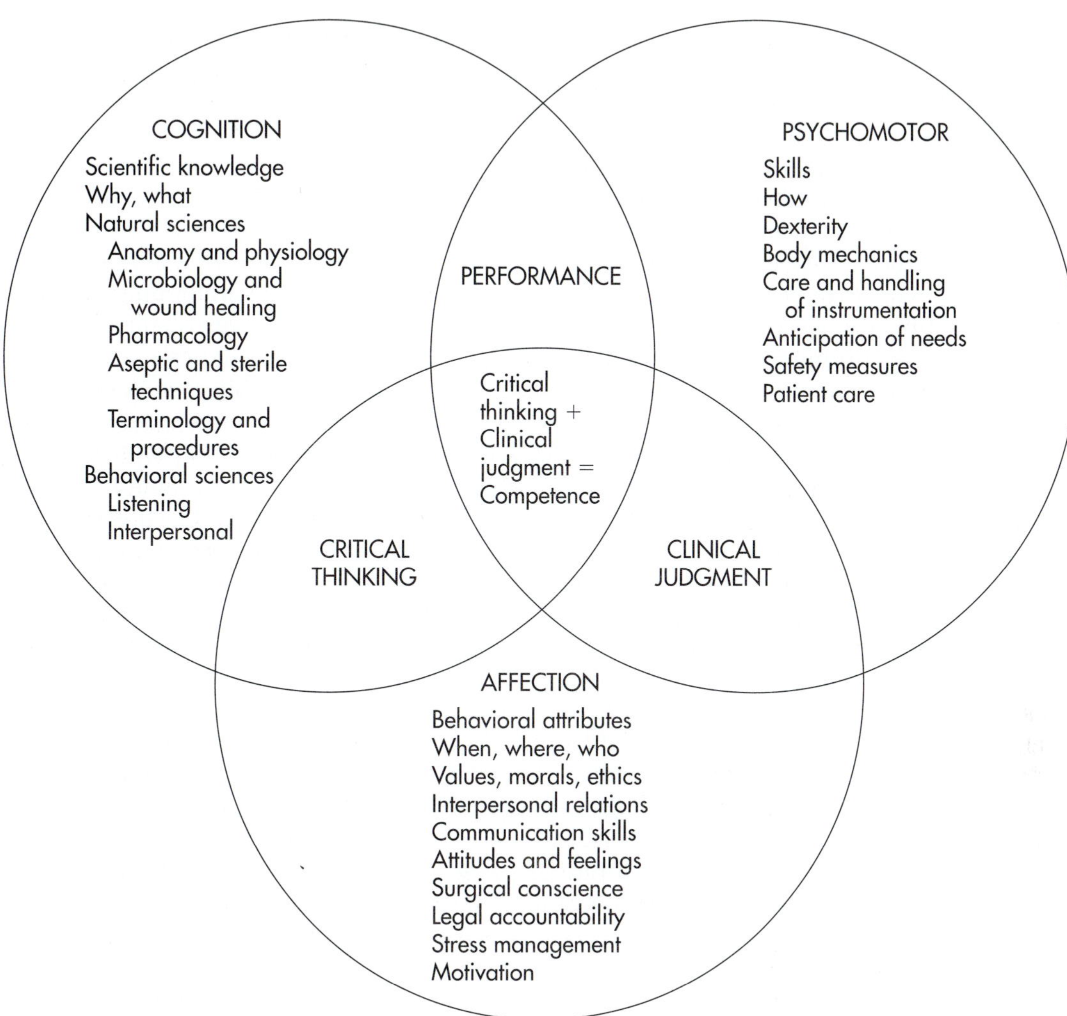

FIGURE 1-1 Performance-based learning takes place on three levels: cognition, psychomotor, and affection.

3. To differentiate between seemingly innocuous occurrences and situations that, if unrecognized and allowed to progress, will lead to injury of the patient or a team member or damage to departmental equipment.
4. To cope with any situation in a calm, efficient manner and to think clearly and act quickly in an emergency.
5. To attend to every pertinent detail, to observe keenly, and to anticipate the needs of the patient and of colleagues.
6. To understand the importance of aseptic and sterile techniques and to comprehensively and conscientiously apply knowledge to practice.

Above all, OR experience teaches that *no surgical procedure is a minor event to the surgical patient!* The only predictable element in the OR is the potential for the unpredictable occurrence. Surgical procedures may be classified as major or minor by hospitals for practical use, but in reality no such distinction exists. Every procedure has a deep personal meaning for each patient, and the possibility of death cannot be ruled out completely. All invasive procedures carry an element of inherent risk. A relatively safe procedure can rapidly become catastrophic, even fatal, if the patient is allergic to a medication or anesthetic drug, if uncontrollable bleeding develops, if irreversible shock occurs, if overwhelming postoperative infection develops, or if he or she experiences cardiac arrest on the operating table. Although every precaution is taken to foresee and prevent adverse reactions, such reactions do occur on occasion. No matter how simple a procedure may be, an experienced OR team member is highly aware of potential problems that may occur and gives undivided attention to the patient at *all* times.

During the learning experience, the learner may participate in or observe the preparation of OR supplies and learn their use. With practice, the learner will gain an appreciation of the precision with which surgical instruments and equipment are made for particular functions. Also, in helping to carry out a daily schedule of surgical procedures, the learner will become aware of the interdependence of the various departments of the hospital and how they work together for the well-being of the patient. One of the most valuable learning experiences in the OR is the opportunity to see and become a part of real teamwork in action.

EXPECTED BEHAVIORS OF OPERATING ROOM PERSONNEL

Nurses are expected to be both human and humane, as well as competent. The standard for the behavior of all OR nursing personnel is no less high. The ability to perform duties successfully contributes to efficient teamwork, but more important, to patients' sense of security. Perceived behavior makes a lasting impression that patients associate with their experiences in the OR. It reveals self-confidence (or lack of it), interest (or indifference), proficiency and authority (or incompetence). In addition to possessing special technical expertise, OR personnel should have personal attributes and communication skills that inspire confidence and trust in patients and team members.

Personal Attributes

Personal attributes are reflected in the manner in which an individual performs his or her duties. These inherent characteristics that contribute to quality of patient care include the following:

1. *Empathy.* Feeling persons can put themselves in another's place to understand what the other person is experiencing. Although caregivers are aware of the emotional needs of patients, the care given is not rendered in a subjective manner. As allies of patients, they convey compassion and a sense of personal worth. They understand and are sensitive to feelings, values, viewpoints, and actions. Yet they do not let emotions indiscriminately obscure or override professional judgment or interfere with care. Caring can be painful for the caregiver too, so caring persons can be vulnerable. To insulate against anxiety, suffering, or even death, nursing personnel sometimes lose their ability to interact with patients or colleagues.

   The sedated patient is not totally unaware of the OR environment. Soft-spoken, reassuring words and a gentle touch are ways to express concern. Members of the team should not hesitate to communicate empathy to a patient. Many patients are not sedated before arrival in the OR. They are acutely aware of their unfamiliar surroundings and are in need of empathy from the OR team.
2. *Conscientiousness.* Persons with this quality will not compromise or sacrifice principles of self-accountability. A *surgical conscience* implies an awareness of the importance of strictly applying knowledge to ensure quality in practice. The entire OR team should take a personal interest in the activities within the OR suite and be alert to potential situations that could compromise integrity. They should approach every procedure in the same way they would want to have it approached if it were being performed on them or their family members.
3. *Efficiency and good organization.* Persons who develop organized work habits are assured that the patients are properly prepared and the OR is ready with the required equipment in working order. They anticipate the needs of patients and team members to save time and energy. They are prepared for the unexpected. Efficiency provides reassurance and comfort to patients, surgeons, and the entire OR team.
4. *Flexibility and adaptability.* Team members react quickly to changing circumstances in a calm, efficient manner and appropriately respond by altering the routine as necessary. Discriminating judgment prepares adaptable people to cope with all situations with professional decorum.
5. *Sensitivity and perception.* Perceptive persons exhibit genuine interest and kindness in caring for patients. Perceptive people are sensitive to the special needs of the people in their environment. OR team members should develop a sense of caring for each other as people and try to understand the subjective aspects of working together in an often tense, fast-paced environment. Patience and kindness should be prevailing attitudes of team members.
6. *Understanding, reassuring, and supportive nature.* In a kind and emotionally controlled way, team members allow others to express their feelings. This approach conveys to the patient the team's ability to relieve physical and emotional discomfort. Holding the patient's hand during the induction of anesthesia is one way of demonstrating support. A nonjudgmental stance while assisting a new team member develop a new skill is very reassuring and leads to successful attainment of competency. Overt anger and hostility are never acceptable at any time in the OR.
7. *Good listening, observation, and communication skills.* People who are attentive, observant, and

listen will act effectively. Aware personnel will not underestimate the importance of communication in their relations with patients and colleagues.

8. *Consideration.* Individuals with this quality respect other people's rights and belief systems and do not automatically reject views different from their own. They convey to patients and colleagues an interest in them as unique persons and act accordingly. All personnel should be aware of ethnocultural differences and demonstrate respect for the personal value systems of others. Consideration extends to all interpersonal relationships. A pleasant smile and active listening can make a difficult situation easier to bear.
9. *Informative and sincere approach.* OR personnel should answer questions and share pertinent information for the mutual benefit of patients, families or significant others, and colleagues. All health care team members should have the same information to deal honestly and factually with patients and their families. Sharing information and forewarning can avoid problems. Nurses should explain procedures before performing them and provide the rationale. Patients must never be permitted to feel lost, confined, or abandoned. Control and trust are enhanced by knowledge. Patients have greater confidence when an open, facilitating approach is used. The OR team should reinforce the physicians' explanations.
10. *Objectivity.* Individuals who are objective assemble factual data before making a judgment. They view situations from all sides before taking action. Objectivity requires experience and self-discipline. This attribute does not exclude concern, but neither is it based on personal, subjective feelings. Team members should remain sensitive to problems without imposing their own values or beliefs on another.
11. *Impartial, nonjudgmental, open-minded approach.* Individuals who take this approach set value judgments aside when making decisions and do not permit their own values and attitudes to distort observations. They accept others as they are without attaching conditions to acceptance.
12. *Versatility.* Persons who are versatile have a comprehensive knowledge of instrumentation and equipment. They are familiar with numerous surgical procedures and the care required for many diverse patients. They approach each procedure as unique and individualized, while maintaining acceptable performance standards.
13. *Analytical nature.* Persons who are analytical are competent in analyzing and correlating significant data about the procedure, the patient, and the needs of the team. They know the *why* as well as the *how* of surgical intervention. Analytical persons are able to anticipate the unexpected and to prevent problems from developing into crises.
14. *Creativity.* Creative individuals are innovative in devising effective methods of approach to meeting the individual needs of patients and colleagues by using available resources. Many major innovations in surgical equipment and supplies have been developed by OR teams that identified a need for something new or different.
15. *Humanistic approach.* OR team members act in a humane way toward others. They consider the patient as a person not as a surgical procedure. The OR team should not make the patient or colleagues the center of jokes and hurtful comments.
16. *Sense of humor.* People with a sense of humor can maintain a balance for their own mental health through their perception of the ironies in life situations. Laughter can ease tension, but not at someone's expense or at an inappropriate time.
17. *Manual and intellectual dexterity.* Dexterous people have quick hands, sharp minds, and keen eyes. Manual dexterity, inherent in most OR team members, is perfected with experience.
18. *Endurance.* Personnel with endurance are able to maximize their physical and emotional capacities and stamina. OR personnel interact in a critical setting under stress, often for prolonged periods. Continual demands are made on them for keen observation, rapid judgment, and fast action. All personnel must be prepared for disaster and work rapidly, often under pressure, without sacrificing competency. Each team member is responsible for maintaining good health habits that enhance personal performance.
19. *Intellectual eagerness and curiosity.* The entire OR team has a legal responsibility to remain current in their knowledge. Documented proof of continuing education and demonstrated competence in performing functions are of value in litigation. Educational development is a dynamic, ongoing process. Continuing education is a shared responsibility of the hospital, the nursing service, and the individual. Learning is not just subject-centered, but problem-centered. Participating in research improves nursing practice and patient care.
20. *Ethical manner.* Persons with this nature use ethical principles, moral values, and professional codes as the basis for making decisions and solving problems. Personal values do influence behavior, but they should not violate the legal or ethical rights of patients or the hospital. Personnel should always be honest and truthful. They should respect the equality of human rights and the dignity of others as human beings but also

"to thine own self be true." Ethical dilemmas should be resolved in the best interest of all involved (see Chapter 4).

Communication Skills

Communication is the basis for the continuum of patient care and for teamwork among the staff. Relationships between people are established through communication. Therefore it is important for the perioperative caregiver to know and understand communication skills.

Communication is a process by which meanings are exchanged between individuals. The process is cyclical. Each communicator influences and is influenced by the other. Communication is both proactive and reactive, causative and purposive. In therapeutic communication the goals are patient-directed and patient-centered. Communication is effective only when the patient and caregivers understand one another. A capacity for sincerity and empathy is the most effective constituent of communication. Communication is necessary for successful interpersonal relations and serves to clarify actions.

Principles of Communication Process

Some principles of the communication process (Figure 1-2) are as follows:

1. Communication incorporates:
   a. Sender (speaker, encoder).
   b. Message sent via a transmission channel (verbal, nonverbal).
   c. Receiver (listener, decoder).
2. Goals are to inform, to obtain information, to release tension, to explore problems.
3. Channels of communication are:
   a. Verbal—words convey content of message through speaking and listening or writing and reading. Verbal communication through language is directed toward patient care, for example, by conferring about patient problems, teaching, and providing interdisciplinary liaison on behalf of the patient.
   b. Nonverbal—body language, including eye contact, facial expression, tone of voice, inflection of voice, gestures, posture, body movements, to convey feelings. Pictures, diagrams, and other visuals also are forms of nonverbal communication. Nonverbal communication provides clues to feelings and attitudes. We often communicate through nonverbal channels without realizing it. Actions often speak louder than words. When the patient is feeling sad, lonely, or isolated, touch is an effective means of communicating empathy, for example.
4. Sender puts thoughts into words or some other channel of communication, then transmits idea in the form of a message to receiver who attempts to understand the thought. The mind decodes messages on the basis of previous experiences, prejudices, culture, moods, values, attitudes, feelings, and current motives.
5. Communication is facilitated by active listening. Listening involves physiologic, cognitive, and psy-

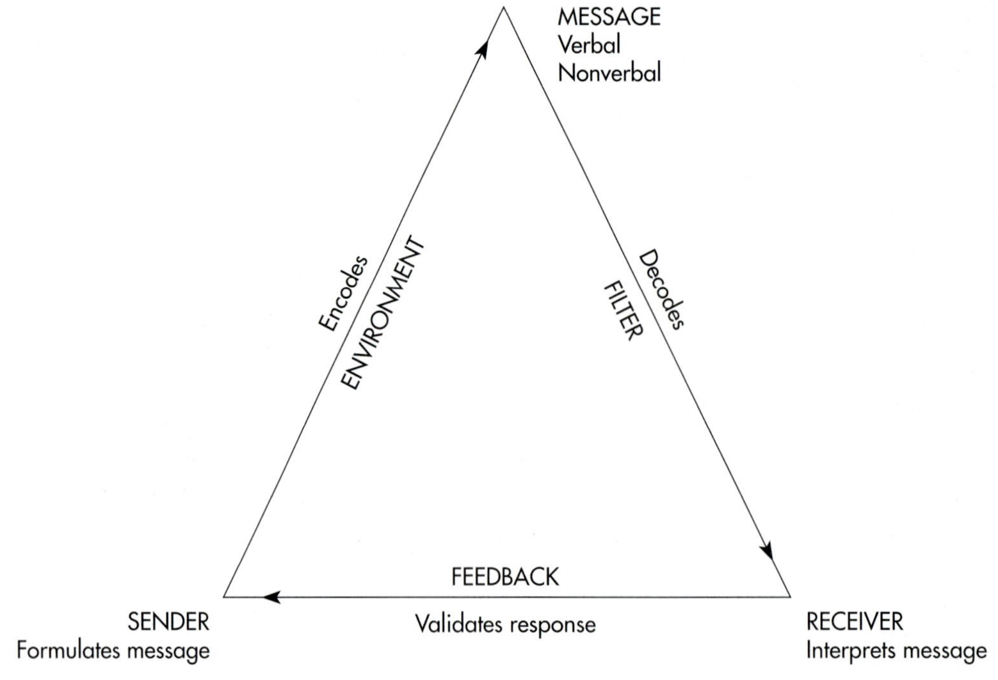

FIGURE 1-2 Communication process.

chologic processes. Physiologically, sounds are heard. Cognitive ability interprets words and influences response to them. The psychologic state of mind and relationship between sender and receiver affect communication interactions. The mnemonic EARS may help to enhance listening skill.

E	*Eye contact:*	Look into speaker's eyes.
A	*Attentive:*	Give speaker your attention.
R	*Receptive:*	Acknowledge message speaker is conveying without judgment.
S	*Sensitive:*	Respond positively to speaker's message.

6. Setting for communication and attitudes of those involved influence the degree of effectiveness. An individual's emotional state affects listening. An anxious patient or learner may not hear, may misunderstand, or may draw erroneous conclusions.
7. Communication should be source-centered rather than message-centered. Unqualified statements are avoided.
8. Prerequisites are to know what you are going to say and to say what you mean. As the speaker, verify or paraphrase until you are convinced the receiver has the message.
9. Variations of meanings that a message can have are:
   a. What the speaker means to say—what the speaker actually says.
   b. What the receiver hears—what the receiver thinks he or she hears.
   c. What the speaker says—what the receiver thinks the speaker said.
10. For accurate interpretation of communication the sender should know the receiver's level of or capacity for understanding and use appropriate language or channel.
11. Barriers to communication can be:
    a. Verbal—changing the subject, having a judgmental attitude (stating one's own opinion about a patient or situation), offering false or inappropriate reassurance, jumping to conclusions or taking things for granted, using medical facts or nursing knowledge inappropriately.
    b. Nonverbal—showing a lack of trust or feeling, disinterest, rejection.

Criteria for Determining Success of Communication

1. Feedback. Let the sender know how you perceived the message so he or she knows if it was understood as intended. A breakdown in communication occurs when the idea of the receiver does not match the idea of the sender. Two people should have mutual understanding about the meaning of a message. Language should convey meaning.
2. Appropriateness of reply. Do not evaluate the receiver's comprehension totally on basis of language. Observe nonverbal behavior also.
3. Efficiency. Is the sender overloading the listener? Is the listener's intrapersonal communication (i.e., silently talking to self or daydreaming) interfering with concentration on the message?
4. Specific results. Behavioral changes indicate that the goal is reached. Through communication the caregiver can influence behavior by encouraging the patient to express feelings or by redirecting actions toward more beneficial behavior.

Teamwork

A *team* is a group of two or more persons who recognize common goals and coordinate their efforts to achieve them. Broadly defined, the *health care team* includes all personnel relating to the patient, those in direct patient contact and those in other departments whose services are essential and contribute indirectly to patient care. Interdependence characterizes a team because without the other members the goals cannot be met.

The team's approach to patient care should be a coordinated effort that is performed with the cooperation of all caregivers. Members of the team should communicate and have a shared division of duties to perform specified tasks as a unified body. The failure of any one member to perform his or her role can seriously impact the success of the entire team. Performing as a team requires that each member exert an effort to attain the common goals in a competent, safe manner. Each team member's actions are important. No one individual can accomplish the goal without the rest of the team's cooperation.

Pride in one's work and in the team as a whole leads to personal satisfaction. High morale is facilitated by adequate staff orientation, staff participation in departmental decision making and problem solving, receipt of deserved praise, opportunity for continuing education, and motivation to reach and practice at the highest potential.

The common goal of the OR team is the effective delivery of care in a safe, efficient, and timely manner. The team should understand the patient's need for the relief of suffering, the restoration of bodily structure and function, and a favorable postoperative outcome. Unified teamwork contributes to the patient's optimal health and return to society or death with dignity.

Teamwork is the essence of patient care in the OR. To function efficiently, effective communication between team members is critical. Patients must be continuously monitored. Problems such as a break in aseptic or sterile technique must be identified and corrective action taken. Team members must be aware of each other's needs for information to fulfill expectations. Efforts of other support services, such as radiology and pathology departments, must be coordinated with the needs of the surgeon.

Mutual respect is the foundation of teamwork. It is also a right. We show respect through collaboration, cooperation, and truthful communication. Verbal abuse, disruptive behavior, and harassment are out of place in an OR. Behavior that inhibits the surgical procedure and the performance of team members or that threatens patient care should be factually documented. Disciplinary action may be justified.

Teamwork is the commitment and effort of team members to increase productivity, to ensure quality performance, and to participate in problem solving by communicating and cooperating with one another. A team approach is necessary for patient-centered care. Surgeons, other attending physicians and assistants, anesthesiologists or anesthetists, nursing staff, and supporting services should coordinate their efforts. Several factors contribute to successful outcomes of surgical intervention.

1. Communication of the OR team with other patient care departments is important for mutual cooperation, consideration, and efficient collaboration.
   a. Nursing unit, emergency department, OR, postanesthesia care unit, and intensive care unit nurses and physicians share pertinent information concerning patients. Collected data are documented by accurate recording, thereby protecting the patient, the medical personnel, and the health care institution.
   b. Personnel work together in a congenial atmosphere of equality with knowledge of and respect and appreciation for each other's unique skills and contributions. Team members benefit from the expertise of each other. Teamwork is at its finest in the OR.
   c. Personnel are considerate of each other and of the patient. For example:
      - Surgeons inform their teammates ahead of time of any anticipated potential deviation from their regular routine or the scheduled procedure. They appreciate thoughtful preparation and assistance.
      - Nurses and surgical technologists do all in their power to provide the best possible atmosphere to ensure the surgeon's uninterrupted concentration. It is always a risk to interrupt the surgeon during any procedure, unless absolutely necessary.
      - The anesthesiologist and circulator assist each other with certain procedures.
2. Adequate preparation and familiarity with the surgeon's preferences and the surgical procedure to be performed are fundamental. If team members are unfamiliar with the routine and equipment, it distracts the surgeon's train of thought. The effort of the team also is distracted from patient care issues and the environment becomes a difficult place in which to work. The surgeon's plea is for dedicated nursing personnel and other assistants who are knowledgeable and caring. Only then can the surgeon, who needs their expertise and cooperation, help the patient. Surgeons want to work in collegial relationships with their team members. By not being properly oriented, assigned, prepared (both the patient and the OR), or attentive (to the patient and the team), both the patient and the surgeon's skill are placed in jeopardy. An adequately experienced and skilled OR team is essential for the effective performance of a safe, efficient procedure.
3. Assignment of adequately oriented and competent personnel, who work together as a team, prevents delays and keeps anesthesia time to a minimum. The potential for complications increases proportionately with the length of anesthesia time and the surgical procedure. Calm, experienced personnel greatly reduce all hazards, especially in critical situations. Lack of knowledge and personnel shortages pose a serious threat to the patient and to the expected outcome of the surgical procedure. The entire interdisciplinary health care team must care about what happens to the patient. The need for communication and cooperation cannot be overemphasized.
4. Attention to the patient's welfare must be constant. The patient has an unconditional right to the team's complete concentration and attention at all times. The members of the team must be concerned with meeting the patient's needs, regarding him or her as a unique individual who is completely dependent on them for survival.

Although the ideologic differences of personnel may at times be a source of conflict, teamwork and the task at hand should overcome any differences in personalities. Also, problems in the OR suite that are caused by complex procedures, heavy operating schedules, or shortages of personnel should not interfere with the delivery of efficient, individualized patient care.

Clinical Competence

A practitioner can be categorized, based on experience and performance, as novice, competent, proficient, or expert. The novice lacks experience but is expected to perform to the best of his or her ability. Assistance must be available. Most employers provide a formal orientation program for new nurses and surgical technologists that lasts from 6 to 12 months. Within this time, the necessary knowledge, skills, and abilities should be developed to function independently at a basic competency level. As experience is gained, competence develops from a minimal level to an advanced level of expertise. Competency requires knowledge for critical thinking and decision making in addition to technical skills. Technical and cognitive skills are complementary and integral components of patient care in all practice settings.

Statements of clinical competency are established by professional organizations such as the Association of Operating Room Nurses (AORN) and the Association of Surgical Technologists (AST). These guidelines are published by each professional organization and made available to practitioners of all disciplines. (Clinical competencies are discussed in Chapter 2 in more detail.)

REALITIES OF CLINICAL PRACTICE

When a formal educational experience is completed, a learner is eager to apply skills and knowledge in an employment setting. However, of necessity, a transition period from dependent learner to independent practitioner occurs. The realities of the work environment and the emotional and ethical dilemmas of some situations must be faced as basic competencies are developed. It can take 6 months to 1 year to feel fully confident as a functioning OR team member.

Reality Shock

Reality is a sense of actuality, a feeling that this is what the real world is all about. Each individual should learn the rules and accepted behaviors and assume responsibilities for personal behavior. Reality shock sets in as the transition takes place from being a beginning learner to becoming an employed graduate professional nurse or surgical technologist. The familiar instructor and peer learners are no longer present to give counsel, advice, and moral support. As caregivers attempt to adapt to new demands, they need to remember:

1. Learning never ends with basic education. It is an ongoing process throughout a caregiver's career for improving skills and mastering new technologies.
2. Everyone has stood in the shoes of the novice (although some may have forgotten those novice days). They have all experienced the feelings and frustrations of being the newest staff member. The experienced caregiver should try to remember these feelings and offer encouragement to new personnel.
3. Patience is an asset while developing work habits and establishing working relationships. Expectations of self and others should be realistic. Feelings of excitement, anticipation, and fear of failure or making mistakes are normal but should be expressed appropriately.
4. Applying the principles and techniques already learned will enable the caregiver to make sound judgments and appropriate decisions in the OR.
5. Ask questions and acknowledge not knowing how to do something. Seeking help promotes professional growth. In the pursuit of knowledge, use human and material resources. Everyone can benefit from constructive criticism.

Everyone wants and needs to become an accepted member of both social and work groups. The OR nursing staff collectively is a social group. The OR team, including the surgeon and anesthesiologist, is a work group. Ambivalent feelings may arise on entering these groups. The pleasures of functioning as a team member may be offset by uncertainty about the ability to perform well. Initial goals will be task/skill-oriented as learning focuses on policies, procedures, and routines. Eventually, insecurity will be replaced with self-confidence. The display of confidence will increase trust, respect, and recognition from others as well as the personal satisfaction of accomplishment. Familiarization with surgeons, anesthesiologists, nursing managers, peers, and subordinates will enable the beginner to learn the expected norms of behavior both from the team and oneself.

Dynamics of Psychologic Climate

Learning to adapt to the variety of tasks and ever-changing demands in the OR environment is difficult. Some anxiety is to be expected, especially in situations in which feelings of insecurity are generated or a sense of intimidation pervades the environment. At times the demands of the job may seem to outweigh the caregiver's personal resources. Confidence develops as skills are learned.

Understanding of expected performance is perhaps the most important element in the transition from basic learner to novice practitioner. The beginner should look for a support system, such as those staff members who are willing to help bridge the gap. Look for role models, those staff members who are respected for their clinical competence and who are emulated. Stick with the winners, those staff members who are reaping personal rewards and self-satisfaction from their work effort. Avoid the losers, those staff members who have negative attitudes, complain, and do not make an effort to solve problems but create them.

Eustress vs. Distress

Physical and emotional stresses are part of daily life. Stress is the nonspecific reaction of the body, physiologically and/or psychologically, to any demand. The demand may be pleasant or unpleasant, conscious or unconscious. The intensity of the stressor will dictate adaptation. Individual perception of a situation will influence reaction to it.

Stress is not only an essential part of life but a useful stimulant. Positive stress, referred to as *eustress,* motivates an individual to be productive and efficient. It forces adaptation to the ever-present changes in the OR environment. The response should be quick, for example, when a trauma victim arrives or a patient has a cardiac arrest. To expect the unexpected is part of OR nursing. Eustress fosters a sense of achievement, satisfaction, and self-confidence.

Stress that becomes overwhelming and uncomfortable is referred to as *distress.* In the OR, behavior of others may be perceived as cause for distress. Policies, or lack of them, can also be a source of distress if they are in conflict with the caregiver's expectations. Through adaptive mechanisms the caregiver can cope with the tensions, conflicts, and demands of the OR environment either in a collaborative way or in an unproductive manner. Even though perceived as distress, some conflict is necessary to stimulate change in work methods and solve organizational problems.

Nursing personnel may be distressed by conduct of other team members. For example, it is uncomfortable to be harshly criticized by a surgeon. Keep in mind that much that is said is not personally directed. Often the surgeon is reacting to his or her distress caused by unanticipated circumstances presented by the patient during the surgical procedure. The reactions of the personnel will be influenced by their attitudes, mood, cultural and religious background, values and ethics, experiences, and concerns of the moment. Outbursts of anger are inappropriate at the operating table at any time. However, constant frustration and inner conflict create the distresses that can lead to job dissatisfaction.

Stress Reduction

Assertive behavior is a useful tool for conflict resolution. Shared professional communication can keep the tension in the environment to a minimum. The caregiver should keep his or her composure at all times and maintain a professional, assertive (not aggressive) attitude. Personal conflicts between team members should be dealt with privately.

Humor can be an effective method of reducing anxiety. It should be used appropriately to defuse tension, however. Laughing at oneself helps to preserve self-esteem while learning from the experience.

At the end of the work shift, the caregiver should evaluate the events of the day, the emotions evoked and how they were handled. What was done effectively? What coping skills may be needed to improve or enhance positive attitudes in the work environment and in interpersonal relations? Teamwork is essential in the OR, with every team member obligated to contribute positively to it.

Stress is a reality that need not create a sense of self-defeat. Despite the source of stress, the body responds; the physiologic and psychologic effects can be subtle or intense. The determination of whether a stressor is good or bad depends on an individual's perception of the circumstances. Any event that creates a feeling of impending danger also creates the perception of loss of control. A major factor in stress management is maintaining control. This can be done by learning to tune in to the balance between the body and the mind. The caregiver can learn to be prepared for life's difficulties by understanding how the perception of stress can affect decision making, self-expression, and subsistence in the world.

Listen to the Body Develop a sense for how the body signals exhaustion, hunger, illness, and/or physical pain. Ignoring physical signals decreases the body's ability to manage stress. The body is a sensory barometer of the environment's effects on the caregiver. Going without sleep or skipping meals creates physical stress that can be avoided. Regular sleep and rest, exercise, adequate dietary practices, and routine health checkups provide a sound basis for care of the body.

Maintain the Mind Mental relaxation can help the caregiver manage stress. Using meditation and mental imagery on a regular basis provides a break from stressful routines and allows the mind to fortify itself against negative perceptions of a situation. Creating time to clear confusing thoughts and align productive thinking enables the body and the mind to support an emotional balance and a sense of well-being. This positive interaction can become an influence in a stressful situation and serve as an example to co-workers.

BIBLIOGRAPHY

Beitz JM: Project Alpha: a nursing elective implemented in a general systems theory, *AORN J* 55(5):1218-1230, 1992.

Boegli EH: Preceptorship: a gift that keeps on giving, *Surg Technol* 26(2):12-14, 1994.

Brazen L, Roth RA: Using learning style preferences for perioperative clinical education, *AORN J* 61(1):189-195, 1995.

Donley DL: Promoting active learning in the classroom: an instructor's challenge, *Surg Technol* 26(8):15, 24, 1994.

Farley MJ: Teamwork in perioperative nursing, *AORN J* 53(3):730-738, 1991.

Farley MJ: Thought and talk, *AORN J* 56(3):481-484, 1992.

Fox V et al: The mentoring relationship, *AORN J* 56(5):858-867, 1992.

Goodall R: Assert yourself: effective communication for nurses, *AORN J* 57(4):894-899, 1993.

Good-Reis DV et al: Structured vs. unstructured teaching, *AORN J* 51(5):1334-1339, 1990.

Grossman D, Taylor R: Cultural diversity on the unit, *Am J Nurs* 95(2):64-67, 1995.

Hierich K, Killeen ME: The gentle art of nurturing yourself, *Am J Nurs* 93(10):41-44, 1993.

Khan K et al: Career guide: from expert to novice, *Am J Nurs* 93(9):53-58, 1993.

Larson BA, Martinson DJ: Words can hurt: dealing with verbal abuse in the operating room, *AORN J* 52(6):1238-1241, 1990.

Lessner MW et al: Orienting nursing students to cost effective clinical practice, *Nurs Health Care* 15(9):458-462, 1994.

Markey BT et al: Perioperative internship for college credit, *AORN J* 51(6):1575-1579, 1990.

Mathias JM: Nurses need good communication skills, *OR Manager* 8(4):19, 1992.

Merrian SB, Caffarella RS: *Learning in adulthood: a comprehensive guide,* San Francisco, 1991, Jossey-Bass.

Middlemiss MA, Van Neste-Kenny J: Curriculum revolution: reflective minds and empowering relationships, *Nurs Health Care* 15(7): 350-353, 1994.

Miller MA, Malcolm NS: Critical thinking in the nursing curriculum, *Nurs Health Care* 11(2):67-73, 1990.

National Committee on Education: *Precepter guide for perioperative nursing practice,* Denver, 1993, Association of Operating Room Nurses.

Pearson D: Getting a handle on stress and distress, *Surg Technol* 25(12):18, 1993.

Pearson D: Overcoming stress through self-esteem, *Surg Technol* 25(5):1, 20, 1993.

Polis SL: Competency-based laser education, *AORN J* 55(2):567-572, 1992.

Radziewicz KM et al: Perioperative education, *AORN J* 55(4):1060-1071, 1992.

Schmaus D: Evaluating computer-assisted instructional software for the OR, *AORN J* 54(6):1296-1301, 1991.

Sherwood G: Planning an educational activity, *AORN J* 51(6):1586-1590, 1990.

Shuman J: Six ways to take this job...and love it! *Am J Nurs* 94(6):59-63, 1994.

Sparks SM: The educational technology network, *Nurs Health Care* 15(3):134-141, 1994.

Stock N: A positive attitude can make the most of OR orientation, *AORN J* 52(1):147-148, 1990.

The revised *essentials* of accredited programs, *Surg Technol* 22(4):15-18, 1990.

Thomas KJ: Whole-brain learning, *AORN J* 51(1):196-203, 1990.

Tolley RG et al: Perioperative nursing: designing, implementing a baccalaureate elective, *AORN J* 52(1):105-112, 1990.

Vestal KW: Failure: making it a positive experience, *AORN J* 51(3):784-786, 1990.

Wolinski K: Self-awareness, self-renewal, self-management, *AORN J* 58(4):721-730, 1993.

Yoder ME: Preferred learning style and educational technology, *Nurs Health Care* 15(3):128-132, 1994.

CHAPTER 2

Foundations of Patient-Centered Care

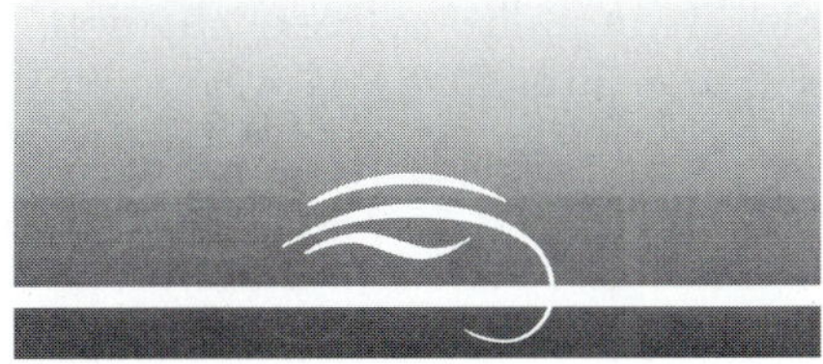

The perioperative experience encompasses a broad scope of scientific yet humanistic activities to provide care for surgical patients. The surgical procedure is the focal point for these patients. It is imperative that patients come to the operating room (OR) optimally prepared both physically and psychologically. The persons concerned directly or indirectly with surgical patient care are many; they are discussed in Chapters 5 and 6.

Both perioperative nurses and surgical technologists work toward the common objective of providing the safest possible care so that patients achieve favorable surgical outcomes. Although surgical technologists make valuable contributions to surgical patient care, qualities of the professional perioperative nurses are needed and used to implement a personalized, patient-oriented approach to care. They do this through creative application of the nursing process, judgment, skills, and interpersonal competencies. This chapter focuses on the perioperative nurse and the surgical technologist who work together to fulfill the patients' needs throughout the perioperative experience.

PROFESSIONAL NURSING

The members of a profession must act responsibly in accord with their commitment to public trust and service. Simply stated the word *profession* implies a combination and coordination of knowledge, skills, and ideals. These are communicated through a highly specialized educational discipline. In this way education sets the standards for practice. However, the characteristics of a profession are that:

1. It defines its own purposes and code of ethics.
2. It sets its own standards and conducts its own affairs and self-regulation; it has autonomy.
3. It identifies and develops its own body of knowledge unique to its role, through research.
4. It requires critical thinking skills in clinical judgment and problem-solving and decision-making skills in application of knowledge.
5. It engages in self-evaluation and peer review to control and alter its practices and accountabilities.

Professional nursing is dedicated to the promotion of optimal health for all human beings in their various environments. Nursing is both a humanistic art and a basic and applied science. Nurses as patient advocates perform many roles including teaching health-seeking behaviors, promoting preventive medicine, taking part in patient rehabilitation, and participating in nursing research. The professional nurse in the acute-care setting performs functions that are primarily curative and restorative in nature. *The Scope of Nursing Practice*, developed by the American Nurses Association (ANA), identifies the essence of clinical nursing practice as nursing diagnosis and treatment of human responses to health and to illness. The science of nursing is based on knowledge and theories about the nature of man, health, and disease. It is the "what and why" of appropriate caregiving measures and the basis for predicting outcomes of nursing interventions. Professional competence relates to the nurse's ability to apply knowledge of principles, theories, and facts to decision making in clinical performance.

Because nursing is a helping profession, the ideal characteristics of the nurse include the ability and commitment to respond with compassion to human needs and society's expectations for health care services. This is the art of nursing. If we deny humanity to others, we dehumanize ourselves as well. Professional nurses are committed to life, health, and death with dignity. In practice, they help each patient to attain his or her highest possible level of general health. Nurses are morally responsible and legally accountable for the quality of their practice.

Professional and legal standards establish measurable criteria for responsibility and accountability. Their purpose is to fulfill the profession's obligation to define, provide, and improve practice. Standards and recommended practices have been established by professional organizations, federal and state governments, the Joint Commission on the Accreditation of Healthcare Organizations (JCAHO), and other voluntary agencies. Definitions, standards, and recommended practices give guidance to nursing service and nursing education. They will be referred to throughout this text.

Nursing education prepares nurses to translate nursing science into relevant therapeutic skills and clinical judgments. Professional nursing education should be built on a solid base of general education in liberal arts, humanities, and natural and behavioral sciences. The nurse, educated to assess the total patient, is an indispensable member of the OR team.

Professional Nursing in Operating Room

A wise physician once said that the physician's role is to cure sometimes, to relieve often, to comfort always. The same can be said for the perioperative nurse who embodies all that the word *nurse* has traditionally meant to a patient—provider of safety and comfort, supporter, and confidante. The patient's safety and welfare are entrusted to the OR nurse from the moment of arrival in the OR until departure and transfer of responsibility for care to another professional health care team member. The primary emphasis of the nurse's responsibility is to the patient. The nurse is accountable and responsible for the care of the patient whether it is accomplished personally or by another perioperative team member.

Professional nursing in the OR has been defined as ``the identification of the physiological, psychological and sociological needs of the patient, and the implementation of an individualized program of nursing care that coordinates the nursing interventions, based on a knowledge of the natural and behavioral sciences, in order to restore, or maintain, the health and welfare of the patient before, during, and after surgical intervention."*

The professional perioperative nurse, a licensed RN, is legally responsible for the nature and quality of the care patients receive during surgical intervention. The scope of perioperative nursing practice encompasses those nursing interventions that assist the individual surgical patient in a conscious or unconscious state. These interventions are directed toward providing continuity of care through preoperative assessment and planning, intraoperative intervention, and postoperative evaluation.

Perioperative Nursing Practice

Perioperative nursing practice includes activities performed by the RN during the *preoperative, intraoperative, and postoperative phases* of the patient's surgical experience. *Perioperative,* therefore, is a term that encompasses the patient's total experience when surgical intervention is accepted as the treatment of choice. *Practice* refers to the expected behavior patterns and technical activities the nurse performs during the three phases of surgical patient care. The *perioperative nurse* possesses a depth and breadth of knowledge that allows for the coordination of care of the surgical patient. The nurse prioritizes interventions based on a comprehensive body of scientific knowledge and variations in patient responses. He or she uses critical thinking skills in applying the nursing process, acting as patient advocate, and exercising judgment in a professionally accountable manner to achieve the best possible patient outcomes. The perioperative nurse designs, coordinates, and delivers care to meet the identified physiologic, psychologic, sociocultural, and spiritual needs of patients whose protective reflexes or self-care abilities are potentially compromised because they are having invasive procedures. The nursing activities address the needs and responses of patients and their families or significant others.†

Perioperative nurses must be flexible and diverse to practice in a technologically complex environment. Their *roles* incorporate both technical and behavioral components of professional nursing. Competent fulfillment of the perioperative nursing role is based on the

*From AORN Statement Committee: Definition and objective for clinical practice of professional operating room nursing, *AORN J* 10(5):48, 1969.

†From AORN Statement Committee: Definition of perioperative nurse, *AORN J* 59(1):86, 1994.

knowledge and application of the principles of the biologic, physiologic, behavioral, and social sciences. Perioperative nurses make decisions about patients' problems, needs, and health status. This is essential information in the identification of expected outcomes and the formulation of a perioperative plan of care.

Patient-Nurse Relationship

The perioperative nurse shares a special experience with the patient at a time of great stress and need in his or her life. Their relationship encompasses feelings, attitudes, and behaviors. It must be humanized in structure. Mutual trust and understanding are vital components. Effective interaction encompasses concern for the unique personhood of both the patient and the nurse. The length of time spent with the patient is not as important as the quality of the interaction. The level of the interaction may directly affect the patient's perception of the perioperative experience.

To achieve and maintain a viable cooperative relationship, the patient must know that the nurse unconditionally cares about his or her well-being both within and outside of the OR. The nurse is aware that personal interaction is often predicated on culture, attitudes, and past experiences. Knowledge of the patient and the impact of surgical intervention on his or her life situation is therefore indispensable.

Perioperative nursing involves patient-nurse interaction through direct patient contact and care. Individualized care, the art of nursing, demonstrates genuine concern for the patient as a person. It is not purely technical or procedure-oriented. Standardized care, the science of nursing, is derived from a body of knowledge that has been developed through research and clinical practice. Perioperative nursing care is a specialized combination of the art of individualized care and the science of standardization. The perioperative nurse delivers care through the use of the nursing process in a cost-effective manner without compromising the quality of care.

NURSING PROCESS

Perioperative patient care requires preplanning and identifying expected outcomes through the nursing process. This process provides a systematic approach to nursing care planning and delivery. The nursing process provides the foundation for the nursing activities used in assessing, planning, implementing, and evaluating patient care. These interventions are:

1. Observation of the patient's signs, symptoms, and reactions
2. Promotion of the patient's physical and emotional health by meeting identified needs
3. Monitoring the physiologic and psychologic status of the patient
4. Supervision of others who contribute to the care of the patient
5. Application and implementation of nursing procedures and techniques
6. Application and implementation of the physician's legal orders
7. Documentation and reporting

A *process* is the act of proceeding through a series of interventions that contribute to an end. It provides a framework for cyclic problem solving in a logical, interrelated sequence of steps. Each step of the nursing process is documented for the purpose of communicating with all health care team members. The steps comprise a rational method of identifying patient problems and needs, determining diagnoses based on health status information, establishing expected outcomes, formulating an individualized plan of care, implementing the plan, and evaluating the effectiveness of the plan in the attainment of the desired outcomes.

A *problem* or *need* may be defined as any condition or situation in which the patient requires help to maintain or regain physical, emotional, spiritual, or social equilibrium. A problem or need may be classified as actual or potential. The scientific process of problem solving furnishes an organized approach to nursing care and a mode of determining expected outcomes resulting from that care, while adhering to the philosophies of nursing. The application of the art and science of nursing is integral in this process. An *independent nursing function* is the selection of priority problems or needs in a given situation. Rationale for the order in which the problems or needs are selected is necessary. Patient input is important for the formulation of mutual goals and gaining cooperation for the fulfillment of expected outcomes.

The nursing process is a systematic approach to nursing practice using problem-solving techniques and has four major components. The nursing process can be associated with the mnemonic *A PIE* for the patient; the four parts make a whole (Box 2-1).

Integration of Nursing Process Into Phases of Perioperative Nursing

The four components of the nursing process are integrated into the three phases of the patient's perioperative experience (see Figure 2-1).

Preoperative Phase

The preoperative phase of the patient's surgical experience begins when the decision is made to undergo surgical intervention. This phase ends when the patient is transferred to the operating table. During this phase, the perioperative nurse performs the assessment and

BOX 2-1

Nursing Process

A Assessment

1. Identify the actual or potential problems, needs, and health status considerations through appraisal of the physiologic, psychosocial, objective, subjective, cultural, and ethnic data related to the patient as an individual.
2. Formulate prioritized actual or potential nursing diagnoses unique to the patient.
3. Develop measurable and attainable expected outcomes and mutual goals in collaboration with the patient, significant others, and other health care providers. Identify realistic time frames in which fulfillment may be accomplished.
4. Assessment is an ongoing process throughout the perioperative experience.
5. Document all pertinent assessment findings.

P Planning

1. Establish and prioritize a working set of interventions for the actual problems, needs, and health status considerations.
2. Establish a contingency plan for the potential problems, needs, and health status considerations that may become actual during the course of the perioperative experience.
3. Include the patient's input for the construction of the individualized plan.
4. Document the plan of care in a retrievable manner.

I Implementation

1. Share the plan with the perioperative team for continuity of care.
2. Activate the interventions in a systematic order of priority.
3. Discontinue any intervention that is ineffective.
4. Document the implementation of the interventions and their effectiveness.

E Evaluation

1. Determine the effectiveness of the plan as the expected outcomes and mutual goals are met.
2. Reformulate the plan and implement new interventions as necessary.
3. Document the effectiveness of the plan of care in an ongoing systematic manner.

planning components of the nursing process. The nurse assesses the patient to identify any actual or potential physiologic, psychosocial, and spiritual needs, problems, or other health status considerations. Then the nurse, in collaboration with the patient and/or significant other, determines the nursing diagnoses and identifies the expected outcomes of the perioperative experience. The perioperative nurse plans and prioritizes the nursing interventions necessary to achieve the desired results.

Intraoperative Phase

The intraoperative phase begins with the placement of the patient on the operating table and extends to the time the patient is admitted to the recovery area. The implementation component of the nursing process is performed during this phase. The perioperative nurse either personally carries out the plan or supervises others in carrying out the plan of care with skill, safety, efficiency, and effectiveness.

Postoperative Phase

The postoperative phase begins with admission of the patient to the recovery area, which may be a postanesthesia care unit (PACU) or an intensive care unit (ICU). Unless the surgical procedure is performed as an ambulatory procedure, the patient will transfer from the immediate postoperative recovery area to progressive stages of self-care on a surgical unit before discharge from the hospital. The postoperative phase ends when the surgeon discontinues follow-up care. Evaluation, the fourth component of nursing process, is completed during this phase. The perioperative nurse appraises the quality of nursing care rendered during the preoperative and intraoperative phases of care. Evaluation determines whether the assessment, planning, and implementation processes were effective in terms of the patient's achievement of the expected outcomes.

STANDARDS OF PERIOPERATIVE CLINICAL PRACTICE

A *standard* is an authoritative statement established and published by a profession by which the quality of practice can be measured. The setting of standards for nursing practice is a means of ensuring the quality of the services nurses offer, *provided nurses implement the standards.*

The ANA *Standards of Clinical Nursing Practice* reflect the nursing process and state the interventions to be performed. They are a description of competent level of practice common to all nurses. The standards are the foundation of all decision making in the provision of care to all patients. The *interpretive statements* that accompany each standard provide definitions of terms and interventions and guidelines to achieve the standards. *Criteria* for achievement of each standard are also stated and remain consistent with current nursing practice. Nursing practice is based on theory and is constantly evolving with the development of new technology and research. The standards are written in behavioral terms so nurses can measure to what degree each standard has been met.

The *Standards of Perioperative Clinical Practice,* originally published in 1981, were revised in 1992 by the As-

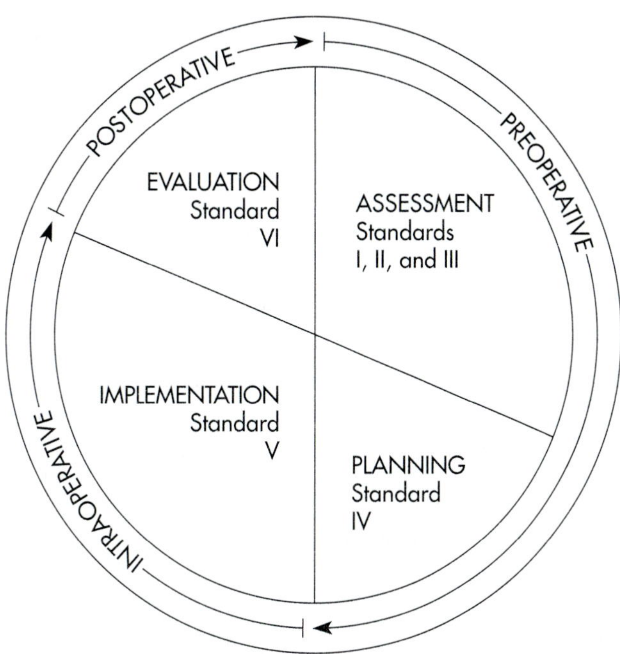

FIGURE 2-1 Nursing process: A PIE for the patient. Three phases of perioperative nursing incorporate four components of nursing process and six standards of perioperative clinical practice.

sociation of Operating Room Nurses (AORN). The nursing activities inherent in each standard are incorporated in the nursing process during the three phases of the surgical patient's experience (Figure 2-1). The six perioperative standards of care will be presented under the four major headings of the nursing process, *A PIE* for the patient.

Preoperative Assessment

A purposeful patient-nurse interaction that continues through all phases of the nursing process begins by the nurse getting to know the patient and what is happening to him or her. *Assessment* consists of appraising the patient and his or her existing and potential nursing care needs. This is the basis for individualized care planning and establishment of expected outcomes related to the identified problems and needs. From specific data collected and analyzed preoperatively, the nurse constructs a database, a composite picture of the patient's condition, to serve as a basis for comparison with subsequent observations and postoperative status. The baseline data includes subjective material (what the patient states he or she is experiencing such as pain or anxiety) and objective material (that which can be observed and validated by another person such as the unit nurse, family member, or social worker).

From the baseline data, the perioperative nurse determines the appropriate nursing diagnoses that are consistent with accepted nursing interventions during the preoperative and intraoperative phases of patient care. A *nursing diagnosis* is a concise, descriptive statement of the patient's health status, based on nursing assessment and amenable to nursing intervention. Analysis and interpretation of the baseline data collected during the assessment phase leads to identification of actual or potential problems, needs, or health status considerations (i.e., nursing diagnoses). For example, a sensory perceptual alteration may be a visual or hearing problem that is caused by a neurologic deficit.

Maslow's hierarchy of basic needs (see Chapter 7 and Figure 7-2, p. 99) can be used as a basis for collecting the information necessary for identification of the appropriate actual or potential nursing diagnoses.

Standard I: Assessment

The perioperative nurse collects patient health data. Data collection is continuous and ongoing. It may be gathered in the preoperative holding area in the OR suite, on the surgical unit, in the clinic, or by a telephone call to the patient at home. Information can be obtained from the patient's chart, by consultation with other members of the health care team (unit nurses, surgeon, anesthesiologist, etc.), through interview with the patient and/or family or significant others, and by observation and physical assessment of the patient. Data collection is a progressive and orderly process to gather meaningful information pertinent to the planned surgical intervention. This includes, but is not limited to, the following:

1. Current medical diagnosis and therapy
2. Diagnostic studies and laboratory test results
3. Physical status and physiologic responses, including allergies and sensory or physical deficits
4. Psychosocial status
5. Spiritual needs, ethnic and cultural background, and lifestyle
6. Previous responses to illness, hospitalization, and surgery
7. Patient's understanding, perceptions, and expectations of the procedure

Pertinent data collected through physiologic and psychosocial assessment must be recorded, and identified problems or needs should be communicated to other team members. Box 2-2 lists the assessments to be considered.

Physiologic Assessment Fulfilling basic life-sustaining needs is of the highest priority during surgical intervention. Therefore, in addition to the physician's physical examination, the perioperative nurse should perform a physical assessment of the patient. Techniques include inspection/observation, auscultation, percussion, palpation, and olfaction. Assessment of major body systems establishes the current health status of the patient. It alerts the nurse to possible complications and/or physiologic manifestations of anxiety. Therefore it provides a basis for planning appropriate preoperative and intraoperative nursing interventions. It also provides a database for postoperative evaluation.

The perioperative nurse must also be familiar with laboratory norms so critical deviations are identified in all phases of surgical intervention. Other important parameters for planning intraoperative care include knowledge of allergies, skin integrity, sensory or physical handicaps, prosthetic devices, nutritional/metabolic status, and chronic illness.

The patient also should be screened for substance abuse that can affect postoperative recovery. A smoker who will have general anesthesia needs to be taught coughing and deep breathing exercises. The patient who is dependent on alcohol or mind-altering drugs can suffer physiologic and psychologic manifestations of withdrawal postoperatively. A recovering chemically dependent person may refuse preoperative sedation and postoperative narcotics for pain.

Psychosocial Assessment Individuals vary in their ability to cope with stressful situations. Illness makes a person vulnerable. Culture, religion, and socioeconomic factors have an impact on the patient's interpretation of illness and impending surgical procedure. Anticipatory apprehension, although normal to some degree, may diminish critical thinking and decision-making abilities. The stress may initiate an exaggerated response of normal coping mechanisms for self-protection. Physiologic secretion of adrenal cortical hormones may delay wound healing and decrease resistance to infection. Surgical patients are in a

BOX 2-2

Preoperative Assessment Parameters

Physiologic

Medical diagnosis
Operative site and procedure
Results of diagnostic studies and laboratory tests (i.e., deviations from norms)
Anatomic or physiologic alterations from previous surgery, injury, or disease
Mobility, range of motion
Prosthetics, internal or external
Sensory impairments
Allergies
Skin condition
Nutritional and metabolic status
Weight and height
Vital signs
Elimination pattern (i.e., continence)
Sleep, rest, exercise patterns
Medications
Substance abuse

Psychosocial

Cognition (i.e., mental status)
Cultural and religious beliefs
Perception of operation
Expectations of care
Knowledge base (i.e., informed consent)
Readiness to learn
Ability to understand and retain teaching
Stress level (i.e., anxiety and fears)
Coping mechanisms
Support from family or significant others
Attitude and motivation (i.e., health management)
Affective responses (i.e., ability to express feelings)
Speech characteristics (i.e., language)
Nonverbal behavior

psychologically perilous situation when they are threatened by loss of life, body parts, or function, and by unfamiliar social relationships. The strangeness of the OR itself—its noise, odors, and equipment—represents a potential hazard. Stress, perceived by the patient as *distress,* may be expressed in one or many ways. These are described in more detail in Chapter 7.

Documentation Immediately after leaving the patient, the nurse writes a summary of the assessment data on the nurses' note or progress sheet in the patient's chart to convey pertinent information to the unit nurses and surgeon. Written documentation is necessary also to correlate the preoperative assessment with the nursing audit, a part of the evaluation phase of nursing process. This information includes the patient's responses to the interview and the teaching given, as well as the patient's needs for further preoperative and postoperative instruction. Identified family attitudes and needs are also included. This becomes a permanent part of the patient's record.

Assessment guidelines or nursing interview forms specifically designed for the perioperative nurse are valuable tools to organize and record data gleaned during preoperative assessments. However, it is inappropriate for patients to see nurses writing during an interview. They may become uncomfortable and less communicative. Nurses should concentrate on remembering pertinent data, observations, and preoperative teaching and to record appropriate information after the interview.

A computer program may be available to establish a computerized patient database. The nurse enters data obtained from physiologic and psychosocial assessments through physical examination, interview, and observation. The computer assigns the signs and symptoms, the defining characteristics, to nursing diagnostic categories. Then the related factors, expected outcomes, and nursing interventions may be selected. A printed copy of the patient care plan is obtained for patient's record.

The perioperative nurse records the data. The mnemonic *SOAP* is helpful to incorporate the basic elements of a nursing assessment.

S *Subjective response:* The patient's perceptions and expectations of the procedure and problems the patient has identified may be recorded in his or her own words in the form of a direct quote.

O *Objective perception:* The nurse's impressions of the patient and the identified problems as determined from the chart data and observation of patient during the preoperative interview.

A *Analysis:* The determination of the patient's basic needs, as outlined in Maslow's hierarchy (see Figure 7-2, p. 99) and defining characteristics of patient's actual, potential, or high risk for health problems. The data collected must be organized, analyzed, and interpreted to formulate the nursing diagnoses.

P *Plan:* The interventions that meet the actual or potential needs or problems are outlined.

Standard II: Diagnosis

The perioperative nurse analyzes the assessment data in determining diagnoses. Nursing diagnoses are conclusions the perioperative nurse makes based on analysis and interpretation of the assessment data. These are concise written statements about a patient's actual or potential problems, needs, or health status considerations amenable to nursing intervention.

A medical diagnosis defines problems on the basis of a patient's pathologic condition(s). A nursing diagnosis identifies a patient's response to this condition(s). The North American Nursing Diagnosis Association (NANDA) has developed a list of nursing diagnoses acceptable for clinical use. This list, known as a taxonomy, classifies human response patterns and standardizes nomenclature for describing them. It includes definitions and defining characteristics for each diagnosis. Because the list is not all-inclusive, the perioperative nurse may identify some actual or potential needs or problems not listed in the NANDA taxonomy. AORN has published a patient classification instrument for perioperative nursing that may be used to measure patient acuity preoperatively and intraoperatively.

A nursing diagnosis has three components:

1. *Defining characteristics.* Human responses to altered body processes and other contributing factors describe the acuity of an actual or potential health status deviation. The nurse identifies those characteristics for which nursing interventions can legally be used to maintain current health status or to reduce, eliminate, or prevent its alteration.
   a. *Problem.* Any health care condition that requires diagnostic, therapeutic, or educational action. Problems can be *active,* requiring immediate action, or *inactive,* having been solved. Problems are *subjective,* reported by the patient, or *objective,* observed by the nurse (e.g., edema suggestive of impaired tissue perfusion related to decreased cardiac output).
   b. *Need.* A lack of something essential for the maintenance of health that may be met by nursing intervention. Needs may be *actual,* in existence at the time of assessment, or *potential,* anticipated to possibly become actual during the length of stay (e.g., knowledge deficit).
   c. *Health consideration.* A personal habit, lifestyle, or influencing agent that if uncontrolled can lead to a decline in physiologic or psychologic

well-being (e.g., occupational hazards, exposure to chemical agent or smoke, or substance abuse).

2. *Signs and symptoms.* Subjective and objective data obtained during the assessment identify the defining characteristics of patient's actual or potential health problems.
3. *Etiology/related factors.* Causes of problems may be related to physiologic, psychosocial, spiritual, environmental, or other factors contributing to the patient's health status. These causes define relevant risk factors to be considered in planning nursing care.

Nursing diagnoses are synonymous with specific patient problems or needs as determined by patient's responses during physiologic and psychosocial assessment. The format of nursing interview forms or assessment guides varies, but all forms or guides elicit essentially the same information as a basis for nursing care planning. Use of the NANDA terminology helps nurses establish communication when documenting nursing diagnoses. A common language facilitates continuity of patient care.

Standard III: Outcome Identification

The perioperative nurse identifies expected outcomes unique to the patient. Expected outcomes are the desired patient objectives following surgical intervention within specified time frames and with specific criteria for evaluation. They direct the nursing interventions to modify or maintain the patient's present or potential physical capabilities and behavioral patterns. The patient's rights and preferences are considered. The expected outcomes should be realistic, attainable through available human and material resources, and consistent with medical regimen and patient outcome standards for perioperative nursing. In formulating expected outcomes as written statements, the perioperative nurse should consider, but not be limited to, the following:

1. Absence of infection
2. Maintenance of skin integrity
3. Absence of adverse effects through proper application of safety measures related to positioning and to chemical, physical, and electrical hazards
4. Maintenance of fluid and electrolyte balance
5. Knowledge and understanding the patient and family or significant others have of the potential physiologic and psychologic responses to surgical intervention and of their participation in the rehabilitative process

The outcomes are prioritized to maximize the therapeutic effect of the nursing interventions. Immediate actual diagnoses must be resolved first by the safest, most efficient approach. Then potential diagnoses are addressed.

Preoperative Planning

From the nursing diagnoses the nurse structures a flexible, individualized plan of care designed to seek ways to solve patient problems. This plan designates key functions (i.e., necessary interventions and possible nursing interventions). Nursing care is based on nursing diagnoses, established patient care standards, and related factors. Plans to assist the family in helping the patient become oriented to reality, as well as supportive, therapeutic, palliative, preventive, and rehabilitative measures to assist the patient, may be included.

NOTE

1. The concept of preoperative planning can be simply thought of as the patient *has* (health data), therefore the patient *needs* (nursing diagnoses) *specific actions* (nursing interventions) to achieve *expected outcomes* (desired results).
2. The mnemonic SOAP applies in gathering individualized information and also for the development of a plan of care. It incorporates the first two components of the nursing process and the first four standards of perioperative nursing practice.

Standard IV: Planning

The perioperative nurse develops a plan of care that prescribes interventions to attain expected outcomes. The perioperative nurse asks creative questions such as: "In what ways can I ensure the safety and welfare of this patient?" "What specific or unusual problems does this patient have?" "What are this patient's needs?" Based on the assessment data, nursing diagnoses, and identified expected outcomes, the perioperative nurse devises a plan of care to fulfill the patient's needs and expedite the surgical procedure in a safe manner for the patient. The plan should include provision for preoperative support and comfort measures, intraoperative intervention, and postoperative evaluation of outcomes specifically related to the total plan of care. Key concepts to consider in planning perioperative nursing care are:

1. Medical diagnosis and impact of surgical intervention on body systems
2. Location of surgical site and required position and comfort measures for the surgical procedure
3. Potential risks of the proposed procedure on other physical needs
4. Psychosocial and spiritual needs of patient
5. Environmental safety and provision of supplies and equipment

The plan of care should reflect current standards, including nursing interventions and key activities, that will facilitate the medical care prescribed and that will restore, maintain, or promote the patient's well-being. The scope of the plan is determined by the assessed needs of the patient. *Any unusual problems must be con-*

sidered for individualized patient care. Alternative options or interventions, not just routine procedures, are a necessary part of the plan. Regardless of format, the plan of care specifies:

1. Nursing interventions necessary to achieve expected outcomes
2. Priorities for nursing interventions
3. Logical sequencing of nursing interventions
4. How nursing interventions are to be performed
5. When nursing interventions are to be performed
6. Where nursing interventions are to be performed
7. Who is to perform nursing interventions

Human and material resources must be available to implement the plan. Therefore the planning phase of the nursing process also includes ensuring that appropriate, properly prepared, and functioning supplies and equipment will be available. Methods for monitoring environmental safety should be delineated, as well as those for psychologic and physiologic monitoring of the patient. Communication of the plan to all personnel involved in providing care to the patient is essential for continuity of care. The plan of care should be communicated to the patient and family or significant others as appropriate.

Documentation

Standardized patient care plans may be developed for common, expected problems of patient populations undergoing similar procedures (e.g., abdominal operations, open-heart surgery, or intracranial surgery). These can be organized on preprinted forms to include the usual, predictable problems/nursing diagnoses and expected outcomes. Space must be provided to note any unique or unusual patient needs. A preprinted perioperative record with standardized care plans for most common needs or problems may include, but is not limited to:

1. Potential for knowledge deficit
2. Potential for impaired skin integrity
3. Potential for hypothermia
4. Potential for fluid and electrolyte imbalance
5. Potential for impaired gas exchange
6. Potential for altered tissue perfusion
7. Potential risk for infection
8. Potential risk for injury

The format of the record may include checklists and spaces for specific patient data. The perioperative nurse who collects assessment data completes sections for individual patient factors relating to the nursing diagnoses and expected outcomes and any unusual nursing interventions that must be taken. This record accompanies the patient to all areas within the OR suite. It serves as a guide for the perioperative team who will provide care for this patient.

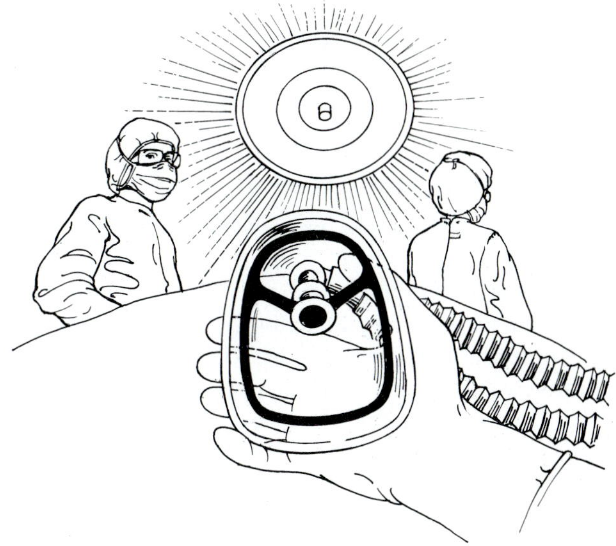

FIGURE 2-2 OR from patient's perspective.

Preoperative and Intraoperative Implementation

Implementation, the third component of nursing process, begins when the plan of care is put into action in the OR suite during the preoperative phase of the patient's experience and continues throughout the intraoperative phase. All interventions focus on the patient and are directed to the expected outcomes. Nursing interventions directly affect patient outcomes.

The perioperative nurse who planned care personally carries it out or communicates the plan to others to ensure that expected outcomes are achieved. The patient's responses are monitored during performance of planned nursing interventions.

Being a surgical patient is perhaps the only way of gaining insight into knowing what it feels like to be on the receiving side of perioperative care. Riding horizontally in an elevator on a stretcher is an extremely different sensation from moving vertically. Although premedication dulls the senses, when the circulating nurse assists the patient to move onto the operating table, the patient is jolted from a sedated calm state by the realization that "This is it—the moment I've dreaded is now actually here." The starkness of the OR is completely obvious (Figure 2-2). The patient looks to the nurse as his or her advocate. It is then that the patient-nurse relationship, the basis of nursing, is revealed. A fundamental element in this relationship is effective communication, both with and for the patient.

The perioperative nurse collaborates with physicians in giving and promoting continuous care to surgical patients. In the OR, the surgeon is in charge of the surgical procedure. The circulating nurse is the organizer, coordinator, stabilizer, and manager of the OR to which he or she is assigned. The surgeon relies on the circulating nurse to prepare for and keep the surgical procedure running smoothly. The nurse coordinates and implements the plan of care with and through the OR team members.

Standard V: Implementation

The perioperative nurse implements the interventions identified in the plan of care. Scientific principles provide the basis for nursing interventions. These interventions are consistent with the plan to foster continuity of nursing care in the preoperative, intraoperative, and postoperative phases. They must be performed with safety, skill, efficiency, and effectiveness.

The patient's welfare and individual needs are paramount in every facet of activity within the OR suite. They must not be compromised. Seemingly routine details have significant importance. For example, taking a defective instrument out of circulation may prevent injury to the patient. Checking the operating light helps to ensure the surgeon of vision in the surgical site. All preoperative preparations within the operating room must provide for the physical safety of the patient in an aseptic, controlled environment. The circulator also provides emotional support to the patient before transfer to the operating table and during induction of anesthesia.

The plan of care is implemented during the intraoperative phase of patient care. The remainder of this text focuses on the many and varied interventions that perioperative nurses and surgical technologists must take to ensure achievement of expected patient outcomes. Implementation of quality nursing care requires application of technical and professional knowledge, sound clinical judgment, and a surgical conscience on the part of all team members. Nurses have a responsibility to monitor constantly the physical and emotional responses of patients to nursing interventions. They also must control environmental factors that affect outcomes of surgical intervention.

Documentation

All nursing interventions, both routine and complicated, and observations of patient responses and resultant outcomes delineated in the care plan are documented as evidence of the care given. This written documentation becomes a part of the patient's permanent record. The RN circulator accountable for the patient's care is responsible for the documentation. Nursing interventions contributing to patient comfort and safety must be identified. Also, activities other than direct nursing care not recorded elsewhere that may affect patient outcomes are included, for example, how tissue specimens were handled.

Writing nurse's notes or progress notes on the patient's chart or completing an intraoperative observation checklist provides a profile of what has happened to the patient. Records and forms must be accurate and specific. State what happened and why. Besides having legal value, records are of value to the postoperative care team in their assessment and interpretation of altered physiologic status (e.g., pain or drainage from the trauma to living tissue occurring during the surgical procedure).

Intraoperative and Postoperative Evaluation

Evaluation is a comparison of actual results with expected outcomes. The evaluation component of nursing process begins after the planned nursing interventions are carried out or, by unanticipated circumstances, during implementation of the plan in the intraoperative phase of care. The effectiveness and appropriateness of expected outcomes, plans, and interventions are measured by the interpretation of the patient's responses to and outcomes of nursing interventions.

Tools used for evaluation include retrospective study of charts, records, and care plans or intraoperative process audit, peer review (see Chapter 3), and/or postoperative visits with patients. The purposes of evaluation are:

1. To provide feedback to providers about the surgical patient's total care.
2. To influence policy making and procedures. New methods are devised from evaluation and research.
3. To reveal areas where in-service education is needed for nursing personnel.
4. To revise the facility's quality improvement program. Evaluation provides an objective means for upgrading nursing care and improving performance.
5. To provide data for self-evaluation. Every nurse is accountable for his or her own actions and those of personnel under the nurse's supervision.

Standard VI: Evaluation

The perioperative nurse evaluates the patient's progress toward the attainment of outcomes. Evaluation is a continual process of reassessing patient needs, modifying expected outcomes and priorities, and revising plans when expected outcomes are not achieved or the patient's condition or adaptive level changes. In the OR a caregiver deals continually with anxiety and stress. A sense of tension more or less prevails from the team's constant need to accommodate to a variety of intense situations within a short time. The OR team is always on the alert and prepared to respond to any eventuality. Therefore the four components of the nursing process are performed concurrently and recurrently during the intraoperative phase as changes occur in the patient's internal and external environments.

The patient is observed during the surgical procedure and evaluated for responses to nursing and medical interventions. Changing conditions may require reassessment for new data and identification of new problems, revision of expected outcomes, implementation of alternative actions, or other modification of the initial plan of care. Ongoing assessment data are used to revise diagnoses, outcomes, and the plan of care as needed. Revisions in diagnoses, outcomes, and the plan of care are documented.

Determination of patient responses and realization of expected outcomes can be verified by direct observation of and/or conversation with the patient. In the narrowest scope, the perioperative nurse observes the patient's responses to nursing interventions during the immediate preoperative and intraoperative phases of care in the OR suite. The nurse may accompany the patient to the PACU to determine results of nursing interventions to the extent that they can be evaluated in the immediate postoperative period.

Ideally, the perioperative nurse visits the patient a day or two postoperatively or phones an ambulatory care patient at home. In the broadest scope of perioperative nursing, the nurse sees the patient for follow-up evaluation of outcomes of surgical intervention after the patient recovers sufficiently to be mentally alert.

Documentation

The patient's permanent record should reflect the ongoing evaluation of perioperative nursing care and its outcomes. This includes a comparison of expected outcomes to the degree of outcome attainment as determined by patient responses to nursing interventions. Documentation provides legal evidence of results of planned nursing interventions and revisions of plan based on reassessment of patient's needs.

CLINICAL COMPETENCY OF PERIOPERATIVE NURSE

Using the framework of the nursing process, AORN published *Competency Statements in Perioperative Nursing* in 1986, and revised them in 1992. These broadly written statements of expected competencies can be used to develop position descriptions, to develop performance appraisals, and to organize orientation and staff development activities. They may serve as guidelines for skills a nurse reasonably should expect to achieve to function as an RN in the OR. They incorporate the many principles, procedures, and practices elaborated throughout this text for competent care of the surgical patient. They include *competency* to:

1. Assess the physiologic health status of the patient.
2. Assess the psychosocial health status of patient and family.
3. Formulate nursing diagnoses based on health status data.
4. Establish patient's expected outcomes based on nursing diagnoses.
5. Develop a plan of care that identifies nursing interventions to achieve expected outcomes.
6. Implement nursing actions in transferring the patient according to the prescribed plan.
7. Participate in patient and family teaching.
8. Create and maintain a sterile field.
9. Provide equipment and supplies based on patient needs.
10. Perform sponge, sharps, and instrument counts.
11. Administer drugs and solutions as prescribed.
12. Physiologically monitor the patient during the surgical procedure.
13. Monitor and control the environment.
14. Respect the patient's rights.
15. Perform nursing actions that demonstrate accountability.
16. Evaluate patient outcomes.
17. Measure the effectiveness of nursing care.
18. Continuously reassess all components of patient care based on new data.

SURGICAL TECHNOLOGY

The activities of registered professional nurses are supplemented and complemented by the services of allied technical health care personnel. Broadly, the term *allied health care personnel* refers to individuals trained in a health care–related science with responsibility for the delivery of health care–related services, but who are not graduates of schools of medicine, osteopathy, dentistry, podiatry, or nursing. About two thirds of the health care work force is designated as allied health professionals. Educational preparation may be offered in colleges, vocational-technical schools, hospital-based programs, or military service schools. Technologists, technicians, and therapists in more than 130 occupational categories work collaboratively with and under the direction of physicians and nurses.

The *surgical technologist*, or ST, works with the surgeon, anesthesiologist or anesthetist, and professional RN as a member of the direct patient care team during surgical intervention. This team is referred to as the *OR team* or *surgical team*. The surgical technologist assists by preparing and handling supplies and equipment to maintain a safe and therapeutic environment for the patient. The surgical technologist performs specific techniques and functions designed to exclude pathogenic microorganisms from the surgical wound.

A surgical technologist completes a 1- to 2-year intensive educational program. This includes courses in anatomy and physiology, pathology, and microbiology as prerequisites to courses involving theory and application of technology during surgical procedures and for care of the OR environment. Other courses in the curriculum, such as pharmacology, help explain the underlying basis for technical tasks to be mastered. Courses in psychology, ethics, and interpersonal communication are fundamental to an appreciation of the humanities. These generic courses are beyond the scope of this text, which focuses on the essentials of OR technique that all OR personnel, professional and technical, should master.

Because they are administratively responsible to nursing service and considered part of the nursing staff complement in the OR, surgical technologists will be included in reference to *nursing personnel* throughout this text.

Standards of Practice for Surgical Technologists

The Association of Surgical Technologists (AST) has developed standards of practice. These provide guidelines for the development of performance descriptions and performance evaluations. The quality of the surgical technologist's practice may be judged by these standards. The six authoritative statements that comprise the standards describe the scope of patient care and serve as a guide on which to base clinical practice.

Standard I

Teamwork is essential for perioperative patient care and is contingent on interpersonal skills. Communication is critical to the positive attainment of expected outcomes of care. All team members should work together for the common good of the patient. Interpersonal skills are demonstrated in all interactions with the health care team, the patient and family, superiors, and peers for the benefit of the patient and the delivery of quality care. Personal integrity and surgical conscience are integrated into every aspect of professional behavior.

Standard II

Preoperative planning and preparation for surgical intervention are individualized to meet the needs of each patient and his or her surgeon. The surgical technologist collaborates with the professional RN in the collection of data for use in the preparation of equipment and supplies needed for the surgical procedure. The implementation of nursing interventions identified in the plan of care will be performed under the supervision of a professional RN.

Standard III

The preparation of the surgical suite/clinical area and all supplies and equipment will ensure environmental safety for patients and personnel. The application of the plan of care includes appropriate attire, anticipating the needs of the patient and OR team, maintaining a safe work area, observing aseptic technique, and following all policies and procedures of the institution.

Standard IV

Application of basic and current knowledge is necessary for a proficient performance of assigned functions. The surgical technologist should maintain a current knowledge base of procedures performed, equipment and supplies used, emergency protocol for various situations, and changes in scientific technology pertinent to his or her performance description objectives. It is the responsibility of the surgical technologist to augment his or her knowledge base by studying recent literature, attending in-service and continuing education programs, and pursuing new learning experiences.

Standard V

Each patient's rights to privacy, dignity, safety, and comfort are respected and protected. Each member of the OR team has a moral and ethical duty to the patient to uphold strict observance of the patient's rights. The surgical technologist, like all members of the health care team, is expected to perform as a patient advocate in all situations. This is an accountability issue that should be part of each aspect of patient care.

Standard VI

Every patient is entitled to the same application of aseptic techniques within the physical facilities. Implementation of the individualized plan of care for every patient includes the application of aseptic or sterile technique at all times while caring for the patient by all members of the health care team. All patients are given the same dedication in their care.

Clinical Competency of Surgical Technologist

The performance description developed by AST identifies performance objectives by which the surgical technologist may measure his or her level of competency. Adapted for this text are measurable competencies derived from the AST performance description for the surgical technologist. These include *competency* to:

1. Apply the principles of asepsis in a knowledgeable manner, assist in the sterilization and disinfection of equipment and supplies, maintain sterile technique at the sterile field, and assist with the terminal care of equipment and supplies after the surgical procedure is completed.
2. Identify emergency situations and institute corrective actions in a calm and efficient manner.
3. Maintain a current knowledge base and seek new learning experiences.

4. Provide a safe, efficient environment for the patient and the OR team.
5. Function in the role of patient advocate in support of the patient's rights, dignity, privacy, and best interest.
6. Perform within safe guidelines in the presence of the administration of anesthetic agents.
7. Maintain organizational skill and manual dexterity in the economy of time, motion, and supplies in a safe and efficient manner.
8. Demonstrate knowledge of anatomy and physiology and the recognition of pathologic deviations.
9. Perform in the role of surgical technologist in a professional manner at all times.
10. Perform as a team member for the common good of the patient and take responsibility for personal actions.

Scope of Practice

AST has identified three roles of the surgical technologist who has had specific education and job-related training. The roles identified are as the scrub person, the circulator, and the first assistant. National certification examinations are available for qualified surgical technologists who meet specific eligibility criteria.

Scrub Person

The scrub person is a team member who is qualified to assemble supplies, to prepare and maintain the sterile field, to anticipate the needs of the sterile team during a surgical procedure, and to provide a safe, efficient environment for the patient and team. On completion of the procedure, the scrub person is responsible for caring for the used equipment and supplies, disposing of contaminated articles in a safe manner, and assisting with patient care as indicated.

Circulating Surgical Technologist

Circulating duties are performed under the supervision of a professional RN. Interventions performed are identified by the established plan of care developed by the professional RN and are within the scope of educational preparation, supervised experience, and legal guidelines for surgical technologists.

Surgical Technologist First Assistant

First assisting duties may include exposure of the surgical site, hemostasis, and technical functions to assist the surgeon carry out a safe procedure with positive expected outcomes for the patient. This role is performed within the additional educational preparation, experience, and institutional guidelines for the surgical technologist first assistant.

CREDENTIALING

Credentialing refers to the processes of accreditation, licensure, and certification of institutions, agencies, and individuals. These processes establish quality, identity, protection, and control for competency-based education and performance of professional and allied technical health care personnel. Credentialing also protects the public.

Accreditation

An accrediting body of a voluntary organization evaluates and sanctions an educational program or an institution as meeting predetermined standards and/or essential criteria. The National League for Nursing accredits schools of nursing. Surgical technology programs are accredited in compliance with the *Essentials for an Accredited Educational Program in Surgical Technology*. The JCAHO accredits hospitals and ambulatory care centers. The American Osteopathic Association also accredits its member hospitals.

Licensure

A license to practice is granted to professionals by a governmental agency, such as the state board of nursing or medicine. On completion of formal academic education, nurses and physicians who successfully pass a state examination receive a license to practice in that state. To maintain this license; they must register with the state as required by law; hence the term *registered nurse*. Practical/vocational nurses also are licensed (LPN/LVN). Many states require evidence of continuing professional education for renewal of a license to practice.

Most states grant a license by reciprocity to applicants who move into their state to practice but who took the examination in another state. Some states require licensure for some categories of allied health occupations; however, surgical technologists and physician assistants are not currently licensed in any state.

Certification

A nongovernmental private organization can award a credential that attests to the competence or high level of knowledge of an individual who meets predetermined qualifications. Certification may be defined as the documented validation of the professional achievement of identified standards by an individual. Certification is voluntary, as opposed to licensure, which is mandatory.

Physicians, nurses, and allied health care personnel may be certified by their professional specialty association as competent in knowledge and skills to practice. Applicants must take an examination that tests knowledge in the area of specialization. Surgical technologists who successfully pass an examination attesting to their theoretical knowledge are certified by the Liaison Council on Certification (LCC), the certifying body for AST. These individuals are *certified surgical technologists* (CST). Similarly, a nurse anesthetist becomes a *certified registered nurse anesthetist* (CRNA) by passing the examination of the Council on Certification of Nurse Anesthetists.

Some nursing associations grant recognition of professional achievement and competence in current practice. A perioperative nurse who has been in clinical practice for 2 years and who has successfully passed an examination is certified by the National Certification Board: Perioperative Nursing, Inc. (NCB:PNI) as a certified perioperative nurse, designated CNOR. Several nursing specialty organizations, such as the National Association of Orthopaedic Nurses (NAON) and the American Society of Plastic and Reconstructive Surgery Nurses (ASPRSN), also offer certification examinations through their certifying bodies as an additional credentialing tool. Certification of nonphysician first assistants is discussed in Chapter 5.

Certification is usually granted for a limited time. To retain this credential, the individual must complete the recertification process established by the certifying body. Some certifying organizations require a specified number of clinical hours, continuing education hours, or a written examination or a combination of these to recertify. Maintaining certification by going through the recertification process established by the certifying body demonstrates a high level of motivation and commitment. To be certified is to demonstrate the attainment of more than minimal competency; it is a statement of certification level knowledge.

BIBLIOGRAPHY

Allen DE, Girard NJ: Attitudes toward certification, *AORN J* 55(3):817-829, 1992.

Allen GJ: Professionalism in the OR, *Surg Technol* 26(4):24-26, 1994.

American Nurses Association: *ANA standards of clinical nursing practice,* Washington, DC, 1991, The Association.

Association of Surgical Technologists: *AST Job description: CST surgical assistant,* Englewood, Colo, 1990, The Association.

Association of Surgical Technologists: *Essentials and guidelines for an accredited educational program in surgical technology,* Englewood, Colo, 1992, The Association.

Association of Surgical Technologists: *Standards of practice,* Littleton, Colo, 1989, The Association.

AST Board of Directors: Changing the paradigm, *Surg Technol* 22(1):7-9, 1990.

Brider P: Who killed the nursing care plan? *Am J Nurs* 91(5):34-39, 1991.

Chana CH: Documenting the nursing process: a perioperative nursing care plan, *AORN J* 55(5):1231-1235, 1992.

Corrigan D: Preparation: the key to success, *Surg Technol* 25(10):1, 19, 1993.

Giger NJ et al: Nightingale & Roy: a comparison of nursing models, *Today's OR Nurse* 12(4):25-30, 1990.

Glawe L: The surgical technologist and ethics, *Surg Technol* 26(2):1, 27, 1994.

Groah LK, Girard N: Professional nursing care delivery model, *AORN J* 57(6):1416-1424, 1993.

Haselfeld D: Patient assessment, *AORN J* 52(3):551-557, 1990.

Kam BW, Werner PW: Self-care theory: application to perioperative nursing, *AORN J* 51(5):1365-1370, 1990.

Lunow K, Jung L: Comprehensive perioperative care: patient assessment, teaching, documentation, *AORN J* 57(5):1167-1177, 1993.

Meyer C: Behind the double doors: the challenge of OR nursing, *Am J Nurs* 93(6):69-70, 1993.

Null S et al: Development of a perioperative nursing diagnoses flow sheet, *AORN J* 61(3):547-557, 1995.

Pobojewski BJ et al: Documenting nursing process in the perioperative setting, *AORN J* 56(1):98-112, 1992.

Proposed recommended practices for documentation of patient care in the perioperative practice setting, *AORN J* 61(3):616-621, 1995.

Rothrock JC: *Perioperative nursing care planning,* St Louis, 1990, Mosby.

Seifert PC, Grandusky RJ: Nursing diagnoses: their use in developing care plans, *AORN J* 51(4):1008-1021, 1990.

Shelly SR: Opinion: is professional nursing in the operating room? *AORN J* 51(1):287-289, 1990.

Shirley MA: Perioperative documentation: a generic care plan, *AORN J* 57(6):1427-1440, 1993.

Standards of perioperative nursing, *AORN J* 55(4):1047-1056, 1992.

Teutsch W: Surgical assisting: an issue for the 90s, *Surg Technol* 22(3):13-15, 1990.

Walsh KC: How to revise printed patient education materials, *Plast Surg Nurs* 12(3):128, 1992.

Watson DS: Opinion: technology in the perioperative environment, *AORN J* 59(1):268-277, 1994.

Weber G: Making nursing diagnosis work for you and your client: a step-by-step approach, *Nurs Health Care* 12(8):424-430, 1991.

Wilson CB et al: NLN accreditation as a marriage of strangers, *Nurs Health Care* 14(9):458-461, 1993.

CHAPTER 3

Accountability and Professional Obligations

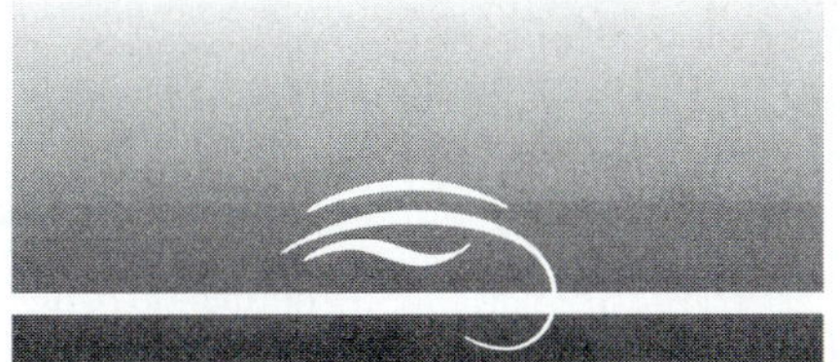

ACCOUNTABILITY

Accountability is the obligation of an individual to account for actions taken, consistent with responsibilities contracted by virtue of employment or learner experience. Stated more succinctly, to be accountable means to answer to someone else for something a person has done. Perioperative nurses and surgical technologists, both practitioners and learners, are accountable to:

1. Patients receiving services.
2. Employer or educational institution providing learning experiences.
3. Profession or vocation to uphold established standards of practice.
4. Self and other team members. Trust, honesty, and confidence are the essence of valid team member relations.

Accountability is concerned with both *efficiency* and *effectiveness*. Patients and the public demand quality care. Quality improvement programs establish methods for evaluating effectiveness by comparing actual care with established standards of practice. Perioperative nursing should include a systematic series of interventions directed toward preoperative assessment of the patient and development and implementation of an individualized intraoperative plan of care. Postoperative evaluation of the patient's responses and of the expected outcomes should be ongoing following nursing care. Patient care should be documented.

Incompetence or inappropriate behavior in the operating room (OR) may result in patient injury or dissatisfaction with care. Health care providers have a legal and moral obligation to identify and correct behaviors that threaten a patient's safety and well-being. An injury may result in pain, disfigurement, prolonged hospitalization or rehabilitation, or both, and may even prove fatal. If malpractice or negligence is established, a nurse or surgical technologist can be held liable for his or her own acts of omission or commission.

The welfare and safety of the patient constitute the principles on which nursing care is built. Efficiency and effectiveness focus on protection of the patient. Provision of safe care of the patient also protects the nurse, the surgical technologist, the surgeon and assistants, the anesthesiologist or anesthetist, and the health care facility from liability. It also upholds the reputation of the professions by maintaining the confidence of the consumer public. Safeguards against the hazards peculiar to care of patients in the OR are stressed throughout this text. Most incidents that could endanger the patient and lead to legal actions can be prevented. Prevention focuses on performance and quality improvement.

PROFESSIONAL OBLIGATIONS TO PATIENT

Inherent in professional practice is the duty to safeguard the well-being and rights of patients. The use of modern technology and the performance of some procedures may present risks to patients. These factors also may present ethical dilemmas for health care providers that are complicated by legal issues. Respect for the patient's autonomy and the right to make informed decisions about his or her own health care should be considered and balanced by professional obligations of beneficence, the duty to benefit, and nonmaleficence, not to harm.

Patient's Rights

The patient as a consumer purchases services to fulfill health care needs. The patient is entitled to certain rights. Access to health care is recognized as a right, not a privilege, for every human being.

In the interest of "more effective patient care and greater satisfaction for the patient, his or her physician, and the hospital organization," the American Hospital Association adopted *A Patient's Bill of Rights* as a national policy statement. Intended to be upheld by the hospital on behalf of its patients, these rights follow:

A Patient's Bill of Rights*

1. The patient has the right to considerate and respectful care.
2. The patient has the right to and is encouraged to obtain from physicians and other direct caregivers relevant, current, and understandable information concerning diagnosis, treatment, and prognosis.

   Except in emergencies when the patient lacks decision-making capacity and the need for treatment is urgent, the patient is entitled to the opportunity to discuss and request information related to the specific procedures and/or treatments, the risks involved, the possible length of recuperation, and the medically reasonable alternatives and their accompanying risks and benefits.

   Patients have the right to know the identity of physicians, nurses, and others involved in their care, as well as when those involved are students, residents, or other trainees. The patient also has the right to know the immediate and long-term financial implications of treatment choices, insofar as they are known.
3. The patient has the right to make decisions about the plan of care prior to and during the course of treatment and to refuse a recommended treatment or plan of care to the extent permitted by law and hospital policy and to be informed of the medical consequences of this action. In case of such refusal, the patient is entitled to other appropriate care and services that the hospital provides or transfer to another hospital. The hospital should notify patients of any policy that might affect patient choice within the institution.
4. The patient has the right to have an advance directive (such as a living will, health care proxy, or durable power of attorney for health care) concerning treatment or designating a surrogate decision maker with the expectation that the hospital will honor the intent of that directive to the extent permitted by law and hospital policy.

   Health care institutions must advise patients of their rights under state law and hospital policy to make informed medical choices, ask if the patient has an advance directive, and include that information in patient records. The patient has the right to timely information about hospital policy that may limit its ability to implement fully a legally valid advance directive.
5. The patient has the right to every consideration of privacy. Case discussion, consultation, examination, and treatment should be conducted so as to protect each patient's privacy.
6. The patient has the right to expect that all communications and records pertaining to his/her care will be treated as confidential by the hospital, except in cases such as suspected abuse and public health hazards when reporting is permitted or required by law. The patient has the right to expect that the hospital will emphasize the confidentiality of this information when it releases it to any other parties entitled to review information in these records.
7. The patient has the right to review the records pertaining to his/her medical care and to have the information explained or interpreted as necessary, except when restricted by law.
8. The patient has the right to expect that, within its capacity and policies, a hospital will make reasonable response to the request of a patient for appropriate and medically indicated care and services. The hospital must provide evaluation, service, and/or referral as indicated by the urgency of the case. When medically appropriate and legally permissible, or when a patient has so requested, a patient may be transferred to another facility. The institution to which the patient is to be transferred must first have accepted the patient for transfer. The patient must also have the benefit of complete information and explanation concerning the need for, risks, benefits, and alternatives to such a transfer.
9. The patient has the right to ask and be informed of the existence of business relationships among the hospital, educational institutions, other health care providers, or payers that may influence the patient's treatment and care.
10. The patient has the right to consent to or decline to participate in proposed research studies or human experimentation affecting care and treatment or requiring direct patient involvement, and to have those studies fully explained prior to consent. A patient who declines to participate in research or experimentation is entitled to the most effective care that the hospital can otherwise provide.
11. The patient has the right to expect reasonable continuity of care when appropriate and to be informed by physicians and other caregivers of available and realistic patient care options when hospital care is no longer appropriate.
12. The patient has the right to be informed of hospital policies and practices that relate to patient care, treatment, and responsibilities. The patient has the right to be informed of available resources for resolving disputes, grievances, and conflicts, such as ethics committees, patient representatives, or other mechanisms available in the institution. The patient has the right to be informed of the hospital's charges for services and available payment methods.

Conclusion

Hospitals have many functions to perform, including the enhancement of health status, health promotion, and the prevention and treatment of injury and disease; the immediate and ongoing care and rehabilitation of patients; the education of health professionals, patients, and the community; and research. All these activities must be conducted with an overriding concern for the values and dignity of patients.

This document gives patients the right to know what is being done to, for, and about them and their illnesses. For those patients not wishing to know the details during a crisis, their wish for only capsule explanations or essential information should be respected. The duty of disclosure is not absolute.

Patient-Physician Relationship

The attending physician should adequately explain—in clear, simple language—the nature, purpose, extent, potential hazards, and expected outcome of the procedure proposed, as well as other available options of therapy. The patient usually wants to know about the anticipated duration of hospitalization, absence from work, and cost of the procedure. Physicians, both surgeons and anesthesiologists, should inform the patient and not delegate this responsibility to a nurse or assistant. Adequate translation should be provided for patients with a language barrier, and interpretation should be provided for deaf patients.

*Reprinted with permission of the American Hospital Association, copyright 1992. *Note:* These rights can be exercised on the patient's behalf by a designated surrogate or proxy decision maker if the patient lacks decision-making capacity, is legally incompetent, or is a minor.

The surgeon is responsible for informing the patient about a proposed surgical procedure and its possible risks or complications. The explanation should include discussion of removal of parts, disfigurement, disability, and what the patient may expect in the postoperative period. It should be meaningful without creating unnecessary anxiety over very rare or insignificant hazards. Preoperative discussion also should include advice to the patient regarding diet, bathing, smoking, and other factors that might affect outcome and rehabilitation. The ultimate responsibility for obtaining consent for the surgical procedure is the surgeon's.

The anesthesiologist also has a responsibility to inform the patient of any potential for unfavorable reactions to a medication or anesthetic agent that may be given during the surgical procedure. The risks of anesthesia should be explained, but without causing the patient undue stress.

Persons facing a proposed surgical procedure are under stress. They often do not listen to or comprehend the physician's explicit information, even if it is repeated. Also, they may misunderstand what is said, or they may have unrealistic expectations of the potential outcome. For this reason, many physicians will, in a nonstressful manner, simply repeat the basic facts on a second occasion preoperatively. For legal protection, a physician should include in the patient's record a brief note covering the explanatory conversation of potential extent and consequences of a surgical procedure and the patient's reaction. Failure to provide full disclosure of the risks of the procedure and alternative modes of therapy has led to successful negligence suits. The physician is liable for misrepresentations, whether by affirmative statement or nondisclosure.

The physician-patient relationship is a contractual one. However, the physician is under no legal obligation to accept any person as a patient. The potential for litigation may influence the surgeon because positive guarantee of a favorable outcome of surgical intervention can never be fully guaranteed. Naturally, the patient wants a favorable outcome. The key to making medical decisions is the risk versus benefit ratio. A black-and-white answer is not possible in medicine. Once the patient has been accepted for treatment, the physician has a duty to perform to the best of his or her ability.

Immediately after the surgical procedure, the surgeon speaks to the patient's family or significant others and discusses with them the procedure performed, the patient's tolerance, and the prognosis. On the rare occasion when a patient dies during the surgical procedure, the attending physician is responsible for informing the family or next of kin. The surgeon has the ultimate responsibility of facing the patient and the family whether the outcome of surgical intervention is satisfactory or unsatisfactory.

Postoperatively the surgeon follows the patient's progress until discharge from his or her care or until return to a referring physician is indicated. At this point the duty to care for the patient is complete.

Second Opinion

If the physician or patient has doubts about the necessity for a procedure, another opinion should be sought from a qualified specialist in the appropriate field of surgery. A second opinion may be particularly indicated if the surgical procedure involves extended disability, such as amputation of an extremity or removal of an eye. Special consultation or consent may be required by hospital policy for procedures to terminate reproductive capability through sterilization and to perform an abortion. Consultation is a common and desirable part of good surgical practice. A second opinion may be required by third-party payers (i.e., insurance carriers).

Informed Consent

The patient should reconcile the need for or weigh the advantages and disadvantages of surgical intervention. Every patient is entitled to receive sufficient information on which to intelligently base a decision. The patient has the right to decide what will or will not be done to him or her. Only after making this decision is the patient asked to sign a written consent for a surgical procedure.

Written *informed consent* is necessary for any procedure that may possibly be injurious to the patient. The surgeon is responsible for making certain that the patient, parent, or legal guardian is adequately prepared to sign the consent document. A written consent is not an infallible legal protection for the surgeon and health care facility, but it does have legal value for all concerned with patient care. It provides evidence of the patient's agreement to allow a procedure(s) to be performed. Consent documents vary. Policies related to informed consent are developed by the medical staff and governing body in accordance with legal requirements. All personnel involved in care of patients should be familiar with these policies. All consent documents become a permanent part of the patient's medical record and accompany him or her to the OR.

Purposes of Informed Consent

An informed consent provides a mechanism to protect a patient's right to self-determination regarding surgical intervention. It also provides a means by which the patient can make an educated choice about having a procedure performed. The surgeon, the OR team, and the facility are protected from claims of unauthorized procedures not agreed to in advance.

General Consent

Most hospitals ask the patient, parent, or legal guardian to sign a *general consent* form on admission.

This form authorizes the physician in charge and the hospital staff to render such treatment or perform such procedures as the physician deems advisable. This general consent is relied on only for routine duties performed in the hospital. Physicians and nurses should be knowledgeable about the statements on the form used in their hospital.

Consent for Surgical Procedure/Operative Permit

The patient has a right to obtain information and to understand all relevant considerations—nature of procedure, benefits, risks, complications, and alternatives—before making a decision to accept or reject treatment. According to the American College of Surgeons, a reasonable approach to informed consent should answer the following patient questions:

1. What do you plan to do to me?
2. Why do you want to do this procedure?
3. Are there any alternatives to this plan?
4. What things should I worry about?
5. What are the greatest risks or the worst thing that could happen?

The patient has the right to waive an explanation of the nature and consequences of the procedure and the right to refuse treatment.

The surgeon and anesthesiologist should explain procedures to the patient or a family member or both, in understandable lay language, without details that might frighten them unnecessarily. When the patient signs an agreement, consent is given for the specific procedure the patient understands will be done. The patient must sign the consent unless he or she is a minor, is unconscious or mentally incompetent, or is in a life-threatening situation. The next of kin, legal guardian, or other authorized person, *not the surgeon,* must sign for these patients. Explanations are given by the physician to the parent of a minor or legal guardian of an incompetent adult. A witness verifies that the consent was signed without coercion after the surgeon explained the details of the procedure.

An informed consent document specifically outlines each procedure to be performed and explains the risks and benefits. The patient's consent is required for:

1. Each surgical procedure to be performed, including secondary procedures such as incision and drainage
2. Any procedure for which a general anesthetic is administered, such as an examination of a child under anesthesia
3. Procedures involving entrance into a body cavity, such as endoscopy
4. Any hazardous therapy, such as radiation or chemotherapy

The surgeon may be approved by the federal Food and Drug Administration (FDA) as a clinical investigator, or by the Department of Health and Human Services (DHHS) as a researcher for controlled experimental use of new drugs, chemical agents, or medical devices. Prior written consent based on an informed decision to participate in the research must be obtained from the patient. The surgeon completes an investigator's report that is returned to the supplier of the drug or device and eventually filed with the FDA. The patient is free to refuse or withdraw at any time from research carried out under DHHS auspices.

Validity of Consent

The document should contain the patient's name in full (a married woman's given name), the surgeon's name, the specific procedure to be performed, the signatures of the patient and authorized witness(es), and the date of signatures.

The patient giving consent must be of legal age and mentally competent. The patient must sign before premedication is given and before going to the OR or other treatment area, except in life-threatening, emergency situations. Before an elective surgical procedure, the patient should be asked to sign at least 1 day preoperatively. This may be done in the surgeon's office, hospital admitting office, or on the nursing unit, but *it must be an informed consent freely given (without coercion).* If the patient is:

1. A minor, a parent or legal guardian must sign.
2. An emancipated minor, married or independently earning a living, he or she may sign.
3. Illiterate, he or she may sign with an X, after which the witness writes *"patient's mark."* Illiteracy implies the inability to read and write. The patient must understand a verbal explanation, however.
4. Unconscious, a responsible relative or guardian must sign.
5. Mentally incompetent, the legal guardian who may be either an individual or an agency must sign. A court of competent jurisdiction may legalize the procedure in the absence of the legal guardian. A spouse or responsible relative of legal age may sign for an adult or an emancipated minor who is mentally incapacitated by chemical substances or alcohol when the urgency of the procedure does not allow time to regain mental competence.

A signed consent is legally regarded as valid for as long as the patient still consents to the same procedure. Institutional policy may vary.

Witnessing a Consent

The patient's or guardian's signature must be witnessed by one or more authorized persons. The witnesses may be physicians, nurses or other hospital employees, or family members as established by policy. Checking or witnessing a form does *not* ensure or validate that the document constitutes informed consent. The witness assumes no liability or responsibility for the patient's understanding. The witness signing a consent document attests only to:

1. Identification of patient or legal substitute
2. Voluntary signature, without coercion
3. Mental state of signatory (i.e., not sedated or confused) at the time of signing

Consent in Emergency Situations

In a life-threatening emergency, consent is desired but not essential. Although every effort should be made to obtain consent, the patient's physical condition takes precedence over an operative permit. The patient's state of consciousness may prevent him or her from verbalizing or signing a consent. Permission for a lifesaving procedure, especially for a minor, may be accepted from a legal guardian or responsible relative by telephone, telegram, or written communication. If it is obtained by telephone, two nurses should monitor the call and sign the form, which is signed later by the parent or guardian on arrival at the hospital. In lieu of these methods, a written consultation by two physicians other than the surgeon will suffice until a relative can sign a consent.

Responsibility for Consent Before a Surgical Procedure

The ultimate responsibility for obtaining consent is the surgeon's. The consent document becomes a permanent part of the patient's medical record and accompanies him or her to the OR. It is the duty of the circulator and the anesthesiologist when checking the patient's identity and chart on arrival in the OR to be certain that:

1. The consent is on the chart and is properly signed.
2. The information on the form is correct.

NOTE Checking or witnessing a form does not ensure that it constitutes informed consent.

The attending surgeon should also check the consent before an anesthetic is administered. If the surgeon intends or wants to perform a procedure not specified on the consent form, the circulator has the responsibility to inform the surgeon and/or proper administrative authority of the discrepancy.

Right to Refuse a Surgical Procedure

The patient has a right to withdraw written consent before the surgical procedure if his or her determination to do so is reached while in a rational state and voluntarily. The surgeon is notified and the patient is not taken to the OR.

The surgeon or referring physician explains to the patient the medical consequences of refusing the surgical procedure. If therapeutically valid, alternative methods of medical management should be offered. The surgical procedure is postponed until the patient makes a final decision.

The physician should inform the hospital administration of the patient's refusal to consent to treatment if the consequences will be substantially adverse. The physician also should obtain a written refusal from the patient, parent, or legal guardian to absolve him or her and the hospital from liability for failure to perform the recommended surgical procedure or other treatment.

Some states have legislated restrictions on rights of patients, or others on their behalf, to refuse surgical or medical treatments. Under a *doctrine of informed refusal*, the physician is required to inform the patient of dangers to his or her health if diagnostic tests or therapeutic procedures are not performed. Patients have the right to refuse to participate in research studies or be subjected to experimental procedures. The patient's right to self-determination may also permit him or her to refuse measures to prolong life. Hospital personnel need to be familiar with laws in their state pertaining to advance directives.

Advance Directives

The Patient Self-Determination Act enacted by the U.S. Congress in December 1991 ensures the patient of the opportunity to participate in decision making in advance of a procedure. This act applies to hospitals, nursing homes, home health care agencies, hospice programs, and health maintenance organizations (HMOs). It does not apply to freestanding ambulatory or office settings. The law requires that patients be informed of their rights to make their own decisions regarding their own health care.

Each patient has the right to determine the care he or she wishes to receive and to participate in the selection of delivery methods. The patient is entitled to the right of *self-determination* in decision making and to be consulted in matters concerning his or her well-being. This right extends to the issue of refusing treatment. The caregiver has the obligation to respect the patient's wishes regarding his or her care. A hospital policy must provide for making the patient aware of his or her right of self-determination. In many institutions policies permit the patient to indicate his or her preferences for treatment in the event that he or she should become disabled or incoherent. This is a legal document called an *advance directive.* The term *advance directive* encompasses durable power of attorney and living wills. The living will concept allows the patient to refuse treatment or nonessential measures to prolong life in a hopeless situation.

Many states require that the patient be asked on admission to the hospital whether he or she has a *durable power of attorney*. This document designates the person authorized to make decisions in the event that the patient is incapacitated. It allows the wishes of the patient to be met concerning his or her care needs if he or she becomes impaired and cannot make decisions. A federal regulation requires that the institution be aware of whether such a document exists and enacts it in the event of impaired cognitive function of the patient. Although the patient is not required by law to have a durable power of attorney, the OR team should be made aware of its existence. A copy, not the original, is placed in the patient's record.

The durable power of attorney does not apply to pediatric patients or to incompetent adults who are already under legal guardianship. These patients already have decision makers available to decide treatment options.

Patient Advocacy

If the perioperative nurse truly believes that *caring* is the essence of nursing, his or her practice will be guided by personal and professional values, beliefs, and standards. The nurse will use discretion and make morally and ethically valid decisions to protect the rights of the patient. The nurse will extend his or her perioperative practice beyond the confines of the OR and will become a patient advocate in the truest sense. Patient advocacy is not only the responsibility of the perioperative nurse but also the responsibility of the entire health care team.

A *patient advocate* recognizes the patient's and the family's needs for information and assistance in coping with the surgical experience regardless of the setting. As an advocate, the perioperative nurse can provide information discovered during patient assessment that identifies specific needs or health concerns that require action. Advance preparation can help the patient and family anticipate events. Assistance in coping acknowledges the anxieties and fears the patient and family are experiencing, regardless of how minimally invasive the procedure may seem. Remember, *no* procedure is minor to the patient! Every person reacts differently. The patient senses some relief in knowing that the caregiver has taken the time to identify needs specific to his or her care. The patient advocate is a caregiver who:

1. Establishes rapport with the patient, family, or significant other that conveys genuine concern and sincere caring.
2. Encourages the patient and family or significant other to express feelings and to ask questions.
3. Helps relieve anxiety and apprehension by providing factual information about what to expect.
4. Helps the patient make informed decisions throughout the perioperative experience.
5. Acts as a patient representative by communicating pertinent information to other team members.
6. Oversees all activities throughout the perioperative experience to ensure the safety and welfare of the patient.
7. Keeps the family informed of significant events throughout the perioperative experience.
8. Protects the patient's rights by compliance with advance directives for care (i.e., living will, durable power of attorney, or both).

In some settings a designated *nurse liaison* is present to maintain communication channels between the patient, the family, and the OR team. This nurse makes frequent rounds to see patients in the preoperative holding area and the postanesthesia care unit and to talk with families or significant others in the waiting area.

PROFESSIONAL OBLIGATIONS TO PERIOPERATIVE TEAM

Professional obligations may conflict with personal values. A perioperative nurse or surgical technologist may refuse to participate in a specific procedure for religious or moral reasons, if these beliefs have been made known. These should be discussed as a condition of employment and noted in the employee's personnel file. From a legal viewpoint, personal beliefs and values do not give nurses and surgical technologists the right to refuse to provide care to specific patients or in emergency situations. However, refusal to accept an assignment on the basis of inadequate preparation or incompetence is not only a right but a legal and ethical responsibility. Caregivers should not assume functions, such as first assisting, that cannot be performed competently without adequate instruction and supervision, and credentialing.

Work Assignments

The nurse manager is accountable for appropriateness of work assignments and for delegation of tasks to qualified personnel. The nurse manager who assigns or delegates tasks ultimately can be held accountable for actions performed. Therefore delegation of duties should be appropriate within the scope of nursing practice, and supervision must be adequate. *Delegation* implies directing a competent person to perform activities and tasks (i.e., duties) in a specific situation under the delegator's supervision. *Supervision* assumes appropriate guidance in the accomplishment of these duties with periodic observance and evaluation of the performance of them and validation that the assignments were performed according to the established standards of practice. Broadly interpreted, supervision includes provision of orientation, in-service and continuing education, policies and procedures, performance appraisal, and assistance as determined by qualifications and competencies. The nurse manager has a responsibility to determine that:

1. The duties are those that a reasonable and prudent nurse manager would delegate either to licensed professional nurses or to unlicensed assistive personnel, based on state statutes and other regulations governing delegation of nursing practice.
2. The assigned person can competently and safely perform tasks without compromising the patient's welfare.
3. The degree of supervision is appropriate.
4. The delegated duties were appropriately and completely performed.

The perioperative nurse or surgical technologist must be aware of his or her own competencies or limitations before assuming responsibility for duties in the circulator, scrub, or first assistant role. A current job description should reflect duties for which employees can be held accountable. Nurses must function within the limitations of the legal scope of nursing practice in their state.

Right to Refuse Assignment

Do not assume responsibility for tasks or duties unless instructed or prepared to perform them. For example, the circulator can refuse an anesthesiologist's request to pump the reservoir bag in the ventilating system of the anesthesia machine. Report requests outside the written job description to the nurse manager. Professional and legal responsibilities as well as the patient's rights dictate this course of action. The patient entrusts his or her well-being to others when undergoing surgical intervention. Nursing personnel should act as patient advocates when patients' rights are compromised.

Physician's Orders

The physician's orders must be understood and evaluated in relation to the patient's condition. If an order is difficult to understand, find out what is required before carrying it out. Always observe the patient closely. If a change is seen in the patient's condition, report it at once to the surgeon, anesthesiologist, or nurse manager. Do not carry out an order without checking or questioning it if it is not in the best interests of the patient. If a patient shows an adverse reaction to a medication or an intervention of any type, report this at once. The caregiver can be held liable for not reporting a patient's symptoms to the appropriate person in a timely manner. The adverse reaction may indicate a need for special medication or intervention. A delay in reporting may result in permanent or irreversible damage to the patient. In some cases, such as in an allergic reaction, the delay could result in death.

Keeping Nurse Manager Informed

Policies pertaining to patients and personnel apply to nursing personnel in the OR suite as well as to those on other units. The OR nurse manager is justifiably disconcerted to learn from someone outside the OR suite about events that should have been communicated to him or her by the OR staff. For the safety and welfare of patients and the efficient management of the OR suite, the nurse manager should learn what goes on in the department through proper channels. The manager must be informed of:

1. Any unexpected complication or change in condition of a patient.
2. Any injury to a patient or staff member.
3. Any unusual incident, including noncompliance with policies or procedures by a surgeon, anesthesiologist, nurse, surgical technologist, or nursing assistant. Every member of the OR team has both a moral and legal obligation to report a flagrant violation of accepted standards of patient care through appropriate administrative channels.
4. Concerns about instruments, equipment, or other supplies. Broken instruments and equipment must be taken out of service, and repaired or replaced.
5. Requests for equipment not available or for change of procedure.
6. Problems that can lead to conflict between team members or departments. The OR nurse manager will discuss problems concerning another nursing unit or department with the respective manager.
7. Any other problems that might impair efficiency within department. Seek advice and discuss minor problems before they develop into major incidents.

Impaired Team Member

To ensure patient safety and to help an impaired colleague, evidence of inability to function competently must be confronted. Impairment is usually caused by the dependency on a chemical substance such as drugs or alcohol. Signs and symptoms of impairment should be carefully documented in an objective manner with specific incidents. Most institutions have a form for the purpose of documenting irregular events. It is advisable to use this form for continuity of information and the ease of flow through the chain of command.

It is against the law to perform in the role of caregiver while under the influence of a mind-altering chemical substance. Rendering patient care while under the influence of alcohol or a mind-altering drug is potentially hazardous to the patient and to the work of the team as a whole. The impaired team member may be the surgeon, an assistant, the anesthesiologist, a nurse, or a surgical technologist. Chemical dependency is self-destructive behavior. The concern of all team members should be for the patient but also for the impaired team member. Incompetence or dangerous performance for whatever reason cannot be tolerated in the OR. Team members are legally and morally obligated to prevent participation by a colleague who is impaired by alcohol or drugs or who is incompetent in any way. Legally, team members are accountable for what they know. The facility can be liable for not taking action on substantial information about the performance of an employee or physician.

Treatment programs are available to assist an impaired professional. After the documentation is carefully evaluated, the impaired professional is confronted by his or her superiors. The impaired professional is given the opportunity to enter a treatment program, followed by a period of routine care after returning to the job. An impaired individual can be barred from practice by the state licensing board. A license to practice may be revoked or suspended for an act committed while impaired.

Working Conditions

The OR environment should be safe for both patients and personnel. Instruments and equipment should be used properly and maintained in good working condition. Broken instruments and malfunctioning equipment should be removed from the area, marked to prevent further use, and reported to appropriate persons. The equipment should be sent for repair or replacement. The surgeon may need to be notified that a piece of equipment he or she routinely uses is unavailable.

The Occupational Safety and Health Act became public law in 1970. Under this law, the Department of Labor created the Occupational Safety and Health Administration (OSHA). The major purpose of OSHA is to ensure safe and healthful working conditions for employees. Reducing the frequency of work-related injuries and illnesses and making the facility as safe as possible benefit both personnel and patients. OSHA regulations and other personnel safety measures are discussed in detail in Chapter 10.

The OR suite is a high-risk area with respect to employee safety. Obvious hazards to the physical well-being of any employee should be brought to attention of the nurse manager. If an employer fails to correct a condition that an employee believes to be in violation of a safety or health standard, physically harmful, or an imminent danger, the employee may request an inspection by an OSHA compliance officer.

Sexual Harassment

The health care team members have the right to work in an environment that is free of sexual hostility, coercion, and harassment. Accusations of sexual impropriety should be studied in terms of human behavior and how it is perceived by others. No two situations are alike. Feelings of harassment are very subjective and may be interpreted by others to be insignificant. The caregiver who thinks that another person in the work environment is imposing sexual advances or uncomfortable innuendoes should document specific incidents by describing the event or the exchange of conversation and the circumstances surrounding the occurrence. The names of witnesses should be included in the report. Documentation should be processed through the chain of command. A copy of all reports should be retained in the caregiver's personal file. If the harassment involves a superior, the documentation may be given to the person at the next higher level above the accused offender. According to Title VII of the Civil Rights Act of 1964 and the Equal Employment Opportunity Commission (EEOC) in 1980, sexual harassment is a barrier to employment. It is illegal and prosecutable by law. No caregiver at any level of the chain of command should tolerate this type of behavior; no offender is exempt from prosecution. The employer also may be held responsible. This is particularly true when an employer is made aware of the situation and nothing is done to remedy the problem.

IMPORTANCE OF STANDARDIZATION

OR nursing personnel should be able to cope with all situations and to give patients the best of their skills and knowledge. The enhancement of each individual's potential will provide the best guarantee of high-quality patient care. Although the use of different techniques may achieve the same results, each hospital establishes policies and procedures for all personnel to follow based on standards and practice guidelines developed by professional organizations. These written guidelines help prevent confusion and foster coordination of activities. Uniform procedures performed without deviation help personnel to develop skill and efficiency because:

1. The main purpose is to ensure the safety and welfare of the patient and personnel.
2. It is easier for the instructor and preceptors to teach learners clearly defined methods of work.
3. Learning is easier if everyone performs procedures in the same way.
4. Deviations show a need for evaluation of the procedures or the staff. Do the procedures need revision? Or have staff members become careless?
5. They provide an efficient check during the preparation for any surgical procedure. They supplement the memory of the OR staff.
6. One person can take over for another at any time during the surgical procedure, if necessary, and know exactly where to find instruments and supplies.

7. Routine procedures establish habits that increase speed in thought and action. Doing work in a certain way promotes a high level of proficiency.

All personnel involved in caring for surgical patients during the critical intraoperative phase should be thoroughly familiar not only with setups, policies, procedures, and surgeons' routines but also with equipment. Inasmuch as types vary, discussion of specific equipment has been minimized in this text. However, certain items and techniques for handling equipment are basic because comparable or identical equipment is in use in all facilities. Efficiency is increased by knowledge of equipment and its use. Many items are used only during the surgical procedure; others are returned to units with patients, and their use carries over to care of patients there.

The following *reference sources* are useful in mastering and carrying out accepted procedures and techniques:

1. *Nursing Practice Standards.* The nursing department establishes standards for appropriate patient care. Optimal standards of nursing practice guide the provision of patient care throughout the institution. Written policies and procedures reflect these standards. Institutional standards are based on standards established at national levels by the Joint Commission on Accreditation of Healthcare Organizations (JCAHO), the Association of Operating Room Nurses, Inc. (AORN), the Association of Surgical Technologists, Inc. (AST), the American Nurses Association (ANA), other nursing organizations, and governmental agencies. Nurses must practice within the limitations of the Nurse Practice Act of the state within which they practice. Copies of these documents are available for perusal from nursing or hospital administration.
2. *Hospital Policy Manual.* This manual contains basic and general administrative and patient care policies that apply to all hospital personnel. A copy is retained on each patient care unit and in all departments of the hospital.
3. *Safety Plan Manual.* The potential hazards and identifiable situations that may cause injury to a caregiver or patient are described in the manual provided by the hospital safety committee. Plans for fire drills and evacuation routes are outlined.
4. *Disaster Plan Manual.* This manual outlines the plans for both internal and external disasters. An *internal disaster* is an event that happens within the facility, such as an explosion or fire, that would require employee assistance for control of the situation and evacuation of personnel and patients. An *external disaster* is an event that happens outside the confines of the facility. An external disaster could be a natural phenomena such as an earthquake or a man-made accident such as a train wreck. Both events could cause injury to many people, requiring the activation of all services within the hospital in a short period. Personnel who are off duty will be called to work and will be assigned as needed.
5. *Infection Control Manual.* This manual contains the policies and procedures designed to minimize the risk of infection and control the spread of disease within the health care facility. It includes state, local, federal, and professional standards for the protection of the patient and the caregiver.
6. *Operating Room Policy Manual.* This manual, usually a hardcover ringed binder, contains the policies pertaining solely to the administration and operation of the OR department. A copy is available for reference either in the manager's office, at the control desk, or in both places.
7. *Operating Room Procedure Manual.* Procedure manuals are assembled for the OR department, as for other hospital departments. The primary purpose of the OR procedure manual is to detail why and how procedures should be specifically performed within the OR suite. It includes those procedures involving direct patient care and supportive procedures.
8. *Orientation Manual.* The orientation manual is designed to aquaint personnel with the environment, policies, and procedures specific to performance and the position descriptions of all personnel in the department.
9. *Instrument Book.* The instruments for each surgical procedure may be listed in a separate book, which is kept in the instrument room or processing area. Photographs or catalog illustrations help learners identify the vast number of instruments used.
10. *Surgeon's Preference Cards.* A preference card is maintained for each surgical procedure that each surgeon performs. A set of cards is kept in a central file under the surgeon's name. The file is kept where it is readily available. Each day the cards are pulled for the surgical procedures scheduled and taken to the appropriate OR. Nurses and surgical technologists consult them, along with the procedure book, as they prepare for each surgical procedure. The surgeon's specific preferences and any variance from the procedures in the procedure book are noted on the card. This information may be computerized. The cards are revised as procedures and personal preferences for new technology change. Figure 3-1 shows a sample surgeon's preference card.

SURGEON:	PROCEDURE:
Glove size: ______ Skin prep:	Position of patient: ______ Drapes:
SUTURES AND NEEDLES	INSTRUMENTS AND EQUIPMENT
Ties: Peritoneum: Fascia: Sub-cu: Skin: Retention: Other:	Basic: Special:
Dressings:	

FIGURE 3-1 Surgeon's preference card. (Reproduced by permission of Ethicon, Inc.)

11. *Directories.* Alphabetic listings of the location of supplies and equipment are maintained for the instrument room, general workroom, sterile supply room, and general OR suite storage areas. Regardless of where the storage areas are located, personnel should know the location of supplies and equipment. Directories save valuable time in trying to locate items.

BOX 3-1

Elements of Quality

- Q *Quality* improvement as an ongoing process
- U *Understanding* regulations, standards, policies, and procedures that provide guidelines for acceptable practices
- A *Accountability* for one's own actions
- L *Legal* rights of patients
- I *Individualized* patient care
- T *Technical* competency
- Y *Your* surgical and ethical conscience

QUALITY IMPROVEMENT AND PERFORMANCE

Perioperative nursing focuses on quality patient care. Quality is a difficult concept to define, measure, and evaluate. (Box 3-1 lists some elements of quality.) Nursing research and experience have shown that quality cannot be ensured, only monitored and improved. The JCAHO has adopted a definition of quality as "continual improvement" in patient care services to increase the probability of desired patient outcomes and to reduce the probability of undesired outcomes. Outcomes can be defined, monitored, and measured. Patient satisfaction is one outcome measurement that is critical in evaluating quality. Satisfied patients are more cooperative and receptive to therapy and teaching.

AORN has operationally defined quality of perioperative patient care as "professional nursing practice that encompasses components of analysis and interpretation."* These components include providing patient care within an environment conducive to effectiveness and efficiency, meeting patient needs in a caring manner and in conformity with established standards, and achieving desired outcomes or reducing the probability of undesired outcomes as perceived by the patient through properly implemented practices. These components imply that quality of care focuses on the service provided to meet the identified needs of the patient, and on the process of performing the necessary tasks to ensure safety and efficiency.

Each patient deserves the best possible care. Without the structure the nursing process provides, health care services would be fragmented and accountability for the quality of services rendered made difficult. Society demands accountability of those who provide services. Patients are protected by laws, standards, and recommended practices (see Chapter 4, pp. 56-58).

Performance should comply with established policies and procedures of the hospital or ambulatory care

*Operational definition of perioperative patient care quality, *AORN J* 49(5):1303-1305, 1989.

facility and with professional standards of practice. Nurses and surgical technologists can be held legally responsible for unethical, illegal, or unsafe practices or for failure to exercise judgment that is considered prudent practice. Nurses are responsible for their own acts in the patient-physician-nurse relationship and are required to exercise skilled judgment in making decisions. Nurses should see that all nursing procedures and techniques are correctly executed with patient outcomes kept in mind.

Quality improvement is important for professionalism, accountability, and cost containment. The mnemonic *SCORE* incorporates the elements of a quality improvement program (Box 3-2). Quality improvement programs provide a means for monitoring the quality of care received by a patient in a particular health care setting. Nursing care in the OR can be evaluated in the context of the total nursing process: assessment, planning, implementation, and evaluation. Quality is measured by identifying observable characteristics, judged according to standards, for an optimum achievable level of competence. For example, postoperatively the patient should be free from infection, skin breakdown, and injury related to positioning, instrumentation, or chemical agents. Effective care and improved patient outcomes result from efforts directed at applying the nursing process. Exemplary performance is achieved by dedicated perioperative nurses who achieve personal satisfaction from practicing quality patient-centered nursing. These nurses also are dedicated to continuously evaluating and improving patient care. Nurses may improve the quality of patient care by:

1. Identifying expected outcomes, providing specialized nursing interventions, and meeting the patient's physiologic and psychosocial needs based on observation and assessment of the patient's responses
2. Helping the patient and family adapt to what happens in the OR in relation to their perceptions and expectations through teaching
3. Delivering and supervising patient care with skilled planned nursing intervention and interdisciplinary collaboration
4. Coordinating all activities in the OR by planning, preparing for, and expediting the surgical procedure, keeping in mind individual patient, surgeon, and team needs

BOX 3-2

SCORE Elements of Quality Improvement Program

S *Standards* Statements of nursing interventions to be performed by health care personnel to achieve outcomes that the patient has the right to expect (e.g., provision for safety).

C *Criteria* Measurable clinical indicators and practice guidelines by which appropriateness of patient care is monitored systematically and outcomes are evaluated. They imply compliance with standards (i.e., requirements).

O *Outcomes* Patient's subjective perception of results of nursing interventions in relation to outcomes and expectations, and objective evidence of specific health status and observable behavioral responses.

R *Reports* Data collected to compare outcomes with criteria as basis for identifying and resolving problems.

E *Evaluation* Ongoing process of assessing maintenance of appropriateness and improvements in effectiveness of nursing interventions in providing patient care according to established standards and criteria.

Quality Improvement Programs

Quality improvement has been defined as the establishment of methods for assessing and measuring the degree of excellence in practice that constitutes quality and the determination that the patient receives this level of care. Although quality cannot be ensured, it can be monitored and effectively improved through performance. *Performance* has been defined as the way in which a health care organization carries out or accomplishes those functions that affect patient outcomes. Dimensions of performance include efficiency, effectiveness, efficacy, appropriateness, timeliness, and safety. Quality of care is a subjective judgment or perception. However, performance can be quantitatively measured to provide objective evidence on which quality judgments can be based. Quality then becomes the degree to which health care services achieve the desired patient outcomes, consistent with current professional knowledge. Quality improvement is a dynamic, ongoing process that focuses on the evaluation of patient outcomes to determine the method of improving care. Activities attempt to identify existing or potential problems in delivery of patient care and to resolve these problems.

The 1972 amendment to the federal Social Security Act creating the Professional Standards Review Organization (PSRO) for medical audits and utilization review in hospitals receiving federal reimbursement mandated the initiation of quality improvement programs in all hospitals. Some states and insurance carriers require hospitals to also have formal risk management programs. During the past two decades the JCAHO has shifted emphasis in its standards from quality assessment of patient care and quality improvement toward performance improvement of actual patient care and in management of health care organizations. AORN published quality improvement standards for perioperative nursing in 1992 that give guidance for monitoring and evaluating aspects of surgical patient care. These aspects include clinical activities that involve a risk for patients or tend to produce problems for patients or providers.

The JCAHO requires an ongoing program designed to objectively and systematically measure and evaluate the quality and appropriateness of patient outcomes, pursue opportunities to improve patient care, and resolve identified problems. In surveying facilities for compliance with its standards, the JCAHO looks for performance-based functional institutional standards and performance indicators that identify processes, systems, and outcomes. An *indicator* is a well-defined quantitative measure of an aspect of patient care that can be used as guide to monitor and evaluate the quality and appropriateness of health care delivery. Process indicators specify actions, events, or functions carried out during course of patient care. System or structure indicators monitor management and environment within the health care facility. Outcome indicators monitor what actually does (or does not) happen as a result of care provided. Each department is responsible for assessing and evaluating patient care and for improving levels of personnel performance and overall quality of care. However, the JCAHO emphasis focuses on performance improvement throughout the organization through a collaborative interdepartmental effort.

Quality and performance improvement are processes. Programs develop the tools to evaluate the quality of care and services that are delivered, to identify problems and opportunities, and to improve performance. Objectives of these programs may include the need to decrease patient dissatisfaction or to increase employee satisfaction and productivity. The quality improvement committee or the coordinator, or the risk manager, oversees established programs and coordinates activities and data analyses.

Indicator Measurement System

Clinical indicators that measure elements in the process or outcome of care are tools to assess quality. Analysis of data related to all patient care activities is essential to performance improvement. An integrated automated system using a single hospital-wide database facilitates indicator measurement, data retrieval, and analysis. The system allows departments to communicate by computer. Data are entered into the patient's medical record at the source (i.e., in the admission office or preoperative testing center, in the laboratory, in the OR, or at the bedside). The computer automatically scans patient data and flags abnormal findings, unexpected outcomes, or inappropriate interventions. Providers can use this information to correct problems immediately or to gather statistics for analysis of quality or performance failures. Postoperative infections can be differentiated, for example, by organism, wound classification, type of surgical procedure, and patient care activities. Incident reports also can be analyzed to identify recurring problems. Use of computerized indicator measurement systems helps document compliance with standards of care and practice guidelines.

Quality Improvement Studies

Most studies are designed to measure compliance with current policies and procedures and to identify need for change in practice guidelines or need for education of staff. Both strengths and weaknesses are identified. Ultimately the purpose is to correct deficiencies and deviations from expected standards. Important aspects that impact the quality of patient care are identified. A measurable indicator is established for each aspect. Data are collected and organized for evaluation. Data sources and methods of data collection must be appropriate for each indicator. The frequency of data collection and sample size must be sufficient to identify trends or patterns in delivery of care. An adequate sample size to obtain reliable data is usually 5% of the monitored patient population selected for study or 25 patients or events, whichever is greater. Data are collected concurrently or retrospectively.

A *concurrent study* begins with a current manifestation and links this effect to occurrences at the same time (i.e., is related to care in progress). Formerly referred to as a process audit, this type of study focuses on a systematic series of actions that brings about an outcome. Through concurrent observation, the implementation component of the nursing process can be monitored during the intraoperative phase of patient care to determine whether interventions performed are consistent with established standards for care and recommended practices. The interventions performed should protect the welfare and safety of the patient and should meet the identified physiologic and psychologic needs of the patient. The environment, including equipment or supplies used in the room, also can be evaluated at this time.

A *retrospective study* focuses on the end result of nursing care or a measurable change in the actual state of the patient's health as a result of care received. This evaluation of outcomes usually is done through review of patient records. The study begins with a current manifestation and links this effect to some occurrence in the past (i.e., is related to care previously given). Complications attributable to intraoperative care may be identified: for example, nerve palsy from poor positioning, infiltration of an intravenous infusion, or postoperative wound infection. The source of these complications may be difficult to identify unless every detail of actual care given and unusual occurrences are recorded in the patient's record. Accurate and complete documentation is essential for meaningful retrospective studies.

Any method that systematically monitors and evaluates the quality of patient care can enable perioperative nurses and surgical technologists to take corrective action for improvement of performance. Quality improvement studies also assist in coordination of plans for patient care with surgeons, improve communications with other departments, identify needs for revision of policies and procedures, and reassess equipment, personnel, and other aspects of patient care.

Intradepartment Quality Teams

Small groups of less than 10 staff members who work in the same department and who are supervised by the same manager meet voluntarily on a regular basis to identify, analyze, and develop solutions to problems in their specific work area. Each member should be committed to improving work methods, patient satisfaction, employee satisfaction, and cost containment. Achievement of these objectives may require data collection and presentations to peers, management, or both. Some problems can be solved directly by the team; others should be presented to management with recommended solutions. The team evaluates the success of its corrective actions and is committed to making them work. Documentation of intradepartmental quality control activities becomes part of the overall hospital quality improvement program.

Interdepartment Focus Groups/Teams

Representatives of all departments that directly or indirectly provide services to a group of patients, such as surgical patients, meet to identify specific problems and to analyze processes or systems that impact personnel performance and ultimately patient care. For example, delivery of supplies from the laundry or materiels management may contribute to delays in the OR. The focus group analyzes current procedures, recommends solutions, and implements changes. This collaborative effort improves personnel performance and enhances patient care. Interdepartmental communication is an essential organizational function.

Peer Review

Peer review differs from other quality improvement programs in that it looks at the strengths and weaknesses of an individual practitioner's performance rather than appraising the quality of care rendered by a group of professionals to a group of patients. An associate with the same role expectations and job description examines and evaluates the clinical practice of a peer. The individual is evaluated by written standards of performance. The review should offer constructive criticism of the performance observed. Through this framework, staff nurses and surgical technologists gain feedback for personal improvement or confirmation of personal achievement related to their effectiveness of technical and interpersonal skills and of decision-making abilities in providing patient care.

Bibliography

AORN quality improvement standards for perioperative nursing, *AORN J* 55(1):212-226, 1992.

Berstein SJ, Hilbane LH: Clinical indicators: the road to quality care? *J Comm J Qual Improve* 19(11):501-509, 1993.

Cushing M: Demystifying informed consent, *Am J Nurs* 91(11):17-19, 1991.

Defining performance of organizations, *J Comm J Qual Improve* 19(7): 215-221, 1993.

DeLong DL: Surgical quality assessment, *AORN J* 54(4):831-836, 1991.

Donabedian A: The role of outcomes in quality assessment and assurance, *QRB* 18(11):356-360, 1992.

Fernsebner B: QA monitoring reflects OR's uniqueness, *OR Manager* 6(5):8-9, 1990.

Fogg D: Discussion of the Joint Commission on Accreditation of Healthcare Organization's Agenda for change, Part I, *AORN J* 58(1):127-130, 1993; Part II, *AORN J* 58(2):390-395, 1993.

Gregory BS: AORN recommended practices: a valuable resource, not policy, *AORN J* 52(2):361-368, 1990.

Horty J: Advance directives give patients a new voice, *OR Manager* 8(2):18-19, 1992.

Hughes TL, Smith LL: Is your colleague chemically dependent? *Am J Nurs* 94(9):30-35, 1994.

Indemoto BK et al: Implementing the Patient Self-Determination Act, *Am J Nurs* 93(1):20, 22-25, 1993.

Jezewski MA: Culture brokering as a model for advocacy, *Nurs Health Care* 14(2):78-85, 1993.

JCAHO: new manual has major changes for 1994 surveys, *OR Manager* 9(10):1, 6-10, 1993.

Julius DJ, DiGiovanni N: Sexual harrassment, *AORN J* 52(1):95-104, 1990.

Krueger NE, Mazuzan JE: A collaborative approach to standards, practices, *AORN J* 57(2):467-480, 1993.

Murphy EK: OR nursing law: advance directives and the Patient Self-Determination Act, *AORN J* 55(1):270-272, 1992.

Murphy EK: OR nursing law: a preceptor's liability; filing reports on impaired colleagues; documenting lack of consent, *AORN J* 51(2):596-599, 1990.

Murphy EK: OR nursing law: at-will employment, *AORN J* 57(3):708-713, 1993.

Murphy EK: OR nursing law: rights of pregnant employees to refuse assignment, *AORN J* 55(4):1043-1046, 1991.

Palmer PN: Learn all you can about "advanced directive" now, *AORN J* 53(4): 901-902, 1991 (editorial).

Patterson P: Peer review promotes professional growth, *OR Manager* 8(2):10-11, 1992.

Rozovsky LE, Rozovsky FA: How nursing quality assurance can set the stage for liability, *Can Oper Room Nurs J* 8(4):19-20, 1990.

Ryan M, Martin J: Surgical nurse liaison, *AORN J* 53(6):1529-1535, 1991.

Schwarz JK: Living wills and health care proxies: nurse practice implications, *Nurs Health Care* 13(2):92-96, 1992.

Selbach KH: Chemical dependency in nursing, *AORN J* 52(3):531-541, 1990.

Shirley MA: Perioperative documentation: a generic OR care plan, *AORN J* 57(6):1427-1440, 1993.

White L: Quality improvement, *AORN J* 58(1):96-101, 1993.

CHAPTER 4

Legal and Ethical Issues

LEGAL ISSUES

Along with the development of *consumerism,* a movement that focuses on consumer rights, a well-informed American public has developed an increasingly litigious attitude, demanding compensation for bodily injuries or damages to personal property. The quality of health care in this country is assessed through the outcome of services rendered. If outcome is unacceptable, patients tend to take grievances to court. The severity of an injury usually determines whether a claim will arise, but other contributing factors include a breakdown of rapport between the patient and the health care team members and unrealistic expectations about the outcome of care.

Historical Background

Hammurabi (circa 1955-1913 BC), the King of Babylon, codified the laws of human behavior. The Code of Hammurabi included penalties for physician/surgeons who did not cure. "If a physician has treated a man with a metal knife for a severe wound and has caused the man to die, or has opened a man's tumor with a metal knife and destroyed the man's eye, his hands shall be cut off." Although this ancient punishment seems severe, it should remind the operating room (OR) team that their primary consideration is still to do patients no harm, *primum non nocere.*

The first recorded medical malpractice suit was tried in England in 1374. The first one in the United States occurred in 1794. Throughout the nineteenth century and the early part of the twentieth century, litigation against physicians was quite uncommon and rarely affected nurses. Malpractice suits began to increase markedly in the 1970s as an increasing number of people sought health care services and became aware of their humanitarian and consumer rights.

Causes for litigation lie in patients' and their families' belief that physicians have not provided appropriate diagnosis, treatment, or results. Although the physician is professionally responsible for patient care, other professionals and allied health care personnel act as part of the health care team. Ancillary personnel and suppliers of equipment and drugs also are indirectly involved in treatment and may be held liable.

Liability

To be *liable* is to be legally bound, as to make good any loss or damage that occurs in a transaction; to be answerable; to be responsible. Every professional RN and surgical technologist should always carry out duties in accordance with standards and practice guidelines established by federal statutes, state practice acts, professional organizations, and regulatory agencies, and those that are common practice throughout the community. Deviation from these standards and practices that cause injury to a patient can result in liability for negligence or malpractice.

Negligence is the lack of care or skills that any RN or surgical technologist in the same situation would be expected to use. It has been legally defined as omission to do something that a reasonable person would do, guided by appropriate considerations that ordinarily regulate human affairs, or as doing something that a reasonable and prudent person would not do. These acts of omission or commission may give rise to tort action, which is a civil liability, as a result of injury to a patient that can be traced directly to the breach of duty.

Malpractice is any professional misconduct, unreasonable lack of skill or judgment, or illegal or immoral conduct. Malpractice claims usually are settled in a civil court, but, depending on the severity of the injury and the extent of the misconduct, they may be taken to criminal court. From the legal point of view of damages or fault, professional negligence usually is synonymous with malpractice in a tort action.

A *tort* is a legal wrong committed by one person involving injury to another person, or loss of or damage to personal property. When a tort has been committed, a patient or family member may institute a civil action against the person or persons believed to have caused the injury, loss, or damage. Factors contributing to a successful lawsuit have been called the *four Ds of malpractice:*

1. *Duty* to demonstrate and deliver a standard of care directly proportional to the degree of specialty training received
2. *Deviation* of that duty by omission or commission
3. *Damage* to a patient or personal property
4. *Direct* cause of a personal injury or damage because of deviation of duty

Statutory laws (laws by legislation) and *common laws* (laws based on court decisions) differ from state to state. Courts differ at times in their interpretation of laws. Any caregiver who is in some manner thought to be responsible for injury to a patient may be sued. The nurse manager or instructor responsible for assigning duties to this individual may be included in the suit. Nurses and surgical technologists are considered employees of the health care facility and, if the court so rules, the facility is considered liable. However, the court may rule a learner or an experienced practitioner liable for his or her own acts. A learner may be held responsible in proportion to the amount and type of instruction received and judged by the standard of other learners in training. An individual can be held responsible for carrying out a wrong procedure if he or she has received sufficient instruction so that the correct procedure should be known.

Medical care and professional liability have become institutional problems. The primary cause of professional liability claims is *iatrogenic medical injury,* an injury or other adverse outcome sustained by a patient as a result of treatment. Many serious incidents brought to suit occur in the OR. In an alleged liability, the court will determine whether the RN or surgical technologist was acting in the course of duty as an employee, rendering independently contracted services, or responding to instructions as a borrowed servant of the surgeon. Control over and supervision of conduct may determine who is liable for any resulting injury to the patient. Lawyers for plaintiffs tend to name all team members and the facility as defendants in a lawsuit.

An unqualified, unconditional general rule of law is that every person is liable for torts he or she commits. *There is no exception to this rule.* However, liability may be imposed under one of several legal doctrines or common law precedents.

Borrowed Servant Rule

In the past, the surgeon was considered the "captain of the ship" in the OR. If the surgeon had supervisory control and the right to give orders during the surgical procedure, then the OR was like a ship and the surgeon like its captain. The captain or master was liable for the negligent acts of servants. Courts held that this doctrine, based on the master-servant relationship, was applicable by the mere presence of the surgeon. Once having entered the OR, the surgeon was considered to have complete control over other team members. Courts now recognize that the surgeon does *not* have complete control over the acts of the RNs and surgical technologists on the OR team. The surgeon usually is not held responsible when an RN or surgical technologist fails to carry out a routine procedure as expected. Courts have decided that certain procedures do not need to be supervised by the surgeon. By the *borrowed servant rule,* the surgeon is liable for acts of team members only when he or she has the right to control and supervise the way in which an RN or surgical technologist performs the work.

Independent Contractor

The employer may be held responsible for employees under the *master-servant rule.* However, the current trend is to hold an individual responsible for his or her own acts under the principle of an *independent contractor.* For example, a private scrub person, biomedical technologist, or a surgeon's assistant may contract with several surgeons to provide services on a fee-for-service basis. These individuals are not employed by the health care facility.

Doctrine of the Reasonable Man

A patient has the right to expect that all professional and technical nursing personnel will use knowledge, skill, and judgment in performing duties that meet standards exercised by other *reasonably prudent persons* involved in similar circumstances.

Doctrine of *Res Ipsa Loquitor*

Translated from Latin, *res ipsa loquitor* means "the thing speaks for itself." Before this doctrine can be applied, three conditions must exist:

1. The type of injury does not ordinarily occur without a negligent act.
2. The injury was caused by the conduct or instrumentality within the exclusive control of the person or persons being sued.
3. The injured person could not have contributed to negligence nor voluntarily assumed risk.

This doctrine applies to injuries sustained by patients while in the OR, as when a foreign object (i.e., sponge, needle, or instrument) is left in a patient's body or a patient sustains a burn. The defendant must prove that a breach did not occur in carrying out a policy and/or procedure, that is, that he or she was not negligent.

Doctrine of *Respondeat Superior*

An employer may be liable for an employee's negligent conduct under the *respondeat superior* master-servant employment relationship. This implies that the master will answer for the acts of a servant. If a patient is injured as a result of an employee's negligent act within the scope of that employment, the employer is responsible to the injured patient. The patient may sue both the facility and the employee.

Doctrine of Corporate Negligence

Under the corporate negligence doctrine, the facility may be liable, not for the negligence of employees, but for its own negligence in failing to ensure that an acceptable level of care is provided. A hospital has a duty to provide services and is responsible for:

1. Screening and verifying qualifications of staff members, including medical staff, according to standards established by the Joint Commission on Accreditation of Healthcare Organizations (JCAHO)
2. Monitoring and reviewing performance of staff members through established personnel appraisal and peer review procedures
3. Maintaining a competent staff of physicians, RNs, and employees
4. Revoking practice privileges of a physician, RN, or surgical technologist when the administration knows or should have known that the individual is incompetent or impaired

Doctrine of Informed Consent

State statutes differ in their interpretation of the *doctrine of informed consent,* but all recognize the physician's duty to inform the patient and to obtain consent before treatment. Failure to do so may be considered a breach of duty. A surgeon or anesthesiologist may be held liable for negligence if the patient can prove failure to disclose significant information that would have influenced a reasonable person's decision to consent. Informed consent is a protective document for the patient and the treating physicians.

Extension Doctrine

If the surgeon goes beyond the limits to which the patient consented, liability for assault and battery may be charged. However, it must be determined whether the patient consented to a specific procedure or generally to surgical treatment of a health problem. By medical necessity and sound judgment, the surgeon may perform a different or an additional surgical procedure when unexpected conditions are encountered during the course of an authorized surgical procedure. The surgeon may extend the surgical procedure to correct or remove any abnormal or pathologic condition under the *extension doctrine.* This doctrine implies that the patient's explicit consent for a surgical procedure serves as an implicit consent for any or all procedures deemed necessary to cope with unpredictable situations that jeopardize the patient's health.

Assault and Battery

In legal terms, *assault* is an unlawful threat to harm another physically. *Battery* is the carrying out of bodily harm, as by touching without authorization or consent. Lack of consent is an important aspect of an assault and battery charge. Consent must be given voluntarily with full understanding of implications. Witnessed written consents for a surgical procedure and anesthesia are obtained before the patient is premedicated and transported to the OR. The purpose of consent is to protect the surgeon, anesthesiologist, OR team members, and facility from claims of unauthorized surgical procedures and to protect the patient from unsanctioned procedures. (See discussion of informed consent in Chapter 3, pp. 37-39.)

If an economically compensable injury or untoward result occurs, an employee or the facility may be held liable for knowingly failing to intercede for an inadequately informed patient. It is not the duty of nursing personnel to give medical information to patients. This is solely the duty of the physician. However, facilities should have written policies pertaining to patient consent issues in compliance with state law. If a discrepancy from policy is identified, it must be brought to the attention of the surgeon and the nurse manager, and the circumstances should be documented.

Invasion of Privacy

The patient's right to privacy exists by statutory or common law. The patient's chart, medical record, videotapes, x-ray films, and photographs are considered confidential information for use by physicians and other health care personnel directly concerned with that patient's care. Lawsuits can and have been brought to the courts by patients for violation of this right. The patient should give written consent for videotaping or photographing his or her surgical procedure for medical education or research; the patient has the right to refuse consent. Unauthorized persons are not permitted to observe, videotape, or photograph surgical procedures or procedures that are of interest only to professional persons without the patient's written consent.

The patient has the right to expect that all communications and records pertaining to individualized care will be treated as confidential and will not be misused. This includes the right to privacy during interview, examination, and treatment. Every health care worker has a moral obligation to hold in confidence any personal or family affairs learned from patients.

NOTE If a patient has been criminally assaulted or is being held in criminal custody, team members are required by law to divulge voluntarily any information concerning the patient to legal authorities. Withholding known information is punishable by law.

Abandonment

Abandonment consists of leaving the patient for any reason when the patient's condition is contingent on the presence of the caregiver. In simpler terms, the danger to the patient by the caregiver's absence was greater in importance than the reason for leaving the patient. If the caregiver leaves the room knowing there is a potential need for care during his or her absence, even under the order of a physician, the caregiver is liable for his or her own actions.

In *Czubinsky v Doctor's Hospital,* the surgeon ordered the circulating nurse to leave the room to help him start another procedure. During the circulating nurse's absence, the patient had a cardiac arrest. The only team members on hand were the anesthesiologist and the surgical technologist. At the trial, the circulating nurse admitted to knowing that it was wrong to leave the patient, because of his condition, but left because of the surgeon's insistence. The expert witness testified that the circulator should not have been ordered away from the patient to work in another room. The court decided that if adequate help for resuscitation had been available in the OR during the patient's crisis, he would not have suffered permanent brain damage. The circulating nurse had a duty to remain with the patient, according to the court. This breach of duty resulted in permanent brain damage.

If an event necessitates leaving a patient, it is important to transfer care to another caregiver of equal status and function. In uncontrollable circumstances, consult with the OR manager or charge person immediately. Do not leave the patient unattended. No one may release a caregiver from a responsibility to a patient. A child or disoriented patient left alone or unguarded in a holding area, for example, may sustain injury by an electric shock from a nearby outlet or by other hazard within reach. The circulator may be considered negligent by reason of abandonment for failure to monitor a patient in the OR. The circulator should be in attendance during induction of and emergence from anesthesia and throughout the surgical procedure to assist as needed.

Liability Insurance

Formerly it was thought that patients did not sue RNs and other health care providers because they had no large assets. Unfortunately, this is no longer true. Increased autonomy increases the risk for liability. Perioperative nurses and surgical technologists work in concert with surgeons to provide care to the patient in the OR. Perioperative nurses make independent nursing decisions based on their assessments, and they are able to carry out nursing interventions without a physician's order. No matter how careful the nurse is, mistakes can happen. An unintentional wrong may cause injury to a patient. Most institutions carry insurance policies to cover incidents that result in harm to a patient when the event happens within the scope of institutional policies and procedures. However, in some instances, the insurance may not adequately cover the event. In this case, the nurse or surgical technologist who accidentally caused the injury can be sued as an individual, or as a codefendant. Carrying personal malpractice insurance protects against a possible discrepancy with the hospital's insurance policy. A policy can be individualized to meet the practice of the insured. The policy costs are tax deductible, and the protection of personal assets may well be worth the price of the coverage. Professional associations recommend individual professional liability insurance.

Safeguards for Operating Room Team

Complex technologies, acuity of hospitalized patients' conditions, short-stay procedures, diverse roles of providers, staffing inadequacies, and other factors present challenges in managing risks of liability. Many surgeons restrict their practices to avoid patients who have complex diseases or who are at high risk of uncertain outcomes. Others practice defensive medicine, ordering tests principally to protect themselves against possible litigation. As lawyers have become increasingly sophisticated in representing injured patients, all health care providers need to take measures to protect themselves from litigation. A preventive strategy includes:

1. Establishment of positive rapport with patients. Patients are less likely to sue if they perceive that they were treated with respect, dignity, and sincere concern. Patients expect information and good communication.

2. Compliance with legal statutes and standards of accrediting agencies, professional associations, and the health care facility.
3. Documentation of assessments, interventions, and evaluations of patient care outcomes.
4. Prevention of injuries by adhering to policies and procedures.
5. Control of further insult or damage if an injury occurs by reporting problems and taking corrective action.
6. Maintenance of good communications with other team members.

In addition to these strategies, the institution or ambulatory care facility as the employer and the RN or surgical technologist as the employee should take steps to avoid malpractice liability. A health care facility protects the patient, its personnel, and itself by maintaining good working conditions for a competent staff. Nursing staff members are hired after careful screening of educational preparation and licensure or certification credentials. The staff should be adequate in size and properly trained and assigned. A continuous program of staff orientation and education should be provided. Policies and procedures are established in a manner consistent with standards for competent nursing performance and patient safety.

Orientation and In-Service Education

Orientation of all new employees and regularly scheduled, ongoing, in-service educational programs are necessary to keep the nursing staff informed of policies, procedures, new techniques, and patient care practices. If the quality improvement programs identify deficiencies in patient care because of lack of knowledge, corrective action should be taken to improve performance. Deficiencies in institutional policies and procedures also should be reviewed by the staff and recommendations made to revise them as necessary.

Formally organized programs of environmental safety should be included in general orientation and inservice education. Personnel must be aware of specific job hazards and be familiar with occupational safety and health programs (see Chapter 10).

Continuing Education

Professional nurses and surgical technologists have a personal responsibility for continued learning through reading and attending workshops, seminars, conferences, and other educational offerings. Education does not end with basic training. Continued learning helps the practitioner keep abreast of current trends and practices. Evidence of continuing education is mandatory in some states for renewal of RN licensure. Certified perioperative nurses and surgical technologists must have evidence of continuing education for recertification. Although continuing education is not a measurement of proven competence in practice, it is the most widely accepted method of self-development. Moreover, it helps maintain and update the individual's body of theoretic knowledge as a basis for sound practice and judgment. (See discussion of clinical competency in Chapter 2, p. 31 and pp. 32-33.)

DOCUMENTATION OF PATIENT CARE

Verbal communication between patients and health care providers does not constitute legal evidence in a court of law. Only the patient's medical records can be subpoenaed as legal evidence of care received or omitted. Entries by nurses and physicians in the record provide a history of the patient's clinical course and responses to treatment. The record identifies what occurred and what did not. It also serves as the means of communication between providers during the course of treatment for continuity of care. Deficiencies in the record can destroy the credibility of the record and of the providers.

Documentation of care that has been given, including teaching provided, and patient's responses to care should be complete and accurate. Communications with the patient's family should be recorded. State facts, not conclusions, in objective terms. Some institutions allow patients access to their records so they can review them for reliability of subjective data and clarity of plans for treatment and teaching. The contents of the record substantiate the level of care for third-party reimbursement to the institution and are potentially open to examination in a court of law.

During a preoperative interview, the perioperative nurse should be alert to signs that a patient does not clearly understand what is going to happen as a result of surgical intervention. This must be brought to the attention of the surgeon. Significant observations should be recorded in the chart. For example, if a patient verbally withdraws consent for surgical procedure or expresses a fear of death in the OR, the perioperative nurse is responsible for communicating this information to the surgeon and anesthesiologist, and for recording the patient's statement.

The professional perioperative nursing role includes preoperative patient assessment and teaching, and postoperative evaluation of intraoperative care and reinforcement of preoperative teaching. All interactions with patients should be documented in the patient's chart, either in the nurses' notes or progress notes. The format for recording varies from institution to institution. Regardless of the format of the patient's record, all entries should be:

1. Written *legibly* in ink without erasures. Charting procedure may be specific, for example, that entries should be made in black ink.
2. Stated factually. Documentation of objective data and services rendered should be very specific. Observations and actions should be stated definitively, objectively, and concisely. Record what is seen, heard, felt, or smelled, that is, the *facts* without judgment or opinion.
3. Stated in complete words. Abbreviations may be permissible *only* for very commonly accepted medical terms, such as, T&A, D&C, OD, and TUR. Most institutions provide a standard list of their accepted medical abbreviations for charting purposes.
4. Dated, including the time note is written and the time action was performed as appropriate for significant events or changes in patient's condition.
5. Signed with full legal signature and status of the writer.
6. Corrected if an error is made. Date, time, and initials of person making a correction should be noted next to correction. A *single* line should be drawn through incorrect information without obliterating it, and the correct information should then be entered.

Types of Patient Records

Some facilities use problem-oriented records; others use integrated patient's progress records or do focus charting of patient care. Many of these are computerized. A plan of care in some format should be included in each patient's record. Flow sheets or standardized checklists may simplify this documentation. A standardized language to describe nursing interventions, such as the Nursing Interventions Classification (NIC) developed by the National Institute of Nursing Research, facilitates automated databases and computerized records.

Problem-Oriented Medical Record

With the problem-oriented, outcome-directed approach to care, the patient's chart is organized on the basis of problems rather than on the source of the data about them, such as radiology and laboratory reports. Each problem is numbered in a problem list with the initial plan for meeting each. Progress notes are charted corresponding to the problem number to facilitate assessment of the patient's response to planned intervention. Briefly, the record uses:

1. A defined database of information from history, physical examination, laboratory reports, and so on, to formulate a complete problem list
2. Plans for diagnostic, therapeutic, teaching, and follow-up care for each problem
3. Progress notes and flow sheets for multiple parameters that contain both subjective (symptoms) and objective (signs) information

Problem-oriented records document information needed to accurately diagnose conditions and treat patients. Specific problems, whether medical or nursing, actual or potential, are identified. A problem produces a change or poses a threat to the patient's health status or environment. It may be caused by a physical or emotional sign or symptom, disease process, or social or economic factor. The plan of interventions outlines specific actions and expected outcomes. The progress notes help physicians and nurses to make sound clinical judgments that ensure a consistent, problem-solving approach to patient care for actual and potential problems.

Integrated Patient's Progress Record

A record of the patient's progress from admission to discharge guides all health care providers in planning and coordinating care. Entry of a progress note may be made by a physician or nurse on the same record. This promotes the team concept of continuity in patient care by sharing knowledge and observations made by each team member who cares for the patient. A note is made after a treatment or procedure is initiated to document the condition and tolerance of the patient. Any change in condition, any unusual incident, complication, or deviation from the usual pattern or course of the patient should be recorded as a progress note. The nurse should document any nursing intervention and management, as well as the time the physician was notified, if this is indicated.

Focus Charting

A *focus* is a statement of significant nursing observations and assessments, that is, a nursing diagnosis. It can indicate a patient concern or behavior, or a significant change or event affecting the patient's status or treatment. Focus charting is helpful for recording the nursing process as described in Chapter 2. Patient care notes are organized by:

1. Data related to patient behaviors and status obtained from subjective information and/or objective observations (assessment, diagnoses, outcomes)
2. Intervention based on immediate care needs or plans for future nursing interventions (planning and implementation)
3. Response elicited by medical and nursing care (evaluation)

Focus charting documents the interventions performed. This may be referred to as *charting by exception.* Focus statements are used to identify the nursing diagnoses; the North American Nursing Diagnosis Association (NANDA) taxonomy may be used as described in Chapter 2, p. 27.

Written Plan of Care

Statements of identified patient needs and planned approaches for patient care to meet these needs are formalized into a plan of care (see Chapter 2). The plan includes:

1. Nursing diagnoses reflecting problems, needs, and health considerations unique to the patient
2. Expected patient outcomes
3. Nursing interventions

If standardized or generic patient care plans are used, they should be individualized to reflect modifications necessary to meet specific needs of each patient. The plan of care becomes a permanent part of the patient's medical record. It is used as a guideline for implementation of patient care, for documentation of care given, and for evaluation of compliance with standards of care and recommended practices.

Intraoperative Nurses' Notes

Specific care given in the OR should be documented on the patient's chart, not only for legal reasons, but also for the benefit of the postanesthetic care unit and unit nurses who provide postoperative care. Most ORs use a preprinted form with a standardized plan of care. Space is provided to add individualized patient needs and to document unusual interventions. Expected outcomes should be specified, for example, that the patient is free from injury. The specific nursing interventions performed to achieve these outcomes and to protect the patient should be accurately and completely documented by the circulator. This information should include, but not be limited to:

1. Patient identification and verification of surgical site, informed consent, allergies, and NPO (nothing by mouth) status of patient.
2. History, physical, laboratory reports, consent form, and other documents in chart per policy.
3. Times that patient arrived in and departed from OR and condition on transfer to and from the OR. Also the method of transport to and from the OR, and by whom, are included.
4. Level of consciousness or anxiety manifested by observable physical responses.
5. Position and types of restraints and supports used for maintaining position of patient on operating table and for protecting pressure areas, and by whom.
6. Personal property disposition, such as hearing aid, eyeglasses, and dentures.
7. Skin condition and antiseptics used for skin preparation, and by whom.
8. Location of electrosurgical dispersive electrode and monitoring devices.
9. Site, time started, solutions administered intravenously, including blood products, and type of needle or cannula, and by whom.
10. Medication types and amounts, including local anesthetic agents, and irrigating solutions used, and by whom.
11. Tourniquet cuff location, pressure, time of inflation duration, and identification of unit, and applied by whom.
12. Estimated blood loss and urinary output, as appropriate.
13. Sponge, sharps, and instrument counts as correct or incorrect.
14. Surgical procedure performed, location of the incision, special equipment used, such as a laser, and prosthetic devices implanted, if applicable, including manufacturer and lot/serial number.
15. Specimens and cultures sent to laboratory.
16. Site and types of drains, catheters, and packing as applicable.
17. Wound classification.
18. Type of dressing applied.
19. Any unusual event or complication and action performed.
20. All personnel in the room and their roles, including physicians, visitors, students, and others as applicable.

Incident Report

An injury may occur to a patient or a caregiver during a surgical procedure. The injury may be caused by a lack of proper care, unintentional mishap, or equipment failure. When an accident or unusual incident occurs, whether or not it involves an injury, the person who knows the factual details should notify the nurse manager at once and write an incident report. Details should be complete and accurate. They should be written as *statements of facts* without interpretation or opinion. For example, state that the area of the patient's skin under the inactive dispersive electrode of the electrosurgical unit was mottled and red when the electrode was removed, rather than writing that the patient's skin appeared burned by the dispersive electrode. Include the details of equipment used, including the serial number or asset tag identification, if appropriate. Describe the action performed, care or treatment given as a result of accidental injury on the incident report and, as appropriate, in the patient's record. The equipment in question should be removed from service and tagged "out of order." It must be tested, repaired, and approved for use according to institutional policy before it is again placed into service.

Incident reports are completed per policy and filed by administration. They should be reviewed as part of the overall institution and departmental quality improvement and risk management programs. Incident reports may be accessible to a plaintiff's attorney in some states; in others, they constitute privileged information. They may serve to refresh an individual's memory of events, however, for preparation of defense in a lawsuit. The fact that an incident report was completed should not be mentioned in the patient's medical record, including in the nurses' notes, or in the OR record.

GUIDELINES FOR PATIENT SAFETY

Patient safety refers to a systematic, institution-wide program designed to minimize preventable iatrogenic physical injuries and undue psychologic stress during hospitalization. Focus is on human behavior: what people are supposed to do and what they actually do. For example, whether or not a nurse or surgical technologist is responsible for an injury to a patient caused by defective equipment might depend on whether or not the defect was noticeable and remained unrepaired when the equipment was used. Could the injury have been prevented by foresight, alertness, and good judgment? Potential hazards can be identified and eliminated, thereby reducing risks to patients. A safe environment implies that risks do not exist; however, risks always exist but are controllable. Many standards, regulations, recommended practices, and practice guidelines have been established to help personnel maintain as safe an environment as possible to minimize risks of harm to patients.

OR nursing personnel should be able to cope with all situations and to give patients the best of their skills and knowledge. The enhancement of each individual's potential will provide the best guarantee of high-quality patient care.

Standards

A standard is an authoritative statement. Legally, a *standard of care* is defined as those acts that a reasonably prudent person with comparable training and experience would perform under the same or similar circumstances. Standards provide a basic model to measure the competence of practitioners and the quality of patient care. A competent level of nursing care is demonstrated by a process of accurate assessment and diagnosis, planning and implementing appropriate interventions, and achieving predicted outcomes (i.e., the nursing process). Professional standards delineate activities related to performance, quality improvement, continuing education, ethical behavior, and accountability.

Standards are broad in scope, relevant, attainable, and definitive. They outline for both practitioner and consumer/public what the quality of health care should be. They are the criteria used to evaluate competency in providing patient care. Standards established by regulatory agencies that are mandated by law must be met. Those established by national associations are recognized norms in most courts of law. Although compliance may be voluntary, because standards delineate either optimal or minimal levels of care or performance required, they should be achieved. For OR practice, these include professional/voluntary and regulated/mandated standards.

Professional/Voluntary Standards

1. *Standards of Perioperative Nursing*
   a. *Standards of Perioperative Administrative Nursing Practice.* These are structural standards that provide a framework for establishing administrative practices. They assist in developing philosophy, purpose and objectives, administrative accountability, policies and procedures, staffing patterns, and environmental control.
   b. *Standards of Perioperative Clinical Practice.* These are process standards based on problem-solving techniques utilizing principles and theories of biophysical and behavioral sciences. They describe how the nursing process is used.
   c. *Standards of Perioperative Professional Performance.* These are process standards that describe a competent level of behavior for the professional role of the perioperative nurse. The activities relate to quality practice performance appraisal, continuing education, collegial relations, ethical conduct, and utilization of resources and research.
   d. *Quality Improvement Standards for Perioperative Nursing.* These are process standards to assist in the development of quality improvement programs to monitor and evaluate the quality of patient care.
   e. *Patient Outcomes: Standards of Perioperative Care.* These are outcome standards that reflect desired observable patient outcomes during preoperative, intraoperative, and postoperative phases of the patient's surgical experience. They focus on common potential problems of patients undergoing surgical, diagnostic, or therapeutic intervention.

NOTE

- These five sets of standards for optimal level of practice are published by the Association of Operating Room Nurses, Inc. (AORN), in *AORN Standards and Recommended Practices for Perioperative Nursing.**
- The Operating Room Nurses Association of Canada has published *Recommended Standards for Operating Room Nursing Practice and Quality Assurance Audit.*
- The Australian Confederation of Operating Room Nurses has published *Standards, Guidelines and Policy Statements.*

**AORN Standards and Recommended Practices for Perioperative Nursing*, Association of Operating Room Nurses, Inc., 2170 South Parker Road, Suite 300, Denver, CO 80231-5711.

- The National Association of Theatre Nurses of Great Britain has published *Codes of Practices* for minimum level of practice.

2. *Association of Surgical Technologists Standards of Practice.** These are process standards that provide guidelines for safe and effective patient care in appropriate preoperative, intraoperative, and postoperative practice settings. They include interpersonal skills, environmental safety, and application of principles of surgical technology.
3. JCAHO standards.[†] These standards are functional, performance-based standards that focus on actual clinical care provided directly to patients and on management of the health care organization providing services. They relate to efficiency, effectiveness, safety, and timeliness; to appropriateness, continuity, and availability of care; and to patient satisfaction. The JCAHO evaluates compliance with these standards and reviews clinical outcomes of care provided as fundamental criteria for accreditation. Selective clinical indicators serve as outcome measurements for the processes of patient care.
4. National Fire Protection Association (NFPA) standards.[‡] These standards apply to environmental safety to reduce to the extent possible hazards to patients and personnel.
5. Association for the Advancement of Medical Instrumentation (AAMI) device standards.[§] These standards provide industry with reference documents on accepted levels of device safety and performance and test methods to determine conformance. AAMI also establishes standards for sterilization, electrical safety, and patient monitoring for health care providers related to evaluation, maintenance, and use of medical devices and instrumentation.
6. Clinically based risk-control standards. These standards are written by medical specialty groups and professional liability underwriters. They establish appropriate benchmarks of acceptable practices and outcomes specifically for controlling liability losses. They may be incorporated into the health care facility's risk management program.

*Association of Surgical Technologists, Inc., 7108-C South Alton Way, Englewood, CO 80112.

†*Accreditation Manual for Hospitals,* Joint Commission on Accreditation of Healthcare Organizations, 1 Renaissance Boulevard, Oakbrook Terrace, IL 60181.

‡Copies of NFPA standards are available from the National Fire Protection Association, 1 Batterymarch Park, Quincy, MA 02269.

§Copies of the AAMI standards and recommended practices are available from the Association for the Advancement of Medical Instrumentation, 1901 North Fort Meyer Drive, Suite 602, Arlington, VA 22209.

Regulatory/Mandated Standards

1. The 1965 Federal Medicare Act and all subsequent amendments to this Social Security Act.* This legislation incorporates provision that institutions participating in Medicare must maintain the level of patient care recognized as the norm. Specific requirements are included.
2. American National Standards Institute (ANSI) standards. These standards concern exposures to toxic materials and safe use of equipment, such as lasers.
3. Federal Food and Drug Administration (FDA) performance standards. Federal Medical Device Amendments regulate manufacture, labeling, sale, and use of implantable medical devices and many products used in or on patients. FDA also controls treatment protocols for use of drugs.

NOTE The label, manufacturer's lot number, and product description of implanted devices should be attached to or included in the patient's chart. If technique of implantation is inadequate, according to the manufacturers' instructions for use as approved by the FDA, the surgeon is liable. If the device fails, the manufacturer is liable.

4. Agency for Health Care Policy and Research (AHCPR) quality standards. These standards include indicators for performance measurement. They are based on research and professional judgment regarding effectiveness and appropriateness of medical care, including safety, efficacy, and effectiveness of technology. This agency was created in provisions of the Consolidated Omnibus Budget Reconciliation Act of 1989.
5. Occupational Safety and Health Administration (OSHA) standards. These legally enforceable standards include permissible levels of toxic substances in the environment. Although explicitly developed to protect employees, patients receive secondary benefits from control of hazards in the environment.

Recommended Practices

Recommended practices are optimum goals for the behavior of health care providers. They may not always be achievable, as standards are, because of limitations in a particular practice setting. Recommended practices state what ideally can be done.

AORN recommended practices for perioperative nursing concern aseptic techniques and technical aspects of nursing practice directed toward providing a safe environment for patients in the OR suite. They are based on principles of microbiology, scientific literature, validated research, and experts' opinions. Although compliance is voluntary, individual commitment, professional conscience, and the practice setting should guide OR nursing personnel in using these recom-

*From Social Security Administration, *Conditions of participation for hospitals,* Washington, DC.

mended practices. They represent what is believed to be an optimal level of practice and are intended to be achievable.

Guidelines and recommended practices of other agencies, including AAMI, Centers for Disease Control and Prevention (CDC), National Institute for Occupational Safety and Health (NIOSH), and Environmental Protection Agency (EPA), also are utilized for environmental, patient, and personnel safety (see Chapter 10).

Policies and Procedures

Policies and procedures reflect variations in institutional environments and clinical situations. They are established to protect employees and learners as well as patients. They establish the institution's standard of care. Policies should be consistent with regulatory and professional standards of practice. Procedures define scope, purposes, and instructions to be carried out and by whom. They should be clearly written, current, dated, and reviewed periodically. Although policies and procedures vary from one institution to another, they provide guidelines for patient care and safety in that specific physical facility. Learning and following policies and procedures are protective measures against potentially litigious actions. Many hospitals document in the employee's personnel file that policies and procedures have been reviewed during orientation to employment setting. Employees may be asked to sign a notation verifying knowledge of a new or revised policy or procedure after its introduction. Some policies and procedures apply to all employees; others are specific to department such as the OR. Because of the potential legal implications, adherence to all policies and procedures is mandatory. Personnel are evaluated on their ability to perform procedures correctly. The following should be included in the OR department manual. These are presented here for emphasis because of their legal ramifications. These procedures are incorporated into discussions in subsequent chapters.

Identification of Patient

When a patient enters the hospital or ambulatory care facility, an identification wristband is put on the patient in the admitting area. The unit nurse and OR nursing assistant check the label on the identification wristband before the patient leaves the unit. To verify accuracy, the patient may be asked to spell his or her name and pronounce it. The circulator and anesthesiologist always check the wristband with the patient and surgeon, the patient's chart, and the operating schedule. The surgeon sees the patient before anesthetic agents are administered.

Protection of Personal Property

Generally, unit personnel are responsible for removing valuables and prostheses before patients go to the OR suite. The circulator is responsible, however, for checking each patient and removing, as necessary, hearing aid(s), contact lenses or eyeglasses, dentures, artificial extremities or eyes, wigs, wristwatches, rings, or religious medals. Besides the danger of losing these items, some can be hazardous to the anesthetized patient.

Any item that is removed should be placed in a rigid container and labeled with the patient's name and number. The patient's personal property should never be wrapped in a paper or linen towel that could inadvertently be discarded in a trash receptacle or laundry hamper. The container may be retained by the circulator during the surgical procedure and sent with the patient to the recovery area. Alternatively, the circulator may immediately ask a nursing assistant to return the container to the patient care unit. This person should obtain a receipt for the patient's personal property from the person receiving it. The receipt is given to the circulator to put in the patient's chart along with a notation of the transaction in the nurses' notes.

Patients value their property. Personnel are liable for the care of it. A caregiver can be held liable for loss or damage to a patient's personal property.

Observation of Patient

Unattended patients may fall from a stretcher or the operating table. Falls are one of the most frequent causes of avoidable injuries. Siderails and restraint straps should be used to protect patients, especially children and disoriented or sedated adults. Observe special care when moving all patients to and from the operating table.

Positioning of Patient

The patient should be positioned on the operating table to ensure adequate exposure of the surgical site for the surgeon. However, the position in which the patient is placed must not compromise respiration and circulation or cause injury to skin, soft tissues, joints, or nerves. Adequate support should be provided during movement into desired position. Pressure areas should be adequately protected. The surgeon determines the appropriate position. The circulator assists in positioning the patient.

Because many patients receive general anesthesia and are therefore unconscious, constant vigilance is essential to safeguard patients unable to protect themselves. If a patient receives an injury while unconscious, such as a brachial nerve palsy from hyperextension of an arm on the armboard, negligence on the part of an individual or all team members may have to be disproved in court. Liability on someone's part would be difficult to dispute. Everyone in the OR has a duty to monitor and protect the patient.

Dedication to Aseptic Technique

Infection is a serious postoperative complication that may become life-threatening for the patient. OR team members must know and apply the principles of aseptic and sterile techniques at all times (see Chapter 12). Meticulously follow established procedures. An emergency situation in which asepsis becomes a secondary concern is a rare occurrence.

Postoperative wound infection can originate in the OR from a break in technique by a team member, from airborne contaminants of improperly cleaned floors, furniture, and ventilating systems, or from inadequately sterilized instruments and supplies. Reuse of disposable items may be indefensible, as can be use of an unsterile endoscope introduced into a body cavity or organ through an incision in tissues. Always carry out strict asepsis and be alert to the technique of other team members. Remember the principle: when in doubt about sterility, consider unsterile.

Execution of Accurate Counts

The responsibility for accounting for all sponges, needles and other sharp objects, and instruments *before the surgical procedure begins and at the time of closure* rests with the circulator and scrub person (see Chapter 20, pp. 425-429). The surgeon and assistant facilitate the count of the items on the surgical field before closure. If they have done their part in the count procedure and a sponge is left in the wound because of a miscount by the circulator, this caregiver may be held solely responsible. In such a case the surgeon, facility, and scrub person may be exonerated. Likewise, the scrub person may be deemed responsible for an incorrect needle or instrument count. Because sponge, needle, sharps, and instrument counts are recognized as essential to safe practice, an OR team that omits counts and a facility that has not established counting procedures would be in a difficult legal position. The circulator should document in writing the outcome of the final counts and any unusual incidents concerning them, including the need for an x-ray film to look for a lost item.

Instruction for Use of Equipment

All instruments, equipment, and appliances should be used and tested according to the recommendations and instructions of the manufacturer. Electrical and laser equipment also should pass inspection by the biomedical engineering department. Electrical equipment should be properly grounded to prevent electric shock and burns. *Do not use equipment or devices that are known or suspected to be faulty.* Nursing personnel who set up and operate institution-owned equipment may be negligent if a patient is injured. Great care is critical to prevent injury when using all equipment in the OR.

Prevention of Skin Injury

Skin injury may be caused by an electrical or thermal device, chemical agent, or mechanical pressure. Pressure necrosis is most common following procedures lasting more than 2 hours, especially cardiovascular procedures that involve decreased peripheral perfusion for a prolonged period.

A burn may occur from the use of a hot instrument such as a mouth gag or a large retractor. The scrub person should immerse a hot instrument in a basin of cool sterile water before handing it to the surgeon.

A patient may be burned during use of the electrosurgical unit. Inadequate skin contact or improper placement of the inactive dispersive electrode can cause an electrical burn. Alcohol and other flammable solutions can be ignited if pooled under the patient or allowed to saturate drapes. A thermal burn also can occur from other types of electrical and laser equipment if improperly used or maintained. The caregiver should be aware that the effects of some types of lasers on tissue are not readily visible until tissue necrosis takes place several days postoperatively.

Administration of Drugs

Any drug that the surgeon uses in the surgical site, such as an antibiotic or local anesthetic, is recorded by the circulator and by the surgeon in the operative note. The drug is checked by two RNs, or the circulator with the anesthesiologist or surgeon if a surgical technologist is scrubbed, before it is transferred to the sterile field. The scrub person repeats the name of the drug to the surgeon when passing it. The surgeon is rarely held responsible if handed the wrong drug. The scrub person frequently has more than one drug on the instrument table. Each must be correctly labeled and administered.

An RN must monitor the cardiac and respiratory status of a patient receiving local anesthesia, with or without intravenous (IV) conscious sedation, if an anesthesiologist is not present. The nurse must initiate interventions promptly if the patient has an untoward reaction. Policies and procedures must be delineated for care of the patient receiving local anesthesia (see Chapter 18).

Preparation of Specimens

With very few exceptions, all tissue removed from a patient is sent to pathology (see Chapter 20, pp. 421-422). The loss of a tissue biopsy could necessitate a second surgical procedure to obtain another. Incorrectly labeled specimens could result in a mistaken diagnosis, with possible critical implications for two patients. Also, the loss of a specimen could prevent determination of a diagnosis and subsequent initiation of definitive therapy. The pathology report becomes part of the patient's record as added documentation of the tissue removed and of the diagnosis.

Care for foreign bodies according to institution policy. They may have legal significance and frequently are claimed by police, especially if the foreign body is a bullet. A receipt from the person taking them protects personnel and the facility.

Patient Teaching

The patient and family members expect to be informed about the illness or condition and how to deal with it to restore or maintain optimum health. The patient has the right to make decisions about his or her own care. The perioperative nurse can assist, however, through preoperative teaching of deep-breathing exercises, for example, which will help the patient's postoperative recovery. Information should be provided so the patient knows how to respond appropriately. This is particularly important for ambulatory surgery patients (see Chapter 41). Patient teaching should be documented in the chart.

ETHICAL ISSUES

Some situations that arise in the OR environment may be contrary to personal morals, values, beliefs, or religion. Nursing personnel assume legal and ethical rights, duties, and obligations by virtue of employment and their relation with patients and other health care professionals. Ethics are influenced externally by laws, policies, and societal codes. Internally, ethics are influenced by life experiences, religious persuasion, and ethnocultural background. Important strategies for a health care provider, when faced with an ethical uncertainty, are to clarify personal values, develop a personal philosophy of caregiving, identify the situation at hand, acquire knowledge of laws and professional codes, and understand the ethical principles and values of others. After identifying these factors, the caregiver can make a rational decision in an ethical dilemma.

Values are operational beliefs an individual chooses as the basis for behavior. They may change over time. They may create conflicts when value systems are not compatible with the expectations of others. Values reflect ethics. *Ethics* refer to standards or principles of moral judgment and action. Ethics as a philosophy defines a systematic method of differentiating right from wrong within a specific belief system. Professional and societal codes and standards offer guidelines in this determination. Ethics and law are closely related. Legal doctrines often interpret ethical concepts.

The Bill of Rights of the Constitution of the United States establishes individual rights based on moral principles that respect human worth and dignity. The courts have upheld the right to individual autonomy in making health care decisions, as evidenced by rulings about such issues as abortion, the right to die, and living wills.

Professions have codes of conduct and documents that include value statements derived from moral concepts. Nurses may refer to the International Code of Nursing Ethics and to a code established by their own professional association, such as the Code for Nurses of the American Nurses Association (ANA) (Box 4-1) or the Code of Ethics for Nursing of the Canadian Nurses Association. The Code of Ethics of the Association of Surgical Technologists (Box 4-2) provides guidance for surgical technologists. In the statement of the nature and scope of nursing practice titled *Nursing, A Social Policy Statement*, developed by the Congress of Practice of the American Nurses Association in 1980, nurses are committed to respect for human beings "unaltered by social, educational, economic, cultural, racial, religious or other specific attributes of human beings receiving care, including nature and duration of disease and ill-

BOX 4-1

Code for Nurses: American Nurses Association

1. The nurse provides services with respect for human dignity and the uniqueness of the client, unrestricted by considerations of social or economic status, personal attributes, or the nature of health problems.
2. The nurse safeguards the client's right to privacy by judiciously protecting information of a confidential nature.
3. The nurse acts to safeguard the client and the public when health care and safety are affected by incompetent, unethical, or illegal practice by any person.
4. The nurse assumes responsibility and accountability for individual nursing judgments and actions.
5. The nurse maintains competence in nursing.
6. The nurse exercises informed judgment and uses individual competency and qualifications as criteria in seeking consultation, accepting responsibilities, and delegating nursing activities.
7. The nurse participates in activities that contribute to the ongoing development of the profession's body of knowledge.
8. The nurse participates in the profession's efforts to implement and improve standards of nursing.
9. The nurse participates in the profession's efforts to establish and maintain conditions of employment conducive to high-quality nursing care.
10. The nurse participates in the profession's effort to protect the public from misinformation and misrepresentation and to maintain the integrity of nursing.
11. The nurse collaborates with members of the health professions and other citizens in promoting community and national efforts to meet the health needs of the public.

From American Nurses Association: *Code for nurses with interpretive statements*, Washington, DC, 1985, The Association.

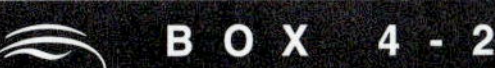

BOX 4-2

Code of Ethics: Association of Surgical Technologists

1. To maintain the highest standards of professional conduct and patient care.
2. To hold in confidence, with respect to patient's beliefs, all personal matters.
3. To respect and protect the patient's legal and moral right to quality patient care.
4. To not knowingly cause injury or any injustice to those entrusted to our care.
5. To work with fellow technologists and other professional health groups to promote harmony and unity for better patient care.
6. To always follow the principles of asepsis.
7. To maintain a high degree of efficiency through continuing education.
8. To maintain and practice surgical technology willingly, with pride and dignity.
9. To report any unethical conduct or practice to the proper authority.
10. To adhere to the Code of Ethics at all times in relationship to all members of the health care team.

Adopted by Board of Directors, Association of Surgical Technologists, Englewood, Colo, 1985.

ness." The ethics of a profession establish the role and scope of professional behavior and the nature of relationships with patients and colleagues.

Universal moral principles guide ethical decision making and activities in clinical practice. These include:

1. *Autonomy.* Self-determination implies freedom of choice and ability to make decisions to determine one's own course of action. Decisions may be made in collaboration with others based on reasonable and prudent information. Decisions should be acknowledged and respected by others.
2. *Beneficence.* Duty to help others seek balance between what is good to do and what might produce harm to another or self.
3. *Nonmaleficence.* Duty to do no harm.
4. *Justice.* Allocation of human, material, and technologic resources a person has a right to receive or claim (i.e., equality of care).
5. *Veracity.* Devotion to truthfulness (i.e., to give accurate information).
6. *Fidelity.* Quality of faithfulness, based on trust and honesty, that protects rights of individuals, such as dignity and privacy.
7. *Confidentiality.* Respect for privileged information received from another person with disclosure only to appropriate others.

Bioethical Situations

An ethical dilemma arises in the work situation when the choice between two or more alternatives creates a conflict between an individual's value system and moral obligation to the patient, to the family or significant others, to the physician, or to the employer and coworkers. Conflicts can be between rights, duties, and responsibilities.

Both legal and ethical considerations can cause conflicts. Legally a patient has the right to choose among treatment alternatives or the right to refuse treatment. Philosophically, the patient's preference may be different from that of the health care provider. The primary responsibility to the patient is to ensure delivery of safe care. This includes use of appropriate and available technology, but only if this is the patient's choice, freely given through informed consent or is known to be the patient's wish. Conversely, the patient and the caregiver may be forced to face court-ordered procedures or treatments. This may impose the need to assist in a surgical intervention, such as a cesarean section on a woman who has moral or religious objections to this form of treatment, but who has been ordered by the court to have the procedure performed for the benefit of the unborn fetus. This example is extreme, but the courts are constantly working to define the rights of the unborn. In the issue of viability vs. possible death, the court usually supports measures necessary to sustain life. The caregiver who participates in a court-ordered procedure is protected by law provided that the performance of his or her duties meets the standards of care.

Health care providers should decide for themselves the appropriate course of action when dealing with an ethical dilemma. By developing a personal philosophy and by understanding both professional and institutional philosophies, the health care provider may better answer many personal ethical questions such as: When does life begin? When does it end? What is my perception of quality of life between conception and death? What is my role in health care? What are my moral rights in relation to my personal beliefs and values and those of others? Where are the dividing lines between a patient's personal rights to privacy and confidentiality and a legal or ethical duty of disclosure?

A few of the ethical dilemmas facing physicians and OR nursing personnel are mentioned for personal consideration. It should also be noted that some of these issues are regulated by state statutes or federal court decisions. Nursing personnel should be familiar with statutes in the state in which they practice, particularly those regarding participation and the right to refrain on the basis of personal beliefs. You may have a right to refuse to participate, but not at the expense of a patient's safety and welfare. The patient cannot be harmed by acts of commission or omission.

Reproductive Sterilization

Voluntary nontherapeutic sterilization as a contraceptive method may be contrary to the moral, ethical, or religious beliefs of a nurse or surgical technologist. A few states have statutes regulating this practice; most do not. Sterilization procedures also may be therapeutic to preserve life or health, or eugenic to prevent procreation by mentally retarded persons, habitual criminals, and sexual deviates. These sterilizations are regulated in many states.

Abortion

Legalized abortion allows the deliberate termination of pregnancy. In the 1973 decision of *Roe v Wade*, the U.S. Supreme Court ruled that any licensed physician can terminate pregnancy during the first trimester with consent of the woman. During the second trimester, the Court requires a state statute that regulates abortion on the basis of preservation and protection of maternal health. During the third trimester, legal abortion should consider meaningful life for the fetus outside the womb and endangerment to the mother's life and health.

Although by law physicians may perform abortions in health care facilities, many persons, individually and collectively, and institutions such as the Roman Catholic Church oppose abortion. Many persons believe abortion is a form of active euthanasia because it takes the life of an innocent victim without consent. By selective abortion, one or more fertilized ova may be aborted so that others may mature properly in a multiple pregnancy, perhaps the result of fertility drugs. Genetic and reproductive biologies have introduced many new procedures to the OR.

In facilities where abortions and other reproductive procedures are performed, employees have the right to refrain from participation because of their moral, ethical, or religious beliefs, except in an emergency that threatens the life of the mother. These beliefs should be made known to the employer. Some states have a protective statute for employees and employers regulating good-faith efforts to accommodate employees' beliefs. In other states, laws protect an employee from being forced by an employer to assist in abortion.

HIV and Other Infections

The prevalence of human immunodeficiency virus (HIV) infection with or without acquired immunodeficiency syndrome (AIDS) has created a catastrophic health problem with many inherent emotional issues. Unlike other communicable diseases, HIV infection is a fatal illness with no known cure at this time, although some drug therapies may slow its progression. We do know its mode of transmission and methods of prevention. Therefore personal biases and prejudices should not discriminate against the infected patient. However, underlying attitudes about homosexuality and IV drug abuse may subconsciously influence care of such patients. Are these patients any different from hemophiliacs or persons who became infected through a contaminated blood transfusion? Should the infant with HIV be treated any differently from an infant with a congenital anomaly? Does the diagnosis make a difference to the health care provider and to the quality of care the patient receives? Should it? Knowing that HIV is transmitted by blood and body secretions, conscientious application of universal precautions for infection control should provide protection against occupational exposure to HIV, hepatitis B, tuberculosis, and other communicable infections. The ANA Code for Nurses emphasizes that care is given regardless of the nature of health problems.

Other ethical questions concern screening and reporting test results vs. confidentiality. Do the same considerations apply to team members as to patients? What constitutes valid reasons for restricting or terminating employment on the basis of health status? This question has broader implications than just the issue of being seropositive for HIV. For example, do pregnant team members have exclusionary rights? No state mandates by law that a health care worker can refuse to provide care for a patient with HIV infection. Risks vs. benefits to self, patients, and team members, plus potential litigation as a result of actions, should be evaluated in making ethical decisions. Confidentiality, privacy, and informed consent are human rights that should be protected, but the right to health care should be protected also.

Both AORN and Association of Surgical Technologists (AST) have published statements encouraging health care facilities to provide policies and procedures to ensure safety of patients and personnel. These organizations believe providers have a right to know the HIV or other infectious status of patients, but providers do not have the right to discriminate against HIV-positive patients. They should follow the CDC guidelines in caring for all patients to prevent transmission of infection.

Human Experimentation

Intrauterine fetal surgery, vital organ transplantation, mechanical or prosthetic device implantation, and other procedures still in developmental stages are performed with the patient's consent, in clinical research-oriented hospitals. Those willing to be pioneers in human experimentation have given, or will give, hope to many patients with poor prognoses. A caregiver should decide if he or she wants to participate in experimental surgery. If not, this individual should seek employment in an OR where only established therapeutic or palliative procedures are performed.

Quality of Life

Surgeons often must make critical decisions before or during surgical interventions regarding quality of patients' lives following surgical procedures. Palliative procedures may relieve pain. Therapeutic procedures may be disfiguring. Life-support systems may sustain vital functions. Life-sustaining therapy may prolong the dying process. Many questions arise regarding care of terminally ill, severely debilitated or injured, and comatose patients. What will be the outcome in terms of mental or physical competence? When should cardiopulmonary resuscitation be initiated or discontinued? Physicians decide, but all team members are affected by the decisions.

How is euthanasia defined? Is mercy killing ethical, legal, or justified? Does the patient, family or guardian, physicians, or courts have the right to decide to abandon heroic measures to sustain life? The patient who is aware of the options and whose decision-making capacity is intact has the right of self-determination. This rarely is feasible in the OR; therefore OR personnel make an ethical decision unless guided by an advance directive.

Euthanasia *Euthanasia,* derived from Greek, means *good* or *merciful death.* Both active and passive euthanasia are intentional acts that cause death, but the methods are different. An act of direct intervention that causes death is active euthanasia. Withholding or withdrawing life-prolonging or life-sustaining measures is passive euthanasia. Death is caused by the underlying disease process, trauma, or physiologic dysfunction. The concept of euthanasia seems to violate traditional principles of medicine to preserve life, but our modern technologies can prolong life without preserving quality. Quality of life can be interpreted as life that has a meaningful value. Most human beings value having cognitive abilities, physical capabilities, or both, and living free of undue pain and suffering. This raises the ethical question of whether physicians should do what they technologically can do.

Right to Die Courts have determined that patients have a constitutional right to privacy in choosing to die with dignity, or a common law right to withhold consent and refuse treatment. A mentally competent adult over the age of 18 can execute a *living will,* an advance directive, directing physicians and other health care providers not to use extraordinary measures to prolong life. Most physicians designate "extraordinary" as those measures that are optional, such as mechanical respiration, hydration, nutrition, medication, or a combination of these, that sustain life. If it is the expressed wish of the patient, the physician writes "no code," "do not resuscitate" (DNR), or "do not attempt resuscitation" (DNAR) orders. A living will relieves family members of decision making when the patient becomes terminally ill, incompetent, or comatose. No laws or court precedents deal specifically with the issue of DNR orders in the OR. Institutional policy should address this matter. Theoretically a patient can attempt to sue for compensation for expenses under a "wrongful life," negligence, or battery charge. In general, courts are reluctant to hold health care workers liable for acts performed to maintain life. In *Anderson v St. Francis,* defibrillation was performed despite a DNR order. The court found that sustaining life was not considered an injury and rejected the compensatory claim on the basis of the wrongful life theory.

A questionable practice would be to automatically suspend the DNR order when a patient has a surgical procedure. A patient who has a standing DNR order may need a procedure to decrease pain or palliate uncomfortable symptoms. Before going to the OR, the DNR order should be reaffirmed with the patient, guardian, or the person who has durable power of attorney. The DNR order must be clarified before the patient goes to the OR. In an emergency, if there is a doubt about the validity of the DNR order or a question of reconsideration of the order, the caregiver should participate in a physician-ordered resuscitation. If there is question about the patient changing his or her mind, a second chance may not be an option during an emergency situation. If the patient or legal guardian is specifically clear about upholding the DNR order in the OR, the OR team has the responsibility to follow the patient's wishes. A caregiver who has a moral objection to upholding a DNR order may request reassignment through the nurse manager of the department.

The issue of discontinuation of life-sustaining measures becomes more difficult in a comatose, mentally incompetent patient who has not executed an advance directive. Family members, in consultation with physicians and other health care team members, may request DNR orders. Many physicians and hospitals will not comply with this request without a court order. Nurses are obligated, however, to follow DNR orders. Exercising the right to die with dignity wish of the patient does not absolve health care providers from the patient's right to receive supportive quality care during the dying process.

Organ Donation and Transplantation

As a result of the Uniform Anatomical Gift Act of 1968, many adults carry cards stating that at death they wish to donate their body organs or parts for transplantation, therapy, medical research, or education. Most states include this information on a driver's license. If this legal authority is not available, some states have a *required request law.* In the event of legally defined brain death, the caregivers are required by this law to ask the family if they wish to allow organ retrieval for transplantation.

Transplant surgeons rely on the OR teams who procure donor organs, eyes, bone, and skin. Organ transplantation has complicated the issue of time of death. Perfusion of oxygenated blood through tissues must be sustained by artificial means during procurement of vital organs with functional viability. Legally, death has occurred when an individual has sustained either irreversible cessation of circulatory and respiratory functions or irreversible cessation of all functions of the entire brain including the brain stem. Therefore the accepted definition of irreversible coma for potential donors includes unresponsivity, no spontaneous movements of respiration, no reflexes, and flat electroencephalogram. When brain death is determined by two physicians who are not part of the transplant team, the donor will be taken to the operating room with artificial support systems functioning to perfuse organs. Some nurses and surgical technologists have difficulty assisting with removal of viable organs from seemingly living bodies. Another difficult scenario occurs at the conclusion of the procedure when the last perfused organ is removed. At this point, ventilatory and circulatory support is discontinued and the anesthesia personnel leave the room. This is a difficult time for the remaining team who may still have the assignment of procuring nonperfused tissues such as skin, bone, or eyes.

Nurses and surgical technologists who believe that donation of organs and body parts is a gift of love find it easier and ethically acceptable to participate in procurement procedures. They may believe that everyone, including themselves and their loved ones, should be donors under appropriate circumstances, or at least has the right to make this decision. Family members of donors have encouraged OR team members not to focus on their grief, but rather to focus on the gifts of life they are giving unselfishly to the recipients. This does not mean the donor's family will not go through the grieving process. They will need support. Similarly, OR team members must cope with feelings related to termination of the life of a donor in a similar manner as dealing with sudden death of a patient in the OR.

Death and Dying

Death is inevitable. Intellectually we know this. But for the health care team, death can be a difficult burden to bear because our education, experience, and philosophy are dedicated to survival. Regardless of religious or cultural beliefs, death is a mystery, a passage from the known to the unknown.

Terminally ill patients and patients with near-fatal traumatic injuries pass through stages of dying. These stages include denial and isolation, anger, bargaining, depression, and acceptance. A therapeutic relationship with a dying patient should be open and caring. The sharing of truth as it is perceived by physicians and nurses is most important. Trust is more important to the patient than efforts to relieve fears associated with dying. Tell the patient what he or she wants to know with sensitivity to minimize psychic trauma. Acknowledge the patient's feelings in a supportive manner that lets the patient know that it is all right to feel and behave the way he or she does. The terminally ill patient should choose how he or she wishes to live in the time remaining. The right to death with dignity should be respected to the extent possible. Facing the reality of death can help an individual understand the meaning of life. Patients fear abandonment. Reassure the patient by words and actions that he or she is not alone. Touch communicates a connection with life.

The mourners, left to grieve the death, go through a process similar to the stages of dying. Family members, friends, and nurses caring for the terminally ill patient may begin to work through the process simultaneously with the patient or within a similar time frame. OR nursing team members rarely are a part of this process. Perhaps, partially for this reason, the death of a patient in the OR is an unsettling experience, especially if it is unexpected.

One of the most difficult aspects of a death in the OR for the nursing team members is after the actual event. The surgeon goes to inform the family. The assistants and anesthesiologist leave the room. Many times the perioperative nurse and the surgical technologist are left alone with the patient's body. The patient should be prepared so the family can view the body if they wish to do so. The family will not be brought to the OR, but to an adjoining area where they can have privacy to express their feelings. The OR nurse may be expected to accompany the family and to lend support during the viewing. A chaplain or nurse manager may not be available, especially at night. Specific departmental policies should be developed to assist the caregiver with this difficult aspect of patient care.

At some point, perioperative nurses and surgical technologists should confront their own feelings regarding death. This is always painful, but it is important for caregivers to work through a grieving process and to acknowledge their own feelings. A sense of failure or helplessness, frustration, guilt, and anger are not uncommon feelings. Neither is detachment, depending on the circumstances. The age of the patient, the patient's condition at the beginning of the procedure, the resuscitative interventions performed to prevent death, and the cause of death all have an impact on emotional reactions. Similarly, personal religious and cultural beliefs, and previous experiences with grief or death affect an individual's coping mechanisms. The OR team expects the patient to leave the OR alive, so it can be devastating when the patient dies. Coping strategies that can help team members may include to:

1. Realize everyone involved is part of a team effort. Recognize personal limitations but also acknowledge efforts.
2. Believe in a power greater than the skills of the team. A fatalistic attitude toward life may help resolve the issue of death.
3. Share feelings with others. It is helpful for team members to talk with each other about what happened. Encourage each other to share feelings associated with the loss. Crying is acceptable behavior. Feelings of grief are expressed in many ways. Expressing personal feelings to peers, family, or friends can be therapeutic.
4. Deal with the patient's death by identifying personally with the loss. Empathy is a positive emotion. Working through the grieving process is also positive. It brings a sense of closure to the relationship.

Some hospitals provide support groups to help staff members and bereaved families deal with death.

Ethical Behavior

Ethics are basic to the establishment of a moral obligation. Key words can be used to help define ethical behavior (Box 4-3).

BOX 4-3

Ethical Behavior

E *Earnestness:* Take seriously responsibilities for which you are legally and morally accountable. Recognize the importance of decisions and the effect they will have on yourself and others.

T *Truthfulness:* State the facts. Autonomy includes being true to yourself. Also respect rights of others who want and need to know the truth as the basis for self-determination or participation in decision making.

H *Honesty:* Express feelings openly. Honest relations foster effective communication and establish trust and confidence.

I *Integrity:* Adhere to your own values, but also to professional standards and codes, institutional policies and procedures, and societal and legal responsibilities. Know what interventions will be beneficial and what will cause harm.

C *Conscientiousness:* Evaluate the alternatives in making decisions and choosing interventions. Differentiate right from wrong, and act accordingly.

S *Sincerity:* Demonstrate a genuine concern and interest in the welfare of others, as well as in yourself. Sincerity builds confidence and self-esteem.

SURGICAL CONSCIENCE

The key words of OR practice are *caring, conscience, discipline,* and *technique.* Optimal patient care requires an inherent surgical conscience, self-discipline, and the application of principles of asepsis and sterile technique. All are inseparably related.

A surgical conscience may simply be stated as a surgical Golden Rule: Do unto the patient as you would have others do unto you. The caregiver should consider each patient as himself or herself or as a loved one. Once an individual develops a surgical conscience, it remains inherent thereafter. In the last century Florence Nightingale summarized what is, in essence, its meaning. She said, "The nurse should keep a high sense of duty in her own mind, must aim at perfection in her care, and must be consistent always in herself."

Surgical conscience involves a concept of self-inspection coupled with moral obligation. Involving both scientific and intellectual honesty, it is self-regulation in practice according to a deep personal commitment to the highest values. It incorporates the caregiver's values and attitudes at a conscious level and monitors behavior and decision making in relation to those values. In short, a surgical conscience is the inner voice for conscientious practice of asepsis and sterile technique *at all times.* This conscientiousness applies to every activity and intervention as well as to personal hygiene and health. An aseptic body image includes an awareness of body, hair, makeup, jewelry, fingernails, and attire. A team member with an infectious process, such as the flu, a cold, or an open skin lesion, clearly cannot work in the OR. Professional responsibility requires that patient safety never be compromised.

Correct practice of asepsis provides a foundation for development of a mature conscience—mastery of personal integrity and discipline. Development of this conscience incorporates knowledge of aseptic principles, perpetual attention to detail, and experience. All are facets of responsibility that involve trust. A surgical conscience does not permit a person to excuse an error but rather to admit and rectify one readily. It becomes so much an automatic part of the caregiver that he or she can see at a glance or instinctively know if a break in technique or violation of a principle occurs. *Conscience dictates that appropriate action be taken, whether the person is with others or alone and unobserved.* A surgical conscience therefore is the foundation for the practice of strict aseptic and sterile techniques (see Chapter 12). Practice according to that conscience results in pride in self and in accomplishment as well as an inner confidence that the patient is receiving quality care.

A very important aspect in assisting the development of a surgical conscience in others is communication skill. Do not criticize a team member for an error, but give credit to that person for admitting it and help him or her correct the violation. Fear of criticism is the primary deterrent in admission of fault. No one should be reluctant to admit a frank or questionable break in technique. However, any individual unmotivated to carry out expected practices as closely to perfection as possible has no place in the OR suite.

Bibliography

Aiken TD: OR nursing law: the OR supervisor's responsibilities in reducing liability, *AORN J* 54(1):136-139, 1991.

American Nurses Association: *Code for nurses with interpretive statements,* Washington, DC, 1985, The Association.

Banja J: Ethical issues: the nurse as patient advocate, *Plast Surg Nurs* 12(4):159-161, 1992.

Barzizza KC: Ethics: ethical questions in organ transplantation still not answered, *AORN J* 53(3):1076-1079, 1990.

Eakes GG: Grief resolution in hospice nurses: an exploration of effective methods, *Nurs Health Care* 11(5):243-248, 1990.

Ericksen JR: Making choices: the crux of ethical problems in nursing, *AORN J* 52(2):394-397, 1990.

Fox V: Ethics: caught between religion and medicine, *AORN J* 52(1):131-146, 1990.

Goodman RS, London-Goodman J: Caught between law and nursing, *Today's OR Nurse* 12(5):25-28, 1990.

Green WP: Ethics: ethical dilemmas in perioperative research, *AORN J* 51(2):612-615, 1990.

Gunby SS: Ethical issues: a framework for ethical analysis, *Plast Surg Nurs* 11(3):123-125, 1991.

Haddad AM: Ethics: the nurse/physician relationship and ethical decision making, *AORN J* 53(1):151-156, 1991.

Halloran J: Taking the risk to care, *Am J Nurs* 93(7):20, 1993.

Hockenberger SJ, editor: Ethical issues: American Nurses Association philosophical statement on ethics and human rights, *Plast Surg Nurs* 13(1):41-44, 1993.

Holzer JF: The advent of clinical standards for professional liability, *QRB* 16(2):71-79, 1990.

Horner J, Miehl JL: Ethics: the deontological decision-making model as a bioethical tool, *AORN J* 54(2):208-218, 1991.

Horty J, Webb P: How do courts determine prudent action? *OR Manager* 6(5):13, 1990.

Husted GL: Ethics: ethical questions nurses can ask potential employers, *AORN J* 53(3):791-792, 1991.

Jacobson BS: Ethical dilemmas of do-not-resuscitate orders in surgery, *AORN J* 60(3):449-452, 1994.

Kaye JS: Ethics: a proper study for the nurse, *Br J Theatre Nurs* 27(9):13-14, 1990.

Keffer MJ, Keffer HL: The do-not-resuscitate order, *AORN J* 59(3):641-650, 1994.

Kemmy J: OR nursing law: legal implications of perioperative documentation, *AORN J* 57(4):954-958, 1993.

Kemmy J: OR nursing law: professional liability insurance coverage for perioperative nurses, *AORN J* 56(3):526-530, 1992.

Kemmy J: OR nursing law: tailoring national guidelines to fit the needs of individual facilities, *AORN J* 55(3):872-878, 1992.

Latz PA: Computerized nursing documentation systems, *AORN J* 56(2):300-311, 1992.

Merriman JA: The American Nurses Association approves, AORN endorses more policy statements on HIV-related issues, *AORN J* 58(4):796-798, 1993.

Merz SM: Clinical practice guidelines: policy issues and legal implications, *J Comm J Qual Improve* 19(8):306-312, 1993.

Morthorst M: OR nursing law: AIDS, HIV infection and health care professionals, *AORN J* 54(3):597-601, 1991.

Murphy EK: OR nursing law: an explanation of the durable power of attorney for health care, *AORN J* 53(5):1267-1269, 1991.

Murphy EK: OR nursing law: applications of the "captain of the ship" doctrine, *AORN J* 52(4):863-866, 1990.

Murphy EK: OR nursing law: are perioperative nurses "borrowed servants"? Are surgeons "captains of the ship"? *AORN J* 60(3):474-477, 1994.

Murphy EK: OR nursing law: do not resuscitate orders in the OR, *AORN J* 58(2):399-401, 1993.

Murphy EK: OR nursing law: incident reports may or may not be privileged information, *AORN J* 51(3):851-854, 1990.

Murphy EK: OR nursing law: intraoperative injury does not always mean liability, *AORN J* 52(1):19-22, 1990.

Murphy EK: OR nursing law: legal concerns of the next decade, *AORN J* 51(1):258-261, 1990.

Murphy EK: OR nursing law: liability for inaccurate counts; assistant circulators, *AORN J* 53(1):157-161, 1991.

Murphy EK: OR nursing law: liability for noncompliance with hospital policies, national standards, *AORN J* 52(5):1060-1064, 1990.

Murphy EK: OR nursing law: nurse liability in administering medications; lack of preoperative assessment, *AORN J* 52(6):1172-1175, 1990.

Murphy EK: OR nursing law: patient's rights vs court orders, *AORN J* 53(3):794-799, 1991.

Murphy EK: OR nursing law: physician actions do not excuse nursing negligence, *AORN J* 55(4):965-967, 1992.

Murphy EK: OR nursing law: US Supreme Court to hear first "right-to-die" case, *AORN J* 51(5):1391-1394, 1990.

Nadzam DM et al: Data-driven performance improvement in health care: the Joint Commission's indicator measurement system (IM-System), *J Comm J Qual Improve* 19(11):492-500, 1993.

Newhouse RP: Ethics: physician, nursing, facility implications of informed consent, *AORN J* 57(2):505-510, 1993.

Ney CA: Nursing ethics: resolution of role conflicts, *Point View* 28(1):3-5, 1991.

O'Leary DS: The measurement mandate: report card day is coming, *J Comm J Qual Improve* 19(11):487-491, 1993.

O'Quinn JL, Hulme P: After HIV testing: what's next? *Nurs Health Care* 14(2):92-94, 1993.

Oxhorn V, Rosen S: Legislation: understanding the regulatory arena, *AORN J* 55(2):623-629, 1992.

Palmer PN, editor: "Immediately available"—two words that require many more to explain them, *AORN J* 51(2):429-430, 1990 (editorial).

Patterson P: Suspension of DNR orders in the OR being questioned, *OR Manager* 8(2):1, 5-8, 1992.

Patterson P: What are an OR manager's primary ethical obligations? *OR Manager* 6(4):1, 8-9, 1990.

Pobojewski BJ et al: Documenting nursing process in the perioperative setting, *AORN J* 56(1):98-112, 1992.

Reeder JM: Ethics: Do-not-resuscitate orders in the operating room, *AORN J* 57(4):947-951, 1993.

Rozovsky LE, Rozovsky FA: Legal woes of incomplete intraoperative charting, *Can Oper Room Nurs J* 8(1):29-30, 1990.

Seifert PC et al: ANA Code for nurses with interpretive statements—explications for perioperative nursing, *AORN J* 58(2):369-388, 1993.

Shannon TA: Ethics: ethical issues involved with in vitro fertilization, *AORN J* 52(3):627-631, 1990.

Steelman VM et al: Toward a standardized language to describe perioperative nursing, *AORN J* 60(5):786-795, 1994.

Today's OR Nurse Round Table Discussion: The malpractice nightmare, *Today's OR Nurse* 12(2):12-17, 1990.

Walleck CA: Ethics: building the framework for dealing with ethical issues, *AORN J* 53(5):1248-1251, 1991.

Zuffoletto JM: OR nursing law: anatomy of a lawsuit, *AORN J* 56(5):933-936, 1992.

Zuffoletto JM: OR nursing law: proving causation damages in malpractice cases, *AORN J* 58(3):589-592, 1993.

Zuffoletto JM: OR nursing law: the doctrine of *res ipsa loquitur* places burden on perioperative personnel, *AORN J* 56(2):342-343, 1992.

SECTION TWO

The Perioperative Health Care Team

CHAPTER 5

The Direct Patient Care Team

OPERATING ROOM TEAM

At no other time during the perioperative experience will the patient be so well attended as during the surgical procedure. The patient is surrounded by a surgeon and one or two assistants, a scrub person, an anesthesiologist or nurse anesthetist, and a circulating nurse or surgical technologist. These individuals, each with specific functions to perform, comprise the operating team. Throughout this text this *direct patient care team* will be referred to as the *operating room (OR) team*. This team literally has the patient's life in its hands. The OR team is like a symphony orchestra; each person is an integral entity in unison and harmony with his or her colleagues for the successful accomplishment of the expected outcomes.

The OR team is subdivided according to the functions of its members:

1. The *sterile* team
   a. Operating surgeon
   b. Assistants to the surgeon
   c. Scrub person, either RN or surgical technologist

These team members scrub (wash) their hands and arms, don sterile gown and gloves, and enter the sterile field. The *sterile field* is the area of the OR that immediately surrounds and is especially prepared for the patient. To establish the sterile field, all items needed for the surgical procedure are *sterilized,* which are the processes by which all living microorganisms are killed. Thereafter the scrubbed, sterile team members function within this limited area and handle only sterile items.

2. The *unsterile* team
   a. Anesthesiologist or anesthetist
   b. Circulator, either circulating nurse or surgical technologist under the supervision of an RN
   c. Others: the OR team may also include biomedical technicians, radiology technicians, or others who may be needed to set up and operate specialized equipment or monitoring devices used during the surgical procedure.

These team members do not enter the sterile field; they function outside and around it. They assume responsibility for maintaining sterile technique during the surgical procedure, but they handle supplies and equipment that are not considered sterile. Using the principles of aseptic technique, they keep the sterile team supplied, give direct patient care, and handle other requirements that may arise during the surgical procedure.

STERILE TEAM MEMBERS

Operating Surgeon

The surgeon must have the knowledge, skill, and judgment required to successfully perform the intended surgical procedure and any deviation necessitated by unforeseen difficulties. The American College of Surgeons (ACS) has stated principles of patient care that dictate ethical surgical practice. Protection of the patient and quality care are preeminent in these principles. The surgeon's responsibilities include preoperative diagnosis and care, selection and performance of the surgical procedure, and postoperative management of care. The care of many surgical patients is so complex that considerably more than technical skill is required of a surgeon. Advance prediction of a simple and uncomplicated surgical procedure is uncertain. A surgeon must be prepared for the unexpected with a knowledge of the fundamentals of the basic sciences and the ability to apply them to the diagnosis and management of the patient before, during, and after surgical intervention.

The surgeon assumes full responsibility for all medical acts of judgment and for the management of the surgical patient. The surgeon is a licensed physician (MD), osteopath (DO), oral surgeon (DDS or DMD), or podiatrist (DPM) especially trained and qualified by knowledge and experience to perform operative procedures.

All physicians complete the equivalent of 4 years of medical school after earning a bachelor's degree. To become a surgeon, the physician completes at least 2 years of general surgical residency training before completing additional years of postgraduate education in a surgical specialty. The surgical residency provides education and experience in preoperative evaluation, operative treatment, and postoperative care of patients. Consultation and supervision are available from faculty and attending surgeons.

Most surgeons, by virtue of their postgraduate surgical education, engage in practice within a specific surgical specialty. Qualification for surgical practice, although not a rigid requirement, is certification by a surgical specialty board approved by the American Board of Medical Specialists. Ten American specialty boards grant certification for surgical practice or include surgery. All 10 boards governing the surgical specialties require at least 3 years of approved formal residency training, and most set the minimum at 4 or 5 years. Any physician who aspires to become a board-certified surgeon must meet these requirements. Highly trained and qualified surgeons limit themselves to their specialty except perhaps in emergency situations.

Surgical procedures may also be performed by physicians who do not meet these criteria. These physicians include a physician who received an MD degree before 1968 and who has had surgical privileges for more than 5 years in a hospital approved by the JCAHO where most of his or her surgical practice is conducted; a physician who renders surgical care in an emergency or in an area of limited population where a surgical specialist is not available; or a physician who by reason of education, training, and experience is eligible for, but who has not yet obtained, certification.

The surgeon must become a member of the medical staff and be granted surgical privileges by each hospital in which he or she wishes to practice. Standards for admission to staff membership and retention of that membership are clearly delineated in the bylaws formulated by the medical staff and approved by the governing body of the hospital. The credentials committee has the primary responsibility for investigating thoroughly not only the training of an applicant but also the surgeon's integrity, technical competence, and professional judgment. In making its recommendations, the committee sets any limitations it deems fit on the surgeon's privileges to ensure that each surgeon performs only those services for which he or she has been deemed competent.

Patients are entitled to protection and assurance that surgical privileges are limited to those for which the surgeon has been trained and in which his or her competence has been demonstrated. The patient's choice of and confidence in a surgeon, as well as adherence to instructions and advice, are factors in the outcome of surgical intervention. A discerning patient will check the surgeon's qualifications preoperatively.

A competent surgeon can be described as a physician who realistically appreciates his or her own cognitive skills and personal characteristics and can intervene effectively in a patient's illness or injury. Appropriate clinical skills, including data gathering, decision making, and problem solving, and appropriate personal characteristics, such as humanistic concern, accountability, and compassionate interpersonal behavior, are important attributes of a surgeon.

Assistants to Surgeon

Under the operating surgeon's direction, one or two assistants help maintain visibility of the surgical site, control bleeding, close wounds, and apply dressings. The assistant handles tissues and uses instruments. The role of and need for an assistant vary with the type of procedure or surgical specialty, the condition of the patient, and the type of surgical facility. For many simple procedures, it would be unreasonable to insist that a second surgeon assist a competent surgeon. However, the characteristics of the surgical procedure should be evaluated: anticipated blood loss, anesthesia time for the patient, fatigue factors affecting the OR team, and potential complications. Procedures requiring considerable judgment or technical skill and those requiring more than one sterile team usually necessitate the assistance of another qualified surgeon. How hazardous a surgical procedure is may depend more on the condition of the patient than on the complexity of the procedure itself. The surgeon should evaluate all factors to determine his or her need for assistance during the surgical procedure. The surgeon should be able to defend his or her decision if challenged or if not in compliance with medical staff bylaws.

Some surgical staffs classify surgical procedures as *major* or *minor*. If policy stipulates that a physician must assist on all major procedures, the surgeon should not be allowed to operate unless another qualified physician is present. Although a surgical procedure may be classified as minor, performing it without complications is sometimes technically difficult. In any surgical procedure that involves unusual hazard to life, a qualified physician must be present and scrubbed as first assistant. Determining what constitutes unusual hazard depends on the operating surgeon's conscience and is part of his or her responsibility to the patient.

Physician First Assistant

Ideally, the first assistant to the surgeon should be a qualified surgeon or a resident in an accredited surgical education program. The first assistant should be capable of assuming responsibility if the operating surgeon becomes incapacitated, which, fortunately, is a rare occurrence. The surgeon may ask another surgeon to be his or her first assistant. This may be an associate with whom surgical practice is shared and to whom part of the patient's care may be delegated. For complex surgical procedures or under exceptional medical circumstances, the services of an assistant proficient in another surgical specialty may be required.

In hospitals that do not have surgical residency training programs, a referring staff physician who is not a surgeon by education and training but has a contractual relationship with the patient may assist the surgeon if granted this privilege by the medical staff. These physicians are usually engaged in general or family practice and have had some training in basic operative principles and techniques. Specially trained nonmedical personnel such as oral surgeons and podiatrists perform or assist with surgical procedures in a hospital or ambulatory care facility only under the authority of the medical staff and the surgeon responsible for the surgical service.

In hospitals with accredited postgraduate surgical residency training programs, the surgical resident in the third or later year usually acts as first assistant. The resident is given increasing responsibilities under supervision at the operating table to acquire skill and judgment. On completion of training, the resident is able to assume responsibility for continuity of surgical patient care in preoperative evaluation, operative treatment, and postoperative rehabilitation.

The staff surgeon who is in charge may delegate the performance of part of a surgical procedure to a resident assistant, provided the surgeon is an active participant throughout the essential part of the surgical procedure. If a senior resident is to operate on and take care of the patient under the general supervision of an attending surgeon who will not participate actively but who is readily available, the patient should be so informed and give consent.

Nonphysician First Assistant

Nonphysician first assistants should successfully complete a formal educational program for first assisting or receive appropriate training that includes both cognitive and psychomotor learning. Whether employed by a surgeon or a health care facility, practice privileges for nonphysician first assistants and for surgical residents and physician assistants must be based on verifiable credentials that attest to essential knowledge and skills. *It is not within the scope of this text to elaborate further on the requisite education and skills of persons who function as first assistants to surgeons.* However, many of the fundamental principles to be discussed are applicable.

Physician Assistant The medical staff may approve privileges for a nonphysician allied health practitioner who is qualified by academic and clinical training to perform designated procedures in the OR and in other areas of surgical patient care. *Physician assistant* (PA) is a generic term with two subcategories: the *assistant to the primary care physician* (PCA or PA-C, physician's clinical assistant) and the *surgeon's assistant* (SA or PSA [physician's surgical assistant]). The PCA must have additional surgical training to first assist at the operating table. Authorization by the medical staff is based on the individual's training, experience, and demonstrated competency. Eligibility for appointment as an allied health nonphysician assistant for specified services is determined by the following criteria:

1. Exercising judgment within areas of competence, with the physician member of the medical staff having the ultimate responsibility for patient care
2. Participating directly in the management of patients under the supervision or direction of a member of the medical staff
3. Recording reports and progress notes on patients' records and writing orders to the extent established by the medical staff
4. Performing services in conformity with applicable provisions of medical staff bylaws, which may include taking medical histories and performing physical examinations

The surgeon's assistant must perform duties under the direct supervision of a surgeon. The assistant may perform tasks delegated by the surgeon for care of patients in any setting for which the surgeon assumes responsibility. The role of the surgeon's assistant cannot be rigidly defined because of variations in geographic, economic, and sociologic factors and state regulations of medical practices. The responsibility an assistant may assume requires that at the conclusion of formal education he or she will possess the knowledge, skills, and abilities necessary to provide those services appropriate to the surgical setting, which may include those of first assistant at the operating table. After completion of a formal academic program, the PAC and SA must pass a national certification examination.

The surgeon's assistant may become highly skilled and specialized in the area in which the immediate supervisor has interest, or he or she may remain a generalist for a wide variety of procedures such as those performed by a family practitioner in a community hospital. The frequency of performance of certain duties will in part determine the degree of special expertise such an individual acquires. A surgeon's assistant may be employed by the surgeon or the hospital but must receive approval from the medical staff. The medical staff bylaws delineate the assistant's practice privileges within the hospital.

Registered Nurse and Surgical Technologist First Assistants The functions of the first assistant are not within the traditional role of an RN or surgical technologist in the OR. These functions are sanctioned and delegated technical medical acts performed to assist the surgeon to carry out a surgical procedure safely with optimal outcomes for the patient. A nurse or surgical technologist may not perform in a role outside the scope of competence or the legal limits of practice. He or she is free to refuse to perform as first assistant out of concern for the well-being of the patient and for his or her professional accountability. Before any nurse or surgical technologist acts as a first assistant, he or she should be certain that a written hospital policy permits this action. If perioperative nurses or surgical technologists are expected to act as first assistants, this function should be part of their written job descriptions and inservice education. Moreover, the individual should be familiar with state statutes and regulations relevant to this role, particularly nurse and medical practice acts. The qualifications to function as first assistants should include, but are not limited to:

1. Demonstrated competency in both scrub and circulator roles
2. Knowledge and skill in applying principles of aseptic and sterile techniques to ensure infection control
3. Knowledge of surgical anatomy, physiology, fluid and electrolyte balance, acid-base regulation, clinical pathology, and wound healing as these factors relate to surgical procedures
4. Comprehension of risk factors and potential intraoperative complications and knowledge of actions to minimize them
5. Technical skill and manual dexterity in handling tissue, providing exposure, using instruments and devices, providing hemostasis, suturing and knot tying, and applying dressings
6. Ability to recognize safety hazards and initiate appropriate preventive and corrective actions
7. Ability to perform cooperatively and effectively with other team members
8. Ability to perform effectively in stressful and emergency situations
9. Certification in perioperative nursing or surgical technology
10. Certification in cardiopulmonary resuscitation

A *certified perioperative nurse* (CNOR [certified nurse operating room]) who has acquired additional knowledge, technical skills, and judgment through structured, organized instruction and supervised practice may serve as a *registered nurse first assistant* (RNFA) under the direct supervision of the surgeon. The RNFA should function solely as the first assistant and not perform the functions of a scrub person in combination with assisting duties. The role of the RNFA is recognized as being within the scope of nursing practice as an expanded role in all states. The National Certification Board: Perioperative Nursing, Inc. (NCB:PNI) has developed a national certification examination for the RNFA who has attained 2000 hours of assisting experience during a period of 5 years and can provide documentation of clinical competency. In 1998, a bachelor of science in nursing (BSN) degree will be required for eligibility to become certified. After successfully passing the examination, the certified RNFA is entitled to use the acronym CRNFA. Every 5 years, the CRNFA must become recertified by examination. Eligibility to take the recertification examination includes maintenance of CNOR status, and documentation of active clinical practice as an RNFA with continued clinical competency for the 2-year period preceding the examination date.

A *certified surgical technologist* (CST) also may be educated or trained to first assist. An associate's degree should be the minimal entry level requirement for a CST to enter a postgraduate first assisting program. A national certification examination is available from the Liaison Council on Certification for the Surgical Technologist (LCC-ST) for the CST who has had at least 2 years of first assisting experience during the previous 4 years. After successfully passing this examination, the CST first assistant may use the acronym CST/CFA. At the time of original certification as a CFA, the CST portion of the certification is adjusted to be of the same time duration as the CFA portion of the certification. In other words, both aspects of the certification will be adjusted for the same period of 6 years. Recertification for the CST/CFA is accomplished by providing documentation of practicing as a CST/CFA for 2 years of the 6-year certification period, and by obtaining 100 continuing education credits in the categories defined by the LCC-ST. Another option is to document 2 years of practice within the 6-year period and take the certification examination again.

Second Assistant to Surgeon

Qualified nurses and surgical technologists may be used as second or third assistants during surgical procedures in which the surgeon deems their assistance is adequate and *for which they have been trained.* The second assistant may retract tissue and suction body fluids to help provide exposure of the surgical site. This assistant is not involved in actual performance of the procedure.

Before they enter postgraduate programs in the surgical specialties, physicians complete at least 1 year of general surgical residency immediately following graduation from medical school. Medical students also receive some exposure to the OR during surgical clerkship. These general surgical residents and medical students usually function as second assistants at the operating table in teaching institutions.

Scrub Person

The scrub person is the nursing staff member of the sterile team. The scrub role may be filled by an RN, a licensed practical/vocational nurse, or a surgical technologist. The term *scrub person* will be used throughout this text to designate this role and to elaborate the specific technical and behavioral functions of the individual performing in this capacity.

The scrub person is responsible for maintaining the integrity, safety, and efficiency of the sterile field throughout the surgical procedure. Knowledge of and experience with aseptic and sterile techniques qualify the scrub person to prepare and arrange instruments and supplies and to assist the surgeon and assistants throughout the surgical procedure by providing the sterile instruments and supplies required. *This demands that the scrub person anticipate, plan for, and respond to the needs of the surgeon and other members of the team by constantly watching the sterile field.* Manual dexterity and physical stamina are required. A stable temperament and ability to work under pressure are also important assets, as well as a keen sense of responsibility and concern for accuracy in performing all duties.

During extremely complicated or hazardous surgical procedures or in teaching situations, two scrub persons may join the team. One may pass instruments and supplies to the surgeon while the other prepares supplies. An experienced preceptor may join the team to teach, guide, and assist the learner to function in the scrub person role. When unexpected, unusual, or emergency situations arise, specific instructions and guidance are received from the surgeon or RN. The surgical technologist provides services under the supervision of an RN at all times.

Some hospitals permit nurses or surgical technologists employed by surgeons to come into the OR to perform the scrub role for their employers. These *private scrub persons* should adhere to all hospital policies and procedures and to approved written guidelines for the functions they may fulfill.

UNSTERILE TEAM MEMBERS

Anesthesiologist or Anesthetist

An *anesthesiologist* is an MD, preferably certified by the American Board of Anesthesiology, or a DO who specializes in the art and science of administering anesthetics to produce the various states of anesthesia. Medical doctors must complete a 2-year residency program to become eligible for certification. An *anesthetist* is a qualified licensed nurse, dentist, or physician who administers anesthetics. When a drug or gas is administered by an anesthetist, this individual works under direct supervision of an anesthesiologist or the surgeon.

A nurse must have a baccalaureate degree in nursing or science for entrance into a school of nurse anesthesia. Graduates of an accredited nurse anesthesia program, which is a minimum of 2 years in length, must pass the certification examination of the Council on Certification of Nurse Anesthetists to become *certified registered nurse anesthetists* (CRNA). They must be recertified every 2 years.

It has been said that no anesthetic agent is safer than its worst administrator. Throughout this text the term *anesthesiologist* will be used to refer to the person responsible for inducing anesthesia, maintaining anesthesia at the required levels, and managing untoward reactions to anesthesia throughout the surgical procedure. Recognizing that anesthesiology is a practice of medicine, the value of well-trained anesthetists is also acknowledged. Medically delegated functions of an anesthetic nature are performed under the overall supervision of a responsible physician or in accordance with individual written guidelines approved within the health care facility.*

Anesthesia and surgery are two distinct but inseparable disciplines; they are the two parts of one. Adequate communication between the surgeon and the anesthesiologist is the greatest safeguard the patient has. The anesthesiologist is an indispensable member of the OR team. Functioning as guardian of the patient, the anesthesiologist should also observe the principles of aseptic technique.

Modern anesthesia is vastly superior to anesthesia of previous years. The number of anesthetic agents available and refinements of administration techniques have broadened its scope. A greater understanding of the pharmacologic action of anesthetic drugs has led to safer anesthesia. The choice and application of appropriate agents and suitable techniques of administration, monitoring of physiologic functions, maintenance of fluid and electrolyte balance, and blood replacement are all essential parts of anesthesiologists' responsibilities. They also share responsibility for minimizing the haz-

*American Association of Nurse Anesthetists: *Guidelines for the practice of the certified registered nurse anesthetist,* Park Ridge, Ill, copyright 1983, The Association.

ards of shock, electrocution, and fire. Appropriate precautions should be taken to ensure the safe administration of anesthetic agents. Anesthesiologists must be able to use and interpret correctly a wide variety of monitoring devices. They are responsible for overseeing the positioning and movement of patients. At no time is an anesthetized patient moved or positioned without the approval of the anesthesiologist.

Anesthesiologists are not confined to the OR, although this is their primary arena. In addition to providing relief from pain for patients and optimal conditions for surgeons during surgical procedures, they oversee the postanesthesia care unit to provide resuscitative care until each patient has regained control of vital functions. They also participate in the hospital's program of cardiopulmonary resuscitation as teachers and team members. They act as consultants or managers for problems of acute and chronic respiratory insufficiency requiring inhalation therapy, and for a variety of other fluid, electrolyte, and metabolic disturbances requiring intravenous therapy. Their advice may be sought in the total care of unconscious, critically ill, or injured patients with acute circulatory disorders or neurologic deficits in the intensive care unit or emergency department. Anesthesiologists also are integral staff members of pain therapy clinics.

Some anesthesiologists prefer to specialize in one area, such as cardiothoracic or obstetric anesthesia. The latter involves care of two lives simultaneously. In some settings they participate in teaching and research as well as in clinical practice. (See Section Seven for a complete discussion of anesthetic agents and techniques.)

Circulator

The *circulator* is preferably an RN, but in certain circumstances may be a surgical technologist who functions under the supervision of an RN. The circulator plays a role that is vital to the smooth flow of events before, during, and after the surgical procedure. Patients undergoing surgical intervention experience physical and psychosocial trauma. They enter an alien environment removed from personal contact with family and friends. Their physical and psychologic needs are great. Because most patients are unconscious or sedated, they are powerless and unable to make decisions concerning their welfare. At this critical time, patients need the professional judgment of others who function on their behalf. These advocates should be within close physical and social proximity at all times.

The surgeon is in charge at the operating table, but he or she relies on the circulator to monitor and coordinate all activities within the room and to manage the care required for each patient. To some extent, the circulator controls the physical and emotional atmosphere in the room, allowing other team members to concentrate on tasks without distraction. This role as the patient's advocate and protector is critical to the safety and welfare of the patient. Therefore a qualified RN is assigned to provide or supervise all circulating duties. The nurse should be continuously knowledgeable about the status of the patient.

In accordance with applicable state laws and approved organizational policies and procedures, licensed practical/vocational nurses and surgical technologists may *assist* in circulating duties under the supervision of a qualified RN who is available to respond to emergencies. "Available" has been interpreted to imply that an RN can supervise an unspecified number of contiguous rooms but should be immediately available to assist in each of these rooms; he or she can leave a room for short periods but can return immediately to supervise or assist if needed. The regulations in several states specify that an RN must circulate in each room. The patient's medical record must identify who provided circulating duties and the name of the qualified RN who supervised them.

The circulating nurse is vital to the provision of care that includes but is not limited to:

1. Application of the nursing process in directing and coordinating all nursing interventions within the OR related to the care and support of the patient. Nursing judgment and decision-making skill are requisites to assessing, planning, implementing, and evaluating the plan of care before, during, and after surgical intervention. This is the *professional perioperative role* of the circulating nurse (see Chapter 2).
2. Creation and maintenance of a safe and comfortable environment for the patient through implementing the principles of asepsis. The circulator must see the OR as a whole and demonstrate a strong sense of surgical conscience. Any break in technique on the part of anyone in the room should be recognized and corrected instantly. Although sterile technique is the responsibility of everyone in the room, the circulator must be on the alert to catch any breaks that others may not have seen. Standing farther away from the sterile field than others, the circulator is better able to observe the entire field and the sterile team members.
3. Provision of assistance to any member of the OR team in any manner in which the circulator is qualified. This requires current knowledge of the legal implications of surgical intervention. The circulator must know the organization of the work and the relative importance of factors involved in accomplishing it. An effective circulator ensures that the sterile team is supplied with every item necessary to perform the surgical procedure efficiently. The circulator must know all supplies, instruments, and equipment, be able to obtain them

quickly, and guard against inadvertent hazards in their use and care. He or she must be competent to direct the scrub person.

4. Identification of any potential environmental danger or stressful situation involving the patient, other team members, or both. This requires constant flexibility to meet the unexpected and to act in an efficient, rational manner at all times.
5. Maintenance of the communication link between events and team members at the sterile field and persons not in the OR but concerned with the outcome of the surgical procedure. The latter includes the patient's family or significant other plus other personnel in the OR suite and in other departments of the hospital. The ability to recognize and effectively communicate situations involving the patient and/or other team members is a vital link in the continuity of patient care.
6. Direction of the activities of all learners. The circulator must have the supervisory capability and teaching skills needed to ensure maintenance of a safe and therapeutic environment for the patient. Assistance kindly given builds up the learner's confidence. In this capacity the circulator acts as supervisor, advisor, and teacher.

DEPENDENCE OF PATIENT ON QUALIFIED TEAM

For the welfare and safety of the patient, the OR team must work efficiently as a functioning single unit. The members should be thoroughly familiar with procedures, setups, equipment, and policies and should be able to cope with the unpredictable. Their qualifications must be beyond reproach. They should have high morale, mutual understanding, trust, cooperation, and consideration. Anyone who cannot function wholeheartedly as a qualified team member has no place in the OR. The OR team works to promote the best interests of the patient every single minute.

All personnel in the OR should have the proven knowledge, skill, and ability to perform at an optimal level at all times. Once each member of the team has passed the novice stage, other criteria demonstrate and document knowledge and skill gained through experience and continuing education. Aligning professionally with the local, state, and nationally recognized organizations that establish the standards of practice provides an opportunity for growth. Certification may include completing a course of instruction and then passing an examination. Other measurements of competence include performance evaluation in a clinical setting. Validation of clinical competence is an important aspect of providing quality patient care.

BIBLIOGRAPHY

Allen DE, Girard NJ: Attitudes toward certification, *AORN J* 55(3):817-829, 1992.

Allmers NM, Verderame JA: *Surgical technology examination,* ed 3, Norwalk, Conn, 1993, Appleton & Lange.

AORN official statement on RN first assistants, *AORN J* 57(6):1319-1321, 1993.

Association of Operating Room Nurses: *Core curriculum for the RN first assistant,* ed 2, Denver, 1994, The Association.

Association of Surgical Technologists: *Core curriculum for surgical technology,* ed 3, Englewood, Colo, 1990, The Association.

Association of Surgical Technologists: *Job analysis, surgical technologist,* Englewood, Colo, 1991, The Association.

AST Board of Directors: Changing the paradigm, *Surg Technol* 22(1):7-9, 1990.

Caruthers B: Continuing education credits for the CST certified first assistant, *Surg Technol* 25(10):15-16, 1993.

Credentialling document format for CST first assistant privileges, *Surg Technol* 24(3):15, 1992.

Gava N: State laws for physician assistants, *J Am Acad Physician Assist* 2(4):303-313, 1989.

Job description: CST surgical assistant, *Surg Technol* 22(6):8-9, 1990.

Lafountain J: The RN first assistant in surgery, *Nurs Manage* 23(12):51-53, 1992.

National Certification Board, Perioperative Nursing: *A job analysis for the perioperative nurse,* Denver, Colo, 1992, NCB:PNI.

National Certification Board, Perioperative Nursing: *A job analysis for the RN first assistant,* Denver, Colo, 1992, NCB:PNI.

National Certification Board, Perioperative Nursing: *CNOR study guide,* ed 2, Denver, Colo, 1993, NCB:PNI.

O'Neale M: Clinical issues: private scrub nurse credentialling; role of the registered nurse first assistant; needle count omissions, *AORN J* 55(6):1575-1578, 1992.

Ponder KS: Opinion: the RN circulator, *AORN J* 60(3):459-462, 1994.

Surgical first assistant curriculum, *Surg Technol* 24(2):8-11, 1992.

Teutsch W: Surgical assisting: an issue for the 90s, *Surg Technol* 22(3):13-15, 1990.

CHAPTER 6

Operating Room Staff and Supporting Services

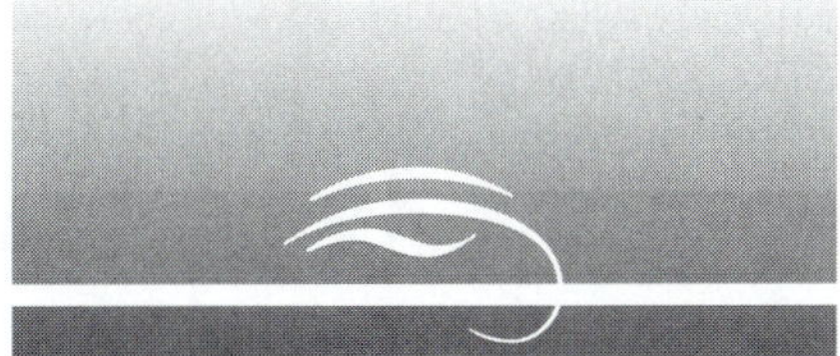

OPERATING ROOM NURSING STAFF

The operating room (OR) team, as described in Chapter 5, immediately surrounds the patient throughout the surgical procedure. This direct patient care team functions within the physical confines of a specific room, *the operating room or theatre.* This room is one part of the physical facilities that comprise the total *OR suite.* Similarly, this team makes up only one part of the human activity directed toward the care of the surgical patient. Many other people function in an indirect relationship with the patient, contributing vital supporting services toward the common goal of ensuring a safe, comfortable, and effective environment for the safety and welfare of the patient within the OR suite. All the nursing personnel assigned to work in the OR suite are collectively referred to as *the OR nursing staff of the OR department.* The relationship and duties of those staff members within the OR department will vary depending on the size and extent of the physical facilities and the number of personnel employed. No one's job is small! Each has important functions to perform, and each is responsible for assuming a part of the total workload.

Job Descriptions

Each OR staff member should understand his or her own functions and responsibilities. A *job description* provides a written summary of the job to be done, lists the duties and requirements of the job as it should be performed, and states to whom the employee is accountable.

The staffing plan should delineate those functions for which nursing service is responsible and indicate all positions to carry out the functions. Job descriptions delineate the functions, responsibilities, and desired behaviors of each classification of professional, allied health care, and assistive personnel. They serve as a guide for individual employees and for the manager; give order to individual work assignments and orderly, intelligent direction to the activities of the department; and prevent duplication of effort or neglect of duties.

Job descriptions should be written by each hospital for its own OR department staff. An employee is not required to assume responsibility not specified in the job description. Work satisfaction is promoted by giving members of the staff basic duties and fixed responsibilities. Because the job description spells out each job requirement, it provides the manager with a means of checking that the employee understands the assignments and carries them out.

Performance-Based Standards

Performance-based standards complement job descriptions. They are precise criteria for evaluating what an employee should do under present working conditions to perform a specific duty satisfactorily. They are the measurements by which the employee's performance is judged in terms of quality, quantity, and manner. Standards of acceptable practice in the OR department are based on sound principles of the natural and behavioral sciences.

A standard developed by a profession or regulatory body is an authoritative statement by which competence can be judged. Standards delineate an optimal achievable level of performance. They serve as a reference and guide by which clinical practice can be evaluated. Standards developed by the Association of Operating Room Nurses, Inc. (AORN), the Association of Surgical Technologists, Inc. (AST), and other professional nursing organizations reflect a systematic approach to practice. They are intended to provide safe individualized patient care, detect inadequacy of care, prevent legal implications resulting from alleged malpractice or negligence, and validate patient care.

OPERATING ROOM NURSING ADMINISTRATIVE PERSONNEL

Personnel should know the direction of the entire organizational effort as a prerequisite for their successful functioning. The administrative personnel interpret hospital and departmental philosophy, objectives, policies, and procedures to the OR staff.

1. *Philosophy.* Statement of beliefs regarding patient care and the nature of perioperative nursing that clarifies the overall responsibilities to be fulfilled.
2. *Objectives.* Statements of specific goals and purposes to be accomplished during the course of action and definitions of criteria for acceptable performance.
3. *Policies.* Specific authoritative statements of governing principles or actions, within the context of the philosophy and objectives, that assist in decision making by providing guidelines for action to be taken or, in some situations, for what is not to be done.
   a. *Basic policies.* Statements of the principles of administration and its approach to functioning.
   b. *General policies.* Guidelines of the principles dealing with everyday situations that affect all personnel within the hospital.
   c. *Departmental policies.* Guidelines structured to meet the needs of a specific work unit (i.e., OR policies).
4. *Procedures.* Statements of task-oriented and skill-oriented actions to be taken in the implementation of policies.

Operating Room Nurse Manager

In some hospitals and ambulatory care settings, ORs are supervised by a doctor of medicine or osteopathy. However, in accredited facilities an RN is responsible for administration and supervision of nursing service. The OR department is a business unit of the hospital, and so should be managed as a business. Therefore the title and functions of the *operating room nurse manager* reflect the extent and complexity of the administrative responsibilities. In large hospitals the nurse may hold some variation of a title of *director of operating rooms, assistant vice president for surgical services, director of perioperative nursing,* or *clinical director of surgery.* Because of the magnitude of the administrative duties, actual supervision of personnel may be delegated to a *coordinator.* In smaller hospitals, where administrative responsibilities are not as time consuming, the OR nurse manager supervises personnel. In other situations one nurse may manage more than one clinical service such as the OR, postanesthesia care unit (PACU), ambulatory care unit, and/or emergency department. The title *OR nurse manager* will be used throughout this text to designate the nurse who is responsible for coordinating nursing care and related supporting services of the OR department.

An OR nurse manager should have general knowledge of nursing theory and practice, specialized knowledge of OR technique and management, and knowledge of business and financial management. The manager should possess leadership skills to supervise and direct nursing care of patients by nursing service personnel within the OR department, according to nursing principles and standards. The main function of the manager is to provide leadership that promotes cooperative effort. To be a leader requires an additional set of skills and knowledge. These concern functions of management that include planning, organizing, staffing, directing, and controlling, plus the processes of problem solving, decision making, coordinating, and communicating.

The manager is responsible for the allocation and completion of work but does not do it all or make all the decisions. Capable personnel are employed, and they are delegated increasing responsibility as they develop competence in their work. The manager creates an organization that can function well in his or her absence.

The OR nurse manager should implement and enforce hospital and departmental policies and procedures. He or she also analyzes and evaluates continuously all nursing services rendered and, through participation in research, seeks to improve the quality of patient care given. The manager retains accountability for all nursing care given, all related activities in the OR department, and all aspects of environmental control in the OR suite. The scope of this accountability includes:

1. Provision of competent staff and supportive services adequately prepared to achieve quality patient care objectives
2. Delegation of responsibilities to professional nurses and assignment of duties to allied health care and assistive personnel
3. Responsibility for evaluating the performance of all departmental personnel and for assessing and improving quality of care and services
4. Provision of educational opportunities to increase knowledge and skills of all personnel
5. Coordination of administrative duties to ensure proper functioning of staff
6. Provision and fiscal control of materials, supplies, and equipment
7. Coordination of activities within OR suite with other departments
8. Creation of an environment that fosters teamwork and provides job satisfaction for all staff members
9. Identification of problems and resolution of them in a decisive, timely manner
10. Initiation of data collection and analyses to develop effective systems and to monitor efficiency and productivity

Clinical Coordinator

An assistant nurse manager aids in administration and supervision of nursing service in the OR department and is directly responsible to the OR nurse manager. This nurse acts as administrative head in the absence of the OR manager. The position usually does not exist in small hospitals. In large hospitals one or more *clinical coordinators* provide leadership and assist with the management of manpower and material resources.

Head Nurse

The *head nurse* functions in a middle management position as liaison between staff members and administrative personnel. In some hospitals the title of head nurse is given to the person whose position is comparable to that of coordinator. In others, usually smaller hospitals, the OR nurse manager functions more or less in the capacity of head nurse.

In large hospitals with many surgical specialty services, a head nurse may be responsible for the administration and direct supervision of nursing service in a designated room or rooms within the OR suite assigned to a particular specialty service, such as ophthalmology, neurosurgery, cardiovascular surgery, or urology. With this structure, there are several head nurses in the department. These head nurses should have the technical proficiency required for the specialty service for which they are responsible and should have sufficient managerial ability to plan for and administer effectively the nursing service activities.

The duties of the head nurse will include but are not limited to:

1. Planning for and supervising the nursing activities within the entire OR suite or specific room(s) to which he or she is assigned
2. Coordinating nursing activities with those of the surgeons and anesthesiologists to provide for the care of patients
3. Maintaining adequate supplies and equipment and providing for their economical use
4. Observing the performance of all staff members pertaining to nursing activities and providing feedback
5. Interpreting to personnel the procedures and policies adopted by the department and hospital administration
6. Informing the OR manager of needs and problems arising in the department and assisting with problem solving
7. Assisting with orientation of new staff members

Functions vary in different hospitals, but the position of head nurse, with its direct and continuous responsibility for both patients and staff, is an important one.

Operating Room In-Service Education Coordinator

Planned educational experiences are provided in the job setting to help staff members perform effectively and knowledgeably. Most hospitals have a nursing staff development department or committee to plan, coordinate, and conduct educational and training programs.

A program is planned to ensure a thorough orientation for each new nursing service employee. All new personnel should become familiar with the philosophy, objectives, policies, and procedures of the hospital and nursing service. This general orientation program assists the new employee to adjust to the organization and environment. It is coordinated with an orientation to the duties in the unit to which the employee is assigned.

The *OR in-service coordinator* may be a member of the staff development department, the OR administrative staff, or both. This person is responsible for planning, scheduling, and coordinating the orientation of new OR staff. This includes review of policies and procedures, personnel duties, and performance standards specific to the OR. Based on an assessment of individual skills, the new employee is given guidance and supervision for a period of weeks to months until basic competencies are adequate to function independently. Head nurses, preceptors, and other experienced staff members assist with the orientation of new personnel.

An in-service educational program should also be planned to keep the nursing staff up to date on new techniques, equipment, and patient care practices. Programs focusing on fire prevention, electrical hazards, security measures, and resuscitation training are important to ensure personnel and patient safety. Professional and technical programs designed to develop specialized job knowledge, skills, and/or attitudes affecting patient care are planned and presented for the appropriate segment of the nursing service department and the OR staff. The OR in-service coordinator is responsible for assessing the educational needs of staff members collectively and individually and then for planning, scheduling, coordinating, and evaluating in-service programs. This individual may also conduct some sessions.

Staff development programs, conducted on a continuous basis, enhance performance by maintaining job knowledge and clinical competence. In-service programs may be supplemented by other appropriate continuing educational programs held outside the health care facility.

Preceptor

The orientation process is facilitated by a one-to-one relationship between the new employee and an experienced staff member. The *preceptor* teaches, counsels, advises, and encourages the orientee until he or she can function independently. The preceptor is legally accountable for assessing the orientee's abilities, assigning activities accordingly, and assisting in carrying out duties safely. Learning needs can be assessed through interview, observation, and a skills checklist. To ensure consistency in teaching, the preceptor coordinates development of appropriate and measurable behavioral objectives for the orientee with the in-service coordinator, management staff, or both. The preceptor should evaluate performance and offer constructive feedback to build the orientee's self-confidence. To be effective, the preceptor should have an interest in teaching and should have acquired the necessary skills. Preceptors are role models and mentors for new staff members or beginning learners.

Operating Room Business Manager

To relieve the OR nurse manager of nonnursing duties, some hospitals employ an *OR business manager,* sometimes titled *unit manager.* This person may report to the OR manager or directly to the hospital administrator. Lines of authority and responsibility between the business manager and the OR manager should be clearly defined regardless of the organizational structure. The OR business manager directs the management of nonnursing and nondirect patient care functions in the OR suite; the OR nurse manager and other administrative nursing personnel direct and supervise patient care and professional and allied health care personnel.

Nonnursing administrative duties should include maintaining a clean, orderly, safe environment within the OR suite for patients and personnel. This entails more than removing visible dust and dirt. A safe environment is one that is free of contamination, free of electrical and fire hazards, and free of negligence. Formulation of procedures is necessary. Personnel should be trained. However, inspection and follow-up are equally important. The business manager coordinates these efforts with the supporting service departments: housekeeping, maintenance, laundry, and materiels management. A business manager may prepare and administrate the department budget. Doing so may include maintaining inventories and evaluating supplies and equipment. If the hospital does not employ an OR business manager, the OR nurse manager or coordinator assumes responsibility for these duties.

OPERATING ROOM STAFF NURSING PERSONNEL

Advanced Nurse Practitioner

Within any organization a formal structure of authority and responsibility exists. However, the evolution of technology and the acute illnesses of patients have changed the focus of functions for many nurses within the hospital organization. With experience and advanced study, a nurse can become capable of organizing and providing complex care and of using initiative and independent judgment. This practitioner may hold the title of *team leader, resource clinical nurse, nurse clinician, clinical nurse specialist,* or *nurse practitioner.* Although the term *practitioner* will be used to describe any or all of these advanced roles, differentiation is made within the profession on the basis of formal academic educational preparation.

In general, minimal preparation for this expanded role is a baccalaureate degree in nursing (BSN). The *clinical nurse specialist,* however, in an advanced role, has been defined as a graduate of a master's program in nursing (MSN) who is an expert in a clinical specialty, a role model for and consultant to other nursing personnel, and a teacher of patients and personnel. He or she conducts research to validate nursing interventions. These skills can be used effectively for advanced practice in perioperative nursing.

The practitioner is capable of exercising a high degree of discriminative judgment in planning, executing, and evaluating nursing care based on the assessed needs of patients having one or more common clinical manifestations. A practitioner may develop the nursing care plan for a group of orthopaedic patients, for example. This plan is coordinated for each patient with the surgeon, other professional nurses, and allied health care personnel who assist in the performance of functions related to the plan of care.

Clinical nursing interventions are not necessarily performed by the practitioner. This advanced practice nurse decides what needs to be done, then determines which nursing interventions can be performed by others and which he or she should do. These decisions are based on personal interaction with each patient and a knowledge of the clinical condition. The practitioner exercises a degree of autonomy and independence within the clinical setting.

Because a practitioner has advanced academic preparation in theoretical knowledge and clinical experience in a particular clinical nursing setting and is an expert in nursing situations in that setting, qualified OR clinical coordinators may function as practitioners. In this role they assist in planning the total nursing care for each surgical patient, coordinating nursing and supportive services and participating in the orientation, development, and evaluation of nursing personnel assigned to direct patient care functions in the OR. Coordinators who also assess individual patient needs through personal patient interviews and who plan for individualized nursing care in the OR truly function as perioperative nurse practitioners. They have the title of *patient care coordinator* or *perioperative clinical nurse specialist* in some hospitals. They make decisions relative to the direct and indirect nursing care of the patient in the OR setting, using specialized judgments and skills. Problem solving and decision making are the heart of professional management and professional leadership.

The OR practitioner may be assigned to work solely or primarily with the surgeons in a specific surgical specialty. This concept of nursing specialization coincides with the specialization of surgeons. With practice and formal or informal study, nurses develop expertise in planning and implementing nursing care for patients with similar surgical problems. Skills and knowledge become highly specialized. Surgeons in that particular specialty rely on these nurses to supervise the nursing care of their patients and to direct less experienced nursing personnel on the OR team. Practitioners may fulfill the circulating nurse duties in one OR or serve as consultant coordinators for several rooms in which patients are having surgical procedures performed by surgeons within a given surgical specialty. The job title for the nurse and the assignment structure vary with the size of the hospital and the manner in which it is organized. With either type of assignment, these nurses are practitioners of narrow scope unless they visit patients preoperatively to assess their individual needs, plan nursing care on the basis of need assessment, and evaluate the quality of nursing care postoperatively through direct patient interaction. Then they are advanced nurse practitioners in the broader context of perioperative nursing.

Registered Nurse/Staff Nurse

Entry into professional OR nursing as the clinical practice setting of choice is as a *staff nurse*. After completing a structured orientation program to develop basic competencies in both scrub and circulating duties, the staff nurse may become either a *generalist* or a *specialist*. A generalist should be competent to provide nursing care for all surgical patients and to ensure a safe environment to achieve desired outcomes of surgical intervention. Size of the facility and nursing staff, types of surgical specialties, complexities of surgical procedures performed, risk factors of patients and procedures, and personal preference of the nurse are considerations in determining the most efficient staffing pattern. In many hospitals, ambulatory care centers, and doctors' offices, staff nurses work only with surgeons in a particular surgical specialty. These nurses become specialists themselves. Some have been trained to first or second assist the surgeon (see Chapter 5, pp. 74 and 75).

Staff nurses should be able to perform either scrub or circulating duties competently. Usually the more experienced nurse functions as the circulator and oversees activities of the OR team as the patient's advocate. If staffing does not permit an RN in both positions, the RN circulates.

Staff nurses work collaboratively with surgeons and anesthesiologists to determine the patient's needs during the surgical procedure and to assume responsibility for patient care. RNs use the nursing process in their nursing practice. Ideally, staff nurses have the opportunity to visit patients preoperatively to assess their unique needs and to plan individualized nursing care that is implemented in the operating room. Postoperative follow-up directly with patients provides opportunities to evaluate outcomes of nursing care. Unfortunately, in reality many OR nurses are not in situations in which this valid theoretical concept is practiced.

As part of their professional practice in the OR, staff nurses should document and evaluate the effectiveness of nursing interventions. To ensure a safe environment for patients, they assist other nursing staff members through teaching and supervising aseptic and sterile techniques and other procedures. They also assist in control and maintenance of drugs, supplies, equipment, and records. Staff nurses assist all members of the OR team. They work cooperatively with nurses and members of other departments to provide continuity of patient care.

Those professional OR nurses who are certified perioperative nurses (CNOR) serve as role models for others to emulate.

NOTE: In the United Kingdom, Australia, and some other countries, an *anesthetic nurse* is also a theatre (OR) staff member. This nurse receives patients, assists the anesthetist with induction of anesthesia and extubation, monitors patients during the surgical procedure, and is responsible for the anesthesia equipment. Ideally, the anesthetic nurse visits its patients preoperatively and postoperatively.

Standards of Professional Performance

AORN has identified eight standards of perioperative practice that may be used to measure professional performance of RNs in the OR.

1. *Quality of Care: The perioperative nurse systematically evaluates the quality and appropriateness of nursing practice.* The perioperative nurse participates in quality assessment and improvement programs to promote quality patient care.
2. *Performance Appraisal: The perioperative nurse evaluates his or her practice in context with professional practice standards and relevant statutes and regulations.* Defining and evaluating professional practice behaviors is an ongoing process. Self-assessment and feedback from health care team members provides a framework for future growth and improvement.
3. *Education: The perioperative nurse acquires and maintains current knowledge in nursing practice.* Professional development builds on experiential and educational opportunities that interlace to facilitate the enhancement of nursing practice. The perioperative nurse has the personal responsibility to continue his or her educational and professional growth.
4. *Collegiality: The perioperative nurse contributes to the professional growth of peers, colleagues, and others.* The support of others in their personal and professional growth is a responsibility of the perioperative nurse. Sharing knowledge and expertise through preceptor programs, role modeling, and mentorships assists colleagues to attain a broader knowledge base.
5. *Ethics: The perioperative nurse's decisions and actions on behalf of patients are determined in an ethical manner.* Care and services should be delivered within the practice parameters without violating the basic human rights of patients.
6. *Collaboration: The perioperative nurse collaborates with the patient, significant others, health care providers, and others in providing care.* Care of the patient is a unified effort supported by internal and external forces that work in concert to move toward the attainment of expected outcomes.
7. *Research: The perioperative nurse uses research findings in practice.* Perioperative nursing derives its scientific knowledge base from research. Research demonstrates the relationship between nursing interventions and patient outcomes. Perioperative nurses should participate in the research process.
8. *Resource Use: The perioperative nurse considers factors related to safety, effectiveness, efficiency, environmental concerns, and cost in planning and implementing patient care.* Resources in the perioperative setting are used economically and efficiently in the delivery of safe and effective patient care.

Clinical Ladder

Competency cannot be assumed based on academic credentials and experience alone. After achievement of basic competency, the staff nurse should strive to progress along the continuum to proficient and then to expert achievement in practice. This takes time, energy, discipline, and commitment. Hard work, physically and emotionally, is required to enhance technical, interpersonal, and critical thinking skills. Nurses should respond positively to challenges and opportunities and show interest and initiative.

Some facilities have a competency-based clinical ladder to recognize and reward clinical expertise. Eligibility to progress up the ladder will be determined by personal performance. Specific criteria are established for advancement to each level of clinical practice. The job description for each level incorporates ascending levels of responsibilities for clinical judgment, leadership and teaching functions, and professional behavior. Advanced skills may be needed for an acceptable level of technical proficiency.

Licensed Practical/Vocational Nurse

Licensed practical/vocational nurses (LPN/LVNs) who are qualified by training, experience, and demonstrated ability may give nursing care that does not require the skill and judgment of an RN. With specialized training in surgical technology, these nurses may be permitted to serve as scrub persons at the operating table. LPN/LVNs are not permitted to function independently as circulators in the OR; they may assist by working with a qualified RN. Throughout this text the functions of the LPN/LVN on the OR staff will be considered the same as those of *surgical technologists.*

> NOTE: An *enrolled nurse* is the equivalent of a practical/vocational nurse in some countries. His or her education is not as comprehensive as that of a professional nurse.

Surgical Technologist

Surgical technologists (ST or, if certified, CST) are responsible for their own acts but should function under the supervision of an RN. They assist with the care of patients in the OR by performing routine and assigned duties according to their scope of educational preparation and experience, the AST standards of practice, the policies of the health care facility, and within applicable legal guidelines. They are not permitted to administer medications, complete patient records, or carry out direct physician orders regarding the treatment of patients. Their primary function is as the scrub person, but they may assist with circulating duties. They may be permitted to first or second assist if they have been adequately trained and credentialed.

Routine duties of STs also include stocking, replenishing, preparing, and/or selecting supplies and equipment for storage or for immediate use during surgical procedures. They also assist with housekeeping duties to maintain cleanliness in the OR suite to ensure a safe patient environment.

NOTE

1. A clinical ladder may give the ST an incentive for personal growth and development and an opportunity for advancement in the employment setting. Each level of the ladder distinguishes differences in experience, continuing education, skills, accountability, and criteria-based education.
2. In the United Kingdom and some other countries that follow the British system, an *operating department assistant* (ODA) is trained by an employing hospital to function in the scrub role and to assist with circulating duties. However, the ODA is also trained to assist the anesthetist and prepare anesthesia equipment. In many hospitals this is the primary function of the ODA.

Assistive Personnel

Assistive personnel are unlicensed staff members trained on the job through an in-service educational program.

Clerical Personnel

One or more assistive workers may perform clerical duties associated with activities within the OR suite. These duties may include assisting with preparation of the schedule of surgical procedures, ordering supplies, and maintaining records and reports, including inputting computer data. Clerical personnel relieve administrative nurses of much paperwork by doing the departmental record keeping.

A control desk is usually located at the entrance to the OR suite, where a clerk-receptionist can see and check all visitors and personnel. Unauthorized persons can be intercepted.

Clerical personnel serve as vital communication links between the OR department and other departments. They receive and send messages by telephone, intercommunication system, and mail. The hospital telephone exchange operators frequently relay messages for surgeons while they are operating. The clerk in the OR suite should be aware of the arrival and departure of the surgeons to be certain that they receive their messages without being disturbed during surgical procedures.

Most hospitals have an intercommunication system between the OR and other areas in the OR suite. Clerical personnel coordinate messages through this system. They can arrange for transportation of patients to and from the OR, obtain supplies or additional personnel for the OR team if needed, and so forth.

Many hospitals have a pneumatic-tube system that provides a quick means for the delivery of written communications and small nonbreakable supplies to all parts of the hospital. The clerk operates this system.

Nursing Assistants

Assistive personnel are employed to perform certain indirect nursing care activities. A *nursing assistant* may be male or female. Most OR departments have both. Their duties include but are not limited to:

1. Assisting with transporting, moving, and positioning of patients
2. Performing errands to other departments as needed
3. Cleaning, processing, and storing instruments and supplies
4. Maintaining assigned work area in a clean and orderly condition

A male assistant, sometimes titled an *orderly,* may be asked to do the heavier work in the department, such as lifting patients and moving or setting up large pieces of equipment.

INTERDEPARTMENTAL RELATIONSHIPS

The OR is one of many departments within the total hospital organization, just as the surgical procedure is one phase of total surgical patient care. To provide continuity in total patient care, the staffs of many departments cooperate. Their efforts are coordinated through the administration of the formal organizational structure of the hospital.

Every hospital has a *governing body* that appoints a chief executive officer, usually titled the *hospital administrator,* to provide appropriate physical resources and personnel to meet the needs of patients. Administrative lines of authority, responsibility, and accountability are defined to establish the working relationships between departments and personnel (Figure 6-1).

The *nurse executive* or director of nursing services reports to the hospital administrator. The OR nurse manager will report to the nurse executive if the OR department is structured as a unit within nursing service. In some hospitals the OR is considered an independent department separate from nursing service. The OR manager then reports directly to the hospital administrator, an assistant administrator, or to the chief of the department of surgery or anesthesia services. Through either channel of administration, many activities in the OR department should be coordinated with other nursing units and hospital departments.

Preoperative Testing Center

An area is designated for the preoperative evaluation and education of elective surgical patients. Patients are given an appointment to visit the preoperative testing center 1 to 7 days before the scheduled surgical procedure. Nursing assessment, anesthesia screening, and patient education are conducted, preferably by perioperative nurses with these skills. Routine laboratory tests, x-ray studies, and electrocardiograms as ordered by the surgeon or dictated by policy are performed. The patient may sign consent forms at this time. This

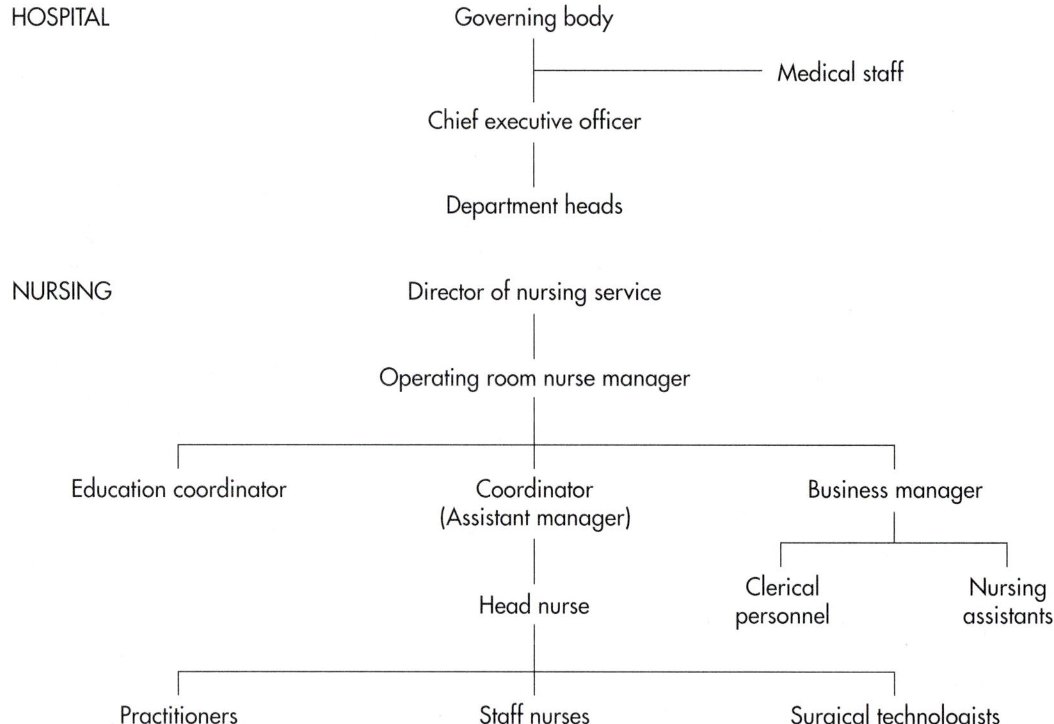

FIGURE 6-1 Management structure. Administrative lines of authority, responsibility, and accountability are defined to establish working relationships between departments and personnel.

center is usually located in the outpatient department of a hospital.

Same Day/Short-Stay Procedure Unit

Many patients are admitted for an elective surgical procedure on the day the procedure is scheduled. Others come to the hospital for a diagnostic or therapeutic procedure and return home the same day. A nursing care unit may be designated to receive these patients. Preparation is completed before the patient is transferred to the OR suite or a special procedure area. After the procedure, the patient is either admitted to the hospital or returned to this unit for discharge to home.

Some patients may need nursing supervision or assistance for up to 72 hours after their procedures; a short-stay unit that provides this care is open 24 hours. Patients are expected to progress rapidly to self-care, including assuming responsibility for taking their medications.

Endoscopy Unit

Many diagnostic and therapeutic procedures are performed through endoscopes. Patients may come to a dedicated unit outside the OR suite for these procedures. This short-stay unit has physical facilities for patient preparation, treatment, and recovery and for equipment storage, cleaning, and preparation. This unit is utilized primarily for gastrointestinal procedures that use sophisticated, complex technology. OR nurses and surgical technologists may staff this unit.

Nursing Units

Patients come to the OR suite directly from a short-stay or inpatient nursing unit, an outpatient ambulatory care area, or the emergency department. Channels of communication should be kept open between OR personnel and nursing personnel in these other nursing units to coordinate preoperative preparation and transportation of patients. Many facilities use a checklist to ensure adequate preparation of surgical patients. An RN or LPN/LVN signs or initials each item accomplished. By the time the patient leaves for the OR suite, all the preparations have been completed.

Emergency Department/Trauma Center

Victims of trauma and acutely ill patients often are seen initially in the hospital emergency department (ED). Cardiopulmonary resuscitative and other equipment is available to initiate prompt triage and treatment. Minor injuries usually can be treated in the ED. Some patients must be scheduled for an emergency surgical procedure, however. These patients may arrive in the OR before the results of all diagnostic tests are confirmed. Therefore communication between OR, ED, laboratory, and x-ray personnel is vital to the success of surgical intervention. OR personnel should be advised of the nature of the injury or illness to prepare all needed equipment and obtain supplies for the emergency surgical procedure.

Designated regional trauma centers should have teams of surgeons, anesthesiologists, and OR nursing personnel who are immediately available in the hospital 24 hours a day. A trauma nurse coordinator is administratively responsible for all personnel and activities to ensure comprehensive trauma care.

Labor and Delivery Suite/Obstetric Unit

The obstetric unit is divided into three separate areas: labor and delivery, postpartum care, and newborn nursery. Some labor and delivery areas have an operating room for delivery by cesarean section (C-section). In other hospitals patients scheduled either for elective or emergency C-section are brought to the OR suite. In addition to supplies needed for the surgical procedure, adequate resuscitative equipment must be available for the newborn.

Postanesthesia Care Unit

The PACU, also referred to as the *recovery room* (RR) or *postanesthesia recovery unit* (PAR), affords maximal care for patients immediately following their surgical procedures. The PACU evolved to meet a need for constant observation of patients by trained personnel within facilities equipped for specialized care until recovery from anesthesia is stabilized sufficiently for safe transfer elsewhere.

The PACU is usually adjacent to the OR suite. In large hospitals the PACU may be open 24 hours a day. In other hospitals, especially if most of the procedures are performed in the morning hours, the PACU may be open only during the day. The extent of use of the ORs will determine the routine hours for recovery care. Special arrangements for constant observation must be made for patients during hours in which the PACU is closed. These arrangements are established by hospital policy.

The PACU is under the supervision of an anesthesiologist in coordination with a nursing supervisor. This supervisor may be the OR nurse manager who has a head nurse assigned to the PACU to directly supervise the activities in this specialized area. The PACU is staffed by specially trained RNs and other nursing personnel. An intercommunication system or emergency call system connects the PACU staff with the OR suite so that additional personnel are readily available in situations that are life-threatening to patients.

A physician is responsible for discharge of the patient from the PACU. The department of anesthesiology and medical staff may approve discharge criteria for the PACU nurse to use to determine readiness for discharge. These should be consistent with accreditation and the professional organizations' standards. Standards for postanesthesia care have been established by the Joint Commission on Accreditation of Healthcare Organizations, the Accreditation Association for Ambulatory Health Care, the American Society of Anesthesiologists, and the American Society of Post Anesthesia Nurses (ASPAN) (see Chapter 26.)

Intensive Care Units

Because surgery has become more specialized and complex, specialized facilities where concentrated treatment can bring the patient to a satisfactory recovery have become a necessity. This care is provided in an *intensive care unit* (ICU), which is open 24 hours a day, 7 days a week. It is staffed by highly trained and specialized RNs. Critically ill patients who need constant care for several days are admitted directly from the OR, PACU, ED, or other nursing unit. Each bedside is equipped with therapeutic and monitoring equipment.

Depending on the size of the hospital and its specialty services, more than one specially designed and equipped ICU may be provided. One ICU may admit only cardiovascular surgical patients, another only burn patients, another only pediatric patients, and another only transplant patients. In addition to surgical ICUs, most hospitals also have a coronary care unit (CCU) and/or a unit for nonsurgical (medical) patients. The increased efficiency these units afford serves the best interests of both the hospital and the patient. They create the most effective use of personnel and equipment and lower morbidity and mortality rates.

Movements of patients to and from the surgical ICUs should be closely coordinated with the surgical schedule, the OR team, and the PACU personnel. If the surgeon anticipates that a patient will need intensive care postoperatively, an ICU bed must be reserved before the patient is scheduled for the surgical procedure. The ICU should be notified promptly when the surgeon determines that an unanticipated bed is needed. Sometimes the patient must wait in the OR or PACU for another patient to be transferred out of the ICU, when the former patient's condition warrants intensive care that was not anticipated. Sometimes elective surgical procedures should be postponed because sufficient ICU beds or staff are not available.

Radiology and Nuclear Medicine Departments

Frequently, personnel from the radiology (x-ray) and nuclear medicine (radiation therapy) departments assist with diagnostic or therapeutic procedures in the OR. For some procedures it may be necessary for OR nursing personnel to go to the x-ray department to assist the surgeon during a procedure requiring sterile technique. Whenever a diagnostic procedure or surgical procedure is scheduled that will require use of x-ray equipment or a radioactive implant, all departments should be notified at least the day before. This facilitates the scheduling of personnel and workload in all departments.

Pharmacy

Many drugs are routinely stocked in the OR suite for the anesthesiologists' use and some for use by the surgeons during surgical procedures. These are obtained by requisition from the pharmacy. When received, narcotics are always kept under lock, and each dosage is recorded as dispensed.

The pharmacy is not an isolated department but an integral part of the hospital. Pharmacists are resource persons who convey drug information to physicians and nurses. They should be responsible for preparation of all admixtures, but often the mixing of medications is done by nursing staff in the OR, PACU, and ICU to expedite administration. The pharmacist is responsible for quality control of drug product services throughout the hospital.

Blood Bank

All hospitals have a blood transfusion service or blood bank. This is a highly technical service for collecting, testing, processing, and distributing blood products. If the hospital does not have its own blood bank, blood may be supplied from a regional blood center. Written policies and procedures for blood transfusion services must conform to the standards of the American Association of Blood Banks. These include criteria for accepting blood donors, laboratory testing of donors' and recipients' blood, and preparing and administering blood products for therapeutic purposes. Blood banks dispense whole blood, plasma, packed cells, or platelets only as they are needed.

If in advance of an elective surgical procedure the surgeon anticipates that blood loss replacement may be necessary, the patient may have his or her own blood *(autologous)* drawn and stored in the blood bank for *autotransfusion,* a blood replacement procedure. Blood bank technicians also may participate on autotransfusion teams for collection of patient's blood intraoperatively and postoperatively.

If autologous blood is not available or additional units of donor blood *(homologous)* are needed, a sample of the patient's blood is sent to the blood bank for type and cross match. In emergency situations this sample may be sent from the ED or the OR. The units of blood products ordered by the surgeon are prepared and labeled with the patient's name and blood data. Suspected or recognized adverse reactions to blood transfusion must be documented on the patient's chart and reported to the blood bank.

Pathology Department

The *pathologist,* a physician who specializes in the cause and effect of disease, may be on call at a few minutes' notice to examine tissue while the patient is anesthetized. This enables the surgeon to proceed immediately with a definitive surgical procedure if malignant tumor cells are found, without subjecting the patient to a second surgical procedure at a later time. A small laboratory may be located within the OR suite with equipment for microscopic tissue examination. This laboratory may be used for other tests and/or for taking photographs of tissue specimens removed from patients. Routinely, all tissue removed during a surgical procedure is sent to the pathology department for examination.

Clinical Laboratory

Samples of blood, urine, or body fluids are taken to the clinical laboratory for analysis. Some analyses are routinely performed preoperatively. Others are done during a surgical procedure, such as blood gas analyses. Samples are obtained and immediately sent to the laboratory, or samples may be obtained during a surgical procedure for analysis later, such as a culture to determine the cause of an infection.

Biologic testing of sterile supplies is done routinely. The OR environment may be biologically tested periodically, and always when a contamination problem is suspected. The *bacteriologist,* who specializes in the study of microorganisms, may come into the OR suite to collect samples for testing, or samples may be collected and sent to laboratory by OR personnel. The results provide a method for evaluating the effectiveness of procedures and the degree of adherence to environmental standards.

Medical Records Department

Clinical records include the admitting diagnosis, the patient's chief complaint, complete history and physical examination, the results of laboratory examinations, and the physicians' and nurses' care plans. Records should state the therapy employed, including surgical procedure(s), and include progress notes, consultation remarks, condition on discharge, or observations in case of death. A summary of the hospitalization experience should be complete. These records are signed by all physicians and nurses attending the patient.

The anesthesia record completed during the surgical procedure by the anesthesiologist also becomes part of the patient's record. Nursing care should also be documented on the patient's chart. Therefore the circulating nurse should write pertinent remarks regarding the nursing care rendered in the OR and the patient's response to care on the nurses' note sheet or the progress notes. *Documentation is a responsibility of all professional team members implementing direct patient care.*

Notes about the surgical procedure should be explicit, dictated promptly after completion of the procedure, and incorporated into the record of each surgical patient. For the surgeons' convenience, many hospitals have dictating machines or a phone hookup with the medical records department installed within the OR suite, usually located in the dressing room or lounge. Details of the preoperative and postoperative diagnosis and the surgical procedure itself may have medical and legal significance. It is the responsibility of the medical records department to transcribe the surgeon's dictation and to maintain the patient's chart after his or her discharge from the hospital. The patient's chart may be put on microfilm for storage.

Environmental/Housekeeping Services

Housekeeping functions are recognized as important preventive measures to eliminate microorganisms from the hospital environment. Each hospital establishes a routine for its particular needs. Usually the environmental/housekeeping services personnel and nursing personnel share housekeeping duties in the OR suite. The amount of cleaning done by the OR personnel varies from one hospital to another. In many hospitals, the members of the housekeeping department clean all furniture, flat surfaces, lights, and floors once a day at the end of the surgical schedule. In others, they also clean the furniture and floors before the schedule starts and between each surgical procedure throughout the day. Whatever plan they follow, housekeeping personnel should have a storage area within the OR suite in which to keep their equipment and supplies. Equipment used for cleaning in the OR is not taken outside the suite.

The *director of environmental/housekeeping services* and the OR nurse or business manager plan the division of work. Personnel in each department should understand their responsibilities. The OR manager checks the work of housekeeping personnel and keeps in touch with the director concerning their performance.

The director evaluates and chooses the proper solutions for effective cleaning, sets up a program and standard of performance for employees, and sees that they are properly oriented and taught the procedures and standards. This includes adherence to procedures for removal and disposal of trash and soiled laundry. Using a checklist helps to cover all areas to be cleaned and inspected on a routine basis, whether it is daily, weekly, or monthly. A weekly or monthly cleaning routine is set up that includes walls and ceilings, in addition to the daily cleaning schedule within the OR suite.

The director impresses on the personnel the importance of the work and the important part they play in enabling the OR personnel to carry out aseptic technique. The housekeeping personnel do indeed function as members of the OR team when working with the scrub persons and circulators between surgical procedures.

Maintenance Department

The maintenance department personnel work in close cooperation with the OR department by providing a continuous preventive maintenance program. This includes routine monitoring of ventilation and heating, electrical and lighting systems, emergency warning systems, and water supply. Humidity is recorded every hour in the maintenance department. All electrical equipment is checked monthly by maintenance department personnel. In addition, they regularly test the autonomous emergency power source and maintain a written record of inspection and performance.

The hospital water supply system should not be connected with other piping systems or with fixtures that could allow contamination of the water supply. The hot water supply and steam lines have temperature control devices and filters regulated by the maintenance department personnel. They are cleaned on a routine schedule, usually weekly, to prevent accumulation of mineral deposits.

Clinical Biomedical Engineering

Competent technical personnel should be available to every area of the hospital to ensure the safe operation of equipment. Nearly every surgical procedure uses some form of powered instrumentation. Because of the variety and complexity of the instrumentation currently in use, most hospitals have a clinical engineer and/or biomedical equipment technician on staff or available. This technical support group assists OR personnel in evaluating and selecting new equipment, in installing and operating it, and in maintaining it.

The *clinical engineer* is systems and applications oriented. This individual can compare different models and manufacturers' specifications and provide recommendations for purchase. The *biomedical equipment technician* is knowledgeable about the theory of operation; the underlying physiologic principles; and the practical, safe clinical applications of biomedical instrumentation. This individual can test, install, calibrate, inspect, service, and repair equipment. Every preventive service or repair is recorded in an instrument history file.

Materiels Management

In an effort to control escalating health care costs, many hospitals belong to contract buying groups. This concept has changed the nature of the purchasing function and the management of supplies. The organizational administrative structure varies, but the basic functions of materiels management are purchasing, processing, inventorying, maintaining proper function, and distributing supplies and equipment. Several departments are responsible for supplies.

Purchasing

The purchasing director coordinates the acquisition of supplies and equipment for the hospital. Standardization of products used throughout the hospital fosters quantity purchases, which provides leverage in negotiating prices with vendors. Items that are too expensive to stock in large quantities or that are used infrequently are ordered through the purchasing department as needed. In some hospitals this department is referred to as *materiels management.*

Central Storeroom

The purchasing director or materiels manager determines the supplies to be stocked for requisition by all the departments of the hospital. Bulk inventories are received and warehoused in the central storeroom. Each department then requisitions supplies as needed, usually on a weekly basis.

Central Service

One area of the hospital is designed specifically for storing, processing, and distributing supplies and equipment used in patient care. This department may be referred to as *central service* or *central supply* (CS), *central processing, supply, processing and distribution* (SPD), or *materiels management.* The functional design and work flow patterns provide for separation of soiled and contaminated supplies from clean and sterile items. Supplies are replenished on the nursing units on a predetermined time schedule to maintain standard inventory levels. This may be done by central service, using an exchange cart system, in which a cart of fresh supplies is exchanged for the one in use. Control of patient charges for supplies also may be coordinated by central service. Inventory control is computerized in most hospitals. Bar code technology on individual packages may facilitate patient charges and inventory management.

Laundry Services

Many disposable nonwoven fabrics are used. However, some woven fabrics are processed daily for use in the hospital, such as patient gowns, bedding, and towels. Hospitals that do not have laundry facilities as part of their physical plant use a commercial laundry service. An adequate inventory should be maintained for daily use. The manager of the laundry services assists in determining appropriate inventories and supervises the laundry processes. Reusable fabrics that must be sterilized before use are packaged and sterilized either in the laundry, central service, sterile processing department, or the OR suite, depending on where the sterilizing equipment is located.

Sterile Processing

Supply needs in the OR are unique. Instruments, reusable products, and many other supplies must be decontaminated and cleaned after use and inspected, packaged, and sterilized before use. Two separated areas must be designated for these functions whether they are performed within the OR suite, in central service, or in a sterile processing department (SPD) designed specifically for this purpose.

Hospitals built or renovated after the mid-1960s usually use a surgery case cart system. Personnel in sterile processing prepare individual carts with the required supplies and instruments for each scheduled surgical procedure. Instrument books and surgeon's preference cards are routinely used to ensure that all the necessary supplies are included. Many of these are commercially prepared one-time-use items and devices that the patient will pay for. Lists for the patient charge items and the instruments provided are usually attached to the cart to assist personnel in appropriately accounting for all items. Each cart is transported to the assigned OR. After the surgical procedure, the cart with soiled supplies is returned to the decontamination area. Usually the decontamination and reprocessing of OR instruments and equipment are done in areas separated from supplies used in other hospital departments. This prevents mixing surgical instruments with those supplied to other units. The personnel assigned to the surgery case cart areas should be familiar with the supplies needed for each surgical procedure, how surgical instruments are used, and the proper method of cleaning and sterilizing each. Surgical technologists frequently are assigned to sterile processing because of their technical background.

Human Resources/Personnel Department

Even though the availability of supplies and equipment and the physical facilities are important, these are secondary to the functioning of the OR department. The efficiency of any department depends on the persons employed there. Therefore the careful selection of capable, highly motivated people contributes to efficiency and effectiveness. The human resources/personnel department helps to screen applicants. Those seen as having potential for available positions are referred to the appropriate department head. If the OR manager reports to nursing service, potential employees may be processed through nursing service before an interview with the OR nurse manager is scheduled, or the OR manager may be contacted directly to arrange an interview with an applicant. In either situation the human resources/personnel department assists in hiring and terminating all employees. This department also provides resources for employee assistance and assists with disciplinary measures.

COORDINATION THROUGH COMMITTEES

A committee is a group of persons delegated to consider, investigate, take specific action, or report on a matter of mutual concern or interest. Many activities within the hospital organization are coordinated by multidisciplinary committees.

Operating Room Committee

The OR committee is a committee of the medical staff. One surgeon is appointed chief or director of the department of surgery. In teaching hospitals a director is appointed chief of each specialty service (e.g., chief of orthopaedics). The anesthesia department also designates a director of this department. These individuals are responsible for professional practice and administrative activities within their respective departments. They should maintain continuing evaluation of the professional performance of all members of the medical staff granted privileges in their specialty. They also serve as liaison representatives between the medical staff and hospital administration.

Vital to the management of the OR suite is an active OR committee. The chief of surgery, the chiefs or representatives of the specialty services, the chief of the anesthesia department, the OR nurse manager, and the coordinator or the OR business manager meet at regular intervals to review OR suite activities. The hospital administrator and director of nursing service may also be members of this committee or may be invited to attend meetings relevant to their concerns.

The OR committee should formulate policies and procedures pertaining to utilization of facilities, schedule of surgical procedures, and maintenance of a safe environment. Evaluation of techniques and selection of new products may require review of reports from other departments or committees in addition to those prepared by OR personnel.

Because this committee determines policy and procedures for efficient functioning within the OR suite, persistent problems are brought before the committee, where recommendations for corrective action are made. For example, if temperature and humidity controls are not being effectively monitored or maintained, the committee may recommend to the hospital administration that procedures be reviewed and revised by the maintenance department or that new equipment be installed. If surgeons are repeatedly late in arriving, thus delaying the surgical schedule, stronger policy may be indicated for the control and better utilization of facilities. If a new product is purchased, a new procedure may need to be written to specify its use and care. Through data collection and a problem-solving approach to decision making, the OR committee seeks to improve the working relationships of all members of the OR team and the supportive services concerned with activities within the OR suite.

Policies and associated directives formulated and approved by the committee serve as guides for governing the actions of surgeons, anesthesiologists, and the OR nursing staff while in the OR suite. The OR nurse manager shares with the OR committee, hospital administration, and nursing service the responsibility for clarification, implementation, and day-to-day enforcement of approved policies and procedures.

Laser Safety Subcommittee

The laser safety committee establishes policies and procedures, standards, documentation systems, and credentialing criteria for the use of lasers in the health care facility. The laser safety committee may also be responsible for the development of training and continuing education programs for physicians, nurses, and surgical technologists. This may be a subcommittee of the OR committee. Members should include, but are not limited to, chief of surgery, chief of anesthesia, physician representatives from each surgical specialty using the laser, OR nurse manager, laser nurse specialists, biomedical technician, and representative of administration.

This committee may delegate safety surveillance duties to a *laser safety officer* (LSO) responsible for identifying problems and safety concerns with the use of lasers. The LSO may be a physician, nurse, or specially trained laser technician. The LSO is usually given the authority to stop any laser procedure if safety is in question.

Infection Control Committee

The infection control committee investigates hospital-acquired (nosocomial) infections and seeks to prevent or control them. Membership may vary but should include representatives of the medical staff, hospital administration, nursing service, and the epidemiologist or infection control coordinator. Representatives from other departments attend meetings when the agenda is relevant to their particular concerns.

The committee meets at least quarterly. Members form a defense against nosocomial infections by reviewing environmental factors and by determining whether the hospital is providing a safe environment for patient care. They review all infection reports and investigate nosocomial infections. Committee members also review policies and procedures and scrutinize the entire chain of asepsis in an effort to determine and then eliminate possible sources of infection.

This committee has the authority to approve changes necessary to eliminate any hazardous practices. Included in its jurisdiction is the education of personnel so that they can provide a high standard of patient care. *A health care facility has a moral duty to provide a safe environment for its patients.* The infection control committee aids the hospital in fulfilling this duty. Surveillance personnel assist in directing infection control policies, procedures, and practices.

Quality Improvement Committee

Members of the quality improvement committee include representatives of both clinical and administrative personnel. This committee monitors routine activities, evaluates clinical outcomes, reviews incident reports, and conducts problem-focused studies in an effort to identify practices deemed substandard. Actual practices may be in violation of policy or not in compliance with accepted standards or governmental regulations. Noncompliance puts a hospital or ambulatory care facility at risk of legal liability. A productive and efficient committee will implement actions designed to eliminate real or potential problems, improve patient care, and reduce financial loss. Because of an emphasis on cost containment, review of utilization of facilities and risk management also may be concerns of this committee.

Many facilities employ a *quality improvement coordinator* and/or a *risk manager* to ensure implementation of committee decisions. The primary function of the person in this position is to assess actual practices and evaluate outcomes of patient care. The quality improvement (QI) coordinator may receive and respond to complaints about patient care or environmental hazards.

Each hospital department and nursing unit may have its own *quality improvement subcommittee.* These unit-based committees monitor performance, identify ways to constructively solve competency problems, and seek opportunities for improvements in practices. Other interdepartmental subcommittees may focus on specific activities or problems requiring input from several disciplines. Reports from these subcommittees are reviewed by the QI coordinator. Mutual problems are shared with the hospital committee.

Ethics Committee

A multidisciplinary ethics committee should represent the hospital and the community it serves. Representatives include physicians, nurses, social workers, patient relations liaison, clergy, lawyers, bioethicists, and laypersons from the community. Their primary purpose is to educate the staff and the community regarding moral principles and processes of ethical decision making when faced with the diverse issues that arise in the care of critically and terminally ill patients. They provide consultation to professional staff, patients, and families. This committee recommends policies and guidelines on such issues as informed consent, research protocols, and advance directives. OR nurses and surgical technologists often are confronted with social, ethical, and legal decisions concerning genetic and reproductive biology, organ transplantation, and death with dignity. The ethics committee can provide a forum for discussion of these issues. Some hospitals have a nursing bioethics committee in addition to the hospital committee. These committees provide education and consultation and develop policies and procedures. They are not decision-making bodies. They do not get involved in disciplinary matters.

Hospital Safety Committee

Representatives from administration, nursing service, medical staff, the engineering and maintenance departments, environmental/housekeeping services, dietary department, and the safety director form the nucleus of the hospital safety committee. This group writes policies and procedures designed to enhance safety within the hospital and on hospital grounds. They exchange information with the infection control and quality improvement committees and conduct hazard surveillance programs. They meet at least every other month to investigate and evaluate reported incidents. Action is taken when a hazardous condition exists that could result in personal injury or damage to equipment or facilities.

Disaster Planning Committee

Health care facilities should have an organized plan for caring for mass casualties if a major disaster occurs. *External disasters* happen outside of the health care facility, such as an airplane crash or an event of nature (e.g., a flood or hurricane). *Internal disasters,* such as a fire or an explosion, happen inside the health care facility. Planning by the intrahospital committee includes consultation with local civil authorities and representatives of other medical agencies to establish an effective chain of command and to make appropriate jurisdictional provisions. This planning results in disaster-site triage to separate and distribute patients to ensure the most efficient use of available facilities and services.

External disaster drills are held at least twice a year to try out the plans developed by the committee, to seek to improve them, and to familiarize personnel with them. Plans for both types of disasters include:

1. An information center within the hospital to facilitate a unified medical command and the movement of patients.
2. A receiving area for the injured. Severely wounded casualties are given emergency care according to their needs and are sent at once to the OR or to other units as indicated or transferred to another facility. Ambulatory patients may be treated in the ED for slight injuries and sent home or admitted to the hospital as indicated.
3. Special disaster medical records or tags that accompany patients at all times.
4. A plan of organization of personnel. As soon as a hospital receives word of a disaster during the evening or night, several key persons are called.

These in turn phone others previously assigned to them, and these call still others, until the full staff has been notified. If the disaster occurs during the day, the full staff is usually on duty, although any off-duty personnel may be called. Other departments are alerted and come on duty as needed; these include personnel for the blood bank, laboratory, pharmacy, materiels management, x-ray department, and the nursing units, including OR, PACU, and ICU. If disposable drape packs are not in use, it may be necessary to alert some laundry personnel. Some key maintenance personnel should be available, especially electricians.

5. Written departmental instructions for personnel. For the OR staff these may include sign-in procedures, checklists of duties, and patient scheduling procedures.

Personnel must know where to report, what to do, and where extra supplies are kept in case of an emergency. Extra supplies are stored in reserve in sufficient quantities to fill possible needs for a minimum of 1 week.

COMMITMENT TO EXCELLENCE

Recognition for expertise is a prime contributor to job satisfaction. Recognition for a job well done fosters self-esteem with positive attitudes about one's abilities. Recognition and respect are earned through a commitment to excellence (i.e., to be the best possible). This should be a personal goal for every staff member. To achieve this goal, personal growth and development should be a continuous process. A patient care provider, either directly or indirectly, may enhance his or her professional career by:

1. Being flexible and open to new ideas
2. Being willing to change and to improve work habits
3. Learning to use new technology safely
4. Participating in organizational activities, such as committees and clinical research
5. Joining professional associations and becoming involved
6. Attending educational programs designed to upgrade skills on own time and at own expense
7. Reading professional journals, listening to audiocassettes, and viewing videotapes and films
8. Becoming certified
9. Being responsible and accountable for own actions with integrity and honesty

BIBLIOGRAPHY

Abbott CA: Intraoperative nursing activities performed by surgical technologists, *AORN J* 60(3):382-393, 1994.

Advance practice nurse competency statement, *AORN J* 61(1):64-69, 1995.

Applegeet C: Standards of practice, recent changes: preparing job descriptions that reflect these standards; how these standards relate to practice, *AORN J* 56(4):739-741, 1992.

Association of Operating Room Nurses: *Preceptor guide for perioperative nursing practice,* Denver, 1993, The Association.

Association of Operating Room Nurses: Standards of perioperative administrative practice. In *AORN standards and recommended practices for perioperative nursing,* Denver, 1995, The Association.

Bell A: The management and utilization of operating departments, *Br J Theatre Nurs* 27(1):5-7, 1990.

Buchanan LM: Therapeutic nursing intervention, knowledge development and outcome measures for advanced practice, *Nurs Health Care* 15(4):190-195, 1994.

Davidhizar RE: Choosing management, *AORN J* 51(3):800-808, 1990.

Ethics committee can be helpful to nurses, *OR Manager* 6(4):10-12, 1990.

Frik SM, Pollack SE: Preparation for advanced nursing practice, *Nurs Health Care* 14(4):190-195, 1993.

Hill EM, Lowenstein LE: Preceptors, *AORN J* 55 (5):1237-1248, 1992.

Job description: Certified surgical technologist, *Surg Technol* 21(6):18-19, 1989.

Jones JE: Clinical ladders, *Surg Technol* 23(3):18-23, 1991.

Krueger NE, Mazuzan JE: A collaborative approach to standards, practices, *AORN J* 57(2):467-480, 1993.

Mark BA et al: Knowledge and skills for nurse administrators, *Nurs Health Care* 11(4):185-189, 1990.

Marousky RT: Disaster planning, *AORN J* 56(4):679-687, 1992.

Patterson P: A manager's challenge: enforcing OR policy, *OR Manager* 6(3):1, 8-11, 1990.

Philosophy of perioperative nursing practice: definition of perioperative nurse; scope of perioperative nursing practice, *AORN J* 59(6): 1188-1191, 1994.

Phippen ML: President's message: nonnurse assistants should complement your work in the OR, not complicate it, *AORN J* 52(1):8-9, 1990.

Phippen ML, Applegeet C: Clinical issues: unlicensed assistive personnel in the perioperative setting, *AORN J* 60(3):455-457, 1994.

Prokopczak D: Bar codes for a more dynamic O.R. inventory system, *Can Oper Rm Nurs J* 8(3):8-14, 1990.

Standards of professional performance, *AORN J* 55(4):1053-1056, 1992.

Wesolowski MS: Practical innovations: admission/discharge unit alleviates overcrowding, *AORN J* 51(3):861-869, 1990.

SECTION THREE

The Patient as a Unique Individual

CHAPTER 7

The Patient

THE REASON FOR YOUR EXISTENCE

PATIENT-CENTERED CARE

Hippocrates (circa 460-377 BC) advocated, "To cure the human body you must have knowledge of the whole thing." His concept is still valid. The human body is a miraculously complex creation that functions as a coordinated unit, an organized entity, and as a person who interacts within the environment and society.

A person facing an impaired health status strives for wellness. As a patient, this person looks to health care providers to fulfill his or her multiplicity of diversified needs. A *patient-centered approach* to perioperative care involves meeting all the surgical patient's basic needs during the preoperative, intraoperative, and postoperative phases. As noted in Chapters 5 and 6, many persons contribute to this care. Each has specific functions in the continuity of care process. The perioperative health care team is dedicated to maintaining optimal health and/or restoring it when it is altered by disease, injury, or deformity. Although the team members may vary with the situation and the patient, the goal is to attain the expected outcomes from surgical intervention.

In viewing the health care team in its broadest scope, one can consider the patient as the central part or hub of a wheel with many persons and departments as the supporting framework (Figure 7-1). All focus their efforts at the hub, meaning that the patient is the center of attention always, not only when under the operating room (OR) spotlight. The ultimate beneficiary of teamwork is the patient. Imperfection in any one part of the wheel imperils the performance and security of all. Each team member makes a unique contribution in reaching the goals. The patient is the reason for the existence of the health care team.

PATIENT AS AN INDIVIDUAL

A *patient* may be defined as an individual seeking help to function or to cope with disease or disability. To effectively meet the patient's requirements and expectations, personnel should have knowledge of his or her needs, understanding of the patient's individuality, and realization of what a surgical procedure means to a patient.

Certain beliefs exist concerning a human being. In our society human beings:

1. Are worthwhile and unique individuals.
2. Respond psychosocially on the basis of personal values and beliefs and ethnic and cultural background.
3. Have the capacity to adapt both to their internal and external environments.

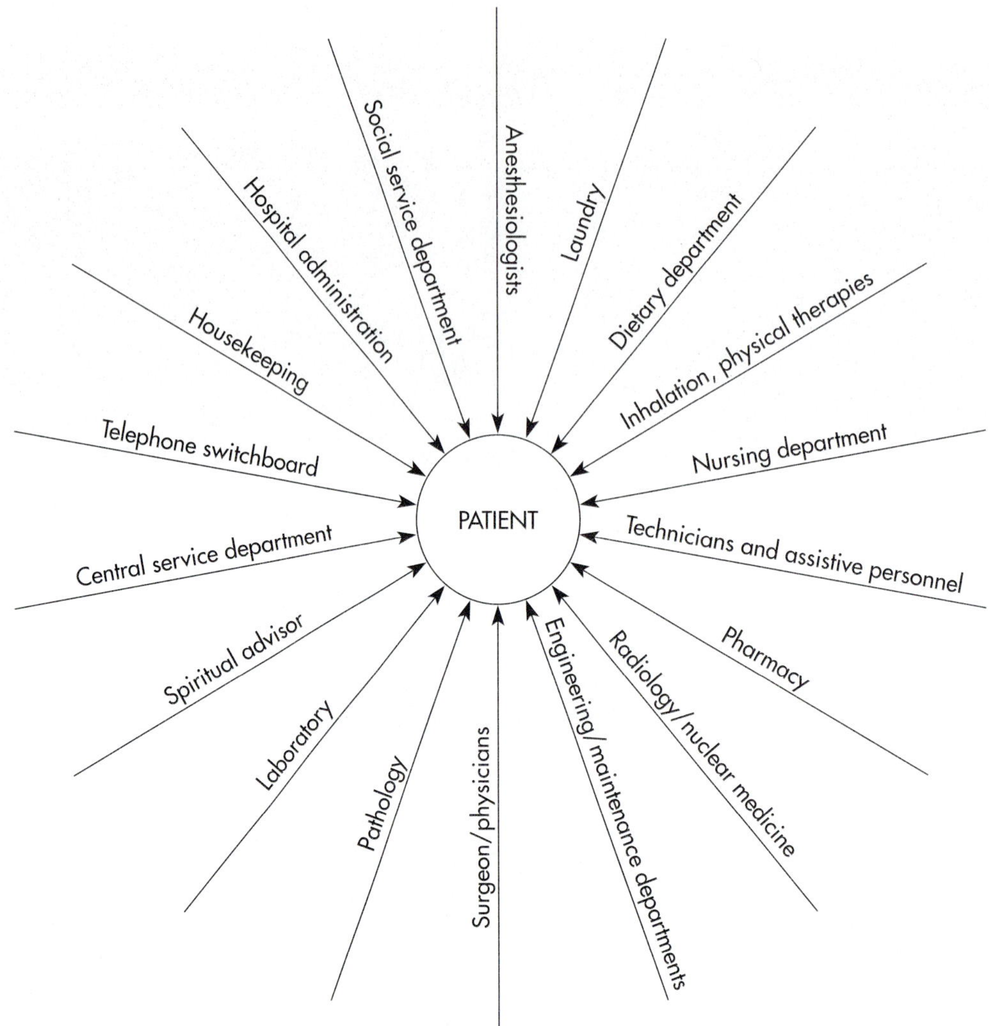

FIGURE 7-1 Patient is focus of attention of entire health care team.

4. Have basic needs that must be met in order to maintain homeostasis.

Homeostasis may be defined as the maintenance of steady or stable states in the organism by coordinated physiologic processes. The body strives to maintain equilibrium within normal limits. This stability depends partly on the structural integrity of the body, the adequacy of its functions, and its surroundings. Change requires adjustment.

PATIENT'S BASIC NEEDS

Needs are factors that must be controlled or redirected to restore altered function. Nursing judgments are based on knowledge of patient needs. It is therefore essential to understand basic human needs of all persons (well or ill) because fulfilling them is an integral part of the nursing process. The surgical patient faces a grave threat to the basic needs classified as physical, emotional or psychosocial, and spiritual.

Physical Needs

Physical needs are the life-sustaining necessities such as food, water, oxygen, sleep, safety, and warmth. In illness, the patient becomes acutely aware of these needs. However, patient care does not focus entirely on bodily needs.

Psychosocial Needs

Concern for the patient's emotional well-being should be as intense as it is for his or her physical health because the two are inseparably intertwined. The society the patient lives in is an integral factor in developing feelings of identity, self-worth, and satisfaction. Thwarted feelings can lead to a state of helplessness or inferiority. Achieving self-actualization, doing the best one is capable of, is the highest level of human development. Examples of *psychosocial* needs that also require fulfillment are:

1. *Security.* People need to feel secure and safe and to trust and to have confidence in those around them. They need to feel comforted, reassured, cared about, and protected.
2. *Acceptance by others.* Individuals need empathetic understanding of their feelings and attitudes, both negative and positive.
3. *Recognition.* People need to be acknowledged as worthy individuals. Cultural values, religious beliefs, race, and socioeconomic status must be respected without judgment. Individuals need consideration of their dignity, rights, and uniqueness. Positive reinforcement enhances self-esteem.
4. *Self-actualization.* People need to be productive, make their own choices and decisions, and control their behavior and environment.

People are social beings who need to establish satisfying meaningful interpersonal relationships and mutual trust and respect and to know that someone cares. Risk is involved in sharing feelings with others, however. Emotional stress develops if individuals do not feel secure. If they are treated with love and kindness, they feel worthy and can respond to others in the same way. Human beings also need a sense of order in their lives.

Spiritual Needs

Spiritual needs include support for a person's religious views or belief in a "higher power" whose guidance influences life. Especially in times of stress and fear, a person reaches out or turns to religious convictions for spiritual sustenance. Because fear of death has a spiritual and a physical dimension, uncertainty about one's relationship with a supreme being can enhance a patient's anxiety. The inner strength derived from a strong religious faith can be a bulwark of hope for the patient facing a surgical procedure.

The hospital chaplain, available to patients of all faiths, or the patient's personal cleric provides the anxious patient with a human element of comfort, warmth, and strength. The giving of sacraments to the ill does not necessarily mean that the patient is dying. The spiritual advisor fulfills a basic need by using the reassuring symbols of the patient's religious experiences. In addition, the chaplain or cleric does more: he or she is able to understand the patient's situation and to help the patient have faith in his or her God, in physicians and caregivers, and in himself or herself. Faith helps to control anxiety. The clergy can be a source of support and encouragement as patients share their fears.

Hierarchy of Needs

In relating Maslow's concept of a hierarchy of needs to set priorities for care (Figure 7-2), basic lower level or physiologic needs—those essential for survival—must be met first. Then satisfaction of the higher level needs—for safety and security, belonging and acceptance, self-esteem, and self-actualization—can be met. Health care personnel should be concerned with a total picture of the patient's needs and consider all of them. In illness, factors such as location of the pathologic condition, type of surgical procedure, and effectiveness of therapy can influence needs. Also, priorities may change with changing situations. Preoperatively, anxiety and nutritional status are two factors that must be addressed. Intraoperatively, the team must concentrate on basic physiologic needs for oxygen, circulation, and prevention of shock and infection. Postoperatively, team members must prevent complications and encourage patient self-actualization. If the patient's needs are not satisfactorily met, undesirable consequences can occur.

PATIENT REACTIONS TO ILLNESS

To meet patient needs, the health care team should be sensitive to patients' feelings about their illnesses. Patients' reactions influence their behaviors and the staff's behavioral responses to them.

Behavior

Health and human behavior are interdependent. Individuals with physiologic problems, regardless of age, experience some emotional change that influences their behavior. Patients react to a new interpersonal environ-

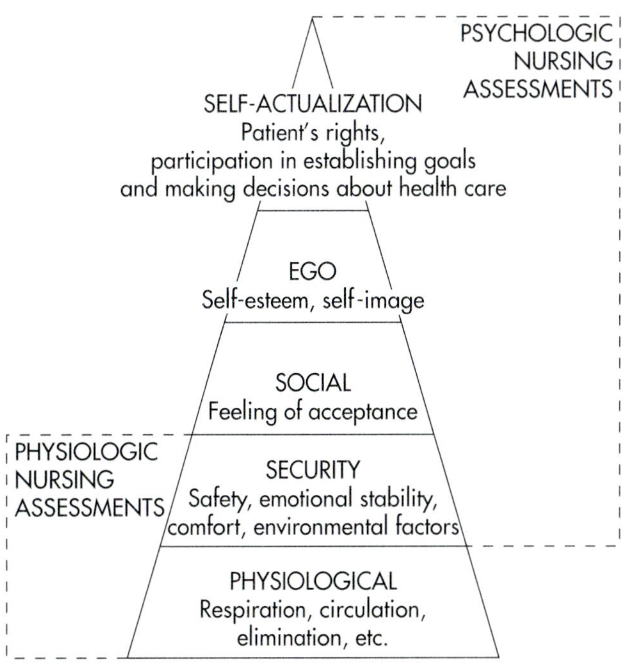

FIGURE 7-2 Maslow's hierarchy of basic needs related to surgical patient's needs during perioperative care.

ment according to their learned behavioral patterns. The following are basic facts about behavior:

1. Perception of interaction within the environment creates individualized differences in personality, behavior, and needs.
2. A person's physical and psychosocial behavior is a response to stimuli in an attempt to maintain homeostasis.
3. Behavior is complex. Behavioral acts have multiple causes in addition to a major precipitating one.
4. A person functions on many levels simultaneously. Many factors determine an individual's response in a given situation.
5. Behavior should be evaluated in light of the person's specific situation and of pertinent social forces such as family, culture, and environment. To understand the meaning of behavior, one must know about the individual.

Patients respond to crises or personal threats in different ways. Some persons face suffering and surgical intervention with extreme courage, dignity, and fortitude. Others may revert to extreme fear or helplessness even when faced with a relatively safe procedure. Overt behavior is not necessarily consistent with one's feelings but often reflects them most accurately. Patients often express frustration and fear behaviorally in an effort to cope with stimuli.

Adaptation

Any deviation from a person's normal daily pattern of living necessitates adaptation through innate or acquired defenses. Adaptation may involve physiologic or psychologic changes.

Personality includes a patient's characteristic responses to anxiety (either calm acceptance or disorganization, depression, and resistance) and to self-image. *Self-image,* an individual's concept or ideas about self and personal philosophy of life, is often affected by other people's reactions. Interpersonal relationships in early childhood are among the most important social determinants of personality formation. A person's adaptive and defensive mechanisms are a basic part of personality and culture. Individuals vary in their adaptive abilities, as demonstrated by varied behavioral responses to illness.

Illness disrupts normal living and equilibrium. It also alters self-image. One may worry about what others think, especially if the illness involves disfigurement, as from severe burns, or is an acquired disease such as syphilis or AIDS. A patient's initial response to illness may be irrational, impulsive behavior requiring patience and understanding from others. He or she may have difficulty thinking clearly, concentrating, or making intelligent, rational decisions. Both mind and body must adapt successfully for the patient to recover. Adaptation requires energy, ingenuity, and persistence.

The adaptive process causes physiologic or psychologic changes that constitute an attempt to counteract stimuli so that the individual can continue to function. If adaptation is interfered with, the effects can be detrimental. Adaptation to illness includes the following three stages:

1. Transition from health: development of symptoms
2. Acceptance: coping and making decisions
3. Convalescence or resolution

Adaptation may be rapid or slow, depending on the nature of the stimuli, the individual's culture, learned responses, and developmental needs. Adaptations may be sensory, motor, or sensorimotor. The extent of adjustment required is contingent on the type of illness, the magnitude of disability, and the patient's personality.

Stress

Stress can be defined as a physical, chemical, or emotional factor that causes tension. It may be a factor in disease causation. It is the result of threat perception and is manifested by changes in physiologic and psychosocial behavior. Tolerance of stress depends on the individual and the intensity of the stressor, its duration, and type—either localized or generalized, as pain.

Inescapable in the process of daily living, some degree of stress can be beneficial *eustress* if it motivates an individual to increased productivity. Conversely, it can be harmful *distress* if increased or simultaneous stressors occur, straining the individual's coping ability. If the individual's adaptive powers are inadequate or malfunctioning, the stress may become overwhelming. In the latter situation, new secondary stressors more incapacitating than the initial one develop, creating a continuous stress-adaptation cycle. Adaptive reserve may become depleted as a result.

Stressful factors can originate from within the individual or from the external environment. *Intrinsic factors,* those originating from within, that affect a patient include:

1. Hereditary or genetic factors, such as hormonic or enzymatic system competency.
2. Nature of the illness or disease process. This may be influenced by nutritional or immunologic status.
3. Severity of the illness or presence of a stigma.
4. Previous personal experiences with illnesses. Chronic illness has a disruptive effect on lifestyle.
5. Age. Children feel threatened. Adolescents resent an interruption of activities and are painfully aware of body changes. Older people think about infirmity and death.
6. Intellectual capacity. Misconceptions can lead to a knowledge deficit about the disease. Impaired cognitive function creates an inability to understand or comprehend.

7. Disturbed sensorium. Hearing or sight loss intensifies a stressful experience.
8. General state of personal well-being.

Extrinsic factors, originating from external sources, include those concerning:

1. Environment. The physical and social environment of the hospital is not the same as that of the home.
2. Family role and status. Expectations and authoritative relationships affect lifestyle, attitudes, and communications.
3. Economic, financial situation.
4. Religion. Beliefs influence attitudes and values toward life, illness, and death. For example, Jehovah's Witnesses will not permit transfusion of whole blood or blood components. Orthodox Jews must follow dietary laws in any environment. The fatalistic attitudes derived from some religious beliefs give a person little control over his or her environment; they can render a patient passive and apathetic.
5. Cultural background, education, and social class. These are closely related to the patient's emotional responses and living habits. Significant elements such as food habits, daily living patterns, hygiene, family organization, child care, orientation to past, present, and future time should be analyzed in relation to culture. An ethnic community is really a larger family. Roles taught by a cultural group influence the mores, beliefs, and social interactions of individuals. Also, responses to pain may vary according to one's cultural or ethnic background. Some groups commonly show an exaggerated emotional response; in others it is more appropriate to conceal suffering and feelings.
6. Social relationships. Family, significant others, and friends help satisfy the need for reassurance and provide a sense of being cared about.

Disability, illness, and hospitalization accentuate feelings of vulnerability and are stress-producing, stress-exaggerating experiences. They threaten a person's security and stability. They may create a crisis state that diminishes defenses and increases emotional responses to threats. The severity of the reaction may be unrelated to the seriousness of the illness. It is often not the problem itself that is devastating, but one's perception of it. Also, the same illness may hold different meanings for different individuals. For many persons hospitalization and surgical intervention represent a critical life experience.

To decrease the potentially traumatic consequences of a surgical procedure, health care personnel must realize that stress and pain are both physiologic and psychologic. Stress can adversely affect appetite and bodily functions such as digestion, metabolism, and fluid and electrolyte balance. Secretion of adrenal cortical hormones may delay wound healing and decrease resistance to infection. In addition, during times of markedly increased stress, one's emotional needs come to the surface. In facing personal threat, a person tends to mobilize defense mechanisms for flight or fight. One's ability to adapt depends in part on the support one receives. Effective nursing intervention at any stage of the adaptation process can alter the exigencies of illness and direct the patient's emotional responses. This will facilitate therapy and recovery through behavior modification.

Anticipatory apprehension, although normal to some degree, may diminish critical thinking and decision-making abilities. It may initiate an exaggerated response. Those surgical patients who are threatened by loss of body parts, function, or life are in a psychologically perilous situation. Some patients feel vulnerable in unfamiliar social relationships and surroundings. The strangeness of the OR itself—its noises, odors, and equipment—represents a potential hazard. A response to stress, perceived by the patient as distress, may be expressed in one or many ways.

Anxiety

Anxiety is an apprehensive uneasiness (tension), a feeling of uncertainty, or a solicitous concern stemming from anticipation of a real or imagined threat. It incites the body's defenses. All patients experience anxieties preoperatively, whether they verbalize them or not. Physiologic manifestations of anxiety may be rapid pulse (usually associated with heart palpitation), rapid respiration, diaphoresis, dry mouth, rapid eye movements and dilated pupils, clammy skin, skeletal muscle rigidity, and, if very severe, even paralysis. The patient may become so anxious that the physiologic manifestation becomes exaggerated. For example, a controlled hypertensive patient may suddenly experience increased blood pressure and electrocardiographic changes that may cause postponement of the surgical procedure. Other indications of increasing tension are stuttering, word blockage, confusion, and distortion of events. Anxiety impairs intellectual functioning. Perception, concentration, feelings of security, and self-image are also disturbed.

Anxiety from prolonged stress is experienced on both physical and emotional levels. *Psychophysiologic reaction* refers to anxiety reactions in which the symptoms center around one organ system, such as the cardiovascular system. Psychosomatic illness results from a combination of physiologic and emotional factors that can cause structural change, such as ulcerative colitis, which may necessitate bowel resection. A person's emotional strength influences one's ability to view oneself objectively. Intensity of feelings is multiform. Sharing a feeling with another often reduces the intensity. Women tend to express anxiety more readily than men. Anxious men and geriatric patients have higher blood pressures.

Anxiety significantly correlates with an alteration in pulse rate.

Varying degrees of anxiety are to be expected preoperatively. Normally, patients are worried to some extent about what will happen during the surgical procedure and consequently may be restless and unable to sleep the night before the scheduled procedure. However, patients who have access to meaningful communication and are able to ask questions are less likely to experience significant emotional disturbances.

Highly anxious patients dwell on the dangers of the surgical procedure and are apparently overwhelmed by them. They may not comprehend what is said or be able to accept reassurance about their magnified fears. They exhibit hyperactive behavior. The perioperative caregiver can help these patients only if a state of calm is achieved. The highly anxious patient should be considered a high-risk patient. Extreme preoperative apprehension predisposes this patient to a more difficult anesthesia induction and intraoperative period, and to more postoperative pain and complications. As less than optimal surgical risks, these patients are more prone to shock, laryngeal spasm, or cardiac arrest. A patient's unresolved severe anxiety or premonition of death should alert the surgeon to delay the surgical procedure until a more favorable time.

Alteration of time perception is not an unusual aspect of anxiety. To a waiting patient a minute may seem like an hour. In addition, the anxious patient experiences a feeling of alienation. Surrounded by unfamiliar people and equipment, separated from loved ones, the patient is expected to adapt to a foreign environment. The patient may feel helpless and alone. Anticipation of surgical alterations of the body produce tremendous anxiety associated not only with the procedure but also with its potential outcomes. The independent, secure individual can cope more easily than the insecure person who has feelings of inferiority. Anxieties originating from reality sources can have a cumulative effect. For example, a young mother facing a surgical procedure with no responsible person to care for her family and home has enhanced feelings of dread. Similar anxiety-inducing factors are:

1. Lack of understanding of instructions for preoperative preparation and postoperative care: "Should I shampoo my hair?" or "What can I eat?"
2. Lack of information about or understanding of test results or diagnostic studies and risks of the surgical procedure: "What did they find?" or "What may happen?" or "What did the surgeon mean?"
3. Confusion about present and future activity: "Will I be able to do all the things I did before?"
4. Worry by a family provider: "Will we go into debt?" or "Will I lose my job?" or "Who will care for my loved ones?"
5. Concern for unfinished projects: "Will I be able to make up my exam?" or "How will I ever regain the lost time?" or "Will I meet my deadlines?"

Relieving contributory stresses helps a patient to cope with the main stress—his or her illness. Specific concerns depend greatly on how illness frustrates the patient's specific needs. The patient with a high level of preoperative anxiety will be very anxious during emergence from anesthesia.

Fear

An emotion marked by dread, apprehension, and alarm, fear is caused by anticipation or awareness of danger. The sympathetic nervous system reacts and stimulates a neurophysiologic response as described for anxiety. This classic *fight-or-flight* response occurs as the patient realizes he or she is vulnerable. As long as the patient perceives fear, it exists.

Many childhood fears remain with a person in various forms throughout life. In illness, anxiety causes repressed fears to resurface from the subconscious and become magnified. The patient may imagine and dread something more frightening than the actual experience. Anticipatory fears are many and varied and include:

1. *Fear of the unknown.* Feelings of uncertainty and suspense are the most common and virulent of the psychologic reactions. The expected is less traumatic than the unexpected. One can more easily deal with feelings when the factors causing them are known and recognized. Fear of what might be discovered in an exploratory surgical procedure augments the patient's anxiety. Advance warning and explanations of stress-producing situations are important for all patients, but especially for those with a low threshold for predanger anxiety.
2. *Fear of pain and discomfort.* Many patients dread pain more than the surgical procedure itself. Pain can be produced by overwhelming fear rather than by a sensation. This type of pain is sometimes indistinguishable from actual physical pain. Both are physically tiring and deleterious to bodily defenses. Although neurologic factors and the brain play a part in pain perception, the psychologic component of pain is very real. Alteration of pain perception can be achieved by attention to psychologic and spiritual needs. Perception can be influenced by circumstances, one's attitude toward health or disability, and one's ethnic or religious beliefs. Cultural differences exist in experiencing and dealing with pain.
3. *Fear of death.* In many instances this is a very valid fear. The patient who fears death in the OR runs

a greater risk of cardiac arrest on the operating table than patients with known cardiac disease. This fear should be dealt with preoperatively to determine its source.

4. *Fear of anesthesia.* Some patients fear loss of consciousness. This is closely aligned with fear of death. The patient who asks, "Will I survive the surgical procedure?" or "Who will care for my family if I die?" may really be asking, "Will I wake up?" General anesthesia invokes complete dependency on the OR team for survival.
5. *Fear of impending procedure and resultant prognosis.* A surgical procedure may be a new experience for the patient. "Will this procedure be successful and help me?" "What will the surgeon find?" "Do I have cancer?" This is a universal fear. Fear also may be caused by the trauma of a previously unpleasant surgical experience. Some patients may grieve before chemotherapy in anticipation of loss of hair. Preoccupation with risks and potential outcomes can heighten anxiety.
6. *Fear of disfigurement, mutilation, or loss of a valued body part.* Patients facing amputation of an extremity or breast, the loss of an eye, or other disfigurement abhor the thought of an incomplete body. "Will my family and society accept me or be revolted by my altered condition?" A surgical procedure on the reproductive organs also may affect self-image and sexuality. This fear provokes real suffering.
7. *Fear of isolation, rejection, neglect, abandonment.* Separation anxiety is common in the elderly, children, immature persons, and those without a family. A sense of being alone and alienated from others accentuates the realization that everyone truly lives life alone. Loved ones cannot protect us from pain, suffering, or death. No one can face uncertainties or adversity for us. Everyone experiences stress and pain personally but, in so doing, may turn to the health care personnel for protection, comfort, and warmth. A threat to one's security reawakens earlier fears of separation or abandonment. Loss of functions and fear of death may be symbolically related to separation.
8. *Fear of depersonalization and loss of self-control.* The patient fears impersonal treatment and dependence on others. Health care personnel strip the individual of identity and a sense of worth by taking away personal possessions, such as clothes, and by invading the body. As a result, the patient may feel insignificant and depersonalized. The patient must be treated with respect and dignity at all times.
9. *Fear of restriction of movement or activity.* Many patients panic when they are restrained by armboard straps or safety belts. An explanation that these are for their personal protection is reassuring. This fear may be future-oriented, such as a fear of institutionalization postoperatively or prolonged rehabilitation.
10. *Fear of invasion of privacy.* Patients must answer personal questions about their bodies and private life; give information about their families; expose their bodies to pain, instrumentation, and examination by strangers; accept help with bodily functions; and be subjected to other indignities. Adolescents and aged persons are especially self-conscious about bodily exposure. Invasive procedures, representing a bodily assault to a patient, must be carried out with minimal embarrassment to the patient.
11. *Fear of loss of livelihood.* Illness can precipitate financial crisis, especially during chronic illness or prolonged rehabilitation.
12. *Fear of burdening others.* Patients experience this fear especially during the course of a severely debilitating condition.
13. *Fear of reliance on a mechanical object or a transplanted organ.* Concern over failure of a device or rejection of an organ may become overwhelming.

Suspicion

Suspicious patients lack complete trust. They do not wholly accept what they are told or believe they have not been told everything. The patient may express a concern about the incompetency of medical personnel by asking questions such as, "Is my surgeon good?" "Am I being experimented on or victimized?" "Will they remove all of the cancer?" These patients take time to adapt because of their "on guard" reaction.

Hearing-impaired patients or those with a language barrier who feel excluded from communication may be suspicious. Allowing the hearing-impaired patient to wear a hearing aid to the OR alleviates some of the tension. An interpreter may be needed to facilitate communication to overcome a language barrier.

Guilt, Shame, Punishment

The patient may feel ashamed of an illness or may think it is a form of punishment for previous behavior or imagined wrongdoing. Invasive procedures involving body orifices may reactivate childhood fears of abuse, deprivation, or punishment that threaten self-image. Consciously, this reaction may be experienced as pain or may precede depression.

Depression

Illness fosters introspection that can depress the patient who wishes to escape an intolerable situation. Depression may be manifested by agitated signs of despair, hopelessness, disinterest, or desolation. Passive depression is characterized by a sad, frowning face or one with little expression, apathy, somatic complaints, impaired thinking and memory, retarded movement and body processes, anorexia, withdrawal from others, and neglect of appearance and body hygiene. Rather than being passive and inert, the agitated depressed person is hyperactive and talkative. Excessive depression may be detrimental to recovery and rehabilitation. This is cause for concern and requires understanding on the part of the nurse to motivate the patient toward acceptance. Depression may be associated with illness, loss of body part or function, or threat of death. Anxious patients seek a reason for their illness. They may ask the question, "Why me?"

Withdrawal

The patient may withdraw from others and from communication. This is a response to feeling that one's physical and emotional privacy has been violated. Withdrawal may accompany depression. Apathetic, detached, evasive, and silent, the patient may ignore the presence of others by feigning sleep or by turning to face the wall. The patient's actions may reveal what cannot be verbalized as a result of mistrusting staff members or of believing they lack interest. In turn, lack of feedback creates a nursing problem.

Dependency

Illness forces the patient to be dependent on others. Many patients feel inadequate because others are making decisions for them. They should be reassured that a normal degree of dependency can be beneficial in providing the rest they need. Illness, however, may provoke a desire for mothering in an overly dependent person as childhood fears resurface. A nurse may be viewed as a mother substitute. Enforced dependency of the disabled (e.g., blind persons) does not fall in this category, however. Emotionally dependent patients center attention on their own helplessness at the present moment. They are overly concerned about their bodily functions. They interpret others' behavior in terms of rejection or acceptance. These patients lack motivation to help themselves. They find peace of mind and security when relieved of making decisions or choices but need explanations related to care.

Regression

A path of least resistance that leads to inertia may accompany dependency. Patients may regress to less mature levels of behavior by crying uncontrollably, failing to respond, or being irritable. They may view staff with ambivalence (i.e., with both affection and resentment).

Denial

To protect their egos, patients may reject reality and danger, thereby reducing anxiety, maintaining stability, and controlling panic. Denial should not be mistaken for courage. Denial can be a dangerous reaction if the patient refuses to recognize a serious illness and to accept appropriate therapy. By denying concern, they repel overwhelming threats to make their difficulties more bearable. These patients divert meaningful conversation and are superoptimistic. They do not want detailed information about procedures or their risks. They block out threats and worries that they recognize they cannot control. They seek hope. Hope is a passive coping mechanism.

Anger, Hostility

Independent self-image is damaged by the passivity caused by illness. Emotional stress may be expressed verbally through open criticism of authority figures, such as physicians and nurses, or nonverbally through physical expressions, such as clenched fists or pursed lips. Patients respond to their feelings of insecurity and dependency by being aggressive and demanding in an attempt to control their environment. They are defensive in an effort to protect themselves. They may be reacting to a feeling of being assaulted or may be rebelling against enforcement of rules.

Shock

In this emotional state, the psyche provokes a sense of unreality that acts as protective insulation. The patient may respond in an automatic manner without thought or feeling or may be unable to answer questions or function coherently. This is a common reaction when a malignancy is first revealed. The immediate need is for understanding and support to face reality.

Grieving and Mourning

Feelings of loneliness, loss, and unhappiness are common with the loss of something valued or with any body disfigurement, be it from severe burns, amputation of a part, or an alteration in body structure. The patient mourns the change or may grieve over impending death caused by advanced malignancy. This reaction occurs especially in "-ostomy," or "-ectomy" patients. The intensity of responses (i.e., fatigue, depression, anxiety, altered sensorium, anger, and/or loneliness) depends on the extent and significance of the loss. Interest in life and living is regained as one's dependence on the lost object decreases. Visits by others who have gone through the same experience can help patients during the period of adjustment.

Coping With Stress Reactions

Each patient's natural inclination toward health or illness influences preoperative response and contributes to postoperative recovery. Psychologic reactions are significant factors affecting the outcome of surgical intervention. To give the patient adequate support during periods of crisis, the health care team should assess the patient's ability to cope with stress. Psychologic preparation is as important as physical preparation. Crisis intervention includes comprehensive nursing care through interactions with patient, family or significant other, and caregivers directed toward controlling crisis behavior in response to stress.

Persons assessing the patient should ascertain his or her needs and share this information with others. All patients' reactions to preoperative stress should be documented, discussed with attending physicians, and reduced by appropriate interventions. Severe or prolonged reactions require psychiatric consultation. Some stress and anxiety are a natural part of surgical patient experience. Specific responses to the stresses of surgical intervention may vary between patient populations and should not be prejudged or predetermined on the basis of race, culture, social status, educational level, or intellectual capacity.

PATIENT PERCEPTIONS OF NURSING CARE

Many factors influence the way the patient views the perioperative nurse. Studies have shown that the patient's perception is based on expectations of high-level care. The patient's belief system defines what he or she considers to be good nursing care. Perceptions of caring behaviors vary according to the degree of illness, type of procedure, level of cognition, and setting. Most patients believe that proficient and efficient perioperative nursing care includes assistance with pain control, warmth, comfort, and a peaceful environment. The nurse is also perceived as an advocate for personal safety and welfare, and a communication link between caregivers and himself or herself, family, and/or significant others.

Preoperatively, research has revealed a need for patient information about the surgical procedure, how it will be performed, and the type of anesthesia to be employed. Intraoperatively, the patient assumes a passive role, entrusting his or her care to the OR team. Before the administration of anesthesia, the patient may be acutely aware of the surroundings and activities. Patients surveyed indicate that during this segment of intraoperative care they want to know what is happening as it takes place and they desire reassurance. Patients expect the nurse to remain in close physical proximity and to provide calming conversation as appropriate. They expect the nurse to remain in the room and act promptly in the event of an emergency. The professional nurse is considered a main source of protection during this period of vulnerability.

During and after the administration of anesthesia, the patient places a strong sense of confidence in the team as a whole with expectations of competence and efficiency. While under local anesthesia, the patient continues to hold the same expectations he or she held before any drugs were given. While under general anesthesia, the patient continues to maintain a passive role, anticipating predetermined positive outcomes.

Postoperatively, the patient is more comfortable if a nurse remains nearby. The patient expects the nurse to monitor his or her condition closely and to provide pain relief as needed. In continuation of the passive role, the patient perceives the nurse as caring, protective, and efficient.

Some studies used to measure patients' opinions of nursing care reveal repetitive themes. The most often identified patient needs met by nursing interventions are:

1. Provision of privacy
2. Sensitivity to the inconvenience of hospitalization
3. Frequent family updates during the surgical procedure
4. Attention to personal and special needs
5. Friendliness
6. Accurate and understandable information about tests and treatments

FAMILY/SIGNIFICANT OTHERS

A discussion of the patient would not be complete without specific mention of the patient's family or others significant in his or her life. Illness often creates an emotional and financial burden on the family. Consequently, family members may have ambivalent feelings toward the patient because of the impact the patient's health status has on their lives. They may experience considerable anxiety over the outcomes of surgery, the feelings of isolation, and the disruption of their own lifestyles.

Families need preoperative instruction to be prepared for postoperative outcomes and rehabilitation. They also need to be kept informed of the patient's progress during the surgical procedure and recovery period. Time passes more slowly when one is waiting. Family members may fear something has gone wrong if the wait is longer than anticipated. Some family members may prefer to wait at home or at work. The surgeon should contact a spouse or significant other when the surgical procedure is over.

Structured information from the health care team may positively alter family members' psychologic responses to surgical intervention, especially for the terminally ill, permanently disabled, or disfigured patient. Fear of malignancy, risks, and complications can be overwhelming.

Consideration must be given to each patient's basic and special needs, both physiologic and psychosocial. Comprehensive care includes adequate preoperative preparation and postoperative rehabilitation for both the patient and his or her family.

Bibliography

Badger JM: Calming the anxious patient, *Am J Nurs* 94(5):46-50, 1994.

Brown M: How do you spell assessment? *Am J Nurs* 91(9):55-56, 1991.

Bryce BE: The operating theatre: strange meeting place for religion and medicine? *Br J Theatre Nurs* 27(4):18, 1990.

Carmody S et al: Perioperative needs of families, *AORN J* 54(3):561-567, 1991.

Donley R Sr: Spiritual dimensions of health care: nursing's mission, *Nurs Health Care* 12(4):178-182, 1991.

Giordano BP: Skilled perioperative care is not enough—customer service is a must, *AORN J* 57(5):1052-1054, 1993, (editorial).

Golder DJ: The power of touch, *Am J Nurs* 93(6):88, 1993.

Leino-Kilpi H, Vuorenheimo J: Perioperative nursing care quality: patients' opinions, *AORN J* 57(5):1061-1071, 1993.

Leske JS: Anxiety of elective surgical patient's family members, *AORN J* 57(5):1091-1103, 1993.

Leske JS: Effects of intraoperative progress reports on anxiety of elective surgical patient's family members, *Clin Nurs Res* 1(8):266-277, 1992.

Messner RL: What patients really want from their nurses, *Am J Nurs* 93(8):38-41, 1993.

Mitchell GJ, Copplestone C: Applying Parse's theory to perioperative nursing: a nontraditional approach, *AORN J* 51(3):787-798, 1990.

Parsons EC et al: Perioperative nurse caring behaviors: perceptions of surgical patients, *AORN J* 57(5):1106-1114, 1993.

Rothenburger RL: Transcultural nursing, *AORN J* 51(5):1349-1363, 1990.

CHAPTER 8

Patients With Special Needs

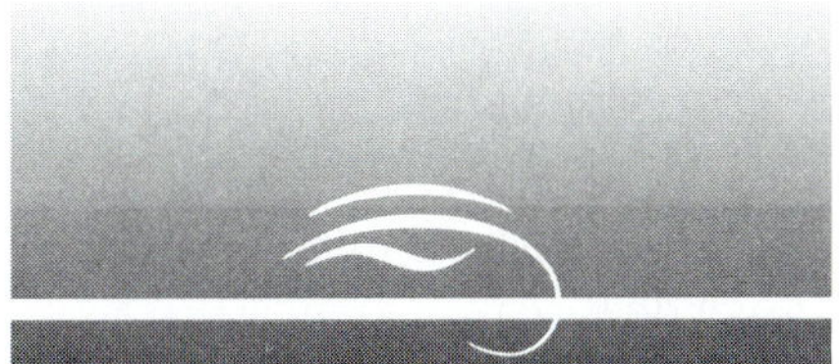

In general, the healthy body can tolerate the trauma of a surgical procedure without serious sequelae. However, the debilitated, chronically ill, or age-extreme patient has increased difficulty combating the stress of trauma to tissues and alteration of physiology from anesthetic agents. An added hazard is the patient's possible concealment from the surgeon of pertinent facts or conditions that, if uncorrected, may predispose to intraoperative complications, postoperative complications, or both.

The importance of sending each patient to the operating room (OR) in the best possible physical and emotional condition must be emphasized. Adequate rest and balanced nutrition are essential factors. Diagnostic and laboratory studies assist in establishing diagnoses and pinpointing areas of deficiencies. Surgical intervention is often postponed until a cardiovascular situation is optimized, for example, by lowering hypertension or correcting cardiac dysrhythmias. Preoperative therapy may be indicated to control diabetes, reduce obesity, or treat infection to decrease the risks of anesthesia and postoperative complications.

Patients of various ages and stages of development have different needs. Ways of meeting these will vary. A family-centered approach to care is valuable. Particularly with elderly patients, family cooperation is essential for communication with, interpretation for, and assistance with the patient.

Many patients have special needs, but space precludes mention of them all. The more common secondary problems associated with surgical intervention will be discussed. These may be encountered in patients coming to the OR for all types of surgical procedures.

AGE-EXTREME PATIENTS

Patients at the extreme ends of the life cycle (i.e., newborn infants and aged persons) present special challenges to surgeons and anesthesiologists. Operative mortality rates are higher in age-extreme patients than in the general population. The mortality rate in newborns is influenced by prematurity, birth weight, and multiplicity of congenital anomalies. Aged persons are prone to multiple organ system failure. Pediatric and geriatric patients must be adequately assessed and prepared preoperatively to minimize the risks of surgical intervention.

Pediatric Patients

Pediatric patients react differently than adults. Infants, especially premature infants, and young children are especially susceptible to the trauma of surgical procedures, physically and emotionally. Responses that are supportive and nurturing can reduce trauma and prevent complications. Accurate information with explanations geared to how the child looks at things, previews of procedures through play techniques, and as much individual care as possible during critical periods preoperatively and postoperatively are the desired protocol.

Modern pediatric surgery has opened new horizons. For example, a newborn infant with a congenital defect who formerly lived only a few days or spent a life of restricted activity now may live a normal active life. Chapter 42 details the special needs of infants and children.

Geriatric Patients

Theoretically, persons older than 65 years of age are considered elderly. However, age is not necessarily an indicator of health status. Many persons in this rapidly increasing population group maintain physical fitness and mental alertness beyond what is expected for their chronologic age. The aging process is a natural one, however. Gradually the physiologic functions of body systems and organs change. Each geriatric patient must be assessed individually for current health status and risk factors.

Surgical risks in geriatric patients are complex, but age alone is not a contraindication. Risks can be attributed to physiologic and psychosocial factors, multiple pathologic conditions, and advanced stages of diseases. Chronic diseases are stabilized to the extent possible before elective surgery. The surgeon, patient, and family should evaluate carefully the potential quality of life postoperatively in considering the necessity for or value of a surgical procedure. Changes in physiologic functioning and adaptability as a result of the aging process potentiate complications. Geriatric patients are prone to infection, poor wound healing, and cardiovascular problems. Chapter 43 details the special needs of geriatric patients.

DISABLED PERSONS

Many persons come to the OR with disabilities unrelated to surgical pathologic conditions. These handicaps influence preoperative anxiety, intraoperative nursing care, and postoperative recovery. Patients, their families, and health care team members should adapt to meet the physical and psychosocial needs of disabled persons, who have the right to be treated with respect and dignity.

Communication is essential to assess needs adequately and to care for these patients. Team members should know about and understand the patient's limitations. The patient has a right to know what will happen during the surgical experience and to participate in decisions about his or her care. The Rehabilitation Act of 1973 states that for an agency to receive federal funds it "must provide, when necessary, appropriate auxiliary aids...to people with impaired sensory, manual or speaking skills to give them an equal opportunity to benefit from services." The complexities of each patient's situation should be evaluated and dealt with appropriately.

Language Barrier

Although not a physical or mental disability, a language barrier can be a psychologic handicap. Anxiety increases in proportion to one's inability to communicate in a stress-producing situation. The inability to understand or to express oneself verbally is frustrating; the patient's behavior may reflect his or her feelings of inadequacy or insecurity. Nonverbal body language through eye contact, pleasant facial expressions, and a gentle touch can comfort the patient who does not speak your language. However, the problem remains unresolved. Every effort should be made to obtain an interpreter to assist the patient and the health care team. Many hospitals employ the services of interpreters for the ethnic groups within the community. Some patients are reluctant to share confidential medical information with a relative or friend. The interpreter should be trusted and accepted by the patient and should be sensitive to the needs of the surgeon and caregivers. The patient must be adequately informed to give consent for a surgical procedure.

Hearing Impairment/Deafness

Hearing impairment varies from inner ear changes that occur during the aging process and affect the distinction of some high-frequency consonant sounds in the geriatric patient to the congenital profound deafness of a newborn. Conductive or sensorineural deafness may result from disease or injury to the ear at any age. The degree of impairment will determine whether the patient communicates through sign language, has a hearing aid, and/or reads lips. Written information is always helpful. An interpreter can assist with the deaf patient who uses sign language.

To communicate with a patient whose hearing impairment is severe enough to make conversation difficult, the room should be quiet and well lit, with minimal distractions. Look directly at the patient. Speak clearly and slowly in a moderate tone of voice, with visible but not exaggerated lip movements. Facial expression, touch, and body gestures can help communicate feelings and instructions.

Allow the patient to wear a hearing aid to the OR. Greet the patient without wearing a face mask. Attract the patient's attention before speaking. Be sure the patient understands and responds appropriately to questions. To help explain your actions, show the patient any equipment (e.g., a safety strap) before placing it on him or her.

Visual Impairment/Blindness

Like deafness, blindness can be a part of the aging process or a congenital anomaly. Cataracts, a frequent cause of loss of visual acuity, may be inherited, but more commonly they are associated with aging. The shape of the eye and other structural factors, as well as diseases and injuries, affect sight.

The blind patient feels insecure in a strange environment. Address the patient by name and introduce yourself. A gentle word followed by a gentle touch can comfort the patient. Always speak to the patient before touching him or her. Raising your voice is inappropriate, however. The blind patient is not necessarily deaf. The patient should be told what is to happen around him or her to avoid a distressful reaction to unexpected noises or sensations. Guiding the patient's hand will help him or her feel secure, such as when he or she is being moved onto the operating table.

A visually impaired patient should be permitted to wear eyeglasses to the OR. The glasses should be sent to the postanesthesia care unit (PACU) so that they are available when the patient wakes up. Sight helps orient the patient to his or her environment. However, contact lenses must be removed before administration of a general anesthetic because they may dry on the cornea or become dislodged.

Physical Disability

The physical needs of disabled persons are as varied as their disabilities. A complete assessment is imperative to prepare adequately for the individual's care. Physical disabilities may make positioning the patient on the operating table difficult. Extra personnel, supports, and positioning aids may be required and additional assistance may be needed to move the patient safely.

Millions of people suffer from some form of arthritis. Children with juvenile rheumatoid arthritis have many systemic problems as a result of the disease process, which continues into adulthood. The onset of this autoimmune disease can occur at any age and can result in stiffness, swelling, and deformity of the joints of the hands, feet, and neck; inflammation of blood vessels; and tissue damage to organ systems. Joints need good support. Long-term treatment with nonsteroidal antiinflammatory drugs or corticosteroid therapy may affect bleeding intraoperatively.

Paralyzed patients, such as persons with spinal cord injury, are unable to move. Patients with involuntary muscle control, such as persons with cerebral palsy, must be protected from falls or injuries during transport or transfer. These patients have decreased sensitivity to heat and cold, so they must be protected from burns or hypothermia.

Physically disabled persons and their families need acceptance and thoughtful care from team members who need to remember that these persons are mentally competent and aware of their surroundings.

Mental Incompetency

Cognitive functions are based on intelligence and the ability to think, learn, remember, and solve problems. These functions are associated with adaptive behavior. Impairment can run the gamut from the educable person who becomes independent as an adult to the severely retarded child or dysfunctional adult who has minimal capacity for independent functioning. Retardation may be congenital; more often, however, mental incompetence develops as a result of brain injury, systemic illness, or senile dementia. A normal infant, for example, can be injured during the birth process or become impaired after a high fever. Hypoxia resulting in inadequate oxygenation to brain cells can cause mental dysfunction, which may be transient or permanent.

The physical needs of these patients must be met. At the same time, their right to dignity and privacy should be protected, such as during positioning, prepping, and draping procedures. Verbal communication should be attempted at the patient's level of understanding and response. Vocal tones and inflections, facial gestures, and body language may be understood by the cognitively impaired patient who is unable to verbalize. This patient needs guidance to adapt to the environment in an effort to conserve energy and retain personal integrity.

NUTRITIONAL NEEDS

Nutrition refers to the sum of the processes concerned in the growth, maintenance, and repair of the body as a whole or its constituent parts. Decreased intake and increased metabolic demands create nutritional problems in surgical patients.

Malnutrition

Perhaps as many as 50% of hospitalized patients are malnourished to some degree. *Malnutrition* in the surgical patient is caused by inadequate intake or use of calories and protein preoperatively and/or postoperatively. This creates a state of impaired functional ability and structural integrity because of a discrepancy between the intake of essential nutrients and the body's demand for them. As a result of malnutrition, the patient may have:

1. Poor tolerance of anesthetic agents
   a. Decreased metabolism of agents by liver
   b. Inadequate excretion of toxins by kidneys
2. Failure of blood-clotting mechanisms
3. Negative nitrogen balance with a serum albumin less than 3 g/dl and blood urea nitrogen (BUN) less than 10 g/dl
4. Altered wound healing potential
   a. Decreased protein synthesis following elective surgery
   b. Increased protein synthesis and breakdown of skeletal muscle following severe traumatic injury
5. Sequential multiple organ failure
   a. Preexisting dysfunction, such as abnormalities in glucose homeostasis associated with liver disease
   b. Following trauma

6. Decreased serum electrolytes associated with anorexia, bulimia, alcoholism, and other chronic metabolic disturbances
   a. Hypokalemia (low potassium level)
   b. Hypomagnesemia (low magnesium level)
   c. Hypocalcemia (low calcium level)
7. Increased susceptibility to infection from immunologic incompetence with a total lymphocyte count less than 1500/mm
8. Increased risk of morbidity and mortality

Biochemical tests help determine nutritional status. These include proteins, albumin/globulin determination and ratio, and blood urea nitrogen (BUN) level. Body weight is significant also. If caloric intake is inadequate, protein is converted into carbohydrate for energy. Protein synthesis then suffers.

The average adult patient needs about 1500 calories daily to spare body protein. Hypermetabolic states can double that requirement to 3000 calories and 18 to 19 g of nitrogen for nitrogen retention if liver function is normal. Depleted reserves of essential elements must be replenished to replace tissue loss and expedite wound healing. Protein deficiency impairs collagen formation, thereby delaying the healing process. Vitamins K, A, and C are also important. The application of principles of aseptic technique, gentle handling of tissues, and physiologic support are preeminent in all surgical patients, but they are not enough for patients with *protein calorie malnutrition.* The surgeon is justifiably concerned about the patient's nutritional status because malnutrition lowers host resistance by impairing lymphocyte and neutrophil functioning. A definite relationship has been demonstrated between hypoproteinemia and terminal postoperative infection.

Metabolism

Metabolism is the phenomenon of synthesizing foodstuffs into complex elements and complex substances into simple ones in the production of energy. It involves two opposing phases:

1. *Anabolism,* or constructive metabolism, the conversion of nutritive material into complex living matter—tissue construction
2. *Catabolism,* or destructive metabolism, the breaking down or dissolution by the body of complex compounds, often with the release of energy

Metabolic disorders and the stress response of traumatic injury can complicate the outcome of surgical intervention. Dietary deficiencies disturb the body's nutritional homeostasis and may markedly alter a patient's nutritional status and needs. Hormonal response to physical stress involves both anabolic and catabolic effects on the body with catabolism predominant. The degree of metabolic reaction may depend greatly on the body's reserve of labile protein. The type and extent of the surgical procedure, the preoperative nutritional state, and the effect of the surgical procedure on the patient's ability to digest and absorb nutrients affect immediate postoperative metabolism.

Biochemical changes accompany surgical intervention. One of the major ones is *protein catabolism.* Limited food intake preoperatively, catharsis, and adrenocortical response to crisis augment a catabolic response. Trauma and blood loss also have a contributory effect. Metabolic disease, dehydration, and fever increase one's need for calories and nutritional substances. This is also true in patients with severe burns, infection, or toxemia in which essential nutrients such as nitrogen are lost. Abnormalities of the gastrointestinal tract and digestive organs may produce malnutrition through incomplete digestion, absorption, or excretion of nutrients. Digestion and absorption are also affected by deviations in digestive secretions, timing of passage through the gastrointestinal tract, and stomach capacity.

Electrolyte and metabolic disturbances other than protein catabolism may accompany surgical intervention and lead to imbalance. Changes in fluid and electrolyte balance affect kidney function, cellular metabolism, and oxygen concentration in circulation. Tissue hydration and distribution of body electrolytes are essential to postoperative recovery.

Drugs also can have an adverse affect on metabolic balance. Broad-spectrum antibiotics, while limiting a disease process, can, in association with dietary inadequacy, cause vitamin K deficiency in older patients by inhibiting the intestinal bacteria that produce that vitamin. Drug detoxification and/or excretion may be altered in patients with kidney or liver damage, leading to possible drug overdose. Metabolism is altered by immunosuppressive drugs and antimetabolites that interfere with nutritional function. Corticosteroids may increase susceptibility to infection and loss of muscle protein. Diuretics and laxatives, often taken without medical supervision, can cause loss of electrolytes with resultant acid-base imbalances.

Nutritional Supplements

Adequate essential nutrients at the cellular level are crucial. Therefore, by dietary management, physicians aim to correct metabolic and nutritional abnormalities before the surgical procedure. In some patients special nutritional supplements are indicated to build up or compensate for a permanent metabolic handicap. Successful therapy is indicated by weight gain, a rise in plasma albumin, and a positive nitrogen balance. A chemically defined elemental diet may be administered via:

1. Oral intake.
2. Nasogastric tube.

3. Gastrostomy tube, with or without constant infusion pump.
4. Intravenous (IV) infusion of protein and dextrose through a peripheral vein. Isotonic fat emulsions also can be administered by this route.
5. Central venous cannulation for hyperalimentation.

Hyperalimentation (Total Parenteral Nutrition [TPN])

Parenteral hyperalimentation is another method of fulfilling nutritional requirements. Essential nutrients are delivered directly into the bloodstream intravenously via an indwelling catheter. This mode of therapy is used for patients with nutritional defects not amenable to oral therapy or nasogastric intubation or those who fail to gain weight by other means. Intravenous infusion by peripheral vein is precluded in some patients because the amount of fluid necessary to supply the adequate calories and nitrogen would exceed the body's fluid tolerance, leading to pulmonary edema and congestive heart failure. For these select patients and for those requiring long-term intravenous therapy, hyperalimentation provides the daily nutrition necessary for protein synthesis.

Hyperalimentation is coordinated with other therapy to establish an adequate nutrition, fluid, and electrolyte balance. Increasing protein nourishment in the preoperative and postoperative periods lessens protein loss and destruction of cell nuclei, skeletal muscle, and connective tissue. It also counteracts the increased catabolism resulting from the stress of surgical intervention. The therapy is beneficial to select patients but is not without danger or complications.

Basic Solution To provide 2500 to 3000 calories daily in small volume, a concentrated hypertonic solution is administered. It usually consists of glucose and fat emulsions to provide calories and amino acids for protein synthesis. The physician orders the solution contents for each patient. Specific serum electrolyte needs determine the essential elements, vitamins, and minerals to be included.

Solutions are prepared in the pharmacy with strict aseptic technique under a laminar airflow hood. The solution is a medium for bacterial and fungal growth, so it must be stored at 4° C (39° F) until used. It is warmed to room temperature before administration and may hang for no more than 12 hours if it is a casein protein hydrolysate solution and no longer than 24 hours if it is an essential amino acid solution.

NOTE

1. Commercial TPN solutions are available. If used, they are modified to meet individual needs. Mixing of additives poses a risk of sepsis.
2. Inspect the admixture for precipitates before and during use. A cloudy solution or one with floating particles should not be used.

Central Venous Cannulation A large-diameter vein in a region of high blood flow must be selected to instantly dilute the irritating hypertonic solution, which has high osmolarity, to prevent thrombus or vein occlusion at the introduction site. A long-term indwelling catheter is inserted through the internal or external jugular, cephalic, or subclavian vein into the superior vena cava or right atrium. Either a single-lumen Broviac, Hickman, Groshong, or other central venous catheter or a double-lumen catheter is used. These catheters are polymeric silicone with a polyester fiber cuff. Under C-arm fluoroscopy, the tip of the catheter is threaded into the vein through a venotomy to the desired position. The distal (external) end is brought through a subcutaneous tunnel with an exit point in the anterior chest wall, usually between the right nipple and the sternum. A Dacron cuff anchors the catheter in the tunnel. The *Broviac catheter* is slightly smaller (1 mm inside diameter) than the Hickman catheter (1.6 mm inside diameter). Therefore the *Hickman catheter* may be used intermittently for infusion of pharmacologic or chemotherapeutic agents, antibiotics, and/or blood products or for withdrawal of blood samples. A double-lumen catheter affords advantages of both: the Broviac port is used for continuous TPN and the Hickman port for other needs.

Infusion Rate A constant infusion rate of the prescribed solution is calculated on the basis of the amount of fluids ordered for a 24-hour period. Slow administration is necessary because bypassing the regulatory mechanism in the gastrointestinal tract and liver places an increased burden of elimination on the cells and kidneys. The flow rate must be maintained as ordered. An overload of hypertonic solution can cause massive dehydration of body cells and heart failure. The solution should not be infused more rapidly than it can be metabolized or hyperglycemia can result. Insulin may then be prescribed. Hypoglycemia may develop from too slow an infusion rate. A decreased flow rate may result from a plugged filter or change in body position. *Constant monitoring is necessary.* The flow rate and patency of the infusion system should be checked every 30 minutes. A filter should be used during infusion of TPN solutions.

Hyperalimentation solutions are usually viscous. A positive pressure pump device may be needed to ensure infusion. Volume may also need to be regulated over a specified time with a volumetric control device. An infusion pump may be implanted subcutaneously for long-term hyperalimentation to deliver fluid automatically at a preselected flow rate. This device attaches to the central venous catheter.

Precautions Maintenance of a closed intravenous system with minimal catheter manipulation is important. Any leaks in external tubing can permit sucking of air into the system during the patient's respiratory inspiration. This can result in air embolus. All connections in the setup should be taped to prevent accidental separation. The patient is instructed not to touch the insertion site and to report any discomfort.

Strict asepsis for catheter insertion, maintenance, and infusion is mandatory. The technique itself introduces a foreign body and exposes the circulation to a potentially dangerous external environment at a time when the patient can least afford complications. Possibility of sepsis is the greatest deterrent to hyperalimentation therapy. Conscientious care is obligatory.

NOTE Every time the line is entered there is risk of contamination. Therefore the parenteral alimentation line should be used *only* for the delivery of nutrition. It should not be used for piggyback intravenous setups as for administration of blood constituents, medications, central venous pressure monitoring, or blood drawing for laboratory analysis. A multilumen catheter may be inserted for these purposes.

Hyperalimentation therapy is discontinued gradually to permit adjustment to a lowered glucose level. Rebound hypoglycemia must be guarded against.

Other Considerations Hyperalimentation therapy is not a contraindication to ambulation. Long-term parenteral hyperalimentation can be accomplished at home with adequate professional instruction, supervision, assistance, and unyielding observance of strict aseptic technique. This therapy is not without risks, however.

PATIENTS WITH DIABETES

Diabetes mellitus is an endocrine disorder affecting glucose tolerance in the body and the production of insulin in the pancreas. Insulin is a hormone that helps break down sugar and carbohydrates. Usually genetic in origin, diabetes mellitus can be triggered in predisposed individuals by environmental stress. Management of the diabetic surgical patient will depend on the type and control of the disorder.

1. *Type I:* Insulin-dependent diabetes mellitus (IDDM). The pancreas produces little or no insulin, thus necessitating regular administration of insulin by injection, infusion, or orally. Onset may be at any age but usually occurs in juveniles (adolescents aged 12 to 16) and adults up to age 40.
2. *Type II:* Noninsulin-dependent diabetes mellitus (NIDDM). The pancreas produces varying amounts of insulin. Onset may be at any age but usually occurs after age 40 in obese persons.
3. Diabetes mellitus associated with other conditions or syndromes. Impaired glucose tolerance may be secondary to pancreatic or hormonal disease, drug or chemical toxicity, abnormal insulin receptors, or other genetic syndromes. Diabetes may be latent, asymptomatic, or borderline.

Stresses caused by physical and emotional trauma, infection, or fever raise the blood sugar level. Stress stimulates the pituitary and adrenal glands. The pituitary gland secretes an *adrenocorticotrophic hormone (ACTH),* which stimulates the production of glucocorticoids. These in turn increase *gluconeogenesis,* the formation of glucose by the liver from noncarbohydrate sources. The resultant extra glucose enters the bloodstream. Coincidentally, the adrenal glands secrete epinephrine, which accelerates the conversion of glycogen in the liver to glucose and also raises the level of blood sugar. More insulin is needed. The primary goal of diabetic control is to maintain a stable internal environment, thereby averting a metabolic crisis. Extreme care must be taken to prevent the following:

1. Hyperglycemia and ketonuria
   a. Rise in blood glucose and ketones can precipitate severe fluid loss, causing dehydration and hyperkalemia from release of potassium from cells.
   b. Some medications (e.g., cortisone) increase blood sugar level and antagonize the effect of insulin.
2. Ketoacidosis and acetonuria
   a. These are caused by insulin insufficiency from natural causes, or reduced or omitted insulin dosage.
   b. If allowed to progress untreated, they may result in coma and ultimately death.
3. Hypoglycemia and hypoglycemic shock
   a. These are caused by too much insulin.
   b. They are of faster onset than ketoacidosis.
   c. Hypoglycemia is especially dangerous. It can occur during major surgical procedures because of omission or delay of oral intake.
   d. These can cause brain damage and stress on the cardiovascular system.

Prevention of these states depends on:

1. Physician's treatment of choice for diabetes
2. Severity and type of disorder
3. Existence of complicating conditions
4. Type of surgical procedure

Preoperative preparation includes laboratory testing, including fasting and postprandial blood sugar determination, urinalysis for sugar and acetone, complete blood count, BUN, and serum electrolyte determinations. A chest x-ray film and electrocardiogram are also advisable.

Common Complications of Diabetes

Surgical intervention upsets the normal regimen of caloric intake and insulin or oral hypoglycemic agents. Anesthesia and reduced activity postoperatively also have disruptive effects. These factors can increase blood glucose and free fatty acids (hyperlipemia) and decrease serum insulin levels. Patients with NIDDM usually withstand surgical intervention without crisis. Intraoperative metabolic control is more difficult in patients with IDDM who have marked unpredictability and greater extremes in blood sugar levels. Lengthy major surgical procedures with extensive tissue trauma present the greatest challenge to regulation. Diabetic patients are prone to:

1. Dehydration and electrolyte imbalance.
2. Infection.
3. Inadequate circulation from vascular disease, causing deficient tissue perfusion. Hyperlipemia affects both coronary and peripheral arteries. Peripheral edema can lead to gangrene.
4. Delayed wound healing as a result of increased protein breakdown or compromised circulation because of obesity. Glycogenesis, the breakdown of glycogen to glucose in the liver, diverts protein from tissue regeneration.
5. Neuropathy or nervous system disorder causing motor and sensory dysfunctions, including cardiopulmonary arrest.
6. Nephropathy, affecting small blood vessels in kidneys.
7. Retinopathy, affecting small vessels in eyes, and blindness.
8. Neuropathic skeletal disease. Severe bone destruction may cause neuropathic fractures.
9. Neurogenic bladder causing incontinence. Urinary tract infections are common.
10. Postoperative blood glucose control may be a problem, especially if the patient remains under stress because of a diagnosis that requires changes in lifestyle or body image.

Diabetes causes many bodily changes that increase in frequency with duration of the disease. Physiologic dysfunctions, as listed in Table 8-1, make the diabetic person a potentially high-risk patient.

Special Considerations

Diabetic patients may come to the OR for implantation of a computerized insulin pump beneath the skin of the abdomen or for pancreatic islet cell transplantation to help control diabetes; for disorders associated with complications of diabetes, such as a gangrenous extremity; for a pathologic condition such as biliary disease; or for any other condition necessitating surgery. Scheduling elective surgical procedures early in the day minimizes the period during which oral intake is restricted. Other special precautions need to be taken in the care of the diabetic surgical patient to minimize the potential risks.

1. Capillary blood for fasting serum glucose test should be obtained preoperatively before induction of anesthesia. The results provide baseline data to assess postoperative control.
2. Preoperative insulin dose may be reduced or eliminated to guard against hypoglycemia or insulin shock during the surgical procedure.
3. Preoperative medication may be reduced by 25% to 50% of a normal dosage. Narcotics may cause vomiting, which predisposes to fluid and electrolyte imbalance. This can precipitate a hypoglycemic reaction from a decreased need for insulin. Adequate glucose is essential to central nervous system function.
4. Continuous intravenous access is vital throughout the surgical procedure in case of a metabolic problem. An infusion of dextrose in water may be started to begin administration of daily carbohydrate requirement before the patient comes to the operating room.
   a. Optional methods of management for insulin-dependent patients are determined by the severity of the disease, preoperative control regimen, and type of surgical procedure. Insulin may be added to the infusion or administered by subcutaneous injection. Amounts are determined by serum glucose levels.
   b. Adequate hydration must be maintained because a rising blood glucose level upsets osmotic equilibrium. Electrolytes may be added to maintain metabolic status.
   c. Fluid intake and output must be monitored to maintain hydration without fluid overload.
5. Metabolic crisis in an unconscious patient is difficult to detect. Therefore, during long surgical procedures, blood glucose levels are monitored for hyperglycemia or hypoglycemia and fractional urine specimens are monitored for ketones. Glucometers accurately measure blood glucose levels. Monitoring is necessary to ascertain the patient's requirements for insulin, glucose, or both.
6. Nasogastric suction may cause acidosis, dehydration, or electrolyte imbalance.
7. Antiembolic stockings usually are worn by the patient during the surgical procedure and postoperatively as a precaution against thrombophlebitis and thromboembolism.
8. Skin integrity must be guarded to avoid sepsis.
   a. Strict aseptic and sterile techniques are extremely important to the infection-prone diabetic patient.
   b. An air, water, or gel mattress should be placed on the operating table for surgical procedures expected to take more than 3 hours to protect

TABLE 8-1

Physiologic Dysfunctions in High-Risk Patients

DIABETES MELLITUS	OBESITY
Integumentary system	
Skin may be dry, itchy	Hirsutism in women
Loss of fat from adipose tissue	Excess subcuticular fat
Injuries heal slowly	Injuries heal slowly
Musculoskeletal system	
Neuropathic skeletal disease with bone destruction	Osteoarthritis
Leg pain, neuropathy	Chronic back pain
Muscular wasting	Strain on joints and ligaments
	Joint pain
	Diminished mobility
Cardiovascular system	
Increased heart rate	Myocardial hypertrophy
Predisposed to coronary artery disease	High blood pressure
Predisposed to thrombophlebitis	Arteriosclerosis
Peripheral edema	Venous stasis
	Varicose veins
Respiratory system	
Predisposed to infection	Shortness of breath
	Decreased tidal volume
	Decrease in lung expansion
Renal system	
Nephropathy	Vascular changes in kidneys
Increased excretion	
Neurogenic bladder	
Gastrointestinal system	
Secretion of glucose by liver	Less intestinal mobility
	Predisposed to liver and biliary disease
Neurologic system	
Neuropathy	
Sensory system	
Retinopathy and blindness	
Endocrine system	
Insulin production poor or nonexistent	Predisposed to diabetes mellitus
Poor metabolic control	Pituitary abnormalities
Adrenal glands increase production of cortisol under stress	Poor metabolic control
Electrolyte imbalance	Dysfunctional uterine bleeding

bony prominences and to prevent pressure sores.

c. Hyposensitive tape is used to affix dressings.

OBESE PATIENTS

Obesity is prevalent in our society. It may be of:

1. *Endocrine origin:* Usually associated with biliary, hepatic, or endocrine disease.
2. *Nonendocrine origin:* Usually associated with excessive caloric intake. It is referred to as *morbid obesity* when weight exceeds 100 lb (45.4 kg) over the ideal weight for one's height.

Common Complications of Obesity

Surgical patients who are 10% or more overweight have an increased incidence of morbidity and mortality caused by concomitant systemic diseases and physical problems. The degree of morbidity varies with the severity of the obese condition. Refer to physiologic dysfunctions in Table 8-1. Obesity predisposes to:

1. Increased demand on the heart. Pulse rate, cardiac output, stroke volume, and blood volume increase to meet the metabolic demands of the adipose tissue (fat). Eventually this overload leads to myocardial hypertrophy (enlargement of the heart). Congestive heart failure may ensue. Coronary artery disease is also common.
2. Hypertension (high blood pressure). Vascular changes in the kidneys, associated with hypertension, affect elimination of protein wastes and maintenance of fluid and electrolyte balance.
3. Varicose veins and edema in the lower extremities. Poor venous return results from pressure on pelvic veins and the vena cava. Venous stasis can ultimately contribute to thrombophlebitis and thromboembolism.
4. Pulmonary function abnormalities. Hypoxemia, inadequate oxygen in blood, may be associated with decreased tidal volume or poor gaseous exchange caused by excessive weight on the thoracic cavity. Patients are susceptible to pulmonary infection and pulmonary embolism postoperatively.
5. Diseases of the digestive system, such as liver or gallbladder disease.
6. Osteoarthritis. This may limit mobility of spine and joints.
7. Diabetes mellitus.
8. Malnutrition. Even though the patient is overweight, the obese patient may have a protein deficiency or other metabolic disturbance such as hyperlipidemia.

Special Considerations

The physical size of obese persons presents problems for the OR and PACU teams. Safety precautions against injury, falls, and burns must be emphasized. Problems include the following:

1. Transporting and lifting the patient. Mechanical patient lifters are desirable. If these are not available, extra persons are needed to ensure safety in lifting.
   a. Tables and stretchers must be stabilized.
   b. In moving the patient from stretcher to operating table, lock the wheels, suggest that the patient feel for the far side of the table, so that he or she does not move too far and fall. Additional personnel should stand at the opposite side of the table to prevent falls.
2. Obese patients are frequently self-conscious; keep exposure to a minimum.
3. Induction, intubation, and maintenance of anesthesia.
   a. Venous cutdown may be necessary to establish an IV line if peripheral veins are invisible.
   b. Mobility of the cervical spine to hyperextend the neck for intubation may be limited.
   c. Inefficient respiratory muscles, poor lung/chest wall compliance, and/or increased intraabdominal pressure in the supine position reduce ventilation capability.
   d. Lower concentrations of gases entering the lungs, caused by inefficient ventilation, prolongs induction time.
   e. Continuous uptake by adipose tissue requires higher concentrations of anesthetic agents to maintain anesthesia. Drug dosages must be calculated by body weight.
   f. Recovery period may be prolonged because adipose tissue retains fat-soluble agents and the poor blood supply in this tissue eliminates agents slowly.
4. Positioning on the operating table.
   a. Extra personnel may be necessary to assist.
   b. Massive tissue and pressure areas must be protected. Protuberances must be padded to prevent bruising and pressure injuries.
   c. Ventilation and circulation must be ensured.
   d. Electrosurgical unit patient dispersive electrode must not be surrounded by overlapping skin folds because tissue could be burned.
5. Mechanics of the surgical procedure may lengthen operating time.
   a. Accessibility of deep organs such as the gallbladder may be a problem.
   b. Large instrumentation may contribute to surgical trauma and postoperative pain.
6. Thromboembolic complications may occur because of venous stasis; erythrocytosis, which increases the viscosity of the blood; and a decrease in fibrinolytic activity. Anticoagulants may be given prophylactically.
7. Healing may be delayed because of poor vascularity of adipose tissue. Obese patients have an increased incidence of postoperative wound infection and disruption.
   a. A sterile closed drainage system is often used to drain accumulated fluid, thereby facilitating healing.
   b. It is harder to eliminate "dead space" in wound closure.

CHRONIC CARDIOPULMONARY ILLNESSES

Many patients come to the OR for surgical procedures unrelated to a chronic cardiopulmonary or pulmonary disease. These conditions, however, may present high risk for physiologic complications. (See section on complications under anesthesia in Chapter 19, pp. 378-395.)

Cardiovascular Disease

The surgeon is particularly concerned about hemostasis and potential for hemorrhage in a patient who is taking anticoagulant medication to treat or prevent thrombophlebitis or thromboembolism. A patient who takes aspirin prophylactically is instructed to discontinue its use for 3 weeks preoperatively.

The anesthesiologist must regulate the medications of a patient with labile (unstable) blood pressure. Blood pressure also is monitored and maintained with appropriate drugs (see intravenous cardiovascular drugs in Chapter 19, pp. 395-399) in a patient with history of hypertension or hypotension. Tissue perfusion and oxygenation are critical to wound healing.

Pulmonary Disease

Any chronic condition that compromises pulmonary function presents a potential risk for a patient undergoing general inhalation anesthesia. Bronchoconstriction, edema, and excess mucus production cause uneven airway narrowing, creating a ventilation/perfusion mismatch. Severe hypoxemia, an abnormal deficiency of oxygen in arterial blood, can trigger life-threatening dysrhythmias and respiratory failure.

Adequate ventilation is difficult in patients with asthma, chronic bronchitis, and pulmonary emphysema. Chronic obstructive pulmonary disease (COPD), which includes these conditions, is characterized by diminished inspiratory and expiratory capacity of the lungs. It is aggravated by cigarette smoking and air pollution. Smokers are advised to stop smoking at least 3 weeks preoperatively. They should be taught to use a spirometer and to practice deep breathing and coughing exercises that will be helpful postoperatively. Mechanical ventilation with a respirator or intermittent positive pressure breathing (IPPB) apparatus may be necessary postoperatively to assist or control respiration. Patients who have trouble breathing are usually highly anxious and need emotional support.

PREGNANT SURGICAL PATIENTS

The pregnant surgical patient who is brought to the OR for reasons other than childbirth presents a unique challenge to the OR team. The plan of care must include consideration for two patients; the mother and her developing fetus. The effects of surgical intervention can be disastrous to a pregnancy, but in some situations it is necessary to save the mother and/or the fetus.

The average gestation, duration of pregnancy, is 38 to 40 weeks or 9 calendar months. This gestation period is divided into trimesters, 3-month segments (Box 8-1). Maternal anatomic and physiologic changes occur during each trimester of pregnancy (Table 8-2). Modifications of the plan of care vary according to these changes. Risks associated with surgical intervention may be specific to the fetus. During the first trimester spontaneous abortion of the developing embryo (until the end of the eighth week) or fetus (from the eighth week) can occur. Preterm labor and/or delivery may be precipitated during the second and third trimesters. The surgeon and anesthesiologist should discuss the risks, benefits, and potential outcome with the patient and her family.

Surgical procedures on pregnant patients are usually performed for an urgent or emergent reason such as incompetent cervix, ectopic pregnancy, cholecystitis, ap-

BOX 8-1

Glossary of Terms Associated With Pregnancy

abortion Spontaneous or induced termination of pregnancy before 20 weeks' gestation of fetus weighing less than 500 g and having crown-to-rump length less than 16.5 cm.

cesarean section Delivery of infant by surgical incision through maternal abdominal and uterine walls.

ectopic pregnancy Nonviable fertilized ovum implanted outside uterine cavity.

embryo Stage of development from implantation of fertilized ovum to 8th week of intrauterine life.

fetus Stage of development from 8th week of intrauterine life to birth.

gestation Period from fertilization of ovum to birth. Average gestation in humans is 266 days (9 calendar months or 38 to 40 weeks).

- **preterm/premature gestation** Pregnancy less than 37 weeks' duration.
- **postterm/postmature gestation** Pregnancy more than 42 weeks' duration.

gravid Carrying a fetus.

gravida Term expressed in numeric form in combination with para (see **para**) to describe number of pregnancies a woman has experienced regardless of duration of gestation or fetal viability (e.g., first pregnancy is Gravida 1 Para 0 [G1P0]; after birth of infant, this is expressed as Gravida 1 Para 1 [G1P1]). Abortion is counted as a pregnancy.

- **primagravida** Woman carrying first pregnancy.
- **multigravida** Woman currently pregnant who has been pregnant before.

neonate Infant in first 28 days of extrauterine life.

organogenesis Differentiation of cells into embryonic organs between 2nd and 8th week of intrauterine life.

para Term expressed in numeric form in combination with gravida (see **gravida**) that indicates how many pregnancies were carried more than 20 weeks' gestation regardless of live birth, stillborn, abortion, or multiple offspring (e.g., first pregnancy resulting in twin infants is Gravida 1 Para 1 [G1P1]; a second pregnancy resulting in stillbirth is Gravida 2 Para 2 [G2P2]).

parturition Process of giving birth.

teratogen Any substance, agent, or process that can cause abnormalities of form or function in exposed fetus. Developing embryo is especially vulnerable to teratogens during first trimester. Known teratogens include ionizing radiation, particularly x-rays; infectious microorganisms, especially *Treponema pallidum* spirochete (syphilis); and chemical agents and drugs, including alcohol and *some* antibiotics, antineoplastic agents, anticoagulants, anticonvulsants, hormones, diuretics, tobacco, and anesthetic agents. Medication should not be taken during pregnancy unless prescribed by physician.

trimester Unit of measurement that divides pregnancy into three segments of approximately 3 months' duration each.

- **first trimester** First day of last menstrual period to end of 12 weeks.
- **second trimester** End of 12th week to beginning of 28th week.
- **third trimester** Beginning of 28th week to birth.

viable Description of neonate who is at least 24 weeks' gestation, weighs 500 g, and is capable of sustaining independent life outside uterus.

zygote Ovum after fertilization until implantation.

TABLE 8-2

Maternal Anatomic and Physiologic Changes of Pregnancy

SYSTEM	FIRST TRIMESTER (1-3 MO GESTATION [1-12 WK])	SECOND TRIMESTER (4-7 MO GESTATION [13-27 WK])	THIRD TRIMESTER (7-9 MO GESTATION [28-38 TO 40 WK])
Cardiovascular	Cardiac output begins to increase at 6th wk. Plasma volume begins to increase.	Cardiac output increased 30%-50% by 16th wk. Plasma volume continues to increase. Hypervolemic and hemodiluted.	Cardiac output decreases slightly by 30th week. Plasma volume increase peaks 50% at 32-36 wk.
		RBC production increases 20%. WBC increases 30%-40%.	RBC increases, peaks at 33%.
	Breast veins dilate. Vasculature increases to vulva and vagina.	Capillary engorgement can cause epistaxis (nosebleeds) and epulis (bleeding gums).	May develop hemorrhoids and varicosities in leg veins. Increased risk for venous thrombosis.
		Heart rate increases 15-20 beats/min.	Factors VII, IX, X increase causes hypercoagulative state. Plasma fibrinogen increases 40%-50%.
		Slight hypotension caused by decreased peripheral vascular resistance.	Normotensive by 26th wk.
		Uterus presses on vena cava when supine.	Uterine circulation is 1L/min 38-40th wk.
		Physiologic anemia: hemoglobin, hematocrit, and platelets decrease.	
Pulmonary			
Lung compliance and pulmonary diffusion remain constant throughout pregnancy.	Vital capacity and partial pressure of oxygen (PO_2) are unchanged.	Diaphragm is displaced upward by rising fundus; thoracic circumference increases by 6 cm.	Diaphragm is displaced 4 cm by rising fundus. Thoracic breathing replaces abdominal breathing.
		Tidal volume increases 30%-40%.	
		Respiratory rate increases 15% to accommodate increasing metabolism.	Venous stasis increases risk for thrombus formation and pulmonary emboli.
		Mild dyspnea. Chronic state of compensated respiratory alkalosis.	
		Nasal congestion caused by estrogen-induced edema.	
Gastrointestinal	Nausea and vomiting. Constipation. Salivation increases.	Nausea and vomiting diminish.	Gastric emptying time is decreased.
		Incidence of cholecystitis is increased.	Gallbladder sluggish, frequently develop gallstones.
		Progesterone causes decreased gastrointestinal motility.	
		Esophageal sphincter tone is decreased; at risk for gastric reflux.	

Continued

TABLE 8-2

Maternal Anatomic and Physiologic Changes of Pregnancy—cont'd

SYSTEM	FIRST TRIMESTER (1-3 MO GESTATION [1-12 WK])	SECOND TRIMESTER (4-7 MO GESTATION [13-27 WK])	THIRD TRIMESTER (7-9 MO GESTATION [28-38 TO 40 WK])
Neurologic	May feel some slight Braxton Hicks contractions starting at 8th wk.	Intraocular pressure decreases. Some temporary visual changes that return to prepregnant state after delivery.	Braxton Hicks contractions increase and become regular.
Endocrine	Human chorionic gonadotropin hormone secreted by corpus luteum of ovary is present in serum 9 days after conception. Progesterone production increases. Basal metabolic rate decreases. Blood glucose level decreases.	Protein binding causes increase in circulating hormones. Thyroid and adrenal hormone levels are elevated. Insulin production increases. Erythropoietin increases by 20th wk. Metabolism increases.	Prolactin increases and peaks at delivery.
Genitourinary Ureters and renal pelves and calyces dilate, increasing risk of urinary tract infection. Dilatation is present throughout pregnancy.	Urinary frequency caused by uterine pressure on bladder.	Bladder pressure decreases as fundus elevates. Bladder is displaced superior to pelvis. Glomerular filtration rate increases 30%-50%. Drugs are excreted faster.	Lateral position facilitates renal blood flow and increases urinary output. Increased frequency as presenting part enters pelvis.
Integumentary	No appreciable change.	Striae gravidarum (stretch marks) appear on breasts and abdomen.	Dark line (linea nigra) appears between umbilicus and pubis. Increased pigmentation of face (cholasma).
Musculoskeletal	Feels fatigue. Weight loss first few weeks caused by nausea and vomiting. Average weight gain 2.2 lb (1 kg) by 10-12 wk.	Feels energetic. Weight gain 1 lb. (0.45 kg) per week; desirable weight gain between 12th and 20th wk is 8 lb (3.62 kg). Gains ½-1 lb (0.24 kg-2.2 kg) per week between 20th and 38th wk.	Energy declines. Ideal total weight gain 25-30 lb (11-13.6 kg) total for entire pregnancy.
		Progressive lordosis to compensate for shifting center of gravity causes backache.	Increased lordosis as uterus expands and protrudes forward.
	Leg cramps.	Leg cramps increase by 24 wk.	Pelvic joints relax and slight separation of symphysis pubis can be seen on x-ray film.

TABLE 8-2

Maternal Anatomic and Physiologic Changes of Pregnancy—cont'd

SYSTEM	FIRST TRIMESTER (1-3 MO GESTATION [1-12 WK])	SECOND TRIMESTER (4-7 MO GESTATION [13-27 WK])	THIRD TRIMESTER (7-9 MO GESTATION [28-38 TO 40 WK])
Reproductive	Menstruation ceases. Progesterone causes uterine lining to thicken. Estrogen causes uterine body to hypertrophy, anteflex, and become globular; by 3rd mo fundus reaches pelvic brim. Cervix softens and vulva and vagina appear blue (caused by increasing vascularity). Vaginal discharge increases.	Uterine fundus elevates halfway between symphysis pubis and umbilicus by 12th-16th wk but rises above umbilicus by 24 wk. Fetal movement is felt by 18th to 20th wk. Lower uterine segment elevates in pelvis.	Uterine fundus elevates halfway between umbilicus and xyphoid process by 28th wk and reaches xyphoid by 32 wk. Fundus decreases in height (caused by uterine weight) by 38th wk. Uterine weight at term is 1100 g.
	Breast tissue enlarges and becomes sensitive.	Areolae darken.	Breasts feel full and tender. May secrete colostrum (precursor to milk).

pendicitis, or trauma. Urgent surgical procedures are delayed until the second or third trimester if possible. Emergency procedures are performed immediately, regardless of gestational stage. If the maternal condition is critical, the primary concern is to save the mother. Elective surgical procedures should be deferred until after delivery of the neonate and the anatomic and physiologic changes of pregnancy have returned to normal.

Anesthesia Considerations in Pregnancy

The surgeon and anesthesiologist collaborate closely because the risks of anesthesia and surgical procedure are high for both the mother and the fetus. Perinatal morbidity and mortality are affected by maternal health, fetal viability, type of anesthetic, and surgical procedure. The incidence of preterm labor, low birth weight, and fetal death increases if general anesthesia must be administered. The objectives of anesthetic management in the pregnant surgical patient include but are not limited to:

1. *Maternal safety.* The pregnant patient should always be treated as if she has a full stomach. Nausea and vomiting are common and place her at risk for aspiration of regurgitated stomach contents during induction of anesthesia, intubation, and extubation. The condition of the mother directly affects the outcome of the pregnancy.
2. *Avoidance of teratogenic drugs.* Many anesthetic drugs cross the placenta and enter the fetus through the uteroplacental circulation. Some drugs that adversely affect the fetus during the first trimester include nitrous oxide, halogenated agents, sedatives, tranquilizers, antidepressants, and amphetamines. Halogenated agents and nitrous oxide have been given without teratogenicity in emergency situations during the second and third trimesters. Only short-acting drugs should be used. The fetal liver is immature and metabolizes tranquilizers and other narcotics slowly. Neonatal respiratory depression is common if these drugs have been used.

   Agents used in local and regional anesthesia have not shown teratogenicity in animal studies and may provide a safer anesthetic alternative than general anesthesia when a surgical procedure must be performed.
3. *Prevention of fetal asphyxia.* Maternal hypoxia rapidly affects the oxygenation of the fetus. The oxygenation capability depends on the hemoglobin content and arterial oxygen tension of maternal blood and uteroplacental perfusion. Maternal hypotension and decreased uterine blood flow cause fetal hypoxia.
4. *Prevention of preterm labor.* Studies have shown no association of any single anesthetic agent to an increase or decrease in preterm labor. Manipulation

of the gravid uterus can cause preterm labor. Use of halogenated agents in advanced pregnancy decreases uterine tone and prevents uterine contractions. Vasopressors and drugs used to reverse muscle relaxants may stimulate the uterus to contract and initiate preterm labor.

Special Considerations

Intraoperative Care of Pregnant Patient

Both the mother and fetus should be monitored during the surgical procedure. (Physiologic monitoring of surgical patient is discussed in Chapter 19.) The mother's physiologic and psychologic condition rapidly affects the well-being of her fetus. Changes in the fetal condition may be the first indicator of a physiologic change in the mother. Intraoperative care and monitoring of the pregnant surgical patient include special considerations to:

1. *Minimize time under anesthesia.* Skin preparation and draping should be done before induction of general anesthesia. Devices for electronic fetal and uterine monitoring should be in position and in proper working order.
2. *Monitor maternal oxygenation.* Pulse oximetry is useful for noninvasive measurement of oxygenation in hemoglobin. Readings should remain above 94% to prevent fetal hypoxia. Continuous oxygen is usually administered.
3. *Monitor fetal heart rate.* An electronic fetal heart monitor (EFM) should be used by appropriately trained personnel for continuous monitoring. Fetal tachycardia may be the first indicator of maternal hypoxia. EFM is most effective after 16 weeks' gestation.
4. *Monitor uterine tone.* Uterine tone should be palpated frequently during the surgical procedure to detect contractions. Uterine manipulation, bladder stimulation, and several anesthetic drugs can cause preterm labor.
5. *Prevent aspiration.* Assist the anesthesiologist during intubation by providing cricoid pressure (Sellick's maneuver) as directed. (See Chapter 17, p. 325, for discussion of cricoid pressure.)
6. *Prevent maternal hypotension.* If the uterus is enlarged to the level of the umbilicus or above (17 to 20 weeks' gestation), place a small pad or folded sheet under the right hip to laterally displace the uterus to the left. This redistributes the weight of the gravid uterus off the vena cava and abdominal aorta and facilitates a normotensive state. Renal perfusion is also improved.
7. *Monitor urinary output.* Minimum urinary output should be 25 ml/hr. Palpate the bladder every 30 minutes. Bladder distention can cause uterine irritability and preterm labor. The bladder is displaced above the pelvis during the second and third trimesters and is easily injured. An indwelling Foley catheter should be inserted if the surgical procedure is anticipated to exceed 1 hour.
8. *Maintain normothermic environment.* Warm the room to 75° F (24° C), and maintain consistent temperature during the surgical procedure. Maternal hypothermia causes decreased uteroplacental perfusion and can cause fetal bradycardia. Use prewarmed blankets and irrigating solutions. Keep the mother's head covered.
9. *Prepare for emergency cesarean birth or preterm delivery.* In the event of untimely rupture of membranes, preterm labor, or fetal distress, it may be necessary to perform a cesarean section or precipitous delivery in an effort to save a viable fetus. A preterm fetus requiring immediate delivery after 24 weeks' gestation or 500 g weight may be considered viable. Fetal viability is individualized by measurement of lung maturity, body weight, and ability to sustain life after removal from the uterus (Box 8-2).
10. *Protect from hazards in the environment.* The pregnant uterus at any stage of gestation should be shielded from ionizing radiation (see Chapter 10, pp. 144 and 146, for discussion of patient safety). During the first trimester, radiation may cause teratogenic damage.
11. *Reassure mother.* Explain that she and her fetus will be monitored closely and they will be carefully protected.

Intraoperative Risks

The enlarging uterus displaces abdominal organs and distorts anatomic landmarks, making diagnoses of trauma or a pathologic condition complex. A motor vehicle accident is a common cause of abdominal trauma. A seat belt (lap belt) without a shoulder restraint can cause compression injury to the enlarged uterus. Spontaneous laceration and/or rupture can occur. Peritoneal lavage, if used to assess for intraabdominal bleeding, should be done through an incision above the umbilicus to avoid injuring the uterus.

Surgical procedures for reasons other than trauma, such as pathologic causes, require careful differential diagnosis. Anatomic and physiologic changes of pregnancy must be considered. For example, the appendix is displaced to the upper right quadrant and may mimic cholecystitis. In advanced pregnancy, chest drainage tubes should be inserted one to two intercostal spaces higher, if needed. Diagnosis is complicated because laboratory tests are altered by the progressing pregnancy, and results vary according to the gestational stage (Table 8-3).

Assessment of the patient's condition is difficult because compensatory mechanisms of pregnancy cause al-

BOX 8-2

Gestational Stages of Fetal Development and Viability Concerns

First trimester (1-3 mo, 1-12 wk)

Zygote implants in uterine wall by 14 days.
Communication of venous sinus and arterial supply of maternal circulation is completed at 17 days.
Teratogens can impair organogenesis until 14th wk.
Primitive placental system with umbilical cord is established by 7th wk.
Heart rate detectable on ultrasound at 10-12 wk.
Facial features and external genitalia are present by 12th wk.
Crown to rump length is 6-7 cm by 12th wk.

Second trimester (4-7 mo, 13-27 wk)

Arms and trunk grow rapidly.
Little muscle tone.
Scalp hair, tiny nipples, and external ears develop by 20th wk.
Meconium present in intestine.
Body weight 300 g.
Skeletal calcification seen on x-ray film.
Sucks thumb and moves freely at will.
Fetal heart rate audible with fetoscope at 120-160 beats/min at 20th wk.
Fingertip pressure causes ballottement (fetal rebound) in amniotic sac during 16th-32nd wk.
Teratogens may cause minor structural and functional abnormalities, especially endocrine, brain, and special senses from 10th wk to term.
Body covered with vernix (gray-white cheeselike substance) and lanugo (soft, downy hair).
Eyebrows and eyelashes present.
Body weight 454-630 g (1-1.4 lb) by 24th wk.
May be viable.

Third trimester (7-9 mo, 28-38 to 40 wk)

Subcutaneous fat begins to develop.
Crown to rump length 25 cm.
Testes are descended in male.
Body weight 1100 g (2½ lb).
Surfactant present in alveoli of lungs by 28th wk.
Increased chance of survival.
Body weight 1361-1814 g (3-4 lb) by 32nd wk.
Body fuller and rounded.
Muscle tone good.
Less vernix and absence of lanugo by 36th wk.
Body weight 3402-3629 g (7½-8 lb) by 38-40 wk.
Crown to rump length 36 cm.

TABLE 8-3

Altered Laboratory Values of Pregnancy

TEST	NONPREGNANT FEMALE	CHANGE IN PREGNANT FEMALE	GESTATIONAL TIMING
Hemoglobin (Hgb)	12-16 g/dl	↓4-7%	Drops to lowest point between 30th and 34th wk, then stable.
Hematocrit (Hct)	37%-47%	↓1.5-2 g/dl	Drops to lowest point between 30th and 34th wk, then stable.
White blood cells (WBC)	5000-10,000/cm^3	↑3.5×10^3	Gradual increase throughout pregnancy.
Platelets	150,000-400,000/mm^3	↓Slightly	Gradual decrease throughout pregnancy.
Fibrinogen	200-400 mg/dl	↑50%	Gradual increase throughout pregnancy.
Calcium (Ca)	9.0-10.5 mg/dl	↓10%	Gradual decrease throughout pregnancy.
Sodium (Na)	136-145 mEq/L	↓2-4 mEq/L	Decreases before 20th wk, then stable.
Chloride (Cl)	90-110 mEq/L	↑Slightly	Gradual rise, almost negligible.
Potassium (K)	3.5-5.0 mEq/L	↓0.2-0.3 mEq/L	Decreases before 20th wk, then stable.
Creatinine clearance	95-125 ml/min	↑40%	Rises through 20th wk, then stable.
Blood urea nitrogen (BUN)	5-20 mg/dl	↓50%	Drops during first trimester, then stable.
Glucose (fasting)	70-115 mg/dl	↓10%	Gradual decrease throughout pregnancy.
Uric acid	2.0-6.6 mg/dl	↓33%	Decreases during first trimester, then stable.
Albumin	3.2-4.5 g/dl	↓1 g/dl	Rapid drop before 20 wk, then stable.

terations in vital signs. The arterial blood pressure is lower than prepregnant values, and the pulse is elevated to accommodate an increase in circulatory volume. Decreased peripheral vascular resistance prevents overt physiologic signs of shock such as cool, clammy skin. Circulating blood volume can be reduced 30% to 35% before the patient shows any signs of hypovolemic shock such as lowered blood pressure and increased pulse rate. In hypovolemic shock, blood is shunted away from the uteroplacental circulation at the expense of the fetus. The fetus becomes hypoxic. Fetal demise is 80% in maternal hypovolemic shock. An EFM can detect early signs of fetal hypoxia and uteroplacental insufficiency. Use of a fetal monitor is recommended during surgical procedures after 16 weeks' gestation. Personnel appropriately trained in fetal monitoring should perform this assessment throughout the perioperative period, including during the surgical procedure and postanesthesia recovery.

In the immediate postoperative period, the pregnant patient must be assessed for uterine irritability, vaginal bleeding, and/or ruptured membranes. Any combination of these signs may signal impending labor and possible preterm delivery and must be reported to the physician immediately. Bladder distention can cause uterine irritability and initiate preterm labor. The bladder should be palpated frequently. A distended bladder is felt as a bulge above the symphysis pubis that is cooler than the surrounding skin.

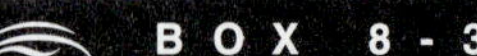

BOX 8-3

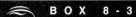

Psychologic Implications of Pregnancy to Mother

First trimester (1-3 mo, 1-12 wk)
Ambivalence and anxiety about pregnancy
Mood swings

Second trimester (4-7 mo, 13-27 wk)
Acceptance of pregnancy as it becomes more concrete
Excited by listening to heart sounds and feeling fetal movement
Considers fetus as real entity
Beginning to dislike physiologic effects of pregnancy by end of 24th wk

Third trimester (7-9 mo, 28-38 to 40 wk)
Feels physically awkward
Tired of being pregnant, but eager to assume motherhood role

Psychologic Considerations

For most patients and their families, pregnancy is a time of joy and excitement (Box 8-3). Their happiness is shattered when they are faced with the prospect of a surgical procedure and its inherent risks. In urgent and emergency situations, there is little time for the family to adjust to the pending procedure. The outcome is uncertain and the risks to the mother and her fetus are great. The patient and family are also facing the possibility of a preterm delivery. The perioperative team should take the special needs of the pregnant patient into consideration and provide as much reassurance as possible.

IMMUNOCOMPROMISED PATIENTS

The immune system protects the body from invasion by pathogenic microorganisms and foreign bodies by creating local barriers and inflammation. Humoral and cell-mediated responses develop if these first-line defenses are inadequate protection. The humoral response produces antibodies to react with specific antigens. The cell-mediated response mobilizes tissue macrophages in the presence of a foreign body. *Immunocompetence* is the ability of the immune system to mobilize and deploy its antibodies and other responses to stimulation by an antigen. Immunocompetence may be compromised by a disease or a virus or by an immunosuppressive agent. Immunocompromised patients have a weakened or deficient immune response with resultant decreased resistance to infection.

Immunosuppression

Immunosuppressive agents include corticosteroid hormones given to prevent or reduce inflammation caused by some diseases. They are frequently prescribed for patients who have an autoimmune collagen disease such as rheumatoid arthritis, systemic lupus erythematosus, and scleroderma or an autoimmune hemolytic disorder such as idiopathic thrombocytopenic purpura or acquired hemolytic anemia. They are also given to patients with adrenal insufficiency.

Immunosuppressants are given following organ transplantation to combat rejection (see Chapter 44, p. 908).

Antineoplastic cytotoxic agents for chemotherapy (see pp. 926-927) and radiation therapy (pp. 922-924) as used in oncology (Chapter 45), for reduction of malignant tumor cells, may cause immunosuppression.

Common Complications

The manifestations and clinical characteristics of the patient depend on the specific disease and the organ or system affected. For example, systemic lupus erythematosus can affect every organ system in the body. Adrenal insufficiency, as caused by Addison's disease, may be characterized by general debility. In contrast, organ transplantation or malignant tumor may affect a single organ. Immunosuppression, however, lowers resistance to infection.

Special Considerations

Many of these patients have skin rashes or lesions, painful joints, poor nutrition, and/or generalized malaise. They need physical and emotional support preoperatively. Aseptic and sterile techniques are important considerations for all surgical patients. They are especially crucial for immunosuppressed patients, who are at high risk for developing a postoperative infection.

Acquired Immunodeficiency Syndrome

Patients with acquired immunodeficiency syndrome (AIDS) test positive for the human immunodeficiency virus (HIV) in serum and exhibit one or more signs and symptoms of an opportunistic disease, including pneumonia, fungal and/or parasitic infection(s), or malignant neoplasm. HIV is a retrovirus that can remain inactive and undetected in the body for many years before causing immunodeficient illness. During this time, although no outward signs of HIV infection are noted, it is possible for the patient to transmit the virus through blood, body fluids, or sexual contact. Males and females, including infants and children, may be HIV positive or diagnosed with AIDS. At one time AIDS was considered to be transmitted only by homosexual behavior among men, intravenous drug use, or tainted blood transfusions. It is now known that the virus is transmitted also by heterosexual contact. An infected mother may transmit the virus to her fetus. (See Chapter 12, pp. 192-193, for further discussion of transmission of HIV.)

The diagnosis of HIV infection must be confirmed by at least two separate tests. One positive test is not a conclusive diagnosis. Initial testing with the enzyme-linked immunosorbent assay (ELISA) is performed to detect the presence of HIV antibodies in the blood. The diagnosis is confirmed with either the Western blot test or the indirect immunofluorescence assay.

Testing seropositive for HIV infection does not mean that the patient has AIDS. HIV invades and destroys T lymphocytes. During this process the patient's immune system is disabled. The normal T lymphocyte level is 1000 mm^3. The severity of the HIV infection is measured by the level of T lymphocyte cells in the blood. When the T cell level decreases to between 200 to 500 mm^3, the patient has seroconverted to an immunodeficient state and is considered to have AIDS. There is no known cure for HIV infection or AIDS. Some medications are available that delay seroconversion in HIV infection and prolong life in seroconverted AIDS patients. Pharmacologic therapy may include broad-spectrum antibiotics, antivirals, antidiarrheals, vitamins, and antineoplastics.

Common Complications

A patient with HIV infection may complain of night sweats, unexplained fevers, dry cough, weakness, diarrhea, and swollen lymph glands. A patient who has seroconverted to AIDS may have *multiple* opportunistic infections and malignancies concurrently and generalized poor health. Extreme muscle and tissue wasting is common.

Many AIDS patients have multiple external and internal lesions. The skin may have open wounds with infectious exudate and/or large swollen purple lesions associated with Kaposi's sarcoma. This is a malignant multifocal neoplasm of reticuloendothelial cells that spreads in the skin and metastasizes to lymph nodes and viscera. Large painful masses of lymph tissue may be present in the neck, axilla, and groin. Mechanical obstruction caused by internal Kaposi's lesions in the esophagus may prevent swallowing of food. Intestinal lesions may prevent absorption of nutrients or cause bowel obstruction. Constant anorexia, nausea, vomiting, and diarrhea also may prevent adequate intake by mouth. Nutritional supplementation by hyperalimentation may be indicated to meet the patients' high caloric needs.

AIDS causes the body to be susceptible to opportunistic infections because of the lowered resistance by the immune system. *Opportunistic infections* are caused by microorganisms that normally are nonpathogenic in a healthy individual. The mucous membranes of the mouth and genital areas may have herpesvirus lesions or white patches of candidiasis, a yeastlike fungus. Neurologically, the patient may have recurrent episodes of cryptococcal meningitis or toxoplasmosis, causing persistent motor dysfunction and mental changes.

The patient with AIDS experiences a continual cycle of acute and chronic respiratory infections. *Pneumocystis carinii pneumonia* (PCP) is the most frequent lung infection, followed by multiple-drug–resistant tuberculosis (MDR-TB). The patient may be in a perpetual state of respiratory distress. Central and peripheral cyanosis may be present. The respiratory effort expends high energy levels causing the patient to deteriorate rapidly.

Special Considerations

Patients with AIDS may be in poor physical condition, depending on how body systems have been affected. Most systems are eventually involved. The plan of care should incorporate the following considerations:

1. Moving the patient from the transport stretcher to the operating table may require additional personnel for total lifting. The patient may not be able to move because of weakness or pain in joints, muscle and tissue wasting, and superficial skin lesions.

2. Bony prominences, areas of decreased muscle mass, and devascularized tissue must be protected throughout the positioning process and the surgical procedure. Blankets, restraints, monitoring devices, electrosurgical dispersive electrodes, drapes, instruments, and routine care devices may cause inadvertent harm to the patient despite best efforts to protect the patient from injury.
3. Intravenous line insertion, induction of anesthesia, and maintenance of the airway may be difficult. A suitable vein for infusion may be hard to identify because of former illicit intravenous drug use or large areas of epidermal Kaposi's sarcoma. In extreme cases the only intravenous site may be a central venous catheter. Endotracheal intubation may be contraindicated because of potential hemorrhage from Kaposi's lesions in the trachea. Placement of an esophageal stethoscope or rectal temperature probe may rupture other internal Kaposi's lesions with the same result.
4. Postoperative wound healing is delayed or absent because of poor nutrition, decreased circulation, poor tissue integrity, and continued immunodeficient condition.

Many of these patients have been rejected by their families, especially if the virus was transmitted through a route not accepted or understood by family members. The diagnosis of AIDS may be the first time the family is made aware of a patient's alternative lifestyle. Psychologic support systems may consist of a small circle of friends who may also be infected with HIV or have AIDS.

Continual counseling should be emphasized in the discharge plan to include provision for physiologic care and psychologic support. Patient, family, and significant other(s) should be educated about the potential routes of transmission, such as exposure to blood and body fluids through sexual contact or sharing intravenous needles. The virus is also potentially transmissible through shared razors, toothbrushes, and tweezers because of the possibility of blood contamination. Dishes and eating utensils are considered safe when washed in hot soapy water, rinsed, and dried. Education should include physical activities that do not pose a risk of transmission, such as hugging, shaking hands, and sitting in close proximity.

Confidentiality is a concern because of the nature of transmission routes of HIV infection. It is an issue of the patient's right to privacy. Testing for HIV is not a routine preadmission laboratory procedure. If a patient is tested, the results should be placed in the appropriate section of the patient's chart with other laboratory results, not displayed on the front of the chart. Reporting of the results should be governed by institutional policy and treated in the same manner as all patient confidentiality issues. Dissemination of confidential patient information to inappropriate persons is a breach of duty to the patient's privacy and may be subject to legal action. Physicians and nurses may face disciplinary action, such as license suspension or revocation by the boards of medicine or nursing, as indicated.

OR personnel should provide care to all patients with equal professionalism, compassion, empathy, and positive regard, despite personal feelings about a patient's lifestyle or disease entity. Nonjudgmental care is essential for the psychologic wellness of AIDS patients.

CATASTROPHIC ILLNESSES

Although OR nursing personnel are most frequently involved with patients who have favorable prognoses, they also care for those of all ages with catastrophic illnesses who are having surgical procedures to relieve a specific problem. The procedure may be palliative rather than curative. Included in this category are patients with:

1. Malignancies who are severely debilitated and terminally ill.
2. Severe traumatic disabilities requiring lengthy hospitalization, such as following spinal cord injury or extensive burns.
3. End-stage of a chronic illness, such as those with renal disease on dialysis or those waiting for an organ transplant.

Maximum patient comfort and relief of physiologic disturbances are the primary concerns. All of these patients require highly individualized care. The manner in which patients are told the diagnosis and prognosis naturally has a great impact on their hope for recovery. Patients who have been thoroughly and considerately informed are easier to talk to, accept therapy more readily, and have greater trust in and communicate more openly with the nursing staff.

Each patient deals with the diagnosis in his or her own way. Although not always so, many persons consider the diagnosis of cancer a death warrant and react accordingly. To be supportive, the nurse should mentally review the stages of dying: denial, isolation, anger, bargaining, depression, and acceptance. These stages do not always occur in this sequence, however. The nurse should emphasize the present, focusing on the patient's strengths and attributes and how these can best be used. It is difficult to find hope when one faces a radical disfiguring procedure. The discerning nurse will offer a philosophy of hope but should not focus on the positive without acknowledging the negative. Listening to the patient is particularly important.

Persons caring for patients with a terminal or catastrophic illness should remember that they are interacting with people who have different priorities and values. These patients are present-oriented because many have a limited future. They review their sense of values and the quality of their lives. A bleak prognosis alters one's perspective. Such persons rearrange their ultimate goals for existence. Some persons appreciate living each day. Others are anxious to end their suffering.

The chronically ill or disabled patient feels especially threatened. Disability requires a reorientation of self-image.

Bibliography

Benz JD: Insulin use in the diabetic surgical patient, *AORN J* 52(5):1055-1059, 1990.

Borkgren MW, Gronkiewicz CA: Update your asthma care from hospital to home, *Am J Nurs* 95(1):26-34, 1995.

Bretin L, Sieh A: Caring for the morbidly obese, *Am J Nurs* 91(8):40-43, 1991.

Cunningham FG et al: *Williams obstetrics,* ed 19, Norwalk, Conn, 1993, Appleton & Lange.

Deakins DA: Teaching elderly patients about diabetes, *Am J Nurs* 94(4):39-42, 1994.

Ekstrom I: Communicating with the deaf patient, *Plast Surg Nurs* 14(1):31-32, 1994.

Gusek A: 10 commonly asked questions about diabetes, *Am J Nurs* 94(2):19-20, 1994.

Harding et al: Confidentiality limits with patients who have HIV: a review of ethical and legal guidelines and professional policies, *J Counsel Devel* 71(5):297-304, 1993.

Holt J: How to help confused patients, *Am J Nurs* 93(8):32-36, 1993.

Janson-Bjerklie S: Status asthmaticus, *Am J Nurs* 90(9):52-55, 1990.

Kelly JU, Kelly TJ: Insulin-dependent diabetes, *AORN J* 54(1):61-68, 1991.

Kendrik JM, Powers PH: Perioperative care of the pregnant surgical patient, *AORN J* 60(2):205-216, 1994.

Kuzmak LI et al: Surgery for morbid obesity: using an inflatable gastric band, *AORN J* 51(5):1307-1324, 1990.

Macheca MKK: Diabetic hypoglycemia: how to keep the threat at bay, *Am J Nurs* 93(4):26-30, 1993.

Mason DS et al: Roux-en-Y gastric bypass: surgical treatment for morbid obesity, *AORN J* 58(6):1113-1135, 1993.

Miles A: Caring for the family left behind, *Am J Nurs* 93(12):34-36, 1993.

Stiesmeyer JK: A four-step approach to pulmonary assessment, *Am J Nurs* 93(8):22-28, 1993.

SECTION FOUR

The Surgical Environment

CHAPTER 9

Physical Facilities

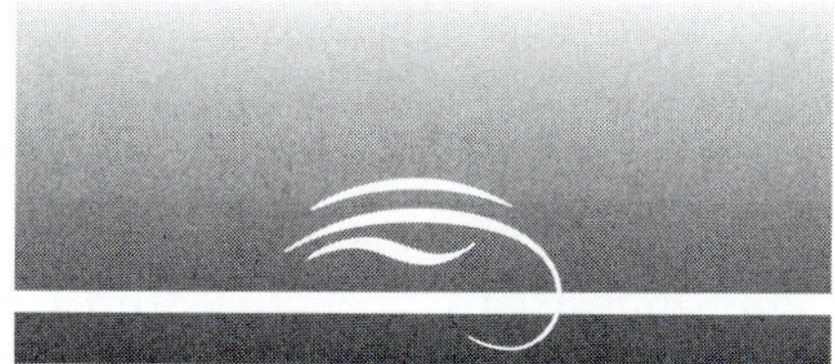

PHYSICAL LAYOUT OF OPERATING ROOM SUITE

Utilization of the physical facilities is important; however, it is secondary to the functioning of the providers of health care services. The design of an operating room (OR) suite offers a challenge to the planning team to optimize efficiency by creating realistic traffic and work flow patterns for patients, personnel, and supplies. Design should also allow for flexibility and future expansion. Architects consult surgeons and OR nursing administrative personnel before allocating space.

No one plan suits all hospitals; each is designed on an individual basis to meet projected specific future needs. The number of rooms required depends on:

1. Number and length of the surgical procedures to be performed
2. Type and distribution by specialties of the surgical staff and equipment for each
3. Proportion of elective inpatient and emergency surgical procedures to ambulatory patient and minimally invasive procedures
4. Scheduling policies related to the number of hours per day and days per week the suite will be in use and staffing needs
5. Systems and procedures established for the efficient flow of patients, personnel, and supplies

Location

The OR suite is usually located in an area accessible to the critical care surgical patient areas and the supporting service departments—the central service or sterile processing department, pathology, and radiology. The size of the hospital is a determining factor because it is impossible to locate every desirable unit or department immediately adjacent to the OR suite. A terminal location is necessary to prevent unrelated traffic from passing through the suite. A location on a top floor is not necessary for microbial control because all air is filtered to control dust. Traffic noises may be less evident above the ground floor. Artificial lighting is controllable so that daylight is not a factor; in fact, it may be a distraction. Many OR suites are underground or have solid walls without windows.

Principles in Design

The universal problem of environmental control to prevent wound infection exerts a great influence on the design of the OR suite. As much as the floor plan will permit, clean and contaminated areas should be differentiated. Architects follow two principles in planning the physical layout of an OR suite:

1. Exclusion of contamination from outside the suite with sensible traffic patterns within the suite
2. Separation of clean areas from contaminated areas within the suite

Physical planning of an OR suite, which separates clean from contaminated areas, makes it easier to carry out good aseptic technique. The clean area is often referred to as the *restricted area.*

Type of Design

Most OR suites are constructed according to a variation of one of these basic designs:

1. Central corridor, or hotel plan
2. Central core, or clean core plan
3. Peripheral corridor
4. Combination central core and peripheral corridor, or racetrack plan
5. Three corridor layout
6. Grouping, or cluster plan

Each design has its advantages and disadvantages. Efficiency is affected if corridor distances are too long in proportion to other space, if illogical relationships exist between space and function, or if inadequate consideration was given to storage space, materiel handling, and personnel areas.

Space Allocation and Traffic Patterns

Space is allocated within the OR suite to provide for the work to be done, with consideration of the efficiency with which it can be accomplished. The OR suite should be large enough to allow for correct technique yet small enough to minimize the movement of patients, personnel, and supplies. Provision must be made for traffic control. The type of design will predetermine traffic patterns. All persons—staff, patients, and visitors—should follow the delineated patterns in appropriate attire. Signs should be posted that clearly indicate the attire and environmental controls required. The OR suite is divided into three areas that are designated by the physical activities performed in each area.

Unrestricted

Street clothes are permitted. A corridor on the periphery accommodates traffic from outside, including patients. This area is isolated by doors from the main hospital corridor or elevators and from other areas of the OR suite. It serves as an outside-to-inside access area, that is, a vestibular/exchange area. Traffic, although not limited, is monitored at a central location.

Semirestricted

Traffic is limited to properly attired personnel. Body and head coverings are required. This area includes peripheral support areas and access corridors to the ORs. The patient may be transferred to a clean "inside" stretcher or wheel base on entry to this area. The patient's hair must be covered. Traffic is limited to properly attired personnel.

Restricted

Masks are required to supplement OR attire. Sterile procedures are carried out in the OR. The area also includes scrub sink areas and substerile rooms or clean core area(s) where unwrapped supplies are sterilized.

VESTIBULAR/EXCHANGE AREAS

Both patients and personnel enter the semirestricted and restricted areas of the OR suite through a *vestibular or exchange area.* This transition zone, inside the entrance to the OR suite, separates the OR corridors from the rest of the facility.

Preoperative Check-in Unit

If a remote same-day procedure unit is not available for admission of patients who arrive shortly before a surgical procedure, facilities must be provided within the unrestricted area of the OR suite for patients to change from street clothes into a gown. The area must ensure privacy. It may be compartmentalized with individual cubicles or be an open area with curtains. The decor should create a feeling of warmth and security. Lockers should be provided for safeguarding patients' clothes. Lavatory facilities must be available.

Preoperative Holding Area

A designated room or area should be available for patients to wait in the OR suite that shields them from potentially distressing sights and sounds. The corridor outside the OR is the least desirable area. The area should provide privacy. Individual cubicles are preferable to curtains. Hair removal and insertion of intravenous lines, indwelling urinary catheters, and/or gastric tubes may be done here. The anesthesiologist may insert invasive monitoring lines and give regional blocks. These procedures require good lighting. Each patient area is equipped with oxygen and suction and devices for monitoring and cardiopulmonary resuscitation.

A nurses' station within the area provides for medication storage and preparation and for interdepartmental and intradepartmental communication. Computer access to patient information, such as laboratory reports, and to nursing care documentation facilitates completion of patients' records, if necessary. Coordination with persons managing the surgical schedule is essential to prevent delays.

NOTE Some hospitals have an induction room adjacent to each OR where the patient waits and is prepared preoperatively, before administration of anesthesia.

Postanesthesia Care Unit

The postanesthesia care unit (PACU) may be outside the OR suite, or it may be adjacent to the suite so that it may be incorporated into the unrestricted area with access from both the semirestricted area and an outside corridor. In the latter design, the PACU becomes a vestibular area for the departure of patients.

NOTE Hospitals and ambulatory care facilities must accommodate both patients and their families. A designated waiting area must be provided for families. This is most conveniently located outside the OR suite adjacent to the recovery area.

Dressing Rooms and Lounges

Dressing rooms must be provided for both men and women to change from street clothes into OR attire before entering the semirestricted area, and vice versa. Lockers are usually provided. Doors separate this area from lavatory facilities and adjacent lounges. Walls in the lounge areas should have an aesthetically pleasing color or combination of colors to foster a restful atmosphere. A window view of the outdoors is psychologically desirable. Dictating equipment and telephones should be available for surgeons in lounges or in an adjacent semirestricted area.

PERIPHERAL SUPPORT AREAS

Adequate space must be allocated to accommodate the needs of OR personnel and support services.

Central Administrative Control

From a central control point, traffic in and out of the OR suite may be observed. This area usually is within the unrestricted area. The clerk-receptionist is located at the control desk to coordinate communications. A pass-through window may be used to stop unauthorized persons, to schedule surgical procedures with surgeons, or to receive drugs, blood, and various small supplies. A computerized pneumatic tube system within the hospital can speed the delivery of small items and paperwork, thus eliminating some messenger services, such as from the pharmacy to the control desk. Tissue specimens or blood samples also can be sent to the laboratory through some tube systems.

Computers may be located in the control area. Automated information systems and computers assist in financial management, statistical recording and analysis, scheduling of patients and personnel, materiels management, and other functions that evaluate the utilization of facilities. An integrated system interfaces with other hospital departments. It may have a modem that allows surgeons to schedule surgical procedures directly from their offices. Retrieval for review of patient records gives the OR nurse manager the opportunity to evaluate the nursing care given and documented by nurses. Personnel records can be maintained. Other essential records can be stored in and retrieved from computer databases. The central processing unit for the OR computer system usually is located in or near the central administrative control area. A facsimile (fax) machine may be available for the electronic transfer of documents, records, and patient care orders between the OR and the surgeons' offices.

Security systems usually can be monitored from the central administrative control area. Alarms are incorporated into electrical and piped-in systems to alert personnel to the location of a system failure. A centralized emergency call system facilitates summoning help. Narcotics must be kept locked up and be signed out. Access to exchange areas, offices, and storage areas may be limited during evening and night hours and on weekends. Doors may be locked. Some hospitals use alarm systems, television surveillance, and/or electronic metal detection devices to control intruders and to prevent vandalism. Computers and records must be secured to protect patients' confidentiality.

Offices

Offices for the administrative nursing personnel and the anesthesia department are best located with access to both unrestricted and semirestricted areas. These staff members frequently need to confer with outside persons and to be kept informed of activities within all areas of the suite.

Conference Room/Classroom

Ideally, a conference room or a classroom is located within the semirestricted area. This is used for nursing staff in-service educational programs and by the surgical staff for teaching. Closed-circuit television and/or videocassettes may also be available for self-study. The departmental reference library may be housed here.

Support Services

The size of the health care facility and the types of services provided determine whether laboratory and radiology equipment is needed within the OR suite.

Laboratory

A small laboratory where the pathologist can examine tissue specimens and perform frozen sections (see Chapter 28, p. 562) expedites the decisions that the surgeon must make during a surgical procedure when a diagnosis is questionable. A refrigerator for storing blood for transfusions also may be located in this room. Tissue specimens may be kept here before they are delivered to the pathology department.

Radiology Services

Special procedure rooms may be outfitted with x-ray and imaging equipment for diagnostic procedures or insertion of catheters, pacemakers, and other devices. The walls of these rooms contain lead shields to confine radiation. A darkroom for processing x-ray films usually is available within the OR suite if the volume of procedures warrants it or if the radiology department is not close by.

Work and Storage Areas

Clean and sterile supplies and equipment must be separated from soiled items and trash. If the OR suite has a clean core area, soiled materials should not be taken into this area. They should be taken to the decontamination area for processing and then storage, or to the disposal area. Work and storage areas must be provided for handling all types of supplies and equipment.

Anesthesia Work and Storage Areas

Space must be provided for the storage of anesthesia equipment and supplies. Gas tanks are stored in a well-ventilated area separated from other supplies. Nondisposable items must be thoroughly decontaminated and cleaned after use. A separate workroom usually is provided for care of anesthesia equipment. Dirty and clean supplies must be kept separated. The storage area includes space for drugs and anesthetic agents.

Housekeeping Storage Area

Cleaning supplies and equipment need to be stored; the equipment used within the restricted area is kept separated from that used to clean the other areas. Therefore more than one storage area may be provided for housekeeping purposes, depending on the design and size of the OR suite. Sinks are provided, as well as shelves for supplies. Trash and soiled laundry receptacles should not be allowed to accumulate in the same room where clean supplies are kept; separate areas should be provided for these. Conveyors or designated elevators may be provided for prompt removal of bags of soiled laundry and trash from the suite.

Central Processing Area

Conveyors, dumbwaiters, or elevators connect the OR suite with a central processing area on another floor of the hospital. If efficient materiel flow can be accomplished, support functions can be removed from the OR suite. Effective communications and a reliable transportation system must be established. Some ORs send all their instruments and supplies to the sterile processing department for cleaning, packaging, sterilizing, and storing. This system eliminates the need for some work and storage areas within the OR suite, but exchange areas must be provided for carts. The movement of clean and sterile supplies must be kept separate from that of contaminated items and waste by space and traffic patterns.

Case Cart Systems Most hospitals built or renovated after the mid-1960s provide facilities for a case cart system. Carts are prepared in a remote area and transported to the OR (Figure 9-1). Ideally, the processing department is located directly below or above the OR suite or immediately adjacent to it. Designated clean and contaminated elevators and dumbwaiters connect these respective areas in the two departments. Clean carts of supplies needed for each surgical procedure are delivered to the clean holding area in the OR suite. After use the cart is taken to the contaminated holding area for return to the decontamination area. Carts may have open or closed shelves. The cart must be enclosed during transport. Some carts are designed to serve as the instrument table during surgical procedure.

Each case cart should be large enough to hold the supplies, both sterile and nonsterile, for use during and cleanup after one surgical procedure. These supplies are selected according to standard routines and the individual surgeon's preferences. For the system to be efficient, good communication must exist between the staff in the OR and the sterile processing departments. Surgeon's preference cards must be kept up to date. Inventory lists that are supplied with the carts may be used for patient charges and inventory control. A bar code or other computer label system may be used to facilitate these functions.

Utility Room

Some hospitals use a closed-cart system and take contaminated instruments to a central area outside the OR suite for cleanup. Some perform cleanup procedures in the substerile room. Many, by virtue of the limitations of the physical facilities, bring the instruments to a util-

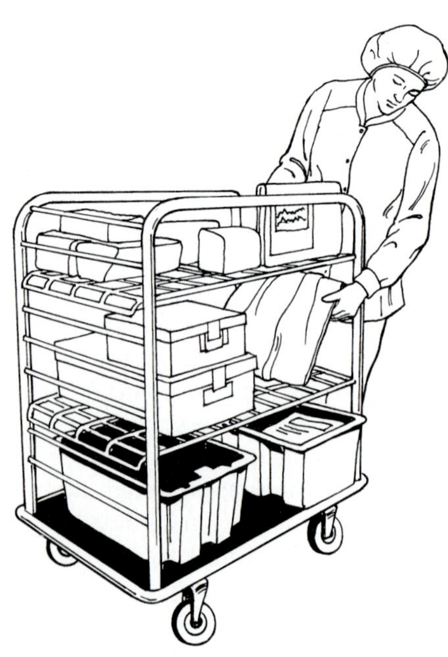

FIGURE 9-1 Surgery case cart being loaded for transport to OR.

ity room. This room contains a washer-sterilizer, sinks, cabinets, and all necessary aids for cleaning. If the washer-sterilizer is a pass-through unit, it opens also into the general workroom, which eliminates the task of physically moving instruments from one room to another.

General Workroom

The general work area should be as centrally located in the OR suite as possible to keep contamination to a minimum. The work area may be divided into a cleaning area and a preparation area. If instruments and equipment from the utility room are received from the pass-through washer-sterilizer into this room, an ultrasonic cleaner should be available here for cleaning instruments that the washer-sterilizer has not adequately cleaned. Otherwise, the ultrasonic cleaner may be in the utility room.

Instrument sets, basin sets, trays, and other supplies are wrapped for sterilization here. The preparation and sterilization of instrument trays and sets in a central room ensures control. This room also contains the stock supply of other items that are packaged for sterilization. The sterilizers that are used in this room may open also into the next room, the sterile supply room. This arrangement helps to eliminate the possibility of mixing sterile and nonsterile items.

Storage

Technology nearly tripled the need for storage space in the decade of the 1980s. Many older OR suites have inadequate facilities for storage of sterile supplies, instruments, and bulky equipment. Storage space should fit logically into the design of the suite.

Sterile Supply Room

Most hospitals keep a supply of sterile drapes, sponges, gloves, gowns, and other sterile items ready for use in a sterile supply room within the OR suite. As many shelves as possible should be freestanding from the walls, which permits supplies to be put into one side and removed from the other; thus older packages are always used first. However, small items must be contained in boxes or bins to prevent them from falling to the floor. Inventory levels should be large enough to prevent running out of supplies, yet overstocking of sterile supplies should be avoided. Storage should be arranged to facilitate stock rotation.

The sterile storage area should be adjacent to or as close as possible to the sterilizing area if sterilizing is done in the OR suite. Access to the sterile storage should be limited—it should be separated from high-traffic areas. Humidity should be controlled at 35% to 50%, and temperature should be 65° to 72° F (18° to 22° C). Ten air exchanges per hour are recommended.

Instrument Room

Most hospitals have a separate room or a section of the general workroom designated for storing nonsterile instruments. The instrument room contains cupboards in which all clean instruments are stored when not in use. Instruments usually are segregated on shelves according to surgical specialty services.

Sets of basic instruments are usually cleaned, assembled, and sterilized after each use. However, special instruments such as intestinal clamps, kidney forceps, and bone instruments may be stored after cleaning. Sets are then made up according to each day's schedule of surgical procedures.

Storage Room

Some large portable equipment must also be stored in the OR suite, readily accessible for use. A storage room for this equipment, such as the orthopaedic table that may not be used daily, keeps equipment out of corridors when not in use. Lasers and video equipment can be damaged if inadvertently bumped by a passing stretcher in a corridor.

Scrub Room

An *enclosed* area for surgical scrubbing of hands and arms must be provided adjacent to each OR (see scrub sink, Chapter 11, p. 170). Water spills on the floor are particularly hazardous if the scrub area is in a traffic corridor. An enclosed scrub room is a restricted area within the OR suite.

OPERATING ROOM ITSELF

All ORs are restricted areas because sterile procedures are carried out here.

Size

The size of individual ORs varies. In the interest of economy and flexibility, it is desirable to have all ORs the same size, so that they can be used interchangeably to accommodate elective and emergency surgical procedures. Adequate size for a multipurpose OR is at least 20 × 20 × 10 feet (400 sq ft or approximately 37 m^2) of floor space; the maximum, beyond which efficiency is lost, is 20 × 30 × 10 feet (600 sq ft, approximately 60 m^2).

A room may be designed for a specialty service if use by that service will be high. The room must accommodate equipment, such as lasers, microscopes, or video equipment, that is either fixed (permanently installed) or portable (movable). Portable equipment may require more floor space—a minimum of 22 × 22 × 10 feet (484 sq ft, approximately 45 m^2). A specialized room, such as one equipped for cardiopulmonary bypass or trauma, may require as much as 600 sq ft (approximately 60 m^2) of useful space.

Some rooms are designated for special procedures, such as endoscopy, radiologic studies, or the application of casts. Other rooms have adjacent areas used for specific purposes, such as visitor viewing galleries, or for installing special equipment such as monitors.

Substerile Room

A group of two, three, or four ORs may be clustered around a central scrub area, work area, and a small substerile room. Only if the latter room is immediately adjacent to the OR and separated from the scrub area will it be considered the *substerile room* throughout this text.

A substerile room adjacent to the OR contains a sink, steam sterilizer, and/or washer-sterilizer. Although cleaning and sterilizing facilities are centralized, either inside or outside of the OR suite, a substerile room with this equipment offers the following advantages:

1. It saves time and steps. Emergency cleaning and sterilization of items can be done here by the circulator. This reduces waiting time for the surgeon, anesthesia time for the patient, and saves steps for the circulator. The circulator, or scrub person if necessary, can lift sterile articles directly from the sterilizer onto the sterile instrument table without transporting them through a corridor or another area.
2. It reduces the need for a messenger service to obtain sterile instruments and allows the circulator to stay within the room.
3. It allows for better care of instruments and equipment that require special handling. Certain delicate or sensitive instruments, or perhaps a surgeon's personally owned set, usually are not sent out of the OR suite. They are handled only by the personnel directly responsible for their use and care: the circulator and scrub person can clean them within the confines of the OR and this adjacent room. (See Chapters 14 and 27 for precautions.)

The substerile room also usually contains a combination blanket and solution warmer, cabinets for storage, and perhaps a refrigerator for blood and medications. Specimen containers with labels may be conveniently stored in this room. Slips for charges or other records may be kept here. Individual hospitals may find it convenient to keep other items in this room to allow the circulator to remain in or immediately adjacent to the OR during the surgical procedure.

Doors

Ideally, sliding doors should be used in the OR. They eliminate the air currents caused by swinging doors. Microorganisms that have previously settled in the room are disturbed with each swing of the door. The microbial count is usually at its peak at the time of the skin incision because this follows disturbance of air by gowning, draping, movement of personnel, and doors. During the surgical procedure, the microbial count rises every time doors swing open from either direction. Also, swinging doors may touch a sterile table or person.

Sliding doors should not recede into the wall but should be of the surface-sliding type. Fire regulations mandate that sliding doors for ORs be of the type that can be swung open if necessary. *Doors do not remain open either during or between surgical procedures.* Closed doors decrease the mixing of air within the OR with that in the corridors, which may contain higher microbial counts. Air pressure in the room also is disrupted if the doors remain open.

Ventilation

The OR ventilation system must ensure a controlled supply of filtered air. Air changes and circulation provide fresh air and prevent accumulation of anesthetic gases in the room. Concentration of gases is dependent solely on the proportion of pure air entering the air system to the air recirculated through the system. Twenty to 30 air exchanges per hour are recommended for rooms with recirculated air. Some state building codes require 100% fresh air; others permit up to 80% recirculation of air. If air is recirculated, a gas scavenger system is mandatory to prevent the buildup of waste anesthetic gases. Various types of scavengers and evacuators are used to minimize air pollutants that are health risks for team members (see Chapter 10).

Ultraclean laminar airflow is installed in some ORs. This high-flow unidirectional air-blowing system is housed in a wall or ceiling enclosure. The value of this system in reducing airborne contamination is inconclusive (see Chapter 12, pp. 196-197). Other types of filtered air-delivery systems that have a high rate of airflow are as effective in controlling airborne contamination. Filtration through *high-efficiency particulate air (HEPA) filters* can be 90% efficient in removing particles that are larger than 0.5 µm. These microbial filters in ducts filter the air, practically eliminating all dust particles. The ventilating system in the OR suite is separate from the hospital's general system.

Positive air pressure (0.005 inch of water pressure) in each OR is greater than that in corridors, scrub areas, and substerile rooms. Positive pressure forces air from the room. The inlet is at the ceiling. Air leaves through the outlets at floor level. If the reverse is true, air is drawn into the room around the doors and through open doors. Microorganisms in the air can enter the room unless positive pressure is maintained.

An air-conditioning system is ideal and valuable. It controls humidity, which helps to reduce the possibility of explosion. High relative humidity (weight of water vapor present) should be maintained between 50% and 60%. A relative humidity of not less than 45% is mandatory. Moisture provides a relatively conductive medium, allowing static charge to leak to earth as fast as it is generated; sparks form more readily in atmospheres of low humidity.

Room temperature is maintained within a range of 68° to 75° F (20° to 24° C). A thermostat to control room temperature can be advantageous to meet patient needs: for example, the temperature can be increased to prevent development of hypothermia in pediatric, geriatric, or burn patients. However, overmanipulation of controls can result in calibration problems; controls should not be adjusted solely for the comfort of team members. Only the maintenance department can regulate temperature in some OR suites.

Even with controls of humidity and temperature, air-conditioning units may be a source of microorganisms that come through the filters. These must be changed at regular intervals. Ducts must be cleaned regularly.

Floors

Floors should be conductive enough to dissipate static from equipment and personnel but not conductive enough to endanger personnel from shock. To prevent the accumulation of electrostatic charges in locations where flammable anesthetic agents are used, conductive flooring must be installed. Conductive floors are available in many materials, including asphalt tile, linoleum, and terrazzo. The electrical resistance of these materials may change with age and cleaning. The surface of the floor provides a path of moderate electrical conductivity between all persons and equipment making contact with the floor.

Flooring in nonflammable anesthetizing locations does not have to be conductive. A variety of hard plastic, seamless materials are used for nonconductive floors. The surface of all floors must not be porous but suitably hard for cleaning by the flooding, wet-vacuuming technique. Personnel fatigue may be related to the type of flooring, which can be too hard or too soft. Cushioned flooring is available.

Walls and Ceiling

Finishes of all surface materials should be hard, nonporous, fire resistant, waterproof, stainproof, seamless, nonreflective, and easy to clean. The ceiling may have acoustic soundproof tiles.

Wall paneling made of hard vinyl materials is easy to clean and maintain. Seams can be sealed by a plastic filler. Laminated polyester or smooth, painted plaster provides a seamless wall; epoxy paint has a tendency to flake or chip, however. Dust and microorganisms can collect between tiles because the mortar between them is not smooth. Most grout lines, including those made of latex, are porous enough to harbor microorganisms even after cleaning. Tiles can also crack and break. A material that is able to withstand considerable impact also may have some value in noise control. Stainless steel cuffs at collision corners help prevent damage.

Walls and ceilings often are used to mount devices, utilities, and equipment in an effort to reduce clutter on the floor. In addition to the overhead operating light, the ceiling may be used for mounting an anesthesia service core, operating microscope, cryosurgery device, x-ray tube and image intensifier, electronic monitor, closed-circuit television, and a variety of hooks, poles, and tubes. Demands for ceiling-mounted equipment are diversified. However, suspended track mounts are not recommended because they engender fallout of dust-carrying microorganisms each time they are moved. If movable or track-ceiling devices are installed, they should not be mounted directly over the operating table but away from the center of the room and preferably recessed into the ceiling to minimize the possibility of dust accumulation and fallout.

Piped-in and Electrical Systems

Vacuum for suction, compressed air, oxygen, and/or nitrous oxide may be piped into the OR. The outlets may be located on the wall or suspended from the ceiling in either a fixed or retractable column. The anesthesiologist needs at least two outlets for oxygen and suction and one for nitrous oxide. To protect other rooms, the supply of oxygen and nitrous oxide to any room can be shut off at control panels in the corridor should trouble occur in a particular line. A panel light comes on and a buzzer sounds in the room and in the maintenance department. The buzzer can be turned off, but the panel light stays on until the problem is corrected.

Electrical outlets must meet the requirements of the equipment that will be used. Some machines require 220-volt power lines; others operate on 110 volts. Permanently mounted fixtures, such as a clock and x-ray viewing boxes, can be recessed into walls and wired rather than plugged into outlets. Outlets suspended from the ceiling should have locking plugs to prevent accidental disconnection. Grounded wall outlets are installed above the 5-foot (1.5 m) level, unless explosion-proof plugs are used. Electrical cords that extend down the wall and/or across the floor are hazardous. Straight or curved ceiling-mounted tracks are satisfactory for bringing piped-in gases, vacuums, and electrical outlets close to the operating table. They eliminate the hazard of tripping over cords, but insulation materials around electrical power sources from mobile, ceiling-mounted tracks must be protected from repeated flexing to prevent cracks and damage to wires. Rigid or retractable ceiling service columns eliminate these hazards.

Multiple electrical outlets should be available from separate circuits. This minimizes the possibility of a blown fuse or a faulty circuit shutting off all electricity at a critical moment.

All personnel must be aware that the use of electricity introduces the hazards of electric shock, power failure, and fire. Faulty electrical equipment may cause a short circuit or the electrocution of patients or personnel (see Chapter 10 for detailed discussion). These hazards can be prevented by:

1. Using only electrical equipment designed and approved for use in the OR. Equipment must have cords of adequate length and adequate current-carrying capacity to avoid overloading.
2. Testing portable equipment immediately before use and grounding correctly.
3. Discontinuing use immediately and reporting any faulty electrical equipment.

Fire safety systems are installed throughout the hospital. *All personnel must know the fire rules.* They must be familiar with the location of the alarm box and the use of fire extinguishers.

Lighting

General illumination is furnished by ceiling lights. Most room lights are white fluorescent but may be incandescent. Recessed lights do not collect dust. Lighting should be evenly distributed throughout the room. The anesthesiologist must have sufficient light, at least 200 footcandles, to adequately evaluate the patient's color.

To minimize eye fatigue, the ratio of intensity of general room lighting to that at the surgical site should not exceed 1:5, preferably 1:3. This contrast should be maintained in corridors and scrub areas, as well as in the room itself, so that the surgeon becomes accustomed to the light before entering the sterile field. Color and hue of the lights also should be consistent.

Illumination of the surgical site is dependent on the quality of light from an overhead source and the reflection from the drapes and tissues. White glistening tissues need less light than dull, dark tissues. Light must be of such quality that the pathologic conditions are recognizable. The overhead operating light must:

1. Make an intense light, within a range of 2500 to 12,500 footcandles (27,000 to 127,000 lux), into the incision without glare on the surface. It must give contrast to the depth and relationship of all anatomic structures. The light may be equipped with an intensity control. The surgeon will ask for more light when needed. A reserve light should be available.
2. Provide a diameter light pattern and focus appropriate for size of the incision. An optical prism system has a fixed diameter and focus. Other types have adjustable controls mounted on the fixture. Most fixtures provide focused depth by refracting light to illuminate both the body cavity and the general operating field. The focal point is where illumination is greatest. It should avoid a dark center at the surgical site. A 10- to 12-inch (25 to 30 cm) depth of focus allows the intensity to be relatively equal at both the surface and depth of the incision. To avoid glare, a circular field of 20 inches (25 cm) in diameter provides a 2-inch (5 cm) zone of maximum intensity in center of the field with one fifth intensity at the periphery.
3. Be shadowless. Multiple light sources and/or reflectors decrease shadows. In some units the relationship is fixed; others have separately maneuverable sources to direct light beams from converging angles.
4. Produce the blue-white color of daylight. Color quality of normal or diseased tissues is maintained within a spectral energy range of 3500° to 6700° Kelvin (K). Most surgeons prefer a color temperature of about 5000° K, which approximates the white light of a cloudless sky at noon.
5. Be freely adjustable to any position or angle by either a vertical or horizontal range of motion. Most overhead operating lights are ceiling mounted on mobile fixtures. Some have dual lights or dual tracks with sources on each track. These are designed for both lights to be used simultaneously to provide adequate intensity and minimize shadows in a single incision. Many fixtures are adapted so that the surgeon can direct the beam by manipulating sterile handles attached to the lamp or by remote control at the sterile field. Automatic positioning facilitates adjustment, and braking mechanisms prevent drift (i.e., a movement away from the desired position). Fixtures should be manipulated as little as possible to minimize dispersion of dust over the sterile field.
6. Produce a minimum of heat to prevent injuring exposed tissues. Most overhead lights dissipate heat into the room, where it is cooled by the air-conditioning system. Halogen bulbs generate less heat than other types. Lamps should produce less than 25,000 $\mu W/cm^2$ of radiant energy. If multiple light sources are used, collectively they must not exceed this limit at a single site. Beyond this range, the radiant energy produced by infrared rays changes to heat at or near the surface of exposed tissues. Some infrared and heat waves are absorbed by a filter globe over the light bulb or by an infrared cylindrical absorption filter of a prism optical system.
7. Be easily cleaned. Tracks recessed within the ceiling virtually eliminate dust accumulation. Suspension-mounted tracks or a centrally mounted fixture must have smooth surfaces that are easily accessible for cleaning.

An auxiliary light may be needed for a secondary surgical site. Some hospitals have portable explosion-proof lights. Others have satellite units that are part of the overhead lighting fixture. These should only be used for secondary sites unless the manufacturer states that the additional intensity is within safe radiant energy levels when used in conjunction with the main light source.

A source of light from a circuit separate from the usual supply must be available for use in case of power failure. This may require a separate emergency spotlight. It is best if the operating light is equipped so that an automatic switch can be made to the emergency source of lighting when the usual power fails.

Some surgeons prefer to work in a darkened room with only stark illumination of the surgical site. This is particularly true of surgeons working with endoscopic instruments and the operating microscope. (This equipment is discussed in Chapter 15.) If the room has windows, lightproof shades may be drawn to darken the room when this equipment is in use. Because of the hazard of dust fallout from shades, the windows may be painted in rooms where this equipment is routinely used. Even though the surgeon prefers the room darkened, the circulator or anesthesiologist must be able to see adequately to observe the patient's color and to monitor his or her condition. A grazing light over the floor can be installed.

Some surgeons wear a headlight designed to focus a light beam on a specific small area, usually in a recessed body cavity such as the nasopharynx. Fiberoptic headlights produce a cool light and reduce shadows. Both the surgeon and first assistant may wear a headlight. Alternatively, a light source that is an integral part of a sterile instrument such as a lighted retractor or fiberoptic cable may be used to illuminate deep cavities or tissues difficult to see with only the overhead operating light.

X-Ray Viewing Boxes

X-ray viewing boxes can be recessed into the wall. The viewing surface should accommodate standard-size films. The best location is in the line of vision of the surgeon standing at the operating table. Lights for x-ray viewers should be of high intensity.

Clock

A time-elapsed clock, which incorporates a warning signal, is useful for indicating that one or more predetermined periods of time have passed. This may be used during surgical procedures for total arterial occlusion, when using perfusion techniques or a pneumatic tourniquet, or during cardiac arrest.

Cabinets or Carts

Each OR is supplied with cabinets unless a cart system is used. Supplies for the types of surgical procedures done in that room are stocked, or every OR may be stocked with a standard number and type of supplies. Having these supplies saves steps for the circulator and helps to eliminate traffic in and out of the OR. Glass shelves and sliding doors provide ease in finding and taking out items. Many cabinets are made of stainless steel or hard plastic, however. Wire shelving minimizes dust accumulation. Cabinets must be easy to clean. One cabinet in the room may have a pegboard at the back to hang items, such as table appliances.

Pass-through cabinets that circulate clean air through them while maintaining positive air room pressure allow transfer of supplies from outside the OR to inside it. They help ensure the rotation of supplies in storage or can be used only for passing supplies as needed from a clean center core. Some pass-through cabinets between the OR and a corridor accommodate supply carts, which are easily removable for restocking.

In lieu of or as an adjunct to cabinets, some hospitals stock carts with special sutures, instruments, drugs, and other items for some or all of the surgical specialties. The appropriate cart is brought to the room for a specific surgical procedure.

Furniture and Other Equipment

Stainless steel furniture is plain, durable, and easily cleaned. Each OR is equipped with:

1. Operating table with a mattress covered with conductive rubber, attachments for positioning patient, and armboards.
2. Instrument tables.
3. Mayo stand. The *Mayo stand* is a frame with a removable rectangular stainless steel tray. The frame slides under the operating table and over the sterile field. The tray serves to bring near the surgical field a supply of instruments that are used frequently during the surgical procedure.
4. Small tables for gowns and gloves and/or patient's preparation equipment.
5. Ring stand for basin(s).
6. Anesthesia machine and table for anesthesiologist's equipment.
7. Sitting stools and standing platforms.
8. Standards (IV poles) or hangers for intravenous solution bags.
9. Suction bottle and tubing, either wall mounted or portable in a low-wheeled base.
10. Laundry hamper frame.
11. Kick buckets in wheeled bases.
12. Wastebasket.
13. Writing surface. This may be a wall-mounted, stainless steel desk or an area built into a cabinet for the circulator to document in the records.

Communication Systems

A communication system is a vital link to summon routine or emergency assistance or to relay information to and from the OR team. Many OR suites are equipped with telephones, intercoms, call-lights, video equipment, and computers. These communication systems may connect the OR with the clerk-receptionist's desk, the nurse manager's office, the holding area, the family waiting room, the PACU, the pathology and radiology departments, the blood bank, and the sterile processing department. These systems make instantaneous consultation possible through direct communication.

Voice Intercommunication System

Either monodirectional or bidirectional voice systems, via telephone or an intercommunication (intercom) system, are useful devices for the OR team but are potentially hazardous for patient. Sounds are distorted to the patient in early stages of general anesthesia. Incoming calls over an intercom should not be permitted to disturb the patient at this time. Also, an awake patient should not receive traumatic information about a pathologic diagnosis, for example, from a strange voice coming through an intercom speaker box after a biopsy has been performed. Installing any type of intercom equipment either in the adjacent substerile room or scrub area rather than in the OR helps to eliminate sounds that could disturb both the patient and the surgeon.

Call-Light System

In addition to or instead of a voice system, a call-light system can summon assistance from the anesthesia staff, pathologist, nursing staff, and/or housekeeping personnel. Activated in the OR by a foot- or hand-operated switch, a light alerts personnel at a central point in the suite or displays at several receiving points simultaneously.

Closed-Circuit Television

Television surveillance is an easy way for the nurse manager to keep abreast of activities in each OR. By means of a black-and-white television camera with a wide-angle lens mounted high in the corner of each OR, the manager may make rounds simply by switching from one room to another by pushing buttons at his or her desk and viewing a screen in the office.

More commonly, television serves a number of useful purposes for the surgeon in the OR. It is widely used for teaching surgical techniques. This keeps visitors out of the OR, which, in the interest of sterile technique, is advantageous. In addition, television provides a better view for more persons to see the surgical procedure from a remote area or through a microscope or endoscope. It can also be used for record keeping and documentation for legal purposes for the surgeon.

As an aid to diagnosis, an audiovideo hookup between the OR and the x-ray department permits x-ray films to be viewed on the television screen in the OR without having to transport the films into the OR and mount them on viewing boxes. With such a hookup, the surgeon gains the advantage of remote interpretive consultation when it is desired.

A two-way audiovideo system between the frozen-section laboratory and the OR enables the surgeon to examine the microscopic slide by video in consultation with the pathologist without leaving the operating table. The pathologist can view the site of the pathologic lesion without entering the OR.

For these purposes the color television camera may be mounted over the operating table in one of a number of ways. Usually it is attached to the stem of the operating light and outfitted with detachable sterilizable handles. An operating light with a television camera mounted in the center is available.

Video screens usually are adapted television sets and may be wall mounted or placed on floor stands that can be moved readily. All pieces of television equipment must be labeled to indicate that they comply with applicable electrical safety regulations for use in the OR. They also must be encased in nonporous materials that can be easily cleaned.

Computers

A computer terminal in each OR affords access to information and allows data input by the circulator. The type of hardware and software programs available dictates the capabilities of the automated information system. A keyboard, light pen, and/or bar code scanner may be used for input. The computer processes and stores information for retrieval on the viewing monitor and by printout from a central processing unit. The computer database assists the circulator to obtain and enter information that may include:

1. Schedule, including patient's name, surgeon, procedure, special or unusual equipment requirements, wound classification, elective or emergency procedure
2. Preoperative patient assessment data, nursing diagnoses, expected outcomes, and plan of care
3. Results of laboratory and diagnostic tests
4. Surgeon's preference card with capability to update
5. Inventory of supplies and equipment provided and used
6. Charges for direct patient billing
7. Intraoperative nursing interventions
8. Timing parameters including anesthesia, procedure, and room turnover
9. Incident reports

The computer terminal may be mounted on the wall or placed on a shelf or a portable table or cart. The computer keyboard can be moved so the circulator can see the patient and the activities of the OR team while documenting intraoperative information, electronically, into the record. The computerized patient information that is generated in the OR may interface with the hospital-wide computer system.

Monitoring Equipment

Monitors and computers are designed to keep the OR team aware of the physiologic functions of the patient throughout the surgical procedure and to record patient data. The anesthesiologist or a perioperative nurse uses monitoring devices as an added means to ensure safety for the patient during the surgical procedure (see Chapter 19).

In some hospitals a central room may be set up to monitor all patients undergoing surgical procedures. More frequently, the monitors are housed in a room immediately adjacent to the OR, separated by a glass partition. These rooms are staffed by well-trained personnel familiar with the types of monitoring or computerized equipment in use. Documentation from computerized monitors becomes a part of the patient's medical record.

SPECIAL PROCEDURE ROOMS

Cardiac Catheterization Room

Cardiac catheterization may be performed within the OR suite in a room equipped for fluoroscopy. Imaging screens are located near the head of the table to allow the surgeon and the team to visualize the coronary arteries during the procedure. Monitors, suction, oxygen, and cardiopulmonary resuscitation equipment are available in this room for each cardiac catheterization procedure. The team must be alert for emergency situations, such as a perforated coronary artery, and be prepared for an emergency thoracotomy or transfer to an OR for an open procedure (see Chapter 39).

Endoscopy Room

Many OR suites have a designated room in which endoscopic procedures, such as bronchoscopy, are performed. Most are equipped for the use of lasers and electrosurgery. Some endoscopy rooms have x-ray and video capabilities (see Chapter 15).

Cystoscopy Room

A cystoscopy room may be available for a urologic endoscopic examination or procedure. This room may be equipped with special floor drains for the disposal of fluids during the procedure. It is also equipped with x-ray and fluoroscopy machines because many procedures require the use of radiopaque contrast media to visualize the kidneys, ureters, and bladder. Imaging screens are located in the room to allow the urologist to visualize the urologic structures during fluoroscopy. Some urologists use ultrasonic waves, lasers, and electrosurgery to perform minimally invasive procedures. (See discussion of urologic endoscopy in Chapter 31, pp. 633-636.)

BIBLIOGRAPHY

Fogg D: Clinical issues: operating room construction requirements, *AORN J* 53(2):496-497, 1991.

Mathias JM: Advanced technology in the operating room, *OR Manager* 8(5):10-13, 1992.

McLean VJ: Computerized preference lists, *AORN J* 52(3):509-522, 1990.

OR design: Profiles of four new surgical suites, *OR Manager* 8(7):10-13, 1992.

Patterson P: OR automation: OR automation pushes into intraop charting, integration; computer linkages help to streamline care; hospitals linking 'Islands of automation'; making management reports work for you, *OR Manager* 9(5):1, 6-9, 11-14, 1993.

Patterson P: OR design: floor plans establish traffic patterns for people and supplies; materials handling systems, *OR Manager* 8(6):10-15, 1992.

Rea CM, Walker GJ: Designing a state-of-the-art operating room complex, *Today's OR Nurse* 12(3):28-32, 1990.

Recommended Practices: traffic patterns in the surgical suite, *AORN J* 57(3):730-734, 1993.

Schmaus DC: Computers in the OR, *AORN J* 52(6):1250-1253, 1990.

Schmaus DC: Computer security and data confidentiality, *AORN J* 54(4):885-890, 1991.

Schrader E: Computer in every room: a growing trend, *OR Manager* 7(9):1, 10-11, 1991.

Smith CD: Clinical Issues: OR temperature, humidity control, *AORN J* 58(5):1023-1025, 1993.

Welch TC: A case cart system, *AORN J* 52(5):993-998, 1990.

CHAPTER 10

Potential Sources of Injury to Caregiver and Patient

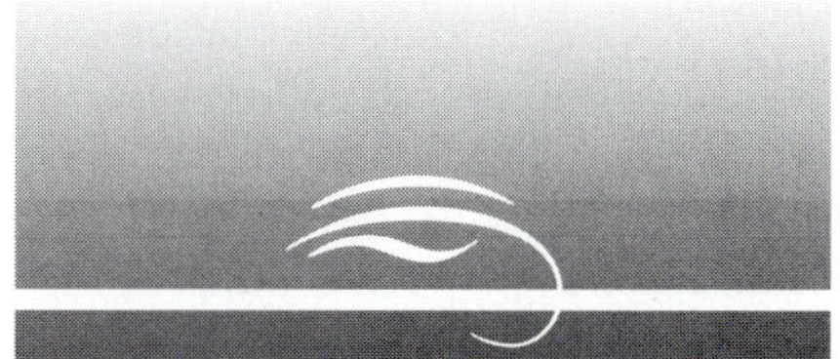

Every employer must provide as safe a working environment as possible for employees. Every employee must make full and proper use of safety and control measures and respect the equipment. Proper care, handling, and use ensure efficient functioning and safety. Patient safety is a prime consideration stressed throughout this text. Personnel safety is equally important. Safety goes hand in hand with competence, efficiency, and productivity.

Literally, the word *safe* is defined as free from risk or harm. Because of the many hazards in the environment, neither patients nor personnel are completely free from risks. However, these risks can be minimized. Potential hazards must be identified and safe practices established. Legally, *safety* refers to conditions for the employee, the patient, and other persons in the health care facility that will not cause injury or harm.

From a risk management perspective, education and training of employees are essential. Personnel should be aware of hazards. No one should be allowed to use equipment until he or she has been properly instructed in its correct use and care. Each employee should use his or her own initiative to seek instruction when needed.

ENVIRONMENTAL HAZARDS

The operating room (OR) is a location fraught with hazards for both patients and personnel. Possibilities for physical injury from electric shock, burns, fire, explosion, and inhalation of toxic substances are ever present. Therefore it is mandatory that staff have knowledge of hazards involved in use of equipment, causes of accidental injury, and sources of health risks. All individuals have a personal responsibility for ensuring a safe environment for themselves and others. Faulty equipment or improper usage increases hazards of potential risk factors.

Concern about fire and explosions caused by anesthetic agents intensified in 1925 with the introduction of ethylene gas, in addition to the already popular use of drop ether. In the following decade cyclopropane, another highly flammable gas, became popular. The potential hazard of static electricity causing combustion of flammable anesthetics has been minimized by elimination of these agents. Ignition from thermal devices is a fire hazard, however. Electric shock, electrocution, burns, exposure to carcinogens and mutagens, inhalation of toxic chemicals, and transmission of pathogenic microorganisms remain potential hazards in the OR.

Classification of Hazards

Injuries can be caused by using faulty equipment or using equipment improperly, by exposing oneself or others to toxic or irritating agents or by contacting harmful agents. Hazards in the OR environment can be classified as:

1. *Physical,* including back injury, fall, noise pollution, radiation, electricity, and fire
2. *Chemical,* including anesthetic gases, toxic fumes from gases and liquids, cytotoxic drugs, and cleaning agents
3. *Biologic,* including patient as host for or source of pathogenic microorganisms, infectious waste, cuts or needlestick injuries, surgical plume, and latex sensitivity

Regulation of Hazards

Standards, guidelines, and recommended practices have been developed by many professional associations and governmental agencies for environmental, patient, and personnel safety. (See Chapter 4, pp. 56-58, for a list of many of these resources.) Policies and procedures of the health care facility should be in compliance with local, state, and federal regulations.

In 1970 the Occupational Safety and Health Administration (OSHA) was created within the U.S. Department of Labor. Initially, OSHA adopted preexisting federal and national consensus standards and guidelines. For example, the U.S. government had issued information, recommendations, and regulations for use of anesthetic agents since 1941. The American Conference of Governmental Industrial Hygienists (ACGIH) developed a list of threshold limit values (TLV) for exposure to toxic materials. The American National Standards Institute (ANSI) continues to develop standards for exposure to toxic materials and use of hazardous equipment. Since its inception, OSHA has issued new standards and amended others. OSHA standards include permissible exposure limits (PEL) to occupational health and safety hazards. OSHA is authorized to enforce its standards. Some of these regulations require:

1. Providing protection from high noise levels for prolonged periods
2. Minimizing exposure to ionizing radiation
3. Safeguarding exposure from instruments that emit sound or radio waves, visible light, infrared, ultraviolet, and nonionizing electromagnetic radiation as recommended by ANSI
4. Meeting standards for laser safety as developed by ANSI
5. Meeting standards of electrical codes and fire safety as developed by the National Fire Protection Association (NFPA)
6. Installing ventilating systems that maintain no more than maximum permissible concentrations of atmospheric contamination from toxic and/or flammable chemical vapors and gases as recommended by National Institute for Occupational Safety and Health (NIOSH)
7. Initiating procedures for safe use, handling, storage, and dispensing of flammable and combustible liquids
8. Monitoring procedures for infection control as recommended by the Centers for Disease Control and Prevention (CDC)
9. Disposing of infectious and hazardous wastes

OSHA standards may require employers to measure and monitor exposure to toxic or harmful agents, to notify employees of overexposure and provide medical consultation or care, and to maintain records of corrective actions. OSHA inspects health care facilities for compliance with standards. The Environmental Protection Agency (EPA) also enforces its recommendations and guidelines.

PHYSICAL HAZARDS AND SAFEGUARDS

Architectural design of the OR suite affects overall efficiency and productivity. As described in Chapter 9, the physical facility is designed to control traffic patterns, decrease contamination, facilitate the handling of equipment and supplies, and provide a comfortable working environment. The worker should be at ease but also should protect himself or herself, other team members, and patients from injury.

Environmental Factors

Several factors contribute to providing a comfortable working environment: ventilation, odor, lighting, color, and noise. Ventilation should provide physical comfort (i.e., it should not be too warm or too cool). It is difficult to concentrate when room temperature causes sweating or shivering. The ventilating system usually evacuates odors fairly quickly. However, heavy perfume can have an annoying, lingering effect. Perfume and other odors can cause nausea or respiratory congestion in sensitive persons. Ventilating systems should help remove toxic fumes and waste anesthetic gases.

Lighting should be adequate; however, excessive glare produces fatigue. Illumination is the product of the light times the reflectance of the target. A bright, highly polished mirror finish on an instrument tends to reflect light and can restrict the vision of the surgeon. Satin- or dull-finished instruments eliminate glare and lessen the surgeon's eye strain. These instruments are made with varying degrees of dullness depending on the manufacturer. Tinted or polarized glasses may save the sterile team members from visual fatigue but should not distort color of tissues.

Soft pastel colors, especially blues and greens, are less reflective for drapes and walls than white. Drapes with dark tones help reduce contrast between most tissues and the surrounding field. Some OR suites have murals on the walls to enhance the visual effect of the environment, particularly if the suite is windowless.

Although attention is given to ventilation, lighting, and color, less attention is given to the design of the OR in terms of auditory effects. Some hospitals have piped-in music. Music can be relaxing for the patient awaiting surgery or undergoing a surgical procedure under local anesthesia and stimulating for personnel. Music with a moderate rhythm and bright tone can motivate muscular activity and increase levels of efficiency. This would not be conducive to relaxation for the patient, however. Selection of music should be appropriate for the intended listener. It can be a distraction and an annoyance, especially for the anesthesiologist who may depend on hearing to aid in monitoring the patient. Music should always be played at low volume in the OR. It should be turned off at the request of the patient, surgeon, or anesthesiologist. Constant playing of music can be more harmful than beneficial for personnel; therefore it should be turned off periodically to help prevent mental fatigue.

Noise can be irritating and potentially dangerous to patients and personnel. It can become intense enough to increase blood pressure and to provoke peripheral vasoconstriction, dilatation of the pupils, and other subtle physiologic effects. It can also interfere with necessary communication and thereby provoke irritation. The EPA recommends that noise levels in hospitals not exceed 45 decibels during daytime hours.

The OR should be as quiet as possible except for the essential sounds of communication between team members directly concerned with the patient's care. When it is necessary to talk, do so in a low voice. Conversation unrelated to the surgical procedure is out of place. Even during deep stages of anesthesia, an anesthetized patient does perceive noises and conversations that occur during the surgical procedure and may remember them. If a regional or local anesthetic is used, remember that the patient can hear the conversation. Patients interpret anything they hear in terms of themselves, so all words should be guarded. Counts or requests for supplies should be done quietly, so the patient cannot hear.

Major sources of noise in the OR involve paper, gloves, objects wheeled across the floor, instruments striking one another, monitors, and high-pitched powered instruments including suction. The scrub person should keep these sources and their effects in mind. Avoid clattering instruments. Clamp off or kink a loop into suction tubing except while in actual use. The circulator should keep doors closed to shut out noise in corridors, of water running in the scrub room, or of the sterilizer operating in the substerile room. Do not crush paper wrappings. Hold a bottle of solution inches, not feet, away from basin when pouring. Monitors with audible signals should be placed as far away from the patient's ears as possible, with the amplifier turned away from the patient.

Working in a pleasantly quiet environment is less fatiguing, with fewer psychologic and physiologic adverse effects, and allows for greater efficiency on behalf of the patient. Monitor alarms also can be distractions for the surgeon and anesthesiologist.

Body Mechanics

The human body was not designed to do many of the things that the job requires of OR personnel. Consequently, backache is a leading cause of work-related lost time, second only to upper respiratory infections. Standing for prolonged periods, often in an awkward position, is a cause of low back pain. Tiring body motions or awkward or strained body posture should be avoided. During standing work, when the heels are together, constant muscular effort is required by the thigh muscles to maintain an erect posture. In contrast, when the heels are apart, the ligaments of the hips and knees support the body without effort. A wide stance while standing at the operating table for prolonged periods will be less fatiguing for the scrub person. The circulator can stand in a location to observe both the surgical procedure and the instrument table with the upper and lower extremities in a resting position. In this standing position the arms are clasped behind the back and the feet are in a wide stance. Weight bearing on only one foot causes additional strain.

The operating table is adjusted to the best height for the surgeon. This may not be the most comfortable position for the other members of the sterile team. Team members should be able to stand erect with their arms comfortably relaxed from the shoulders, without stooping, and should not have to raise their hands above the level of their elbows for the majority of their work motions. Foot platforms (standing stools) may be needed to elevate the scrub person and/or the assistant surgeon to a feasible working height. Platforms should be long enough to allow a wide stance.

Correct posture in the sitting position is equally important. The back is strongest when it is straight. When seated, sit well back in the chair or on a stool with the body straight from hips to neck. Lean forward from the hips, not from the shoulders or waist. This position puts the least strain on muscles, ligaments, and internal organs. Before and after the surgical procedure, the circulator and scrub person(s) should rest in a sitting position between periods of standing. If work is done in a sitting position, the stool or chair should be adjusted to the correct height for the working surface.

Sprains and strains are common injuries sustained to back, arms, or shoulders from lifting patients or moving equipment. Several principles of body mechanics should be observed to minimize physical injury.

1. Keep the body as close as possible to the person or equipment to be lifted or moved, maintaining a straight back
2. Lift with the legs and abdominal muscles, not the back
3. Bend the knees to get body weight under load, then straighten the legs to lift with heels flat on floor
4. Lift with a slow, even motion, keeping pressure off the lumbar (lower back) area
5. Push, do not pull, stretchers, tables, and heavy equipment on wheels or casters
6. Use large body muscles to maneuver the base of portable equipment, such as lasers or microscopes
7. Stand for prolonged periods in a wide stance with heels apart, so the ligaments of the hips and knees support the body without effort
8. Distribute weight evenly on both feet, but shift the body occasionally during prolonged periods of standing
9. Sit with back straight from the hips to the neck, and lean forward from the hips
10. Align the head and neck with the body when standing or sitting, maintaining lumbar curve
11. Change position, stretch, or walk around occasionally if possible
12. Pivot the entire body to avoid twisting at the waist
13. Bend forward with hip flexion and hand support
14. Avoid overhead reaching or overstretching; keep materials in chest-to-knee range if possible; use foot platforms as appropriate

A lifting frame or Davis roller helps relieve the potential strain of moving unconscious or obese patients. Do not try to move these patients alone. Assistance may also be needed to position patients on the operating table. The physical therapy department or occupational health director can be a resource to teach nursing staff proper techniques for lifting, bending, reaching, and pivoting.

Ionizing Radiation

Radiation cannot be seen or felt. However, ionizing radiation produces positively and negatively charged particles that can change the electrical charge of some atoms and molecules in cells. These changes can alter enzymes, proteins, cell membranes, and genetic material. This can cause death of cancer cells when radiation is used in therapeutic doses; however, exposure to radiation also can cause cancer, cataracts, injury to bone marrow, burns, tissue necrosis, genetic mutations, spontaneous abortion, and congenital anomalies.

OR nursing personnel may assist with invasive x-ray studies. If unprotected, they are exposed to scatter radiation from patient during intraoperative procedures when x-rays are taken or fluoroscopes and image intensifiers are used. Team members are exposed during implantation or removal of radioactive elements. Patients exposed to radioactivity for therapeutic purposes or by accident may emit radiation. The effect of radiation is directly related to the amount and length of time of exposure. Exposure is cumulative with an extended latency period. The effects may not be evident for years. Therefore constant vigilance for personal safety is essential to avoid excessive exposure to ionizing radiation. Protection implies understanding basic terminology and adhering to strict policies and procedures.

Definitions Pertaining to Radiation

The terms defined in Box 10-1 are sequenced to help the learner understand the concept of ionizing radiation. Its use for diagnostic and therapeutic procedures is discussed in detail later in the text (see Chapters 28 and 45).

Safety Considerations in Use of Ionizing Radiation

Because of adverse and cumulative effects of ionizing radiation on body tissues, safety precautions are taken to protect patients and personnel from potential hazards.

Patient Safety The patient is exposed to the primary beam of x-rays and radioactivity of implants and to scatter radiation. Any exposure to radiation has biologic risks. Therefore exposure should be as low as possible.

1. Fluoroscope should be turned off when not in use. The patient is continuously exposed to radiation during fluoroscopy.
2. Every effort to reconcile an incorrect sponge, sharp, or instrument count should be taken. An x-ray film should be taken as a last resort to locate an item that is unaccounted for.
3. Body areas should be shielded from scatter radiation or focused beam whenever possible. A lead shield can be positioned between patient and radiation source if it will not interfere with the sterile field or visualization for the x-ray study. This is placed before the patient is draped. A shadow shield connected to the x-ray tube may be a preferable alternative if a lead shield cannot be used.

BOX 10-1

Glossary of Terms Related to Ionizing Radiation

radiation Process of emitting radiant energy in form of electromagnetic waves or atomic particles or combined process of emitting and transmitting radiant energy.

ionizing radiation Sufficient radiant energy to yield ions from disintegration of nuclei of unstable or radioactive elements. These ions disrupt electronic balance of atoms. This occurs naturally from cosmic rays. Manmade x-rays and nuclear power are capable of modifying molecules within body cells as they pass through tissue. They can be mutagenic, that is, cause mutations of DNA in somatic body cells predisposing to cancer and in germ cells predisposing to spontaneous abortion or congenital malformations.

nonionizing radiation Radiant energy does not produce ions but can produce hyperthermic conditions harmful to skin and eyes. Wavelengths from electromagnetic spectrum do not alter DNA in body cells, with possible exception of ultraviolet rays.

emissions Electromagnetic waves or atomic particles spontaneously given off by ionizing radioactive elements.

alpha particles Relatively large particles with dense ionization within short distances emitted from disintegrating radioactive atoms. They are easily stopped by thin sheet of paper.

beta particles Relatively small particles with greater penetration at faster speed than alpha particles. They also are easily stopped.

gamma rays High-energy, short electromagnetic wavelengths emitted spontaneously from nucleus of radioactive atom. They have no mass, but they can be stopped by dense material such as lead.

x-rays High-energy electromagnetic waves capable of penetrating various thicknesses of solid substances and affecting photographic plates. They are generated from high-velocity electrons only when machine that produces them is turned on. They can be stopped by dense material such as lead or concrete.

exposure Total quantity of radiation body receives. This is cumulative over a lifetime.

external exposure X-rays and gamma rays originate from outside body, pass through it, and then are gone. Extent of exposure depends on amount of radiation, time of exposure, distance from source, and shielding of body.

internal exposure Radiation source is placed within body or directed to exposed body tissue. Alpha or beta particles or gamma rays may be emitted from elements that are intentionally implanted or injected or inadvertently inhaled, ingested, or absorbed by body. Internal sources of radiation within patient become external source of exposure for health care providers.

latency period Long-term effects of cumulative exposure may not be evident for several years, perhaps as long as 20 years.

scatter radiation X-rays travel in a straight, focused beam from generating tube until they strike obstacle, usually the patient. Most of beam penetrates through patient, but some radiation randomly scatters around patient through room air until it is absorbed. Densest areas of scatter radiation are within 45-degree angles on each side of patient.

inverse square law Amount of radiation received is decreased in proportion to square of the distance from *small* source, such as focused beam from x-ray tube. For example, when distance away from source is doubled, dose rate is decreased by 25%; at 2 feet from source, exposure is one fourth that at 1 foot. If radiation source is large, inverse square law may not apply, but exposure will decrease significantly with distance.

sources Alpha or beta particles are emitted from different sources than those that generate gamma rays and x-rays. Sources used in OR include:

fluoroscope Fluorescent light reproduces optical images of body structures identified by x-rays onto luminescent screen. These images can be amplified with *image intensifier*. They can be projected on television monitor. Radiation exposure can be as much as 10 times greater during 1 minute of fluoroscopy than that of single x-ray.

x-ray machine Fixed or portable generator projects x-rays through enclosed tube directed at patient. Focused beam passes through patient to photographic film only when generator is activated for single exposure.

radioactive implants Radioactive elements continuously emit alpha and beta particles and/or gamma rays. All radiation sources for therapeutic implantation are prepared by nuclear medicine department. They require very special handling in OR for safety of both patients and personnel (see Chapter 45, p. 925). *Radionuclides* have primarily replaced therapeutic use of radium and radon. Radionuclide is element that has been bombarded in nuclear reactor with radioactive particles. As it disintegrates, it emits radiation.

external beam Gamma or x-rays are generated from orthovoltage (low) or megavoltage (high) linear accelerators or betatrons for preoperative, intraoperative, or postoperative radiation therapy (see Chapter 45, pp. 925-926).

measurements Intensity of radiation is expressed in different units of measurement.

roentgen (R) Roentgens are measures of pairs of ions (charged particles) produced in air by gamma rays and x-rays, used in calibration of radiation-producing sources.

radiation absorbed dose (rad) Rad is unit of absorbed dose from all types of ionizing radiation, calculated as 100 units of energy per gram.

Continued

BOX 10-1

Glossary of Terms Related to Ionizing Radiation—cont'd

roentgen equivalent man (rem) Rem is unit of equivalent dose derived by multiplying rads by quality factors for relative biologic effects of type of radiation. Rem is measurement used in occupational monitoring: 1 rem = 1 R = 1 rad; 1 milliroentgen (mR) = 1/1000 rem.

sievert (Sv) Sievert is international unit of measure for equivalent dose, that is, absorbed dose weighted by quality factor for type of radiation: 1 Sv = 100 rem; 1 millisievert (mSv) = 1/1000 Sv = 100 mR.

curie Curie measures radioactivity or number of spontaneous nuclear transformations per unit of time. It has no direct relationship to ionization, absorption, and dose equivalent.

half-life Half-life is time required for radioactive element to lose 50% of its activity by disintegration or time required for body to eliminate one half of administered dose. Each radionuclide has its own half-life.

permissible dose National Council on Radiation Protection and Measurements has formulated government standards for certification of x-ray equipment and for human exposure. Permissible doses of radiation are based on *units of equivalent dose*—quantity that expresses all radiations on common scale for purpose of calculating their biologic effects. *Maximum permissible doses per year* for occupationally exposed persons over 18 years of age varies by body parts:

- Whole body, including blood-forming organs, bone marrow, and gonads = 5 rem, 50 mSv
- Lenses of eyes = 15 rem, 150 mSv
- Other organs and tissues = 50 rem, 500 mSv
- Fetus in utero = 0.5 rem, 5 mSv; no more than 50 mR, 0.5 mSv in any 1 month of gestation during pregnancy

Exposure should not exceed 100 mR, 1 mSv per week. With protective precautions OR personnel rarely, if ever, exceed this limit.

monitors Monitoring devices measure rems or sieverts of occupational exposure to ionizing radiation. These are recommended for each person with probability of exceeding 25% of maximum permissible dose of 5 rem (50 mSv) per year as result of frequent proximity to radiation sources.

shields Lead shields provide best protection from gamma and x-rays to halt and absorb radiant energy. Lead in thickness of 0.5 mm reduces scatter radiation exposure by 80% to 90%. Lead aprons, eyeglasses, gloves, gonadal shields, and thyroid collars can be worn. Lead screens and walls absorb radiation.

time Shorter the exposure, less the amount of radiation absorbed.

a. Thyroid/sternal shield should be used during x-rays or fluoroscopy of the head, upper extremities, and chest. Lymphatic tissue, thyroid, and bone marrow of the sternum are especially sensitive to radiation.
b. Gonadal or ovarian shield should be used during x-rays or fluoroscopy of the hips and thighs to protect the testes or ovaries.
c. Lead shield should always be used to protect the fetus of a pregnant patient. X-rays to the abdomen and pelvis are avoided, especially during the first trimester. Even low levels of scatter radiation may be harmful to the fetus.

Intraoperative documentation should include anatomic location of direct beam x-rays or fluoroscopy, type and location of radioactive implants, and shielding measures to protect the patient from scatter radiation. Other factors to be considered for the welfare of the patient when x-rays are taken or fluoroscopy is used in the OR are discussed in Chapter 28, p. 571. Safety rules for handling radioactive elements used for radiation therapy are discussed in Chapter 45, p. 925.

Personnel Safety Safety precautions should be taken to protect oneself and team members from potential hazards of ionizing radiation. Always remember key factors: *time, distance,* and *shielding*.

TIME Overexposure and unnecessary exposure of any person, especially one of child-bearing age, must be avoided. Changes that may occur in reproductive cells leading to future genetic defects are potential hazards.

1. Nursing personnel should rotate assignments on procedures that involve radiation.
2. Staff member may request relief from exposure during pregnancy. If this is not possible, a pregnant staff member should leave the room or be adequately shielded when x-rays are taken or fluoroscopy is used.
3. Radiation from an x-ray tube, fluoroscope, and image intensifier is present only as long as the machine is energized. Machines should be turned off when not in use.
4. Radioactive elements should remain in lead-lined containers until ready for implantation. They should

be handled as quickly as possible, and always with special forceps, by trained personnel.

5. Patient who has received radioactive substances for diagnostic studies may emit up to 2 milliroentgen (2 mR) per hour. If possible, the surgical procedure should be delayed for at least 24 hours posttest.
6. Personnel should limit time in close proximity to the patient who has had a diagnostic study with or implantation of radioactive elements until disintegration reaches low level.
7. Body tissues and fluids removed from patients with radioactive emissions should be contained quickly.

DISTANCE Automatic or manual collimators that confine the x-ray beam to the precise size of the x-ray film or fluoroscopic screen are required for all equipment. Most image intensifiers have a lead shield as part of the installation. A single-frame videodisc recording device incorporated into the fluoroscopy system also helps reduce exposure. Fluoroscopy produces more scatter radiation than direct x-ray beams. Personnel should distance themselves as far as possible from the radiation source.

1. Unsterile team members who can safely do so should leave the room during each single x-ray exposure.
2. Holding devices should be used to maintain the position of x-ray film and patient.
3. Sterile team members and others who cannot leave room should stand 6 feet (2 m) or more from patient, if possible, and out of direct beam during exposure. Remember the inverse square law of distance: double distance equals one fourth intensity.
4. Stand behind or at a right angle to the beam on the side of patient where beam enters, not exits, if possible.
5. Lateral or oblique x-rays increase scatter radiation. Positioning the beam in a plane vertical to the pelvis or thighs helps reduce scatter. Supine and upright x-rays direct beam at floor or walls.

SHIELDING Lead, at least 0.5 mm thick, is the most effective protection against gamma and x-rays to halt and absorb radiation scatter. Alpha and beta particles do not require shielding.

1. Walls of rooms with fixed radiation equipment usually are lead lined. Gamma rays can penetrate lead to a depth of 12 inches (30.7 cm). X-rays may be stopped by lead or thick concrete.
2. Portable lead screens should be available.
   a. Sterile team members and others who cannot leave the room should stand behind a screen while x-rays are taken or the patient is exposed to intraoperative radiation therapy. Screen(s) should be positioned behind a portable machine.
   b. Screen should be positioned behind the x-ray film cassette when a lateral exposure is taken to absorb rays that penetrate through or scatter from the cassette.
   c. Person preparing radioactive implants emitting gamma rays should do so from behind a lead screen that is up to 12 inches (30.7 cm) thick. A sterile drape can be put over the screen so the scrub person or other sterile team member can stand behind the screen and reach around it.
3. Lead aprons can be worn by sterile and unsterile team members.
   a. Apron is worn under sterile gown.
   b. If the apron does not wrap around the body, face the radiation source so the apron provides protection between the source and the body.
   c. Team members should wear aprons during fluoroscopy and for lateral or oblique x-rays to protect against beam and scatter radiation. Levels of scatter radiation are greater at lateral and oblique angles, and exposure time is prolonged during fluoroscopy.
   d. Lead aprons should be hung or laid flat when not in use. They should *never* be folded. Folding can crack the lead, making the shield ineffective.
4. Lead-impregnated rubber gloves can attenuate (reduce intensity) of rays by 15% to 25%.
   a. Sterile gloves should be worn by sterile team members when the hands will be in direct exposure, as during fluoroscopy, for injecting radioactive dyes or elements and while handling radioactive implants.
   b. If it is necessary to hold a cassette in position for a single x-ray exposure, lead gloves should be worn.
   c. Lead gloves may be supplied sterile or be sterilized by ethylene oxide gas for reuse. Aeration should be adequate from rubber to avoid skin irritation of wearer.
5. Lead thyroid/sternal collars or shields should be worn during fluoroscopy and exposure to oblique angle x-rays. Personnel, including the anesthesiologist, within 6 feet (2 m) of the radiation source risk exposure of the head and neck.
6. Leaded glasses may be worn to protect eyes during fluoroscopy.

Lead shields should be tested routinely by the radiology department every 6 months or whenever damage is suspected. Defects may not be visually detected.

Monitoring Radiation Exposure

All personnel who will be exposed to ionizing radiation with any frequency or during prolonged procedures should wear a monitoring device. The purpose of the device is to measure total rems of accumulated exposure. Therefore the monitor is worn only by the person to whom it is issued and at all times of exposure for the designated period. Exposure data on the monitor are recorded for each individual, either monthly or weekly, depending on the type of monitor.

Film badges are the most widely used monitors. These contain small pieces of photographic film sensitive to different types of radiation: beta, gamma, and x-rays. Thermoluminescent badges and pocket dosimeters also are available. More than one monitor, of the same or a different type, may be worn.

Placement of the monitor determines the body parts being monitored. The monitor should be consistently worn at the same area. A single monitor can be worn outside a lead apron at the level of the neck to measure exposure of head and neck, especially during fluoroscopy. Another monitor may be worn under the apron to measure exposure of the whole body and gonads.

Nonionizing Radiation

Radiant energy, in the form of heat and/or light, is emitted from radiowaves, microwaves, televisions, computers, radiant warmers, and light sources. For example, overhead operating lights produce heat. Fiberoptic light cables are cool, although the light transmitted is intense and can produce heat. Radiation from these sources is nonionizing, with the exception of ultraviolet lights that can produce radiant energy in sufficient wavelengths and intensity to alter DNA in cells. Nonionizing radiation is not accumulative in the body and therefore does not require monitoring. Nonionizing radiation per se is not hazardous when properly controlled.

Lasers concentrate very high-energy light beams within a small circumference to produce intense heat. Laser is an acronym for *light amplification by stimulated emission of radiation.* Laser equipment must be used in accordance with established regulatory standards, guidelines, and the manufacturer's instructions for laser safety. Lasers vaporize, cut, or coagulate tissues directly exposed to beams. However, they can cause thermal burns from indirect exposure. Fire, explosion, eye and skin exposure, and laser plume also are potential hazards for patients and personnel. Safety measures must be taken. Laser surgery is described in detail in Chapter 15, pp. 270-279, and its many uses are discussed by surgical specialty.

Electricity

Appropriate use of electronic devices is a prime concern of health care providers and industry personnel seeking safer patient care. Underlying this concern is the rapidly expanding use of electronic equipment. The marketing and safety standards of medical electronic devices used in the OR are federally regulated. The standards and practices recommended by the Association for the Advancement of Medical Instrumentation (AAMI) are helpful to both manufacturers and users. Standards of the Joint Commission on Accreditation of Healthcare Organizations (JCAHO) must be met for hospital accreditation as well. Inadequately trained personnel or malfunctions in equipment that cause short-circuiting of devices such as heart monitors, defibrillators, and x-ray machines are responsible for the fatalities and near-fatalities that occur.

Definitions Pertaining to Electrical Safety

Electrical safety is neither a major problem nor a complicated one if personnel understand the appropriate terminology and a few simple principles of electricity (Box 10-2).

Parameters of Electricity

Electricity is the flow of electrons along a path. It consists of three basic parameters.

Voltage Voltage forces electrons to move through material in one direction and causes current to flow. It is measured in *volts.* The greater the number of volts, the more direct the path of the current.

Resistance Resistance is the measurement of opposition to flow of electrons through material. It is measured in *ohms.* Electricity flows easily through conductors (i.e., metals, carbon, water). Flow is difficult through insulators (i.e., rubber, plastic, glass). Insulators prevent equalization of potential differences. The resistance of the human body is more similar to a conductor than an insulator.

Current Current is the rate of flow of electrons through a conductor. It is measured in *amperes,* the number of electrons passing a given point each second. The type of current may be:

1. *Direct current* (DC), as from a battery. This is a low-voltage current.
2. *Alternating current* (AC), as from a 110- or 220-volt line. The current has an alternating directional flow. AC is considered low voltage, but it is three times more dangerous than low-voltage DC.

Current flow is proportional to voltage and inversely proportional to resistance.

Grounding

Grounding of all electrical equipment is essential for safety and prevention of stray leakage current. Ground-

BOX 10-2

Glossary of Terms Related to Electrical Safety

anesthetizing location Any area of hospital or ambulatory care facility in which it is intended to administer any inhalation anesthetic agents in course of examination or treatment.

- **flammable anesthetizing location** Any location used or intended for use of flammable anesthetic agents where static electricity is potential hazard.
- **hazardous location** Space extending 5 feet (1.5 m) above floor during administration of flammable anesthetic agent.
- **nonflammable anesthetizing location** Any location used for, or intended for the *exclusive* use of, administration of nonflammable anesthetic agents.*

combustible Flammable substance capable of reacting with oxygen to burn if ignited.

conductive materials Not only those materials that are commonly considered as electrically conductive, such as metals, but also class of materials that, when tested in accordance with *NFPA standard 99C,* have resistance to passage of electricity not exceeding 1,000,000 ohms. Such materials are required where electrostatic interconnection is necessary.†

flammable Any gas or liquid, including oxygen, that will burn or is capable, when ignited, of maintaining combustion.

grounding Equipotential system of conductors that establishes conducting connection, whether intentional or accidental, between electrical circuit in equipment and earth or to some connecting body that serves in place of earth to divert stray currents.

isolated power system Assembly of electrical devices that provides local isolated power, single grounding point, and distinctive receptacles.

leakage current Any current not intended to be applied to a patient but that may be conveyed from exposed metal or other accessible parts of appliance to ground.†

line isolation monitor Instrument that continually checks hazard current from isolated circuit to ground.‡

macroshock Effect of large electric currents (milliamperes or larger) on body.‡

microshock Effect of small electric currents (as low as 10 microamperes) on body.†

nonflammable anesthetic agent Inhalation agents that, because of their vapor pressure at 98.6° F (37° C) and at atmospheric pressure (760 mm Hg), cannot attain flammable concentrations when mixed with air, oxygen, or mixtures of oxygen and nitrous oxide.

patient ground Terminal bus that serves as single focus for grounding all electric devices serving individual patient that are not connected by power cord to reference grounding point and for grounding conductive furniture or equipment within reach of person who may touch him or her.*

path of least resistance Return path for current to ground with minimal resistance or through leakage current.

*Modified from *NFPA 99C standard for medical gas,* National Fire Protection Association, Quincy, Mass, 1990.
†Excerpted from *NFPA 99C standard for medical gas,* National Fire Protection Association, Quincy, Mass, 1990.
‡From *NFPA 99C standard for medical gas,* National Fire Protection Association, Quincy, Mass, 1990.

ing systems are designed to prevent inadvertent passage of electric current through the patient by discharging any harmful potentials directly to the ground without including the patient in the circuit, thereby preventing shock or burn. Electric power is supplied through two wires: *hot* and *neutral.* These wires transmit current to the three-wire outlets in the building. The third wire is the ground wire. When the cord from an electrical device is plugged into an outlet, the hot and neutral wires deliver the current. The ground wire is attached to a copper pipe driven into the ground at the point where power enters the building. An electrical connection to the ground provides a means for current to flow through the ground wire or any other conductive surface connected to the ground rather than going to the neutral wire. The copper ground wire is used to prevent the metal housings of electrical equipment from becoming electrically "hot." The ground wire within the three-wire power plug and cord connects the equipment (instrument) housing to the ground contact in the receptacle (wall outlet). This provides a constantly available return path for current to the electrical source. If insulation on wires is defective, such as broken or frayed cords or plugs, some current will leak or flow to other nearby conductors, for example, the equipment housing. When an instrument is grounded, leakage current returns through the ground wire to earth, causing no damage. If the ground path is absent or broken, leakage current will seek another path to ground.

Equipotential Grounding System Current flows between points only when a voltage difference exists between them. Therefore electric shock can be minimized by eliminating voltage differences. One system designed to do this is the equipotential grounding system, which maintains an equal potential or voltage between all conductive surfaces near the patient. To achieve equipotential grounding, all exposed conductive surfaces within 6 feet (2 m) of the patient are electrically connected to a single point that is itself connected by a copper conductor to the ground tie point at the electrical distribution center serving the area. Consequently, all exposed metal surfaces are electrically tied together and to the ground.

Isolation Power System Isolated power systems are used in hazardous locations such as ORs. An isolation transformer isolates the OR electrical circuits from grounded circuits in the power mains; thus the isolated circuit does not include the ground in its pathway. The current seeks to flow only from one isolated line to the other. As a result, accidental grounding of persons in contact with the hot wire does not cause current to flow through the individual. A *line isolation monitor* checks the degree of isolation maintained by an isolated power system by continually measuring resistance and capacitance between the two isolated lines and the ground. The meter reading is called the *hazard index*. The monitor, a wall-mounted meter, has an alarm that is activated at the 2 milliampere level. This warning system indicates when inadvertent grounding of isolated circuits has occurred and alerts personnel to a dangerous situation. Because grounding can take place only when faulty equipment is plugged into ungrounded circuits, maximum safety is afforded by use of the isolation transformer. Ungrounded circuits fed through isolation transformers are required in OR and obstetric suites. Permanently installed overhead operating lights and receptacles in anesthetizing locations must be supplied by ungrounded electrical circuits.

In the event that the line isolation monitor alarm is activated during a surgical procedure:

1. Unplug the last piece of electrical equipment that was plugged into the power system.
2. Continue to unplug all equipment in the OR, including the anesthesia machine, to identify the faulty equipment. A battery-operated backup system may be needed.
3. Close the OR suite until a biomedical engineer can check for current leakage.

Electric Shock, Electrocution

Electrocution occurs when an individual becomes the component that closes a circuit in which a lethal current may flow. Lethal levels may be attained by currents through the intact body via skin or by currents applied directly to the heart. Electric shock occurs when a current is large enough to stimulate the nervous system or large muscle masses, for example, when the body becomes the connecting link between two points of an electrical system that are at different potentials. The physiologic effect of shock may range from a mere tingling sensation to tissue necrosis, ventricular fibrillation, or death. This is an electrical response of sensory cells, nerves, or muscles to electrical stimuli originating either intrinsically (within the body) or extrinsically (outside the body). The severity depends on the magnitude of the current flow and path taken through the body. Macroshock and microshock are the two types of shock.

Macroshock Macroshock occurs when the current flows through a relatively large surface of skin. It usually results from inadvertent contact with moderately high voltage sources, expressed in milliamperes (1/1000 ampere). A current intensity of 1 to 5 amperes through the chest can cause severe burn at the point of contact. However, if the cardiac conduction system is involved, a current intensity of 50 to 100 milliamperes through the chest can cause ventricular fibrillation because the heartbeat is electrically controlled. Macroshock occurs through the trunk of the body, with the current following many paths, each path carrying a fraction of the current. It may or may not be harmful, depending on how much current flows through a susceptible heart along its path. Common sources of macroshock are electrical wiring failures that allow skin contact with a live wire or surface at full voltage. Never touch the victim, instrument, or surface with your bare hands in a case of shock. Disconnect the power supply or use an insulating material to push the victim away from the source of electricity.

Microshock Microshock occurs when current is applied to a very small contact area of skin. The development of medical techniques permitting application of electrical impulses directly to the heart muscle drew awareness of the extreme danger of microshock to an electrically sensitive patient. Cardiac microshock is a potential hazard from indwelling catheters filled with conductive fluid, probes inserted into the great vessels, and electrodes implanted about the heart. These devices multiply the potential for electrocution because they can be conductors of electricity. The external portion of a cardiac catheter generally consists of two parts: an inner conductor(s) of wires or conductive fluid and an outer insulating sheath. When there is a highly conductive pathway from outside the body to the great vessels and heart, small electric currents may cause ventricular fibrillation and cardiac arrest. When a shock has an internal route to the heart, it takes only one thousandth as much electricity to be fatal as when the shock is transmitted through the surface of the skin. Microshock occurs only if current from an exterior source flows through the cardiac catheter or conductor. Conductive intravascular catheters that disperse current at skin level diminish the risk of microshock. The most important precaution is to protect the exposed end of the cardiac conductor from contact with conductive surfaces, including your body. Always wear rubber or plastic gloves when handling the external end of a cardiac catheter or conductor.

Safeguards Although the value of electronic devices is unquestionable, their use must not be allowed to cause needless electric shock or electrocution. Cardiac fibrillation and arrest may occur if a patient encounters an excess of accumulated small currents while connected to the ground through implanted electronic devices or by contact with other grounded objects, such as electrocardiograph (ECG) leads. Faulty electrical equipment may cause short circuit or electric shock or cause severe sparks that may be a source of ignition.

1. Particular care should be used when operating high-voltage equipment such as x-ray, electrosurgical unit, laser, and electronic monitoring devices. These machines should be checked for frayed or broken power cords, for properly functioning power switches, and for grounding.
2. Power cables should not be stretched taut or across traffic lanes.
3. Liquids should never be placed on an electrical unit. A spill could cause an internal short circuit.
4. Electrosurgical and laser units should be located on the operator's side of the table as far as possible from the monitoring equipment. These units may interfere with operation of other equipment. Preferably, these units are plugged into separate circuits to avoid overloading power lines. They should not be plugged into extension cords.
5. Equipment must be properly grounded to prevent small extraneous leakage currents.
6. Needle electrodes for ECG should be avoided because they can transmit leakage currents into the body.
7. Machine should be turned off when plugging into or unplugging from the power receptacle and when attaching cords to the machine.
8. Power cords should be unplugged by pulling on plugs, never cords, to prevent breakage of wires.
9. All electrical equipment, including a surgeon's personal property, should be inspected by the biomedical engineering department before initial use. Every piece must meet Underwriters Laboratories (UL) or other electrical safety requirements. All equipment should be inspected, preferably monthly but at least quarterly, and verified to be safe for use. It should be used according to the manufacturer's instructions.

Electrical and Thermal Burns

Electricity supplied by a defective system may cause burns. Monitors and all high-powered equipment are hazardous. Current that is concentrated or has a high density at the point of contact can result in an electrical burn severe enough to require debridement.

Electrical energy is converted into thermal energy. The amount of heat produced depends on current density, contact time, and tissue resistance. As little as 300 milliamperes of current for 20 seconds can produce enough heat at 113° F (45° C) to burn intact skin.

Electrosurgical units generate high-frequency current. Current flows to an active electrode used to cut or coagulate tissue (see Chapter 15, pp. 266-270). The patient is protected by grounding with a dispersive electrode. This provides a low current density pathway for the high-frequency current present at the active electrode back to the generator. Proper connections from the dispersive electrode to the patient and to the unit are essential to prevent burns. Burns can occur at the site of a dispersive electrode if it does not have adequate surface contact with skin or body tissue. Burns also can occur at the site of rings or other metal jewelry, ECG electrodes, or other low resistance points from invasive monitor probes, such as temperature probes, if current diverts to alternate grounds.

Conductive surfaces should be capable of providing a return path for current other than through the operating table or its attachments. If the return circuit of high-frequency equipment is faulty, the ground circuit may be completed through inadvertent contact with metal parts or attachments of the operating table. If the ground area is small, the current passing through the exposed area of skin contact will be relatively intense, causing a burn to the patient. For example, one such contact point may be the thigh touching the leg stirrup when the patient is in the lithotomy position.

Surface burns can occur when battery-operated equipment, such as a peripheral nerve stimulator, is used with external electrodes. Tetanic stimuli should be limited to 1 or 2 seconds.

Other potential sources for burn include malfunctioning controls on heat-generating devices that are in contact with the patient, such as radio-frequency diathermy or hypothermia/hyperthermia machines. Factors such as the patient's nutritional state, the amount of body fat that acts as insulation, and the circulation in the body part in contact with the device influence individual reaction to a hazard.

Static Electricity

Static electricity consists of high voltage and low ampere. An electrostatic spark develops from friction and accumulates on physical objects. When two static-bearing objects come in contact, the one bearing the higher potential discharges to the one with the lower potential. Air is a nonconductor. However, a high enough potential can overcome air resistance, jump the gap between it and a lower-potential object, causing an arc across air gaps seen as a spark(s) from the heat thus generated. Sparks can ignite flammable materials or gases. Objects accumulate static in inverse proportion to their conductivity. The aim is to provide adequate channels for dissipation of static. Because earth has a zero potential, a charge brought directly, or indirectly, through a conductor, into contact with it is discharged to earth. A spark between two objects can occur only when an electrical path of good conductivity does not exist between them. Moderate conductivity has a tendency for gradual spread of charge over both objects so they come to the same potential. Generation of static electricity cannot be prevented absolutely because its intrinsic origins are present at every interface. For static electricity to be a source of ignition, there must be:

1. An effective means of static generation
2. A means of accumulating the separate charges and maintaining a suitable difference of electrical potential
3. A discharge of energy adequate to make a spark in an ignitable mixture

Fire and Explosion

Fire should be a matter of prime concern in the OR. Fires in an oxygen-enriched atmosphere (OEA) are fundamentally different in character than those occurring in normal atmosphere. The fire severity potential should be regarded as serious, with extensive damage potential and endangerment to lives of patients and personnel. The presence of flammable and combustible liquids, vapors, and gases in an OEA can result in ultrarapid combustion of surrounding materials with explosive violence.

Anesthesiologists have discontinued use of highly flammable anesthetic agents, such as cyclopropane and ether, in favor of halogenated agents. However, these are mixed with air, oxygen, or nitrous oxide. Although oxygen and nitrous oxide are nonflammable gases, they support and accelerate combustion. A fire or explosion is the result of a combination of three factors:

1. A flammable gas, vapor, or liquid, such as ethylene oxide, alcohol, ether, methane gas, or collodion
2. A source of ignition, such as laser, electrosurgery, or static electricity
3. Oxygen (pure or in air) or some other substance providing oxygen, such as nitrous oxide

Safeguards

Standards of the NFPA, AAMI, and JCAHO safeguard against fire and explosion in anesthetizing locations. Requirements are less stringent where *only nonflammable inhalation agents are used.* Nonconductive flooring and footwear are acceptable, for example. The factors that can cause fire must be controlled, however.

Flammable Agents Spontaneous combustion can occur when flammable agents are exposed to an ignition source in the presence of oxygen.

1. Anesthesia machines, cylinders of compressed gas, and flammable liquid containers must be kept away from any source of heat and must not touch each other. A mixture of gases under high pressure is hazardous.
2. Oil or grease is not used on oxygen valves or parts of anesthesia machines. Oil or grease should not contact any cylinders, including those containing ethylene oxide, compressed air, or nitrogen.
3. Flammable antiseptics and fat solvents are not applied for preoperative skin preparation before laser or electrosurgery. Pooling on or around the skin or vapors under drapes can ignite.

Ignition Sources Minimum ignition temperatures of combustible materials in an OEA are lower than in air.

1. Lasers and other heated objects can cause fire or explosion.
   a. Precautions must be taken to prevent the laser beam, either directly or indirectly, from igniting drapes, sponges, and gowns or melting endotracheal tube. Refer to Chapter 15 (pp. 274-278) for safety factors with lasers.
   b. Electrosurgical unit should not be used on the neck, nasopharynx, and adjacent areas if a flammable inhalation agent was used for induction of anesthesia.
   c. Inadvertent activation of laser and electrosurgical units must be avoided. When not in use, handpieces should be placed in a holder, not left loose, on the sterile field.
   d. Beam from fiberoptic light carriers should not be directed onto a drape. Heat can build up until it is sufficient to produce burning or smoldering.
   e. Lights and sources of heat must be kept at least 4 feet (more than 1 m) away from the anesthesia machine and cylinders.
   f. Heat-generating equipment, such as the operating microscope and the projection lamp for fiberoptic lighting, must not be completely enclosed. Heat can build up under covering.
   g. Hypothermia/hyperthermia machine must be at least 3 feet (1 m) away from the anesthesia machine, and both must be adequately grounded.
   h. Only approved photographic lighting equipment with suitable enclosures can be used. Sparks and hot particles, as from a burst flash bulb, could be an ignition source.
2. Electrostatic (incendiary) spark can be an ignition source.
   a. Relative humidity (weight of water vapor present) should be maintained between 50% and 60%. Moisture provides a relatively conductive medium, allowing static electricity to leak to

earth as fast as it is generated. Sparks form more readily in low humidity.

b. Explosion-proof electrical receptacles or locking plugs cannot be pulled apart accidentally. Grounded outlets are installed above the 5-foot (1.5 m) level. Grounding adapter plugs, multiple-outlet plugs, and extension cords are prohibited.
c. Power cords should be rubber-coated and switches explosion-proof. Electrical equipment should be plugged into the power receptacle before the anesthetic is administered, and before the power switch is turned on.
d. Static charges should be dissipated before contact with the patient or anesthesiologist. This can be done by first touching the anesthesiologist's back or stool, the operating table, or the patient at least 2 feet (60 cm) from face mask. This provides for discharge of any charge in that person.
e. Patient and anesthesiologist should be grounded. An impedance conductive strap in contact with the patient's skin should have one end of strap fastened to the metal frame of operating table. Mattresses are covered with conductive material. A stool with smooth rounded feet and a bare metal top or conductive cushioning will ground the anesthesiologist.
f. Motion in the area around the anesthesia equipment and the patient's head should be minimal. Avoid friction on the reservoir bag. Watch that drapes do not touch the bag or cover the machine.
g. Patients are covered with cotton blankets. Woolen or synthetic blankets are prone to produce static electricity.
h. Hair of patients, personnel, and visitors is covered to avoid static discharge.
i. Antistatic outer garments are worn. Hose and undergarments in close contact with the skin may be of synthetic material.
j. Antistatic liners in kick buckets are handled with caution.
k. Metals should not make contact with a force sufficient to produce percussion sparks.
l. Anesthesia is discontinued as soon as possible if the ground monitoring system indicates a warning. Following completion of the surgical procedure, the room is not used until the electrical defect is corrected.

Flammable anesthetic agents are used *only* in areas where a conductive pathway can be maintained between the patient and a conductive floor. Conductive flooring is a means of electrically connecting people and objects to prevent accumulation of electrical charges and to equalize potentials. Conductive footwear should be worn.

Fire Safety

All health care facilities have fire warning and safety systems. Staff members should be familiar with the location and operation of fire alarms and fire extinguishers and with evacuation routes and procedures. Fire drills are held quarterly. Personnel should know the uses of fire extinguishers, be able to distinguish among the three classes of them, and how to operate them.

1. *Class A:* Pressurized water for combustibles such as paper, cloth, wood
2. *Class B:* Carbon dioxide or dry chemical to smother flammable liquids, oil, gas
3. *Class C:* Halon (bromochlorodifluoromethane halogenated compressed gas) to smother electrical or laser fire without leaving a residue on equipment

When a fire extinguisher is used, the mnemonic *PASS* may aid in remembering how to operate the device.

P Pull the safety ring out of the handle
A Aim the nozzle
S Squeeze the handle
S Sweep the spray over the base of the fire

If fire should occur in an OR during a surgical procedure, the first concern is for the safety of the patient and personnel. Immediately move the burning article from proximity of the oxygen source and the anesthesia machine or outlet of piped-in gases to prevent explosion. Smother fire on the field with wet towels. Remove burning drapes from the patient. Turn off the shutoff valves for piped-in gases, and unplug electrical power cords. The mnemonic *RACE* may aid in preventing panic and should enable the team to act quickly in the event of fire in the OR.

R Rescue anyone who is immediately in danger
A Activate the fire alarm
C Contain the fire if possible
E Evacuate the area

The fire should be extinguished in the room, if possible, but the patient must be removed immediately from any danger. If the patient is anesthetized, evacuate the patient on the operating table. Assist anesthesia personnel with life-support equipment, such as breathing bags and tubing. Refer to the departmental policy and procedure manual for evacuation and safety protocol specific to the facility.

CHEMICAL HAZARDS AND SAFEGUARDS

Health care providers are exposed to many hazardous chemicals on a daily basis. The hazards range from irritation of eyes or mucous membranes, contact dermatitis or burns, toxicity causing renal or liver disease, to exposure to carcinogens or mutagens. These or other effects may be immediate, delayed, or chronic. Hazardous chemicals in the workplace are controlled by government regulations, such as those of OSHA and EPA in the United States, or the Control of Substances Hazardous to Health (COSHH) regulations in Great Britain.

Chemicals must be labeled by the manufacturer with the identity of the agent(s) and appropriate warnings of hazards. The latter may be symbolic, that is, pictures added to words. Labels must not be removed or defaced. Employees should read labels and understand procedures for safe handling and use. OSHA incorporated "right-to-know" regulations in its standards. One part of this *Hazard Communication Standard* requires that employees should have access to *material safety data sheets* (MSDS) supplied by the manufacturer for each hazardous chemical in the workplace. The MSDS specifies:

1. Chemical by composition and common names
2. Chemical and physical properties
3. Known acute and chronic health effects, such as carcinogenic, mutagenic, or allergenic
4. Exposure limits
5. Protective measures
6. Antidote or first-aid measures

OSHA standards are legally enforceable. Although not legally enforceable, NIOSH and ACGIH recommendations for exposure limits to hazardous gases and vapors in ambient air should be adopted for personnel safety.

Anesthetic Gases

Air-conditioning or ventilating systems aid in prevention of pockets of anesthetic gases in the OR, although concentration around the anesthesia machine and the patient's head may not be remarkably reduced. Substantial amounts of gases can escape during surgical procedures. Heavy gas can accumulate and channel along the floor for as far as 50 feet (15 m). Confining agents by the use of a closed carbon dioxide absorption technique tends to restrict gases from getting into air streams. However, the patient's exhalations also can pollute the air in the OR and the postanesthesia care unit (PACU).

Waste anesthetic gases refer to gases and vapors that escape from the anesthesia machine, hoses, and connections, from around the face mask on the patient, and those released through the patient's expirations. Although not conclusive, data from studies indicate that personnel chronically exposed to waste anesthetic gas may incur health hazards. Stress, long working hours, and other unknown related factors may contribute to this occupational risk. Possible health hazards include the risk of spontaneous abortion, congenital abnormalities in offspring of male and female personnel, cancer, and hepatic and renal disease. Significant behavioral changes, including decreased perception, cognition, and manual dexterity, have been observed. Personnel also may complain of fatigue or headache.

Studies of retention of anesthetic agents in anesthesiologists following administration of clinical anesthesia have demonstrated traces of gas in expired air for varying lengths of time, from 7 hours following nitrous oxide administration to 64 hours after halothane administration. It has been shown that high doses of nitrous oxide block vitamin B_{12} metabolism. Chronic exposure to trace levels of this gas may lead to neurologic problems or neuropathy.

Because an estimated multimillion inhalation anesthetics are administered annually, a substantial number of OR staff are occupationally exposed to these gases. OSHA enforces the NIOSH recommendations that room air should not be contaminated by more than 0.5 parts per million (ppm) of halogenated agents per hour when used in combination with nitrous oxide or by more than 2 ppm per hour when used alone. Nitrous oxide should be controlled to less than 25 ppm during an 8-hour time-weighted exposure.

Proper and consistently conscientious use of scavenging equipment and procedures is strongly recommended. Scavenging involves removal of waste anesthetic gases, mainly by trapping them at the site of overflow on the breathing circuit followed by disposal to the outside atmosphere, and good dilution. The rate of removal of gases by the disposal system depends on the rate at which fresh air enters the OR and the patterns taken by air currents as they circulate through the room. Exposure to trace concentrations of gas can thus be reduced by 90% to 95%.

Personnel exposure should be reduced to the lowest practicable limits by reducing waste gas to the most technically feasible level. A waste-gas control program to ensure the continuing purity of environmental air includes the following measures:

1. Good work practices of anesthesiologists. The major source of waste gas in the OR is the intentional outflow of gases from the anesthesia breathing system. The quantity of gases discharged varies, depending on the type of breathing system, gas-flow rate, and gas concentration.
2. Use of a well-designed, well-maintained scavenging system. Inexpensive, practical, effective exhaust systems are available. The gas evacuation system should be attached to every anesthesia machine and ventilator to scavenge excess gases directly into a vacuum line with a minimum flow rate of 440 ppm.
3. Use of proper anesthesia technique.
   a. Different techniques of administration result in different exposure levels. Some leakage is uncontrollable.
   b. Components of the breathing system should fit well. Masks should fit facial contours to ensure a good seal. An airway may reduce the escape of gas from around the mask.

c. Liquid halogenated agents should not be spilled. Gas flow should not be turned on until the mask is in place or the patient is intubated and the endotracheal tube is connected to the breathing circuit.
d. Masks, tubing, reservoir bags, and endotracheal tubes should be inspected after each cleaning for leaks, holes, and abnormalities. Disposable equipment is preferable to recycled equipment.

4. Proper maintenance of anesthesia equipment through:
   a. Daily routine checking of anesthesia machines for leaks. NIOSH recommends that the total leak rate of each machine should not exceed 100 ml/min at 30 cm of water pressure. Leaks can be detected by use of a gas analyzer or a bubble test.
   b. Periodic preventive maintenance of all machines and fittings by a manufacturer's representative every 6 months with in-house monitoring at least quarterly.
5. Maintenance of a high flow rate of fresh air into the air-conditioning system through engineering control procedures. A good ventilating system (preferably not a recirculating one) is also important in the PACU. The ventilation system should comply with minimum requirements for 20 air changes per hour.
6. Use of an OR atmospheric monitoring program to record trace anesthetic levels and to determine the effectiveness of the above measures. Specialized monitoring equipment, such as an infrared analyzer, is the only way to detect leaks. Dosimeters are available for each individual to wear to provide an indication of exposure.

Sterilizing Agents

Chemical agents used for sterilization of heat-sensitive items are described in Chapter 13. Some of these are toxic or vaporize to emit noxious fumes that are irritating to the eyes and nasal passages even at low levels of exposure.

Ethylene Oxide

Used in a gaseous form for sterilization, residual products can be toxic in direct contact with the skin or by inhalation of ethylene oxide (EO) gas. Exposure can cause dizziness, nausea, and vomiting. EO is known to be a mutagen and carcinogen. Ethylene glycol and ethylene chlorohydrin are by-products of a reaction with moisture, as on hands. All porous items sterilized in EO must be aerated to dissipate the gas (see Chapter 13, pp. 227-228). The permissible exposure limits (PEL) for EO are 5 ppm for a short-term exposure of 15 minutes and 1 ppm time-weighted average (TWA) over 8 hours.

Formaldehyde

Formaldehyde may be used in a gaseous or liquid form (see Chapter 13, pp. 229 and 231). Vapors are toxic to the respiratory tract. Formaldehyde is a potent allergen, mutagen, and carcinogen, and it can cause liver toxicity. The PEL is 1 ppm TWA (NIOSH recommendation) to 3 ppm TWA (OSHA standard) over 8 hours.

Glutaraldehyde

The least toxic of these three agents, the fumes from liquid glutaraldehyde may be irritating to the eyes, nose, and throat. Contact dermatitis has been reported. PEL is 0.2 ppm per exposure. Glutaraldehyde should be used only in a closed container and in a well-ventilated area (see Chapter 13, pp. 231 and 232). A dosimeter is available to determine airborne concentration of fumes.

Disinfectants

Some of the disinfectants used for cleaning or decontaminating equipment and furniture (see Chapter 13, pp. 238-240) can be irritating to the skin and eyes. Gloves and goggles should be worn when using these chemicals. Agents must be used in proper dilution. Fumes from some agents can be irritating to nasal passages. OSHA has set exposure limits for:

1. Isopropyl alcohol: 400 ppm TWA
2. Phenol: 5 ppm TWA
3. Sodium hypochlorite: 1 ppm per exposure

Methyl Methacrylate

Commonly referred to as *bone cement,* methyl methacrylate is a mixture of liquid and powder polymers. It must be mixed at the sterile field just before use (see Chapter 24, pp. 507-508). Vapors released during mixing are irritating to the eyes and can damage soft contact lenses. Vapors are also irritating to the respiratory tract. They can cause drowsiness. Methyl methacrylate may be a mutagen, a carcinogen, or toxic to the liver. The liquid solvent can cause corneal burns if splashed in the eyes. It also can diffuse through latex gloves to cause an allergic dermatitis. Gloves are available that are impermeable to solvent. A scavenging system should be used to collect vapor during mixing and to exhaust it to the outside air or absorb it through activated charcoal. PEL for methyl methacrylate has been established at 100 ppm TWA.

Drugs and Other Chemicals

Antineoplastic cytotoxic drugs used for chemotherapy can be hazardous, as can laser dyes and other pharmaceuticals. All chemical agents must be prepared and administered to minimize unnecessary exposure for both patients and personnel. Chemicals should be combined or mixed with dilutants only when this is known to be a safe practice, as specified by the manufacturer.

Safe Handling of Cytotoxic Agents

Antineoplastic cytotoxic agents have carcinogenic and mutagenic properties, and most can cause local and/or allergic reactions. Personnel should avoid inadvertent direct skin or eye contact, inhalation, and ingestion of these agents during handling. Written precautions and procedures for handling, preparing, administering, and disposing of cytotoxic agents should be followed. Some basic guidelines include:

1. Protect self from skin and respiratory contact. Preferably, prepare agents under a vertical laminar flow hood. Whether or not a containment hood is available, wear thick gloves, mask, eye protection, and gown.
2. Wash hands after handling agents and all items that have been in contact with them, including those used for administration.
3. Place all cytotoxic waste in sealed, leakproof bags or containers. Incineration is recommended for all materials used in preparing and administering cytotoxic agents.

BIOLOGIC HAZARDS AND SAFEGUARDS

Transmission of infection and disease within the health care facility is a concern of consumers and providers. Biologic hazards do exist in the environment. Most diseases (e.g., cardiovascular disease) are not communicable, but others are caused by or secondary to transmission of microorganisms, as elaborated in Chapter 12. Every effort should be made by health care providers to protect patients and themselves. Universal precautions are a necessity (i. e., treating all body fluids and materials as infectious). Employers must ensure that appropriate protective equipment is available and that *employees are trained to and do use it.*

Infectious Wastes

Infectious medical waste is an environmental concern both within and outside the health care facility. The EPA defines infectious waste as *waste capable of causing an infectious disease*. This waste contains pathogens with sufficient virulence and quantity so that exposure to them by a susceptible host could result in an infectious disease. Disposal of potentially infectious waste generated in health care facilities is regulated by governmental mandates. Although *regulated medical waste* refers to the portion of waste that has the potential to transmit infectious disease, a uniform definition of what constitutes regulated medical waste has not been universally adopted. Factors that should be considered include:

1. Presence of pathogenic organisms in sufficient numbers to be capable of causing infection in living beings. Many microorganisms are incapable of causing infection.
2. Presence of a portal of entry into a susceptible host. A cut, needlestick, puncture wound, or skin lesion provides a portal of entry, but not all living beings are susceptible hosts to infectious diseases.

Because of these two factors, medical waste that poses public health and environmental risks and creates aesthetic concerns for the public is regulated. Potentially infectious waste is considered to be blood and blood products, pathologic waste, microbiologic waste, and contaminated sharps. This includes items contaminated by blood, such as sponges, drapes, gowns, and gloves. These items should be segregated from general waste, such as wrappers. They are placed in leakproof containers or bags strong enough to maintain integrity during transport, and should be closed and labeled or color coded. Red bags, for example, may be used to differentiate infectious waste. Needles and sharps must be put in puncture-resistant containers. If the outside of the container(s) is contaminated, double-bagging is necessary for safe handling during transport to disposal area.

Waste can be steam sterilized or decontaminated with microwaves before compaction and disposal in a landfill, or it can be incinerated. Federal, state, or local regulations must be followed for disposal.

Biohazards

All patients are potential sources of infection. OSHA defines *occupational exposure* as reasonably anticipated skin, eye, mucous membrane, or parenteral contact with blood or other potentially infectious materials during course of duties. This contact includes blood, tissues and organs, and all body fluids except urine, feces, and vomitus unless they contain visible blood. Careful handling of and adequate protection from potentially contaminated equipment also is important. Handwashing is a must after every patient contact or removal of gloves. Personal exposure should be a concern of all team members.

To be in compliance with the OSHA standard, every health care facility must develop a written exposure control plan that includes procedures for determining when exposure has occurred and for evaluating an incident. Engineering controls include safety devices or equipment designed to minimize or eliminate a biohazard. Likewise restrictions or changes in work practices should ensure the safety of all patients and personnel in the environment. For example, food must not be stored in the same refrigerator with blood products or specimens. Eating and drinking are prohibited in areas where contact with blood or other potentially hazardous material is possible. Eating should never be allowed in the OR during a surgical procedure.

Bloodborne Disease

A penetrating injury, such as a needlestick or cut, or a splash as in the eye or onto mucous membranes with fluid contaminated with blood or body fluids must not be ignored. Hepatitis, human immunodeficiency viruses, and other bloodborne pathogens can be transmitted through breaks in the skin or contact with mucous membranes. Universal precautions to prevent injury are discussed in Chapter 12, pp. 198-199. Hepatitis B vaccine is recommended for all high-risk health care workers. If you become injured:

1. Stop what you are doing immediately or as soon as possible.
2. Squeeze the skin around the needlestick or cut to expel blood and contaminants.
3. Cleanse the puncture site or rinse the eye.
4. Report the incident and seek medical attention promptly.

Surgical Plume

Plume is generated by thermal destruction of tissue or bone. Bloodborne pathogens, mutagens, carcinogens, and other toxic substances can be aerosolized by lasers (see laser plume, Chapter 15, p. 277), electrosurgery, and powered surgical instruments. Masks capable of filtering particles at least as small as 0.1 μm are recommended to prevent inhalation. Face shields, goggles, or eyeglasses with side shields should be worn to protect the eyes.

A smoke evacuator should be used to suction laser and electrosurgical plumes. The evacuator has a filtration system that incorporates a prefilter to trap particles, an ultralow penetrating air filter for particles in the 0.1 μm range, and a charcoal filter to absorb odor and hydrocarbons. The nozzle should be held close to the surgical site. Wall suction is not recommended for smoke evacuation because an in-line filter is necessary to avoid clogging the system. OR personnel can change the filters in some evacuators; others require maintenance by the biomedical technician. Filters are contaminated with biohazardous material and must be disposed of in the same manner as items contaminated with blood and body fluids. Gloves, masks, and protective eyewear must be worn when changing filters because the connecting couplers have been contaminated with plume and the material may be released into the air when the connection is disengaged.

Latex Sensitivity/Allergy

Many items used in the OR, such as surgical gloves, catheters, drains, medication vial stoppers, tubing, anesthesia breathing circuits, endotracheal tubes, breathing bags, and syringe plungers, contain latex (Table 10-1). Latex is manufactured from sap obtained from rubber trees. A water-soluble protein in the latex contains an antigen that can cause a potentially fatal allergic response. Two types of responses have been identified, *local* and *systemic*. Local reactions are less severe and occur when latex comes in contact with the skin, causing skin rash, itching, redness, and burning. The patient may have a systemic reaction when a latex product comes in contact with mucous membranes, serosa, or peritoneum during a surgical procedure. This reaction is more severe, causing anaphylactic shock or death. The signs of severe anaphylaxis are hypotension, tachycardia, bronchospasm, and generalized erythema.

Studies by the U.S. Food and Drug Administration (FDA) have shown that 6% to 7% of nursing personnel and surgeons are sensitive to latex. Health care personnel who are frequently exposed to latex products can become sensitized. Several items used in the OR contain latex but are not identified as having latex as a product content, for example, the elastic bands on caps and shoe covers or mattress and pillow covers. The manufacturer should be consulted to determine whether a product in use contains latex and if a latex-free substitute is available. Latex proteins can contaminate the starch on prepowdered gloves, thus providing a potential route of airborne exposure to allergens during donning. Sterile surgical nonlatex gloves are available commercially but are more expensive. They should be used only when an allergy is confirmed or is highly suspected in the user or in a patient receiving care.

Testing procedures are available for the detection of latex allergy. Testing of all personnel and patients would be a costly endeavor, but testing of persons suspected of having a latex sensitivity should be considered. Patients should be asked preoperatively if they have a known sensitivity (i.e., a history of a reaction after handling a toy balloon or wearing rubber gloves). Children with spina bifida, a congenital defect in the vertebral column, are known to be prone to latex allergy.

RISK MANAGEMENT

The OR suite is a high-risk environment. The risks can be minimized by adhering to the many safeguards discussed in this chapter. An effective risk management program continuously seeks to provide working conditions that will not jeopardize the health and safety of employees. Such a program has at least four key elements.

1. *Administration*
   a. Regulations, recommendations, guidelines, and laws must be enforced to prevent disastrous consequences of occupational hazards.
   b. Policies and procedures must be written, reviewed periodically, and updated as appropriate. All employees should have access to them.
   c. Protective attire and safety equipment must be made available to employees, as appropriate.

TABLE 10-1

Care of Latex-Sensitive Patient

COMMONLY USED LATEX PRODUCTS	LATEX-FREE ALTERNATIVES	PATIENT TEACHING	CONSIDERATIONS
Anesthesia breathing circuit, endotracheal tube, breathing bag	Disposable plastic breathing circuits and endotracheal tubes	NA (not applicable)	Disposal of used equipment
Bite blocks for oral surgery	Dental rolls, rolled gauze squares, silicone blocks	NA	Avoid using counted radiopaque sponge
Catheters, enema tips, and drains	Silicone catheters and drains	Instruct patient to report irritation or discomfort in area of drain or catheter	Patients rarely have silicone sensitivity; check product for content in manufacturer's enclosed literature
ECG leads, dispersive electrodes, pulse oximeter leads	Nonlatex gel pads	Instruct patient to report irritation at application site	Patient may have sensitivity to conductive gel; may need to use water-soluble lubricant
Elastic bandages, antiembolism stockings	White cotton bandages	Instruct patient to report any sensory changes in bandaged part, such as tingling, pain, or loss of sensation	Nonelastic bandages or stockings may restrict movement and have less expansion properties; circulation may become impaired if applied too tightly
Elastic and adhesive tape	Plastic, paper, or silk tape	Instruct patient to report irritation around or under area of tape	Some patients have sensitivity to adhesive rather than tape backing
Elastic bands on surgical caps, shoe covers, urinary catheter leg bags, plastic pants, disposable diaper	Cloth towel or paper caps with ties to cover hair; cloth hook and loop leg bands, cloth diapers	Instruct patient to report irritation around hairline or leg(s)	Cloth diapers will not be impervious to leaks; cloth hook and loop bands may impair circulation to leg
Embolectomy catheters	Silicone catheters	NA	Check composition of entire catheter and balloon
Hypothermia/hyperthermia blanket, hot water bottle, heating pad, mattress cover	Disposable plastic warming blankets and pads	Instruct patient to report irritation or discomfort	Observe for temperature control of device to avoid skin injury
Latex gloves, finger cots	Plastic or other nonlatex gloves	Instruct patient that utility gloves used at home may contain latex	Use nonlatex sterile gloves; vinyl utility gloves for nonsterile activities
Positioning devices, such as eggcrate, donuts, wedges, rolls	Rolled blankets and towels	NA	Roll blankets around larger objects, such as plastic water bags, for more height
Rubber shods	Silicone catheter or plastic tubes	NA	May not be radiopaque; plastic shods are not as pliable
Syringe plungers in plastic syringes	Glass syringes	Plungers in plastic syringes used for self-administered injectable medications contain latex	Air-powered autoinjector device or implantable medication dispensing mechanism are options at home
Tubing as on blood pressure cuffs and endoscopic insufflators	Disposable plastic tubing and cuff covers	NA	Wrap limb with cotton sheet wadding to avoid contact

d. Monitoring devices should be used in all hazardous locations, as recommended by regulatory agencies.
e. Employee health services must be provided for immunizations and in event of injury.

2. *Prevention*
   a. Regular in-service programs should be conducted to keep employees informed about hazards and safeguards.
   b. Employees must be taught how to use and care for new equipment before it is put into service.
   c. Employees must know the location and use of emergency equipment, such as fire extinguishers and shut-off valves.
   d. Employees must wear protective attire, as appropriate.
   e. Routine preventive maintenance should be provided for all potentially hazardous equipment.
3. *Correction*
   a. Faulty or malfunctioning equipment must be taken out of service immediately.
   b. Any injury should be reported and medical attention sought as soon as possible.
   c. Unsafe conditions should be reported.
4. *Documentation*
   a. Records of preemployment medical examination and periodic examinations for surveillance and early detection of disease should be maintained for each employee. These records should be retained in a permanent file after termination of employment in the event of a future health problem.
   b. New employees may be given a letter explaining occupational risks at the time of employment.
   c. Incident reports should be filed with administration for injuries to personnel and patients.

Prevention of injuries is vital to maintaining a safe environment. This is everyone's responsibility.

Pregnant Employee

Excessive exposure to ionizing radiation, waste anesthetic gases, and ethylene oxide during pregnancy may cause a spontaneous abortion or congenital fetal anomaly. Pregnant employees may be more susceptible to fatigue from prolonged periods of standing, lifting heavy items, and irregular meals and breaks. Exposure to infectious diseases also is a hazard. The health care facility should have a policy for pregnant employees. This may include transferring a pregnant employee from a hazardous area such as the OR. When possible, assignments should limit exposures for the safety of the fetus. For example, a pregnant woman should not assist with implantation of radioactive elements.

The pregnant employee is personally responsible for her own welfare and the safety of her fetus. Immunizations should be current, especially for hepatitis B and rubella. Safeguards, as previously described in this chapter, should be taken to limit her exposures to lowest levels possible. Ultimately, the pregnant employee should decide for herself whether or not she wishes to continue working.

Bibliography

Addington C: All the right moves: a program to reduce back injuries for OR nurses, *AORN J* 59(2):483-488, 1994.

Barlow R, Handelman E: OSHA's final bloodborne pathogens standard. Part I, *AAOHN J* 40(12):562-567, 1992; Part II, *AAOHN J* 41(1):8-15, 1993.

Bauman N: Some ET tubes fail fire-resistance test, *OR Manager* 6(9):13-14, 1990.

Beezhold DH et al: The transfer of protein allergens from latex gloves, *AORN J* 59(3):605-613, 1994.

Bloodborne infections: a practical guide to OSHA compliance, Arlington, Tex, 1992, Johnson & Johnson Medical.

Botsford J et al: Environmental issues committee creates collaborative document on "regulated medical waste," *AORN J* 58(1):106-114, 1993.

Curry J: New devices claim to reduce injuries from needlesticks, *OR Manager* 9(2):1,12-14, 1993.

Fay MF: Hand dermatitis: the role of gloves, *AORN J* 54(3):451-467, 1991.

Fay MF et al: Medical waste: the growing issues of management and disposal, *AORN J* 51(6):1493-1508, 1990.

Guidelines for prevention of latex allergic reactions, *OR Manager* 8(7):15, 1992.

Guidelines for protecting the safety and health of health care workers, Department of Health and Human Services (NIOSH) pub. no. 88-119, Washington, DC, 1988, US Government Printing Office.

Halstead MA: Fire drill in the operating room: role playing as a learning tool, *AORN J* 58(4):697-706, 1993.

Harris HR: Anesthetic gas: danger in the OR, *Surg Technol* 26(10):14-15, 1994.

Holloway J: Safety from sharps, *Br J Nurs* 1(8):389-390, 1992.

Jacobson E: New hospital hazards: how to protect yourself. Part I, *Am J Nurs* 90(2):36-41, 1990; Part II, *Am J Nurs* 90(4):48-53, 1990.

Klein BR, editor: *Health care facilities handbook,* ed 4, Quincy, Mass, 1993, National Fire Protection Association.

Lagier F et al: Prevalence of latex allergy in operating room nurses, *J Allergy Clin Immunol* 90(3):319-322, 1992.

Lynch P, White MC: Surgical blood exposures after the OSHA bloodborne pathogens standard: frequency and prevention, *Today's OR Nurse* 15(5):34-39, 1993.

McAbee RR et al: Adverse reproductive outcomes and occupational exposures among nurses: an investigation of multiple hazardous exposures, *AAOHN J* 41(3):110-119, 1993.

Murphy EK: Rights of pregnant employees to refuse assignment, *AORN J* 53(4):1043-1046, 1991.

National Fire Protection Association: *Life safety code,* Quincy, Mass, 1991, The Association.

National Fire Protection Association: *Standard for health care facilities,* Quincy, Mass, 1990, The Association.

Newton C: Hazards of N_2O exposure, *Nurs Times* 88(39):54, 1993.

O'Neale M: Clinical issues: environmental issues, *AORN J* 55(2):606-608, 1992.

Patterson P: OR air pollution: OSHA steps up action on waste anesthetic gases; OR exposure to electrosurgical smoke a concern; efficiency of evacuators depends on filtration system, *OR Manager* 9(6):1, 6-11, 1993.

Patterson P: OSHA issues rules to protect workers from HIV, hepatitis B, *OR Manager* 8(1):1, 5-7, 1992.

Pediani R: Hazards and safety in theatre, *Br J Theatre Nurs* 2(12):19-21, 1993.

PlumeFacts buyers' guide for ultimate plume protection, PlumeFacts, 1995, AORN Congress Edition.

Popejoy SL, Fry DF: Blood contact and exposure in the operating room, *Surg Gynecol Obstet* 172(6):480-483, 1991.

Proposed recommended practices: reducing radiological exposure in the practice setting, *AORN J* 58(3):599-608, 1993. (Adopted in 1994.)

Quebbeman EJ et al: Risk of blood contamination and injury to OR personnel, *Ann Surg* 214(11):614-620, 1991.

Recommended practices: environmental responsibility in the practice setting, *AORN J* 58(4):789-794, 1993.

Recommended practices: safe care through identification of potential hazards in the surgical environment, *AORN J* 51(4):1050-1055, 1990.

Recommended practices: sanitation in the practice setting, *AORN J* 56(6):1089-1092, 1992.

Reflections—some hazards in anaesthesia, *Br J Theatre Nurs* 2(12):24-25, 1993.

Regulated medical waste definition and treatment: a collaborative document, *AORN J* 59(6):1176-1183, 1994.

Regulations, the law, standards—what is the real status? *PlumeFacts* 4(3):1-4, 1994.

Reis JG: Latex sensitivity, *AORN J* 59(3):615-621, 1994.

Robaire B, Hales BF: Paternal exposure to chemicals before conception, *Br Med J* 307(6900):341-342, 1993.

Rogers B, Travers P: Nursing can be hazardous to your health, *RN* 55(3):67-74, 1992.

Roncarti JW, Naylor S: Fire safety: a JCAHO requirement—an approach for OR/P.A.C.U., *Point View* 27(2):4-5, 1990.

Rozovsky LE, Rozovsky FA: Legal implications of high tech surgery, *Can Oper Room Nurs J* 8(2):15-16, 1990.

Siegel JF et al: Latex allergy and anaphylaxis, *Int Anesth Clin* 31(1):141-145, 1993.

Spaeth D: Protective eyewear must meet ANSI standards, *PlumeFacts* 1(3):1-4, 1990.

US Department of Labor, Occupational Safety and Health Administration: *Occupational exposure to bloodborne pathogens,* Final rule, Federal Register 29, CFR Part 1910.1030, 1992.

Valenti WM: Infection control and the pregnant health care worker, *Nurs Clin North Am* 28(3):673-686, 1993.

Walker B: High efficiency filtration removes hazards from laser surgery, *Br J Theatre Nurs* 27(6):10-12, 1990.

Waywell L: Contact dermatitis due to surgical latex gloves—a personal experience, *Br J Theatre Nurs* 3(4):18-21, 1993.

Weaver VM et al: Occupational chemical exposures in an academic medical center, *J Occup Med* 35(7):701-706, 1993.

Young MA et al: Latex allergy: a guide for perioperative nurses, *AORN J* 56(3):488-502, 1992.

Zaza S et al: Latex sensitivity among perioperative nurses, *AORN J* 60(5):806-812, 1994.

SECTION FIVE

Surgical Asepsis, Instrumentation, and Equipment

CHAPTER 11

Attire, Surgical Scrub, Gowning, and Gloving

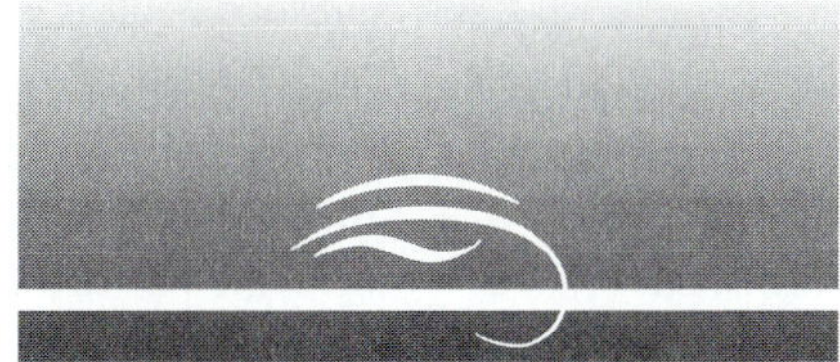

HISTORICAL BACKGROUND

The evolution of special operating room (OR) attire as an adjunct to asepsis paralleled the development of aseptic techniques in the latter half of the nineteenth century. In spite of the advances in technique, many surgeons of that time still operated while wearing street clothes under pus- and blood-encrusted aprons.

One of the earliest mentions of specific OR attire appeared in a nurse's training handbook that advised the nurse to bathe before a surgical procedure, to take a carbolic bath before laparotomy, and to wear long sleeves and a clean apron for the surgical procedure. As late as 1900, the surgeon often relied on his nurse to have the necessary instruments in her apron pocket. Although the apron has long since given way to the present scrub attire, long sleeves are again recommended for anesthesiologists and circulators to reduce the shedding of microorganisms.

The first use of caps and sterile gowns occurred in Germany while the value of Joseph Lister's principle of antiseptic surgery to exclude putrefactive bacteria from wounds was still being debated. In some operating theatres, bacteria-laden, infection-causing woolen suits and Prince Alberts were replaced by OR garb made of sterilizable material that lessened the introduction of pathogenic organisms into the wound, as advocated by the German surgeon Gustav Neuber. The use of sterile gowns antedated the routine use of caps, gloves, and masks, although in 1883 Neuber insisted on personnel wearing caps also.

Hunter Robb, a gynecologist at Johns Hopkins Hospital in Baltimore, insisted on OR cleanliness and on the wearing of caps and sterile gowns in the OR. In 1897 Dr. William Halsted, chief of surgery at Johns Hopkins, designed a semicircular instrument table to separate himself, in sterile gown and gloves, from observers in street clothes who watched him operate.

Emphasis on personal cleanliness expedited acceptance of special OR attire, but these standards were not rigidly practiced in all hospitals. Various styles of turbans and shower cap–style head coverings were worn from about 1908 to the 1930s, when hair was generally acknowledged to be an attraction for and shedder of bacteria. Some photographs taken in the early twentieth century show only the surgeon and instrument nurse wearing special head covering, although hair had been recognized as a contaminant. In a 1900 photograph, the team was operating in short surgical gowns and rubber gloves but without caps or masks. Charles Mayo and team were photographed in 1913 operating in surgical gowns, caps, and masks. The onlookers, however, wore only white coats over street attire. Another photo showed the surgeon in gown, cap, gloves, and a mask below his nose, the instrument nurse in gown and head cover but no mask, and the anesthetist and other nurses in gowns but regular nurses' caps. Universal standards of attire did not exist at that time.

In 1924 one of the first OR nursing texts described the OR nurses: the circulator wears an OR cap, but no mask, and a gown with a pocket for pad and pencil; the scrub nurse wears both mask and gown. By the 1930s and 1940s, scrub dresses began to replace nurses' regular uniforms, heretofore worn under the sterile gown. Observers in the OR were gowned, capped, and masked. In the 1960s full skirts were replaced by close-fitting scrub dresses and pantsuits that reduced the hazard of brushing against a sterile table when near or passing by it.

Rubber surgical gloves were introduced, not to protect the patient but to protect the wearer's hands from harsh, irritating antiseptic solutions and hand soaks of the 1870s and 1880s. Their use was not popularized until the 1890s, when Halsted's nurse complained of dermatitis. One of his assistants began to wear gloves routinely for clean surgical procedures in 1896, although Halsted himself is known for popularizing the use of gloves to protect patients from the bacteria of ungloved hands. Johann von Mikulicz, a pioneering German surgeon, advocated the wearing of cotton gloves in 1896 also, but these were soon found to lack the qualities of impermeable rubber gloves for infection control. Disposable latex gloves, introduced about 1958, were a welcome innovation that saved countless hours of daily glove reprocessing, repairing, and sterilizing. Today the universal use of disposable gloves is well established.

Gauze masks were advocated by Mikulicz in 1897, when the droplet theory of infection was demonstrated. However, it was not until 1926, when wound infections yielded the same organisms as found in noses and throats of surgeons and nurses, that masks became obligatory. Although gauze masks were routinely worn, their efficiency decreased rapidly during wearing from saturation with saliva. Often the nose was not properly covered. Modern protocol demands that both mouth and nose be completely covered to exclude bacterial spray as a potential source of contamination. The most efficient masks are disposable ones containing a high-efficiency filter.

In 1950, as restrictions became more rigid, OR personnel were required to change shoes when entering the OR suite and to wear only those shoes when within the suite. Currently disposable shoe covers are commonly worn.

The Association of Operating Room Nurses (AORN) has published recommended practices for OR surgical attire (wearing apparel) and aseptic barrier materials for surgical gowns and surgical hand scrubs.

OPERATING ROOM ATTIRE

Purpose

Sebaceous and sweat glands and hair follicles contain microorganisms that are continually shed (dispersed) from the skin into the environment. The purpose of OR attire is to provide effective barriers that prevent the dissemination of these microorganisms to the patient. However, these barriers coincidentally protect personnel from infected patients. The barriers prohibit contamination of the surgical wound and sterile field by direct body contact. OR attire has been shown to reduce particle count of shedding from the body from over 10,000 particles per minute to 3000 per minute, or from 50,000 microorganisms per cubic foot to 500.

Definition

OR attire consists of body covers, such as a two-piece pantsuit, head cover, mask, and shoe covers. Each has an appropriate purpose to combat sources of contamination *exogenous* (external) to the patient. Sterile gown and gloves are added to this basic attire for scrubbed team members. Proper attire is one facet of environmental control. It also protects personnel against exposure to communicable diseases and hazardous materials. Eyewear and other protective attire are worn by personnel as appropriate for anticipated exposure.

Dress Code

The OR should have specific written policies and procedures for proper attire to be worn within the semirestricted and restricted areas of the OR suite. The dress code should include aspects of personal hygiene important to environmental control. Protocol must be strictly monitored so that *everyone* conforms to established policy.

1. Dressing rooms located in the unrestricted area adjacent to the semirestricted area of the OR suite are reached through the outer corridor. Street clothes are *never* worn beyond the unrestricted area.
2. Only approved, clean, and/or freshly laundered OR attire is worn within the semirestricted and restricted areas. This policy applies to *anyone* entering the OR suite, both professional and nonprofessional personnel and visitors.
   a. Clean, fresh attire is donned each time on arrival at the OR suite and as necessary at other times, if it becomes wet or grossly soiled. Blood-stained attire, including shoe covers, is not only unattractive but can be a source of cross infection.
   b. An adequate supply of clean attire should always be available. Attire is laundered daily *only*

in the hospital's laundry facilities. It should not be taken home for laundering.

c. Masks and head covers should be changed between patients.

3. OR attire *should not be worn outside* the OR suite. This protects the OR environment from microorganisms inherent in the outside environment and protects the outside from contamination normally associated with the OR. Before leaving the OR suite, everyone should change to street clothes.
   a. On occasion, such as for lunch breaks, a single-use cover gown or coverall may be worn over OR attire outside the suite. This practice is *not* encouraged and is *acceptable only when a clean gown with a back closure is worn one time.* It is discarded, if disposable, or put in a laundry hamper after wearing. Some hospitals provide laboratory coats. These must be completely buttoned and worn only once.
   b. A clean, fresh scrub suit should be put on after return for reentry to the suite.
   c. OR attire should not be hung or put in a locker for wearing a second time. It should be discarded in the trash or put in a laundry hamper after one use, as appropriate.
4. Impeccable personal hygiene must be reemphasized.
   a. A person with an acute infection, such as a cold or sore throat, should *not* be permitted within the OR suite. Persons with cuts, burns, or skin lesions should not scrub or handle sterile supplies because serum, a bacterial medium, may seep from the eroded area. An open skin lesion may be a portal of entry for cutaneous contact with bloodborne pathogens.
   b. Sterile team members who are known carriers of pathogenic microorganisms should routinely bathe and scrub with an appropriate skin antiseptic agent and shampoo their hair daily.
   c. Fingernails should be kept short, that is, should not extend past the fingertips. Routine manicures prevent cracked cuticles and hangnails. Subungual areas harbor the majority of microorganisms on hands. Nail polish on short healthy nails may not alter microbial count on fingernails. Polish may seal crevices. However, damaged nails and chipped or peeling polish may provide a harbor for microorganisms. Studies have shown that artificial nails and other enhancers harbor organisms, especially fungi and gram-negative bacilli. These devices that cover fingernails *cannot* be worn.
   d. Jewelry, including rings and watches, should be removed before entering semirestricted and restricted areas. Organisms may harbor under rings, thus preventing effective handwashing. Necklaces or chains can grate on the skin, increasing desquamation. They might fall into a wound or contaminate a sterile field. Jewelry also harbors organisms. Pierced-ear studs must be confined within head cover. Dangling earrings are inappropriate in the OR.
   e. Facial makeup should be minimal. Mascara, false eyelashes, and dried or caked makeup can flake off into the wound or environment.
   f. Eyeglasses should be wiped with a cleaning solution before each surgical procedure.
   g. External apparel that does not serve a functional purpose should not be worn.
   h. Hands must be washed frequently and thoroughly. Using hand cream regularly helps prevent chapped, dry skin.
5. Comfortable, supportive shoes should be worn to minimize fatigue and for personal safety. Shoes should have enclosed toes and heels; clogs and sandals should not be worn. Cloth shoes do not offer protection against spilled fluids or sharp items that may be dropped or kicked. Shoes must be cleaned frequently, whether or not shoe covers are worn.

Components of Attire

Each item of OR attire is a specific means for containment of, or protection against, the potential sources of environmental contamination, including skin, hair, and nasopharyngeal flora and microorganisms in air, blood, and body fluids. Body (scrub suit) and head covers are worn by all personnel in the semirestricted areas of the OR suite. Masks are also worn in the restricted areas. Additional items are worn only during a surgical procedure and for protection during hazardous exposure.

Body Cover

Everyone must don a *scrub suit* before entering a semirestricted or restricted area. A variety of scrub suits, either two-piece pantsuits or one-piece coveralls, are available in either a solid color or attractive print. All should fit the body snugly. Pantsuits confine organisms shed from the perineal region and legs more effectively than dresses; 90% of bacterial dissemination originates from the perineum. Pantyhose does not contain this shedding.

Shirt and waistline drawstrings are tucked *inside* pants to avoid their touching sterile areas and to reduce fallout of skin debris shed from thoracic and abdominal areas. Microorganisms multiply more rapidly beneath a covered area. A tunic top that fits snugly may be worn on the outside of pants. The scrub suit should be changed as soon as possible whenever it becomes wet or visibly soiled.

Persons who will not be sterile team members should wear long-sleeved jackets over a scrub suit. The sleeves help contain bacterial shedding from axillae and arms. The jacket should be closed to prevent a bellows effect and the possibility of brushing against the sterile field during movement.

One-piece coveralls with attached hoods and boots are convenient garb for visitors whose presence in the OR will be brief (e.g., pathologists).

Head Cover

Since hair is a gross contaminant, a cap or hood is put on *before* a scrub suit to protect the garment from contamination by hair. All facial and head hair must be *completely* covered in the semirestricted and restricted areas. Various types of lightweight caps, helmets, and hoods are available. Most of them are made of disposable, lint-free, nonporous, nonwoven fabrics. Reusable head covers should be made of a densely woven material and laundered daily. Net caps are too porous to be acceptable. If hair is long, a helmet or hood must be worn to cover the neck area. Headgear should fit well so it confines and prevents escape of any hair. Hair should not be combed while wearing a scrub suit. Persons with scalp infection should be excluded from the OR and treated.

Hair is also a source of electrostatic spark. Some anesthesiologists wear a full coverage hood with ear slits. The slits facilitate use of a stethoscope.

Caps of different colors are helpful to differentiate personnel. For example, students may wear pink caps, and graduate staff members may wear blue. Easy identification helps to avoid asking someone to do something that they are not qualified to do.

Shoe Covers

Shoe covers may be worn in the semirestricted and restricted areas. They will protect the wearer from spills into or onto shoes during procedures when extensive fluid irrigation and/or blood loss can be anticipated. Some surgeons wear plastic or rubber boots. The legs of scrub pants are tucked into boots.

Studies have not shown a significant correlation between footwear and wound infection. However, the flow of traffic is one critical factor in dispersal of microbes from the floor into the air. Unprotected street shoes can increase floor contamination. Shoes restricted to wear in the OR suite or shoe covers over shoes are preferable in reducing microbial transfer from the outside into the OR suite. Protective gloves should be worn to change shoe covers whenever they become wet, soiled, or torn. Shoe covers can inadvertently become soiled and harbor microorganisms. They should be removed before entering the dressing room area and must be removed before leaving the OR suite.

Mask

A mask is worn in the restricted area to contain and filter droplets containing microorganisms expelled from the mouth and nasopharynx during breathing, talking, sneezing, and coughing. Some tight-fitting masks also effectively reduce exposure to submicron particles by filtration of inhaled air. Many masks filter about 99% of particulate matter larger than 5.0 μm in diameter, but only about 45% to 60% of particles of 0.3 μm diameter. Aerosolized particles and viruses dispersed in laser and electrosurgical plume or by power instruments may be this small. Masks provide some protection to the sterile team members from bloodborne pathogens that may splash or spray toward the nose or mouth.

Reusable cotton masks are obsolete; they filter ineffectively as soon as they become moist. Contemporary disposable masks of soft, clothlike material in very fine synthetic fiber mats, fulfill essential criteria:

1. They are at least 95% efficient in filtering microbes from droplet particles in exhalations and also filter inhalations. A fluid-resistant mask is advantageous.
2. They are cool, comfortable, and nonobstructive to respiration.
3. They are nonirritating to the skin. Disposable masks are made of polypropylene, polyester, or rayon fibers. Some have fiberglass filters. If a person is sensitive to one type, he or she should try another brand.

Some experts believe masks should be worn to protect team members rather than to protect patients from moisture droplets. Current AORN recommended practice, however, advocates that masks be worn at *all* times in the restricted area of the OR suite—where sterile supplies will be opened and scrubbed persons may be present—including areas where scrub sinks are located. Masks always should be worn in the OR itself whether or not a surgical procedure is in progress. Masks are worn on entering the room before, during, and after the surgical procedure (i.e., during setup and cleanup). This includes terminal cleaning at the end of the day and restocking of supplies. Policy in some OR suites may be less restrictive. Written policy should be followed by all team members, departmental staff, and visitors.

To be effective, a mask must filter inhalations and exhalations. Therefore *it must be worn over both nose and mouth.* Air must pass only through the filtering system, so the mask must conform to facial contours to prevent leakage of expired air. Venting, the drawing of air back and forth, can occur along the sides, top, and bottom of the mask. Double-masking is not recommended because the extra thickness can cause venting from the effort to breathe through it. Ejected droplets must not escape the filter action.

Masks are designed for close fit, but improper application can negate their efficiency. Always tie the strings tightly, if this is the method of securing the mask, to prevent the strings from coming loose during the surgical procedure. Tie upper strings at the back of the head; tie lower strings behind the neck (Figure 11-1). Strings are never crossed over the head because this distorts the contours of the mask along the cheeks. Some types of masks have an exterior pliable strip or noseband that can be bent to contour the mask over the bridge of the nose. A close-fitting mask or a small strip of tape over the nose piece also helps to avoid steaming of eyeglasses. To prevent cross infection, masks should:

1. Be handled only by the strings, thereby keeping the facial area of a fresh mask clean and the hands uncontaminated by a soiled mask. Do not handle the mask excessively.
2. Never be lowered to hang loosely around the neck, be placed on top of the cap, or put in a pocket. Avoid disseminating microorganisms.
3. Be promptly discarded into the proper receptacle on removal. Remask with a fresh mask between patients.
4. Be changed frequently. Do not permit the mask to become wet. Talking should be kept to a minimum.

Protective Attire

Personnel must be protected from hazardous conditions in the semirestricted and restricted areas. Depending on the exposure that will be encountered, protective attire should be worn. The type and characteristics of this attire depend on the task and degree of exposure anticipated. Protective attire does not allow blood or other potentially injurious materials to reach inner clothing, skin, or eyes.

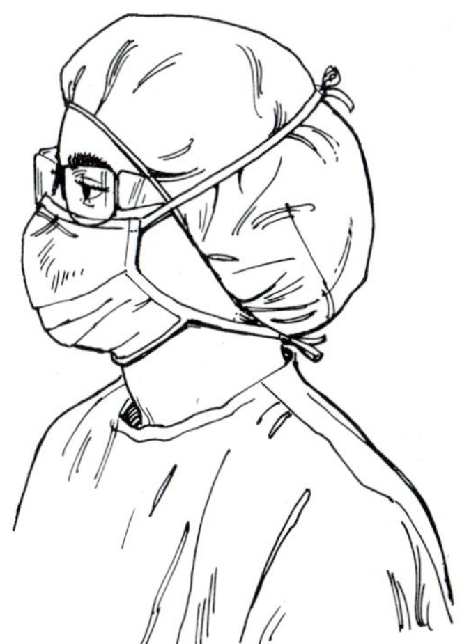

FIGURE 11-1 Mask covers nose and mouth and conforms to facial contours. Upper strings are tied at back of head; lower strings are tied behind neck.

1. Aprons
   a. A decontamination apron worn over the scrub suit protects against liquids and cleaning agents during cleaning procedures. It should be a full-front barrier.
   b. Fluid-proof aprons are worn by sterile team members under permeable reusable sterile gowns when extensive blood loss or irrigation is anticipated. They should be lightweight and full front.
   c. Lead aprons worn under sterile gowns protect against radiation exposure during procedures performed under fluoroscopy or image intensification or when handling radioactive implants (see Chapter 10, p. 147).
2. Eyewear
   a. Eyewear or a face shield is worn whenever a risk exists of blood or body fluids from the patient splashing into the eyes of sterile team members. Bone chips and splatter can be projected from bone-cutting instruments. Several styles of goggles and eyeglasses with side shields fit securely against the face. Antifog goggles fit over prescription eyeglasses. A combination surgical mask with a visor eye shield or a chin-length face shield are other options.
   b. Laser eyewear must be worn for eye protection from laser beams. Lenses of the proper optical density for each type of laser must be available and worn (see Chapter 15, p. 277).
   c. Protective eyewear, preferably a face shield, should be worn by personnel handling or washing instruments when this activity could result in a splash, spray, or splatter to the eyes or face.
   d. Eyewear or a face shield that becomes contaminated should be decontaminated or discarded promptly.
3. Gloves
   a. Nonsterile latex or vinyl gloves are worn to handle any material or items contaminated by blood and body fluids. Gloves should be worn only during the period of contact, not continuously. Clean objects and sterile packages should not be handled with contaminated gloves.
   b. Sterile gloves are worn by sterile team members and for all invasive procedures. Liners may be worn under gloves to protect the hands from cuts and seepage through punctures (p. 169).
   c. Lead gloves may be needed for protection from radiation exposure. The surgeon may wear latex gloves impregnated with lead for procedures performed under fluoroscopy.
   d. Thick gloves should be worn for skin protection from ethylene oxide exposure if sterilized

packages must be handled before aeration (see Chapter 13, p. 226).

e. Utility gloves are worn for cleaning and housekeeping duties. (Refer to universal precautions, Chapter 12, p. 198.)

NOTE

- Sterile and nonsterile single-use disposable latex and vinyl gloves are discarded after use. They should not be washed and reused.
- Hands must be washed after removing gloves.

Gown

A sterile gown is worn over the scrub suit to permit the wearer to come within the sterile field. It differentiates sterile (scrubbed) from unsterile (unscrubbed) team members. The gown must provide a protective barrier from strike-through, that is, migration of microorganisms from the skin and scrub suit of the wearer to the sterile field and the patient, and penetration of blood and body fluids from the patient to the scrub suit and skin of the wearer.

Both reusable and disposable gowns, in a variety of styles, are in use. Although the entire gown is sterilized, the back is not considered sterile, nor is any area below table level, once the gown is donned. Wraparound sterile gowns that provide coverage to the back by a generous overlap are recommended. These gowns are secured at the neck and waist before the sterile flap is brought over the back and secured by ties or grips at the side or front. If the gown is closed merely by ties along the back, a sterile vest put on over the gown covers any exposed back area of scrub attire. The cuffs of gowns are stockinette (rib-knit) to tightly fit wrists. Sterile gloves cover the cuffs of the gown.

Gowns should be resistant to penetration by fluids and blood and should be comfortable, without producing excessive heat buildup. Most single-use disposable gowns are made of spun-laced fiber or nonwoven, moisture-repellent materials. Some of these are reinforced with plastic on the forearms and front. Reusable gowns must be made of a densely woven material. Loosely woven, 140-thread count all-carded cotton muslin or similar quality permeable material is *not* a barrier to microbial migration. Some 180-thread count cotton gowns have insets of 270-thread count fluid-resistant fabric or plastic film to reinforce sleeves from cuff to elbows and front from the midchest to below the waist. Pima cotton with a 270- to 280-thread count per square inch treated with a moisture-repellent finish is an acceptable woven textile. Some reusable gowns are a cotton-polyester blend. Tightly woven 100% polyester gowns are impervious to moisture. Seams of the gowns should be constructed to prevent penetration of fluids.

Sterile team members may not need a reinforced barrier gown for every procedure; the scrub person usually can safely wear a single-layer impervious gown. The surgeon and first assistant are at greatest risks during procedures within the abdominal or chest cavity, when blood loss will be more than 200 ml, or when time will exceed 2 hours. The amount of blood and fluid on the outside of the gown is a critical factor in strike-through by wicking. Bloodborne pathogens can penetrate fabric without visible strike-through. Forearms are the most frequently contaminated areas. Therefore the surgeon and first assistant should wear a gown with at least reinforced or plastic-coated sleeves for these procedures.

Woven textile gowns withstand about 75 launderings and sterilizing cycles before appreciable deterioration of the finish occurs. Monitoring the number of uses is necessary to remove the gown from use at the sterile field when it is no longer an effective barrier. Also, an additional rinse cycle may be required in the laundering process to remove residual detergent that could adversely affect the fabric. Mechanical damage from sharp instruments or snags will destroy the integrity of the gown, jeopardizing its purpose. The gown must be changed if punctured or torn during the surgical procedure. Textile gowns can be patched only with heat-applied vulcanized mending fabrics.

All woven and some nonwoven gowns are not flame-retardant. Fire-resistant gowns should be worn for laser surgery and preferably when electrosurgery is used (see Chapter 15).

Special attire often is worn with ultraclean laminar airflow systems (see Chapter 12, pp. 196-197). A body exhaust gown envelops the wearer from the top of the head to within about 16 inches (40 cm) of the floor. If a gown that fits closely at the neck is used, a rigid face mask or helmet must be worn. With both types of gowns, an exhaust system is attached for body cooling and air flow.

Gloves

Sterile gloves complete the attire for sterile team members. They are worn to permit the wearer to handle sterile supplies and tissues of the surgical wound. Surgical gloves are made of natural latex rubber, synthetic rubber, vinyl, or polyethylene. Disposable latex gloves are worn most frequently. Latex is a polymeric membrane of natural rubber with an infinite number of holes between lattices. However, it is a better barrier than vinyl, which may allow permeation of blood and fluids over prolonged exposure. Latex gloves of varying thickness, with a minimum of 0.1 mm, can be chosen to meet the needs of the surgeon for tactile sensation. Latex contains protein antigen and is cured with agents that may cause an allergic dermatitis or systemic anaphylaxis (see Chapter 10, p. 157). Hypoallergenic milled gloves that do not contain these sensitizers are available. Latex gloves labeled "hypoallergenic" do not always prevent reaction in a highly sensitive person. Several varieties of synthetic nonlatex sterile gloves, for example, those made of neoprene, are available commercially. Sterile team members must not wear latex gloves if the patient has a known latex sensitivity or allergy.

Gloves are packaged in pairs with an everted cuff on each to protect the outside of the sterile glove during donning. The inner paper wrap of the disposable glove package protects the sterility of the gloves when they are removed from the outer wrap. Glove packages are generally the peel-apart type. Before opening, the package should be inspected for damage or wetness, which indicates contamination. When the inner paper is unfolded, the wearer finds the right glove to the right, the left glove to the left, palm side up (Figure 11-2).

Both inner and outer surfaces may be prelubricated with an absorbable dry cornstarch powder before the sterilization process to facilitate donning, to decrease loose powder in the OR air, and to prevent adhesion of glove surfaces. Although considered absorbable and inert in tissue, this lubricant may cause serious complications, such as granulomas, adhesions, or peritonitis, if it is introduced into wounds. Consequently, it is important to remove the lubricant from the outside of the gloves. To do this, the gloves should be thoroughly wiped with a sterile damp towel or sterile terry washcloth after donning and before touching instruments or other sterile items. Simple rinsing in most solutions is ineffective because the particles of starch clump together. Povidone-iodine solution seems to be the most effective for removing starch, if a basin of solution is used for rinsing gloves. This practice has been eliminated in most ORs. Latex coated on the inside with a hydrogel lubricant allows smooth donning of gloves without the hazard of glove powder. Latex protein allergens can adhere to powder, thus providing another potential route of exposure or sensitization.

Surgeons frequently puncture their gloves, most often on the index finger of the nondominant hand. Glove puncture and minute holes in unworn gloves are hazardous to both patients and team members. Shedders present a special threat to patients. Seepage under a glove poses a threat to a team member if his or her skin is not intact. The risk of blood contamination of the fingers increases the longer a glove is worn. Antiseptic-impregnated latex gloves may minimize microbial colonization if punctured. High-molecular-weight polyethylene gloves resist punctures and tears. Some surgeons prefer to double glove (wear two pairs of latex gloves). Double gloving may be prudent when the patient has a known or suspected transmissible bloodborne virus and for procedures involving blood loss of more than 100 ml or lasting more than 2 hours. *If a sterile glove is punctured or torn, it must be changed immediately* to prevent escape of microorganisms from wearer's skin and seepage of blood and body fluids from the patient into the glove.

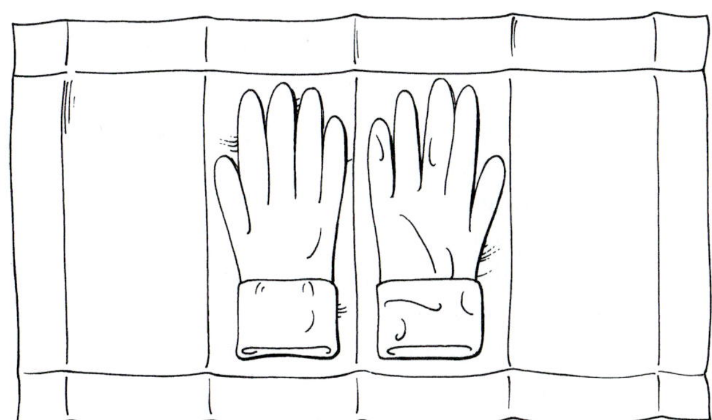

FIGURE 11-2 Gloves on unfolded open wrapper, right glove to right, left glove to left, palm sides up.

Many sterile team members wear glove liners for protection from scalpel cuts or instrument tears. These do not protect the hands from punctures, such as needlesticks, however. Liners are usually worn between two pair of latex gloves, usually a half-size larger than usual so that they will not constrict circulation. The liners may be made of polymer fibers or a metal mesh. Some are disposable; others may be sterilized with steam or ethylene oxide.

NOTE Petrolatum-based lotions or lubricants should not be used on the hands before donning latex gloves. Hydrocarbons will penetrate latex, causing a change in its physical characteristics, including tear resistance.

Criteria for Operating Room Attire

Attire should be:

1. An effective barrier to microorganisms. Both reusable woven and disposable nonwoven materials are used. Design and composition should minimize microbial shedding.
2. Closely woven material void of dangerous electrostatic properties. The garment must meet National Fire Protection Association Standards (NFPA-56A), including resistance to flame.
   a. Undergarments of synthetic material such as nylon are permissible when in close contact with the skin, such as hosiery.
   b. Nylon and other static spark-producing materials are forbidden as outer garments.
3. Resistant to blood, aqueous fluids, and abrasion to prevent penetration by microorganisms.
4. Designed for maximal skin coverage.
5. Hypoallergenic, cool, and comfortable.
6. Nongenerative of lint. Lint can increase the particle count of contaminants in the OR.
7. Made of a pliable material to permit freedom of movement for the practice of sterile technique.
8. Able to transmit heat and water vapor to protect the wearer.

9. Colored to reduce glare under lights. Various types of clothes in colorful prints that fulfill the necessary criteria are both attractive and functional.
10. Easy to don and remove.

SURGICAL SCRUB

Definition

The *surgical scrub* is the process of removing as many microorganisms as possible from the hands and arms by mechanical washing and chemical antisepsis before participating in a surgical procedure. The surgical scrub is done just before gowning and gloving for each surgical procedure.

Microorganisms

The skin is inhabited by:

1. *Transient organisms* acquired by direct contact. Usually loosely attached to the skin surface, they are almost completely removed by thorough washing with soap or detergent and water.
2. *Resident organisms* below the skin surface in hair follicles and in sebaceous and sweat glands. They are more adherent and therefore more resistant to removal. Their growth is inhibited by the chemical phase of the surgical scrub. Resident skin flora represent the microorganisms present in the hospital environment. They are predominantly gram-negative, but some are coagulase-positive staphylococci. Prolonged exposure of skin to contaminants yields a more pathogenic resident population (i.e., capable of causing infection).

In freeing the skin of as many microorganisms as possible, two processes are used:

1. *Mechanical:* Removes soil and transient organisms with friction.
2. *Chemical:* Reduces resident flora and inactivates microorganisms with a microbicidal or antiseptic agent (i.e., an inorganic chemical compound that inhibits growth of microorganisms without necessarily killing).

Purpose

The purpose of the surgical scrub is to remove soil, debris, natural skin oils, hand lotions, and transient microorganisms from the hands and forearms of sterile team members. More specifically, the purposes are:

1. To decrease the number of resident microorganisms on skin to an irreducible minimum
2. To keep the population of microorganisms minimal during the surgical procedure by suppression of growth
3. To reduce the hazard of microbial contamination of the surgical wound by skin flora

Scrub Sink

Adequate scrubbing and handwashing facilities should be provided for all operating team members. The scrub room is adjacent to the OR for safety and convenience. Individually enclosed scrub sinks with automatic controls or foot- or knee-operated faucets are preferred to eliminate the hazard of contaminating hands after cleansing.

The sink should be deep and wide enough to prevent splash. Aerated faucets prevent splatter. A sterile gown cannot be put on over damp scrub attire without resultant contamination of a reusable woven gown by strike-through of moisture.

Scrub sinks should be used *only* for scrubbing or handwashing. They should not be used to clean or rinse contaminated instruments or equipment.

Equipment

Sterilized reusable scrub brushes or disposable sponges may be used. Single-use disposable products may be a brush-sponge combination. Some are impregnated with antiseptic-detergent agents. Disposable products are individually packaged. If reusable brushes are taken from the dispenser in which they were sterilized, each brush must be removed without contaminating the others. Brushes may be wrapped to provide sterile individual packages. The brush should not cause skin abrasion. The scrubbing solution is dispensed onto the brush or sponge by foot pedal from a container attached or adjacent to the sink. Six drops, about 2 to 3 ml (2 cc), of solution is sufficient to generate a lather for the scrub procedure. Avoid waste of antiseptic solution.

Debris must be removed from the subungual area under the nail of each finger. Metal or plastic single-use disposable products are available. Reusable nail cleaners must be sterilized between uses.

NOTE Orangewood sticks are not used to clean under the fingernails because the wood may splinter and harbor *Pseudomonas* organisms.

Agents for Antisepsis

Various antimicrobial (antiseptic) detergents are used for the surgical scrub. The agent must be:

1. A broad-spectrum antimicrobial agent
2. Fast-acting and effective
3. Nonirritating and nonsensitizing
4. Prolonged-acting, that is, leaves an antimicrobial residue on the skin to temporarily prevent growth of microorganisms
5. Independent of cumulative action

Although the action of the agent is important in relation to its efficacy, mechanical friction and effort while scrubbing are equally important. Frequent scrubbing with the same agent tends to inhibit reestablishment of resident flora. Some agents have more residual effect than others. Variables in effectiveness of the scrub are mechanical factors, chemical factors, and individual differences in skin flora. More than one agent usually is available in the scrub room for personnel allergic or sensitive to a particular agent.

Antiseptics

Products are chosen from among those approved by the Food and Drug Administration (FDA) for surgical hand scrubs. Each product has a specific antimicrobial agent. Antiseptics alter the physical or chemical properties of the cell membrane of microorganisms, thus destroying or inhibiting cellular function.

Chlorhexidine Gluconate A 4% aqueous concentration of this agent exerts an antimicrobial effect against gram-positive and gram-negative microorganisms. Residues tend to accumulate on the skin with repeated use and produce a prolonged effect. This agent produces effective, immediate, and cumulative reductions of resident and transient flora. The residual effect is maintained for more than 6 hours. Chlorhexidine gluconate is rarely irritating to the skin, but it is highly irritating if splashed in the eye. It can cause corneal damage. Caution must be observed when scrubbing with this agent.

An alcohol-based chlorhexidine preparation is available that is effective if the hands are bathed in solution for 20 to 30 seconds after mechanical cleansing.

Iodophors A povidone-iodine complex in detergent fulfills the criteria for an effective surgical scrub. Iodophors are rapidly antimicrobial against gram-positive and gram-negative microorganisms. They slowly release iodine for some residual effect, but this is not sustained for a prolonged period (over 6 hours). Iodophors can be irritating to the skin. Persons allergic to iodine should not scrub with these agents.

Triclosan A solution of 1% triclosan is a nontoxic, nonirritating antimicrobial agent that inhibits growth of a wide range of both gram-positive and gram-negative organisms. It develops a prolonged cumulative suppressive action when used routinely. The agent is blended with lanolin cholesterols and petrolatum into a creamy, mild detergent. It may be used by personnel sensitive to other antiseptics, although it can be absorbed through intact skin. Triclosan is less effective than chlorhexidine gluconate and iodophors.

Alcohol Ethyl or isopropyl alcohol (60% to 90%) is rapidly antimicrobial. It does not have residual activity. It is nontoxic but has a drying effect on skin. Alcohol preparations, usually in a foam, contain emollients to minimize drying. If other agents cannot be used because of skin sensitivity, mechanical cleansing with soap to remove transient organisms may be followed by vigorous rubbing with an alcohol-based skin cleanser.

Hexachlorophene In concentrations up to 3%, this agent is most effective after buildup of cumulative suppressive action. However, its high potential for toxicity makes it unsuitable for routine use. Hexachlorophene is available by prescription only.

Parachlorometaxylenol Used in a concentration of 1% to 3.75%, this agent does not substantially reduce microorganisms immediately. It does not produce sustained residual activity. Its antimicrobial activity can be altered significantly by the composition of the antiseptic product. Efficacy data should be reviewed before these products are used for surgical scrubs.

Preparation for Surgical Scrub

General Preparations

1. Skin and nails should be kept clean and in good condition, and cuticles should be uncut. If hand lotion is used to protect the skin, a non–oil-based product is recommended.
2. Fingernails should not reach beyond the fingertip to avoid glove puncture.
3. Fingernail polish should not be worn. The lacquer may chip and peel, thereby providing a harbor for microorganisms in crevices.
4. Artificial devices must not cover natural fingernails.
5. Remove *all* jewelry from fingers, wrists, and neck. Jewelry harbors microorganisms.

Preparations Immediately Before Scrub

1. Inspect the hands for cuts and abrasions. Skin integrity of the hands and forearms should be intact (i.e., without open lesions or cracked skin).
2. Be sure *all* hair is covered by headgear. Pierced-ear studs *must* be contained by the head cover. They are a potential foreign body in the surgical wound.
3. Adjust disposable mask snugly and comfortably over nose and mouth.
4. Clean eyeglasses if worn. Adjust protective eyewear or face shield comfortably in relation to mask.
5. Adjust water to a comfortable temperature.

Length of Scrub

The length of the surgical scrub varies, as does the scrub procedure. Variations may depend on the frequency of scrubbing, the agent used, and the method. A vigorous 5-minute scrub with a reliable agent may be as effective as a 10-minute scrub done with less mechanical action. Prolonged scrubbing raises resident microbes from deep dermal layers and is therefore counterproductive. Care must be taken not to abrade the skin during the scrub process. Denuded areas allow the entry of microorganisms. Too short a scrub may be equally ineffectual.

Everyone should scrub according to a standardized written procedure. The time required may be based on the manufacturer's recommendations for the agent used and documentation of product efficacy in the scientific literature. A copy of the procedure should be posted in every scrub room.

Subsequent scrubs should follow the same procedure as the initial scrub of the day. When gloves are removed at the end of the surgical procedure, the hands are contaminated. Resident microorganisms multiply rapidly in the warm, moist environment under the gloves. Hands should be washed as soon as the gloves are removed, but they will become contaminated as soon as contact is made with any inanimate items.

Surgical Scrub Procedure

The surgical scrub procedure may be either the *time method* or counted *brush-stroke method*. If properly executed, they are both effective and each exposes all surfaces of the hands and forearms to mechanical cleansing and chemical antisepsis. One should think of the fingers, hands, and arms as having four sides or surfaces. Both methods follow an *anatomic pattern of scrub:* the four surfaces of each finger, beginning with the thumb and moving from one finger to the next, down the outer edge of the fifth finger, over the dorsal (back) surface of the hand, the palmar (palm) surface of the hand, or vice versa, from the small finger to the thumb, over the wrists and up the arm, in thirds, ending 2 inches (5 cm) above the elbow. Since the hands are in most direct contact with the sterile field, all steps of the scrub procedure begin with the hands and end with the elbows.

NOTE During and after scrubbing, keep the hands *higher* than the elbows to allow water to flow from the cleanest area, the hands, to the marginal area of the upper arms.

Time Method

Fingers, hands, and arms are scrubbed by allotting a prescribed amount of time to each anatomic area or each step of the procedure.

Five-Minute Scrub

1. Wet the hands and forearms.
2. Apply 2 to 3 ml (6 drops) of antiseptic agent from the dispenser to the hands.
3. Wash the hands and arms several times thoroughly to 2 inches (5 cm) above the elbows. Rinse thoroughly under running water, with the hands upward, allowing water to drip from flexed elbows.
4. Take a sterile brush or sponge (from a package or dispenser) and apply an antiseptic agent (if it is not impregnated in the brush). Scrub each individual finger, nails and hands, a half minute for each hand.
5. Hold the brush in one hand and both hands under running water, and clean under the fingernails with a metal or disposable plastic nail cleaner. Discard the cleaner after use.
6. Again scrub each individual finger, nails, and hands with the brush a half minute for each hand, maintaining lather.
7. Rinse the hands and brush, and discard the brush or sponge.
8. Reapply the antimicrobial agent, and wash the hands and arms with friction to the elbow for 3 minutes. Interlace the fingers to cleanse between them.
9. Rinse the hands and arms as before.

Brush-Stroke Method

A prescribed number of brush strokes, applied lengthwise of the brush or sponge, is used for each surface of the fingers, hands, and arms. A short prescrub wash loosens surface debris and transient organisms. Scrub by brush or sponge removes resident flora.

1. Wet the hands and arms.
2. Wash the hands and arms thoroughly to 2 inches (5 cm) above the elbow with an antiseptic agent.
3. With the hands held under running water, clean under the fingernails carefully with a metal or disposable plastic nail cleaner. Discard the cleaner after use.
4. Rinse the hands and arms thoroughly under running water, keeping the hands up and allowing water to drip from the elbows.
5. Take a sterile brush or sponge from a dispenser or package. Apply an antiseptic agent to the brush or sponge (if not previously impregnated).
6. Scrub the nails of one hand 30 strokes, all sides of each finger 20 strokes, the back of the hand 20 strokes, the palm of the hand 20 strokes, the arms 20 strokes for each third of the arm, to 2 inches (5 cm) above the elbow.
7. Repeat step 6 for the other hand and arm.
8. Rinse the hands and arms thoroughly.

GOWNING AND GLOVING

The sterile gown is put on immediately after the surgical scrub. The sterile gloves are put on immediately after gowning.

Purpose

Sterile gown and gloves are worn to exclude skin as a possible contaminant and to create a barrier between the sterile and unsterile areas.

General Considerations

1. The scrub person gowns and gloves self, then may gown and glove the surgeon and assistants.
2. Gown packages preferably are opened on a separate table from other packages to avoid any chance of contamination from dripping water.

3. Avoid splashing water on scrub attire during surgical scrub because moisture may contaminate the sterile gown.

Drying Hands and Arms

After scrubbing, hands and arms must be thoroughly dried before the sterile gown is donned to prevent contamination of the gown by strike-through of organisms from wet skin.

The gown package for the scrub person contains one sterile gown, folded before sterilization, with the inside out, so that the bare scrubbed hands will not contaminate the sterile outside of the gown. A towel for drying the hands is placed on top of the gown during packaging. The hands are dried as follows:

1. Reach down to the opened sterile package and pick up the towel. Be careful not to drip water onto the pack. Be sure no one is within arm's reach (Figure 11-3).
2. Open the towel full-length, holding one end away from nonsterile scrub attire (Figure 11-4). Bend slightly forward to avoid letting the towel touch the attire.
3. Dry both hands thoroughly but independently. To dry one arm, hold the towel in the opposite hand and, using an oscillating motion of the arm, draw the towel up to the elbow.
4. Carefully reverse the towel, still holding it away from the body. Dry the opposite arm on the unused (now uppermost) end of the towel.

NOTE Often the towel is an absorbent, disposable one. Two absorbent washcloths may be used in lieu of a towel. They are crisscrossed on top of the gown to separate them. To use them, reach down to the sterile package and pick up one washcloth, being careful not to drip water. Holding the arms away from the washcloth, dry one hand, then the arm, as with the towel. Discard the washcloth. Use the second washcloth to dry the other hand and arm in the same manner.

Gowning and Gloving Techniques

Sterile gloves may be put on in two ways: by *closed glove technique*, or by *open glove technique*. If properly done, gloves can be put on safely either way. *The method of gloving determines how the gown is donned.*

Closed Glove Technique

The closed glove method is preferred, except when changing a glove during a surgical procedure or when donning gloves for procedures not requiring gowns. Properly executed, the closed glove method affords assurance against contamination, when gloving oneself, because no bare skin is exposed in the process.

Gowning for Closed Glove Technique

1. Reach down to the sterile package and lift the folded gown directly upward (Figure 11-5).
2. Step back away from the table, into an unobstructed area, to provide a wide margin of safety while gowning.
3. Holding the folded gown, carefully locate the neckband.
4. Holding the inside front of the gown just below the neckband with both hands, let the gown un-

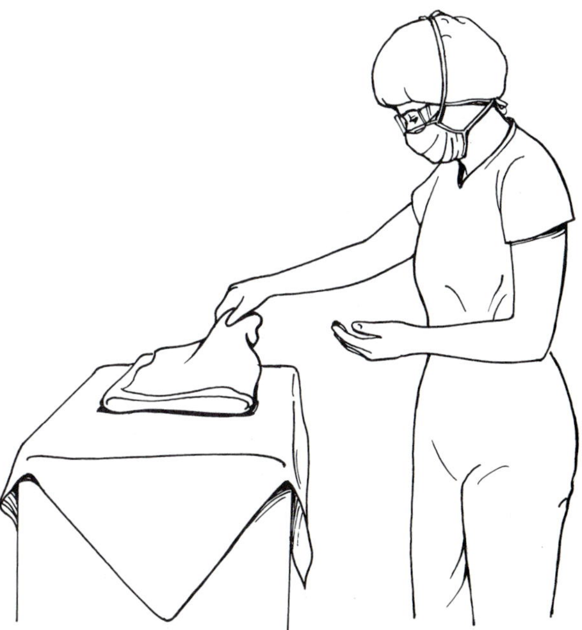

FIGURE 11-3 Scrub person preparing to gown removes hand towel on top of gown from opened package.

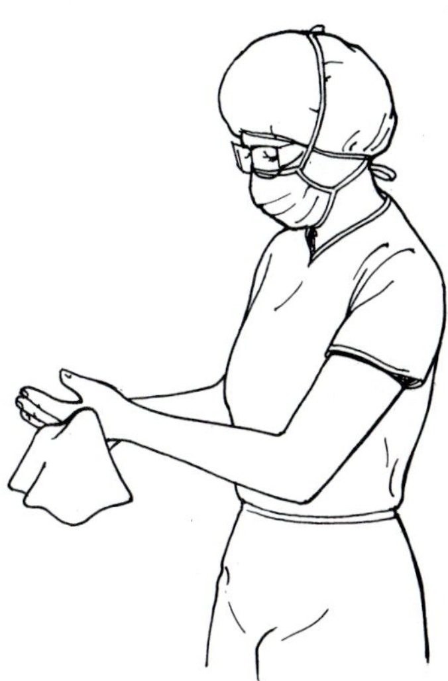

FIGURE 11-4 Scrub person, holding towel out away from body, dries only scrubbed areas, starting with hands. He or she avoids contaminating hands on areas proximal to elbows, then discards towel.

fold, keeping the inside of the gown toward the body. Do not touch the outside of the gown with bare hands.

5. Holding the hands at shoulder level, slip both arms into the armholes simultaneously (Figure 11-6).
6. The *circulator* brings the gown over the shoulders by reaching inside to the shoulder and arm seams. *The gown is pulled on, leaving the cuffs of the sleeves extended over the hands.* The back of the gown is securely tied or fastened at the neck and waist; touching the outside of the gown at the line of ties or fasteners, in the back only (Figures 11-7 and 11-8).

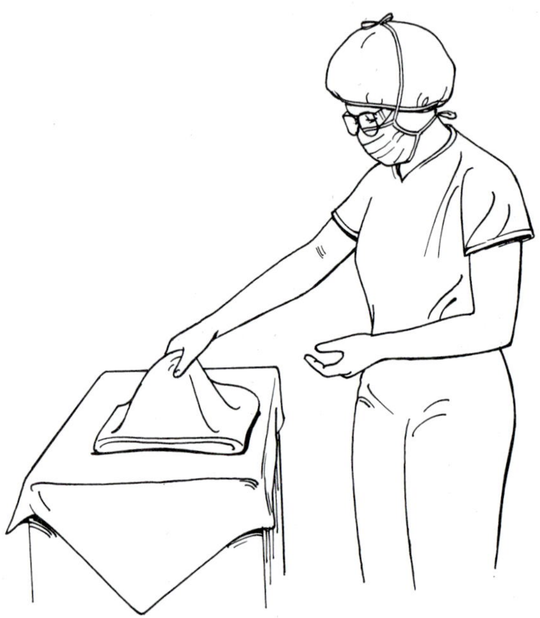

FIGURE 11-5 Scrub person, picking up gown below neck edge, lifts it directly upward and steps away to avoid touching edge of wrapper. Note that sterile inside of wrapper covers table. Gown is folded inside out.

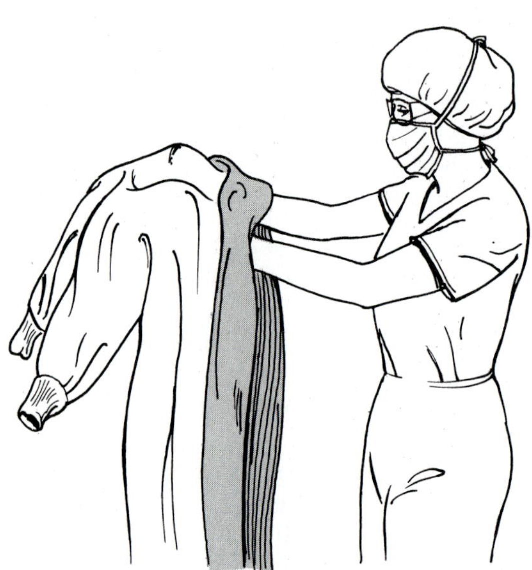

FIGURE 11-6 Scrub person, putting on gown, gently shakes out folds, then slips arms into sleeves without touching sterile outside of gown with bare hands.

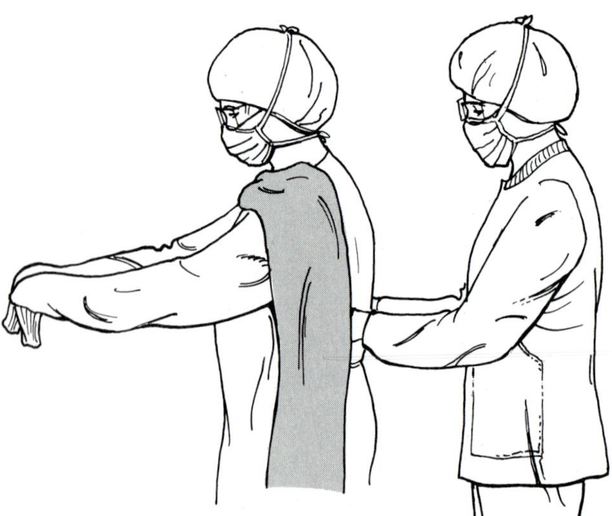

FIGURE 11-7 Circulator, pulling gown on for closed gloving technique, reaches inside gown to sleeve seams and pulls gown on, leaving cuffs of sleeves extended over hands.

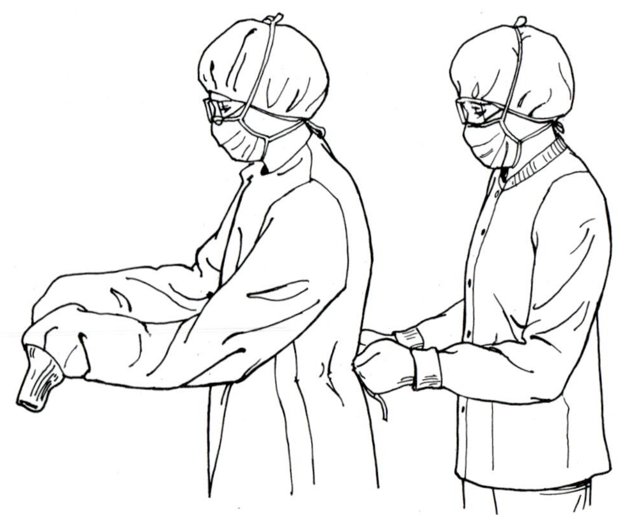

FIGURE 11-8 Circulator completes pulling on scrub person's gown, secures ties on inside of back, and closes fastener at neck.

NOTE

- If the gown is wraparound style, the sterile flap to cover the back is not touched until the person has gowned and gloved. A sterile gown may be wrapped around in various ways:
  1. With gloved hands, release the fastener or untie the ties at the front or side of the gown. Hand the tie on the right to a sterile team member who remains stationary. Allowing a margin of safety, turn around to the left, thereby completely covering the back with the extended flap of the gown. Accept the tie from the assistant and secure the ties at the left side of the gown.
  2. If you are the first person to gown and glove and other sterile team members are not available to assist, snap a sterile instrument such as an Allis's forceps (*never* a hemostat or clamp for hemostasis) to the tie on the right. Carefully hand the instrument to the circulator. While he or she remains stationary, turn to the left, thereby covering the back. Take the tie in hand. The circulator then releases and places the instrument aside; it is considered contaminated. Tie the ties at the left side.
  3. Some disposable gowns have the end of one tie covered by a disposable strip. Hand the strip to the circulator, taking care to protect the hands. Turn around toward the opposite side, thereby closing the gown. Grasp the tie at a distance from the end. The circulator pulls the strip, releasing it from the still-sterile end of the tie, and discards it. Tie the ties at the front or side of the gown as indicated.
- If the top of the gown drops downward inadvertently, discard the gown as contaminated. Never reverse a sterile gown or drape if the wrong end is dropped toward the floor.

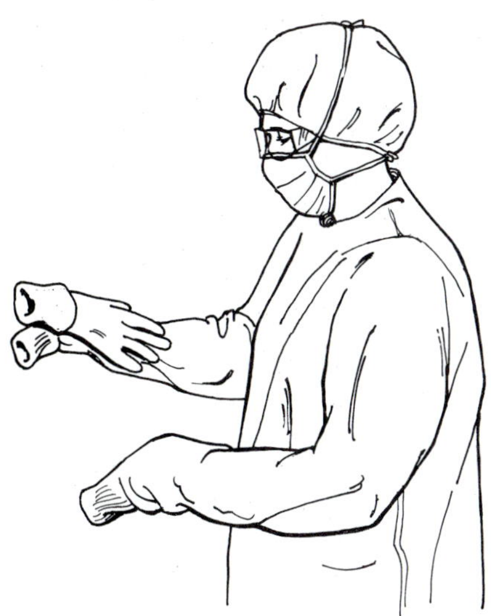

FIGURE 11-9 For closed gloving technique, using left hand and keeping it within cuff of sleeve, gowned scrub person picks up right glove. Palm of glove is placed against palm of right hand, grasping top edge of glove cuff above palm.

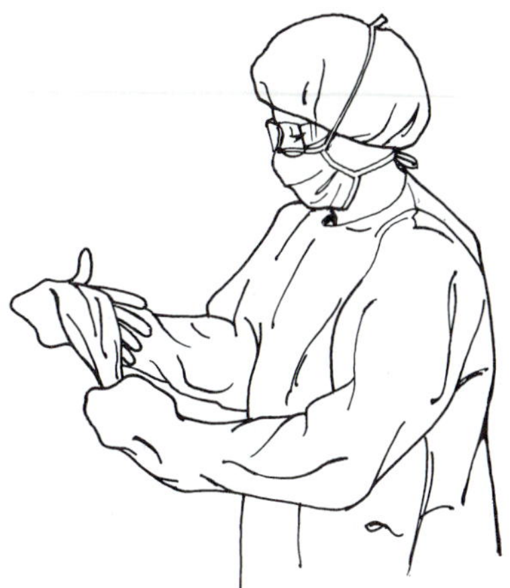

FIGURE 11-10 Back of cuff is grasped in left hand and turned over right sleeve and hand.

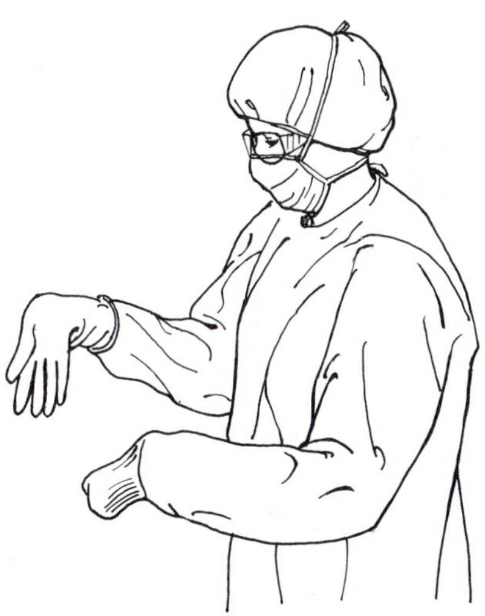

FIGURE 11-11 Cuff of glove is now over stockinette cuff of sleeve, with hand still inside sleeve.

Gloving by Closed Glove Technique

1. Using the left hand and keeping it within the cuff of the left sleeve, pick up the right glove, from the inner wrap of the glove package, by grasping the folded cuff.
2. Extend the right forearm with the palm upward. Place the palm of the glove against the palm of the right hand, grasping in the right hand the top edge of the cuff, above the palm. In correct position, glove fingers are pointing toward you and the thumb of the glove is to the right. The thumb side of the glove is down (Figure 11-9).
3. Grasp the back of the cuff in the left hand and turn it over the end of the right sleeve and hand. The cuff of the glove is now over the stockinette cuff of the gown, with the hand still inside the sleeve (Figures 11-10 and 11-11).

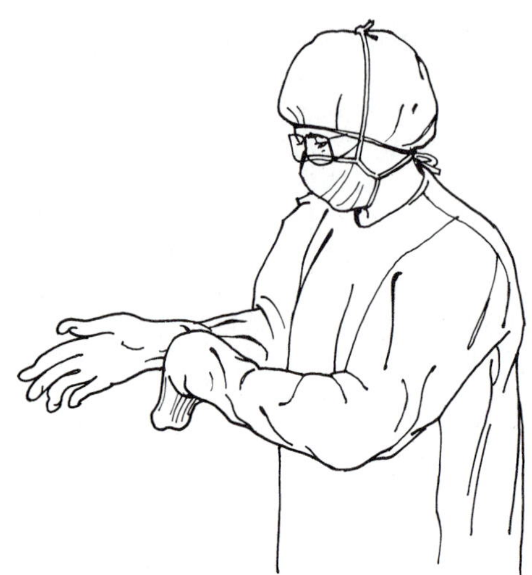

FIGURE 11-12 Top of right glove and underlying sleeve of gown are grasped with left hand. By pulling sleeve up, glove is pulled onto hand.

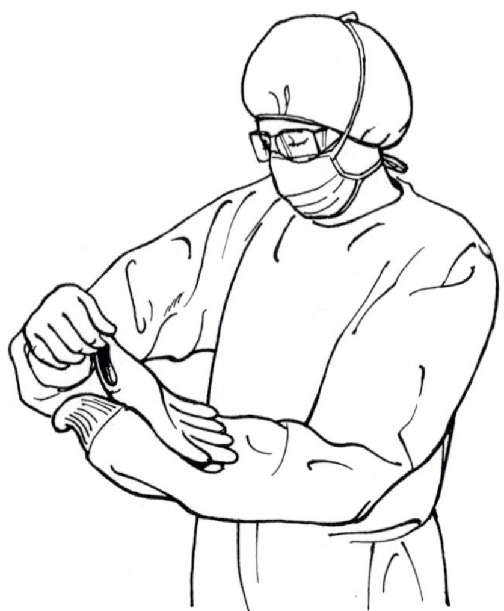

FIGURE 11-13 Using gloved right hand, left glove is picked up and placed with palm of glove against palm of left hand. Back of cuff is grasped, above palm in right hand and turned over left sleeve and hand.

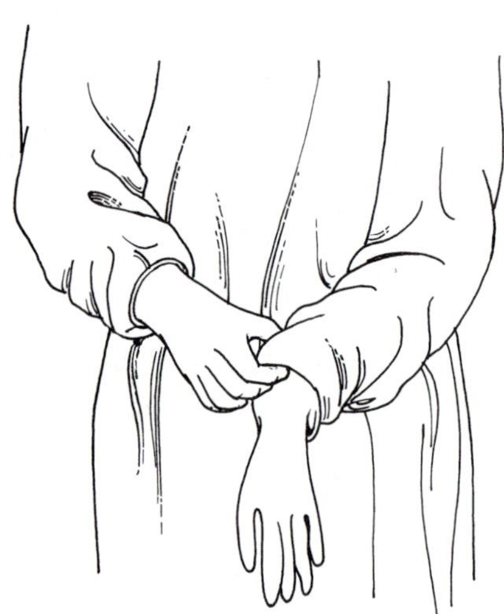

FIGURE 11-14 Cuff of left glove is now over stockinette cuff of sleeve, with hand still inside sleeve.

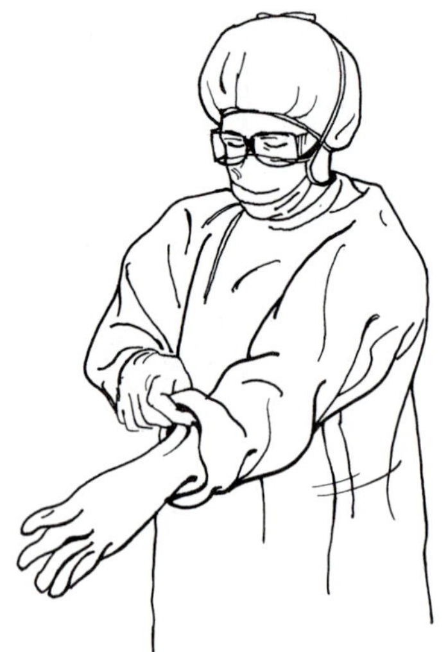

FIGURE 11-15 Top of left glove and underlying gown sleeve are grasped with right hand, and sleeve is pulled up, pulling glove onto hand.

4. Grasp the top of the right glove and underlying gown sleeve with the covered left hand. Pull the glove on over the extended right fingers until it completely covers the stockinette cuff (Figure 11-12).
5. Glove the left hand in the same manner, reversing hands. Use the gloved right hand to pull on the left glove (Figures 11-13 through 11-15).

Open Glove Technique

Open glove technique is used for changing a glove or gown and gloves during a surgical procedure. It also is used when only sterile gloves are worn, as for intravenous cutdown or administration of spinal anesthesia or in the emergency department when donning sterile gloves as for suturing lacerations.

Gowning for Open Glove Technique

1. Reach down to the sterile package and lift the folded gown directly upward.
2. Step back away from the table, into a clear area, to provide a wide margin of safety while gowning.
3. Holding the folded gown, carefully locate the neckband.
4. Holding the inside front of the gown just below the neckband with both hands, let the gown unfold, keeping the inside of the gown toward the body.
5. Holding the hands at shoulder level, slip them into the armholes simultaneously, without touching the sterile exterior of the gown with bare hands.
6. The *circulator* reaches inside the gown to the sleeve seams and *pulls the sleeves over the hands* to the wrists. Then the back of the gown is securely closed at the neck and waist with ties or fasteners, touching the outside of the gown at the line of ties or fasteners in the back only (Figure 11-16).

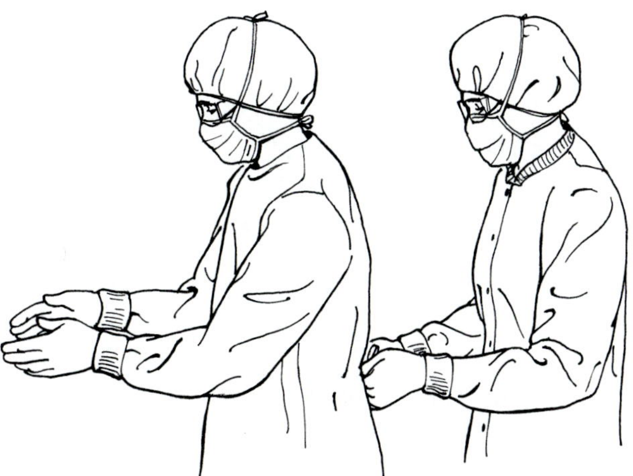

FIGURE 11-16 Circulator fastens back of scrub person's gown for open gloving technique. Note that hands extend through stockinette cuffs.

Gloving by Open Glove Technique

This method of gloving uses a skin-to-skin, glove-to-glove technique. The hand, although scrubbed, is not sterile and must not contact the exterior of the sterile gloves. The everted cuff on the gloves exposes the inner surfaces. The first glove is put on with skin-to-skin technique, bare hand to inside cuff. The sterile fingers of that gloved hand then may touch the sterile exterior of the second glove, that is, glove-to-glove technique.

1. With the left hand, grasp the cuff of the right glove on the fold. Pick up the glove and step back from the table. Look behind you before moving.
2. Insert the right hand into the glove and pull it on, leaving the cuff turned well down over the hand (Figure 11-17).
3. Slip the fingers of the gloved right hand *under* the everted cuff of the left glove. Pick up the glove and step back (Figure 11-18).
4. Insert the hand into the left glove and pull it on, leaving the cuff turned down over the hand.
5. With the fingers of the right hand, pull the cuff of the left glove over the cuff of the left sleeve. If the stockinette is not tight, fold a pleat, holding it with the right thumb while pulling the glove over the cuff. Avoid touching the bare wrist (Figure 11-19).
6. Repeat step 5 for the right cuff, using the left hand, and thereby completely gloving the right hand (Figure 11-20).

Gowning Another Person

A team member in sterile gown and gloves may assist the surgeon or another team member in gowning and gloving by taking the following steps:

1. Open the hand towel and lay it on the surgeon's hand, being careful not to touch the hand.
2. Unfold the gown carefully, holding it at the neckband.
3. Keeping your hands on the outside of the gown under a protective cuff of the neck and shoulder area, offer the *inside* of the gown to the surgeon. He or she slips the arms into the sleeves.
4. Release the gown. The surgeon holds arms outstretched while the circulator pulls the gown onto the shoulders and adjusts the sleeves so the cuffs are properly placed. In doing so, only the inside of the gown is touched at the seams.

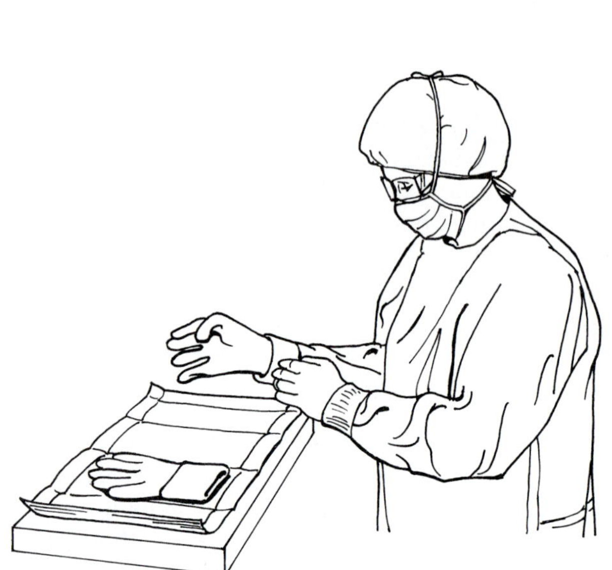

FIGURE 11-17 Scrub person gloving right hand with open gloving technique. With left hand, person grasps right glove on folded-back cuff and lifts it directly up and away from wrapper. Right hand is inserted in glove. Note that left hand touches only cuff or inside of glove, which is skin-to-skin technique.

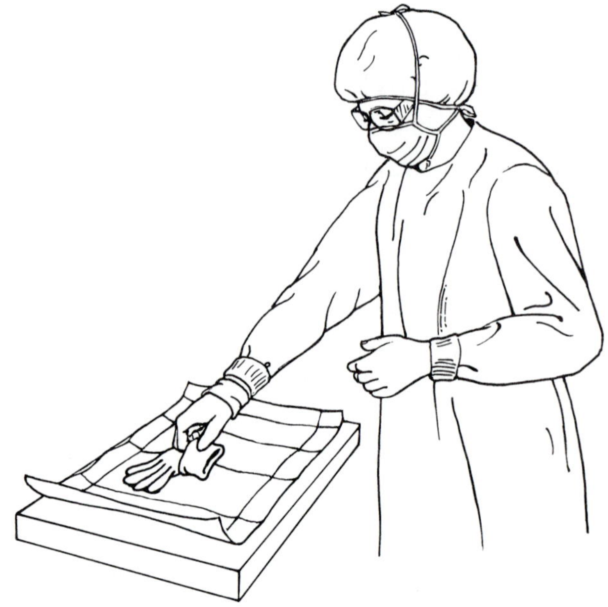

FIGURE 11-18 Picking up left glove, scrub person lifts glove from wrapper by slipping gloved right fingers under protective cuff, using glove-to-glove technique. Bare hand does not touch outside of glove.

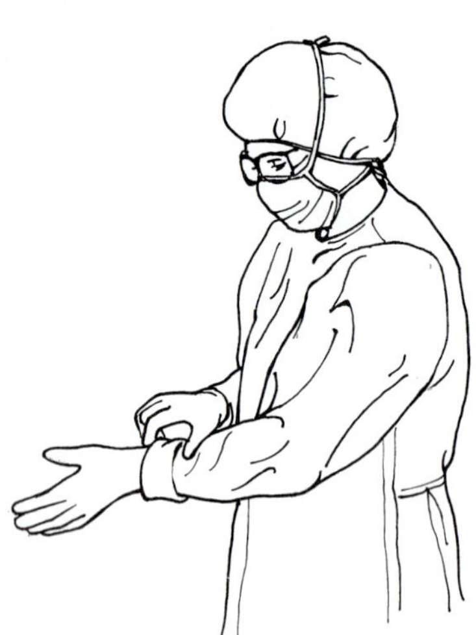

FIGURE 11-19 As cuff of left glove is pulled up over cuff of sleeve, gloved fingers of right hand touch only outside of left glove, near wrist. If stockinette is not tight, fold a pleat, holding it with right thumb while pulling glove over cuff. Contact with exposed skin would contaminate right glove. (A pleat cannot be held if *regloving* because cuff is contaminated.)

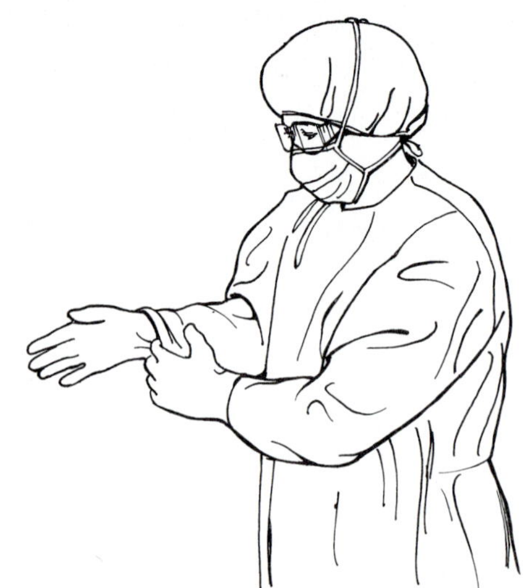

FIGURE 11-20 With completely gloved left hand, left fingers are inserted under folded-back cuff of right glove and glove cuff is pulled up over right sleeve cuff, using glove-to-glove technique.

Gloving Another Person

1. Pick up the right glove, grasp it firmly, with the fingers under the everted cuff. Hold the *palm* of the glove toward the surgeon.
2. Stretch the cuff sufficiently for the surgeon to introduce the hand. Avoid touching the hand by holding your thumbs out (Figure 11-21).
3. Exert upward pressure as the surgeon plunges the hand into the glove.
4. Unfold the everted glove cuff over the cuff of the sleeve.
5. Repeat for the left hand.
6. If a sterile vest is needed, hold it for the surgeon to slip the hands into the armholes. Be careful not to contaminate gloves at the neck level. If the gown is a wraparound, assist the surgeon.

Changing Gown During Surgical Procedure

Occasionally a contaminated gown must be changed during a surgical procedure. The circulator unfastens the neck and waist. Grasped at the shoulders, the gown is pulled off inside out. The gown is always removed first. The gloves are removed using glove-to-glove and then skin-to-skin technique. If only the sleeve is contaminated, a sterile sleeve may be put on over the contaminated one.

Changing Glove During Surgical Procedure

If a glove becomes contaminated for any reason during a surgical procedure, it must be changed immediately. If you cannot step away immediately, hold the contaminated hand away from the sterile area. To change the glove:

1. Turn away from the sterile field.

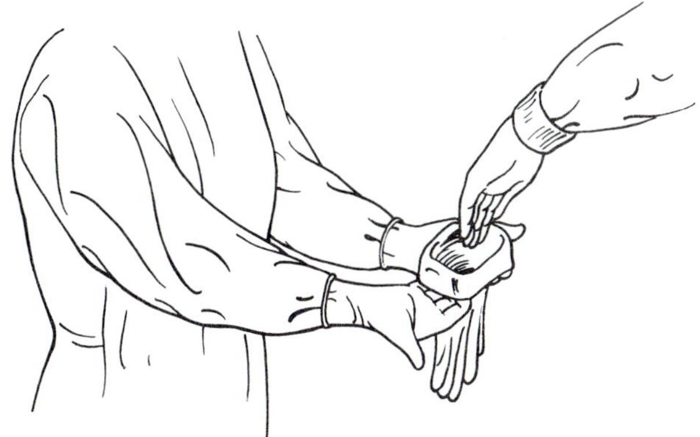

FIGURE 11-21 In gloving surgeon or another person, scrub person holds glove with palm toward him or her. Scrub person keeps thumbs extended outward to avoid being touched by bare hands of person donning gloves.

2. Extend the contaminated hand to the circulator who, wearing protective gloves, grasps the outside of the glove cuff about 2 inches (5 cm) below the top of the glove and pulls the glove off inside out.
3. Preferably a sterile team member gloves another. If this is not possible, step aside and glove the hand using the open glove technique.

NOTE

- The closed glove technique cannot be used for glove change during a surgical procedure without contamination of the new glove by the sleeve of the gown or without contamination of the hand by the cuff of the gown. The cuff must not be pulled down over the hand. If this method is used, gloves and gown must be removed and another sterile gown donned before gloves.
- The scrub person should change own gloves, before gowning and gloving another team member.

Removing Gown and Gloves

The gown is always removed before the gloves at the end of the surgical procedure.

Removing Gown

The circulator unfastens the neck and back closures of the gown so the wearer does not contaminate his or her scrub suit. If wearing a wraparound gown, the wearer unfastens the waist closure in front. The gown is always removed inside out to protect the arms and scrub suit from contaminated outside of the gown. To remove:

1. Grasp the right shoulder of the loosened gown with the left hand and pull the gown downward from the shoulder and off the right arm, turning the sleeve inside out (Figure 11-22, *A*).
2. Turn the outside of the gown away from the body with flexed elbows (Figure 11-22, *B*).
3. Grasp the left shoulder with the right hand and remove the gown entirely, pulling it off inside out (Figure 11-22, *C*).
4. Discard in a laundry hamper or in a trash receptacle (if disposable).

Removing Gloves

The cuffs of gloves usually turn down as the gown is pulled off the arms. Use glove-to-glove, then skin-to-skin technique to protect the clean hands from the contaminated outside of the gloves, which bear cells of the patient (Figure 11-23).

1. Grasp the cuff of the left glove with gloved fingers of the right hand and pull it off inside out.
2. Slip the ungloved fingers of the left hand under the cuff of the right glove and slip it off inside out.
3. Discard gloves in a trash receptacle.
4. Wash hands.

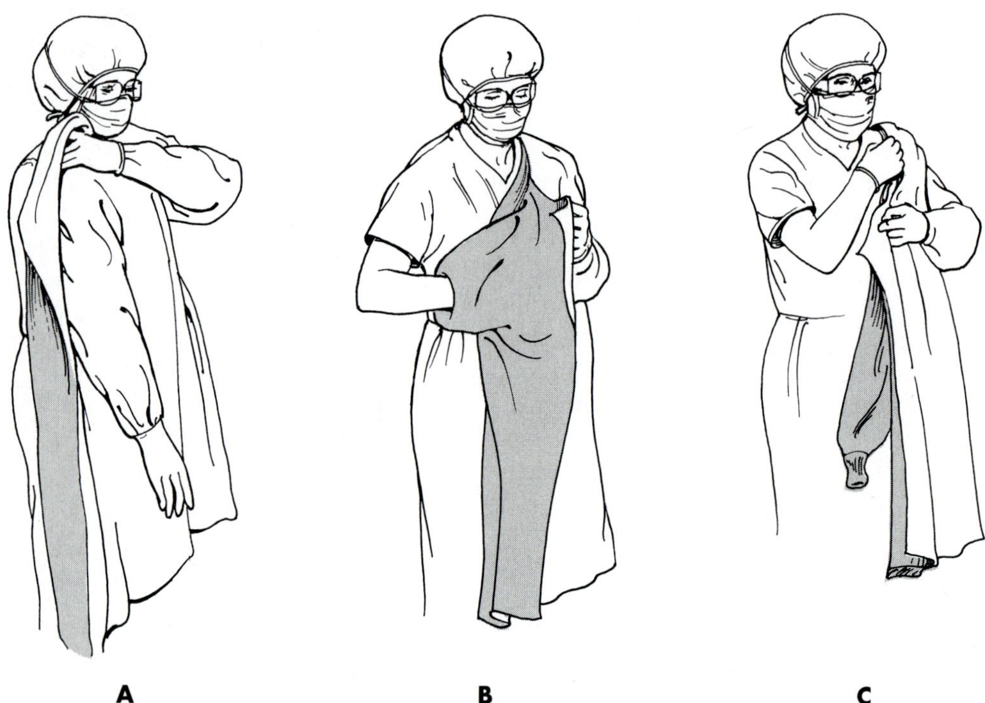

FIGURE 11-22 Sequence of scrub person removing soiled gown at end of surgical procedure. Clean arms and scrub suit are protected from contaminated outside of gown. **A,** With gloves on, cuffs of gown are loosened and shaken down over wrists. Then right shoulder of gown (unfastened or untied) is grasped with left hand. **B,** In pulling gown off arms, arm of gown is turned away from body with flexed elbow. **C,** Other shoulder is grasped with other hand and gown is removed entirely by pulling it off inside out and keeping arms clean.

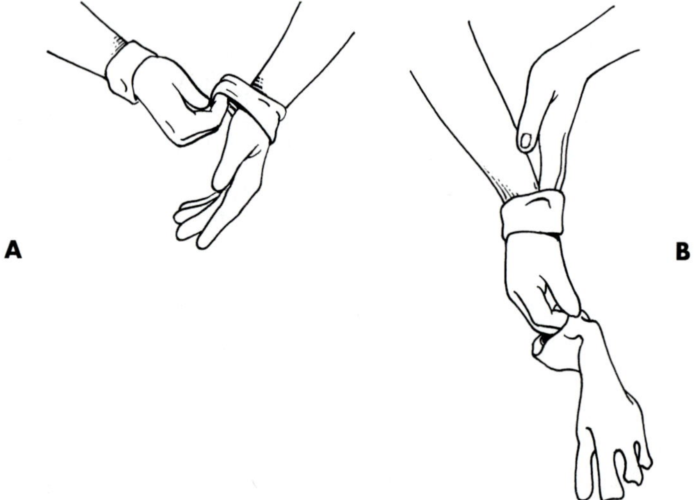

FIGURE 11-23 Sequence of scrub person removing soiled gloves at end of surgical procedure. First, glove-to-glove technique **(A)**, then skin-to-skin technique **(B)** is used to protect "clean" hands from contaminated outside of gloves, which bear cells of patient. Gloves are turned inside out for removal.

Bibliography

Baumgardiner CA et al: Effects of nail polish on microbial growth of fingernails: dispelling sacred cows, *AORN J* 58(1):84-88, 1993.

Beck WC: Guest editorial: the surgical mask: another "sacred cow"? *AORN J* 55(4):955-957, 1992.

Beezhold D, Beck WC: Surgical glove powders bind latex antigens, *Arch Surg* 127(11):1354-1357, 1992.

Belkin NL: Gowns are "protective"—not barriers, *Nurs Manage* 24(1):79-80, 1993.

Belkin NL: Personal protective equipment in aseptic technique and universal precautions, *Today's OR Nurse* 14(6):15-20, 1992.

Bendig JW: Surgical hand disinfection, *J Hosp Infect* 15(2):143-148, 1990.

Bowell B: Operation clean-up: hands for cleanliness, *Nurs Standards* 6(15-16):24-25, 1992.

Breeze W: It is time to standardize surgical hand scrubs, *AORN J* 60(2):294-295, 1994.

Chen CC, Willeke K: Aerosol penetration through surgical masks, *Am J Infect Control* 20(4):177-184, 1992.

Chiu KY et al: The use of double latex gloves during hip fracture operations, *J Orthop Trauma* 7(4):354-356, 1993.

Eccleston SB: Gloving, *AORN J* 56(2):265-269, Aug 1992.

Fay MF, Dooher DT: Surgical gloves, *AORN J* 55(6):1500-1519, 1992.

Fogg DM: Clinical issues: glove removal, *AORN J* 60(1):106, 1994.

Harris HR: Contaminated shoe covers: an overlooked risk, *Surg Technol* 25(7):14-20, 1993.

Heenan A: Handwashing practices, *Nurs Times* 88(34):70, 1992.

Hubbard MS et al: Reducing blood contamination and injury in the OR, *AORN J* 55(1):194-201, 1992.

Korniewicz DM et al: Do your gloves fit the task? *Am J Nurs* 91(6):38-40, 1991.

Leclair J: A review of antiseptics, *Today's OR Nurse* 12(10):25-28, 1990.

Mathias JM: Experts discuss merits of surgical masks, *OR Manager* 9(11):1, 8-10, 1993.

Mathias JM: Is it time to shorten the five-minute scrub? *OR Manager* 10(4):1, 9, 12, 1994.

Mitchell NJ, Hunt S: Surgical face masks in modern operating rooms—costly and unnecessary ritual? *J Hosp Infect* 18(3):239-242, 1991.

Olsen RJ et al: Examination gloves as barriers to hand contamination in clinical practice, *JAMA* 270(3):350-353, 1993.

O'Neal M: Clinical issues: changing scrub clothes; hand scrub policies, *AORN J* 58(4):785-787, 1993.

O'Shaughnessy M et al: Optimum duration of surgical scrub time, *Br J Surg* 28(6):685-686, 1991.

Patterson P, Schwanitz L: Flexible OR eyewear policy okay, OSHA says, *OR Manager* 9(4):1, 18-19, 1993.

Paulson DS: Comparative evaluation of five surgical hand scrub preparations, *AORN J* 60(2):246-256, 1994.

Proposed recommended practices for surgical attire, *AORN J* 60(2): 282-292, 1994.

Proposed recommended practices for surgical hand scrubs, *AORN J* 60(2):270-279, 1994.

Quebbeman EJ et al: In-use evaluation of surgical gowns, *Surg Gynecol Obstet* 174(5):369-375, 1992.

Recommended practices: Protective barrier materials for surgical gowns and drapes, *AORN J* 55(3):832-835, 1992.

Sadler C: A necessary spectacle? *Nurs Times* 87(23):21, 1991.

Schwanitz L: What to wear when going outside to smoke, *OR Manager* 9(9):22-23, 1993.

Tanner M: Increasing use, power of lasers make eye protection essential, *Occup Health Safety* 59(7):44-46, 1990.

Tests evaluate barrier effectiveness of gowns, *OR Manager* 9(5):1,7, 1993.

Webb JM, Pentlow BD: Double gloving and surgical technique, *Ann R Coll Surg Engl* 75(4):291-292, 1993.

Wynd CA et al: Bacterial carriage on the fingernails of OR nurses, *AORN J* 60(5):796-805, 1994.

Zinner NL: How safe are your gloves? *AORN J* 59(4):876-882, 1994.

CHAPTER 12

Essentials of Asepsis

APPLICATION OF PRINCIPLES OF ASEPTIC AND STERILE TECHNIQUES

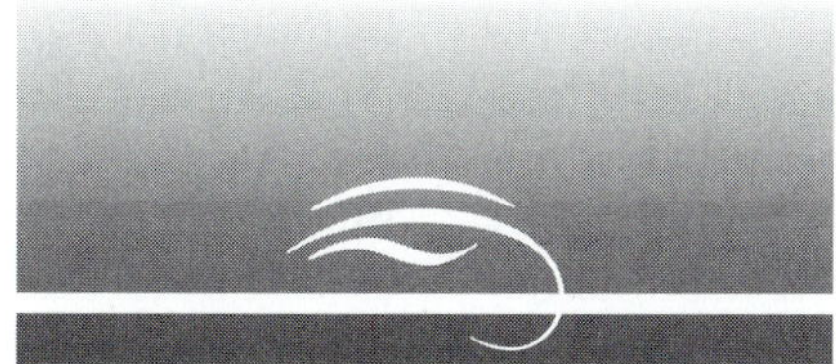

HISTORICAL BACKGROUND

In ancient times demons and evil spirits were thought to be the cause of pestilence and infection. Strange methods to drive them away were replaced by purification with fire. Today we still use heat as one means of destroying microorganisms.

In the pre-Christian era Hippocrates (460-377 BC) advocated irrigation of wounds with wine or boiled water, foreshadowing asepsis. Galen (130-200 AD), a Greek who practiced medicine in Rome and was the most distinguished physician after Hippocrates, boiled instruments used in caring for wounded Roman gladiators. His writings and those of Hippocrates were the established authority for medicine for many centuries.

Not until after Ignaz Semmelweis (1818-1865) advocated the value of handwashing and Louis Pasteur (1822-1895) taught his germ theory in the mid-nineteenth century did physicians begin to study the cause of infections and means to control them. Robert Koch (1843-1910), who isolated the tubercle bacillus, advocated the use of bichloride of mercury as an antiseptic. These events triggered interest in antisepsis.

During the mid-nineteenth century Florence Nightingale (1820-1910) advocated the use of pure air, pure water, efficient drainage, cleanliness, and light to promote health. Her nursing experience during the Crimean War proved the efficacy of these practices. She believed that the environment had a direct bearing on prevention of disease. Her tenets remain the foundation of nursing care. Indeed nurses have had a major influence during the twentieth century in preventing infection and the spread of communicable diseases. Some of the practices became ritualistic, but the principles supporting most are scientifically sound.

Surgical technique has advanced since the nineteenth century when the surgeon operated in a Prince Albert coat. He unwound sutures from a spool and hung them in a buttonhole. He kept a household pincushion nearby for his needles. He used the same blood- and pus-absorbent sponges for every patient. During a surgical procedure he may have held the scalpel between his teeth to protect the blade.

Joseph Lister (1827-1912), the English surgeon who became known as the father of modern surgery, pursued Pasteur's work. Because the relationship between bacteria and infection was known, he searched for a chemical to combat bacteria and surgical infections. He was the first to use a carbolic solution on dressings, which reduced the mortality of his patients somewhat. Lister believed infections were airborne. He wanted to kill them in the wound and the surrounding area. In 1865 he started to use carbolic spray in the OR. Then he used it in the wound, on articles in contact with the wound, and on the hands of the operating team. The result was a notable decrease in mortality. However, the carbolic solution caused wound necrosis and skin irritation in both patients and operators. It was said to "favour hemorrhage," making hemostasis difficult. Although unable to decide whether putrefaction was "germinal or chemical," some surgeons were convinced of the value of antiseptics. However, Lister was derided by other surgeons. It was not until 1879 at a medical meeting in Amsterdam that Lister's antiseptic principle of surgery was truly accepted by the medical profession.

German surgeons played a role in the transition from antisepsis to asepsis. Gustav Neuber (1850-1932) introduced mercuric chloride in 1886 to clean his apron. He advocated scrubbing the furniture with disinfectant and wearing gowns, boots, and caps. He eventually sterilized everything in contact with wounds.

The concept of asepsis further evolved with the development of sterilization. The first steam sterilizer also was introduced in Germany in 1886. Surgeons learned that all things that came in contact with a wound should be sterile (i.e., free from microorganisms and spores). Subsequent to the development of sterilization, other aspects of aseptic technique evolved. These included refinement of surgical technique, use of controlled environment, precise housekeeping methods, and universal precautions to protect patients and personnel from infection.

The development of passive and active immunization and antibiotic therapy had revolutionary effects on surgical practice. Nevertheless the ideal state of infection-free surgical procedures is not always a reality. Wound and systemic infections continue to occur.

Community-acquired infections have plagued society throughout history. The devastating effects of syphilis once filled mental institutions. Epidemics such as the bubonic plague of 1348 and the influenza epidemic of 1918 took their toll on human lives. Tuberculosis, once prevalent in the general population, remains a major health problem in some parts of the world and is on the increase again in the United States. Viral hepatitis has been a concern for decades.

Vaccines have been developed to prevent many communicable diseases. The first of these was developed by Edward Jenner (1749-1823), an English physician. In 1796 he inoculated a child with a cowpox vaccine to prevent smallpox. Subsequently vaccines and antitoxins have been developed to provide passive acquired immunity against such infectious diseases as diphtheria, rubella, and poliomyelitis. Although nearly eradicated, these and other infectious diseases still occur, sometimes in epidemic proportions.

The human immunodeficiency virus (HIV) clearly represents a worldwide threat to public health that is unprecedented in modern times. Since this virus was introduced into the United States in the late 1970s, the resultant infection has spread at an alarming rate via contaminated blood and infected persons. Clinical problems in patients with seropositive sera began appearing in 1978. Because of its effect on the immune system and its unknown origin when first reported in 1981, this infection became known as acquired immunodeficiency syndrome (AIDS). In 1983 researchers at the Institut Pasteur in Paris isolated the lymphadenopathy-associated virus (LAV). In 1984 a similar retrovirus called human T-cell lymphotropic virus type III (HTLV-III) was reported by the National Institutes of Health in Bethesda, Md. Since 1986, LAV and HTLV retroviruses causing AIDS or related illnesses have been known collectively as HIV.

Because of the prevalence of community-acquired infections and the potential for development of nosocomial infection (acquired during the course of health care), careful attention to the creation and maintenance of a safe and therapeutic environment is mandatory. Knowledge of causative microorganisms, their modes of transmission, and methods of control is the basis of prevention of infection. The Centers for Disease Control and Prevention (CDC) issue guidelines for prevention of transmission of infections. Whether in a surgical wound or systemic in the body, infection is a serious and potentially fatal postoperative complication (see Chapter 25).

DEFINITIONS

To effectively apply the principles of asepsis, environmental control, and sterile techniques to be discussed in this chapter, the meaning of terms related to microbiology must be understood (Box 12-1).

INFECTION

Aseptic and sterile techniques, based on sound scientific principles, are carried out primarily to prevent transmission of microorganisms that can cause infection (Table 12-1). Microorganisms are invisible, but they are present in the air and on animate and inanimate objects. To prevent infection, all possible measures are taken to create and maintain a therapeutic environment for the patient. Infection that is acquired during the course of health care is known as a *nosocomial infection.* The infection may occur in the postoperative wound or as a complication unrelated to the surgical site. Postoperative infection is a very serious, potentially fatal complication that may result from a single break in technique. There-

BOX 12-1

Glossary of Terms Related to Microbiology

aerobe Microorganism that requires air or presence of oxygen for maintenance of life (adj., *aerobic*).

aerosol Dispersion of fine mist, droplets, or particulate matter into air (vt., *aerosolize;* to become airborne).

anaerobe Microorganism that grows best in oxygen-free environment or one that cannot tolerate oxygen (e.g., *Clostridium* species that causes gas gangrene) (adj., *anaerobic*).

antibiotics Substances, natural or synthetic, that inhibit growth of or destroy microorganisms. Used as therapeutic agents against infectious diseases; some are selective for a specific organism; some are broad-spectrum.

antimicrobial agent Chemical or pharmaceutical agent that destroys or inhibits growth of microorganisms (syn., *antiseptic, disinfectant, antibiotic, antiviral drugs*).

antisepsis Prevention of sepsis by the exclusion, destruction, or inhibition of growth or multiplication of microorganisms from body tissues and fluids.

antiseptics Inorganic chemical compounds that combat sepsis by inhibiting growth of microorganisms without necessarily killing them. Used on skin and tissue to arrest growth of endogenous microorganisms (resident flora), they must not destroy tissue.

asepsis Absence of microorganisms that cause disease; freedom from infection; exclusion of microorganisms (adj., *aseptic;* without infection).

aseptic body image An awareness of body, hair, makeup, clothes, jewelry, fingernails, and attire. Team members must be aware of proximity to areas considered sterile vs. those that are contaminated.

aseptic technique Methods by which contamination with microorganisms is prevented (alternate term: *aseptic practice,* to maintain asepsis).

bacteriostasis Inhibition of growth of bacteria. Bacteria are undamaged to extent that they will grow if placed in a favorable medium, away from action of chemicals (adj., *bacteriostatic;* most antiseptics are bacteriostatic because they do not kill bacteria).

barrier Material used to reduce or inhibit migration or transmission of microorganisms in the environment. Barriers include attire of personnel, drapes over furniture and patients, packaging of supplies, and filters in ventilating system.

bioburden Degree of microbial contamination on a device or object before sterilization or disinfection.

carrier Apparently healthy person who harbors and can transmit a pathogenic microorganism.

contaminated Soiled or infected by microorganisms.

cross contamination Transmission of microorganisms from patient to patient and from inanimate objects to patients and vice versa.

decontamination Cleaning and disinfecting or sterilizing processes carried out to make contaminated items safe to handle.

disease Specific entity that is the sum total of numerous characteristics of one or more pathologic processes; failure of the body's adaptive mechanisms to counteract adequately the stress to which it is subjected, resulting in disturbance in function or structure of any part, organ, or system of the body.

disinfectants Agents that kill all growing or vegetative forms of microorganisms, thus completely eliminating them from inanimate objects (syn., *germicide* [the suffix *-cide* means to kill]; adj., *germicidal*). Reference is made frequently to the specific action of the following disinfectants:

- **bactericide** Kills gram-negative and gram-positive bacteria unless specifically stated to the contrary (adj., *bactericidal*). Action may be specific to a species of bacteria (e.g., pseudomonacide kills *Pseudomonas aeruginosa;* tuberculocide kills *Mycobacterium tuberculosis*).
- **fungicide** Kills fungi.
- **sporicide** Kills spores.
- **virucide** Kills viruses.

disinfection Chemical or physical process of destroying most forms of pathogenic microorganisms except bacterial spores; used for inanimate objects, but not on tissue. Degree of disinfection depends primarily on strength of agent, nature of contamination, and purpose for the process.

- **high-level disinfection** Process that destroys all microorganisms except high numbers of bacterial spores.
- **intermediate-level disinfection** Process that inactivates vegetative bacteria, including *M. tuberculosis* and most fungi and viruses, but does not kill bacterial spores.
- **low-level disinfection** Process that kills most bacteria, some viruses, and some fungi, but does not destroy resistant microorganisms such as *M. tuberculosis* or bacterial spores.

droplet Minute particle of moisture, as expelled from respiratory tract by talking, sneezing, or coughing, which carries microorganisms.

endogenous Source of infection from within the body (i.e., disruption of balance between potentially pathogenic organisms and host defenses causing infection).

epidemiology Study of occurrence and distribution of disease; the sum of all factors controlling presence or absence of a disease.

exogenous Source of infection from outside the body (i.e., from environment or personnel).

flora Bacteria and fungi normally inhabiting the body, often delineated as *resident* or *transient.*

fomite Inanimate object that may be contaminated with infectious organisms and serves to transmit disease.

Gram's stain Bacteriologic test to classify species of bacteria. Bacteria are stained with solutions of crystal violet and iodine, followed by exposure to alcohol, and then counterstained. Bacteria that stain blue are *gram-positive;* those that remain pink are *gram-negative.*

Continued

BOX 12-1

Glossary of Terms Related to Microbiology—cont'd

infection Invasion of the body by pathogenic microorganisms and the reaction of tissues to their presence and to toxins generated by the organisms (adj., *infectious*).

community-acquired Infectious disease process that developed or was incubating before patient entered the health care facility.

cross infection Infection contracted by a patient from another patient or staff member, and/or contracted by a staff member from a patient.

droplet infection Infection transmitted from one person to another by airborne droplets.

nosocomial infection Hospital-associated or acquired infection not present when patient was admitted to health care facility. Infection may occur in postoperative wound or as complication unrelated to surgical site.

superinfection Secondary subsequent infection caused by a different microorganism that develops during or following antibiotic therapy.

infectious material Blood, serum, or other human body fluids that potentially may be hazardous to another person.

isolation Special precautions taken to prevent transmission of microorganisms from specific body substances.

microaerophilic Pertaining to microorganisms that require free oxygen for growth but thrive best when oxygen is less in amount than that in the atmosphere.

microorganisms Living organisms, invisible to the naked eye, including bacteria, fungi, viruses, protozoa, yeasts, and molds (syn., *microbe;* adj., *microbial*).

opportunists Microorganisms that do not normally invade tissue but are capable of causing infection or disease if introduced into the body mechanically through injury, such as tetanus bacillus, or when resistance of host may be lowered, as by HIV infection.

pathogenic Producing or capable of producing disease.

pathogenic microorganisms Microorganisms that cause infectious disease. They can invade healthy tissue through some power of their own or can injure tissue by a toxin they produce.

sepsis Severe toxic febrile state resulting from infection with pyogenic microorganisms, with or without associated septicemia.

septicemia Clinical syndrome characterized by significant invasion of microorganisms from a focus of infection in tissues into the bloodstream. Microorganisms may multiply in the blood. Infection of bacterial origin carried through the bloodstream is sometimes referred to as *bacteremia*.

spatial relationships An awareness of sterile, unsterile, clean, and contaminated areas and proximity to each. This would include height of scrubbed team members in relation to each other and the sterile field. The circulator must be aware of closeness to sterile field and of appropriate means to control environmental contaminants.

spores Inactive but viable state of microorganisms in the environment. Certain bacteria and fungi sustain themselves in this form until environment is favorable for vegetative growth. The spore stage is highly resistant to heat, toxic chemicals, and other methods of destruction.

sterile Free of microorganisms, including all spores.

sterile field Area around the site of incision into tissue or introduction of an instrument into a body orifice that has been prepared for use of sterile supplies and equipment. This area includes all furniture covered with sterile drapes and personnel who are properly attired.

sterile technique Methods by which contamination with microorganisms is prevented to maintain sterility throughout the surgical procedure.

sterilization Processes by which all pathogenic and nonpathogenic microorganisms, including spores, are killed. This term refers *only* to a process capable of destroying *all* forms of microbial life, including spores.

sterilizer Chamber or equipment used to attain either physical or chemical sterilization. Agent used must be capable of killing all forms of microorganisms.

surgically clean Mechanically cleaned but unsterile. Items are rendered surgically clean by the use of chemical, physical, or mechanical means that markedly reduce the number of microorganisms on them.

terminal sterilization and disinfection Procedures carried out for the destruction of pathogens at end of surgical procedure in the OR or in other areas of patient contact (i.e., PACU, ICU, nursing unit).

universal precautions Policies and procedures followed to protect personnel from contact with blood and body fluids of *all* patients.

unsterile Inanimate object that has not been subjected to a sterilization process; outside wrapping of package containing sterile item; person who has not prepared to enter sterile field (syn., *nonsterile*).

virulence Infectious disease evoking power of a microorganism. Pathogens are not equally capable of causing infection.

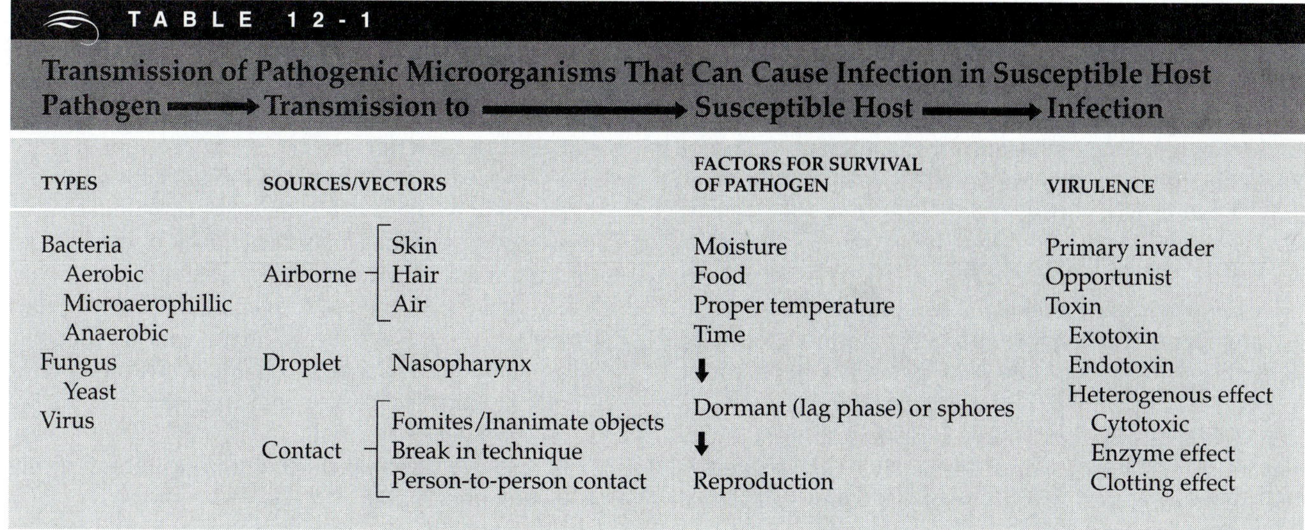

TABLE 12-1

Transmission of Pathogenic Microorganisms That Can Cause Infection in Susceptible Host
Pathogen ——→ Transmission to ——→ Susceptible Host ——→ Infection

TYPES	SOURCES/VECTORS		FACTORS FOR SURVIVAL OF PATHOGEN	VIRULENCE
Bacteria		Skin	Moisture	Primary invader
Aerobic	Airborne	Hair	Food	Opportunist
Microaerophillic		Air	Proper temperature	Toxin
Anaerobic			Time	Exotoxin
Fungus	Droplet	Nasopharynx	↓	Endotoxin
Yeast			Dormant (lag phase) or sphores	Heterogenous effect
Virus		Fomites/Inanimate objects		Cytotoxic
	Contact	Break in technique	↓	Enzyme effect
		Person-to-person contact	Reproduction	Clotting effect

fore knowledge of causative agents and their control as well as the principles of aseptic and sterile techniques is the basis of prevention.

Microbial Etiology

Infections may be caused by one or several types of microorganisms. Types are numerous and vary in incidence and significance of infection produced. The reader is referred to a standard textbook of microbiology for in-depth study.

Pathogens

Pathogenic microorganisms are those that cause sepsis, a severe toxic febrile state. They can invade healthy tissue through some power of their own or can injure tissue by a toxin they produce. Pathogens can cause either a bacterial or nonbacterial infection.

Bacterial Infections Bacteria are classified by the environment that sustains their life with oxygen (aerobic) or without oxygen (anaerobic), and as gram-positive or gram-negative. Gram's stain is a laboratory technique for identifying a primary characteristic of bacteria. Gentian violet is put on bacteria. Those that stain blue are gram-positive; those that do not stain are gram-negative. Infections may be caused by aerobic, microaerophilic, or anaerobic bacteria or can be mixed bacterial infections. Microaerophils require less oxygen than present in air. The following are the most common bacterial pathogens:

1. Aerobic bacteria (require oxygen)
   a. Gram-positive cocci, such as *Staphylococcus aureus, Staphylococcus epidermidis, Streptococcus* Group B, *Streptococcus* Group D, methicillin-resistant *Staphylococcus aureus* (MRSA)
   b. Gram-negative cocci, such as *Neisseria gonorrhoeae*
   c. Gram-positive bacilli, such as *Bacillus* species, *Mycobacterium tuberculosis*
   d. Gram-negative bacilli, such as *Escherichia coli, Klebsiella* species, *Pseudomonas aeruginosa, Pseudomonas cepacia, Proteus* species, *Serratia marcescens, Citrobacter* species, *Salmonella* species, *Alcaligenes faecalis, Hemophilus influenzae, Enterobacter aerogenes, Enterobacter cloacae, Legionella pneumophilia*
2. Microaerophilic bacteria (require oxygen less than in the atmosphere)
   a. Gram-positive cocci, such as hemolytic and nonhemolytic streptococci
3. Anaerobic bacteria (grow in the absence of oxygen)
   a. Gram-positive cocci, such as peptostreptococcus, peptococcus
   b. Gram-positive bacilli, such as *Clostridium tetani, Clostridium welchii*
   c. Gram-negative bacilli, such as *Bacteroides* species, *Bacteroides fragilis*

This list is incomplete but includes the organisms that most frequently cause nosocomial infections. Some organisms are primary invaders; others are opportunists that secondarily invade or superimpose on an already infected host with inhibited resistance. Identification of causative organisms will direct the investigation (e.g., streptococcus or *Staphylococcus aureus* from personnel, mycobacterium from inanimate objects). Epidemics caused by gram-negative microorganisms may be spread from environmental sources. Every bacterium is a potential pathogen given dense enough contamination and a susceptible host.

Nonbacterial Infections Infections may be caused by fungi, protozoa, or viruses. Specific infections are discussed later in this chapter. Nonbacterial microorganisms are as follows:

1. Fungi, such as *Candida albicans, Histoplasmosis capsulatum, Phycomycosis* species, wild yeasts
2. Protozoa, such as *Entamoeba histolytica, Trichomonas vaginalis, Pneumocystis carinii*
3. Viruses, such as hepatitis virus, human immunodeficiency virus, herpesvirus, cytomegalovirus, Epstein-Barr virus

Viability of Organisms

Microorganisms need moisture, food, proper temperature, and time to reproduce. When transferred from one place to another, they pass through a dormant or lag phase of about 5 hours or longer. Then each organism divides itself about every 20 minutes. Most bacteria, fungi, and viruses are killed easily by the processes of sterilization and disinfection (see Chapter 13), but bacterial spores are not.

Spores are the resting, protective stage of some rod-shaped bacilli. Dense layers of protein form within the cells; they can be compared to the shell of a nut. The thicker the wall or shell, the more resistant the spore is to destruction. When conditions suitable for bacterial growth are reestablished, the spore releases cells for active growth and reproduction. In the vegetative state spore-bearing bacteria are no more difficult to kill than nonspore-forming bacteria. Although spores are formed by only about 150 species of bacilli, they are universally present in the environment.

Toxins of Microbial Origin

Pathogenic microorganisms produce substances that adversely affect the host locally and/or systemically on invasion. Toxic substances affecting tissues, cells, and possibly enzyme systems diffuse from the microbial cells. The cellular substance of a wide variety of organisms is toxic also. In addition, harmful effects may be produced indirectly by activation of tissue enzymes by bacteria. Such toxic substances include:

1. *Exotoxins.* These classic bacterial toxins are the most potent toxins known. As little as 7 oz (200 ml) of crystalline botulism type A toxin is said to be able to kill the world's entire population. Exotoxins appear to be proteins, are denatured by heat, and are destroyed by proteolytic enzymes, which break down protein. The formation of exotoxins is relatively uncommon, but their actions are multiple.
2. *Endotoxins.* These are contained within the cell wall of bacteria. They are heat stable and are not digested by proteolytic enzymes. On parenteral inoculation they cause a rise in body temperature and are known as *bacterial pyrogens.* They increase capillary permeability with the resultant production of local hemorrhage. Although causing injury to body cells at the site of infection, endotoxins more importantly cause serious, often lethal, effects by dissemination and widespread injury to many tissues throughout the body. Endotoxic shock may occur in bacteremia caused by gram-negative bacteria.
3. *Heterogeneous substances.* Microorganisms also form a variety of other heterogeneous (dissimilar) toxic substances, which may contribute to the disease process directly or facilitate the establishment of foci of infection. Toxins, which diffuse from the intact microbial cell, have the following various effects:
   a. *Cytotoxic effect* affects red and white blood cells, e.g., causing leukopenia (reduction of leukocytes below normal).
   b. *Clotting effect* interferes with the clotting mechanism of blood.
   c. *Enzymatic effect* causes bacterial hemolysins to dissolve red blood cells or fibrin, thereby inhibiting clot formation. *Coagulase,* a substance of bacterial origin, is causally related to thrombus formation. Coagulase-positive staphylococcus, *Bacillus subtilis, Escherichia coli,* and *Serratia marcescens* accelerate clotting of blood and induce intravascular clotting.
4. *Viral substances.* Toxic substances are also associated with viruses.

Some bacteria are encapsulated, a defense mechanism against phagocytic activity of leukocytes. These bacteria may be ingested by white blood cells, but instead of being killed and digested they remain within the phagocyte for a time, then are extruded in a viable condition. The presence of a capsule is associated with virulence among pathogenic bacteria.

SOURCES OF CONTAMINATION

In spite of many variables associated with sepsis, people remain the major source of microorganisms in the environment. Everything on or around a human being is contaminated by him or her in some way. In addition, the action and interaction of personnel and patients contribute to the prevalence of organisms.

OR personnel are primarily concerned with protecting the OR suite environment. Surgical procedures should be performed under optimal conditions within the limits of professional capability. The two most critical areas for the introduction and spread of microorganisms are as follows:

1. Semirestricted area, open to properly attired authorized personnel
2. Restricted area, occupied by OR teams and patients

Many sources contaminate the OR environment. Most microbes grow in a warm, moist host, but some aerobic bacteria, yeasts, and fungi can remain viable in the air and on inanimate objects.

Skin

Skin of patients, OR team members, and visitors constitutes a hazard. Hair follicles and sebaceous and sweat glands (sudoriferous) contain abundant resident microbial flora. An estimated 4000 to 10,000 viable particles are shed by an average individual's skin per minute. Some people disperse up to 30,000 particles per minute. *Shedders* are persons who present an additional hazard. They are densely populated with virulent organisms that they shed with skin cells into the environment. These organisms usually are *Staphylococcus aureus.* Shedders have a much higher incidence of wound infection. True shedders are estimated to be 1 in 50 persons. Major areas of microbial population on all persons are the head, neck, axillae, hands, groin, perineum, legs, and feet. Cosmetic detritus is also laden with skin bacteria. Microbial shedding is contained most effectively by maximum skin coverage (see Chapter 11).

Hair

Hair is a gross contaminant and major source of species of *Staphylococcus*. The extent to which the microbial population is attracted to and shed from hair is directly related to the length and cleanliness of the hair. Hair follicles and filaments harbor resident and transient floras.

Nasopharynx

Organisms forcibly expelled by talking, coughing, or sneezing give rise to bacteria-laden dust and lint as droplets settle on surfaces and skin. Persons known as *carriers* harbor many organisms, notably Group A *Streptococcus* and *Staphylococcus aureus,* which may be carried pharyngeally or rectally. They usually are transmitted by direct contact. More surgeons and anesthesiologists are carriers than nurses because of intimate contact with patients' respiratory tracts. Carriers do not usually present a real threat in the absence of an overt lesion. However, when clusters of infection break out postoperatively, shedders and carriers who disseminate organisms and whose organism matches that of infected patients are sought.

Fomites

Contaminated particles are present on inanimate objects such as furniture, OR surfaces (walls, floors, cabinet shelves), equipment, supplies, and fabrics. Covert contamination may result from improper handling of equipment such as anesthesia apparatus or intravenous (IV) lines and fluids. Contamination may result from the administration of unsterile medications or use of unsterile water to rinse sterile items.

Air

Thousands of submicron sized particles per cubic foot of air are present in the OR. During a long surgical procedure particle count can rise to more than a million particles per cubic foot. Air and dust are vehicles for transporting microorganism-laden particles. Air movement and thermal currents entrain dust and microbial particulates. The OR lights and other heat-generating equipment produce convective upcurrents. Particulates that become airborne can then settle on an open wound. Between 80% and 90% of microbial contamination found in an open surgical wound comes from ambient (room) air. Because airborne contamination is generated by personnel, every movement increases potential for wound infection.

Microorganisms have an affinity for horizontal surfaces, of which the floor is the largest. From it, they are projected into the air. Endogenous flora from the patient's skin, oropharynx, tracheobronchial tree, and gastrointestinal tract, as well as exogenous flora, are significant. Microorganisms from patients or carriers settle on equipment and flat surfaces, then become airborne. Airborne particles increase significantly during activity before incision and after wound closure.

An effective ventilation system is essential to prevent patients and staff from breathing contaminated air, which would predispose them to respiratory infection and could increase the incidence of microbial carriers among OR personnel.

Human Error

Although air is a major vehicle for transmission of pathogens, direct person-to-person contact is the most frequent means by which infection is spread. Human error is an exogenous source of contamination not to be underestimated. If breaks in technique occur through lack of knowledge or lack of adherence to the principles of technique and their applications, the patient is exposed to a risk that could have been prevented. Errors must be readily admitted and corrected.

Cross Infection

Every patient in the OR should be considered potentially infected. Specific precautions, in addition to routine aseptic techniques, are observed whether an infectious or communicable disease or specific organism is known to be present at the time of the surgical procedure or not. Care, caution, and conscientiousness are essential on the part of all team members. A mnemonic, Search Every Source To Provide Safe Care For Health, may be helpful to remember the most common pathogens in the environment (Table 12-2).

Breaks in aseptic technique can be a source of cross infection. *Universal blood and body fluid precautions* (see pp. 198-199) *must be followed in the care of all patients.* Thorough handwashing after every patient contact also is important.

TABLE 12-2

Common Pathogens in OR Environment, Using Mnemonic *Search Every Source To Provide Safe Care For Health*

MICRO-ORGANISM	USUAL ENVIRONMENT	MODE OF TRANSMISSION
Staphylococci	Skin, hair	Direct contact
	Upper respiratory tract	Airborne
Escherichia coli	Intestinal tract	Feces, urine
	Urinary tract	Direct contact
Streptococci	Oronasopharynx	Airborne
	Skin, perianal	Direct contact
Mycobacterium tuberculosis	Respiratory tract	Airborne, droplet
	Urinary tract	Direct contact
Pseudomonas	Urinary tract	Direct contact
	Intestinal tract	Urine, feces
	Water	Water
Serratia marcescens	Urinary tract	Direct contact
	Respiratory tract	Water
Clostridium	Intestinal tract	Direct contact
Fungi	Dust, soil	Airborne
	Inanimate objects	Direct contact
Hepatitis virus	Blood	Bloodborne
	Body fluids	Direct contact

Some specific infectious diseases are worthy of mention because they present significant nosocomial hazards to both patients and personnel in the environment.

Tuberculosis

Tuberculosis (TB) is caused by *Mycobacterium tuberculosis,* an aerobic, acid-fast gram-positive bacteria. Tubercle bacilli usually infect the lungs (pulmonary TB), but they may be present in joints, kidneys, or other organs. Acute miliary tuberculosis may be seen in an abdominal procedure as generalized peritonitis. *M. tuberculosis* is an opportunistic organism. Individuals at high risk include persons immunosuppressed from human immunodeficiency virus (HIV), corticosteroid therapy, chemotherapy, or malnutrition. Others with diabetes mellitus, cirrhosis, alcoholism, silicosis or other lung disease and persons with prolonged exposure and contact with an actively infected person are also at risk. The tubercle bacillus can remain dormant, encased in a hard shell for years after exposure. Because the bacillus may become airborne by droplets from the respiratory tract, the disease must be monitored and controlled to prevent cross infection. Unsuspected active cases and inactive carriers represent a particular hazard. Patients with acute disease are isolated and placed on respiratory secretion precautions for approximately 2 weeks following initiation of treatment.

Therapy is long term, usually 6 to 12 months of drug therapy. Isoniazid (INH) and rifampin most effectively kill reactive bacilli and prevent reactivation. Pyrazinamide, ethambutol, and streptomycin also may be used for multidrug therapy; some other drugs that are less effective and have more side effects may be indicated. *M. tuberculosis* mutates and may become resistant to a single- or multidrug therapy regimen. Multidrug-resistant tuberculosis (MDR-TB) can be fatal, especially in HIV-infected persons.

For care of surgical patients who have active TB:

1. Postpone elective surgical procedures, if possible, until patient shows response to drug therapy (i.e., is no longer infectious as confirmed by a negative sputum smear).
2. Use disposable anesthesia equipment to the extent possible. Reusable equipment must be sterilized or high-level disinfected immediately after use. A bacterial filter on the endotracheal tube or at the expiratory side of the breathing circuit may be useful in reducing the risk of contamination of anesthesia equipment or the discharge of tubercle bacilli into ambient air.
3. Use respiratory isolation precautions for patients with positive sputum. This includes putting a mask on the patient during transport to the OR. The transporter also wears a mask. OR team members should wear face-fitting masks that filter particles of 1 µm at a 95% efficiency level (i.e., a disposable high-efficiency particulate air [HEPA] filtered mask, valveless dust-mist respirator, or dust-fume-mist filtered respirator). A powered respirator mask (approved by the National Institute for Occupational Safety and Health) equipped with HEPA filter may be worn during high-risk procedures such as bronchoscopy, endotracheal intubation, and tracheal suctioning.
4. Perform the surgical procedure at a time when other patients and a minimum number of staff members are present in the OR suite (i.e., at end of day's schedule if possible). Keep OR doors closed and traffic to a minimum.
5. Sterilize critical items (i.e., those entering the bloodstream or body cavity); semicritical items (i.e., those in contact with mucous membranes only) may be sterilized or high-level disinfected with a tuberculocide.
6. Move patient into an isolation room that has negative pressure ventilation with local exhaust and HEPA air filtration and/or ultraviolet radiation lamps.
7. Screen high-risk patients and test personnel at least annually. Testing includes chest x-ray film and skin test. Exposed personnel should be retested every 6 months.

TB is the number one fatal infectious disease in the world. In many facilities yearly TB testing of all OR personnel is mandatory. The most accurate test is the *Mantoux* method. The Mantoux test is administered by injecting 0.1 ml of *purified protein derivative* (PPD) of tubercle bacillus subcutaneously in the forearm to form a small wheal under the skin. The site is examined in 24 to 72 hours. Redness, itching, and induration of 8 to 10 mm at the site of injection are considered a positive or a significant reaction. Further testing and chest x-ray films may be performed before treatment can begin. Reaction of less than 8 mm at the site of injection is considered an insignificant or negative reading, and no further action is needed.

Viral Hepatitis

Viruses can produce acute inflammation of the liver. The pathogens causing viral hepatitis create an occupational hazard to health care providers. A patient may be in an acute stage of the infection but more commonly is an unknown carrier of one of the viruses that cause hepatitis.

Hepatitis A Formerly called infectious hepatitis, hepatitis A is an acute illness that is usually brief but can last for several months. It is spread by oral ingestion of contaminated water and food, especially shellfish, and by fecal contaminants. The hepatitis A virus (HAV) is most infectious during the 2 weeks before the onset of symptoms and until after the first week of jaundice. The incubation period is 15 to 90 days, with an average of 28 days. Immune globulin may be effective if given within 2 weeks of exposure. HAV infection is the most common type of viral hepatitis. However, HAV is not a major nosocomial problem because it does not have a chronic carrier state.

Hepatitis B Formerly called serum hepatitis, the hepatitis B virus (HBV) is a major nosocomial problem. Carriers are a main source of cross infection. Hepatitis B surface antigen is the carrier state of HBV. This can be harbored for prolonged periods of up to 15 years and has been found in practically all body fluids of infected persons. It is transmitted percutaneously or permucosally by blood, serum, and other body fluids. The incubation period is 6 weeks to 6 months, with an average of about 60 days, before mild to severe symptoms become apparent. Chronic hepatitis, cirrhosis, or liver carcinoma may develop.

Serologic tests are used to diagnose infection, detect carriers, and monitor high-risk persons. Patients who have undiagnosed hepatitis, who fail to reveal they have chronic hepatitis, or who are asymptomatic carriers can transmit the virus to health care providers. Personnel in the OR, emergency department, blood bank, laboratory, and hemodialysis unit are especially at risk. HBV surface antigen is easily transmitted by direct contact with blood and body fluids via a needlestick or scalpel cut, via a break in the skin such as a minor cut or hangnail, or via a splash into mucosa of the eye, nose, or mouth. Fomites also can transmit HBV. HBV can be transmitted by sexual intercourse and from an infected mother to a neonate during birth.

Immunization against HBV is recommended for high-risk health care workers. HBV vaccination is given before exposure. After exposure, such as following an accidental needlestick, both the vaccine and hepatitis B immune globulin are given. Hospitals are required to make these immunizations available to personnel.

NOTE Any accidental exposure, such as self-puncture with a contaminated needle or splash in the eye, should be reported and followed up as soon as possible for immunizations, even if the patient is not known to have hepatitis.

Hepatitis C Formerly known as transfusion-associated or non-A, non-B hepatitis, the hepatitis C virus (HCV) is responsible for about 90% of posttransfusion hepatitis. HCV is a bloodborne ribonucleic acid (RNA) virus. Recipients of multiple transfusions or chronic hemodialysis, intravenous drug users, and health care workers are at risk. Persons with acute hepatitis C are asymptomatic. A worldwide, bloodborne infection, HCV is transmitted predominantly by transfusion of blood and blood products. However, it can also be transmitted by needlestick injuries. A screening test detects the presence of antibodies in the blood. Incubation varies from 2 weeks to 6 months. The infection may progress insidiously in a carrier for as long as 25 years. HCV infection can precipitate chronic hepatitis, cirrhosis, and liver cancer.

Hepatitis D Also known as *delta hepatitis,* hepatitis D coexists with a HBV infection or superinfects a HBV carrier. A defective RNA virus, hepatitis D virus (HDV) requires HBV for its survival and replication in both acute and chronic forms. HDV is communicable during all phases of active infection. It can lead to necrotizing liver disease and death. The majority of patients developing this complication of HBV infection are intravenous drug abusers who used contaminated needles. Immunization against HBV will also prevent hepatitis D.

Hepatitis E The hepatitis E virus (HEV) is a form of non-A, non-B virus common in Asia, Africa, and Mexico. HEV can cause an epidemic of hepatitis E. The incubation period is 15 to 64 days, with an average of 25 to 42 days in different epidemics. Similar to HAV in characteristics, there are no specific serologic tests for HEV at this time. HEV is spread via the fecal-to-oral route through contaminated water or food or from poor sanitation conditions. Current immunoglobulins do not provide protection. HEV has no known chronic carrier state, and full recovery in infected persons can usually be expected. The best protection is proper handwashing.

Human Immunodeficiency Virus Infection

The human immunodeficiency viruses, known collectively as HIV, are RNA retroviruses. A retrovirus synthesizes deoxyribonucleic acid (DNA) from its RNA, a reversal of the usual process. Normally when a virus enters the body, T-helper lymphocytes (T cells) release proteins that activate the immune system to produce antibodies against the virus and macrophages to attack the virus. HIV is different from other viruses in that this retrovirus attacks the cell membrane of these white blood cells. HIV has a protein coat surrounding its RNA and the enzyme reverse transcriptase. RNA controls chemical activity within cells. When the virus passes through the T-cell membrane, the RNA and enzyme are released into the cell cytoplasm and convert into DNA. This DNA penetrates the T-cell nucleus causing production of more HIV viruses. These new viruses kill the cell and then are released into the bloodstream to attack other T-helper lymphocytes and macrophages, thus compromising the immune system.

Although the immune system produces some antibodies, HIV can live and reproduce in macrophages without stimulating production of antibodies. HIV will survive in blood and any body fluid that contains white cells, including semen, cervical and vaginal secretions, saliva, tears, cerebrospinal fluid, synovial fluid, pleural fluid, pericardial fluid, peritoneal fluid, amniotic fluid, and breast milk. The primary routes of transmission are through sexual intercourse and by direct contact with blood and blood products. It may be transferred to the fetus by the blood of an infected mother or to the neonate via breast milk. *HIV is not transmitted by casual contact with an infected person.* The virus is relatively fragile and easily destroyed outside the body.

After exposure antibodies may not be identified through serologic testing for 6 to 12 weeks but can be delayed for up to 18 months or longer. Enzyme immunoassays (EIA) and the Western blot analysis are used to measure presence of antibodies. Blood banks test donor blood for HIV antibodies. Transplant donors also are tested. Seropositive blood or tissue from donors is destroyed. Blood screening has been routine in the United States since 1985, thus decreasing the potential for transmission by blood transfusion.

The incubation period before symptoms of infection develop ranges from 6 months to 5 years or longer. Persons in whom the antibody is identified are considered infected and infective. They are classified by physical findings.

Acute Infection The acute stage of HIV infection lasts 2 to 3 weeks. Symptoms may be specific to an opportunistic infection or disease, but marked fatigue, prolonged diarrhea, weight loss, dry cough, enlarged lymph nodes, fever, and night sweats are striking features. Infections are primarily viral, mycobacterial, and fungal in origin. Oral candidiasis lesions (thrush) may be the first observable symptoms. *Pneumocystis carinii* pneumonia, an unusual lung infection caused by a protozoan parasite, is quite common. Other common infections are cytomegalovirus, herpes simplex, cryptococcosis, and *Mycobacterium avium* complex disease. The patient may survive one infection only to succumb to another. Prophylactic drug therapy aims to prevent or delay onset of infections. Malignancies and lymphomas also may develop.

As the syndrome progresses, the cell-mediated immune system is irreversibly compromised. As concentration of the virus gradually increases, the patient becomes symptomatic for clinical manifestation of AIDS. Clinical diagnosis of AIDS requires a positive test for HIV antibodies and one of the specified opportunistic infections. AIDS is not a well-defined disease but rather a state of immune dysfunction. AIDS is a persistent proliferative destruction of the T-helper lymphocytes (white blood cells that stimulate production of antibodies) resulting in profound immunosuppression (diminished resistance to infection and disease). The acronym AIDS helps to define the disease process.

A *Acquired:* HIV has passed from one person to another by blood or body fluid in direct blood cell-to-cell contact; infection is not hereditary except through transplacental transfer from an infected mother to a fetus.

I *Immune:* The normal defense system protects the body against certain diseases and opportunistic infections; immunity depends on production of antibodies.

D *Deficiency:* The immune system becomes compromised (i.e., immunosuppressed against opportunists); the host is unable to protect the person with no previous history of immunodeficiency against opportunists.

S *Syndrome:* A group of symptoms or laboratory evidence indicates the presence of a particular disease, abnormality, or infection; seroconversion is positive for HIV antibodies. *Pneumocystis carinii* pneumonia is the most common opportunistic infection. *Mycobacterium avium* complex, the most common AIDS-related bacterial infection, is a leading cause of the wasting syndrome (i.e., loss of body fat and weight). Human papilloma virus infection in women can lead to cervical carcinoma. Kaposi's sarcoma, a vascular tumor, is the most common malignancy. Neurologic disease may cause dementia. Lymphomas and opportunistic infections of the brain, spinal cord, and peripheral nerves are not uncommon.

Asymptomatic Infection Patient may be completely asymptomatic of infection, but tests seropositive for HIV antibodies, which confirms the presence of virus in the body.

Persistent Generalized Lymphadenopathy Swelling or enlargement of lymph nodes suggests cellular immune dysfunction. Prolonged infection with HIV may occur without formation of HIV antibodies.

HIV-Related Clinical Manifestations Originally referred to as *AIDS-related complexes,* a variety of health conditions suggest an impaired immune system. The patient who does not have one of the specific opportunistic infections but is seropositive for HIV antibodies does not technically have AIDS. An infectious disease, such as tuberculosis, and some cancers may be the result of a deteriorating immune system. AIDS usually develops within a year of seroconversion.

Patients with known HIV infection or AIDS or those who test positive for HIV antibodies may come to the OR for diagnostic or palliative procedures. Otherwise asymptomatic patients or those who have not been tested may be operated on for an acute illness, such as cholecystitis, or a traumatic injury. A patient may be infected but may not yet test positive. Health care providers who have a valid reason to be concerned that they may have been infected may request to be tested. Few health care providers seroconvert from a single needlestick or splash of blood on mucous membranes. Handling all needles and sharp instruments carefully and using barriers to avoid direct contact with blood and body fluids are the best measures to prevent work-related transmission of HIV. An HIV inhibitor such as zidovudine may be given immediately after exposure. A vaccine has not been developed for immunization. Antiviral agents interfere with the life cycle of the virus. Immune-modulating agents stimulate function of the suppressed immune system.

Herpesvirus Infection

Related DNA viruses that form eosinophilic intranuclear inclusion bodies are collectively called *herpesvirus.* The viral infections they cause may be acute and highly contagious, or they may remain latent for many years even if antibodies are in circulation.

Herpes Simplex The herpes simplex virus (HSV) is the pathogen of herpes simplex infections. These cutaneous infections may cause localized eruptions, similar to blisters, on the border of the lips or external nares, in the mouth, or in the genital or anal region. Transmission is by direct contact with vesicle fluid from lesions or with saliva. The infection may be transmitted to the neonate during passage through an infected birth canal. HSV also can cause cutaneous eczema, acute stomatitis, keratoconjunctivitis, acute retinal necrosis, and meningoencephalitis. Herpes simplex infections are common in HIV-infected and other immunocompromised patients.

Herpetic Whitlow Herpetic whitlow, a herpesvirus infection of the fingers, is transmitted by direct contact with oral secretions from a person with active herpesvirus or from an asymptomatic carrier. Entry of the virus into the host is via a cut or break in the skin or in nail folds. Herpetic whitlow is an occupational hazard to nurses, physicians, dentists, and anesthesiologists.

Cytomegalovirus Infection Cytomegalovirus (CMV) may infect salivary glands or viscera, causing enlargement of cells. Transmission can be by direct contact with body fluids, secretions, and excretions. CMV usually is asymptomatic in a healthy person, but it is an opportunistic pathogen in immunosuppressed HIV-infected and AIDS patients. Lymphadenopathy, enteritis, and pneumonitis may persist. Chorioretinitis and blindness may result in the end stage of infection. CMV also may be associated with hepatitis. CMV may infect arterial smooth muscle cells, stimulating them to proliferate, which can contribute to the formation of atherosclerotic plaque. CMV is the most common cause of congenital viral infection; it may be transmitted from an asymptomatic mother during pregnancy. A CMV-infected infant may develop neurologic problems. Latent CMV may become reactivated following organ transplantation. The incidence of primary and reactivated CMV infection is fairly high after renal, cardiac, and bone marrow transplantation.

Sexually Transmitted Diseases

Any sexually active person who has multiple partners is at risk for acquiring a sexually transmitted disease. In addition to those previously discussed—hepatitis B, HIV infection, and herpes simplex—gonorrhea, syphilis, and chlamydia are transmitted by sexual contact. Transmission can also occur from contact with secretions containing the causative organism, such as a health care provider might encounter through a cut or broken skin.

Gonorrhea *Neisseria gonorrhoeae* most often infects the genitourinary tract, but it may infect the rectum, pharynx, or conjunctiva. Burning, itching, or pain around the vaginal or urethral orifice with purulent discharge are characteristic symptoms. If untreated, the infection can spread to cause inflammation within the peritoneal cavity and septicemia. Disseminated infection is more common in women than men. Gonorrhea is treated with penicillinase-inhibiting antibiotics. Generally patients should be treated simultaneously for presumptive chlamydial infections.

As a prophylactic measure a one-time instillation of silver nitrate, erythromycin 0.5% ophthalmic ointment, or tetracycline 1% ophthalmic ointment may be administered within 1 hour after birth to protect the neonate against potential contamination by vaginal secretions of an infected mother. Single-use tubes or ampules are preferable to multiple-use tubes to prevent cross contamination between newborns. A newborn with a known gonorrheal infection will need further antibiotic treatment.

Syphilis Routine screening for syphilis in hospitalized patients and couples applying for marriage licenses is a thing of the past. However, the incidence of syphilis is on the increase again. *Treponema pallidum* is a bloodborne spirochete that may infect any organ system. Syphilis is characterized by distinct stages of effects over a period of years if untreated by antibiotics. Congenital syphilis results from prenatal infection unless the infected mother is treated within the first 4 months of pregnancy.

In the first stage (primary syphilis) a lesion on the skin or mucous membrane, most commonly around the anogenital region, quickly forms a chancre. This is a painless ulceration that exudes fluid laden with spirochetes. The chancre heals spontaneously within 40 days. During the second stage (secondary syphilis) spirochetes migrate from the chancre throughout the bloodstream. The disease can remain contagious for as long as 2 years during this stage. The third stage (tertiary syphilis) may not develop for many years. When it does, secondary lesions may damage or destroy tissues and body structures, including the heart and central nervous system with ensuing mental disability or death.

Chlamydia Chlamydial infection is caused by a *Chlamydia trachomatis* bacteria. It is the most prevalent sexually transmitted disease, more common than gonorrhea and syphilis. It is transmitted only by person-to-person contact. It occurs more often in men than in women but is more frequently asymptomatic in women than in men. Chlamydia can cause epithelial tissue inflammation, ulceration and scarring of the urethra and rectum, and damage to reproductive organs. Pelvic inflammatory disease (PID) is a serious complication in women. Asymptomatic salpingitis is a major cause of tubal infertility or ectopic pregnancy. Exposure of infants to chlamydia in the birth canal can cause neonatal conjunctivitis and pneumonia.

Creutzfeldt-Jakob Disease

Although rare, Creutzfeldt-Jakob disease (CJD) is a progressive, fatal disease characterized by dementia, myoclonus (muscle spasms), and multifocal neurologic symptoms. Thought to be associated with genetic factors that influence susceptibility, the virus may be dormant for more than 20 years before onset of symptoms. The disease then progresses rapidly, leading to coma and death usually within 2 years.

The mode of transmission of the virus is unknown. However, ocular infection following corneal transplantation and intracerebral infection from contaminated stereotactic electrodes have been documented. Blood, cerebrospinal fluid, organs (especially corneas and brain tissue), and other body substances are considered hazardous. The CJD virus is particularly virulent and resistant to destruction. Instruments should be steam sterilized for 1 hour in a gravity displacement sterilizer or for 18 minutes in a prevacuum sterilizer (longer than normal cycles) before routine cleaning. Universal blood and body fluid precautions must be strictly observed. Percutaneous exposure to blood, cerebrospinal fluid, or tissue should immediately be followed by irrigation of the wound with 0.5% sodium hypochlorite solution.

Toxic Shock Syndrome

Toxic shock syndrome (TSS) is an acute condition caused by toxins secreted by strains of *Staphylococcus aureus*. The pathogen can invade any part of the body. TSS is characterized by fever over 102° F (38.9° C), hypotension, erythematous rash, and derangement of function and injury to multiple organ systems. Diagnosis is based on the presence of abnormal clinical and laboratory findings. Prompt supportive treatment and antibiotic therapy are crucial. Desquamation, peeling of skin usually from the palms of the hands and soles of the feet, occurs 1 to 2 weeks after onset. Recovery is usually complete, but TSS is potentially fatal. It can originate from a surgical wound, burn, postpartum infection, or septic abortion infected or colonized with the implicated toxin. TSS can afflict any age group of either sex.

ENVIRONMENTAL CONTROL

Control of the environment is a necessary part of overall infection prevention. The inanimate and animate environment of the OR suite presents a risk for transmission of microorganisms. The aim of a microbiologically controlled environment is to keep contamination to a minimum and to maintain the balance in favor of the patient, not the microorganisms.

Recommended practices developed by the Association of Operating Room Nurses (AORN) provide guidelines for aseptic practices in the perioperative care of surgical patients. These are recommendations for optimal level of *achievable* technical and aseptic practices. They are intended to give direction and information for formulation of institutional policies. Individual hospital policies and procedures reflect variations in physical environment and/or clinical situations that determine the degree to which the recommended practices can be implemented. The recommendations may not necessarily reflect current practice in individual institutions. Throughout this text referral is made to specific appropriate guidelines, and/or their content is incorporated in the material presented. The AORN recommended practices are listed in the bibliography for the applicable chapters in the text.

The recommendations for infection control from the CDC and regulations for exposure to bloodborne pathogens from the Occupational Safety and Health Administration (OSHA) should be incorporated into policies and procedures of all health care facilities.

Asepsis literally means *without infection*. This implies the absence of microorganisms that cause infection. However, it is impossible to exclude all microorganisms from the environment. Every effort is made to minimize and control them for the safety of both patients and personnel. The methods by which microbial contamination is prevented in the environment are referred to as *aseptic techniques*. These practices are the key to containment of microorganisms.

OR suites are designed with optimal function and safety in mind and to protect patients from sources of contamination. The suite includes specific areas for traffic, support systems, administration, communication, and storage (see Chapter 9). Clean and soiled activities, areas, personnel, and sterile and unsterile supplies should be distinctly separated. Traffic patterns are designed to flow smoothly and to prevent backtrack and crossover traffic.

Aseptic Barriers

Contact contamination plays a major role in bacterial spread. Therefore barriers are established to create a safe environment. They protect sterile areas, isolate surgical wounds from infectious contaminants, and keep the number of microorganisms to a minimum. To retard or prevent transfer of organisms, barriers must be impervious to their passage under ordinary operating conditions. Procedures are established to provide barriers against the migration of microorganisms from potential sources of microbial contamination in the OR.

Skin

Skin normally harbors resident organisms below its surface and transient organisms on the surface that are acquired by direct contact. Both types of flora are constantly shed into the environment. Procedures to control those shed and those potentially acquired by sterile team members are discussed in detail in Chapter 11. Key points are mentioned here for *all* personnel entering the OR.

1. Daily bathing with soap containing an antibacterial agent.
2. Donning of clean OR attire for *each* entry into the OR suite. Long sleeves are worn by unsterile team members.
3. Covering abrasions or cuts on hands and skin. Persons with infected skin lesions should not be permitted in the OR suite.
4. Thorough handwashing before initial entry into restricted area of the OR suite.
5. Impeccable handwashing after every direct contact with the patient or items in contact with the patient's blood, body fluids, or excretions.
6. Wearing of gloves when handling blood, excreta, drainage, and secretions or items contaminated with body substances, including tissue specimens. Hands are washed after removing gloves.

NOTE Handwashing cannot be overemphasized. This is *vigorous* rubbing together of all surfaces of well-lathered, soapy hands, followed by rinsing under a stream of water.

Hair

Hair should be shampooed frequently. Caps or hoods are worn to completely cover hair, including beards.

Nasopharynx

Masks are worn to cover the nose and mouth. They should be changed after caring for each patient. Persons with respiratory infection should not be permitted in the OR suite. Coughing and sneezing explode droplets into the environment. Talking should be kept to a minimum.

Fomites

Inanimate objects collect dust, lint, droplets, and particles from the air. Surfaces of furniture, equipment, and floors may be contaminated by spills or contact with organic debris. In addition to the housekeeping practices listed below and those discussed in Chapter 27, the following key points should be considered:

1. Proper packaging and storing of supplies. External shipping cartons should be removed before bringing supplies beyond the unrestricted area in the OR suite.
2. Placement of dust covers over sterile items during transport and in prolonged storage.
3. Separation of clean and soiled items. Sterile storage areas are physically separated from decontamination areas.
4. Prompt decontamination of used equipment and reusable supplies.
5. Prompt disinfection of OR surfaces (i.e., furniture and floors, and disposal of waste and laundry).

Environmental Services/Housekeeping

Housekeeping practices using the most effective supplies, techniques, and equipment available are a most important aspect of infection control. *Housekeeping* procedures include cleaning and disinfecting the operating rooms and suite, handling soiled laundry, and disposing of solid wastes. They are carried out according to established practices, policies, and schedules. These procedures are performed by environmental service personnel under supervision. Good housekeeping cleaning techniques should reduce microbial flora by about 90%. *Detergent-disinfectants alone are no substitute for thorough mechanical cleaning,* the proverbial "elbow grease." Locations that by design or construction are difficult to clean and areas that may be touched by patients or personnel are of primary concern.

Any equipment or procedure requiring water in its operation presents a hazard, especially if the water is not frequently changed or the sinks are not cleaned. Unsterile water, the universal solvent and transporter, can support, maintain, and protect almost every contaminant produced by human beings. The numbers, types, and species of microorganisms in a water supply are limited only by the attention paid to the equipment containing it. Water especially supports the growth of certain gram-negative bacilli, including *Serratia, Pseudomonas, Alcaligenes,* and *Flavobacterium* genera. Aerosols produced during hand scrubs become airborne and contaminate. Disinfectants reduce the contamination of cleaning water.

Points in housekeeping, especially relevant to infection control and prevention of cross infection, are listed to emphasize the importance of OR environmental control:

1. Faucet heads should be of a type that does not hold water. They should be removed for sterilization. Handwash antiseptic containers should be sterilized before refill.
2. No surface should remain wet, thereby supporting microbial growth.
3. Organic debris should be promptly removed from walls and OR surfaces with a disinfectant to prevent drying and airborne contamination.
4. Lights and overhead tracks should be cleaned at least twice daily, before first scheduled surgical procedure and on completion of the schedule.
5. Entrance to the OR suite and floors in corridors and rooms should be cleaned with the wet-vacuum system. Dry debris is removed with a dry vacuum; the floor is sprayed with a detergent-disinfectant solution and wet-vacuumed.
6. Housekeeping equipment should be kept clean and dry and never stored moist in a dark area conducive to microbial growth.
7. Disposable waste/trash should be put in impervious receptacles.
8. Service elevators rather than chutes should be used to remove soiled laundry and waste/trash from the OR suite. Chutes become grossly contaminated and are an airborne contamination hazard and a fire hazard.
9. Waste should be contained at the source of origin to prevent aerosol generation during handling. Contaminated waste must be decontaminated and/or sterilized before compaction or disposal in the general environment. Incineration is the most effective means of waste disposal, especially of infectious wastes. Health care facilities must comply with local, state, and federal regulations for contamination control measures and waste disposal, however.
10. *Adequate time must be allowed between patients for proper terminal disinfection of the OR* (see Chapter 27, pp. 549-553). A patient must not be assigned to an inadequately cleaned OR, which could be a source of a wound infection.
11. All areas and equipment throughout the OR suite should be cleaned on a regular basis. These areas include grills, vents, and filters of the air-conditioning system, storage shelves and cabinets, lighting fixtures, walls, etc. in offices, lounges, dressing rooms, storage areas, workrooms, and corridors. Handles of cabinets and push plates of doors should be cleaned daily.

Control of Airborne Contamination

Air currents and movement in the OR should be kept to a minimum to prevent airborne contamination. Viable microorganisms from the air settle on horizontal surfaces. Proper cleaning of these surfaces helps control this contamination. The ventilating system and efforts to minimize air turbulence and contaminants also are important factors.

Air-Conditioning System

When properly designed, installed, and maintained, a conventional air-conditioning system effectively reduces the number of airborne organisms by removing dust and aerosol particles. As fresh, clean outside air is supplied, air contaminated by dust and lint is removed. Recirculation of filtered air at a minimum rate of 20 volume exchanges per hour, at least four of fresh air, is considered safe and economical. Fire codes in some states require 100% outside fresh air. All air, recirculated or fresh, is filtered before entering the OR. Using *HEPA filters,* the system reduces particles larger than 0.5 µm to 1 to 5 per cubic foot. The dilution principle is used. Air enters from a ceiling vent, is diluted, and passes out through vents at floor level. Filters are located downstream from air-processing equipment so microorganisms will not be drawn into the room. The system maintains a positive pressure.

Ultraclean Air System

Frequently referred to as *laminar airflow,* a special air-handling system for filtration, dilution, and distribution of air may be installed in one or more ORs. High-risk procedures such as total joint replacement, cardiac surgery, or organ transplantation are performed here. Laminar airflow is a controlled, unidirectional, positive-pressure stream of air. From a ceiling diffuser, clean air flows downward at a high velocity, progressively decreasing as it flows radially outward. The controlled airstream entraps particulate matter and microorganisms. The flow returns to the system and passes through a prefilter to remove gross particles. It then passes through a HEPA filter that traps and eliminates more than 99% of all particles larger than 0.3 μm. This includes virtually all bacteria and most viruses. A rate of 100 to 400 air changes per hour is possible; most systems deliver about 240.

To complete the system, the sterile team members wear a total body exhaust gown. It resembles a spacesuit and covers the entire body. Air, piped into the headpiece, is removed through filtered tubes. The hood or helmet is equipped for hearing and speaking. Negative pressure is maintained under the gown by a vacuum hose. The system provides body cooling for the wearer.

Laminar airflow with a total body exhaust system reliably reduces bacterial contamination at the wound site. Although an ultraclean air system provides microbe-free air (no more than one organism per cubic foot) with minimal air turbulence, *it is not a substitute for meticulous surgical technique.* The decrease in particle count does not significantly reduce the rate of surgical wound infection. It is an adjunct to controlling airborne contamination.

Doors

OR doors should be kept closed except as necessary for passage of the patient and personnel or supplies and equipment. Disrupted pressurization mixes inside (positive pressure) OR clean air with outside (negative pressure) corridor air of higher microbial count. Cabinet doors should remain closed.

Traffic and Movement

Traffic in and out of the OR must be kept to a minimum. Only the OR team and authorized and essential personnel should be allowed inside the OR. As the number of people present increases, the amount of activity in the room increases, which increases potential contamination from shedding and air turbulence that carries microbes to the wound. Movement in the OR should be reduced to a minimum.

Lint

Textile lubricants added to the final rinse during laundering minimize lint that results from friction of woven fibers against each other. Disintegrated paper from disposable products is another source of lint on fabrics. Paper products should not be discarded with soiled reusable woven fabrics.

Isolation Precautions

Isolation of patients by diagnosis or body substance is related to mode of transmission of pathogenic microorganisms (i.e., contact, droplets, air, or fomites). Isolation precautions and guidelines are detailed in hospital procedure books and in the CDC *Guideline for Isolation Precautions in Hospitals.* Different methods of isolation technique are described:

1. Category-specific isolation precautions for patients with suspected or confirmed diagnosis of infectious disease transmitted by droplets via airborne route, such as pulmonary tuberculosis, or by enteric excretions, drainage, or secretions.
2. Disease-specific isolation precautions for contact with patients known to be infected with bloodborne and nonbloodborne pathogens, such as HBV.
3. Body substance isolation incorporating universal precautions (see p. 198) for contact with *all* moist body substances, including blood, urine, feces, saliva, sputum, tears, wound drainage, etc., of all patients, regardless of diagnosis. All patients harbor microorganisms (i.e., are colonized); therefore they are potentially infectious to the environment. Body substance isolation is interaction-driven rather than diagnosis-driven.

The purpose of these precautions is to prevent transmission of pathogenic microorganisms from the patient to personnel, from one patient to another patient, and from personnel to the patient. Isolation techniques separate an infected patient from other noninfected, susceptible patients. Barrier techniques protect personnel and other patients.

Each hospital may incorporate into its procedures whichever method is most appropriate for its particular needs and patient population. The OR staff should be informed about a patient requiring isolation precautions before the patient comes to the OR. A sticker on the patient's chart indicates the type of hospital isolation. For most patients the same precautions apply in the OR as on the unit. A commonsense approach is used. In all types of isolation the most important control measure is *thorough handwashing* before and after close patient contact, after handling contaminated objects, body fluids, or excretions, and between patients. Isolation techniques must not be implemented in a way that causes the patient to feel victimized. The patient should be educated to accept the regimen.

UNIVERSAL PRECAUTIONS

Transmission of infection requires a source, a method, and a susceptible host. *Every patient is considered a source when blood and body fluids containing blood will be encountered,* as in invasive diagnostic or therapeutic procedures. Other sources may be skin, hair, secretions, excretions, and fomites. Direct contact with blood and body fluids, airborne contamination, or fomites may infect patients or personnel. In addition to measures to prevent microbial contamination, OR policies and procedures follow *universal precautions.* As established by the CDC and enforced by OSHA, these precautions protect health care workers from contact with blood and body fluids of *all* patients, not just of patients diagnosed or suspected of being infected with hepatitis B, HIV, or other bloodborne pathogens. These precautions supplement other procedures for environmental control. They are the minimum precautions for *all invasive procedures.*

NOTE An invasive procedure involves entry into tissues, organs, or body cavities in the OR, delivery room, emergency department, physician's or dentist's office, radiology department, or cardiac catheterization laboratory. It is any procedure during which bleeding occurs or the potential for bleeding exists.

1. *Protective barriers.* Appropriate barriers prevent skin and mucous membrane contact with blood and body fluids. The characteristics of the attire depend on the task and degree of anticipated exposure. Barrier materials must prevent blood and other fluids from passing through or reaching the wearer's clothing or body.
   a. *Gloves* reduce contamination of hands.
      (1) Sterile gloves are worn for procedures involving invasion of body tissues when a sterile field is created.
      (2) Unsterile latex or vinyl examination gloves are worn for procedures that do not require a sterile field, such as procedures on intraoral mucous membranes, and for handling specimens, placentas, newborns, and contaminated items such as sponges.
      (3) General-purpose utility gloves are worn for cleaning instruments and for decontaminating and housekeeping procedures involving potential blood contact.
      (4) Gloves are changed after every contact with patients or contaminated items. Latex and vinyl gloves are discarded; intact utility gloves may be decontaminated and reused. The hands are washed immediately after removal of the gloves.

   NOTE
   - Persons with exudative skin lesions or weeping dermatitis should not have direct patient contact or handle contaminated items and medical devices used during invasive procedures.
   - Potential for becoming infected through skin exposure depends on concentration of the virus, duration of contact, presence of skin lesions on the hands, and immune status. The concentration of HBV is much higher in blood than is HIV.
   - Vinyl may be more permeable to viruses than latex.

   b. *Masks* protect personnel from aerosols and patients from droplets. They are worn for all invasive procedures. If grossly contaminated by a splash of blood or body fluid, the mask should be changed immediately.
   c. *Eyewear or face shields* protect mucous membranes of the eyes, nose, or mouth. They are worn for procedures in which blood, bone chips, amniotic fluid, or aerosol of other body fluids may splash or be projected into the eyes. Goggles with enclosed sides and chin-length face shields offer better protection than eyeglasses.
   d. *Gowns or aprons* made of fluid-resistant material protect the wearer from a splash with blood and body fluids. A plastic apron may be worn under a textile gown. Impervious gowns offer better protection.
   e. *Shoe covers or boots* protect the wearer when gross contamination on the floor can be anticipated, as during some head and neck, abdominal, extremity, and perineal procedures. Grossly soiled shoe covers or knee-high disposable boots are removed before the wearer leaves the room. If the boots are not disposable, they may be wiped off with a detergent-disinfectant.
2. *Prevention of puncture injuries.* Needles, knife blades, and sharp instruments present a potential hazard for the handler and user. Skin may be punctured or cut if caution is not taken. Specific recommendations for handling disposable surgical needles, syringes and needles, and knife blades include:
   a. Do not manipulate by hand. Use an instrument to attach the blade to the knife handle. Arm the needle directly from suture packet when possible. Pass needles in a needleholder. Do not bend or break an injection needle. Sharp instruments and needles may be passed on a tray or a magnetic mat for a hand-free technique rather than from hand to hand. Remove instruments from the surgical site after use, that is, return them to the instrument table promptly.
   b. Do not recap used injection needles, except with a recapping safety device.
   c. Do not remove the needle from a disposable syringe after use.

d. Place all used blades and needles in a puncture-resistant container.

NOTE
- If a glove is torn or punctured, remove the puncturing needle, blade, or instrument from the sterile field immediately and change the glove promptly.
- If the skin is punctured or cut, remove the glove immediately. Squeeze skin to release blood. Wash out contaminants under running water with an antiseptic, then irrigate with a virucidal disinfectant such as an iodophor, bleach, or peroxide. Report the incident immediately.
- Electrosurgery, lasers, and staplers reduce the use of cutting instruments and surgical needles.
- Double gloving does not prevent puncture wounds. Glove liners (see Chapter 11, p. 169) may provide protection from skin cuts. Double gloving may substantially reduce the risk of exposure from blood and fluid seepage through gloves onto hands during long procedures or in the presence of voluminous blood loss.

3. *Oral procedures.* Although transmission by saliva is unlikely, contact with blood-contaminated saliva and gingival fluid is expected during dental and surgical procedures in the oropharyngeal cavity. Mouth protection, resuscitation bags, and other ventilation devices should be available for emergency mouth-to-mouth resuscitation.
4. *Care of specimens.* All specimens of blood, body fluids, and tissues should be contained to prevent leaking during transport to the laboratory. The outside of the container should be clean. The circulator, wearing gloves, will need to disinfect the outside of a culture tube handed from the sterile field or a container if it has been contaminated.

   NOTE Because blood and body fluids from *all* patients are considered infective, warning labels are not necessary on specimens.

5. *Decontamination.* All instruments must be thoroughly cleaned before sterilization or high-level disinfection (see Chapters 13 and 14). Surfaces of furniture and floors are cleaned and decontaminated with detergent-disinfectant. Spills of blood or body fluids on the floor during a procedure should be wiped up immediately and the area decontaminated. Gloves are worn for cleaning procedures.
6. *Laundry.* Soiled woven fabrics should be handled as little as possible. They are transported to the laundry in leak-proof bags. Bags or transport containers should be appropriately color coded or labeled to alert laundry workers to wear gloves while handling contaminated laundry.
7. *Waste.* Blood and suctioned fluids may be safely poured down a drain connected to a sanitary sewer. Trash is disposed of by incineration or sent to a sanitary landfill in sealed containers, as required by local ordinances or state regulations. Trash bags must be leakproof and of sufficient thickness and strength to ensure integrity during transport. Waste may be differentiated as either infectious or noninfectious for disposal purposes. Bags may be color coded (e.g., red for infectious waste), or biohazard labeled.
8. *Handwashing.* Thorough handwashing following every contact with a patient, blood, and items in contact with blood and body fluids cannot be overemphasized.

All health care providers must be familiar with policies and procedures and must understand the need for universal precautions for their own protection and the safety of patients. The risk of exposure for the patient is greater in those procedures designated as *exposure-prone,* such as suturing in a confined area. Surgeons and first assistants who are infected with HBV or HIV should not perform these procedures unless they have sought counsel of an expert review panel and informed the patient of their seroconversion status. A health care provider should report exposure by inoculation with blood or body fluid of a patient; the surgeon and first assistant usually are at greatest risk. Similarly, the patient should be informed of an incident in which he or she is exposed to the blood of a health care provider.

STERILE TECHNIQUES AND THEIR APPLICATIONS

Strict aseptic and sterile techniques are needed at all times in the OR. The aseptic techniques discussed control the environment. *Sterile techniques* prevent transfer of microorganisms into body tissues. Freshly incised or traumatized tissue can become infected easily. Intact skin and mucous membranes are the body's first line of defense against infection. Infraction of their integrity creates a portal of entry for microorganisms. Therefore anything in contact with body tissues is potentially dangerous. Depending on their intended purpose and body contact, items are classified as:

1. *Critical.* Items entering body tissues underlying skin and mucous membranes *must be sterile* (i.e., free of microorganisms, including spores). They are handled to maintain sterility.
2. *Semicritical.* Sterility is less critical for items that come into contact with intact skin or mucous membranes. These items are *surgically clean* (i.e., mechanically cleaned and disinfected to reduce microorganisms but unsterile). Some items are disinfected immediately before use and are handled to prevent contamination before use. Other items are terminally sterilized, but sterility is not maintained during use.

3. *Noncritical.* Items that will come in contact only with intact skin or mucous membranes in an area remote from the surgical site may be cleaned, terminally disinfected, and stored unsterile between patient uses.

Surgical procedures are performed under sterile conditions; contamination with microorganisms is prevented to maintain sterility throughout the procedure. A *sterile field* is created around the site of incision into tissues or for introduction of sterile instruments into a body orifice. Conversely, all material and equipment used during a surgical procedure are terminally decontaminated and sterilized with the assumption that *every patient is a potential source of infection for other persons.*

It is essential that all members of the OR team know the common sources of contamination by microorganisms in the OR and the means by which they reach the sterile field and surgical wound. Sterile technique is the responsibility of everyone caring for the patient in the OR. *All members of the OR team must be ever vigilant in safeguarding the sterility of the sterile field. Any contamination must be remedied immediately.*

Principles

The patient is the center of the sterile field, which includes the areas of the patient, operating table, and furniture covered with sterile drapes and the personnel wearing sterile attire. Strict adherence to sound principles of sterile technique and recommended practices is mandatory for the safety of the patient. This adherence reflects one's surgical conscience. *Principles remain the same; it is the degree of adherence to them that varies.* The principles of sterile technique are applied:

1. In preparation for an invasive procedure, by sterilization of necessary materials and supplies
2. In preparation of the sterile team to handle sterile supplies and intimately contact the surgical site, by scrubbing, gowning, and gloving
3. In creation and maintenance of the sterile field, including skin preparation and draping of the patient
4. In maintenance of sterility and asepsis throughout the surgical procedure
5. In terminal sterilization and disinfection at the conclusion of the surgical procedure

If the principles are understood, the need for their application becomes obvious. Sterile technique is the basis of modern surgery.

Only Sterile Items Are Used Within Sterile Field

Some items such as drapes, sponges, or basins may be obtained from a stock supply of sterile packages. Others, such as instruments, may be sterilized immediately preceding the surgical procedure and taken directly from the sterilizer to the sterile tables. Every person who dispenses a sterile article must be sure of its sterility and of its remaining sterile until used. Proper packaging, sterilizing, and handling should provide such assurance. *If you are in doubt about the sterility of anything, consider it not sterile.* Known or potentially contaminated items must not be transferred to the sterile field, for example:

1. If a sterilized package is found in a contaminated area (e. g., the general unsterile workroom).
2. If uncertain about the actual timing or operation of the sterilizer. Items processed in a suspect load are considered unsterile.
3. If an unsterile person comes into close contact with a sterile table and vice versa.
4. If a sterile table or unwrapped sterile items are not under constant observation.
5. If the integrity of the packaging material is not intact.
6. If a sterile package wrapped in a material other than plastic or another moisture-resistant barrier becomes damp or wet. Humidity in the storage area or moisture on hands may seep into the package.
7. If a sterile package wrapped in a pervious woven material drops to the floor or other area of questionable cleanliness. These materials allow implosion of air into package. A dropped package is considered contaminated. If the wrapper is impervious and the area of contact is dry, the item may be transferred to the sterile field. Packages that have been dropped on the floor should not be put back into sterile storage.

Sterile Persons Are Gowned and Gloved

Gowns are considered sterile only in front from chest to level of sterile field, and the sleeves from above elbows to cuffs. When wearing a gown, consider sterile only the area you can see in front down to the level of the sterile field. Usually this does not extend below waist level. The following practices must be observed:

1. Self-gowning and gloving should be done from a separate sterile surface to avoid dripping water onto sterile supplies or a sterile table.
2. Stockinette cuffs of the gown are enclosed beneath sterile gloves. Stockinette is absorbent and will retain moisture, thus this part of the gown does not provide a microbial barrier.
3. Sterile persons keep their hands in sight at all times and at or above the waist level or the sterile field (Figure 12-1).
4. Hands are kept away from the face. Elbows are kept close to the sides. Hands are never folded under arms because of perspiration in axillary re-

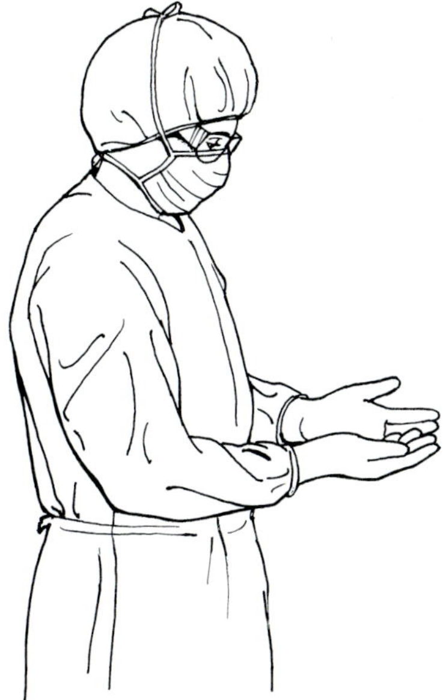

FIGURE 12-1 Sterile persons keep hands in sight at or above waist or level of sterile field. Gowns are considered sterile only in front from chest to level of sterile field, and the sleeves from above elbows to cuffs.

gion. Neckline, shoulders, and back also may become contaminated with perspiration.

5. Sterile persons are aware of the height of team members in relation to each other and the sterile field. Changing levels at the sterile field is avoided. The gown is considered sterile only down to the highest level of the sterile tables. If a sterile person must stand on a platform to reach the surgical site, the platform should be positioned before this person steps up to the draped area. Sterile persons should sit only when the entire procedure will be performed at this level.

Tables Are Sterile Only at Table Level

The result is that:

1. Only the top of a sterile, draped table is considered sterile. Edges and sides of the drape extending below table level are considered unsterile.
2. Anything falling or extending over the table edge, such as a piece of suture, is unsterile. The scrub person does not touch the part hanging below table level.
3. In unfolding a sterile drape, the part that drops below the table surface is not brought back up to table level. Once placed, the drape is not moved or shifted.
4. Cords, tubing, etc. are secured on the sterile field with a nonperforating device to prevent them from sliding over the table edge.

Sterile Persons Touch Only Sterile Items or Areas; Unsterile Persons Touch Only Unsterile Items or Areas

For example:

1. Sterile team members maintain contact with the sterile field by means of sterile gowns and gloves.
2. Unsterile circulator does not directly contact the sterile field.
3. Supplies are brought to sterile team members by the circulator, who opens wrappers on sterile packages. The circulator ensures a sterile transfer to the sterile field. Only sterile items touch sterile surfaces.

Unsterile Persons Avoid Reaching Over Sterile Field; Sterile Persons Avoid Leaning Over Unsterile Area

For example:

1. Unsterile circulator *never* reaches over a sterile field to transfer sterile items.
2. In pouring solution into a sterile basin, the circulator holds only the lip of the bottle over the basin to avoid reaching over a sterile area (Figure 12-2).
3. Scrub person sets basins or glasses to be filled at the edge of the sterile table; the circulator stands near this edge of the table to fill them.
4. Circulator stands at a distance from the sterile field to adjust the light over it to avoid microbial fallout over the field.

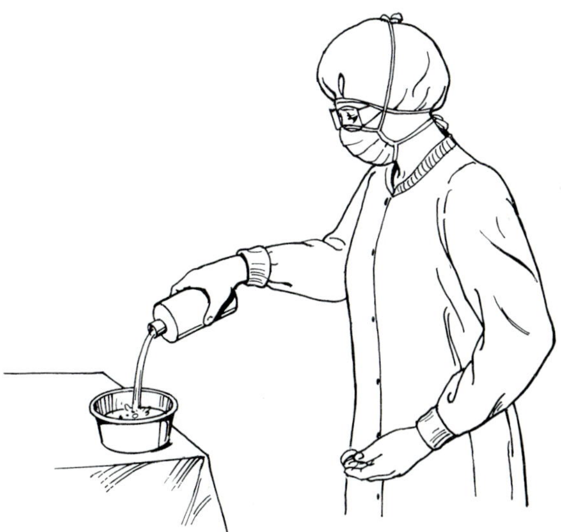

FIGURE 12-2 Circulator pouring sterile solution into sterile basin. Note that only lip of bottle is over the basin. Unsterile person avoids reaching over sterile field.

5. Surgeon turns away from the sterile field to have perspiration removed from the brow.
6. Scrub person drapes an unsterile table toward self first to protect the gown. Gloved hands are protected by cuffing a drape over them (Figure 12-3).
7. Scrub person stands back from the unsterile table when draping it to avoid leaning over an unsterile area (Figures 12-4 to 12-6).

Edges of Anything That Encloses Sterile Contents Are Considered Unsterile

Boundaries between sterile and unsterile are not always rigidly defined, for example, the edges of wrappers on sterile packages and caps on solution bottles. The following precautions should be taken:

1. In opening sterile packages, a margin of safety is always maintained. The inside of wrappers is considered sterile to within 1 inch of the edges. The circulator opens the top flap away from self, then turns the sides under. Ends of flaps are secured in the hand so they do not dangle loosely. The last flap is pulled toward the person opening the package, thereby exposing the package contents away from the unsterile hand.
2. Sterile persons lift contents from packages by reaching down and lifting them straight up, holding their elbows high.
3. Flaps on peel-open packages should be pulled back, not torn, to expose sterile contents. Contents should be flipped or lifted upward and not permitted to slide over edges. The inner edge of the heat seal is considered the line of demarcation between sterile and unsterile.
4. If a sterile wrapper is used as a table cover, it should amply cover the entire table surface. Only the interior and surface level of the cover are considered sterile.

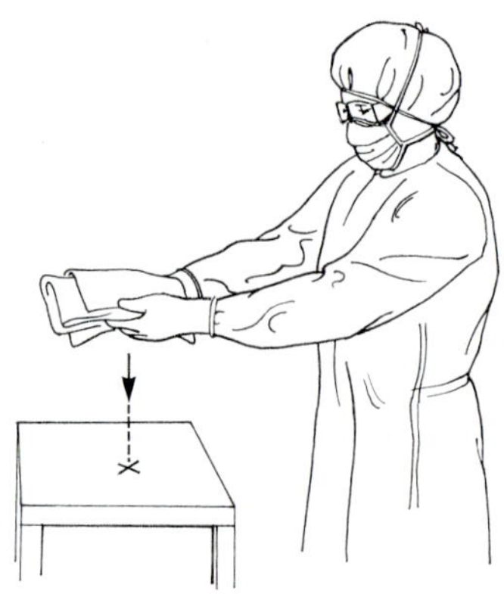

FIGURE 12-4 Draping large unsterile table. Scrub person holds the sterile fan-folded table drape high and drops it on the center of the table, standing back from the table to protect gown.

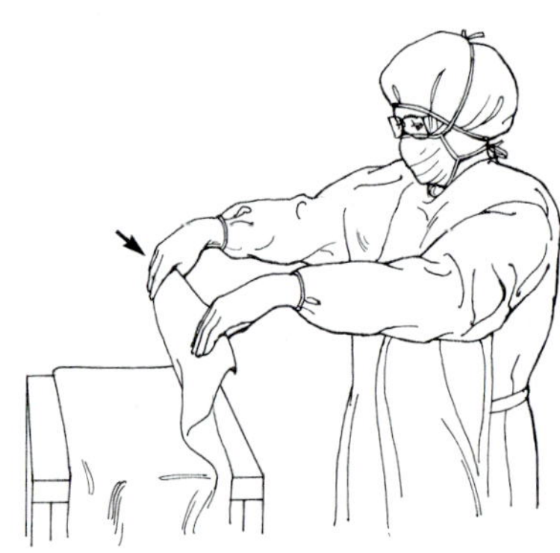

FIGURE 12-5 Scrub person unfolding sterile table drape. Scrub person stands back from unsterile table and unfolds drape first toward self. Note that hands are inside sterile cover to protect them.

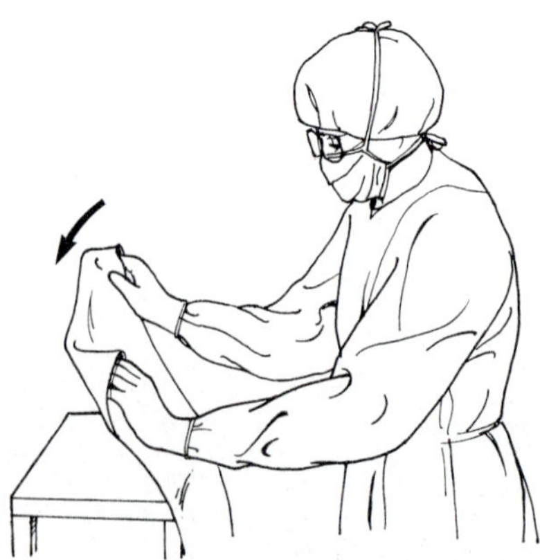

FIGURE 12-3 Sterile scrub person draping a small table. Sterile persons avoid reaching over unsterile field. The scrub person therefore drapes unsterile table first toward self, then away. Gown is protected by distance. Hands are protected by cuffing drape over them.

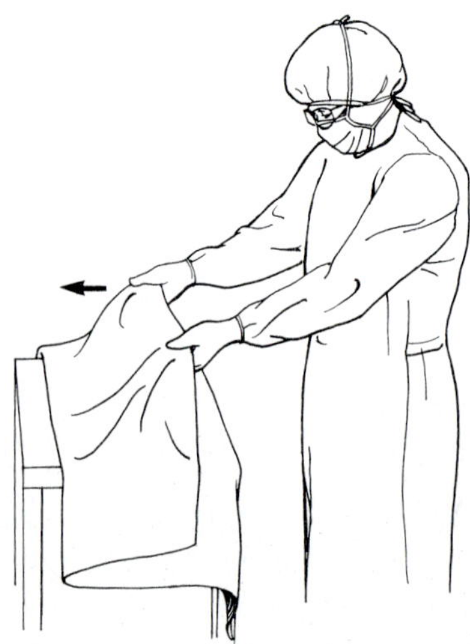

FIGURE 12-6 Scrub person continuing to unfold sterile table drape. Hands are inside sterile cover for protection. Scrub person may now move closer to the table, since the first part of unfolded drape now protects gown.

5. After a sterile bottle is opened, the contents must be used or discarded. The cap cannot be replaced without contaminating the pouring edges.
6. Steam reaches only the area within the gasket of a sterilizer. Instrument trays should not touch the edge of the sterilizer outside the gasket.

Sterile Field Is Created as Close as Possible to Time of Use

Degree of contamination is proportionate to length of time sterile items are uncovered and exposed to environment. Precautions must be taken as follows:

1. Sterile tables are set up just before the surgical procedure (see Chapter 20, p. 410).
2. It is virtually impossible to uncover a table of sterile contents without contamination. *Covering sterile tables for later use is not recommended.*

Sterile Areas Are Continuously Kept in View

Inadvertent contamination of sterile areas must be readily visible. To ensure this principle:

1. Sterile persons face sterile areas.
2. When sterile packs are open in a room or a sterile field is set up, someone must remain in the room to maintain vigilance. Sterility cannot be ensured without direct observation. An unguarded sterile field should be considered contaminated.

Sterile Persons Keep Well Within Sterile Area

Sterile persons allow a wide margin of safety when passing unsterile areas and follow these rules:

1. Sterile persons stand back at a safe distance from the operating table when draping the patient.
2. Sterile persons pass each other back to back at a 360-degree turn (Figure 12-7).
3. Sterile person turns back to an unsterile person or area when passing.
4. Sterile person faces a sterile area to pass it.
5. Sterile person asks an unsterile individual to step aside rather than risk contamination.
6. Sterile persons stay within the sterile field. They *do not walk around* or go outside the room.
7. Movement within and around a sterile area is kept to a minimum to avoid contamination of sterile items or persons.

Sterile Persons Keep Contact With Sterile Areas to Minimum

The following rules are observed:

1. Sterile persons do not lean on sterile tables or on the draped patient.
2. Sitting or leaning against an unsterile surface is a break in technique. If the sterile team sits to operate, they do so without proximity to unsterile areas.

Unsterile Persons Avoid Sterile Areas

Unsterile persons maintain an awareness of sterile, unsterile, clean, and contaminated areas and their proximity to each. They must be aware of their closeness to the sterile field. A wide margin of safety must be maintained when passing sterile areas by following these rules:

1. Unsterile persons maintain a distance of at least 1 foot (30 cm) from any area of the sterile field.
2. Unsterile persons face and observe a sterile area when passing it to be sure they do not touch it.
3. Unsterile persons never walk between two sterile areas (e.g., between sterile instrument tables).
4. Circulator restricts to a minimum all activity near the sterile field.

Destruction of Integrity of Microbial Barriers Results in Contamination

Integrity of a sterile package or sterile drape is destroyed by perforation, puncture, or strike-through. *Strike-through* is the soaking of moisture through unsterile layers to sterile layers or vice versa. Ideal barrier materials are abrasion resistant and impervious to permeation by fluids or dust that transport microorganisms. The integrity of a sterile package and appearance of process monitor must be checked for sterility just before opening (see control measures in Chapter 13, pp. 233-235).

To ensure sterility:

1. Sterile packages are laid on dry surfaces.
2. If a sterile package wrapped in absorbent material becomes damp or wet, it is resterilized or discarded. The package is considered unsterile if any part of it comes in contact with moisture.
3. Drapes are placed on a dry field.
4. If solution soaks through a sterile drape to an unsterile area, the wet area is covered with impervious sterile drapes or towels.
5. Packages wrapped in woven fabric or paper are permitted to cool after removal from the sterilizer and before being placed on cold surface to prevent steam condensation and resultant contamination.
6. Sterile items are stored in clean, dry areas.
7. Sterile packages are handled with clean, dry hands.
8. Undue pressure on sterile packs is avoided to prevent forcing sterile air out and pulling unsterile air into the pack.

Microorganisms Must Be Kept to Irreducible Minimum

Perfect asepsis in the surgical wound is an ideal to be approached; it is not absolute. All microorganisms can-

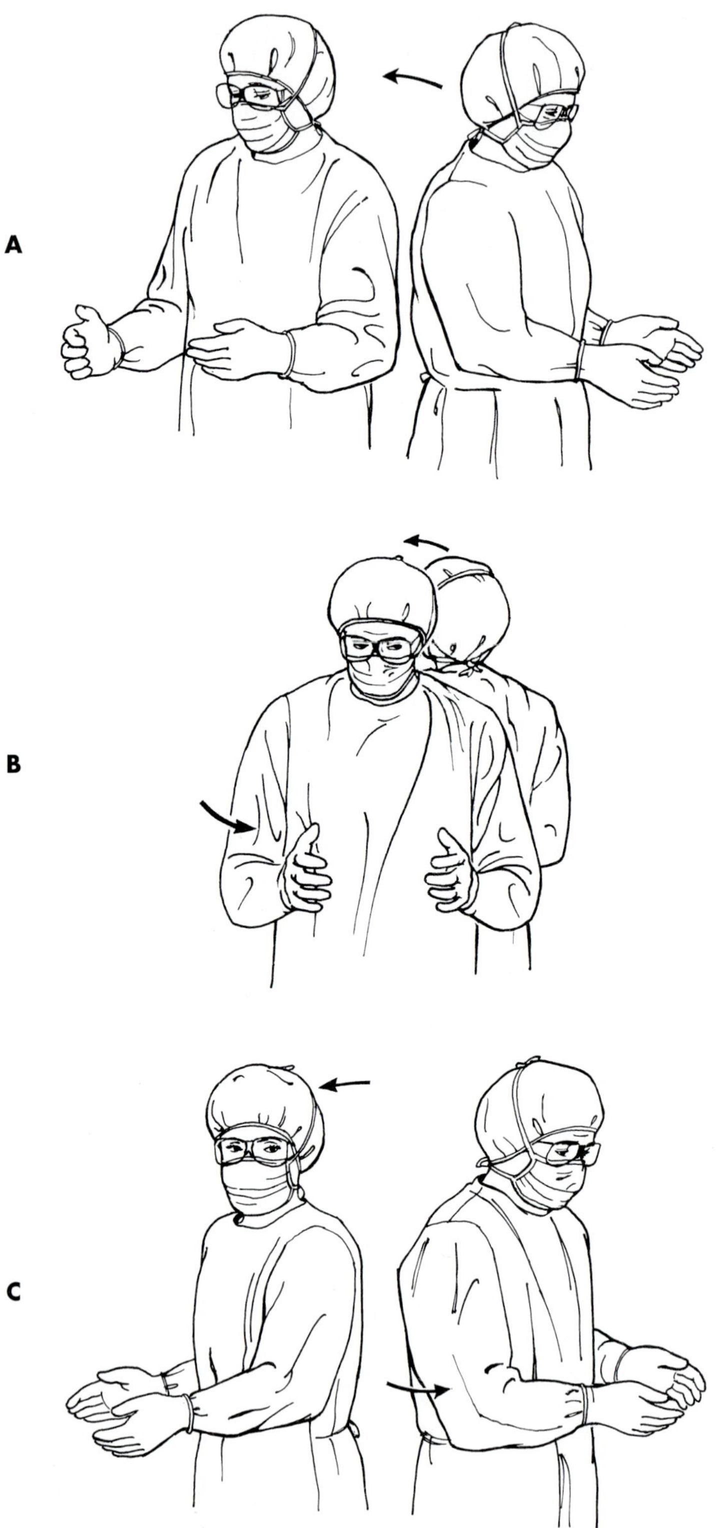

FIGURE 12-7 Sequence of one sterile person going around another. They pass each other back to back, keeping well within the sterile area and allowing a margin of safety between them.

not be eliminated, but this does not obviate the necessity for strict sterile technique. It is generally agreed that:

1. *Skin cannot be sterilized.* Skin is a potential source of contamination in every invasive procedure. Inherent body defenses usually can overcome the relatively few organisms remaining after the patient's skin preparation. Organisms on the hands and arms of the OR team are a hazard. All possible means are used to prevent entrance of microorganisms into the wound. Preventive measures include:
   a. Transient and resident floras are removed from the skin around the surgical site of the patient (see Chapter 22) and hands and arms of sterile team members (see Chapter 11) by mechanical washing and chemical antisepsis.
   b. Gowning and gloving of the OR team is accomplished without contamination of the sterile exterior of gowns and gloves.
   c. Sterile gloved hands do not directly touch skin and then deeper tissues. Instruments used in contact with skin are discarded and not reused.
   d. If a glove is torn or punctured by a needle or instrument, the glove is changed immediately. The needle or instrument is discarded from the sterile field.
   e. Sterile dressing should be applied before drapes are removed to reduce the risk of the incision being touched by contaminated hands or objects.
2. *Some areas cannot be scrubbed.* When the surgical site includes the mouth, nose, throat, or anus, the number of microorganisms present is great. Various parts of the body, such as the gastrointestinal tract and vagina, usually are resistant to infection from floras that normally inhabit these parts. However, the following steps may be taken to reduce the number of microorganisms present in these areas and to prevent scattering them:
   a. Surgeon makes an effort to use a sponge only once, then discards it.
   b. Gastrointestinal tract, especially the colon, is contaminated, so measures are used to prevent spreading this contamination (see Chapter 29, p. 578 and p. 591).
3. *Infected areas are grossly contaminated.* The team avoids disseminating the contamination.
4. *Air is contaminated by dust, droplets, and shedding.* Environmental control measures are used. In addition to those discussed on pp. 194-199:
   a. Drapes over the anesthesia screen or attached to IV poles separate the anesthesia area from the sterile field.
   b. Movement around the sterile field is kept to a minimum to avoid air turbulence.
   c. To avoid dispersion of lint and dust, drapes are not flipped, fanned, or shaken.
   d. Talking is kept to a minimum in the OR. Moisture droplets are expelled with force into the mask during the process of articulating words.
   e. Attire is worn properly: mask covers the nose and mouth; hair is completely covered; body covers are close fitting. Unsterile persons wear long sleeves.

NO COMPROMISE OF STERILITY

Sterility is never taken for granted. It must be maintained and checked. Chapter 13 details the procedures for sterilization and handling of sterile supplies.

Basically there is no compromise with sterility. In clinical practice an item is considered sterile or unsterile. Always be as certain of sterility as possible. That certainty rests on the fact that the necessary conditions have been met and that all factors in the sterilization process have been observed. Obviously it is impossible to prove that every package is free from bacteria, but a single break in technique can compromise the life of a patient. OR personnel must maintain the high standards of sterile technique they know are essential. Every individual is accountable for his or her own role in infection control.

BIBLIOGRAPHY

Anastasi JK, Rivera J: Understanding prophylactic therapy for HIV infections, *Am J Nurs* 94(2):36-41, 1994.

Avey MA: TB skin testing: how to do it right, *Am J Nurs* 93(9):42-44, 1993.

Bailes BK: Creutzfeldt-Jakob disease, *AORN J* 52(5):976-985, 1990.

Bruning LM: The bloodborne pathogens final rule, *AORN J* 57(2):437-441, 1993.

CDC drafts new guidelines on tuberculosis, *OR Manager* 9(12):15-16, 1993.

Centers for Disease Control: Recommendations for preventing transmission of human immunodeficiency virus and hepatitis B to patients during exposure-prone invasive procedures, *MMWR* 40:1-9, July 12, 1991.

Compliance with universal precautions high in OR, *OR Manager* 9(10):20-22, 1993.

Crow S: It's second nature to me now, *Today's OR Nurse* 12(10):6-8, 1990.

Curry J: Hepatitis C poses another risk to the surgical team, *OR Manager* 9(3):1, 14-15, 1993.

Cuzzell JZ: Clues: recurrent, punched-out lesions, *Am J Nurs* 90(5):21-22, 1990.

Erickson MJ: Chlamydial infections: combating the silent threat, *Am J Nurs* 94(6):16B-16F, 1994.

Fox VJ: Clinical issues: preventing glove tears, sharp injuries, *AORN J* 57(3):703-706, 1993.

Gerberding JL: Procedure-specific infection control for preventing intraoperative blood exposures, *Am J Infect Control* 21(12):364-367, 1993.

Herrera JL: Hepatitis E as a cause of non-A, non-B hepatitis, *Arch Intern Med* 153(6):773-775, 1993.

Hubbard MS et al: Reducing blood contamination and injury in the OR, *AORN J* 55(1):194-201, 1992.

Jackson MM, Lynch P: In search of a rational approach, *Am J Nurs* 90(10):65-74, 1990.

Jackson MM, McPherson DC: Hepatitis A through E: current and future trends, *Today's OR Nurse* 13(10):7-11, 1991.

Jackson MM, Pugliese G: The OSHA bloodborne pathogens standard, *Today's OR Nurse* 14(7):11-16, 1992.

Jackson MM, Rymer TE: Viral hepatitis: anatomy of a diagnosis, *Am J Nurs* 94(1):43-48, 1994.

Kelly PJ, Holman S: The new faces of AIDS, *Am J Nurs* 90(3):26-32, 1993.

King CA: Clinical issues: risks of donor organs; tuberculosis in the OR; unexplained immunodeficiency states; the HIV-infected health care worker, *AORN J* 56(6):1102-1108, 1992.

Larkin MA: Aseptic technique adherence never goes out of style, *AORN J* 54(2):353-355, 1991.

Lisanti P, Talotta D: Hepatitis update: the delta virus, *AORN J* 55(3):790-800, 1992.

McQuarrie DG et al: Laminar airflow systems, *AORN J* 51(4):1035-1048, 1990.

National Institute for Occupational Safety and Health: *NIOSH recommended guidelines: personal respiratory protection of workers in health-care facilities potentially exposed to tuberculosis,* Cincinnati, 1992, NIOSH.

Nettina SL: Syphilis: a new look at an old killer, *Am J Nurs* 90(4):68-70, 1990.

O'Brien LM, Bartlett KA: TB plus HIV spells trouble, *Am J Nurs* 92(5):28-34, 1992.

Palmer PN: This tuberculosis epidemic cannot be silent, *AORN J* 56(2):211-212, 1992 (editorial).

Patterson P: Hepatitis proves a greater threat than HIV, *OR Manager* 10(4):1, 6, 1994.

Patterson P: New OSHA rules for TB prevention are controversial, *OR Manager* 10(3):1, 10-11, 14-15, 1994.

Patterson P: OSHA issues rules to protect workers from HIV, hepatitis B, *OR Manager* 8(1):1, 5-7, 1992.

Patterson P: Programs to help prevent TB transmission in the OR, *OR Manager* 11(2):14-15, 1995.

Patterson P: Sacred cows: must that dropped package be discarded? *OR Manager* 6(4):1, 4-6, 1990.

Programmed instruction in asepsis II: microbiology and health care, Arlington, Tex, 1991, Johnson & Johnson Medical.

Radke SR, Ford DA: Aseptic technique monitoring, *AORN J* 58(2):312-323, 1993.

Rathkowski PL: Traffic control, *AORN J* 59(2):439-448, 1994.

Recommended practices: aseptic technique, *AORN J* 54(4):819-824, 1991.

Recommended practices: universal precautions in the perioperative nursing setting, *AORN J* 57(2):554-558, 1993.

Ronk LL, Girard NJ: Risk perception, universal precautions compliance: a descriptive study of nurses who circulate, *AORN J* 59(1):253-266, 1994.

Scherer P: How AIDS attacks the brain, *Am J Nurs* 90(1):44-52, 1990.

Scherer P: How HIV attacks the peripheral nervous system, *Am J Nurs* 90(5):66-70, 1990.

Stelck MJ: Tuberculosis: a resurging health care issue, *Surg Technol* 25(2):8-11, 1993.

Taylor M: Universal precautions in the operating department, *Br J Theatre Nurs* 30(1):4-7, 1993.

US Department of Health and Human Services, Centers for Disease Control and Prevention: *Draft guidelines for isolation precautions in hospitals,* Federal Register 59:55552-55570, Nov 7, 1994.

US Department of Health and Human Services, Centers for Disease Control and Prevention: *Draft guidelines for preventing transmission of tuberculosis in health-care facilities,* ed 2, Federal Register 58:52827, Oct 12, 1993.

US Department of Labor, Occupational Safety and Health Administration: *Occupational exposure to bloodborne pathogens: Final Rule, 29 CFR Part 1910.1030,* Federal Register, Dec 1992.

Wright JG et al: Mechanisms of glove tears and sharp injuries among surgical personnel, *JAMA* 266(12):1668-1671, 1991.

CHAPTER 13

Sterilization and Disinfection

HISTORICAL BACKGROUND

By the end of the nineteenth century, the concepts of Semmelweis, Pasteur, Lister, Nightingale, Neuber, and others were established to control the operating room (OR) environment. Surgeons had moved out of their front parlors into hospitals. Disinfectants were used to clean furniture, floors, and walls. Antiseptics, or soap at least, were used to clean the skin of patients and team members. The team wore gowns and gloves. Methods of sterilization were known.

"Sterilization" by boiling was introduced in the 1880s. Everything used during a surgical procedure, including linens, dressings, and gowns, was boiled, although some surgeons still believed Lister's method of using carbolic spray to be adequate.

In 1876, heat-resistant bacteria were demonstrated. About 1886, Ernst von Bergmann and his associates introduced the steam sterilizer, a great improvement over von Bergmann's previous method of soaking surgical supplies in bichloride of mercury. However, surgeons soon learned that steam in itself is inadequate for sterilization. Steam must be under pressure to raise the temperature sufficiently to kill heat-resistant microorganisms. Pressure steam sterilizers were developed to kill resistant spores. Vacuum-type pressure sterilizers and hot-air sterilizers followed.

Used as a fumigant for insects in the early twentieth century, ethylene oxide was recognized as an antibacterial agent around 1929, when it was used to sterilize imported spices. It has been employed as a sterilizing agent in industry and hospitals since the 1940s. Sterilization by irradiation, developed thereafter, is used for commercial sterilization of surgical supplies.

Coincidental with the development of sterilization, the efficacy and effectiveness of chemical agents for disinfection were recognized. Lister's carbolic acid, with its caustic effects, and Neuber's mercuric chloride, with its limited effectiveness, were replaced by other agents. Not only did hot water boilers give way to steam sterilizers, but green soap gave way to detergent-disinfectants. Glutaraldehyde, introduced in 1963, was the first chemical solution approved by the Environmental Protection Agency (EPA) as a sterilant for heat-sensitive instruments.

STERILIZATION VS. DISINFECTION

Pathogenic microorganisms and those that do not normally invade healthy tissue are capable of causing infection if introduced mechanically into the body. Therefore specific standardized procedures, based on accepted principles and practices, are necessary for the sterilization or disinfection of all supplies and equipment used in the operating room. *Sterilization* renders items safe for contact with tissue without transmission of infection as long as sterility is maintained. *Disinfectants* are used to kill as many microorganisms in the environment as possible on items and materials that cannot be sterilized.

Surgical instruments and many other items are prepared on site (i.e., in the health care facility) for use in the sterile field. Many supplies are purchased already sterilized by the manufacturer. The term *sterile* has different meanings depending on the control of the sterilization process.

1. *User's theoretical definition:* A sterile item has been exposed to a sterilization process to render it free of all living microorganisms, including spores. This is the absolute definition of sterility. Unfortunately this condition cannot be scientifically proven. Therefore it is accepted that the sterilization process provides the highest level of assurance that an item can be expected to be free of known viable pathogenic and nonpathogenic microorganisms, including spores.
2. *Manufacturer's probabilistic definition:* An item is sterile if the probability of living microorganisms is less than one in one million. This can be statistically validated.
3. *Regulatory agency's definition:* An item may be labeled and sold as sterile if the manufacture of the item includes cleaning, packaging, and sterilizing processes that ensure product quality, stability, and sterility. These processes are rigidly controlled and validated.

Items that will penetrate or separate tissue or invade the intravascular system must be sterile. Theoretically, all items used in the sterile field should be sterilized. Practically, some specialized instruments and equipment cannot be sterilized between each patient use or will not withstand a sterilization process. Disinfection may be the only alternative. *Disinfection is the process of destroying or inhibiting growth of pathogenic microorganisms on inanimate objects.* It reduces the risk of microbial contamination, but it does not provide the same level of assurance as sterilization. Disinfection can be classified by the effectiveness of the process, that is, the ability of the agent to kill microorganisms.

1. *High-level disinfection:* Kills all bacteria, viruses, and fungi. The process may kill spores if contact time is sufficient and other conditions are met. A high-level disinfectant should be used if a semicritical item must be disinfected rather than sterilized for use in contact with nonintact skin or mucous membranes.
2. *Intermediate-level disinfection:* Kills most bacteria, viruses, and fungi. The process does not attack spores. It does inactivate *Mycobacterium tuberculosis.*
3. *Low-level disinfection:* Kills most vegetative bacteria, fungi, and the least resistant viruses, including human immunodeficiency virus (HIV).

To be effective, specific requirements must be met for each sterilization and disinfection process. The purpose of the process may determine the method.

Terminal sterilization and *disinfection* are the procedures carried out for the destruction of pathogens at the end of an invasive procedure. Organic debris and microbial bioburden are substantially reduced so that items are safe to handle. Further cleaning may be required before items are prepared or packaged for sterilization.

Bioburden

Bioburden is the relative number of actual or suspected microorganisms that may be found on a specific item or in the environment at a specific time. This number may be reduced through the environmental control measures and sterile techniques described in Chapter 12.

Sterilization kills microorganisms in their vegetative and spore stages. For the process to be effective, however, the bioburden on items must be relatively low. All items must be thoroughly cleaned before sterilization or high-level disinfection. The cleaning process physically removes some microbes and all organic debris that harbors microorganisms.

Some porous materials or internal mechanisms cannot be thoroughly cleaned after use. Items or devices whose physical characteristics, function, or safety will be altered should not be reprocessed or resterilized. *Most single-use disposable items should not be reprocessed.* Many materials deteriorate during sterilization. Manufacturers' written instructions for cleaning and sterilizing limited-use items must be followed. *Limited-use items* are those designed to be reprocessed only the number of times specified by the manufacturer. On-site sterilization places the burden of proof and responsibility for sterility, safety, and efficacy on the health care facility and user, not the original manufacturer of a single- or limited-use item.

Microbiologic Safety

Before availability of commercially packaged and sterilized products, all items were prepared in the hospital for use in a sterile field and for implantation in body tissues. Traditionally, sterility was considered by users to be the absolute absence of all microorganisms. This concept is not held today because it is known that microorganisms are killed according to a logarithmic order of death when subjected to a sterilization process. A given percentage of surviving population is killed in a unit of time; that is, a percentage of the initial concentration will die and a percentage will survive during each subsequent unit of time of exposure. Absolute sterilization cannot be attained because it is impossible to reach zero.

The rate at which microorganisms die is expressed as the decimal reduction value (D value). The D value is the time required at a constant temperature and/or dose of agent to destroy 90% of the microbial population or the time required for the survivor curve to complete a logarithmic cycle. The D value is independent from the initial logarithmic reduction. The same time-agent ratio is required to reduce the microbial population tenfold: 1 million (10^6) to 100,000 (10^5) to 10^4, and so on to 1 to 0.1.

Sterility actually refers to the probability that an item is not contaminated. Manufacturers of sterile products employ quality control procedures to ensure at least a probability that no more than one in 1 million products will be unsterile. Expressed scientifically as 1×10^6, this generally accepted standard refers to the level of assurance that 99.9999% of items are sterile. A higher level of sterility assurance is sought by some manufacturers of critical implants. A manufacturer may label a product *sterile* following compliance with Federal Food and Drug Administration (FDA) and United States Pharmacopeia (USP) testing procedures. These include tests of presterilization bioburden (degree of contamination) and control tests of sterilization process variables with biologic indicators or dosimeters.

A *microbiologic safety/survival index* (MSI) was developed in Canada as a quality control measurement for sterile products to counter the differences in user, industry, and regulatory definitions of sterility. MSI is defined as the absolute value of the logarithm (negative common logarithm) of the probability that an item is unsterile, contaminated with a viable microorganism. An MSI of 6, for example, indicates 0.000001 or 1×10^6 probability of nonsterility, 99.9999% probability of sterility. As the MSI value increases, so does assurance of sterility. An increase or decrease of one in the MSI increases or decreases the probability tenfold. Although not required, manufacturers may include the MSI on labeling of their sterile products.

Although sterility cannot be guaranteed, all items brought into the sterile field must be microbiologically safe for their intended uses. The in-hospital sterilization of supplies should be performed only by individuals who demonstrate knowledge of the principles of microbiology as they pertain to containment of contamination and of the sterilization processes.

STERILIZATION PROCESS

Bacterial spores are the most resistant of all living organisms because of their capacity to withstand external destructive agents. Although the physical or chemical process by which all pathogenic and nonpathogenic microorganisms, *including spores,* are destroyed is not absolute, supplies and equipment are considered sterile when necessary conditions have been met during a sterilization process.

Parameters of Sterilization

Two types of parameters must be considered for all sterilizing methods. These parameters are product and process associated.

Product-Associated Parameters

1. *Bioburden:* Degree of contamination with microorganisms and organic debris
2. *Bioresistance:* Factors such as heat and/or moisture sensitivities and product stability
3. *Biostate:* Nutritional, physical, and/or reproductive phase of microorganisms
4. *Bioshielding:* Characteristics of packaging materials
5. *Density:* Factors affecting penetration and evacuation of the agent

Process-Associated Parameters

1. Temperature
2. Humidity/moisture/hydration
3. Time
4. Purity of the agent and air, and residual effects or residues
5. Saturation/penetration
6. Capacity of sterilizer and position of items within the chamber

Methods of Sterilization

Reliable sterilization depends on contact of the sterilizing agent with *all* surfaces of the item to be sterilized. Selection of the agent to achieve sterility depends primarily on the nature of the item to be sterilized. The time required to kill spores in the equipment available for the process then becomes critical. Each method of sterilization has its advantages and disadvantages. Sterilization processes are either physical or chemical. The sterilizing agents (sterilants) are:

1. Thermal (physical)
   a. Steam under pressure—moist heat
   b. Hot air—dry heat
   c. Microwaves—nonionizing radiation
2. Chemical
   a. Ethylene oxide gas
   b. Formaldehyde gas and solution
   c. Hydrogen peroxide plasma/vapor
   d. Ozone gas
   e. Acetic acid solution
   f. Glutaraldehyde solution
   g. Peracetic acid solution
3. Ionizing radiation (physical)

Sterilization Cycle

The time required to achieve sterilization is referred to as the *process cycle.* This includes:

1. Heat-up and/or penetration of the agent

2. Kill time (i.e., exposure to the agent)
3. Safety factor for bioburden
4. Evacuation or dissipation of the agent

Monitoring of Sterilization Process

To ensure that instruments and supplies are sterile when used, monitoring of the sterilization process is essential. General considerations are mentioned here. Specific tests are discussed with each process.

Administrative Monitoring

Work practices must be supervised. Written policies and procedures must be strictly followed by all personnel responsible and accountable for sterilizing and disinfecting items and for handling sterile supplies. If sterility cannot be achieved or maintained, the system has failed. Policies and procedures pertain to:

1. Decontaminating, terminally sterilizing, and cleaning of all reusable items; disposing of disposable items
2. Packaging and labeling of items
3. Loading and unloading the sterilizer
4. Operating the sterilizer
5. Monitoring and maintaining records of each cycle
6. Adhering to safety precautions and preventive maintenance protocol
7. Storing of sterile items
8. Handling sterile items ready for use
9. Making sterile transfer to a sterile field

Mechanical Indicators

Sterilizers have gauges, thermometers, timers, recorders, and/or other devices that monitor their functions. Most sterilizers have automatic controls and locking devices. Some have alarm systems that are activated if the sterilizer fails to operate correctly. Records are reviewed and maintained for each cycle. Test packs are run at least daily to monitor functions of each sterilizer, as appropriate. These can identify process errors in packaging or loading.

The sterilizer manufacturer provides a manual for the comprehensive care and maintenance of the sterilizing device. Reliable operation is dependent on:

1. Routine maintenance consisting of daily inspections and scheduled cleaning per manufacturer's recommendation. All gaskets, gauges, graph pens, drain screens, and charting devices should be repaired or replaced by qualified personnel as needed.
2. Preventative maintenance including periodic calibration, lubrication, and function checks by qualified personnel on a scheduled basis.

Chemical Indicators

A chemical indicator on a package verifies *exposure to a sterilization process*. An indicator should be clearly visible on the outside of every on-site sterilized package. This helps differentiate sterilized from unsterilized items. More important, it helps monitor physical conditions within the sterilizer to alert personnel if the process has been inadequate. An indicator may be placed inside a package in a position most likely to be difficult for the sterilant to penetrate (Table 13-1). A chemical indicator can detect sterilizer malfunction or human error in packaging or loading of the sterilizer. If chemical reaction of the indicator does not show the expected results, the item should not be used. Several types of chemical indicators are available:

1. Glass tube with pellet that melts when a specific temperature is attained in sterilizer. This is a single-parameter process monitor.
2. Tape, labels, and paper strips printed with an ink that changes color when exposed to one or more process parameters.
3. Encapsulated chemical tablet that migrates along a wicking paper gauge as it melts during exposure to the sterilization process. An integrator of this type has defined end points to assess the effect of variables in the process. When all process parameters are met, the color bar reaches the "accept" area on the gauge.

Biologic Indicators

Positive assurance that sterilization conditions have been achieved can be obtained only through a biologic control test. The biologic indicator *detects nonsterilizing conditions in the sterilizer.* A biologic indicator is a preparation of living spores resistant to the sterilizing agent. These may be supplied in a self-contained system, in dry spore strips or disks in envelopes, or in sealed vials or ampules of spores in suspension. Each of these units contains the spores to be sterilized and a control that is not sterilized. Some incorporate a chemical indicator also. The sterilized units and controls are incubated for 24 hours for *Bacillus stearothermophilus* at 131° to 140° F (55° to 60° C) to test steam under pressure, and for 48 hours for *Bacillus subtilis* var *niger strain globigi* at 95° to 98.6° F (35° to 37° C) to test dry heat and ethylene oxide. If sterilization conditions have not been met, the processed incubated unit and the unprocessed control unit will display the same conditions (e.g., coloration, usually a bright yellow).

A rapid readout biologic indicator specifically for monitoring a high-speed pressure steam sterilizer with a gravity displacement cycle (see p. 214) is based on the fluorometric detection of a *B. stearothermophilus*–bound enzyme, rather than on spore growth. The enzyme becomes fluorescent yellow within 60 minutes as the spores are killed.

TABLE 13-1

Guidelines for Use of Chemical and Biologic Indicators

AAMI	AHA	AORN	CDC	JCAHO
Chemical				
Purpose: to indicate items exposed to sterilization process; to monitor one or more sterilization parameters; to detect failures in packaging, loading, or sterilizer function. Indicators do *not* verify sterility.				
Placement				
External: On all packages except if internal indicator is visible *Internal:* In center or area least accessible to sterilant within each package	With each package; can be used inside or on outside	*External:* Visible on every package *Internal:* Inside each package	*External:* Attached to each package *Internal:* Inside large pack	With each package, no designation to inside or outside
Biologic				
Purpose: to document efficacy of sterilization process by killing resistant spores; to ensure that all process parameters are met; to detect nonsterilizing conditions in sterilizer.				
Steam				
Frequency: At least weekly, preferably daily *Placement:* In test pack positioned in cold point, normally front bottom of sterilizer	*Frequency:* Once a day	*Frequency:* At least once a week, preferably daily, and each load of implantables	*Frequency:* At least once a week, and each load of implantables	*Frequency:* At least weekly, recommend daily, or with each load if sterilization activities are performed less frequently or load contains implantable or intravascular material
Ethylene oxide				
Frequency: Each load *Placement:* Inside pack in geometric center of load	*Frequency:* Each load	*Frequency:* Every load	*Frequency:* At least once a week, and each load of implantables	*Frequency:* At least weekly, recommend daily, each load if sterilization activities are performed less frequently or load contains implantable or intravascular material

NOTE: All organizations require that indicators be used routinely.
AAMI, Association for the Advancement of Medical Instrumentation; *AHA,* American Hospital Association, *Guidelines for the Hospital Central Service Department; AORN,* Association of Operating Room Nurses, Inc.; *CDC,* Centers for Disease Control and Prevention; *JCAHO,* Joint Commission on Accreditation of Healthcare Organizations.

A biologic indicator must conform with USP testing standards. A control test must be performed at least weekly in each sterilizer (Table 13-1). Many hospitals monitor on a daily basis; others test each cycle. Every load of implantable devices must be monitored, and the implant should not be used until negative test results are known. Biologic indicators also are used as a challenge test before introducing new products or packaging materials, after major repairs on the sterilizer, or after a sterilization failure. All test results are filed in a permanent record for each sterilizer.

THERMAL STERILIZATION

Heat is a dependable physical agent for destruction of all forms of microbial life, including spores. It may be used dry or moist. The most reliable and frequently used method of sterilization is steam under pressure.

Steam Under Pressure—Moist Heat

Heat destroys microorganisms, but this process is hastened by the addition of moisture. Steam in itself is inadequate for sterilization. Pressure, greater than atmospheric, is necessary to increase the temperature of steam for thermal destruction of microbial life. Death by moist heat in the form of steam under pressure is caused by the denaturation and coagulation of protein or the enzyme-protein system within cells. These reactions are catalyzed by the presence of water. Steam is water vapor; it is saturated when it contains a maximum amount of water vapor, that is, 98% steam and 2% water droplets.

Direct saturated steam contact is the basis of the steam sterilization process. Steam, for a specified time at a required temperature, must penetrate every fiber and reach every surface of items to be sterilized. When steam enters the sterilizer chamber under pressure, it condenses on contact with cold items. This condensation liberates heat, simultaneously heating and wetting all items in the load, thereby providing the two requisites: moisture and heat. *This sterilization process is spoken of in terms of degrees of temperature and time of exposure,* not in terms of pounds of pressure. Pressure increases the boiling temperature of water but has no significant effect on microorganisms or steam penetration.

Vegetative forms of most microorganisms are killed in a few minutes at temperatures ranging from 130° to 150° F (54° to 65° C); however, certain bacterial spores will withstand a temperature of 240° F (115° C) for more than 3 hours. No living thing can survive direct exposure to saturated steam at 250° F (121° C) for longer than 15 minutes. As temperature is increased, time may be decreased. A minimum temperature-time relationship must be maintained throughout all portions of the load to accomplish effective sterilization.

Exposure time depends on the size and contents of the load and the temperature within the sterilizer. At the end of the cycle, revaporation of water condensate must effectively dry contents of the load to maintain sterility.

Advantages of Steam

1. Steam sterilization is the easiest, safest, and surest method of on-site sterilization. Heat- and moisture-stable items that can be steam sterilized without damage should be processed with this method.
2. Steam is the fastest method; its total time cycle is the shortest.
3. Steam is the least expensive and most easily supplied agent. It is piped in from the facility's boiler room. An automatic, electrically powered steam generator can be mounted beneath the sterilizer for emergency standby when steam pressure is low.
4. Most sterilizers have automatic controls and recording devices to eliminate the human factor from the sterilization process as much as possible when operated and cared for according to the recommendations of the manufacturer.
5. Many items such as stainless steel instruments withstand repeated processing without damage. Steam leaves no harmful residue.

Disadvantages of Steam

1. Precaution must be used in preparing and packaging items, loading and operating the sterilizer, and drying the load.
2. Items must be clean, free of grease and oil, and nonheat-sensitive.
3. Steam must have direct contact with all areas of an item. It must be able to penetrate packaging material, but the material must be able to maintain sterility.
4. Timing of the cycle must be adjusted for differences in materials and sizes of loads; these variables are subject to human error.
5. Steam may not be pure. Steam purity refers to the amount of solid, liquid, or vapor contamination in steam. Impurities can cause wet or stained packs and stained instruments.

Types of Steam Sterilizers

Sterilizers designed to use steam under pressure as the sterilizing agent frequently are referred to as *autoclaves* to distinguish them from sterilizers employing other agents. Personnel charged with the responsibility of operating steam sterilizers must fully understand the principles and operation of each type. They must be aware of problems that cause malfunction, involving such things as attaining the sterilization temperature and maintaining it for the required period of time, trapped air, and dirty traps.

Gravity Displacement Sterilizer The metal construction contains two shells, either round or rectangular, to form a jacket and a chamber. Steam fills the jacket that surrounds the chamber. After the door is tightly closed, steam enters the chamber at the back, near the top, and is deflected upward. Air is more than twice as heavy as steam. Thus, by gravity, air goes to the bottom and steam floats on top. Steam, entering under pressure and remaining above the air, displaces air downward both in the chamber and in the wrapped items and forces it out through a discharge outlet at the bottom front. The air passes through a filtering screen to waste line. A thermometer located at this outlet below the screen measures the temperature in the chamber. When steam has filled the chamber, it begins to flow past the thermometer (Figure 13-1). Timing of sterilizing period starts only when the thermometer reaches the desired temperature.

When air is trapped in the chamber or wrapped items, the killing power of steam is decreased in direct proportion to the amount of air present. Because the vital discharge of air from the load always occurs in a downward

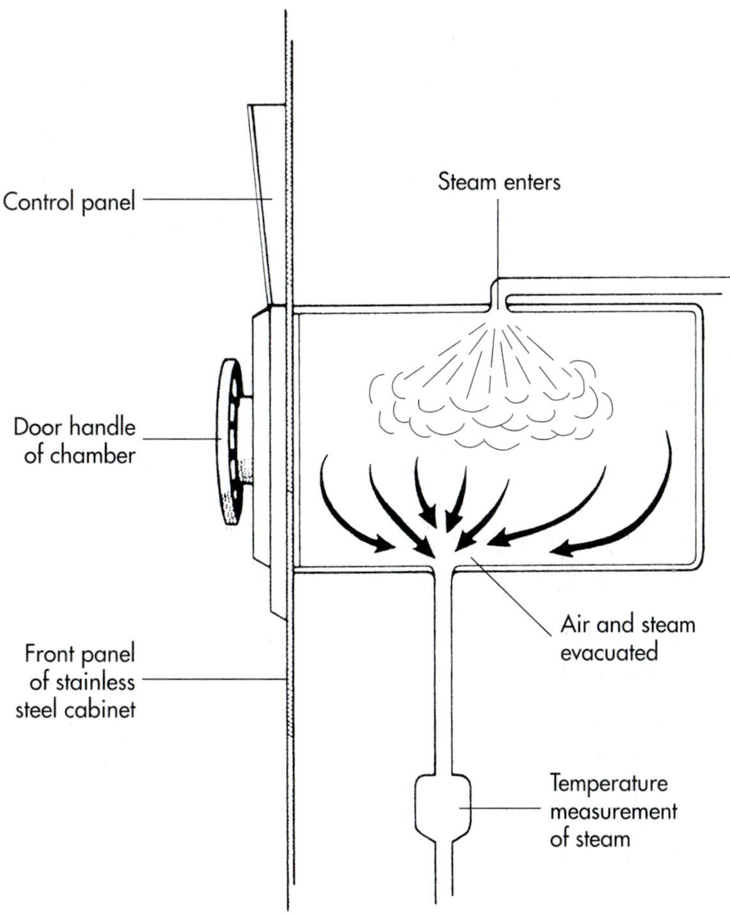

FIGURE 13-1 Schematic cross section of steam under pressure sterilizer. Steam enters at top of chamber to displace air or after air is withdrawn by vacuum. Air and steam are evacuated at bottom of chamber. Temperature of steam is measured in air-steam drain line near vent.

direction, never sideways, all supplies must be prepared and arranged to present the least possible resistance to the passage of steam through the load from the top of the chamber downward. Also, air and steam discharge lines must be kept free of dirt, sediment, and lint.

Many gravity displacement steam sterilizers operate on a standard cycle of 250° to 254° F (121° to 123° C) at a pressure of 15 to 17 psi. The size of the chamber and the contents will determine the exposure period; the minimum is 15 minutes. Exposure time may vary if a closed sterilization container system is used. Some air-powered instruments may require longer exposure periods. Consult the manufacturer's instructions included with the instrumentation for recommended times and settings for steam sterilization.

Prevacuum Sterilizer In this high-vacuum sterilizer, air is almost completely evacuated from the chamber before the sterilizing steam is admitted. This is accomplished to the desired degree of vacuum by means of a pump and a steam-injector system. A prevacuum period of 8 to 10 minutes effectively removes the air to minimize steam penetration time. The steam injector preconditions the load and helps eliminate air from packages. When the sterilizing steam is admitted to the chamber, it almost instantly penetrates to the center of the packages. Provided items making up the load are easily penetrable and the sterilizer is functioning properly, there is no demonstrable time differential between complete steam penetration of large or small, tight or loose packages. Air is not displaced by steam. Therefore maximum capacity can be used. A postvacuum cycle draws moisture from the load to shorten drying time.

Temperatures are controlled at 270° to 276° F (132° to 135.5° C) at a pressure of 27 psi. Some prevacuum sterilizers with computer-controlled pulsing air evacuation systems reach temperatures between 275° and 285° F (135° and 141° C). All items must be exposed to a temperature of at least 270° F (132° C) for a minimum of 4 minutes. A complete cycle takes approximately 15 to 30 minutes depending on sterilizer capacity.

Flash/High-Speed Pressure Sterilizer Usually called a *flash sterilizer,* this sterilizer may have either a gravity displacement or a prevacuum cycle; the gravity displacement cycle is the most common. It operates at a pressure of 27 psi at sea level to a maximum of 22 psi at 5000 feet above sea level to increase the temperature in the chamber to 270° to 275° F (132° to 135° C). *The minimum exposure time at this temperature is 3 minutes for unwrapped nonporous items without lumens only.* When porous items or instruments with lumens are included in the load, timing must be increased to 4 minutes or longer in a prevacuum sterilizer and to 10 minutes or longer in a gravity displacement sterilizer. With these cycles, the entire time for starting, sterilizing, and opening the sterilizer is a minimum of 6 to 7 minutes. Steam should be maintained in the jacket at all times.

Flash sterilization in a high-speed pressure sterilizer should only be used in urgent, unplanned, emergency situations, such as for individual items inadvertently dropped or forgotten for which no alternative method exists. This sterilizer should *not* be used for routine sterilization of complete instrument sets. Items to be permanently implanted in the body are *never* flash sterilized for immediate use. Sterility is not ensured without results of biologic test indicators. This process takes 24 hours for a spore test or 60 minutes with a rapid readout indicator.

Some pulsing gravity displacement and prevacuum high-speed pressure sterilizers have a modified sterilization cycle that mechanically evacuates air and infuses steam. A single wrapper may be placed on a perforated or mesh-bottom instrument tray to protect nonporous items (i.e., metal instruments without lumens). The cycle includes a brief drying period at the end of the cycle that dries the wrapper. Wrappers should not be used in flash sterilization cycles unless the sterilizer is specifically designed and labeled for their use.

Container systems are available for flash sterilization to protect items during transfer from the sterilizer to the sterile field. The manufacturer of the container should provide scientific evidence of its suitability for the sterilizer in use.

A high-speed pressure sterilizer to be used for flash sterilization of unwrapped instruments must be physically located in or immediately adjacent to the OR, as in the substerile room. A sterile transfer must be made from the sterilizer to the sterile field. A pass-through, two-door sterilizer loaded in a work area and unloaded in the OR facilitates a safe transfer. However, extensive condensation poses a problem as does heat in making this transfer. Transferring the sterilized item to the sterile field is difficult without contaminating it. The following methods may be used as a means of transporting the sterilized instrument to the sterile field:

1. If the OR is connected to the substerile room containing the sterilizer, the sterile scrub person may enter the substerile room, retrieve the sterilized item, and return to the sterile field. Great care must be taken by the sterile scrub person not to contaminate his or her gown or gloves in the process. The scrub person uses sterile towels for protection from contact burns from the hot tray.
2. The circulator may use a special open flash-sterilization tray with a detachable handle. The tray is sterilized with the instrument inside. When the cycle is complete, the circulator attaches the nonsterile handle to the outside front of the tray and carries it to the scrub person, who in turn, retrieves the sterile item without touching the edges of the tray. The inside is considered sterile. The outside surface is considered contaminated and is not placed in direct contact with the sterile field. Closed varieties are commercially available that allow an item to be flash sterilized in a covered container. The outside is considered contaminated, but the inside is considered sterile. The circulator removes the lid toward self, touching only the edges. The scrub person reaches inside to remove the sterile item.
3. A single item may be brought to the sterile field from the sterilizer by the circulator with a single-use sterile transfer forceps.
4. A less desirable method is for the circulator to don sterile gloves and use a sterile towel to prevent contact burns to transport the sterilized tray containing the sterile instrument to the scrub person, who only removes the contents without touching the exterior of the tray.
5. If the tray is too large to be lifted by one end, the circulator may attach sterile handles or don sterile gown and gloves and remove the tray from the sterilizer using a sterile towel to protect the hands from contact burns. The scrub person removes the item from the interior of the tray without touching the edges.

Washer-Sterilizer This sterilizer is designed to wash and terminally sterilize instruments and some other items immediately after operation. Because heat is involved in the process, gross debris should be removed before placing instruments in the washer-sterilizer. Organic material can literally become cooked on, making it almost impossible to remove.

Washer-sterilizers differ in efficiency. Automated sterilizers with a spray arm clean more efficiently than units in which instruments are submerged initially. Cold water enters the chamber and mixes with a neutral detergent to dissolve and loosen blood and debris. Steam and air, injected through powerful jet streams located near the bottom of the chamber, create turbulence in the water to continue the washing process. As water is heated, it rises and carries debris to the water line. Steam then enters at the top of the chamber to force the wash water out through the bottom drain. Steam under pressure floods the chamber to sterilize items at 270° F (132° C). Although designed specifically for the combination of washing and sterilizing cycles, some units can be programmed and used as flash sterilizers.

Precautions

With all four types of steam sterilizers, the following precautions must be taken to ensure safe operation:

1. Turn the valve on for steam in the jacket before use. Steam may be kept in the jacket throughout the day. (It may be turned off at the end of the surgical schedule.) The jacket maintains heat, so do not touch the inside of the chamber when loading. (Check the sterilizer; not all have a steam jacket.)
2. Never put heat-sensitive items in a steam sterilizer of any type; they will be destroyed.
3. Close the door tightly before activating either automatic or manual controls.
4. Do not set a manually operated timer, unless it is an automatically controlled device, until desired temperature registers on the thermometer and recording graphic chart. *Thermometers, not pressure gauges, are the guides for sterilization.*
5. Open the door only when the exhaust valve registers zero. Stand behind the door and open slowly to avoid the steam that may be escaping around the door.
6. Wash the inside of the chamber with Calgonite or trisodium phosphate solution, rinse with tap water, and dry with a lint-free cloth every day.
7. Remove and clean the filtering screen daily.
8. Flush discharge lines weekly with a hot solution of trisodium phosphate: 1 oz (30 ml) to 1 qt (1000 ml) of hot water. Follow flush with a rinse of 1 qt (1000 ml) of tap water.
9. Wipe the gasket daily with a lint-free cloth, and check for signs of wear and defects.
10. Provide routine preventive maintenance including evaluation of steam and air purity. The amount of solid, liquid, or vapor contamination in the steam must be minimal. An ineffective air filter may contaminate a load when air is drawn into the chamber at the end of the cycle. A defective steam trap or clogged exhaust line can cause malfunction. The thermometer must be correctly calibrated.

Preparing Items for Steam Sterilization

For effective steam sterilization, organic debris must be removed. After cleaning, items must be thoroughly rinsed and dried.

Surgical Instruments Special attention must be given to cleaning surgical instruments before sterilization. Most instruments are made of metal, but many are difficult to clean. Because of the complexities of caring for and preparing them for sterilization, Chapter 14 discusses surgical instruments in detail.

Basin Sets If they are nested, basins and solid utensils must be separated by a porous material to permit permeation of steam around all surfaces and condensation of steam from the inside during sterilization. Sponges or drapes are not packaged in basins; steam could be deflected from penetration through fabrics.

Drape Packs Freshly laundered woven textile drapes and gowns must be fanfolded or rolled loosely to provide the least possible resistance to penetration of steam through each layer of material. Packs must not exceed a maximum size of 12 × 12 × 20 inches (30 × 30 × 50 cm) and not weigh more than 12 lb (5.5 kg). Drapes are loosely crisscrossed so they do not form a dense, impermeable mass. Pack density should not exceed 7.2 lb/cu ft. See Box 13-1 for the calculation of density. The outside wrapper becomes the table drape when the pack is opened (see Chapter 20, p. 411).

Rubber Goods and Thermoplastics A rubber sheet or any other impervious material should not be folded for sterilization because steam cannot penetrate it nor displace air from the folds. It should be covered with a piece of fabric of the same size, both loosely rolled and then wrapped. For example, a layer of roller gauze is rolled between layers of an Esmarch's bandage.

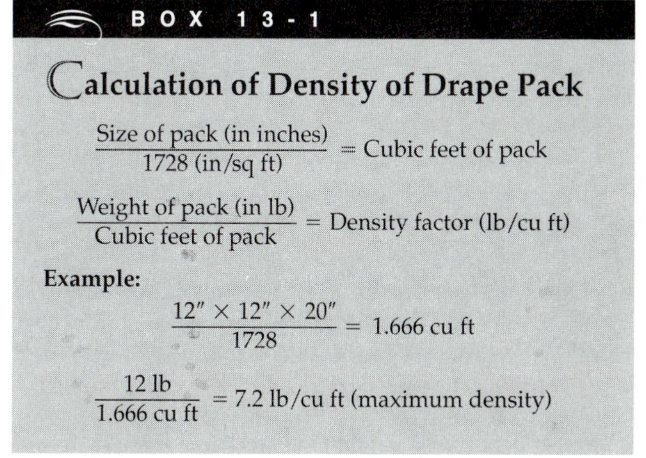

BOX 13-1

Calculation of Density of Drape Pack

$$\frac{\text{Size of pack (in inches)}}{\text{1728 (in/sq ft)}} = \text{Cubic feet of pack}$$

$$\frac{\text{Weight of pack (in lb)}}{\text{Cubic feet of pack}} = \text{Density factor (lb/cu ft)}$$

Example:

$$\frac{12'' \times 12'' \times 20''}{1728} = 1.666 \text{ cu ft}$$

$$\frac{12 \text{ lb}}{1.666 \text{ cu ft}} = 7.2 \text{ lb/cu ft (maximum density)}$$

The mechanical cleaning of tubing, including catheters and drains, is a factor in reducing microbial count inside lumen. A residual of distilled water should be left in the lumen of any tubing to be steam sterilized by gravity displacement. This becomes steam as the temperature rises and helps to displace air in the lumen and to increase the temperature within it. (This is not necessary in a prevacuum sterilizer.) Tubing should be coiled without kinks.

Suction tips must be removed from tubing. Detachable rubber or plastic parts should be removed from instruments and syringes for cleaning and sterilizing. Rubber surfaces should not touch each other, metal, or glassware during sterilization to avoid melting or sticking and to permit steam to reach all surfaces. Rubber bands must not be used around solid items because steam cannot penetrate through or under rubber.

Wood Products During sterilization, lignocellulose resin (lignin) is driven out of wood by heat. This resin may condense onto other items in the sterilizer and cause reactions if it gets into the tissues of a patient. Therefore wooden items must be individually wrapped and separated from other items in the sterilizer.

NOTE Repeated sterilizing dries wood so that during sterilization it will adsorb moisture from the saturated steam. As the water content of saturated steam decreases, steam becomes superheated and loses some of its sterilizing power. Because of this problem, the use of wood products that require steam sterilization should be minimized and their repeated sterilization avoided.

All Items Whether washed by hand, in a washer-sterilizer or washer-decontaminator, or in an ultrasonic cleaner (see Chapter 14, pp. 255-257), all items with detachable parts or parts that can be separated must be disassembled for cleaning, packaging, and sterilizing. Items must be clean and dry, except perhaps the lumen of tubing, before sterilization. Manuals, often with photographs, or index file cards are available in the room in which supplies are packaged for ready reference during preparation and wrapping of single items, packs, or trays. Instructions must be strictly followed to ensure safety in sterilizing items.

Packaging

The packaging materials for *all* methods of sterilization must:

1. Permit penetration of the sterilizing agent to achieve sterilization of all items in the package.
2. Allow release of the sterilizing agent at the end of the exposure period and allow adequate drying or aerating.
3. Withstand physical conditions of the sterilizing process.
4. Maintain integrity of the package at varying atmospheric and humidity levels.

   NOTE In geographic areas of high altitude or dry climates, some packaging materials are susceptible to rupture during sterilization or will dry out and crack in storage.

5. Provide an impermeable barrier to microorganisms, dust particles, and moisture after sterilization. Items must remain sterile from the time removed from the sterilizer until used.
6. Cover items completely and easily, and fasten securely with tape or heat seal that cannot be resealed after opening. Seal integrity should be tamperproof.

   NOTE
   - At least a 1-inch (2.5 cm) margin is considered standard for safety on all sealed packages.
   - Pins, staples, paper clips, or other penetrating objects must never be used to seal packages. These cannot be removed without destroying the integrity of the package and contaminating the contents. If a staple, for example, is used to secure the end of a package, it is impossible to remove it without tearing the package. Scissors should not be used to cut off the end of a package. Contents cannot be drawn out over this cut end because the item would be contaminated by the edge of the packaging material. For the same reason, packages are never torn open below a seal.

7. Resist tears and punctures in handling. If accidental tears and holes do occur, they must be visible.
8. Permit identification of the contents and evidence of exposure to a sterilizing agent.

   NOTE Chemical indicator tapes or strips on the outside of packages change color during exposure to a sterilization process. They do not indicate sterility, only that the package has been sufficiently exposed to a given parameter to turn the color. Integrators indicate that all parameters are met.

9. Be free of toxic ingredients and nonfast dyes.
10. Be lint free or low linting.
11. Protect the contents from physical damage.
12. Permit easy removal of the contents with transfer to the sterile field without contamination or delamination (separation into layers).
13. Be economical.

Wrapping of packages should be done far enough away from sterile storage areas so mixing sterile and nonsterile packages is not possible. Nonsterile cabinets should be labeled conspicuously. A procedure for sending items to the sterilizer and receiving them from it should be set up so that sterile and nonsterile packages can never be confused en route. The procedure must be understood by everyone.

Packaging materials must be compatible with the sterilization process. The following materials may be safely used for wrapping items for *steam sterilization* because they permit steam penetration, adequate air removal, and adequate drying.

Woven Textile Fabrics Reusable woven fabrics are commonly referred to as muslin or linen. Woven fabrics may be:

1. *140-thread count carded cotton muslin.* Steam sterilizer cycles are based on a time-temperature profile of 140-thread count muslin. This is not moisture resistant. It is used in a double thickness. Two pieces are sewn together *on the edges only,* with a blind hem and without cross-stitching, so the wrapper is free of holes. This wrapper should withstand between 50 and 75 launderings before it becomes too worn to be a microbial barrier. A laundering mark-off system is helpful to monitor the number of times a wrapper is used.
2. *180-thread count blend of 50% combed cotton and 50% polyester.* This is somewhat more moisture resistant than 140-thread count muslin but also is used in a double thickness.
3. *270- or 280-thread count combed pima cotton with a water-repellent finish.* A single-thickness wrapper of this fabric is moisture retardant and a more effective barrier to microbial penetration.

Packages are wrapped sequentially in two layers (four thicknesses of double-thickness 140- and 180-thread count fabrics) to serve as a sufficient dust filter and microbial barrier. Items are enclosed with all corners of the wrapper folded in. Either a square or envelope fold may be used (Figures 13-2 and 13-3). After the item is wrapped in one wrapper, the package is turned over and wrapped in the second wrapper. A cuff turned back on first fold of each wrapper provides a margin of safety to prevent contamination when opening after sterilization. Packages can be securely fastened with pressure-sensitive indicator tape.

The *advantages* of woven fabric wrappers are:

1. Textile fabric may be the most economical material, after the initial investment, because it can be used many times.
2. A package wrapped in woven material may be opened on a table so that the wrapper becomes a sterile field drape. Woven fabric is memory-free so will lie flat.

   NOTE *Memory* is the ability of a material to retain a specific shape or configuration.

3. Danger of tearing or gouging holes is minimal. Small holes (not rips) can be heat-sealed with double-vulcanized patches; they should never be stitched. A sewing machine will leave needle holes in fabric. Not more than 20% of surface area should be occluded if the wrapper will be used in a gravity displacement sterilizer. As a general rule, wrappers should be discarded after four to six patchings.
4. Woven material is flexible and easy to handle.

The *disadvantages* of woven fabric wrappers are:

1. Woven fabrics must be laundered to rehydrate, inspected on an illuminated table, patched if necessary, delinted, and folded after each use.

   NOTE
   - Woven materials should be maintained at a room temperature of 64° to 72° F (18° to 22° C) and in relative humidity of 35% to 70%.
   - Moisture content of woven material affects steam penetration and prevents superheating during the sterilization process. Wrappers should be laundered between uses and sterilization cycles.

2. Fabric may create free-floating lint in the OR.
3. Opacity prevents the contents from being seen.
4. Woven material has limited storage life after sterilization: 30 days maximum in closed cabinets, 21 days or less on open shelving. Sterility is not maintained for prolonged periods unless a wrapped package is hermetically sealed in a plastic overwrap, a dust cover.
5. Woven material wets easily and dries quickly so that water stains may not be obvious. A 270- or 280-thread count fabric may overcome this disadvantage.

   NOTE Heavy, tightly woven fabrics, such as canvas, duck, or twill, will retard penetration of steam so that sterility cannot be ensured.

Nonwoven Fabrics A combination of cellulose and rayon with strands of nylon randomly oriented through it, or a combination of other natural and synthetic fibers bonded by a method other than weaving, has the flexibility and handling qualities of woven materials. Nonwoven fabric is available in three weights. Lightweight is used in four thicknesses like 140-count muslin; medium weight is the most economical for wrapping items in two thicknesses; and heavy-duty weight is desirable for wrapping linen packs and basin sets when the wrapper will become the table drape. Packages are wrapped in the same manner as with woven fabrics.

The *advantages* of a nonwoven fabric wrapper are:

1. It is disposable, eliminating the need for inspection, laundering, and repair.
2. It provides an excellent barrier against microorganisms and moisture during storage after sterilization.
3. It is strong enough to be tear-resistant yet is easy to handle and has very little memory.

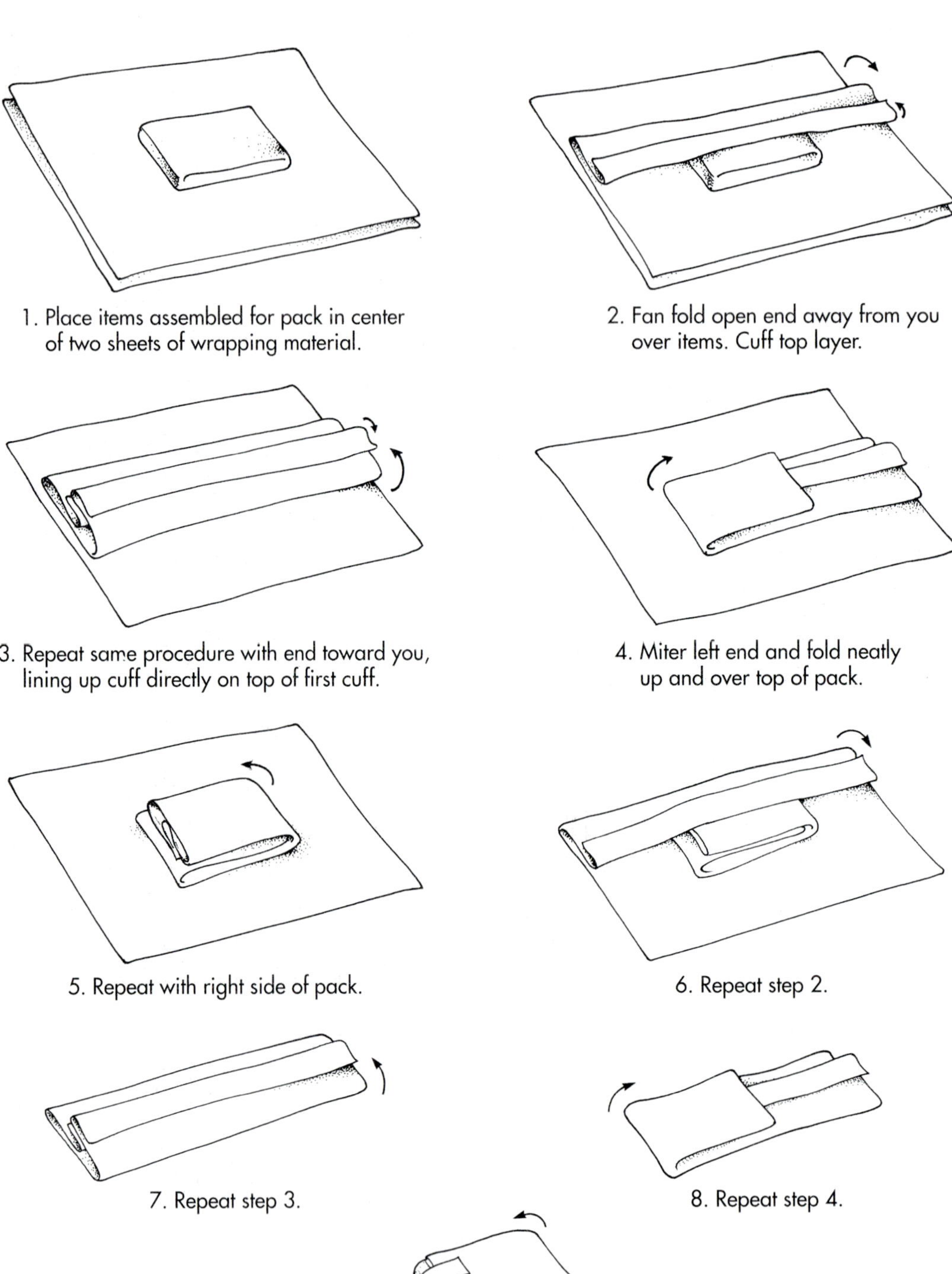

1. Place items assembled for pack in center of two sheets of wrapping material.
2. Fan fold open end away from you over items. Cuff top layer.
3. Repeat same procedure with end toward you, lining up cuff directly on top of first cuff.
4. Miter left end and fold neatly up and over top of pack.
5. Repeat with right side of pack.
6. Repeat step 2.
7. Repeat step 3.
8. Repeat step 4.
9. Repeat step 5 and securely affix with pressure-sensitive indicator tape over end.

FIGURE 13-2 Square fold for wrapping item for sterilization. (Modified from Association for the Advancement of Medical Instrumentation: *Good Hospital Practice: Steam Sterilization and Sterility Assurance;* ANSI/AAMI ST46-1933, Arlington, Va, 1993, AAMI, American National Standards Institute.)

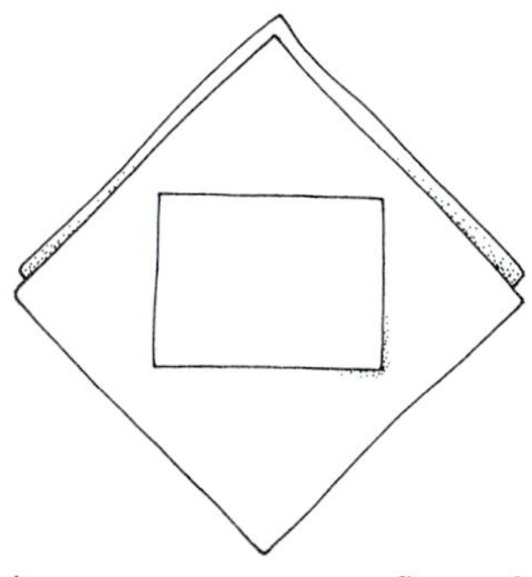

1. Place two wrappers on flat surface with one point toward you. Place item to be wrapped in center of wrapper with its length parallel to you.

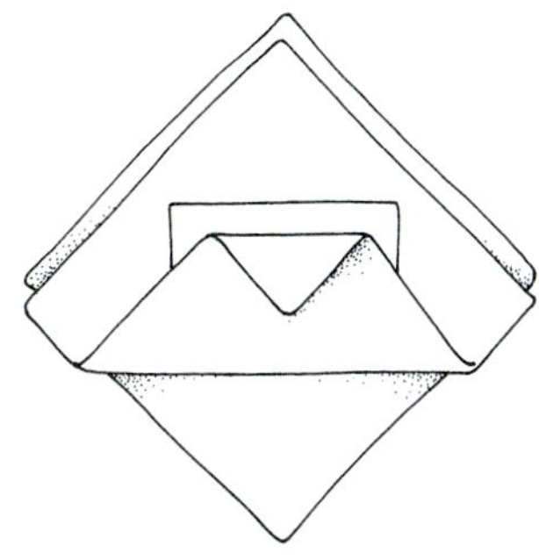

2. Fold corner nearest you over item until it is completely covered. Fold corner back toward you 2 to 3 inches.

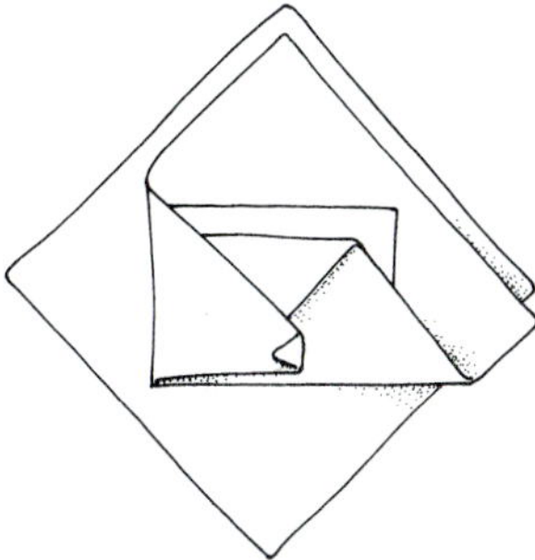

3. Fold left side of wrapper over and parallel to item. Fold end of corner back 2 to 3 inches.

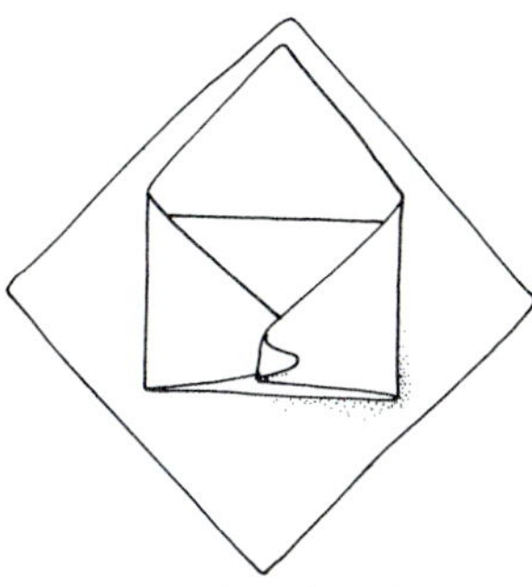

4. Repeat with right side. Lap center folds at least one-half inch.

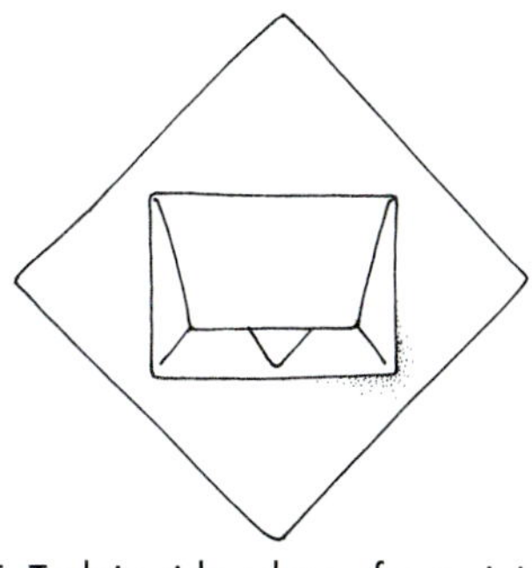

5. Tuck in side edges of remaining corner to eliminate any direct opening to item. Bring top corner down to bottom edges and tuck in, leaving point for opening.

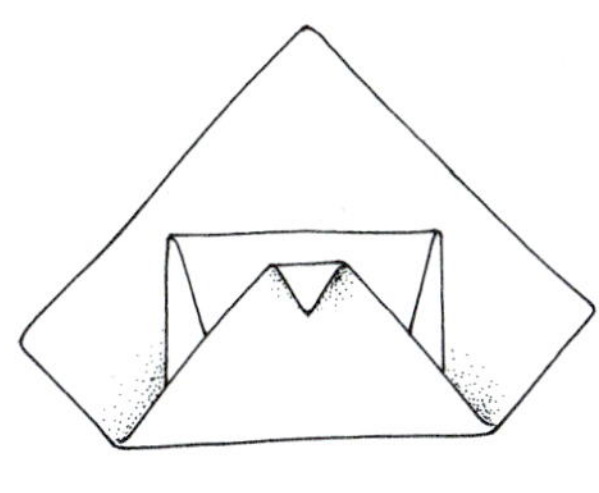

6. Repeat step 2.

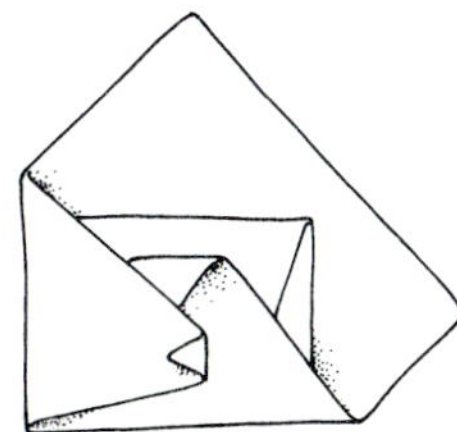

7. Repeat step 3.

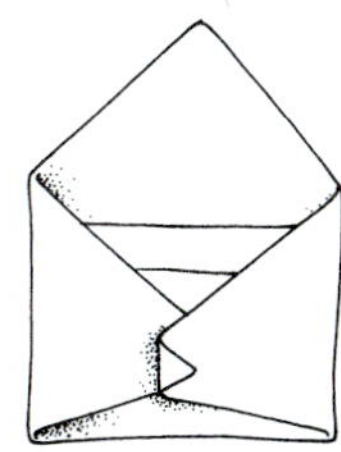

8. Repeat step 4.

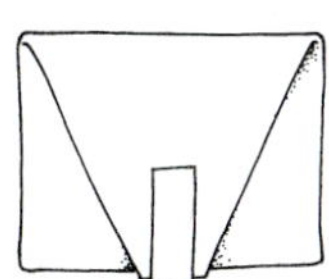

9. Bring point of wrapper completely around package and seal with appropriate tape.

FIGURE 13-3 Envelope fold for wrapping item for sterilization. (Modified from Association for the Advancement of Medical Instrumentation: *Good Hospital Practice: Steam Sterilization and Sterility Assurance;* ANSI/AAMI ST46-1933, Arlington, Va, 1993, AAMI, American National Standards Institute.)

4. It is virtually lint free.

The *disadvantages* of a nonwoven fabric wrapper are:

1. Nonwoven wrappers may have a different time-temperature profile for steam sterilization than woven textile wrappers. This must be predetermined before sterilizing cycles are established. The manufacturer should supply data for time-temperature equivalents compared with 140-count muslin profiles.
2. It is expensive because it is a one-use item. Breaks in fibers that are difficult to detect in the folds may occur after more than one sterilization cycle; therefore the wrapper should be disposed after use.
3. Opacity prevents contents from being seen.
4. The heavy-duty type may retain droplets of water caused by steam condensing on the surface of instruments during the initial phase of prevacuum sterilization. Damp or wet packages may result but may not be noticed until the package is opened. An absorbent towel or foam placed in the bottom of an instrument tray and another under the tray during the wrapping procedure will help absorb moisture for thorough drying of instruments.

Paper If paper products are used, acceptability for steam penetration must be proved. Most craft, parchment, crepe, and glassine papers are acceptable. Water-repellent paper is preferable, but it must have sufficient porosity to allow access and egress of steam and air. Heavily coated paper hinders steam penetration. Available in sheets or envelopes, paper is sealed with pressure-sensitive tape.

The *advantages* of a paper wrapper are:

1. It is disposable and inexpensive as a one-use item. (Reuse is unsafe because quality may not be consistent with repeated exposure to heat.)
2. It provides a good, long-term, poststerilization contamination barrier.
3. It is lint free.

The *disadvantages* of a paper wrapper are:

1. It is difficult to spread open for removal of the contents; it has memory and flips back easily and may not open flat to provide a sterile field.
2. Paper is relatively easy to puncture or tear; it is impossible to see small holes and cracks.
3. Some paper wets easily and dries quickly, making contamination difficult to detect.
4. Opacity prevents the contents from being seen.

Plastic Spunbonded polypropylene wrappers or polypropylene film of 1 to 3 mil thickness is the only plastic acceptable for steam sterilization. Film is usually used in the form of pouches presealed on two or three sides. The open sides must be self- or heat-sealed after the item is placed in the pouch.

NOTE Polyethylene melts in steam. Nylon (polyamide) will not permit adequate escape of condensate when the package is cooling, thereby creating moisture within the contents of the package. Nylon may adhere itself to the contents in prevacuum sterilizer so that sterile transfer is impossible after sterilization.

The *advantages* of a polypropylene pouch are:

1. Transparency allows the contents to be seen.
2. Polypropylene provides an excellent barrier against microorganisms and moisture for prolonged poststerilization storage.

The *disadvantages* of a polypropylene pouch are:

1. It may be difficult to seal to avoid rupture during sterilization; it requires a high heat-sealing temperature.
2. Limited flexibility makes it difficult to handle.

Combination of Paper and Plastic Pouches and tubes made of a combination of paper on one side and plastic film on the other are satisfactory for wrapping single instruments, catheters, drains, and small items. A peel-open seal, for sterile presentation, may be preformed on one end. The other end is either heat-sealed or closed with tape after the item is inserted in the pouch or tube. Self-sealing pouches that do not require heat sealing are also available.

NOTE

1. If a package does not have a preformed, peel-open seal and a heat-sealing machine is not used, the ends must be folded to create a sterile edge for presentation of sterile contents and sealed with a closure tape that is easily removed without tearing the package.
2. A double peel-open package (an item packaged inside a peel-open package that is placed into a slightly larger outer peel-open pouch) is not routinely necessary. However, it may be useful to keep multiple small items together, such as a set of bone screws. Double peel-open pouches should be sequentially sized and sealed to avoid folding the inner pouch.

The *advantages* of the paper and plastic package are:

1. It provides good permeability on the paper side with good visibility of contents on the plastic side.
2. It is generally easy to seal, with peel-open access for sterile presentation.
3. It is economical and durable.
4. It provides an excellent barrier against microorganisms for poststerilization storage.

The *disadvantages* of the paper and plastic package are:

1. The sterilizer must be loaded paper side to paper side, plastic to plastic.
2. Air acts as a barrier to heat and moisture. As much air as possible should be evacuated before the package is sealed.
3. Materials may delaminate during sterilizing or opening procedures.
4. Heat seals may rupture during sterilization.

NOTE A double heat seal should be applied to ensure against accidental opening. The seal must not reseal itself if opened.

Rigid Sterilizer Containers Metal or plastic rigid containers may be used for sterilizing instruments singly or in sets (see Chapter 14, p. 259).

Loading Sterilizer

All packages must be positioned in the chamber to allow free circulation and penetration of steam and to prevent entrapment of air or water. A gravity displacement sterilizer must be loaded in such a way that steam can displace air downward and out through the discharge line. Wire mesh or perforated metal shelves separate layers of packages. Shelves may be contained within the chamber on sliding racks or on a transfer carriage. The shelves are loaded and rolled into the sterilizer. Floor loaders are easier to manage than off-floor carriage racks. Steam sterilizers should be loaded as follows:

1. Flat packages of textiles are placed on the shelf *on edge* so flat surfaces are vertical as shown in Figure 13-4. Instrument trays with perforated bottoms may be laid flat.
2. Large packs are placed 2 to 4 inches apart in one layer only on a shelf. Small packages may be placed on the shelf above with 1 or 2 inches between them. If small packages are placed one on top of another, they should be crisscrossed.
3. Packages must not touch the chamber walls, floor, or ceiling.
4. Rubber goods are placed on edge, loosely arranged, one layer to a shelf, to allow free steam circulation and penetration. No other articles should be with them.
5. Basins or any solid containers are placed on their sides to allow air to flow out of them. They should be placed so that if they contained water, it would all flow out. In a combined load with fabrics, they should be placed on the lowest shelf.
6. Solutions are sterilized alone. At the completion of the sterilization cycle, the steam should be turned off and the temperature allowed to drop to 212° F (100° C) before the exhaust is opened; set the selector to "slow exhaust." Otherwise the solutions will boil over. Allow the pressure gauge to reach zero before opening the door so caps will not pop off.

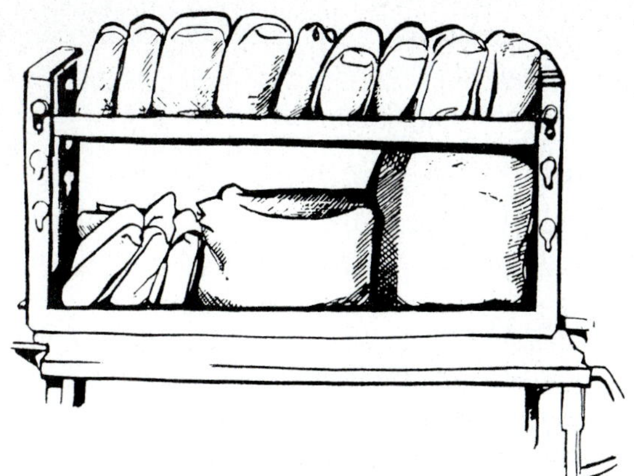

FIGURE 13-4 Proper loading of gravity displacement steam sterilizer; place packs on edge and do not overload rack. Steam must completely surround and penetrate every package in all sterilizers.

Timing Load

Timing of a sterilization cycle begins when the desired temperature is reached throughout the chamber. If the sterilizer does not have an automatic timing device with a buzzer that sounds at the end of the cycle, an oven timer can be set after the proper temperature has been reached to time the load and to alert personnel when the cycle is completed.

Materials that need exposure for different lengths of time to ensure sterilization in a gravity displacement sterilizer should not be combined in the same load if the maximum time needed will be destructive to some items. Items may be sterilized wrapped or unwrapped, alone or combined with other items. Time of exposure varies depending on these factors and on the temperature of the steam. Minimum time standards, calculated after effective steam penetration of porous materials and rate of heat transfer through wrapping materials, are listed in Table 13-2.

Most sterilizers are equipped with automatic electromechanical or microcomputer time-temperature controls and a graphic recorder. Some sterilizers print out a computer record to document each load. Time and temperature for each load are recorded for a 24-hour period. Check the record of each load before unloading it to be certain that the desired temperature was achieved. Also, the temperature being recorded should be checked daily with the thermometer to see that the recording arm is working properly.

Drying Load

After the sterilizer door is opened, a load of wrapped packages is left untouched to dry for 15 to 60 minutes. The time required depends on the type of sterilizer and supplies in a load; large packages require a longer time

TABLE 13-2

Minimum Exposure Time Standards for Steam Sterilization After Effective Steam Penetration and Heat Transfer

	GRAVITY DISPLACEMENT		PREVACUUM
MATERIALS	250° F (121° C)	270° F (132° C)	270° F (132° C)
Basin sets, wrapped	20 min	Not applicable	4 min
Basins, glassware, and utensils, unwrapped	15 min	Not recommended	3 min
Instruments, with or without other items, wrapped as set in double-thickness wrappers	30 min	Not applicable	4 min
Instruments, unwrapped but with other items including towel in bottom of tray or cover over them	20 min	10 min	4 min
Instruments, completely unwrapped	15 min	3 min	3 min
Drape packs, 12 × 12 × 20 inches (30 × 30 × 50 cm) maximum size, 12 lb (5.5 kg) maximum weight	30 min*	Not applicable	4 min
Fabrics, single items wrapped	30 min*	Not applicable	4 min
Rubber and thermoplastics, including small items and gloves, but excluding tubing, wrapped	20 min*	Not applicable	4 min
Tubing, wrapped	30 min	Not applicable	4 min
Tubing, unwrapped	20 min	Not applicable	4 min
Sponges and dressings, wrapped	30 min	Not applicable	4 min
Solutions, flasked	(Slow exhaust)	Not applicable	Automatic selector determines correct temperature and exposure period for solutions
75 ml flask	20 min		
250 ml flask	25 min		
500 ml flask	30 min		
1000 ml flask	35 min		
1500 ml flask	45 min		
2000 ml flask	45 min		

*Fabrics and rubber deteriorate more rapidly with repeated sterilization for prolonged periods in gravity displacement sterilizer.

than small ones. Packages are then unloaded onto a table or cart with wire mesh shelves padded with absorbent material. Warm packages laid on a solid, cold surface become damp from steam condensation and thus contaminated. If the rack of loaded shelves can be rolled onto a transfer carriage or a floor loader pulled out, packages are not handled while they cool.

Packages must be observed for water droplets on the exterior or interior of the package or absorbed moisture in the package. Packs wrapped in moisture-permeable materials that have water droplets on the outside or inside are unsafe for use because the moisture can be a pathway for microbial migration into the package. This is not a problem with moisture-impermeable wrapping materials. However, any package should be considered contaminated if wet when opened for use. Packages should be completely dry after cooling at a room temperature of 68° to 75° F (20° to 24° C) for a minimum of 1 hour.

Biologic Testing for Steam Sterilization

Biologic indicators carrying spores of *B. stearothermophilus* are used to monitor steam sterilization (i.e., to detect nonsterilizing conditions). Each steam sterilizer is tested at least weekly for routine monitoring and as needed for a challenge test. Many hospitals test sterilizers daily. Because of the variables in sterilizers, the correct test must be used for each type of sterilizer.

Gravity Displacement The test pack is placed *on edge* in the lower front of the load. This is the coldest area, representing the greatest challenge. The chamber is *fully loaded*. The contents of the test pack may be either:

1. The equivalent of three woven fabric gowns, 12 towels, 30 gauze sponges (4 × 4 inches), five laparotomy tapes (12 × 12 inches), and one woven fabric drape sheet. Two biologic indicators are placed in

the center with a chemical indicator one towel above or below them. The pack is double-wrapped. It should be approximately 12 × 12 × 20 inches (30 × 30 × 50 cm) and weigh 10 to 12 lb.
2. The equivalent of 16 freshly laundered reusable huck towels or absorbent towels in good condition, each approximately 16 × 26 inches (40 × 66 cm), folded 9 × 9 inches (23 × 23 cm) and stacked with a biologic indicator in the center. They are taped to provide pack density of 12 lb/cu ft. The pack should weigh 3 lb.
3. An equivalent commercial test pack.

Prevacuum The contents of the test pack with biologic indicators can be the same as for a gravity displacement sterilizer. In addition, to check for air entrapment in the prevacuum sterilizer, a *Bowie-Dick test* is conducted daily, usually on the first run of the day. A biologic indicator may be put into this test pack. Test packs must be placed *horizontally* on the bottom shelf at the front, near the door, and over the drain of an *empty prevacuum chamber.* The test pack consists of:

1. Between 24 and 44 absorbent towels folded in a stack no smaller than 9 × 12 × 11 inches (23 × 30 × 28 cm)
2. One Bowie-Dick test sheet placed in the center of the stack
3. One double-thickness wrapper

A Bowie-Dick test sheet can be made by crisscrossing three pieces of chemical indicator tape, about 8 inches (20 cm) long, on a sheet of paper that can be maintained as the test record. If residual air remains in the pack, inhibiting steam penetration during the cycle, the tape does not change color. Commercially prepared test records and preassembled, disposable test packs are available.

Flash/High-Speed Pressure A biologic indicator can be put in the bottom of a tray of unwrapped instruments. It should be positioned in the lower front of the chamber.

Hot Air—Dry Heat

Dry heat in the form of hot air is used primarily to sterilize anhydrous oils, petroleum products, and talcum powder that steam and ethylene oxide gas cannot penetrate. Death of microbial life by dry heat is a physical oxidation or slow burning process of coagulating the protein in cells. In the absence of moisture, higher temperatures are required than when moisture is present because microorganisms are destroyed through a very slow process of heat absorption by conduction.

Advantages of Dry Heat

1. Hot air penetrates certain substances that cannot be steam or gas sterilized.
2. Dry heat is the only acceptable on-site method for sterilizing talcum powder.
3. Dry heat can be used in laboratories to sterilize glassware.
4. Dry heat is a protective method of sterilizing some delicate, sharp, or cutting-edge instruments. Steam may erode or corrode cutting edges.
5. Instruments that cannot be disassembled may be sterilized in hot air.
6. Carbon steel does not become corroded or discolored in dry heat as it may in steam.

Disadvantages of Dry Heat

1. A long exposure period is required because hot air penetrates slowly and possibly unevenly.
2. Time and temperature vary for different substances.
3. Overexposure may ruin some substances.
4. It is destructive to fabrics and rubber goods.

Types of Dry Heat Sterilizers

Mechanical Convection Oven The most efficient and reliable sterilizer is an electrically heated mechanical convection hot air oven. A blower forces hot air in motion around items in the load to hasten the heating of substances and to ensure uniform temperature in all areas of the oven.

Early models operated at 340° to 320° F (171° to 160° C) for a period of 1 to 2 hours. Faster portable tabletop models are available that run at 375° to 400° F (190.5° to 204° C) with total cycle times of 6 minutes for unwrapped items and 12 minutes for wrapped ones. Optional cooling chambers are also available.

Gravity Convection Oven A conventional gravity displacement steam sterilizer chamber can be used for dry heat sterilization. Steam only in the jacket provides heat, but this heat may not be evenly distributed throughout the chamber. Hot air rises initially and by gravity displaces cooler air at the bottom of the chamber. The maximum temperature that can be obtained is 250° F (121° C) or 270° F (132° C) in a high-pressure gravity displacement sterilizer. To ensure adequate conduction of heat through all items, the exposure period must be a minimum of 6 hours and preferably overnight.

Preparing Items for Dry Heat Sterilization

Oils The amount of oil, including mineral oil and lubricating oil for electric or air-powered instruments, put in a container should not exceed 1 oz (30 ml). Preferably the layer depth of the oil is not more than ¼ inch (6.35 mm). The greater the depth, the longer the exposure period must be.

Impregnated Gauze Strips of gauze bandage covered with no more than 4 oz (120 ml) of melted petroleum jelly or other oil-based liquid should be arranged in a stainless steel container to provide a maximum layer depth of ½ inch (12.5 mm).

NOTE Most hospitals purchase sterile packages of impregnated gauze products to eliminate hazards inherent in preparation and sterilization of these products.

Powders One ounce (1 oz) of powder may be spread out in a container so the layer depth does not exceed ¼ inch (6.25 mm).

Talc A maximum of 5 g to 1 oz of talcum powder may be spread out in a glass container so the layer depth does not exceed ¼ inch (6.25 mm). The lid is secured; the cap is screwed tightly on a bottle or jar. A dry heat process chemical indicator is affixed to the bottle. The sterilizing cycle for a gravity convection oven (steam sterilizer with steam in *the jacket only*) should be a minimum of 9 hours at 250° F (121° C) or 6 hours at 270° F (132°).

An average quantity of 2 g of talc usually is needed as a sclerosing agent. This smaller quantity may be evenly distributed inside a sealed glassine envelope or peel-open pouch, which is inserted into a second envelope or pouch. The talcum powder should not accumulate into a mass exceeding ¼ inch (6.25 mm); the package should lie flat in the sterilizer.

NOTE Sterile talc is commercially available.

Packaging Materials for Dry Heat

Glass Petri dishes, ointment jars, flasks, small bottles, or test tubes can be used. Cotton plugs or aluminum foil are used to cover the tops of flasks and tubes. Caps or lids are screwed tightly onto jars.

Stainless Steel Boats or Trays Covers must fit tightly. They can be held in place with indicator tape.

Aluminum Foil Foil conducts heat rapidly.

Woven Textile and Paper These materials can be used for wrapping instruments if the temperature in the chamber will not exceed 400° F (204° C). Powders and talc can be put in double glassine envelopes.

Loading Sterilizer

It is necessary to allow space between items and along the chamber walls so hot air can circulate freely. The chamber never is loaded to full capacity.

Timing Load

Time of exposure varies depending on the characteristics of individual items, layer depth in containers, and temperature in the sterilizer. If the amount in each container is kept to a minimum and the sterilizer is loaded according to the manufacturer's recommendations, items are exposed for a *minimum* period of:

1. Six minutes unwrapped at 400° F (204° C)
2. Twelve minutes wrapped at 375° F (190.5° C)
3. One hour at 340° F (171° C)
4. Two hours at 320° F (160° C)
5. Three hours at 285° F (140° C)
6. Six hours at 250° F (121° C)

Biologic Testing

Biologic indicators with spores of *B. subtilis* are used to monitor the dry heat process. Commercially prepared spore strips in glassine envelopes should be used. Each load should be tested and items quarantined until negative results are confirmed at 48 hours.

Microwaves

The nonionizing radiation of microwaves produces hyperthermic conditions that disrupt life processes. This heating action affects water molecules and interferes with cell membranes. Microwave sterilization uses low-pressure steam with the nonionizing radiation to produce localized heat that kills microorganisms. The temperature is lower than conventional steam and the cycle faster, as short as 30 seconds. Metal instruments can be sterilized if placed under a partial vacuum in a glass container. Small tabletop units may be useful for rapid sterilization of a single or small number of instruments. Current models have a small chamber size 1 to 3 cu ft.

CHEMICAL STERILIZATION

Only chemicals that are registered as a sterilant by the U.S. Environmental Protection Agency (EPA) are used for sterilization. They may be approved for use in either a gaseous, plasma, or liquid state.

Ethylene Oxide Gas

Ethylene oxide gas is used to sterilize items that are heat or moisture sensitive. *Ethylene oxide* (EO or EtO) is a chemical alkylating agent that kills microorganisms, including spores, by interfering with the normal metabolism of protein and reproductive processes, resulting in the death of cells. Used in the gaseous state, EO gas must have direct contact with microorganisms on or in the items to be sterilized. Because ethylene oxide is highly flammable and explosive in air, it must be used in an explosion-proof sterilizing chamber in a controlled environment. When handled properly, EO is a reliable and safe agent for sterilization, but toxic emissions and residues of EO present health hazards to personnel and patients.

Ethylene oxide gas sterilization is dependent on four parameters. Each parameter may be varied. Consequently, ethylene oxide sterilization is a complex multiparameter process. Each variable affects the other dependent parameters.

1. *EO gas concentration.* Liquefied EO is supplied in high-pressure metal cylinders or disposable cartridges. In the sterilization process, air is withdrawn from the chamber and the EO enters as gas under pressure. The only means for controlling EO concentration is to operate the sterilizer according to the manufacturer's instructions. The operating pressure of the cycle influences the gas diffusion rate through the items to be sterilized. The absorbency of the items and packaging materials will influence gas concentration. EO gas may be diluted or used in pure form.
   a. CFC-12, also referred to as 12/88. This is a mixture of 12% ethylene oxide in 88% chlorofluorocarbon (CFC) by weight. Most EO gas sterilizers currently in use utilize this mixture.
   b. HCFC-124, tradenamed Oxyfume 2000 Sterilant Gas. This gas mixture can be used in sterilizers that formerly used CFC. Conversion to this replacement gas requires minor changes in the sterilizing pressure and time. It uses more gas than with CFC.

      NOTE Chlorofluorocarbons cause destruction of the stratospheric ozone shield protecting the earth. Twenty-four nations, including the United States, signed the Montreal Protocol agreeing to reduce production of CFCs. By the year 2000 no CFCs will be produced in the United States. Manufacturers of EO gas sterilizers are researching alternative ozone shield–compatible flame retardants that can be used with minimal or no change in procedures or equipment.

   c. One hundred percent EO. Unit dose cartridges of 67 g or 134 g pure EO are used in small, self-contained sterilizers. Because pure EO is highly flammable, only a small number of cartridges are kept in inventory.
   d. EO/CO_2, referred to as 10/90. This is a mixture of 10% ethylene oxide in 90% carbon dioxide. The pressure differential is great between EO and carbon dioxide, so maintaining a uniform mix is difficult. Because a higher pressure cycle must be used, not all devices can be sterilized safely in this mixture.
2. *Temperature.* Temperature influences the destruction of microorganisms and affects the permeability of EO through cell walls as well as through the packaging materials. Higher density items and loads require longer heat-up time. As temperature is increased, exposure time can be decreased. Gas sterilizers operate at temperatures ranging from 85° to 145° F (29° to 63° C). The uppermost limit for many heat-sensitive plastic materials is 140° F (60° C). The temperature in the chamber is raised by injection of saturated steam.
3. *Humidity.* Moisture is essential in achieving sterility with EO gas. Desiccated or highly dried bacterial spores are resistant to EO gas. They must be hydrated. Moisture content of the immediately surrounding atmosphere and water content within organisms are important to the action of EO gas. Consequently, relative humidity of room atmosphere where items are packaged and held for sterilization should be at least 50% but must not be less than 30% to hydrate them during preparation. The ability of the item and packaging material to absorb moisture will affect humidification and diffusion of gas during the sterilization process. Excessive moisture will inhibit sterilization. Humidity of 30% to 80% is maintained throughout the cycle. Saturated steam provides the necessary humidity.
4. *Time.* Time required for complete destruction of microorganisms is primarily related to gas concentration and temperature. However, cleanliness of items, type of materials, arrangement of load, and rate of penetration also influence exposure time. Drawing an initial vacuum at the start of the cycle aids penetration of gas.

Advantages of EO Gas

1. It is an effective substitute agent to use with most items that cannot be sterilized by heat, such as plastics with low melting points.
2. It provides an effective method of sterilization for items that steam and moisture may erode; it is noncorrosive and does not damage items.
3. It completely permeates all porous materials.

   NOTE
   - EO gas does not penetrate metal, glass, and petroleum-based lubricants. Whether or not it penetrates oils, liquids, or powder depends on the amount in the containers. If the material is spread thin, the gas will penetrate, but it will not go through bulk. EO gas sterilization is *not* recommended for oils, liquids, and powder including talc.
   - Glass ampules can be sterilized in EO since the gas does not penetrate glass. But a glass vial with a rubber stopper must not be put in the sterilizer because the gas will penetrate the rubber and may react with the drugs in solution and cause a potentially harmful chemical reaction.

4. Automatic controls preclude human error by establishing proper levels of pressure, temperature, humidity, and gas concentration. The sterilizer must be operated according to the manufacturer's instructions.
5. It leaves no film on items.
6. EO gas sterilization is used extensively in prepa-

ration of packaged, presterilized items commercially available because packaging materials that prolong storage life can be used.

Disadvantages of EO Gas

1. EO gas sterilization is a complicated process that must be carefully monitored.
   a. *Never gas sterilize an item that can be safely steam sterilized.*
   b. Biologic tests, chemical indicators, sterilizer operation, and maintenance records should be reviewed to verify the adequacy of *every* cycle.
   c. Implants should not be used until results of biologic testing are known—a minimum of 48 hours.
   d. Items must be completely aerated before use to eliminate harmful residues.
2. EO sterilization takes longer than steam sterilization; it is a long, slow process.
3. EO gas requires special, expensive equipment. Gas is somewhat expensive per cycle.
4. Items that absorb EO gas during sterilization, such as rubber, polyethylene, or silicone, require an aeration period (see Table 13-3). Air admitted to the sterilizer at the end of the cycle only partially aerates the load.
5. Toxic by-products can be formed in the presence of droplets of moisture during exposure of some plastics, particularly polyvinyl chloride.
6. Repeated sterilization can increase the concentration of the total EO residues in porous items. These increased levels can be hazardous unless gas can be dissipated.
7. EO is a vesicant in contact with skin and mucous membranes.
   a. Liquid EO may cause serious burns if not removed immediately by thorough washing.
   b. Gloves made of neoprene, polyvinyl fluoride, nitryl or butyl rubber, or other material known to be impermeable to EO penetration should be worn for handling sterilized packages before aeration. If thick cotton gloves are worn, they should be placed in the aerator between uses.
   c. Personnel who wear contact lenses, especially soft lenses, should wear protective goggles when working around EO sterilizers to avoid eye irritation.
8. Inhaled EO gas can be irritating to mucous membranes. Its presence is easily detectable by odor; it is a colorless gas. Overexposure causes nasal and throat irritation. Prolonged exposure may result in nausea, vomiting, dizziness, difficulty breathing, and peripheral paralysis.
   a. Immediately following completion of each cycle, the sterilizer door should be opened approximately 2 inches and the area cleared of all personnel for 15 minutes before unloading.
   b. Loading carts should be pulled, not pushed, from the sterilizer to the aerator. Air currents flowing over the load may accumulate residual gas that could be inhaled.
9. Long-term exposure to EO is known to be a potential occupational carcinogen, causing leukemia. It is a mutagen causing spontaneous abortion, genetic defects, chromosomal damage, and neurologic dysfunction.
   a. Occupational Safety and Health Administration (OSHA) standards limit an employee's exposure to ethylene oxide to one part per million (ppm) of air averaged over an 8-hour period to an action level of 0.5 ppm, and a short-term limit of 5 ppm averaged over a 15-minute period. The short-term limit addresses exposure to bursts of gas, as when opening a sterilizer. Breathing zone sampling must be done daily throughout an 8-hour shift from at least one employee for each job classification of exposed personnel. Passive dosimeter badges are the most popular personnel monitoring devices. Chromographs and other types of detectors are used for continuous gas analysis of the environment.
   b. EO gas must be vented from the sterilizer to the outside atmosphere to avoid personnel exposure. Audible and visual alarm systems should be installed to indicate a failure in the ventilation system. Most sterilizers have an exhaust hood over the sterilizer door.
   c. Sterilizer door has locking and sealing mechanisms. The integrity of the seals must be checked regularly. Automatic controls must function properly so the door cannot be opened until gas is evacuated from chamber.

Types of Gas Sterilizers

The capacity of EO chambers varies from approximately 2 cu ft (57.5 L) in a tabletop size of 12 × 12 × 24 inches (30 × 30 × 60 cm) to very large floor loading units 28 × 67 × 78 inches (72 × 170 × 198 cm). These chambers automatically control gas concentration, temperature, humidity, and time. Most models have vacuum pumps to evacuate air from the chamber and steam ejectors for humidification and to increase temperature. Microcomputer controls and digital printouts of cycle parameters provide evidence of proper operation. A purge cycle follows the timed gas exposure cycle to vent the chamber of airborne residual gas. Some chambers are a combination sterilizer/aerator. These eliminate the need for personnel handling the load immediately after sterilization; the load is removed following aeration.

Preparing Items for Gas Sterilization

All Items All items must be thoroughly cleaned and dried. Detachable parts are disassembled. Syringes are separated. Impermeable items such as caps, plugs, and stylets are removed.

Lumens Any tubing or other item with a lumen should be blown out with air to force it dry before packaging as water combines with EO gas to form a harmful acid, ethylene glycol.

Lensed Instruments Endoscopes (see Chapter 15, p. 283) with cemented optical lenses require special cement for EO gas sterilization.

Lubricated Instruments Remove all traces of lubricant, especially a petroleum-based lubricant. EO cannot permeate the film.

Camera Some cameras and film can be EO gas sterilized. As a permanent record or a teaching aid, photographs are sometimes taken with a sterile camera at the surgical site. An especially constructed camera is used. The film is loaded before packaging for sterilization.

Packaging for Gas Sterilization

Type and thickness of the wrapper used influence the time it takes for gas to penetrate. Size and shape of the package and porosity of the contents also influence penetration time. Items wrapped for gas sterilization should be tagged "for gas" to avoid their inadvertently being steam sterilized and damaged. Materials used for wrapping items must be permeable to EO gas and water vapor and allow effective aeration. The following materials are acceptable.

Woven Textile Fabric Reusable double-thickness woven fabrics are used as for steam with the same advantages and disadvantages (see p. 217).

Nonwoven Fabric Tyvek spunbonded olefin and other high-density polyethylene fabrics are highly permeable to EO and moisture. These single-use disposable wrappers offer the same advantages as the nonwoven fabrics described for use in steam, but not all of them can be used interchangeably; the cellulose/nylon/rayon combination should be used only for steam sterilization (see pp. 217 and 220). Packages should be sequentially double-wrapped or the material used according to the manufacturer's recommendations.

Paper Double-thickness paper is used as for thermal sterilization with the same advantages and disadvantages (see p. 220).

Plastic Both polypropylene and low-density polyethylene of 3 mil or less thickness in film or pouches may be used. Polyethylene is easier to handle than polypropylene, and EO penetrates it more rapidly. Some peel-open pouches are constructed with Tyvek on one side and coated Mylar on the other side. These are durable during storage and have strong seals that peel open smoothly. With all types of pouches, as much air as possible should be expressed before sealing to avoid rupture when the vacuum is drawn in sterilizer.

Combination of Paper and Plastic Pouches and tubes can be used as described for steam (see p. 220) except that double wrapping may not allow adequate penetration of gas and moisture. Peel-pack pouches with either coated or uncoated paper on one side and coated Mylar on the other are generally acceptable for most gas sterilizers. They allow visualization of contents.

NOTE Materials *not* to be used for EO sterilization because of inadequate permeability include nylon, polyvinyl chloride film, saran, polyester, polyvinyl alcohol, cellophane, and aluminum foil. Combinations of materials that make a package insufficiently permeable for adequate humidification, gas penetration, and aeration must be avoided.

Loading Sterilizer

All packages are positioned in the chamber to allow free circulation and penetration of gas. Overloading creates conditions whereby EO, moisture, and heat penetration can be retarded. Air space should be provided between the chamber ceiling and the topmost packages in the load. Also, packages should not touch the chamber walls and floor. Packages should not be stacked tightly; space must be allowed between them. Packages are placed on edge with the plastic side of one facing the paper side of another if paper/plastic pouches are used.

Timing Cycle

Timing is variable depending on the size of the chamber, contents of the load, gas concentration, temperature, and humidity. For example, a cool cycle at 99° F (37° C) may require over 5 hours, whereas the same load at 131° F (55° C) may take less than 3 hours. Closely follow the instructions provided by the manufacturer of the sterilizer.

Aerating Items Following EO Sterilization

Adequate aeration for all absorbent materials that will come in contact with skin or tissues, either directly or indirectly, is absolutely essential. EO exerts toxic effects on living tissue. Residual products after sterilization can include:

1. *Ethylene oxide.* Porous materials, such as plastic, silicone, rubber, wood, and leather, absorb a cer-

tain amount of gas that must be removed. The thicker the walls of items, the longer the aeration time must be. Residual EO in plastic tubing or parts of a heart-lung pump oxygenator causes hemolysis of blood. Rubber gloves or shoes worn immediately after exposure can cause irritation or burns on skin. Acceptable limits for residual EO are:
   a. 25 ppm for blood dialysis units, blood oxygenators, heart-lung machines, and all implants
   b. 250 ppm for all topical medical devices
2. *Ethylene glycol.* Ethylene glycol is formed by a reaction of EO with water or moisture that leaves a clear or brownish oily film on exposed surfaces. This film on plastic or rubber endotracheal tubes or airways can cause irritation to mucous membranes. Acceptable limits of ethylene glycol are:
   a. 250 ppm for blood dialysis units, blood oxygenators, heart-lung machines, and all implants
   b. 1000 ppm for all topical medical devices
3. *Ethylene chlorohydrin.* This by-product is formed when a chloride ion is present to combine with EO, such as in polyvinyl chloride plastic. Rubber, soft nylon, and polyethylene items that have been in contact with saline solution or blood can retain enough chloride ion to cause this reaction in the presence of moisture. Disposable products should be discarded after use to avoid this hazard. Acceptable limits of ethylene chlorohydrin are:
   a. 25 ppm for blood dialysis units, blood oxygenators, heart-lung machines, and all implants
   b. 250 ppm for all topical medical devices

NOTE
- Residuals are expressed as the weight of EO remaining in the item divided by the weight of the item. For example, 25 ppm in a device weighing 2500 g (approximately 5 ½ lb) equals 0.01 mg of EO.
- Residues *cannot* be removed by rinsing in water or liquids.

Air is admitted into the chamber at the end of the sterilization cycle to purge residual gas. Air is admitted and then immediately removed as many as six times in 30 minutes in sterilizers with a pulse-purge cycle. Additional aeration still is required for all wrapped and porous items. Aeration to diffuse any residual products may be accomplished with ambient (room) air or preferably in an aerator chamber designed for this purpose. Manufacturers of products suitable for EO sterilization should provide written instructions for the sterilizing cycle and for aerating. Available recommendations must be followed.

Polyvinyl chloride is one of the most difficult materials to aerate. If the composition of an item is not known, the minimum time for polyvinyl chloride should be followed (Table 13-3). Aeration time depends on:

1. Composition, density, porosity, weight, and configuration of the item
2. Packaging material
3. Sterilizing conditions, such as the size of the load, nature of items in it, and variable required factors
4. Aeration conditions, such as ambient vs. mechanical airflow and temperature
5. Acceptable limits of residual products for the intended use of the item, such as external application or internal implantation

NOTE Items cannot be safely used until completely aerated.

Aeration at an elevated temperature enhances the dissipation rate of absorbed gas, resulting in faster removal. The entire load on the sterilizer carriage can be transferred into an *aerator.* A blower system draws air in from outside to the heater in upper part of the chamber to maintain a minimum rate of four air changes per minute. The aerator must be vented to the outside atmosphere.

All materials remain in the aerator for 8 hours at 140° F (60° C) to 12 hours at 120° F (50° C) or longer, depending on temperature and instructions of the manufacturer of the aerator or the item. In a combination sterilizer/aerator, aeration time will vary according to temperature and airflow (e.g., 12 hours at 130° F (55° C) or 32 hours at 100° F (38° C)).

If an aerator is not available, packages may be moved on a cart or in a basket from the sterilizer into a well-ventilated clean storage area. This area should have at least 10 air changes per hour. Aeration time must be prominently noted on the cart or basket. At room temperature, controlled between 65° and 72° F (18° and 22° C), minimum aeration of 168 hours (7 days) is required for polyvinyl chloride and plastic and rubber items sealed in plastic packages and for porous items that will come in direct contact with blood; will be implanted, inserted, or applied to body tissues; or will be used for assisted respiration. Unwrapped, nonporous metal and glass may be handled immediately. Wrapped metal should be aerated for at least 2 hours. Intravenous or irrigation fluids in plastic containers must *not* be stored in a room where gas sterilized items are aerating. Residual diffusing gas could be absorbed through the plastic.

Biologic Testing for EO Sterilization

Biologic indicators carrying spores of *B. subtilis* var *niger strain globigi* are used to monitor EO sterilizers. Each sterilizer is tested at least weekly. Every load containing implantable devices should be tested. An implant should not be used until the test is negative at 48 hours. Biologic test packs for EO consist of:

1. Routine weekly test pack
   a. One biologic indicator placed in a 20 ml syringe so that the plunger does not touch it

TABLE 13-3

Minimum Aeration Times Following Ethylene Oxide Sterilization at Different Temperatures

	AMBIENT ROOM AIR	MECHANICAL AERATOR	
MATERIAL	65°-72° F (18°-22° C)	122° F (50° C)	140° F (60° C)
Metal and glass			
Unwrapped	May be used immediately		
Wrapped	2 hr	2 hr	2 hr
Rubber for external use—not sealed in plastic	24 hr	8 hr	5 hr
Polyethylene and polypropylene for external use—not sealed in plastic	48 hr	12 hr	8 hr
Plastics except polyvinyl chloride items—not sealed in plastic	96 hr (4 days)	12 hr	8 hr
Polyvinyl chloride	168 hr (7 days)	12 hr	8 hr
Plastic and rubber items—sealed in plastic and/or will come in contact with body tissues	168 hr (7 days)	12 hr	8 hr
Internal pacemaker	504 hr (21 days)	32 hr	24 hr

when the plunger is inserted in the barrel; the needle end of the syringe must be open with the guard removed

   b. A syringe and a chemical indicator placed in the folds of a towel
   c. A towel placed in peel-pouch or nonwoven fabric wrapper

2. Challenge pack
   a. Four absorbent towels fanfolded in thirds
   b. A 10-inch length of latex tubing
   c. One plastic airway or syringe
   d. Two biologic indicators in a syringe as described above
   e. One chemical indicator
   f. Two double-thickness wrappers for sequential wrapping

The biologic test pack should be placed *on its side in the center of the load* in an EO sterilizer. The test pack must be aerated before or after indicators are removed.

Formaldehyde Gas

Formaldehyde kills microorganisms by coagulation of protein in cells. Used as a fumigant in gaseous form, formaldehyde sterilization is complex and less efficacious than other methods of sterilization. It should only be used if steam under pressure will damage the item to be sterilized and ethylene oxide and glutaraldehyde are not available. Its use for sterilization has been almost abandoned in the United States, Canada, and Australia. The method dates back to 1820, and it is still used in Europe and Asia.

Formaldehyde sterilization depends on gas concentration, temperature, humidity, and time. Formalin solution is heated in the Chemiclave sterilizer to produce fumes. The temperature is raised to at least 122° F (50° C) and may be as high as 176° F (80° C) by introducing saturated steam. The steam also humidifies the load. Humidity must be close to 100% for gas penetration. A filtering system removes residual condensate and formaldehyde and the odor of residual aeration vapors. Type of items, size of load, and exchange of air and gas influence the time of the cycle. A cycle with a gas concentration of 40 to 80 mg/L (0.23% formaldehyde) at 131° F (55° C) will take 2 to 12 hours. Time may be decreased as temperature is increased.

Advantages of Formaldehyde Gas

1. Formaldehyde can be used for heat-sensitive items.
2. It is nonexplosive and nonflammable.
3. It is noncorrosive.

Disadvantages of Formaldehyde Gas

1. Formaldehyde is toxic. It is a potent allergen and is mutagenic and carcinogenic. An 8-hour exposure of 1 ppm in air is the accepted limit in several countries.
2. It has an unpleasant odor, and its fumes are irritating to eyes and mucous membranes.
3. Residue of a gray or white film must be removed to prevent tissue irritation. Porous items must be aerated.
4. Microorganisms must be hydrated.

Considerations for Formaldehyde Sterilization

1. All items must be thoroughly cleansed of organic material. Lumens of endoscopes and woven catheters should be blown out with air to force dry them.
2. Paper, plastic, and combination of paper and plastic pouches and tubes may be used as for ethylene oxide gas sterilization.
3. Loading the sterilizer, timing the cycle, and aerating items should be carried out according to instructions provided by the manufacturer of the sterilizer.
4. Either *B. stearothermophilus* or *B. subtilis* biologic indicators can be used to monitor the process.

Hydrogen Peroxide Plasma/Vapor

Hydrogen peroxide is activated to create a reactive plasma or vapor. Plasma is a state of matter distinguishable from a solid, liquid, or gas. It can be produced through the action of either a strong electric or magnetic field, somewhat like a neon light. The cloud of plasma created consists of ions, electrons, and neutral atomic particles that produce a visible glow. Free radicals of the hydrogen peroxide in the cloud interact with cell membranes, enzymes, or nucleic acids to disrupt life functions of microorganisms. The plasma and vapor phases of hydrogen peroxide are highly sporicidal even at low concentration and temperature.

Types of Hydrogen Peroxide Sterilizers

The sterilizer chambers are simple in design, but the process of the sterilization cycle differs depending on the method used to convert hydrogen peroxide into plasma or vapor.

Plasma Sterilizer The patented Sterrad sterilization system activates hydrogen peroxide by radiofrequency energy to create a reactive plasma. The sterilizer connects to a standard electrical outlet. Air is evacuated from the chamber. Then hydrogen peroxide is introduced and vaporized. Electricity generates radiofrequency energy to produce glow discharge plasma within the chamber. The reactive particles in the plasma, maintained at 104° F (40° C), sterilize the load in about 1 hour.

Gas Plasma Sterilizer Plasma is created outside the sterilizer chamber and then flows into it. Liquid hydrogen peroxide put through an electromagnetic field creates a glow discharge. As the activated fluid flows into the chamber, free radicals permeate the packages to react with microorganisms. Plasma sterilizes nonporous, unwrapped items using dry, low-heat settings in less than 30 minutes. Wrapped supplies take 90 minutes. The fluid is exhausted at the end of the cycle by a vacuum pump.

Vapor Phase Sterilizer A vacuum is created in the chamber for delivery of a cold vapor of hydrogen peroxide at 39° to 46° F (4° to 8° C). A vacuum exhausts vapor at the end of the cycle.

Advantages of Hydrogen Peroxide

1. Process is dry and nontoxic.
2. By-products of oxygen and water vapor are safely evacuated into room atmosphere.
3. Aeration is not necessary.
4. Low temperature allows safe sterilization of some heat-sensitive items, including endoscopes and fiberoptic devices.
5. Plasma has significantly less effect on metal than steam sterilization; corrosion does not occur on moisture-sensitive microsurgical and powered instruments.
6. Sterilizer is simple in design and connects to standard electrical outlets.

Disadvantages of Hydrogen Peroxide

1. Metal trays block radio-frequency waves.
2. It is not compatible with cellulose (i.e., woven textiles with cotton fibers and paper products).
3. Nylon becomes brittle after repeated exposure.

Considerations for Hydrogen Peroxide Sterilization

1. All items must be thoroughly clean, free of organic debris, and *dry*.
2. Items must be wrapped in nonwoven polypropylene. Tyvek peel-pouches may be used.
3. Timing of the cycle varies with the process, capacity of the chamber, and contents of the load. The manufacturer's instructions must be followed.
4. Biologic indicators with spores of *B. stearothermophilus* are used to monitor hydrogen peroxide process.

Ozone Gas

Ozone sterilizes by oxidation, a process that destroys organic and inorganic matter. It penetrates membrane of cells, causing them to explode. Ozone is an unstable gas but can be generated easily from oxygen.

Types of Ozone Sterilizers

A generator converts oxygen from a source within the hospital to ozone. A 6% to 12% concentration of ozone continuously flows through the chamber. Penetration of ozone may be controlled by a vacuum in the chamber or enhanced by adding humidity. At completion of the exposure time oxygen is allowed to flow through the chamber to purge the ozone. Cycle time may be up to 60 minutes depending on the size of the chamber or load.

Advantages of Ozone Gas

1. The sterilizer generates its own agent, using hospital oxygen, water, and electrical supply. It is simple and inexpensive to operate.
2. Ozone provides an alternative for EO sterilization of many heat- and moisture-sensitive items.
3. It does not affect titanium, chromium, silicone, neoprene, and Teflon.
4. Aeration is not necessary; ozone leaves no residue and converts to oxygen in a short time.

Disadvantages of Ozone Gas

1. Ozone can be corrosive. It will oxidize steel, iron, brass, copper, and aluminum.
2. It destroys natural gum rubber, such as latex, and some plastics.

Considerations for Ozone Sterilization

Preparing items, packaging, loading the sterilizer, and timing the cycle must be done according to the instructions provided by the manufacturer of the sterilizer. *B. stearothermophilus* biologic indicators can be used to monitor the process.

Chemical Sterilants in Solution

Liquid chemical agents registered by the EPA as sterilants provide an alternative method for sterilizing minimally invasive, heat-sensitive items if a gas or plasma sterilizer is not available or the aeration period makes ethylene oxide sterilization impractical. Items are categorized as critical, semicritical, and noncritical according to the risk of infection to the patient. Items that enter tissue or the vascular system are considered critical and should be sterile. To sterilize items with a liquid sterilant, they must be immersed in solution for the required time specified by the manufacturer to be *sporicidal,* that is, to kill spores. All chemical solutions have advantages and disadvantages; each sterilant has specific assets and limitations.

Advantages of Chemical Sterilants

1. The solution has a low surface tension; it penetrates into crevices and is readily rinsed from items.
2. It is noncorrosive, nonstaining, and safe for instruments that can be immersed in a chemical solution.
3. It does not damage lenses or cement on lensed endoscopes.
4. It is not absorbed by rubber or plastic.
5. It has low volatility and is stable for the time specified by the manufacturer.

Disadvantages of Chemical Sterilants

1. Even though the chemical has low toxicity and irritation, items must be thoroughly rinsed in sterile distilled water before use.
2. Sterile transfer is difficult because items are wet.
3. Items cannot be held in long-term sterile storage.
4. The solution can become diluted during use if an item is wet when placed in it.

Chemical Sterilants

In addition to EPA registration, chemical sterilants are approved by the FDA for marketing as a method of sterilization for critical items that are heat sensitive and that can be immersed. The manufacturer is responsible for providing processing instructions on the container label. The user is obligated to follow these instructions.

Acetic Acid Acetic acid mixed with a solution of salts (Bionox) kills microorganisms by a process of oxidation to denature proteins. The process takes 20 minutes at room temperature. The solution is supplied in unit doses for each cycle.

Formaldehyde A 37% aqueous solution (Formalin) or 8% formaldehyde in 70% isopropyl alcohol kills microorganisms by coagulation of protein in the cells. Solution is effective at room temperature. Formaldehyde has a pungent odor and is irritating to eyes and nasal passages. Its vapors can be toxic.

Glutaraldehyde A 2% aqueous solution of activated, buffered alkaline glutaraldehyde kills microorganisms by denaturation of protein in cells. The solution is activated by adding powdered buffer to liquid. Alkaline glutaraldehyde solution changes pH and gradually loses effectiveness after the date of activation. The expiration date specified by the manufacturer must be marked on the container when activated (e.g., 14 or 28 days for aqueous Cidex activated dialdehyde solution). *The solution is reusable until this date, after which it must be discarded.* These solutions are effective at room temperature.

Glutaraldehyde vaporizes rapidly. The fumes may have a mild odor and can be irritating to eyes, nose, and throat. OSHA has established an exposure limit of 0.2 ppm in room air averaged over 8 hours. Gloves must be worn to prevent skin sensitivity and contact dermatitis.

The concentration of glutaraldehyde in solution should be monitored. A test strip or kit of reagents is used for testing the concentration before and after each use. If the solution has become diluted, it should be discarded, that is, not used for the full period of activation.

Peracetic Acid A proprietary (Steris) chemical formulation of 35% peracetic acid, hydrogen peroxide, and water inactivates critical microbial cell systems. Peracetic acid is an acetic acid plus an extra oxygen atom that reacts with most cellular components to cause cell death. The mechanism may vary with each type of cell (e.g., vegetative bacterial spores, mycobacterium). The sterilant is supplied in unit doses for each cycle and is diluted during the sterilization process to 0.2% peracetic acid solution. During the 20- to 30-minute sterilization process, the solution is heated to 122° to 131° F (50° to 55° C) as it passes through the self-contained processing chamber. All items and internal components of the Steris unit are submerged in the heated sterilant.

On completion of the sterilizing cycle, the sterilant is discharged into the sanitary drain. The used chemical is not considered a hazardous material by the EPA. The instruments are automatically rinsed in tap water that is filtered through two external prefilters and a 0.22 µm internal microfiltration system. The smallest known bacterium, *Pseudomonas diminuta,* is unable to pass through the pores in this filter system. (This is the same method used by pharmaceutical manufacturers to make sterile injectable medication.)

The Steris unit uses a standard tap water supply, a sanitary drain, and a 110 volt electrical connection. This tabletop unit has a printout to document each cycle. Periodic maintenance includes filter changes based on the chemical components of the external water supply. Biologic monitoring, according to the manufacturer's recommendation, is done daily with a commercially prepared spore strip containing *B. subtilis* or *B. stearothermophilus.*

Containers/Sterilizers

Items must be completely immersed in solution and lumens filled with solution. The container must be deep enough for total immersion. Trays or buckets with perforated liners and lids are convenient for solutions used at room temperature. A sterile container is preferable to facilitate removal of items without contamination. The inside of the container and its lid should be kept sterile throughout duration of use of the solution. Containers should also be kept covered to prevent evaporation and to minimize the odor of the solution. Formaldehyde and glutaraldehyde solutions must be used in a well-ventilated room.

Preparing Items for Sterilization by Immersion

Items should be clean and free of organic debris and blood. Glutaraldehyde will attack some organic materials. It remains highly active in the presence of protein matter in serum, mucus, and soap films. The human hepatitis virus cannot be isolated, so removal of blood is critical. Items should be washed thoroughly in a nonfilming solution, rinsed, and dried before immersion. Items must be dry before submersion so the solution will not become diluted.

Timing Immersion Cycle

The time required for sterilization varies with the sporicidal activity of the chemical agent.

1. Acetic acid: 20 minutes at room temperature
2. Formalin, formaldehyde, and other glutaraldehydes: 12 hours at room temperature
3. Cidex solution: 10 hours at room temperature
4. Peracetic acid: 12 minutes at 131° F (55° C)

A load control record of the items sterilized in solution must be kept as for other methods of sterilization (see sample record in Box 13-2).

Rinsing Following Immersion

All items must be thoroughly rinsed in sterile distilled water before use, except in the Steris unit. Sterile gloves must be worn to transfer items from the solution to the container for rinsing. Items then should be dried with a sterile towel before being transferred to or placed on a sterile field.

IONIZING RADIATION

Some products commercially available are sterilized by *irradiation.* Ionizing radiation produces ions by knocking electrons out of atoms. These electrons are knocked out so violently that they strike an adjacent atom and either attach themselves to it or dislodge an electron from the second atom. The ionic energy that results becomes converted to thermal and chemical energy. This energy causes the death of microorganisms by disruption of the DNA molecule, thus preventing cellular division and propagation of biologic life.

The principal sources of ionizing radiation are beta particles and gamma rays. Beta particles, free electrons, are transmitted through a high-voltage electron beam

BOX 13-2

Record for Sterilization or High-Level Disinfection With Chemical Solutions

Date: ______
Solution: Type/agent ______
Strength ______
Activation date ______
Expiration date ______
Temperature ______
Immersion: Time in ______
Time out ______
Load: Control number ______
Location ______
Contents ______
______
______
______

from a linear accelerator. These high-energy free electrons will penetrate into matter before being stopped by collisions with other atoms. Thus their usefulness in sterilizing an object is limited by the density and thickness of the object and by the energy of the electrons. They produce their effect by ionizing the atoms they hit, producing secondary electrons that, in turn, produce lethal effects on microorganisms.

Cobalt 60 is a radioactive isotope capable of disintegrating to produce gamma rays. Gamma rays are electromagnetic waves. They have the capability of penetrating to a much greater distance than beta rays before losing their energy from collisions. Because they travel at the speed of light, they must pass through a thickness measuring several feet before making sufficient collisions to lose all of their energy. Cobalt 60 is the most commonly used source for irradiation sterilization.

Irradiation sterilization with beta or gamma rays is limited to industrial use. The product is exposed to radiation for 10 to 20 hours, depending on the strength of the source. Ionizing radiation penetrates most materials to sterilize reliably. However, physical properties of some materials are altered by exposure to ionizing radiation, thus limiting its use. Rays have a very low temperature effect on materials. This process is dry, so it can be used to sterilize heat- and moisture-sensitive items. Gamma rays can penetrate large bulky objects, so cartons ready for shipment can be sterilized in the cobalt 60 irradiator. This is cost effective for the manufacturer.

Ionizing radiation is the most effective sterilization method. No residual radiation is generated. The process may be monitored with biologic indicators using *Bacillus pumilus*. However, products can be released for use on the basis of dosimetry, measurements of radiation dose, without quarantine periods required for biologic testing.

CONTROL MEASURES

With the exception of items sterilized in a high-speed pressure "flash" steam sterilizer or by immersion in a chemical solution, all items are wrapped before sterilization. The integrity of the packaging material must be maintained before use and during storage. Packages must be labeled so the contents will be known, unless they are visible through the packaging material. The label also includes the conditions of sterilization. A chemical indicator on each package verifies exposure to a sterilization process.

Load Control Number

A load control number should be imprinted on or be part of the label on every package of sterile items, whether sterilized on or off site. This number designates the sterilization equipment used, the cycle, and the sterilization date. For sterilizers with microcomputer processor printouts, a label gun correlates the same control number for every package put in the load. Load control numbers are used to facilitate identification and retrieval of supplies, if necessary, in the event of a sterilization failure.

The sterilization date can be recorded as a Julian date (day 1 through 365) or as a Georgian date (month, day, year). The date the package is sterilized may be stamped on it as it is removed from the sterilizer; thus an undated package is not considered sterile. Or the date may be written or affixed on the package when it is wrapped. Monthly, color-coded, machine-labeling systems may be used. Peel-off bar-coded labels also help control inventory and patient charges for items.

A load control number should also be assigned to items immersed in a chemical sterilant.

Wet Packs

All sterilizing methods in which humidity, usually steam, is a parameter of the process potentially present the hazard of producing wet packages. Microorganisms migrate easily through moisture when a pathway is provided from outside to inside a package. Water droplets may be visible on the outside or inside, or absorbed moisture may be seen or felt. *A pack should be considered unsterile and unacceptable for use if it is wet,* unless the wrapper is completely impermeable to water. A stain on a wrapper may indicate moisture was present and has dried. The cause of wet packs must be investigated and promptly corrected. Reprocessing is necessary for a wet package or a load with one or more wet or suspect packages.

Causes/Conditions

Excessive moisture may be related to the steam itself, to the load, or to the sterilizer.

Wet Steam If steam is abnormally wet, water droplets may form on the outside or inside of packages. Absorbent materials will become soaked with moisture. At the boiling point, water becomes steam. Saturated steam contains as much water in the vapor state as physically possible (98%) and minimal liquid water (2% water droplets). In a steam sterilizer, pressure increases the temperature to raise the boiling point to 250° F (121° C) or above at a pressure of 15 lb or more above atmospheric pressure at sea level. The temperature of steam does not increase above the boiling point at normal atmospheric pressure in other types of sterilizers. If steam loses water vapor, it can achieve a higher temperature at the same pressure, thus becoming *superheated.* In steam sterilization, superheating decreases the effectiveness of steam to kill microorganisms.

The dryness (purity) of steam depends on the amount of water in the vapor state in proportion to the amount of solid, liquid, or vapor contamination. This contamination can come from particles in the boiler, steam lines, or sterilizer; from chemical additives in the water; or from moisture in the load. When steam contacts cold surfaces, a lowering of its temperature reverts steam to water, producing condensation on surfaces and raising the temperature of the remaining vapor, causing superheating of the steam. Dry, dehydrated textiles and other porous materials will absorb water from steam, also changing the proportion of the water content of steam, thus causing superheating. The water content of steam should not fall below 97% during the sterilization cycle. Below this level, items in the load can become supersaturated with water. Subsequent drying will be inadequate.

Characteristics of Load Many factors affect penetration of the sterilant throughout the load. A few are reiterated for emphasis.

1. Items must be clean before they are packaged. Nonporous items must be dry. Porous materials, such as woven fabrics, must be hydrated (i.e., humidified) but not wet.
2. Basins must be separated by absorbent material and positioned so water condensate will drain out.
3. Heat penetrates materials at different rates. For even heating of the load, it is preferable not to mix materials. For example, a load may contain only instrument sets and metals or only packs of fabrics.
4. Density of a pack must allow circulation of air, moisture, and sterilant within the pack. Porous items should not be wrapped tightly. The pack should not exceed 12 × 12 × 20 inches (30 × 30 × 50 cm), 12 lb (5.5 kg), and a density of 7.2 lb/cu ft.
5. Permeability of packaging materials varies. A water droplet on an impermeable wrapper may not be a problem, but it can be absorbed by an adjacent package with a permeable wrapper.
6. Condensation diffuses at different rates so that the drying and cooling cycle depends on the materials in the load. Packages should not be handled until this cycle is complete.

Sterilizer Malfunctions Clogged drains, steam traps and air filters, inoperable control valves, worn gaskets, and a dirty chamber can cause malfunction of the sterilizer. Routine cleaning and preventive maintenance are imperative.

Guidelines for Evaluating Wet Packs

Two guidelines are recommended for determining whether or not to use a package with obvious retained moisture.

1. Water droplets or dampness *outside:*
   a. Package is considered unsterile if packaging material is absorbent (i.e., water permeable).
   b. Contents are considered sterile if packaging material is nonabsorbent (i.e., water repellent, water impermeable).
2. Water droplets or dampness *inside:*
   a. Package is considered unsterile if water droplets are formed or contents are damp when opened, unless wrapped in water-impermeable film such as polyethylene or polypropylene.
   b. Contents in combination paper/plastic peel-pouches are considered wet if water droplets are present.
   c. Contents are considered sterile if wrapped in nonabsorbent, water-impermeable film.

Reprocessing Wet Packs

Wet packs must be disassembled and items properly dried and repackaged before they are resterilized. Reusable woven fabrics should be sent to the laundry. They must be hydrated, but damp or wet fabrics will cause superheating during steam sterilization.

Shelf Life

Sterility is event related, not time related. Packaging material must keep items sterile until the time of use. Storage conditions must maintain the integrity of the package. *Shelf life* is the duration for which sterility is assumed to be maintained. This is the maximum time a sterile package may be kept in storage. Many variables preclude setting a universal standard of time for all packages. As time passes, the likelihood of contamination may increase. The length of time an item is considered sterile depends on the following events:

1. Handling of the package during transport and storage (i.e., prevention of contamination and physical damage)
2. Integrity, type, and configuration of packaging material
3. Conditions of storage

Specific written policies must address shelf life of all stored sterile supplies (i.e., determine expiration dates). An "indefinitely sterile" policy may be adopted for double peel-packed items and those with sealed dust covers. The label should state that the package will be considered sterile until it is opened or damaged or the dust cover is removed. Prolonged storage in most facilities for on-site sterilized items in hermetically (airtight) sealed packages is arbitrarily determined to be from 6 to 12 months.

Most commercially sterilized products are considered sterile indefinitely or as long as the integrity of the package is maintained. An expiration date put on the label by the manufacturer indicates the maximum time the manufacturer can guarantee product stability and sterility based on test data approved by the FDA.

Integrity of Packaging Material

The method of sterilization establishes the type of packaging material that may be used. The permeability and density of the material, the type of closure used, and how packages are handled affect shelf life.

1. An item is no longer considered sterile after accidental puncture, tear, or rupture of the package. Paper may become brittle and crack.
2. Squeezing or crushing a package may force air out and draw unsterile air in, thus contaminating the contents. Packages wrapped in woven fabrics should be handled carefully and not be packed tightly together for storage.
3. Accidental wetting of a package, except one that is hermetically sealed in plastic, contaminates the contents. It is necessary to avoid:
   a. Handling with moist or wet hands
   b. Placing on a wet surface
4. Density of nonwoven fabrics and plastic materials prolongs shelf life.
5. Heat- or self-sealed pouches are airtight, so they can be stored longer than tape-sealed packages.
6. Commercially packaged, sterilized items are usually considered sterile until the package is opened or damaged, or stability of the product becomes outdated.

Dust Cover

A sealed, airtight plastic bag protects a sterile package from dust, dirt, lint, moisture, and vermin during storage. After sterilization, immediately following cooling to room temperature or aerating, infrequently used items may be sealed in plastic 2 to 3 mil thick. Low-use items are those that routinely are stored for more than 30 days. A dust cover will prolong an item's shelf life as long as it remains sealed and does not have cracks or holes in it. The dust cover is removed before the sterile package is taken from a storage area into the OR.

Storage Conditions

Time may be more easily controlled than events. How sterile packages are handled and stored is as important as how long.

1. Storage areas must be clean and free of dust, lint, dirt, and vermin. Routine cleaning procedures must be followed for all areas.
2. All sterile items should be stored under conditions that protect them from extremes of temperature and humidity. Prolonged storage in a warm environment at high humidity can cause moisture to condense inside packages and thus destroy the microbial barrier of some packaging materials. Ventilating and air-conditioning systems with filtered air should maintain temperature below 80° F (26° C) and relative humidity between 30% and 60%. Ten air exchanges per hour are recommended.
3. Packages should be allowed to cool to room temperature before being put into storage to avoid condensation inside the package.
4. Woven fabric- and paper-wrapped items may be stored in closed cabinets and in enclosed or covered carts for up to 30 days, as opposed to on open shelving for up to 21 days.

   NOTE These are the generally accepted arbitrary times for woven fabrics and paper. Other factors may limit or extend these times.

5. For open shelving, the highest shelf should be at least 18 inches (46 cm) below the ceiling and 8 to 10 inches (20 to 25 cm) above the floor.
6. Sterile storage areas should have controlled traffic patterns.

Rotation of Supplies

Shelf life can be minimized by inventory control and the rotation of sterile supplies. With the adjustment of the standard number of packages kept sterile to daily needs, packages seldom need to be held for prolonged storage periods. In the interest of economy and good management, a stock supply of day-to-day items should be regulated to have enough for the busiest day with used items replenished daily. Many items are seldom used yet several must be kept sterile at all times. These supplies should be sterilized, or commercially sterilized items ordered, only in quantities sufficient to ensure prompt use and rapid turnover.

Sterile supplies should be checked daily for the integrity of the packages. Some items deteriorate with repeated sterilization or prolonged storage (e.g., latex items). Any packages that become contaminated must be resterilized. Older supplies should always be used first to minimize storage. The acronym FIFO, *first in/first out,* is helpful to remember for rotation of supplies, particularly sterile supplies.

Opening Sterile Supplies

Sterility must be maintained during the sterile transfer from the package to the sterile field. Refer to Chapters 12 and 20 for opening sterile supplies. A package wrapped in woven fabric that is wet, becomes soiled or dusty, is dropped, or is contaminated while being opened should not be used. A reusable item can be repackaged and resterilized. Any package should not be used if sterility is suspected of being compromised. The integrity of a package should be inspected before opening.

DISINFECTION

Surfaces of items that cannot be sterilized must be disinfected to eliminate as many microorganisms from the environment as possible. Disinfection differs from sterilization by its lack of sporicidal power. Disinfection can be accomplished with *chemical* and *physical* agents. The application of these agents depends on the level of risk of infection or environmental contamination.

1. *Low- to intermediate-level:* Housekeeping disinfection of surfaces such as floors, walls, furniture, and large equipment, and *noncritical* items that ordinarily do not touch the patient or contact only intact skin.
2. *High-level:* Disinfection of *semicritical* items that come in contact with nonintact skin or mucous membranes but do not penetrate body tissues (i.e., endoscopes, respiratory equipment, and thermometers).

Sterilization is *always* preferable for critical items. *High-level disinfection must not be confused with chemical sterilization.* A record of the agent and time of exposure should be maintained for semicritical items that have been high-level disinfected (see sample in Box 13-2). The level of disinfection that can be achieved depends on the type and concentration of the agent, contact time, and bioburden. Items that are disinfected must be "patient safe" for their intended uses to minimize risks of infection for the patient. An all-purpose disinfectant does not exist. The best housekeeping agents are not the best instrument disinfectants and vice versa.

Chemical Disinfectants

Chemical agents, including sterilants, must be registered with the Pesticide Regulation Division of the EPA to be sold in interstate commerce. An EPA registration number is granted only when requirements of laboratory test data, toxicity data, product formula, and label copy are approved. The product must do what the label says it does. To be labeled for hospital use, a chemical disinfectant must be proven effective against *Staphylococcus aureus* (gram-positive), *Salmonella choleraesuis* (gram-negative), and *Pseudomonas aeruginosa* (gram-negative), the most resistant gram-positive and gram-negative organisms. The agent can be classified as a hospital disinfectant without being pseudomonacidal, but the label must say whether or not it is effective against this organism.

The EPA defines a *disinfectant* as an agent that kills growing or vegetative forms of bacteria. The terms *germicide* and *bactericide* may be used synonymously with disinfectant according to this definition. However, *Mycobacterium tuberculosis* has a waxy envelope that makes it comparatively resistant to aqueous germicides. Effective agents against *M. tuberculosis* should be labeled *tuberculocidal.* Agents also are labeled if they kill fungi *(fungicide)*, viruses *(virucide)*, and/or spores *(sporicide).* Agents effective enough to be labeled tuberculocidal will kill HIV. Those that meet the EPA testing requirements may be labeled specifically as HIV virucides. Hepatitis B virus (HBV) cannot be adapted to laboratory testing, but it is known to survive exposure to many disinfectants.

The safest products for use in the OR suite include all categories of biocidal action (Table 13-4). With the exception of the few cold sterilants previously discussed, chemicals in solution are *not* sporicides. Analysis of the label statements helps determine whether a product is appropriate for a specific purpose in the OR. Factors to be considered in the selection of an agent include:

1. Microorganisms differ markedly in their resistance to chemicals.
   a. *Low-level:* most vegetative bacteria, fungi, and lipoprotein (lipid- and protein-coated) viruses including HIV are susceptible to chemicals.
   b. *Intermediate: M. tuberculosis* and nonlipid viruses including HBV are significantly more resistant.
   c. *High-level:* bacterial spores are tremendously resistant.
2. Disinfectants differ widely in level of biocidal action they produce and mechanisms involved. All are protoplasmic poisons that either coagulate or denature cell protein, oxidate or bind enzymes, or alter cell membranes. In-use culture testing must determine the number of viable microorganisms after an agent is used for the intended purpose.
3. Nature of microbial contamination influences the results of chemical disinfection. Bacteria, spores, fungi, and viruses are present in air and on surfaces throughout the environment. However, organic soil, such as blood, plasma, pus, feces, and tissue, absorbs germicidal molecules and inactivates some chemicals. Therefore good physical cleaning before disinfection helps reduce the numbers of microorganisms present and enhances biocidal action.
4. Requirements of the chemical agent vary.
   a. Housekeeping products should be *detergent-disinfectants* that meet the requirements for both cleaning and disinfection:
      (1) Must be effective against a broad spectrum of microorganisms, including *P. aeruginosa* and *M. tuberculosis,* preferably in the presence of organic soil.
      (2) Must be compatible with tap water used for use-dilution.
      (3) Must not leave a residual insulating film that will affect electrical conductivity.
      (4) Should be nontoxic and nonirritating to patients and personnel.
      (5) Should be virtually odorless.
   b. Instrument and equipment disinfectants should kill as many species of microorganisms as possible to decontaminate items effectively for

TABLE 13-4

Activity of Disinfectants in Addition to Being Bactericidal, Pseudomonacidal, and Fungicidal*

DISINFECTANT	ACTIVITY LEVEL	VIRUCIDE HIV	VIRUCIDE HBV†	IMMERSION TIME TUBERCULOCIDE	HOUSE-KEEPING	HAZARDS
Chemicals*						
Alcohol, 70%-95%:						
ethyl	Intermediate	Yes	Yes	15 min	Yes	Flammable
isopropyl	Intermediate	Yes	No	15 min	Yes	Flammable
Chloride compounds	Low	Yes	Yes	N/A	Yes	
Formaldehyde:						
37% aqueous	High‡	Yes	Yes	15 min	No	Toxic fumes
8% in alcohol	High‡	Yes	Yes	10 min	No	Toxic fumes
Glutaraldehyde, 2%	High§	Yes	Yes	45-90 min§	No	Irritating fumes
Iodophors:						
450 ppm	Intermediate	Yes	Yes	20 min	Yes	
100 ppm	Low	No	No	N/A	Yes	
Mercurial compounds	None	No	No	N/A	No	Bacteriostatic only
Phenolic compounds	Low	Yes	No	20 min	Yes	Skin irritant
Quaternary ammonium	Low	Yes	No	N/A	No	
Physical						
Boiling water	Low	Yes	No	N/A	No	
Ultraviolet irradiation	Low	Yes	No	N/A	Air and water	Skin and eye irritant

*Manufacturer's instructions for use and dilution must be followed.
†Probability cannot be tested.
‡Sporicidal in 12 hr.
§Formulation varies. Immersion time for tuberculoide (45-90 min) and sporicide (10-12 hr).
N/A, no activity.

handling by personnel or for preparing semicritical items for patient use, such as stethoscopes and monitors.

5. Kill time is correlated with the concentration of the agent and the number of microorganisms present. Most chemicals are used in aqueous solution. Water brings the chemical and microorganisms together. Without this water reaction, the process stops. Increasing the concentration of the chemical may shorten exposure time but not necessarily.
   a. All tap water has *Pseudomonas* bacteria in it. The pH, calcium, and magnesium in hard tap water can inactivate disinfectants. Therefore distilled water may be recommended for use-dilution.
   b. Temperature of hot water may make chemical agent unstable.
   c. Disinfectants should be premixed in required concentration and stored in properly labeled containers to ensure that personnel use the product in the correct concentration.
   d. Instruments must be completely submerged for the maximum time recommended by the manufacturer of the product used.
   e. All instruments should be clean and dry when put into solution. Drippy, wet items will dilute the solution and change the concentration of a chemical agent.
6. Composition of items to be disinfected varies. Nonporous items such as metal instruments are more easily disinfected than porous materials.

   NOTE Seepage of disinfectant solution into an ampule can occur if the ampule has a microscopic hole or crack in it. If this material is injected or implanted, serious reactions can result. If ampules cannot be sterilized in steam or ethylene oxide gas, a color dye must be added to a disinfectant solution. If color seeps into an ampule or the solution becomes cloudy, it must be discarded. Do not use any suspicious ampule.

7. Method of application influences the effectiveness of the chemical agent.

a. Direct application of a liquid disinfectant, either by mechanical action for housekeeping purposes or by immersion for instrument disinfection, is the most effective method of applying chemicals to the surface of inanimate objects.
b. Aerosol spray from a pressurized container is an effective method of spot disinfection on smooth surfaces and into crevices not otherwise accessible.
c. *Fogging* is the process of filling the air in a room with an aerosolized disinfectant solution in an attempt to control microbial contamination. Action on airborne contaminants is temporary because the agent dispersed through the air settles on surfaces or is exhausted through the ventilating system. This method is potentially toxic to personnel and patients. Unless all surfaces are completely covered by a layer of the disinfectant solution for the minimum exposure period, disinfection is incomplete. Fogging is impractical and too ineffective to be an acceptable method of disinfection in OR suites.

8. Disinfection should be done immediately before and after use or contamination. All patients are considered to be potential carriers of HIV and HBV. Therefore adequate bactericidal and virucidal disinfection is needed before and after every invasive procedure.

Chemical agents are used in solution for disinfection. They must be labeled with the chemical properties and appropriate warnings of hazards. Directions for dilution and/or use must be followed; read the label. Material Safety Data Sheets (MSDS), supplied by the manufacturer as required by OSHA for hazardous chemicals, must be available to users. Isopropyl alcohol, sodium hypochlorite, formaldehyde, glutaraldehyde, and phenol are considered hazardous chemicals. Some other chemicals can cause contact dermatitis. Gloves should be worn when handling chemical agents.

Alcohol

Ethyl or isopropyl alcohol, 70% to 95%, kills microorganisms by coagulation of cell proteins.

Effectiveness

1. It may be used as a housekeeping disinfectant for spot cleaning, such as damp-dusting furniture and lights or wiping electrical cords, without leaving a residue on treated surfaces.
2. It can disinfect semicritical instruments. To prevent corrosion of metal, 0.2% sodium nitrite must be added.
3. It is bactericidal, pseudomonacidal, and fungicidal in a minimum of 10 minutes' exposure by total immersion.
4. It is tuberculocidal and virucidal for most viruses, including HIV, in a minimum of 15 minutes' exposure; 70% to 95% ethyl alcohol is effective against HBV.

Hazards

1. Pattern of effectiveness of 95% isopropyl alcohol on HBV is irregular. It should *not* be used for cleaning up blood or body fluid spills.
2. It is volatile; it will act only as long as it is in solution. Alcohol becomes ineffective as soon as it evaporates and loses its biocidal activity below a concentration of 50%; it should be discarded at frequent intervals.
3. It is inactive in the presence of organic soil. It does not penetrate skin oil that lodges on instruments through handling.
4. It will blanch asphalt floor tiles.
5. It cannot be used on lensed instruments with cement mountings because it dissolves cement.
6. With long exposure, it will harden and swell plastic tubing and items, including polyethylene.
7. It is flammable so it must be stored in a cool, well-ventilated area.

Chlorine Compounds

Inorganic chlorine is valuable for the disinfection of water. Chlorine compounds kill microorganisms by the oxidation of enzymes. Sodium hypochlorite (household bleach), 1:10 dilution of 5.25%, is a low-level disinfectant. Concentration may range up to 1:100, 500 ppm. Sodium dichloroisocyanurate (Presept disinfectant tablet) has a lowered pH so its biocidal action is enhanced. Chloride compounds are limited to housekeeping disinfection.

Effectiveness

1. Chlorine compounds are housekeeping disinfectants for spot cleaning of blood and body fluid spills and for cleaning of floors and furniture.
2. They are bactericidal, fungicidal, and tuberculocidal and have a virucidal effect on HIV, HBV, and other viruses.

Hazards

1. Sodium hypochlorite is unstable and dissipates rapidly in the presence of organic soil. A dilution must be prepared daily.
2. Odor may be objectionable.
3. Chlorine is corrosive to metal; it *cannot be used for instrument disinfection and decontamination.*
4. Chlorine compounds are potentially carcinogenic if combined with formaldehyde.

Formaldehyde

Formaldehyde kills microorganisms by coagulation of protein in cells. The solution may be 37% formaldehyde in water (Formalin) or 8% formaldehyde in 70% isopropyl alcohol. Formaldehyde is not used for housekeeping purposes.

Effectiveness

1. It is a high-level instrument disinfectant. To prevent corrosion of metal, 0.2% sodium nitrite must be added.
2. It is bactericidal, pseudomonacidal, and fungicidal in a minimum of 5 minutes' exposure.
3. It is tuberculocidal and virucidal in a minimum of 10 minutes in alcohol solution and in a minimum of 15 minutes in aqueous solution.
4. It is sporicidal in a minimum of 12 hours.

Hazards

1. Fumes are irritating to eyes and mucous membranes.
2. Fumes are potentially carcinogenic.
3. It is toxic to tissues, so instruments must be thoroughly rinsed with sterile distilled water before use.
4. Rubber and porous materials may absorb formaldehyde so they should not be disinfected in this agent.

Glutaraldehyde

An aqueous solution of glutaraldehyde kills microorganisms by denaturation of protein. It is most commonly used in an activated 2% solution that can be reused for the specified period of activation. Both alkaline and acid solutions are available for high-level disinfection of critical and semicritical items. A 1:16 dilution is not considered a high-level disinfectant; 2% solution is. Glutaraldehyde is not used for housekeeping purposes.

Effectiveness

1. It is a noncorrosive high-level disinfectant for endoscopes and lensed instruments.
2. It is a safe high-level disinfectant for most plastic and rubber items such as those used for administering anesthesia or respiratory therapy.
3. It is bactericidal, pseudomonacidal, fungicidal, and virucidal, including against HIV and HBV, in a minimum of 10 minutes' exposure at a temperature between 68° and 86° F (20° and 30° C).
4. It is tuberculocidal. Variations in formulations of products available affect exposure time and temperature of solution, especially after reuse. A 2% solution at 77° or 86° F (25° or 30° C) may be 100% tuberculocidal in 45 to 90 minutes, depending on the formulation. Label instructions of the manufacturer should be followed.
5. It is sporicidal in a minimum of 10 hours' exposure at room temperature for most of the products labeled as cold sterilants.
6. Some products can be reused in closed containers or in an automatic machine for a period of activation specified by manufacturer.
7. It remains active in the presence of organic matter; it does not coagulate protein material.

Hazards

1. Thorough and careful cleaning in a mild detergent is essential to remove organic debris and reduce microbial contamination. Detergent must be rinsed off and the item dried before immersion.
2. Items must be completely immersed and lumens filled with solution for no longer than 24 hours.
3. Items must be thoroughly rinsed before use.
4. Glutaraldehyde may be retained by woven polyester catheters and be an irritant to mucous membranes.
5. Odor and fumes may be irritating to eyes, throat, and nasal passages. The solution should be kept covered and used in a well-ventilated area.
6. Shelf life is limited after activation.

Iodophors

A complex of free iodine with detergent kills microorganisms through a process of oxidation of essential enzymes. An iodophor is an effective low- to intermediate-level disinfectant. The iodine-detergent complex enhances the biocidal activity of free iodine and renders it nontoxic, nonirritating, and nonstaining when used as directed. Concentration varies among the products available. The manufacturer's instructions for use must be followed.

Effectiveness

1. Iodophors are used as housekeeping disinfectants for surfaces such as floors, furniture, and walls. Iodine is effective as long as it is wet. An aqueous solution is more effective for cleaning than an alcohol solution because it dries more slowly.
2. An iodophor may be used as a semicritical instrument disinfectant. To prevent corrosion of metal, 0.2% sodium nitrite must be added.
3. Iodophors are bactericidal, pseudomonacidal, and fungicidal in a minimum of 10 minutes' exposure in a concentration of 450 ppm of iodine or a minimum of 20 minutes' exposure in a concentration of 100 ppm of iodine.
4. They are tuberculocidal and virucidal, including against HIV and HBV, in a minimum of 20 minutes' exposure with a minimum concentration of 450 ppm of iodine.

Hazards

1. Some iodophors are unstable in the presence of hard water or heat or are subject to inactivation by organic soil.
2. Iodine stains fabrics and tissue; however, this is reduced or is temporary when used as an iodophor.

Mercurial Compounds

Mercurial compounds bind enzymes of bacteria but inhibit growth rather than kill the organisms. Therefore these agents are bacteriostatic, not germicidal. They have little if any value in hospital disinfection.

Phenolic Compounds

Derivatives of pure phenol kill microorganisms mainly by coagulation of protein. Depending on the phenol coefficient and species of organisms, phenolic compounds may cause rapid lysis of cells, leakage of cell constituents without lysis, or death by denaturing enzymes. Pure phenol, obtained from coal tar, is an extremely caustic agent and dangerous to tissue. Derivatives are used as low-level disinfectants, usually with a minimum of a 2% phenolic compound in an aqueous or detergent solution. Phenolic compounds are used for housekeeping purposes primarily.

Effectiveness

1. Phenolic compounds may be used as housekeeping disinfectants for cleaning surfaces such as floors, furniture, and walls. Phenolics retain a safe level of activity in the presence of heavy organic soil.
2. They are disinfectants of choice when dealing with fecal contamination. They have good stability and remain active after mild heating and prolonged drying. Subsequent application of moisture to dry surfaces can redissolve the chemical so it becomes bactericidal again.

Hazards

1. Tissue irritation precludes use for instruments that will come in contact with skin and mucous membranes (e.g., anesthesia equipment).
2. Personnel should wear gloves when cleaning with these products to avoid skin irritation.
3. Rubber and plastics may absorb phenol derivatives.
4. Product may have an unpleasant odor.

Quaternary Ammonium Compounds

Quats, as these compounds often are called, cause gradual alteration of cell membranes to produce leakage of protoplasm of some microorganisms, primarily vegetative bacteria. These compounds possess detergent properties. Benzalkonium chloride, one of the most widely used of these compounds, should be used in a concentration of 1:750.

Effectiveness

1. They are rarely used as housekeeping disinfectants for surfaces such as floors, furniture, and walls.
2. For low-level, noncritical instrument disinfection, 0.2% sodium nitrite must be added to the solution to prevent corrosion of metal.
3. They are bactericidal, pseudomonacidal, fungicidal, and lipid virucidal in a minimum of 10 minutes' exposure.

Hazards

1. Biocidal effect can be reversed by adding a neutralizer, such as soap.
2. Hard water used for dilution reduces active concentration.
3. Active agent can be selectively absorbed by fabrics, thus reducing the strength perhaps to an ineffectively low level. Gauze or a towel must not be put in the basin used for immersing instruments.
4. Compounds are subject to inactivation in the presence of organic soil.

NOTE Mercurial compounds and quaternary ammonium compounds are *not* recommended for hospital use because the hazards outweigh their effectiveness in the hospital environment. Other agents discussed are more efficacious.

Physical Disinfectants

Boiling Water

Boiling water cannot be depended on to kill spores. Heat-resistant bacterial spores will withstand water boiling at 212° F (100° C) for many hours of continuous exposure. Inactivation of some viruses, such as those associated with hepatitis, is uncertain.

If no other method of sterilization or disinfection is available, boiling water can be rendered more effective by adding sodium carbonate to make a 2% solution, which reduces the hydrogen-ion concentration. At sea level the recommended boiling time for disinfection is 15 minutes. Rubber goods and glassware must not be boiled in sodium carbonate as it is destructive to both. If sodium carbonate is not used, the minimum boiling period is 30 minutes. At high altitudes the boiling time must be increased to compensate for the lower temperature of boiling water.

Boiling water is a nontoxic, high-level disinfection process, sometimes referred to as pasteurization, that can be used for items such as metal utensils and breathing circuits. For sanitization, the reduction or destruction of microbial contaminants to a relatively safe level for handling, the temperature of hot water ranges from 140° to 203° F (60° to 95° C).

Ultraviolet Irradiation

Ultraviolet (UV) rays at wavelengths of 240 to 480 nanometers (nm) photochemically transform nucleic acid bases to denature DNA and proteins. Generated by low-pressure mercury vapor bulbs, UV lights produce nonionizing radiant energy in sufficient wavelengths and intensity for low-level disinfection. The rays can kill vegetative bacteria, fungi, and lipoprotein viruses on contact in air or water. The practical usefulness of UV irradiation is very limited, however, because the rays must make direct contact with the organisms. Microorganisms are in a constant state of motion in the air currents of the ventilating system and in water. Moving across the ray of UV light, pathogens may be exposed for too short a time for effective contact with the radiant energy.

UV lights have been installed in a few ORs to decrease airborne microorganisms to low levels. UV rays can cause skin burns, similar to sunburn, and conjunctivitis of the eyes. Therefore, when working under exposure to UV irradiation, protective skin coverings and goggles or a visor over the eyes must be worn. These lights may be turned on only when the room is unoccupied to reduce airborne and surface contamination.

UV irradiation is used in conjunction with activated carbon filters for water purification. UV irradiation kills bacteria but does not remove impurities. The filtration process is followed by exposing water to a UV lamp. This produces purified water, *not* sterile water. UV irradiation is not sporicidal and HBV can survive exposure to it.

BIBLIOGRAPHY

AMSCO technique manual, Erie, Pa, 1991, American Sterilizer.

Are you complying with equipment standard? *OR Manager* 10(7):16-19, 1994.

Association for the Advancement of Medical Instrumentation: *AAMI standards and recommended practices for sterilization,* vol 1, *Sterilization,* Arlington, Va, 1992, American National Standards Institute.

Association for the Advancement of Medical Instrumentation: *Chemical sterilants and sterilization methods: a guide to selection and use* (TIR7-008-HM), Arlington, Va, 1990, American National Standards Institute.

Association for the Advancement of Medical Instrumentation: *Good hospital practice: flash sterilization—steam sterilization of patient care items for immediate use,* Arlington, Va, 1992, American National Standards Institute.

Block SS: *Disinfection, sterilization, and preservation,* ed 4, Malvern, Pa, 1991, Lea & Febiger.

Bubik JS: Preparation of sterile talc for treatment of pleural effusion, *Am J Hosp Pharm* 49(3):562-563, 1992.

Crow S: Peracetic acid—asking the right questions, *Today's OR Nurse* 15(3):47-49, 1993.

Crow S: Peracetic acid sterilization: a timely development for a busy healthcare industry, *Infect Control Hosp Epidemiol* 13(2):111-113, 1992.

Frey KB: The new alternative: plasma sterilization, *Surg Technol* 26(9):8-10, 1994.

Fuller A: Infection control: sterilizing instruments, *Nurs Times* 88(50): 64-65, 1992.

Haney PE et al: Ethylene oxide: an occupational health hazard for hospital workers, *AORN J* 51(2):480-486, 1990.

Harris MH: Flash sterilization: is it safe for routine use? *AORN J* 55(6):1547-1551, 1992.

Hart ML et al: Ethylene oxide sterilization: an evaluation of a test pack, *AORN J* 57(6):1389-1396, 1993.

Kirkwood ME, Crowe L: In-house sterilization of implants, *AORN J* 58(5):971-978, 1993.

Mathias JM: Sterility assurance replaces expiration dating, *OR Manager* 8(3):1, 20-22, 1992.

Mathias JM: Why use double-barrier sterile packaging? *OR Manager* 7(11):5, 9, 1991.

McWilliams RM, Lange CA: An answer to glutaraldehyde containment, *Today's OR Nurse* 15(3):51, 1993.

O'Connor LM: Event-related sterility assurance, *Surg Technol* 26(1):8-11, 1994.

Oliver PA: Resterilization, *Br J Theatre Nurs* 27(3):18-19, 1990.

O'Neal M: Clinical issues: retrieving flash sterilized items, *AORN J* 55(4):1091, 1992.

O'Neal M: Clinical issues: sterilization, high-level disinfection, *AORN J* 58(4):786, 1993.

Patterson P: AAMI releases new guidelines for flash sterilization, *OR Manager* 8(3):1, 12, 1992.

Patterson P: Controversy prompts revision of AAMI's flash sterilization standard, *OR Manager* 10(8):1, 12, 16, 1994.

Patterson P: New technique needed as CFCs are taken off market, *OR Manager* 10(8):1, 6-9, 1994.

Patterson P: Recommendations for flash sterilizing implants differ, *OR Manager* 8(3):1, 13-14, 1992.

Patterson P: Regulators cracking down on flash sterilization, *OR Manager* 9(12):1, 6-8, 1993.

Proposed recommended practices for chemical disinfection, *AORN J* 60(3):463-466, 1994.

Proposed recommended practices for practices for selection and use of packaging systems, *AORN J* 61(3):605-613, 1995.

Proposed recommended practices for sterilization in the practice setting, *AORN J* 60(1):109-119, 1994.

Recommended practices: Selection and use of packaging systems, *AORN J* 56(6):1096-1100, 1992.

Recommended practices: Steam and ethylene oxide (EO) sterilization, *AORN J* 56(4):721-730, 1992.

Reichert M: Glutaraldhyde: monitoring for safe use, *Today's OR Nurse* 15(3):50, 1993.

Reichert M, Young J: *Sterilization technology for the health care facility,* Gaithersburg, Md, 1993, Aspen.

Rutala WA: APIC guideline for selection and use of disinfectants, *Am J Infect Control* 18(4):99-117, 1990.

Rutala WA: Disinfection in the OR, *Today's OR Nurse* 12(10):30-38, 1990.

Rutala WA et al: Evaluation of a rapid readout biological indicator for flash sterilization with three biological indicators, *Infect Control Hosp Epidemiol* 14(7):390-394, 1993.

Sansom A: Activated glutaraldehyde, *Br J Theatre Nurs* 30(10):28, 1993.

Schroeter K: Implementation of an event-related sterility plan, *AORN J* 60(4):595-602, 1994.

Smith CD: Clinical issues: high level disinfection practices; sterilizing talcum powder, *AORN J* 56(1):125-128, 1992.

Steelman VM: Ethylene oxide: the importance of aeration, *AORN J* 55(3):773-787, 1992.

Steelman VM: Infection control, *AORN J* 59(2):476-482, 1994.

Steelman VM: Issues in sterilization and disinfection, *Urol Nurs* 12(40):123-127, 1992.

Sterilizing talcum powder used in surgery, *OR Manager* 8(7):18-19, 1992.

Wilhelm-Hass E: Breaking the time barrier: learning from a new product evaluation, *AORN J* 56(6):1074-1081, 1992.

CHAPTER 14

Surgical Instrumentation

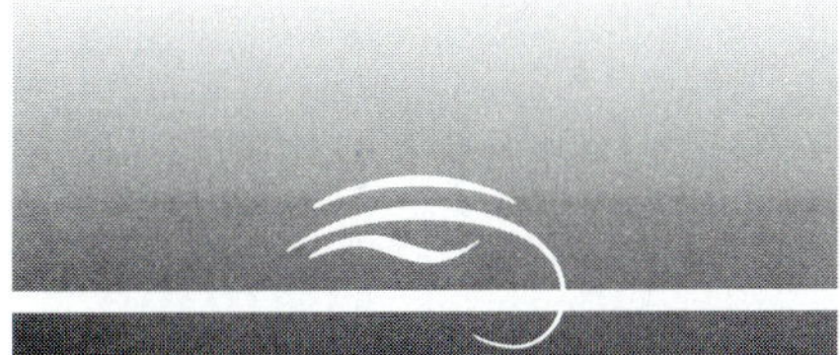

HISTORICAL BACKGROUND

Perhaps as early as 10,000 BC, prehistoric man fashioned tools to cut human flesh for the purpose of either inflicting wounds or repairing them. Early writings describe cutting tools. The Incas of Peru used razor-sharp flint and sharpened animal teeth. The Code of Hammurabi (circa 1900 BC) describes a bronze lancet. The Egyptian Ebers papyrus mentions blades made of flint, reed, and bronze used around 1900 to 1200 BC. Hippocrates (460-377 BC) advocated heating the tips of rounded and pointed blades.

In India in the pre-Christian Era, Shusruta made grasping tools designed for extracting objects such as arrowheads. Many of these tools were in the form of animal or bird heads, such as a toothed forceps that resembled a crocodile or a smooth forceps that was shaped like the beak of a heron. He described more than 100 instruments including scalpels, lancets, saws, bone cutters, trocars, and needles.

In the first century AD, Celsus described the use in Rome of scalpel handles with blunt dissecting ends, knives, saws, forceps and clamps with locking handles, probes, and hooks for retraction. These crude and often heavy instruments were the armamentarium of medicine through the Dark and Middle Ages. Ambroise Paré (1509-1590) was the first to grasp blood vessels with a pinching instrument that was the predecessor of the hemostat used today.

Amputations were the surgical trademark of the American Civil War (1861-1865). In some instances these amputations were performed on kitchen tables with crude heavy knives and instruments. Even table forks were used as retractors.

Through the eighteenth and nineteenth centuries, surgical tools were made by skilled silversmiths, coppersmiths, and woodworkers. Some instruments had beautifully carved ivory, bone, or wood handles. The surgeon kept them in velvet-lined cases. When sterilization became accepted around the turn of the twentieth century, instruments made entirely of metals such as carbon steel, silver, and brass replaced those with ornate but dirt-filled handles. The velvet cases gave way to sterilizer trays.

The development of stainless steel in the 1900s enhanced the art and craft of precision surgical instruments. Craftsmen primarily in Germany, Sweden, France, England, Pakistan, and the United States continue to provide surgical instruments needed to extend the capabilities of the surgeons' hands.

Hippocrates wrote that all instruments ought to be well suited for the purpose in hand as regards their size, weight, and delicacy. Consequently, instrument modifications vary from the strength needed for bone work, to the length needed to reach depths of body cavities, to the delicacy needed to handle structures even under the microscope. All instruments are designed to provide a tool the surgeon needs to perform a basic surgical maneuver. The variations are numerous.

FABRICATION OF METAL INSTRUMENTS

Although some are made of titanium, cobalt-based alloy (Vitallium), or other metals, the vast majority of surgical instruments are made of stainless steel. The alloys used must have specific properties to make them resistant to corrosion when exposed to blood and body fluids, cleaning solutions, sterilization, and the atmosphere. The manufacturer chooses the alloy for its durability, functional capacity, and ease of fabrication for the intended purpose.

Stainless Steel

Stainless steel is an alloy of iron, chromium, and carbon. It may also contain nickel, manganese, silicon, molybdenum, sulfur, and other elements to prevent corrosion or add tensile strength. The formulation of the steel plus heat treatment and finishing processes determine the qualities of the instrument. Chromium in the steel makes it resistant to corrosion. Carbon is necessary to give steel its hardness. However, carbon reduces the corrosion-resistant effects of chromium. Iron alloys in the 400 series, low in chromium and high in carbon, are most commonly used for the fabrication of surgical instruments.

Steel is milled into blanks that are forged, spun, drawn, die-cast, molded, or machined into component shapes and sizes. These components are hand assembled then heat hardened (tempered) and buffed. X-ray and/or fluoroscopy techniques are used to detect defects that may occur as a result of forging or machining operations. The stress and tension must be in balance. The temper of the steel determines this balance, that is, the flexibility to withstand the stresses of normal use.

The instrument is then subjected to processes that protect its surfaces and minimize corrosion. Oxidation of the surface chromium by a process called *passivation* forms a hard chromium oxide layer. Nitric acid both removes carbon particles and promotes formation of this surface coating. Polishing creates a smooth surface for the continuous layer of chromium oxide. Passivation continues to form this layer when the instrument is exposed to the atmosphere and oxidizing agents in cleaning solutions.

The term *stainless* is a misnomer. Steel does not tarnish, rust, or corrode easily; however, with normal use some staining and spotting will occur.

Stainless steel instruments are fabricated with one of three types of finishes before passivation.

1. A mirror finish is shiny and reflects light. The glare can be a distraction for the surgeon or an obstruction to visibility. This highly polished finish tends to resist surface corrosion.
2. An anodized finish is dull and glare-proof. Protective coatings of chromium and nickel, deposited electrolytically, reduce glare. This is sometimes referred to as a *satin finish.* It is somewhat more susceptible to surface corrosion than a highly polished surface. This corrosion is usually easily removed.
3. An ebony finish is black. This eliminates glare. The surface is darkened by a process of chemical oxidation. Instruments with an ebony finish are used in laser surgery to prevent beam reflection. In other surgical procedures, instruments with an ebony finish may offer the surgeon better color contrast because they do not reflect color of tissues.

Titanium

The metallurgic properties of titanium are excellent in comparison to stainless steel for the manufacture of microsurgical instruments. Titanium is nonmagnetic and inert. Titanium alloy is harder, stronger, lighter in weight, and more resistant to corrosion than stainless steel. A blue anodized finish of titanium oxide reduces glare.

Vitallium

Vitallium is the trade name for an alloy of cobalt, chromium, and molybdenum. This inert alloy has the strength and corrosion-resistant properties suitable for some orthopaedic devices and maxillofacial implants. When these devices are implanted, instruments made of Vitallium must be used. In an electrolytic environment such as body tissues, metals of different potential in contact with each other can cause corrosion. Therefore an implant of a cobalt-based alloy is not compatible with instruments that are iron-based alloys (stainless steel) and vice versa.

Other Metals

Although most instruments are made of steel alloys, other metals are used. Some instruments are fabricated from brass, silver, or aluminum. Tungsten carbide is an exceptionally hard metal used to laminate some cutting blades or as inserts on the functional tips or jaws of some instruments.

Plated Instruments

A shiny finish can be put on a basic forging or tooling of an iron alloy. Chromium, nickel, cadmium, silver, and copper are used for coating or flash plating. Any of these metals deposited directly on the steel is prone to rupturing, chipping, and spontaneous peeling. It is difficult to keep plated instruments from corroding. Rust can form beneath the plating. Plated instruments are used infrequently today.

Classification of Instruments

Various basic maneuvers are common to all surgical procedures. The surgeon dissects, resects, or alters tissues and/or organs to restore or repair bodily functions or parts. In the process, bleeding must be controlled. Surgical instruments are designed to provide the tools the surgeon needs for each maneuver. Whether they are small or large, short or long, straight or curved, sharp or blunt, *all instruments can be classified by their function.* Nomenclature is not standardized, however. The names of specific instruments must be learned in the clinical practice setting. All instruments should be used for their intended purpose only and should not be abused.

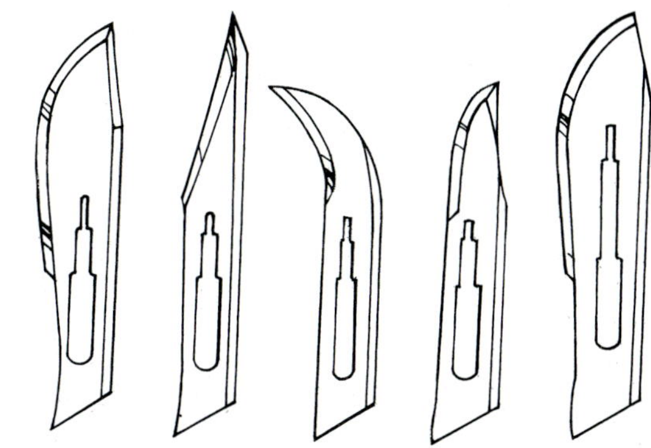

FIGURE 14-1 Scalpel/knife blades: No./sizes 10, 11, 12, 15, 20 (actual size).

Cutting and Dissecting

Cutting instruments have sharp edges. They are used to dissect, incise, separate, or excise tissues. Sharp edges should be protected during cleaning, sterilizing, and storing. These instruments should be kept separate from other instruments. They demand careful handling at all times to prevent injury to the handler and damage to sharp edges.

Scalpels

The type of scalpel most frequently used has a reusable handle with a disposable blade. Most handles are made of brass; blades may be made of carbon steel. The blade is attached to the handle by slipping the slit in the blade into the grooves on the handle (see Figure 20-5, p. 414). An instrument, *never fingers,* is used to attach and detach the blade. The instrument, usually a needle-holder, should not touch the cutting edge. Blades vary by size and shape (Figure 14-1); handles vary by width and length.

1. No. 10 blade is used most frequently. This blade has a rounded cutting edge along one side and fits on No. 3, 7, and 9 handles. No. 20, 21, and 22 blades are the same shape but larger. They fit on No. 4 handles.
2. No. 11 blade has a straight edge that comes to a sharp point. It fits on No. 3, 7, and 9 handles.
3. No. 12 blade is shaped like a hook with the cutting edge on the inside curvature. It fits on No. 3, 7, and 9 handles.
4. No. 15 blade has a smaller and shorter curved cutting edge than a No. 10 blade. This blade also fits on No. 3, 7, and 9 handles. A No. 15C blade has the same shape but is smaller for tiny incisions, such as those for some pediatric procedures.
5. No. 23 blade has a curved cutting edge that comes to more of a point than No. 20, 21, and 22 blades. The No. 23 blade fits on a No. 4 handle.

An assortment of blades with angulations and configurations for specific uses, such as a Beaver rhinoplasty blade, are also used. These blades attach to a universal handle designed specifically for these small blades.

Disposable scalpels also are available. Proper precautions are necessary to take during handling and when disposing of all blades or scalpels (see Chapter 12, pp. 198-199, and Chapter 27, p. 550).

Knives

Knives come in various sizes and configurations. They usually have a blade at one end, like a kitchen paring knife. The blade may have one or two cutting edges. These knives are designed for very specific purposes, such as a cataract knife. Other types of knives have detachable and replaceable blades, such as an adenotome and dermatome. A knife blade may be incorporated into a disposable instrument, such as a stapler that cuts tissue and then staples it.

Scissors

The blades of scissors may be straight, angled, or curved and pointed or blunt at the tips (Figure 14-2). The handles may be long or short. Some scissors are used only to cut or dissect tissues; others are used to cut materials. To maintain sharpness of the cutting edges and proper alignment of the blades, scissors should be used *only* for their intended purpose.

1. *Tissue/operating scissors* must have sharp blades. However, the type and location of tissue to be cut will determine which scissors the surgeon will use. Blades needed to cut tough tissues are heavier than those needed to cut fine, delicate structures. Curved or angled blades are needed to reach under or around structures. Handles to reach deep into body cavities are longer than those needed for superficial tissues.

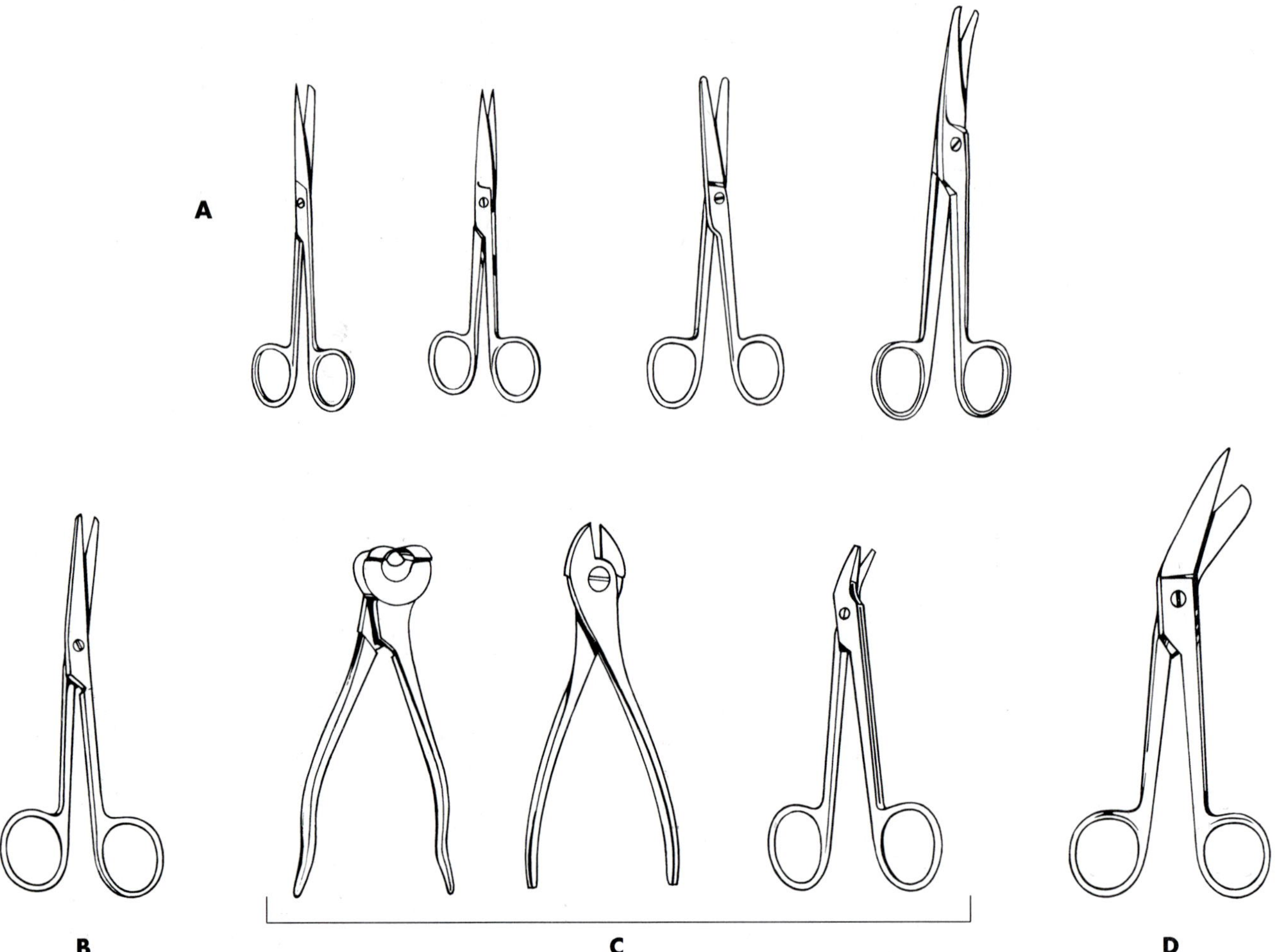

FIGURE 14-2 Scissors. **A,** Tissue/operating scissors. Blades may be pointed/blunt, pointed/pointed, or blunt/blunt, straight, or curved. **B,** Suture scissors. **C,** Wire cutters and scissors. **D,** Dressing/bandage scissors.

2. *Suture scissors* have blunt points to prevent cutting structures close to the suture being cut. The scrub person may use scissors to cut sutures during preparation if needed.
3. *Wire scissors* have short, heavy blades. Wire scissors are used instead of suture scissors to cut stainless steel sutures. Heavy wire cutters are used to cut bone fixation wires.
4. *Dressing/bandage scissors* are used to cut drains and dressings and to open items such as plastic packets.

Bone Cutters

Many types of instruments have cutting edges suitable for cutting into or through bone. These instruments include chisels, osteotomes, gouges, rasps, and files (see Figure 32-5, p. 660). Some have moving parts, such as rongeurs and rib cutters. Others are air or electric powered, such as drills, saws, and reamers.

Other Sharp Dissectors

Sharp dissection to cut tissue apart or to separate tissue layers may be accomplished with other types of sharp instruments.

Biopsy Forceps and Punches A small piece of tissue may be removed for pathologic examination with a biopsy forceps or punch. These instruments may be used through an endoscope.

Curettes Tissue or bone is removed by scraping with the sharp edge of the loop, ring, or scoop on the end of a curette.

Snares A loop of wire may be put around a pedicle to dissect tissue such as a tonsil. The wire cuts the pedicle as it retracts into the instrument. The wire is replaced after use.

Blunt Dissectors

Friable tissues or tissue planes can be separated by blunt dissection. The scalpel handle, blunt sides of tissue scissors blades, and dissecting sponges may be used for this purpose.

Grasping and Holding

Tissues should be grasped and held in position so the surgeon can perform the desired maneuver, such as dissecting or suturing, without injuring surrounding tissues.

Tissue Forceps

Forceps are used, often in pairs, to pick up or hold soft tissues and vessels (Figure 14-3).

Smooth Forceps Also referred to as *thumb forceps* or *pick ups,* smooth forceps resemble tweezers. They are tapered with serrations (grooves) at the tip. Smooth forceps will not injure delicate structures. They may be straight or bayonet (angled), short or long, and delicate or heavy.

Toothed Forceps Toothed forceps differ from smooth forceps at the tip. Rather than being serrated, they have a single tooth on one side that fits between two teeth on the opposing side or a row of multiple teeth at the tip. Toothed forceps provide a firm hold on tough tissues, including skin.

Allis Forceps An Allis forceps has a scissors action. Each jaw curves slightly inward with a row of teeth at the end. The teeth hold tissue gently but securely.

Babcock Forceps The end of each jaw of a Babcock forceps is rounded to fit around a structure or to grasp tissue without injury. This rounded section is fenestrated.

Forceps used to grasp and hold soft tissues and organs are too numerous to elaborate on further. The configuration of each is designed to prevent injury to tissues.

Stone Forceps

Either curved or straight forceps are used to grasp calculi such as kidney stones or gallstones. These forceps have blunt loops or cups at the end of the jaws.

Tenaculum

The curved or angled points on the ends of the jaws penetrate tissue to grasp firmly, such as when a uterine tenaculum is used to manipulate the uterus. Tenaculums may have a single tooth or multiple teeth.

Bone Holders

Grasping forceps, vice-grip pliers, and other types of heavy holding forceps stabilize bone.

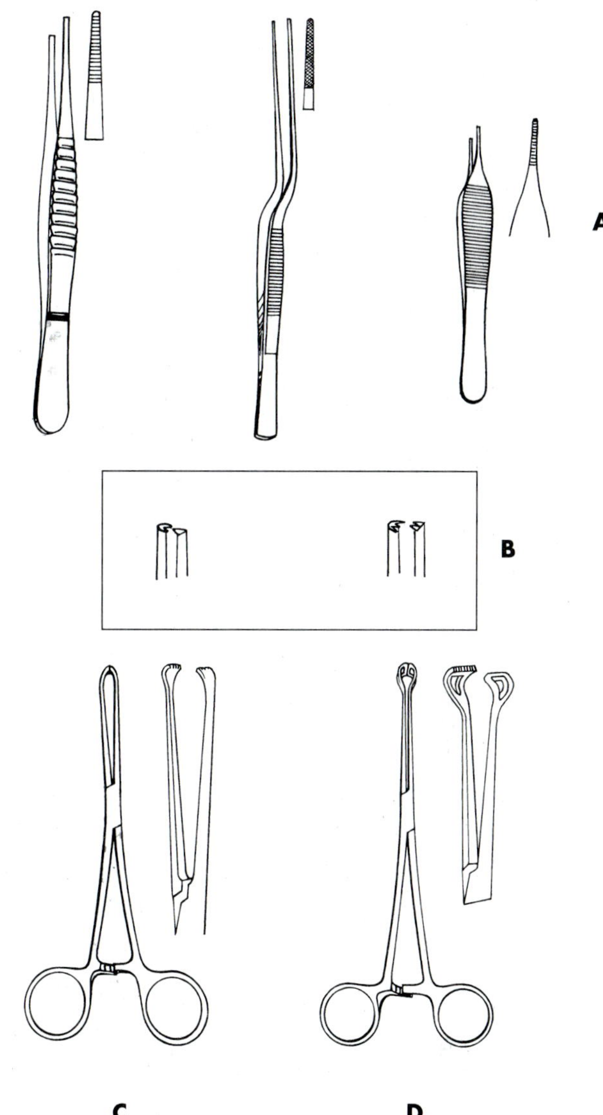

FIGURE 14-3 Tissue forceps. **A,** Smooth thumb forceps may be straight, bayonet, or short and delicate. **B,** Toothed forceps tips. **C,** Allis forceps. **D,** Babcock forceps.

Clamping and Occluding

Instruments that clamp and occlude are used to apply pressure.

Hemostatic Forceps

Most clamps for occluding blood vessels have two opposing serrated jaws that are stabilized by a box lock and controlled by ringed handles. When closed, the handles remain locked on rachets (Figure 14-4).

Hemostat Hemostats are the most commonly used surgical instruments. Hemostats have either straight or curved slender jaws that taper to a fine point. The serrations go across the jaws. Hemostats are used primarily to clamp blood vessels.

Crushing Clamps Many variations of hemostatic forceps are used to crush tissues or clamp blood vessels. The jaws may be straight, curved, or angled. The serrations may be horizontal, diagonal, or longitudinal. The tip may be pointed or rounded or have a tooth (Figure 14-5). The length of the jaws and handles vary. Many forceps are named for the surgeon who designed the style, such as the Kocher or Ochsner forceps. Some are designed to be used on specific organs, such as intestinal forceps or kidney forceps. The features of the instrument will determine its use. Fine points are needed for small vessels and structures. Longer and sturdier jaws are needed for larger vessels, dense structures, and thick tissue. Longer handles are needed to reach structures deep in body cavities.

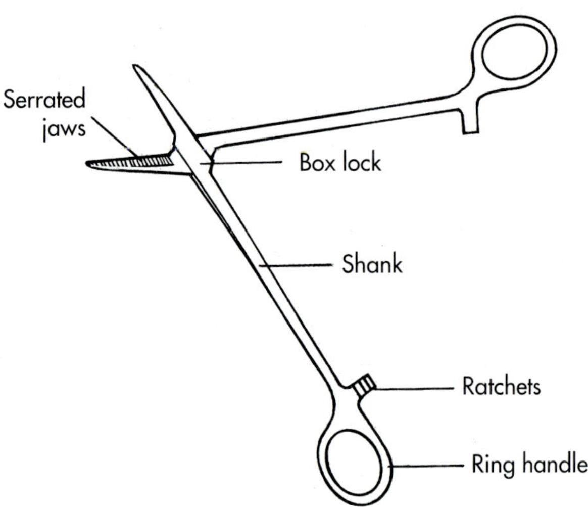

FIGURE 14-4 Hemostatic forceps.

Noncrushing Vascular Clamps

Used to occlude peripheral or major blood vessels *temporarily*, noncrushing clamps minimize tissue trauma. Their jaws have opposing rows of finely serrated teeth. The jaws may be straight, curved, angled, or S shaped.

Exposing and Retracting

Soft tissues, muscles, and other structures should be pulled aside for exposure of the surgical site.

Handheld Retractor

Most retractors have a blade on a handle (Figure 14-6). Blades vary in width and length to correspond with the size and depth of the incision. The curved or angled blade may be solid or pronged like a rake. These blades are usually dull, but some are sharp. Some retractors have blades at both ends rather than a handle on one end. Handheld retractors are usually used in pairs. They are held by the first or second assistant.

Malleable Retractor A flat length of low-carbon stainless steel, silver, or silver-plated copper may be bent to the desired angle and depth for retraction.

Hooks Single, very fine hooks with sharp points are used to retract delicate structures.

Self-Retaining Retractor

Holding devices with two or more blades can be inserted to spread edges of incision and hold them apart (Figure 14-7). A rib spreader, for example, holds the chest open during a thoracic or cardiac procedure. A self-retaining retractor may have shallow or deep

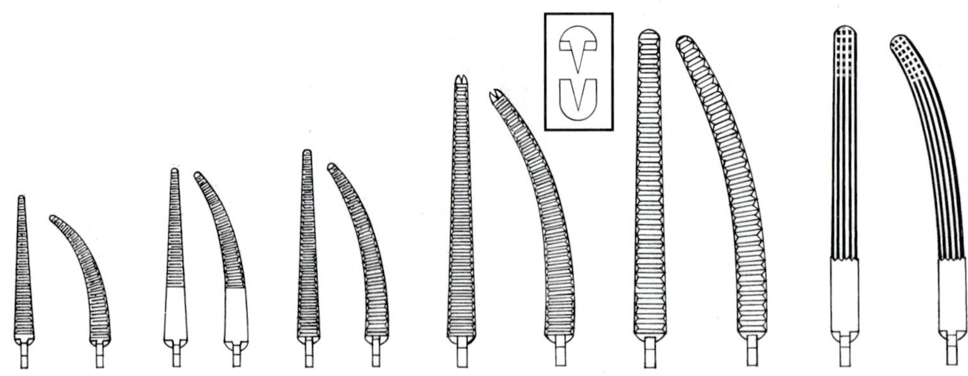

FIGURE 14-5 Crushing clamps. Jaws may be straight or curved. Tips may be pointed, rounded, or have a tooth *(inset)*. Serrations may be horizontal or longitudinal. Jaws and handles may be long or short.

blades. Some retractors have ratchets or spring locks to keep the device open; others have wing nuts to secure the blades. Some retractors have interchangeable blades of different sizes. Some self-retaining retractors can be attached to the operating table for stability.

Suturing or Stapling

Suture materials, surgical needles, and surgical staples are discussed in detail in Chapter 24. Only the instruments required for their placement are mentioned here.

Needleholder

A needleholder is used to grasp and hold curved surgical needles. Most needleholders resemble hemostatic forceps; the basic difference is the jaws (Figure 14-8). A needleholder has short, sturdy jaws for grasping a needle without damaging it or the suture material. The size of the needleholder should match the size of the needle, that is, heavy jaws for large needles and slim jaws for small needles. The jaws are usually straight, but they may be curved or angled and the handles may

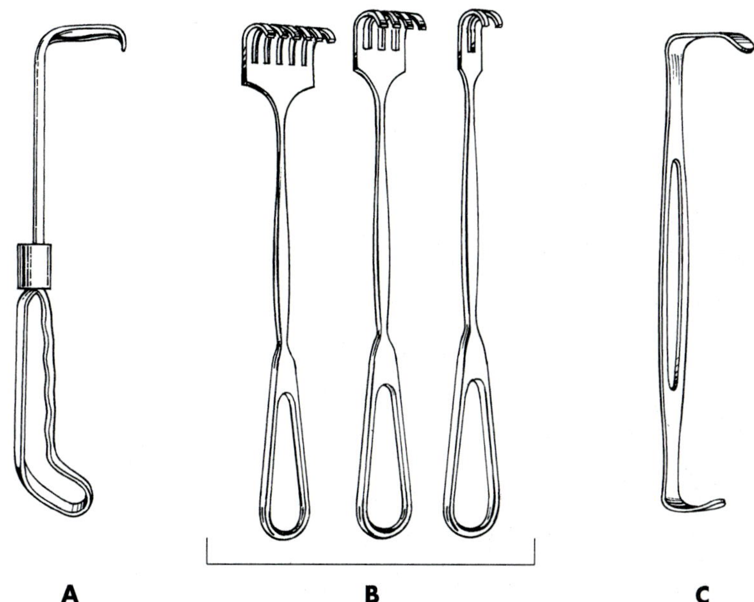

FIGURE 14-6 Handheld retractors. **A,** Solid blade. **B,** Pronged/rake. **C,** Double-ended.

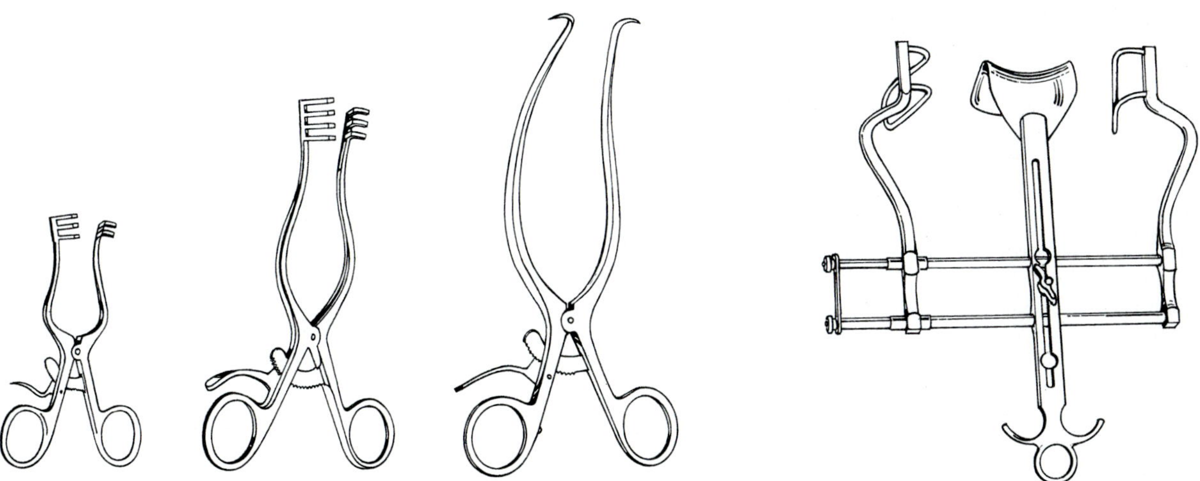

FIGURE 14-7 Self-retaining retractors.

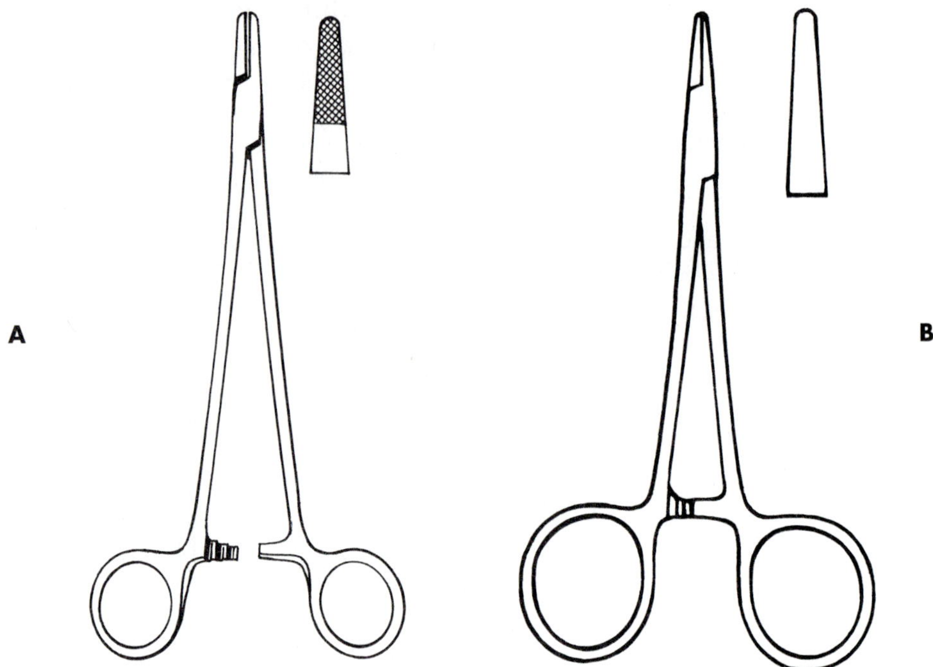

FIGURE 14-8 Needleholders. **A,** Crosshatched serrations on jaws. **B,** Smooth jaws.

be long to facilitate needle placement in surgical sites such as the pelvis or chest. The inside surfaces of the jaws may differ.

Tungsten Carbide Jaws Jaws with an insert of solid tungsten carbide with diamond-cut precision teeth are specifically designed to eliminate twisting and turning of the needle in the needleholder (Figure 14-9). Tungsten carbide is a hard metal. Diamond-jaw needleholders can be identified by the gold plating on the handles.

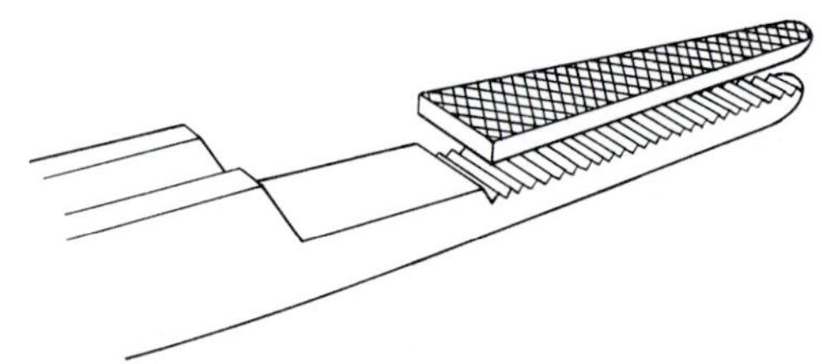

FIGURE 14-9 Tungsten carbide insert in jaws of needleholder, with diamond-cut teeth, is designed to eliminate needle twisting and turning.

Crosshatched Serrations The serrations on the inside surface of the jaws are crosshatched rather than grooved, as in a hemostat. This provides a smoother surface and prevents damage to the needle.

Smooth Jaws Some surgeons prefer needleholders that have jaws without serrations. These needleholders are used with small needles, such as those used for plastic surgery.

NOTE The fine jaws of ophthalmic and microsurgery needleholders may be either diamond-cut or crosshatched. However, the configuration of the handles is different. The jaws are squeezed together by a spring action (see Figure 15-9, p. 292).

Staplers

Reusable staplers have many moving parts. These staplers must be disassembled for cleaning and assembled at the sterile field before use. They are bulky, heavy instruments. Sterile, single-use, disposable staplers that are completely assembled eliminate the many problems associated with reusable instruments.

Viewing Instruments

Surgeons can examine the interior of body cavities, hollow organs, or structures with viewing instruments and can actually operate through some of them.

Speculum

The hinged, blunt blades of a speculum enlarge and hold open a canal, such as the vagina, or a cavity, such as the nose. An ear speculum is like a funnel.

Endoscopes

The round or oval sheath of an endoscope is inserted into a body orifice or through a small skin incision. Each scope is designed for viewing in a specific anatomic location. Endoscopes are discussed in detail in Chapter 15, pp. 279-285. Many accessory instruments are used through endoscopes. Endoscopic procedures are discussed by surgical specialty.

Hollow Endoscopes The rigid hollow metal sheath, made of either brass or stainless steel, permits viewing in a forward direction through the endoscope. A light carrier provides illumination.

Lensed Endoscopes Lensed endoscopes have either rigid or flexible sheaths with an eyepiece that has a telescopic lens system for viewing in several directions. Lensed instruments are complex and require careful handling to avoid damage.

Suctioning and Aspirating

Blood, body fluids, tissue, and irrigating solution may be removed by mechanical suction or manual aspiration. Reusable suction tips and aspiration devices have lumens that are difficult to terminally clean and sterilize. Many of these items are available in disposable models.

Suction

Suction is the application of pressure (less than atmospheric pressure) to withdraw blood or fluids, usually for visibility at the surgical site. An appropriate style tip is attached to sterile tubing; many tips are disposable. The style of the suction tip will depend on where it is to be used and the surgeon's preference (Figure 14-10).

Poole Abdominal Tip The Poole abdominal tip is a straight hollow tube with a perforated outer filter shield. It is used during abdominal laparotomy or within any cavity in which copious amounts of fluid or pus are encountered. The outer filter shield prevents the adjacent tissues from being pulled into the suction apparatus.

Frazier Tip The Frazier tip is a right-angle tube with a small diameter. It is used when little or no fluid except capillary bleeding and irrigating fluid is encountered, such as in brain, spinal, plastic, or orthopaedic procedures. The Frazier tip keeps the field dry without the need for sponging. One model has a connection for an electrosurgical unit, and the tip can be used for fulguration. A fiberoptic cable can be attached to another model.

Yankauer Tip The Yankauer tip is a hollow tube that has an angle for use in the mouth or throat.

Aspirating Tube An aspirating tube is a long, straight tube used through an endoscope.

Autotransfusion A double-lumen suction tip is used to remove blood for autotransfusion (see Chapter 23, p. 486).

Aspiration

Blood, body fluid, or tissue may be aspirated manually to obtain a specimen for laboratory examination or to obtain bone marrow for transplantation. This is frequently done with a needle and syringe.

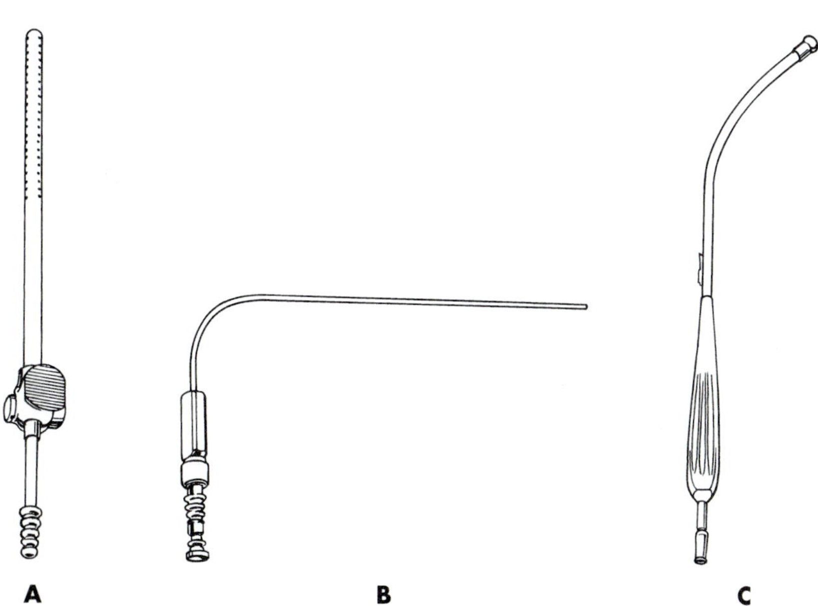

FIGURE 14-10 Tips of suction tubes. **A,** Poole abdominal tip. **B,** Frazier tip. **C,** Yankauer tip.

Trocar A trocar may be needed to cut through tissues for access to fluid or a body cavity. A trocar has sharp cutting edges at the end of a hollow tube. A cannula with a blunt end fits inside the trocar to keep fluid or gas from escaping until the cannula is removed. Endoscopic instruments may be manipulated through special trocars that have valves.

Cannula A cannula with a blunt end and perforations around the tip may be used to aspirate fluid without cutting into tissue. Cannulas also are used to open blocked vessels or ducts for drainage or to shunt blood flow from the surgical site.

Dilating and Probing

A dilator is used to enlarge orifices and ducts. A probe is used to explore a structure or to locate an obstruction.

Accessory Instruments

Many accessories are used in addition to the aforementioned basic instruments. For example, a mallet may be needed to drive a cutting instrument into bone. Screwdrivers are used, as the name implies, to affix screws in bone. Each surgical specialty has its own accessories. Many of these are described in the specialty chapters.

Of the thousands of instruments available, surgeons choose those that are most suitable to meet their particular needs. Differences in size, curvature, or angulation of jaws or blades, length of handles, weight, and shape can simplify, improve, and even shorten surgical time. This ultimately benefits the patient. Instruments should be maintained, however, to provide the specific function each was designed to do.

HANDLING OF INSTRUMENTS

Surgical instruments are expensive and represent a major investment. As surgical procedures have become more complicated and intricate, instruments have become more complex, more precise in design, and more delicate in structure. When abused, misused, or subjected to inadequate cleaning or rough handling, the life expectancy of even the most durable instrument is reduced. Cost of repair or replacement becomes unnecessarily high. With proper care an instrument should have a life of 10 years or more. Instruments do deteriorate from normal use. However, most damage and reduced life is caused by improper cleaning, processing, and handling.

Setting Up Instrument Table

Standardized basic sets of sterile instruments are selected for each specific surgical procedure. A *set* is a group of instruments that may include all appropriate classifications of instruments or the instruments needed for a specific part of the procedure, such as a gallbladder set. The assembly of sets is discussed later in this chapter (pp. 259-260). The surgeon may prefer some specific instruments that are wrapped separately or added to the instrument set.

Instruments are usually prepared, wrapped, and sterilized several hours before the surgical procedure so that they are dry and cool for safe handling. However, sometimes instruments must be steam sterilized immediately before use. They may be kept in an enclosed rigid container, or they may be sterilized in an unwrapped tray. *Uncovered, exposed instruments are never transported through corridors.* The sterilizer may be located in the substerile room or in the OR. The scrub person or the circulator may lift the tray from the sterilizer, depending on its physical location in relation to the OR. *The scrub person should not go beyond the confines of the room,* but this is the practice in some suites in which the sterilizer is immediately adjacent to the door of the substerile room. In lifting a tray from the sterilizer, the scrub person must not brush the sleeves or the front of his or her gown against the sterilizer. The circulator must not reach over the sterile instruments when lifting the tray or over the sterile table when placing it. These instruments are hot. Condensate must not contaminate the sterile table cover. The tray can be set on the large basin in the ring stand.

The scrub person counts all instruments and sharps with the circulator before setting up the Mayo stand and instrument table (see Chapter 20, p. 413). Key points in handling instruments include the following:

1. Handle loose instruments separately to prevent interlocking or crushing.
   a. Never pile one instrument on top of another on an instrument table; lay them side by side.
   b. Microsurgical, ophthalmic, and other delicate instruments are vulnerable to damage through rough handling.
   c. Metal-to-metal contact should be avoided or minimized.
2. Inspect instruments such as scissors and forceps, for alignment, imperfections, cleanliness, and working conditions.
   a. Blades must be properly set.
   b. Exact alignment of teeth and serrations is necessary.
   c. Set aside or remove any defective instrument.
3. Sort instruments neatly by classifications.
4. Keep ring-handled instruments together, with curvatures and angles pointed in the same direction.
   a. Hang ring handles over a rolled towel or over the edge of the instrument tray or container.
   b. Remove instrument pins or holders if used to keep box locks open.
   c. Close box locks on the *first* ratchet.

5. Leave retractors and other heavy instruments in a tray or container or lay them out on a flat surface of the table.
6. Protect sharp blades, edges, and tips. They should not touch anything.
   a. Sets of instruments, such as osteotomes or microsurgical instruments, may be in sterilization racks so that blades and tips are suspended. These instruments can remain in racks during the initial table setup and until they are needed during the surgical procedure.
   b. Tip-protecting covers or instrument-protecting plastic sleeves should be left on until the instruments are actually used.
   c. If they are not in a rack or tip guard, support handles on a rolled towel or gauze sponge to keep blades and tips of microinstruments suspended in midair.

During Surgical Procedure

Efficient instrument handling throughout the surgical procedure is the hallmark of an efficient scrub person.

1. Know the name and use of each instrument.
2. Handle instruments individually.
   a. If several instruments of the same type will be needed in rapid succession, such as hemostats to clamp subcutaneous vessels, three or four may be picked up at one time, but they are passed individually to the surgeon and/or assistant.
   b. Instruments with sharp edges and fine tips are more susceptible to damage than standard instruments. Edges are easily dulled and tips bent or broken.
   c. Extreme caution is necessary not to catch tips of microinstruments on any object that could bend them.
3. Hand the surgeon or assistant the correct instrument for each particular task. Remember the principle: *use for intended purpose only!*
   a. Avoid placing fingers in the instrument rings as the instrument is passed. The instrument may inadvertently drop or snag on drapes, causing an untoward injury to the patient or a team member. The instrument may fall to the floor, thus becoming damaged and contaminated.
   b. Many surgeons use hand signals to indicate the type of instrument needed. An understanding of what is taking place at the surgical site makes these signals meaningful.
   c. Select appropriate instruments for location of surgical site; short instruments will be used for superficial work, and long ones will be used for work deep in a body cavity. Experience will facilitate instrument selection according to the surgeon's preference and need.
   d. Many instruments are used in pairs or in sequence. When the surgeon clamps and/or cuts tissue, he or she will usually request suture. After using suture, the surgeon or assistant will need scissors to cut or a hemostat to hold the end of the strand.
4. Pass instruments decisively and firmly. When the surgeon extends his or her hand, the instrument should be slapped or placed firmly into his or her palm in the proper position for use. Generally, when passing a curved instrument, the curve of the instrument aligns with the direction of the curve of the surgeon's hand. In passing an instrument to the surgeon:
   a. If the surgeon is on the opposite side of the table, pass across right hand to right hand or with the left hand to a left-handed surgeon.
   b. If the surgeon or assistant is on the same side of the table and to the right, pass with your left hand; if the surgeon or assistant is to your left, pass with your right hand.
   c. Hemostatic forceps are held near the box lock by the scrub person and passed by rotating the wrist clockwise to place the handle directly into the surgeon's waiting hand (Figure 14-11).
   d. Sharp and delicate instruments may be placed on a flat surface for the surgeon to pick up. This technique avoids potential contact with items such as cutting blades, sharp points, and needles in hand-to-hand transfer. Always protect hands when manipulating sharp instruments.

   NOTE Some surgeons prefer to have all instruments placed on a magnetic pad or other flat surface to avoid hand-to-hand transfers (i.e., a free-hand technique).

5. Watch the sterile field for loose instruments. Remove them promptly after use to the Mayo stand or instrument table. The weight of instruments can injure the patient or cause postoperative discomfort. Keeping instruments off the field also decreases the possibility of their falling to the floor.
6. Wipe blood and organic debris off instruments *promptly after each use* with a moist sponge.
   a. Demineralized sterile distilled water should be used to wipe instruments. Saline or other solution can damage surfaces, causing corrosion and ultimately pitting.
   b. Blood and debris allowed to dry on surfaces, in box locks, and in crevices increase bioburden that could be carried into the surgical site.
   c. A nonfibrous sponge should be used to wipe off microsurgical, ophthalmic, and other delicate tips. This type of sponge prevents snagging and breaking of delicate tips. Commercial microsurgical instrument wipes are available.

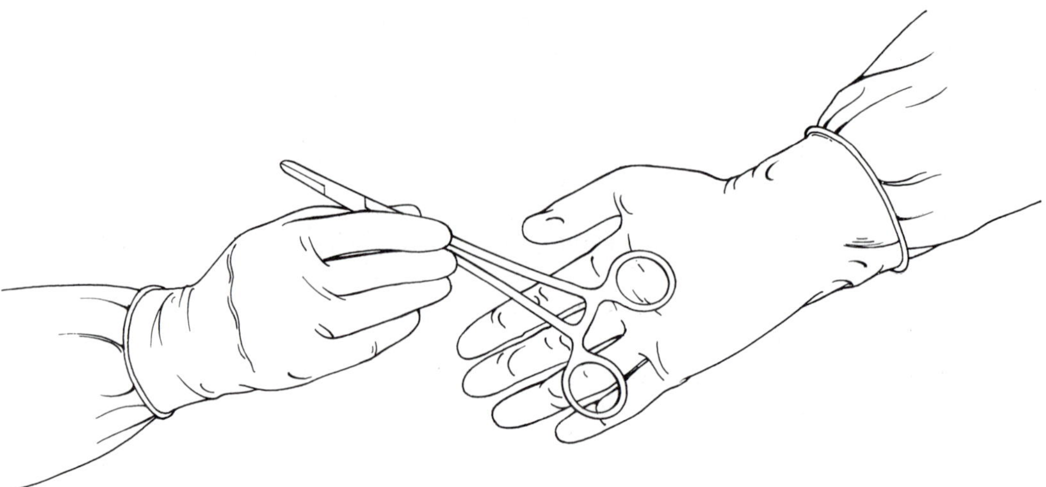

FIGURE 14-11 Passing an instrument. Tip is visible; hand is free. Handle is placed directly into waiting hand.

7. Flush the suction tip and tubing with sterile distilled water periodically to keep the lumens patent. Use only a few milliliters of solution if using irrigating fluids from the surgical field. Keep a tally of the amount used to clear the suction line and deduct this amount from the total used to irrigate the surgical site. Accurate accounting of the solutions used for patient irrigation is necessary when determining blood loss from the surgical procedure.
8. Remove debris from electrosurgical tips to ensure electrical contact. Disposable abrasive tip cleaners are helpful for maintaining the conductivity and effectiveness of the surface of the tip. Avoid using a scalpel blade to clean electrosurgical tips because the debris may become airborne and contaminate the surgical field.
9. Place used instruments not needed again (*except cutting, delicate, or powered ones)* into a tray or basin during or at the end of the surgical procedure.
   a. Blood and gross debris must be removed first.
   b. *Careless dropping, tossing, or throwing of instruments into a basin is absolutely prohibited.*
   c. Bloody instruments should not soak in a basin of solution for a prolonged period. Blood can damage surfaces. Instruments that have been wiped can be immersed in a basin of sterile demineralized distilled water, *not saline solution.* The sodium chloride in saline solution and blood is corrosive.
   d. Heavy instruments such as retractors should not be placed on top of tissue and hemostatic forceps and other clamps. Place them in a separate tray.
   e. Keep instruments accessible for final counts.

Dismantling Instrument Table

All instruments on the instrument table, *used and unused,* are considered contaminated. They must be promptly and properly decontaminated/cleaned, inspected, terminally sterilized, and prepared for subsequent use. Wearing gloves, gown, mask, and protective eyewear, the scrub person prepares instruments for the cleaning process. Instruments are cleaned in a designated instrument processing area, not in the OR.

1. Check drapes, towels, and table covers to be sure that instruments do not go to the laundry or into the trash. A final quick count is a safeguard.
2. Collect instruments from the Mayo stand and any other small tables, and collect those that may have been dropped or passed off the sterile field.
3. Separate delicate, small instruments and those with sharp or semisharp edges for special handling.
4. Disassemble all instruments with removable parts to expose all surfaces for cleaning.
5. Open all hinged instruments to expose box locks and serrations.
6. Separate instruments of dissimilar metals. Instruments of each type of metal should be cleaned separately to prevent electrolytic deposition of other metals.
7. Flush cold distilled water through hollow instruments or channels, such as suction tips or endoscopes, to prevent drying of organic debris.
8. Rinse off blood and debris with demineralized distilled water or an enzymatic detergent solution.
9. Follow procedure for preparing each instrument for decontamination or terminal sterilization. Procedures vary depending on the type of instrument

and its components and the equipment available and its location. Decontamination includes mechanical cleaning and a physical or chemical biocidal process to make instruments safe for handling. This is done in a designated area, not in the OR, immediately after completion of the surgical procedure.

CLEANING

The decontamination process includes prerinsing, washing, rinsing, and sterilizing. Instruments may be prerinsed or presoaked and then cleaned manually or mechanically.

Prerinsing/Presoaking

The purpose of prerinsing or presoaking is to prevent blood and debris from drying on instruments or to soften and remove dried blood and debris. The circulator can prepare a basin of solution for the scrub person. For a *short* immersion period, instruments may be presoaked in the following:

1. Dual proteolytic enzymatic detergent. Proteolytic enzymes dissolve blood and debris, and the detergent removes dissolved particulate from surfaces of the instruments, including otherwise inaccessible areas such as lumens.
2. An enzymatic agent diluted per manufacturer's instructions.
3. Water with a low-sudsing, near-neutral detergent. The detergent should be compatible with the local water supply.
4. Plain, clean, demineralized distilled water.
5. Noncorrosive detergent-disinfectant. Sodium hypochlorite (bleach) is corrosive. Instruments should *not* be soaked in any chlorine compound. Soaking in an iodophor should not exceed 1 hour. A phenolic or quaternary ammonium product with corrosion inhibitors is most suitable.

Instruments can be transported to the decontamination area in the soak basin or washer-sterilizer tray. The basin or tray should be enclosed in a plastic bag to keep the instruments moist and to contain contamination. Prerinsing or presoaking in the OR can make further processing more efficient.

Manual Cleaning

Even if a washer-sterilizer or decontaminator is available, some precleaning of instruments is necessary to remove gross debris. If a washer-sterilizer is not available, instruments must be washed by hand. Delicate and sharp instruments should be handled separately. Microsurgical and ophthalmic instruments should be cleaned and dried by hand; they are never put in a washer-sterilizer. These instruments should not remain wet for long periods of time because moisture is conducive to corrosion. Some complex instruments require disassembly and precleaning before being put in a washer-sterilizer. Others require special care. For example, the outside surfaces of powered instruments must be cleaned, but these instruments cannot be immersed in liquid.

Instruments may be prerinsed in the OR by the scrub person; however, they should not be cleaned in scrub sinks or utility sinks in the substerile room. They may be covered and taken to a decontamination area in the OR suite or returned to sterile processing on the case cart. Personnel in these latter areas must wear protective gloves, waterproof aprons, and face shields to prevent accidental spray from contaminated solutions.

The purpose of manual cleaning is to remove residual blood and debris before terminal sterilization or high-level disinfection. The following steps should be followed to clean instruments manually:

1. Obtain clean, warm water to which a noncorrosive, low-sudsing, free-rinsing detergent has been added.
   a. Detergent should be compatible with the local water supply. Mineral content varies from one area to another. A water softener may be used in the system routinely to minimize mineral deposits. Regardless of the water content, the detergent should be anionic or nonionic and have a pH as close to neutral as possible. Alkaline detergent (pH over 8.5) will stain instruments; acid (pH below 6) will corrode or pit them.
   b. Proteolytic enzymatic detergents dissolve blood and protein and remove dissolved debris from crevices. These detergents are effective in a wide range of water qualities.
   c. Liquid detergents are preferable because they disperse more completely than solids. Always dilute the concentration before contact with instruments to avoid corrosion and staining. Do not pour liquid or put solid detergents directly on instruments.
2. Wash instruments carefully to guard against splashing and creating aerosols.
   a. Use a soft brush to clean serrations and box locks. A soft-bristled toothbrush may be used to clean ophthalmic, microsurgical, and other delicate instruments. Keep instruments submerged while brushing to minimize aerosolizing microorganisms.
   b. Use a soft cloth to wipe surfaces. A nonfibrous cellulose sponge will prevent damage to delicate tips.
   c. Remove bone, tissue, and other debris from cutting instruments.
   d. *Never* scrub surfaces with abrasive agents such as steel wool, wire brushes, scouring pads, or

powders. These agents will scratch and may remove the protective finish on metal, thus increasing the likelihood of corrosion. The finish on stainless steel instruments protects the base metal from oxidation.
3. Rinse instruments thoroughly in hot distilled or deionized water. Inadequate rinsing can leave residue on surfaces that can stain instruments.
4. Load instruments into appropriate trays for terminal sterilization or into containers for high-level disinfection.
   a. Put instruments back into sterilization racks or replace protective guards as appropriate.
   b. Arrange instruments that can be steam sterilized in sterilizer trays for the washer-sterilizer or decontaminator. The tray may be steam sterilized unwrapped or enclosed in a steam-penetrable plastic bag.

      NOTE Hand-washed stainless steel instruments may be placed into a solid basin, covered with a 2% solution of trisodium phosphate, and steam sterilized for 45 minutes at 250° F (121° C).

   c. Lensed instruments that are heat-sensitive are immersed in high-level disinfectant after manual cleaning, unless an automatic cleaning and disinfecting machine is available.
   d. Manufacturers' instructions should be followed for the proper cleaning and sterilizing of powered instruments, which are discussed later in this chapter (see p. 263).

Washer-Sterilizer or Washer-Decontaminator

Mechanical cleaning and automated decontamination can be accomplished in a washer-sterilizer or washer-decontaminator. However, gross debris must be removed before instruments are put in these machines.

The function of the washer-sterilizer is described in Chapter 13 (see pp. 214-215). A washer-decontaminator cleans by impingement, a spray-force action. It is similar to the washer-sterilizer in that the cycle includes a cold water prerinse to dissolve blood and protein, a detergent wash, rinse, and finally steam and heat. Unlike the washer-sterilizer, detergent solution enters under pressure through fixed or rotating arms for the wash cycle. Deionized or softened water is used for the rinse cycle to remove detergent residues. The final cycle includes drying with heated air. These automated thermal units are capable of consistent cleaning and disinfection. A single cycle in a washer-sterilizer or decontaminator does not prepare instruments for immediate use, however.

Instruments should be arranged in perforated trays for processing in the washer-sterilizer or washer-decontaminator.

1. Place heavy instruments in a separate tray or in the bottom of a tray with smaller, lightweight instruments on top.
2. Turn instruments with concave surfaces, such as curettes and rongeurs, with the bowl side down to facilitate drainage of the concave surface. Be certain that bone and tissue is removed from these surfaces.
3. Open box locks and pivots of hinged instruments to expose maximum surface area.
4. Disassemble instruments that can be disassembled without tools.
5. Sharp or pointed instruments should be carefully positioned on top of other instruments to prevent contacts that could damage cutting edges or surfaces of other instruments. An alternative would be to either place sharp instruments in a separate tray or sterilize them after manual cleaning. Fine, delicate instruments should never be put in a washer-sterilizer or decontaminator because the mechanical agitation will damage them.
6. *Always arrange instruments neatly.* They should not be randomly piled on top of one another.

If the washer-sterilizer or washer-decontaminator is not located in an immediately adjacent room, the scrub person, with assistance from the circulator, encloses trays in plastic bags for transport to the decontamination area. The outside of the bags should remain clean.

An indexed washer-decontaminator has several chambers. The instrument tray automatically passes from chamber to chamber, that is, is indexed for the prerinse, ultrasonic cleaning, wash, rinse and lubrication, and drying cycles. The multiple chambers can process several trays simultaneously.

Ultrasonic Cleaning

Surgical instruments vary in configuration from plane surfaces, which respond to most types of cleaning, to complicated devices that contain box locks, serrations, blind holes, and interstices that are difficult to clean. Ultrasonic energy, using high-frequency sound waves, thoroughly cleans by a process of cavitation. These sound waves generate tiny bubbles in the solution in the *ultrasonic cleaner.* The bubbles expand until they are unstable and then collapse. The *implosion* (exact opposite of explosion) of these bubbles generates minute vacuum areas that dislodge, dissolve, or disperse soil. These bubbles are small enough to get into the serrations, box locks, and crevices of instruments that are impossible to clean by other methods.

Instruments should be completely immersed in cleaning solution. The tank should be filled to a level of 1 inch (2.5 cm) above the top of the instrument tray. Suitable detergent, as specified by the manufacturer, is added. The temperature of the water should be 100° to 140° F (37.7° to 60° C) to enhance the effectiveness of the detergent, but it should not coagulate protein on instruments. Instrument trays should be designed for maximum transmission of sonic energy. An important relationship exists between wire gauge, opening size, and sonic frequency. A large mesh of small wire size transmits more energy than heavy wire with narrow spacing.

Solution is degassed by turning on the ultrasonic energy. Gas, present in most tap water, impedes the transmission of sonic energy. An electric generator supplies electrical energy to a transducer. The transducer converts the electrical energy into mechanical energy in the form of vibrating sound waves that are not audible to the human ear because they are of such high frequency. If excess gas is present, it prevents the cleaning process from being fully effective because the cavitation bubbles fill with gas and the energy released during implosion is reduced. Tap water should be degassed for 5 minutes or longer each time it is changed. Solution should be changed or filtered at least once per shift or whenever the detergent solution is visibly soiled. The inside of the tank should be cleaned between fillings.

An ultrasonic cleaner is not a sterilizer. Instruments must be cleaned initially and terminally sterilized *before* immersion in the ultrasonic cleaner. Most surgical instruments, including ophthalmic instruments, microinstruments, glassware, rubber goods, and thermoplastics, can be definitively cleaned by this method to remove the tiniest particles of debris from crevices. The manufacturer's instructions must be carefully followed. In general, these include the following:

1. Arrange instruments as for sterilization, with heavy instruments at the bottom of the tray and lightweight instruments on top.
2. Open box locks and pivots of hinged instruments. Leave the parts disassembled as appropriate.
3. Protect cutting edges from other instruments. Fine, delicate microsurgical and ophthalmic instruments may be damaged by vibrations or contact with each other. Some small units may be suitable for delicate instruments.
4. Separate dissimilar metals. Do not mix stainless steel instruments with other metals. Electrolysis with resultant etching may occur.
5. Do *not* clean plated instruments in an ultrasonic cleaner. Cavitation will accelerate rupture and flaking of plating.
6. Rinse instruments thoroughly in hot demineralized water after the cleaning cycle to remove surface debris and detergent residue.
7. Dry instruments promptly and completely before reassembling or storing. Instruments will corrode if they are stored with trapped moisture.

Lubricating

After they are cleaned, all instruments with moving parts should be lubricated. This is particularly important following ultrasonic cleaning because the sonic energy removes all lubricant. Instruments are immersed in an antimicrobial, *water-soluble* lubricant that is steam penetrable. Its antimicrobial properties help prevent microbial growth in a lubricant bath that can be reused for up to 7 days. A water-soluble lubricant deposits a thin film deep in box locks, hinges, and crevices but will not interfere with sterilization. Some lubricants also contain a rust inhibitor to prevent electrolytic mineral deposits.

Use a lubricant according to manufacturer's instructions for dilution, effectiveness, and exposure. To use most lubricants, instruments are completely immersed for 30 to 45 seconds, that is, dipped and then allowed to drain dry. The solution is *not* rinsed or wiped off; any excess solution can be shaken off. The thin film will evaporate during steam sterilization.

NOTE

1. Mineral oil, silicones, and machine oils are *never* used to lubricate instruments because they leave a residue that interferes with steam or ethylene oxide sterilization. Oiling any surgical instrument is a break in technique.
2. Manufacturer's instructions for lubricating an instrument must be followed to keep the instrument in good working condition.

INSPECTING AND TESTING

Each instrument must be critically inspected after each cleaning. Instruments with movable parts should be inspected and tested following lubrication. Each instrument should be completely clean to ensure effective sterilization and inspected for proper function.

1. Check hinged instruments for stiffness. Box locks and joints should work smoothly. Stiff joints are usually caused by inadequate cleaning. Lubrication eases stiffness temporarily. If box locks are frozen, leave the instruments in a water-soluble lubricant bath overnight, and then gently work the jaws back and forth. Reinspect for cleanliness.
2. Test forceps for alignment. A forceps that is out of alignment can break during use. Close the jaws of the forceps slightly; if they overlap, they are out of alignment. Teeth of forceps with serrated jaws should mesh perfectly. Hold the shanks in each hand with the forceps open and try to wiggle them. If the box lock has considerable play or is very loose, the forceps will not hold tissue securely. If a surgeon continues to use it, jaw misalignment will occur and the forceps' effectiveness is impaired.

3. Check the ratchet teeth. Ratchets should close easily and hold firmly. Clamp the forceps on the first tooth only. Hold the instrument at the box lock and tap the ratchet teeth lightly against a solid object. If the forceps springs open, it is faulty and should be repaired. Ratchet teeth are subject to friction and metal-to-metal wear by the constant strain of closing and opening. A forceps that will spring open when clamped on a blood vessel or duct is hazardous to the patient and an annoyance to the surgeon. The ratchets must hold.
4. Check the tension between the shanks. When the jaws touch, a clearance of $\frac{1}{16}$ to $\frac{1}{8}$ inch (1.5 to 3 mm) should be visible between the ratchet teeth of each shank. This clearance provides adequate tension at the jaws when closed.
5. Test needleholders for needle security. Clamp an appropriately sized needle in the jaws of the needleholder and lock on the second ratchet tooth. If the needle can be turned easily by hand, the needleholder needs repair.
6. Test scissors for correctly ground and properly set blades. The blades should cut on the tips and glide over each other smoothly. Cut tissue/operating scissors through four layers of gauze at the tip of the blades, through two layers if the scissors are less than 4 inches (10 cm) in length. They should cut with a fine, smooth feel and a minimum of pressure.
7. Inspect edges of sharp and semisharp instruments such as chisels, osteotomes, rongeurs, and adenotomes for sharpness, chips or dents, and alignment.
8. Test the penetration of cataract knives, keratomes, and other fine cutting instruments on a small kidskin drum. Slide the blade by gravity through the kidskin with the handle resting on the palm of your hand. The blade should penetrate the drum as though it were passing through butter; it should not stick or tear.
9. Inspect microsurgical instruments under a magnifying glass or microscope to detect burrs on tips and nicks on cutting edges and to check alignment. Exact alignment of teeth on fine-toothed forceps is an absolute necessity. Microscopic teeth are very easily bent. Be certain that instruments are thoroughly dry. A chamois is useful for drying to prevent snagging delicate tips.
10. Checks pins and screws to be sure that they are secure and intact. They can become loose or fall out during ultrasonic cleaning as a result of vibration.
11. Check plated instruments for chips, sharp edges, and worn spots. Chipped plating may harbor debris. Sharp edges will damage tissue or tear gloves. Worn spots will corrode.
12. Flatten or straighten malleable instruments such as retractors and probes.
13. Demagnetize instruments by passing them back through a magnetic field. Instruments can become magnetized, although this is a rare occurrence.

Return unclean instruments to the cleaning area for ultrasonic cleaning. Remove instruments in poor working condition from the processing area. A place is usually designated in the OR suite or in the central service department for collection of instruments for repair. Do not allow a defective instrument to remain in circulation.

New instruments may be marked for identification of ownership before they are put in circulation. They can be imprinted with an electro-etch device. A vibrating or impact-type marking tool breaks the finish on the instrument and can cause hairline cracks. Electro-etching should be done on the shank rather than on the box lock to prevent it from fracturing. Some manufacturers will imprint identification when their instruments are purchased.

Some facilities affix colored tapes to instruments to differentiate them by sets or specialty. These tapes must withstand cleaning and sterilizing without peeling. They must be replaced if they loosen. The presence of marking tape allows debris to accumulate in the folds.

Instruments that will be stored for a period of time before they are packaged and sterilized must be thoroughly dry. Trapped moisture in hinges, box locks, serrations, and crevices will cause corrosion and rust. Stains or spots can appear on surfaces.

PACKAGING AND STERILIZING

To be effective the sterilizing agent must come in direct contact with all surfaces of every instrument. Therefore instruments must be packaged, individually or in sets, to allow adequate exposure to sterilant, to prevent air from being trapped and moisture from being retained during the sterilization process, and to ensure sterile transfer to the sterile field.

The majority of surgical instruments are made of stainless steel and can be sterilized by steam under pressure. This discussion is limited to steam sterilization. Other methods of sterilization for heat- and moisture-sensitive items, including some instruments, are discussed in Chapter 13. Instruments should be steam sterilized when possible.

Effective steam sterilization involves direct contact of *all* surfaces with steam and revaporization of water condensate to produce a dry, sterile instrument. Retained moisture can cause corrosion that inhibits future sterilization of an instrument. A dry, sterile instrument set depends on distribution of weight, density of instruments, and their design.

Instrument Packaging

Instruments are put in a container or tray, or wrapped in a small set or individually, for sterilizing and transporting. Instruments may be sterilized unwrapped immediately before use in a high-speed pressure sterilizer, they may be prepared in advance as for a case cart, or they may be retained in storage until needed. The type of containment will depend on these variables to maintain sterility.

Rigid Containers

Metal or plastic containers provide the outermost enclosure for a set of instruments. The instruments are contained in a removable wire mesh tray or basket that can be lifted out of the rigid container. Air is evacuated from and steam enters into the container through filtered perforations or vents. The bottom of the container may be solid with perforations in the top or side vents along the top for sterilization *only* in porous load cycles of a pulsing prevacuum sterilizer. For sterilization in a gravity displacement sterilizer, the container must have perforations in the top and bottom to allow air removal, steam penetration, and drying of contents.

Filter(s) on the inside cover the perforations. If disposable, these are changed after each use. The filter may have a chemical sterilization indicator in it. A textile or nonwoven liner may be necessary to absorb condensate from the instruments. However, this is not recommended for containers with valves. Containers may have sealing gaskets, locking devices, identification tags, and other accessories. Rigid containers ensure sterility if instruments are properly cleaned and loaded, the correct container is used in each type of sterilizer, and other sterilizing conditions are met. Sterility will be maintained during transport and storage.

Rigid containers usually have a locking mechanism on the lid latches to ensure the integrity of the seal. The locking mechanism is secured with a tamper-proof tag that is applied before the sterilization process. During sterilization the tag shrinks, creating a tight band around the latch. Many varieties of tamper-proof tags have chemical sterilization indicators imbedded on the surface. The tag serves as a break-away lock. An intact tag is reasonable proof that the container has not been opened.

To open a rigid container, detach the tamper-proof tag by pulling the latch to the open position, lift the lid straight up, and then tilt it back toward self. The scrub person lifts the inner tray out by handles on the ends of the tray. If an inner wrapper is packaged between the tray and container, the scrub person opens the wrapper to cover the container and the table. Clips may be provided to hold this drape in place at the corners of the container.

Rigid containers designed specifically for high-pressure flash sterilization are also available. These containers provide enclosed protection during transport and transfer to the sterile field. They must be used according to manufacturer's instructions (e.g., whether to keep the lid open or closed during sterilization).

Wrapped Trays

Instruments are placed in open trays with mesh or perforated bottoms. To allow steam penetration around instruments and to prevent air from being trapped in the tray, trays cannot be solid. Absorbent towels or foam may be placed in the bottom and over instruments to absorb condensate and to protect instruments from snagging in the perforations. Trays are sequentially double-wrapped in woven or nonwoven wrappers. They must be allowed to cool and dry at the end of the sterilizing cycle before they are handled.

Prepackaged Instruments

A single instrument or a small set of instruments may be sequentially double-wrapped in a woven or nonwoven wrapper. A single instrument may also be put in a peel-pouch. Because a hinged instrument must be open during sterilization, wrapping must ensure sterile transfer without contamination or damage to the instrument. A double pouch usually contains disassembled parts. Instruments should *never* be tossed onto a sterile table. The circulator presents them to the scrub person.

Some presterilized disposable instruments, such as staplers, are contained in sealed trays. The circulator peels back the cover for presentation to the scrub person.

The manufacturer may supply a fitted case or rack for a set of instruments or implants, such as orthopaedic devices. These cases or racks help protect the instruments and keep them separated for sterilization and use. These cases or racks must be wrapped before sterilization; they are not rigid containers, as described previously.

Assembly of Instrument Sets

The weight of instruments and density of metal mass must be distributed in the tray to allow steam penetration for sterilizing and revaporization for drying. A large tray distributes instruments so they make minimum contact with one another. The size, design, and density of instruments are more important than their weight. However, conditions necessary for steam sterilization are difficult to achieve in exceedingly heavy sets. Trays should not be overloaded. To assemble, perform the following steps:

1. Make sure instruments are thoroughly dry.
2. Place an absorbent towel or foam in the bottom of the tray to absorb condensate, unless contraindicated, as for a rigid container with vacuum valves.

3. Count instruments as they are placed in the tray and record the number of each type. A preprinted form is often used for this purpose. The form may accompany the tray to the OR for the circulator to verify the count, or it may remain in the processing area to verify that all instruments have been returned.
4. Arrange the instruments in a definite pattern to protect them from damage and to facilitate their removal for counting and use. Follow the instrument book or other listing of instruments to be included.
5. Place heavy instruments, such as retractors, in the bottom of the tray.
6. Open hinges and box locks on *all* hinged instruments.
7. Place ring-handled instruments on pins or holders designed for this purpose. Curved jaws of hemostatic forceps and clamps should be pointing in the same direction. Instruments should be grouped together by style and classification, for example, six straight hemostats, six curved hemostats. Do not band instruments together with rubber bands. Steam cannot penetrate through or under bands to make contact with instrument surfaces.
8. Place sharp and delicate instruments on top of other instruments. They can be separated with an absorbent material or left in a sterilizing rack with blades and tips suspended. Blades of scissors, other cutting edges, and delicate tips should not touch other instruments. If the instrument has a protective guard, leave it on. Tip-protecting covers or instrument-protecting plastic sleeves must be made of material that does not melt or deform with heat and is steam permeable.
9. Place concave or cupped instruments with these surfaces down so that water condensate does not collect in them during sterilization and drying.
10. Disassemble all detachable parts. Some parts, such as screws, can be put in a pouch that is left open.
11. Separate dissimilar metals. For example, brass knife handles and malleable retractors should be separated from stainless steel instruments. Preferably, put each metal in a separate tray or separate metals with absorbent material.
12. Place instruments with a lumen, such as a suction tip, in as near a horizontal position as possible. These instruments should be tilted as little as possible to prevent pooling of water condensate.
13. Distribute weight as evenly as possible in the tray. Some trays have dividers, clips, and pins that attach to the bottom, which help prevent instruments from shifting and keep them in alignment.
14. Wrap the tray or place it in a rigid container. Check woven textile wrappers for holes or abrasion. Sequentially double wrap in woven or nonwoven material.
15. Place a chemical indicator on the outside wrapper or container. Optionally, an indicator may also be placed inside the tray.
16. Label appropriately for intended use, for example, basic set, the date sterilized, and the control number.

Steam Sterilization

Because sterilizers vary in configuration, size, and performance, the sterilizer manufacturer's written instructions should be followed for the specific sterilizer used to sterilize instrument sets. If a rigid container system is used, the manufacturer should provide written instructions and supportive scientific data for maximum weight, assembly, sterilizer loading procedures, exposure times, and drying. In general, the most common time and temperature parameters for wrapped instrument sets are as follows:

1. In a gravity displacement steam sterilizer, a 30-minute exposure time at 250° F (121° C).
2. In a prevacuum steam sterilizer, a 4-minute exposure time at 270° to 275° F (132° to 135° C).
3. High-speed pressure (flash) steam sterilizers are not recommended for wrapped instrument sets. In an emergency, *unwrapped* sets of metal instruments can be sterilized at 270° F (132° C) for 3 minutes in a gravity displacement or prevacuum sterilizer if the load does not contain items with lumens or porous material. For sets with these items, exposure time is extended to 10 minutes in a gravity displacement sterilizer or 4 minutes in a prevacuum sterilizer.

Loading Sterilizer

Rigid containers are loaded flat on the sterilizer rack and can be stacked one on top of another. Wrapped trays with mesh bottoms can be loaded flat but should not be stacked in the gravity displacement sterilizer. The chamber must not be overloaded. Air and steam must circulate. If porous items are in the load, the instrument sets should be on the bottom shelf to prevent condensate from dripping on porous packages during the drying cycle. Preheating instruments by allowing them to sit in the chamber before the cycle is started will help minimize condensation.

Drying

Wrapped instrument sets must dry and cool before the sterilizer door is opened. Drying can take 20 to 25 minutes. After removal from the sterilizer, they should be allowed to cool for another 30 minutes before they are handled.

REPAIRING OR RESTORING VS. REPLACING INSTRUMENTS

Instruments in poor working condition are a handicap to the surgeon and a hazard for the patient. Instruments should be repaired at first sign of damage or malfunction.

Repair

Even with normal usage, over time the blades of scissors and the edges of other cutting instruments will become dull just as kitchen knives do at home. Cutting instruments must be sharp. For this reason, many blades are disposed of after a single patient use. Osteotomes, chisels, gouges, and meniscitomes can be sharpened by OR personnel with handheld hones or a honing machine designed for this purpose. Most manufacturers provide a service for sharpening and repairing instruments. Scissors, curettes, rongeurs, and reamers should be returned to them for sharpening. Small drill bits and saw blades usually are discarded when dull.

Misalignment of hinged instruments is a common problem primarily as a result of misuse. The instrument must be repaired if the teeth or serrations do not mesh perfectly or the jaws overlap.

Stiff joints or frozen box locks are the result of inadequate cleaning or corrosion caused by trapped moisture. The instrument should be repaired before the box lock cracks and the instrument must be replaced.

Parts such as screws or springs may need to be replaced. Worn or loose inserts can be replaced. The life of many instruments can be extended by preventive maintenance or prompt repair. After repeated use, instruments will eventually wear, misalign, and stiffen.

Restoration

Instruments may become spotted, stained, corroded, pitted, or rusted. Some surface discoloration will appear with normal usage. Unusual or severe buildup of deposits may impair function or sterilization. The color of a stain may help identify a problem that needs to be corrected.

1. Light or dark water spots: from mineral content in tap water or condensate in sterilizer caused by inadequate drying
2. Rust-colored film: from iron content or softening agents in steam pipes
3. Bluish-gray stain: from some chemical sterilizing or disinfecting solutions
4. Brownish stain: from polyphosphate cleaning compounds that are incompatible with local water supply, leaving a chromic oxide film on instruments
5. Purplish-black stain: from detergents that contain ammonia or from amines in steam lines
6. Rust deposits: from inadequate cleaning or drying, from agents not thoroughly rinsed off, from electrolytic deposits from exposed metal under chipped chrome plating onto stainless steel, or from residues in textile wrappers

Blood, saline solution, or detergents that contain chloride can cause pitting if they are not thoroughly and promptly rinsed off. Detergents with high or low pH can destroy the protective chromium oxide layer on stainless steel.

If an instrument has been damaged, the surface can be repolished and passivated by the manufacturer to restore the finish. A plated instrument can be replated; this should be done as soon as plating is chipped or begins to peel.

Replacement

Broken instruments that are beyond repair or restoration must be replaced. With normal use, good-quality surgical instruments have an expected life of at least 10 years. Using these precise tools for their intended purpose *only* cannot be overemphasized. Misuse and abuse are the most common causes of instrument breakage. Replacing instruments that were needlessly damaged is an unnecessary expense for the OR.

POWERED SURGICAL INSTRUMENTS

Most surgical instruments have movable parts that are manipulated by the surgeon. However, some instruments are pneumatically powered by compressed air or nitrogen or are electrically powered by battery or alternating current. Powered surgical instruments are complex assemblies of gears, rotating shafts, and seals. They require special handling during preparation and use and special considerations for cleaning and sterilizing. (This discussion does not include other technologies that use an electrical power source; see Chapter 15.)

Powered instruments are used primarily for precision drilling, cutting, shaping, and beveling bone. They also may be used for skin grafts and to abrade skin. Powered instruments increase speed and decrease the fatigue caused by manually driven drills, saws, and reamers. The instrument may have rotary, reciprocating, or oscillating action. Rotary movement is used to drill holes or insert screws, wires, or pins. Reciprocating movement, a cutting action from front to back, and oscillating cutting action from side to side are used to cut or remove bone or skin. Some instruments have a combination of movements and can be changed from one to another by adjusting controls.

Depending on the function desired, the surgeon chooses a drill, burr, blade, reamer, or abrader of appropriate size. These accessories attach securely into the handpiece. Small drill bits, burrs, cutting blades, and abraders may be disposable.

Blood loss from bone is reduced by the tiny particles that these high-speed instruments pack into the cut surfaces. However, the heat generated can damage bone cells. The speed of these instruments may disperse a fine mist of blood and bone cells. For this reason, OSHA, CDC, and the American Academy of Orthopaedic Surgeons recommend wearing at least protective eyewear; a face shield or spacesuit-type headgear should be considered if splatter is anticipated.

Normal tissue, including the operator's or assistant's finger, can be caught in a rapidly spinning drill or oscillating saw unless the instrument is carefully controlled. The instrument may cut more than desired. When a powered instrument is being used, particularly with a rotating movement, all team members must be very careful to keep their hands away from the blade. Most powered instruments have a safety mechanism on the handpiece. Some are operated by foot pedals.

Power Sources

The type of power used determines the accessories that will be needed to operate the instrument.

Air-Powered Instruments

Medical-grade compressed air or pure (99.97%) dry nitrogen is either piped into the OR or supplied from a cylinder on a stable carrier. The pressure must be set and monitored by the operating pressure gauges of the regulator. The correct pounds per square inch (psi), as determined by the manufacturer, is set after the instrument is assembled and turned on. The operating pressure is usually within a range of 70 to 160 psi, with storage pressure in the cylinder at least 500 psi. Excessive pressure can damage the instrument and the hose connecting it to the regulator. A broken air hose under pressure can whip out of control and injure personnel or the patient.

Air-powered instruments are small, lightweight, free of vibration, and easy to handle for pinpoint accuracy at high speeds. Because they operate at a faster and higher speed, they cause minimal heating of bone compared with electric instruments.

Electric-Powered Instruments

Electrically powered instruments such as saws, drills, dermatomes, and nerve stimulators are potential explosion hazards in the OR. Most of the motors are designed to be explosion proof. All must have sparkproof connections.

Battery Power Some battery-operated instruments are cordless with rechargeable batteries in the handpiece. Others have cords that attach to a battery charger, which is plugged into an electrical outlet. The battery charger may be sterilizable for use on the sterile table.

Alternating Current Power switches should be off when cords are being plugged into electrical outlets. The power supply cord should be connected to the outlet before anesthetic gases are administered and should not be removed during anesthesia administration. The anesthesiologist should be alerted that electrical equipment will be used. The scrub person may be able to disconnect the instrument from its power source when it is not in use so a team member cannot inadvertently activate it. Many of these instruments are activated by foot pedals. The circulator can move the foot pedal away from the operator until needed.

Sonic Energy Some instruments are activated by sonic energy to move cutting edges in a linear direction. This is a power assist without the rotary motion and high speed of other electric-powered instruments.

Because of the heat generated when using electrical instruments, the surgeon usually has the assistant drip saline solution on the area from a bulb syringe to cool the bone and wash away particles. Care must be taken so that the syringe does not touch the blade, especially if it is glass. Plastic syringes are less hazardous.

Handling Powered Instruments

Before any new or repaired powered instrument is put into use, the biomedical technician should verify that the instrument is functioning according to manufacturer's specifications. Powered instruments are not without some inherent dangers.

1. Set the instrument and attachments on a small sterile table alone when not in use. This is an added protection from inadvertent activation.
2. Handle and store the air hose or electrical power cord with care. A broken air hose can whip out of control. A broken electrical cord can short-circuit the instrument. Always inspect the hose or cord for cracks or breaks.
3. Assemble the appropriate handpiece, attachments, (e.g., blades, drills, and reamers), and power source with the safety mechanism in position to prevent activation. Always be certain that attachments are completely seated and locked in the handpiece.
4. Test whether the instrument is in working condition before the surgeon is ready to use it and before it is applied to the patient. The safety mech-

anism must be set in position to prevent inadvertent activation until ready to use and when changing attachments.

Cleaning and Sterilizing Powered Instruments

Always operate, clean, and sterilize powered instruments according to the manufacturer's manual with directions for use and care. Each instrument has different cleaning, lubricating, packaging, and sterilizing requirements because of its various component parts. The bioburden is a function of the size, design, complexity, and condition of the instrument, degree of contamination during use, and subsequent decontaminating and cleaning procedures. Microorganisms can become entrapped around seals on rotating shafts. Manufacturers test instruments with a specific biologic challenge in the most difficult area to sterilize and recommend sterilization cycles accordingly. The following general guidelines apply to the care of all powered instruments:

1. Decontaminate and clean immediately after use to maintain optimal function.
   a. Scrub person should wipe off any organic debris between uses during the surgical procedure.
   b. Accessories are disassembled for cleaning.
   c. Air hose should remain attached to the handpiece during cleaning. This or an electrical cord should be wiped with detergent, damp cloth, and dry towel.
   d. *Do not immerse the motor in liquid.* The power mechanism cannot be cleaned in a basin of solution or put in washer-sterilizer or washer-decontaminator or in an ultrasonic cleaner. Wipe the surface with a mild detergent. Use caution to avoid solution from entering the internal mechanism. Wipe off the detergent with a damp cloth and dry with a lint-free towel.
2. Lubricate as recommended by the manufacturer.
   a. Some air-powered instruments can be lubricated with sterile lubricant after sterilization just before use.
   b. Some manufacturers supply lubricant, usually a silicone oil.
   c. Some instruments must be run after lubrication to disperse lubricant through the mechanism.
3. Wrap for sterilization.
   a. Some manufacturers supply sterilizing cases. These cases can be wrapped in woven or nonwoven material.
   b. Instrument must be disassembled.
   c. Protect sharp edges of accessories.
   d. Hoses or cords should be loosely coiled.
4. Sterilize in steam unless contraindicated by the manufacturer.
   a. Prevacuum sterilizer removes entrapped air and allows access of steam into the internal mechanism; therefore it is preferred to a gravity displacement sterilizer.
   b. Exposure time depends on the type of sterilizer, design and complexity of the instrument, and packaging. In a gravity displacement sterilizer at 250° F (121° C), exposure time may be as long as 1 hour.
   c. Sterilization of an unwrapped instrument in a gravity displacement sterilizer at 270° F (132° C) must provide exposure for long enough to sterilize the internal mechanism, usually at least 15 minutes.
   d. Ethylene oxide gas sterilization should only be used if the instrument cannot withstand the heat or moisture of steam sterilization. The instrument must be free of all traces of lubricant. The manufacturer should specify aeration time.

SURGEON'S ARMAMENTARIUM

The surgeon relies on surgical instruments to enhance his or her skill in the art and science of surgery. The nursing staff must ensure that these instruments function properly and are sterilized adequately. Instruments are selected on the basis of safety for their intended use. They must be inspected, maintained, and used appropriately.

BIBLIOGRAPHY

Becker GE: Washer-sterilizers vs indexed washer-decontaminators: a cost comparison, *J Healthcare Materiel Manage* 10(2):44-48, 1992.

Cowlard DM: Annotated tray lists save time, decrease errors, *AORN J* 55(1):286-292, 1992.

Crow S: Protecting patients, personnel, instruments in the OR, *AORN J* 58(4):771-774, 1993.

ECRI: Medical devices and the law: the hospital's responsibility, *Today's OR Nurse* 12(5):39, 1990.

Fox V: Clinical issues: passing surgical instruments, sharps without injury, *AORN J* 55(1):264-266, 1992.

Harrison SK: Cleaning and decontaminating medical instruments, *J Healthcare Materiel Manage* 8(1):36-42, 1990.

Kneedler JA, Darling MH: Using an enzymatic detergent to prerinse instruments, *AORN J* 51(5):1326-1332, 1990.

Recommended practices: care of instruments, scopes, and powered surgical instruments, *AORN J* 55(3):838-848, 1992.

Tighe SMB: *Instrumentation for the operating room: a photographic manual,* ed 4, St Louis, 1994, Mosby.

CHAPTER 15

Specialized Surgical Equipment

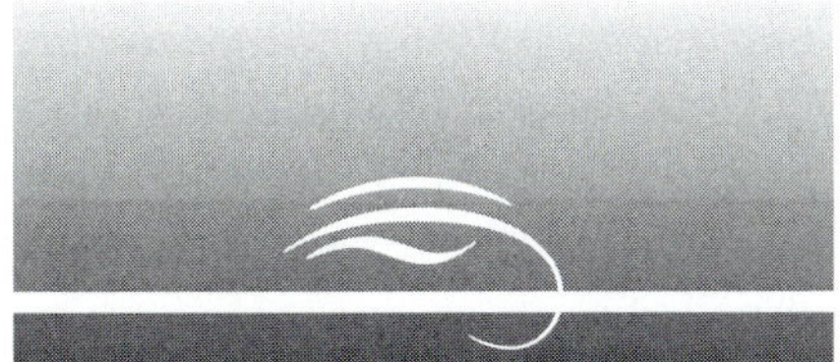

Advances in technology have made possible the complex surgical techniques of the present. *Technology* may be defined as the branch of knowledge that deals with the creation and use of technical means for scientific purposes. In the context of surgery technology refers to a system that uses both devices and people to perform specific tasks. Continuing research will further enhance technology in the future. New devices are usually adjuncts to or extensions of devices or techniques already in use. To enhance their use in patient care, operating room (OR) team members must constantly learn appropriate applications.

Surgical residency programs include education and training in electrosurgery, laser surgery, endoscopy, and microsurgery. Therefore, on completion of postgraduate education, surgeons today are skilled in the use of these advanced technologies. Continuing surgical educational courses, including laboratory study, are available so that practicing surgeons can learn to use the newest technology. Before handling new equipment, nursing personnel who function on the OR team must be knowledgeable about its care and use. Some surgical procedures utilize more than one of these technologies, for example, laser surgery through an attachment to the operating microscope directed through an endoscope. Preparing and handling these expensive pieces of equipment are major responsibilities of perioperative nurses and surgical technologists. In addition, all OR personnel must be aware of and safeguard against hazards associated with equipment. The OR environment must be safe for patients and personnel.

ELECTROSURGERY

The ancient practice of pouring boiling oil into a wound or searing it with hot irons to stop bleeding and infection was extreme. Patients usually were crippled if they survived. However, surgeons continued to use these techniques long after Ambroise Paré discredited their use in the sixteenth century. They recognized that application of heat accelerates the natural chemical reaction of blood to hasten clotting. This eventually led to the development of *electrocautery,* direct contact of an electrically heated wire with tissue. Still in use, pencil-sized, battery-operated units provide hemostasis by using a self-contained battery to heat a cauterizing wire. These are primarily used in plastic surgery. *Electrosurgery,* by contrast, delivers high-frequency oscillating electric currents through tissue between two electrodes to coagulate or cut tissue.

In 1906 Lee DeForest, the physicist commonly known as the father of radio, discovered by accident that a high-frequency electric current could sever tissue with only slight traces of generated heat. In conjunction with his vacuum-tube generator, he patented an electrode that cut tissue with an electrical arc created at the point of a dull blade. Referred to as cold cautery, the device was used unsuccessfully by pioneers like Harvey Cushing.

Working with Dr. Cushing, W.T. Bovie, also a physicist, developed the first spark-gap tube generator in the 1920s. This became the universal basis of electrosurgical units, often still referred to as "the Bovie," before the 1970s when solid-state units became available. These solid-state units use transistors, diodes, and rectifiers to generate current. The spark-gap generator continues to be an acceptable unit, however.

Definitions

A glossary of terms pertaining to electrosurgery is included in Box 15-1.

Principles of Electrosurgery

Electric current can be used to cut or coagulate most tissues. The initial incision must be made by scalpel, however, to prevent charring and scarring of skin. Electrosurgery can then be used on fat, fascia, muscle, internal organs, and vessels. High-frequency alternating or oscillating electric currents move at more than 20,000 cycles per second (10,000 for radio-frequency). Electrosurgical units operate at frequencies between 100,000 and 10,000,000 Hz. This current can be passed through tissue without causing stimulation of muscles or nerves. The heat produced is a direct result of resistance to its passage through tissue. The density of electric current flowing through a point of contact in tissue elevates temperature sufficiently to cause destruction of cells by dissolution of their molecular structure. The amount of heat produced by any amount of resistance is proportional to square of current. For example, doubling the current increases the heat produced fourfold. Conversely, the amount of heat produced by any amount of current is directly proportional to resistance; doubling the resistance doubles the heat produced. Therefore current must be concentrated in a small area of high resistance to produce the high temperature required for electrosurgery.

BOX 15-1

Glossary of Electrosurgery Terms

active electrode Apparatus used to deliver electric current to the surgical site.

current Flow of electric energy.

- **blended current** Current that divides tissue and controls some bleeding.
- **coagulating current** Current that passes intense heat through the active electrode used to sear vessels and control bleeding.
- **cutting current** Current that arcs between tissue and active electrode to divide tissue without coagulation.

electrosurgical unit (ESU) Generator, foot pedal, cords, active electrode, and inactive dispersive electrode designed to safely deliver electric current through tissue.

- **bipolar unit** Current is delivered to the surgical site and returned to the generator by forceps. One side of the forceps is active; the other side is inactive. The current passes only between the tips of the forceps.
- **monopolar unit (unipolar)** Current flows from the generator to active electrode, through patient to inactive dispersive electrode, and returns to generator.

generator Machine that produces electric current by generating high-frequency radio waves.

ground Conducting connection between generator, patient, and the earth.

inactive dispersive electrode Apparatus used to direct current from the patient back to the generator. Also referred to as inactive electrode, return electrode, patient plate, or grounding pad.

Electrosurgical Unit

To complete the electric circuit to coagulate or cut tissue, current must flow from a generator (electrosurgical power unit) to an active electrode, through tissue, and back to the generator via an inactive dispersive electrode. Electrosurgery is utilized to a greater or lesser extent in all surgical specialties. Several different units are available. Some have selective uses; others are adaptable to many types of surgical procedures. Personnel must be familiar with the manufacturer's detailed manual of operating instructions for each type used.

Generator

The machine that produces high-frequency or radiofrequency waves is the generator or power component of the electrosurgical unit. Some generators are *grounded*. This means that the machine acts as a ground to earth. Current returns to the machine, but if the circuit is broken, the current will find an alternate route back to earth, as through metal in contact with body. A balanced output generator is referenced to earth. An *isolated generator* offers the advantage of a non-ground-seeking circuit. The flow of current is isolated and restricted to active and dispersive electrodes, and the current returns directly back to the generator. With an isolated generator, if the circuit is broken, current will not flow.

Solid-state generators are transistorized and use diodes and rectifiers to produce current. They usually operate at a lower output than spark-gap generators and have safety features such as return monitors to prevent burns and electrocution. Both solid-state and spark-gap generators provide two separate circuits within the housing of the machine. Controls on the outside of the housing allow selection of desired characteristic of current. The current may be identical in frequency, power (voltage), and amount (amperage) but vary in quality. Quality depends on the difference in *damping,* the pattern of waveforms by which oscillations diminish after surges of power. This difference determines tissue reaction to the current.

Coagulating Current A damped waveform has a continuous pattern of surges of current that rapidly diminishes to short time periods, gaps, in which no current is delivered. This is produced by the spark-gap circuit. Damped current coagulates tissue. As it approaches the active electrode, the density of current increases to produce an intense heat, which sears the ends of small or moderate-sized vessels to control bleeding on contact. Attempts to coagulate large vessels can result in an extensive burn and necrosis. Excess charring interferes with wound healing and may provide a medium for infection.

Cutting Current An undamped waveform, which is produced by a vacuum tube oscillator, does not diminish but retains a constant output of high-frequency current. *Undamped* current cuts tissue. This continuous current forms an arc between tissues and an active electrode that is intense enough to divide fibrous tissue as it moves along lines of incision (reference is not to skin incision) before sufficient heat builds up to coagulate adjacent tissues.

Blended Current Undamped current can be blended with damped current to add a coagulating effect to the cutting current. At the same time that it cuts through or across tissue, cutting current accomplishes some coagulation of cells on the surface of the incision and prevents capillary bleeding. Some solid-state generators have a setting for "blend"or "hemostasis" for this function. This blend can also be achieved by a slightly damped waveform from a spark-gap generator.

Controls The type and amount of current are regulated by controls on the generator. Most units provide up to 400 watts of power. It is seldom necessary to use full-power settings. A safe general rule for the circulator is to start with the lowest setting of current that accomplishes the desired degree of coagulation or cutting, then increase current at the surgeon's request. The surgeon selects the type of current to be used with either a foot or hand control switch. The circulator verbally confirms the power settings before the generator is activated. The generator should be designed to minimize unintentional activation.

In solid-state units the power output is isolated to prevent overheating and is equipped with a warning buzzer and/or light to warn of too high a setting or a break in the circuit. Flow of current to and from the generator must be balanced. A return electrode monitoring system measures and compares current flowing from the active electrode with current returning from the inactive dispersive electrode. The generator deactivates if continuity in electric circuit is disrupted or inadequate in some units. Safety features should be tested before each patient use, and the generator should be periodically inspected by the biomedical engineering department.

The generator may be mounted on a portable stand. It must be moved carefully to avoid tipping. The machine must be cleaned before and after use. Unintentional activation or failure may occur if liquid or debris enters the generator. The facility may be held responsible for a defect causing patient injury. The generator should have an identification number. This should be recorded in the patient's record to verify the equipment used. This ID number also provides a means of maintaining records of routine inspections and maintenance. Operational instructions should be on or attached to every unit.

Active Electrode

The sterile active electrode directs flow of current to the surgical site. The style of the electrode tip (i.e., blade, loop, ball, or needle) will be determined by the type of surgical procedure and current to be used. The electrode tip may be fixed into or detachable from a pencil-shaped handle, or it may be incorporated into a tissue forceps or suction tube. It is attached to a conductor cord, which is connected to the generator. The scrub person hands the end of the conductor cord off the sterile field to the circulator, who attaches it to the generator. The cord must be long and flexible enough to reach between the sterile field and the generator without stress. It must be free of kinks and bends that could deviate current flow. When the unit is not in actual use, although connected, the electrode tip should be kept clean, dry, and visible. It may be kept in an insulated holster/container attached to the drape over the patient to avoid the possibility of a fire being started by someone on the team inadvertently stepping on the foot switch or activating hand control.

The surgeon places the active electrode tip on tissue and then activates the foot switch or hand control to transfer electric current from the generator to tissue. Some hand switches are color-coded to identify coagulating and cutting functions. Some generators produce a buzzing sound that varies in pitch, depending on which current is being used. Charred or coagulated tissue should be removed from the tip because charred tissue absorbs heat and decreases the effectiveness of current. This can be done by wiping the tip with a damp sponge or scraping it on a disposable tip cleaner. Avoid using a scalpel blade because the debris may become airborne, creating a biologic hazard.

Rather than placement of the tip directly on tissue, bleeding vessels may be clamped with hemostats or smooth-tipped tissue forceps. As little extraneous tissue as possible should be clamped to minimize damage to adjacent tissue. Vessels are coagulated when any part of the metal instrument is touched with the active electrode; this is frequently referred to as "buzzing." The electrode should be in contact with the instrument before activation to avoid arcing. The person holding it should have a firm grip on as large an area of instrument as possible and avoid touching the patient. The active current should not be applied for more than 3 seconds. Inadvertent patient injury can occur if the metal instrument is in contact with retractors or other instrumentation placed in the surgical field. Low voltage should be used. Current can burn through surgical gloves if these precautions are not taken.

The electrode and cord may be disposable. Reusable electrodes should be inspected for damage before reprocessing and before use at the sterile field.

Inactive Dispersive Electrode

Electric current will flow to ground or a neutral potential. Therefore a proper channel must be provided to disperse current and heat generated in tissue. The inactive electrode disperses high-frequency current released through the active electrode and provides low current density return from tissues back to the generator. Resistance from the patient to the generator and from the generator to the wall electrical outlet must be less than 1 ohm. Electrosurgical units have either monopolar or bipolar mechanisms or both to direct the flow of electric current.

Bipolar Units With bipolar units the dispersive electrode is incorporated into forceps used by the surgeon. One side of the forceps is the active electrode through which current passes to tissues. The other side is inactive. Output voltage is relatively low. Current flows only between the tips of the forceps, returning directly to the generator. Current does not disperse itself throughout the patient, as in monopolar units. This provides extremely precise control of the coagulated area. A grounding pad or plate is not needed because current does not flow through the patient.

Monopolar/Unipolar Units With monopolar/unipolar units current flows from the generator to the active electrode, through the patient to an inactive dispersive electrode, and back to the generator. Power is greater than through bipolar forceps. Because current supplied by the generator is dispersed from the active electrode, it seeks completion of the electrical circuit to ground or a neutral potential through the patient's body. *An inactive dispersive electrode must be used to ground the patient.* This is in the form of a patient grounding pad or plate placed in direct contact with skin. The contact area must exceed 100 mm or a diameter greater than 1.2 cm. The most commonly used types are disposable. Some are flexible to mold to any body surface. They must maintain uniform body contact. Some are prelubricated. If a metal plate is placed under the patient, a conductive electrode lubricant (gel) must be spread evenly over the entire plate to thoroughly wet the skin and thus reduce its electrical resistance to a minimum. Some pads also must be lubricated. Prelubricated pads should be checked for dry spots before placement.

Current flows from the active electrode through the body to the inactive dispersive electrode. It then returns to the generator via a conductor cord. This cord must be long and flexible enough to reach without stress on attachments to the electrode or generator. Attachments must be secure. The plug or adapter at the end of the cord fastens into the receptacle on generator. This may be labeled and/or color coded to help ensure correct attachment of the dispersive electrode. Unless disposable, the cord should be checked before use for wire breakage or fraying by grasping the connecting plug and pulling firmly on the cord. If it stretches, wires inside are broken and must be repaired. Reusable cords should be inspected by the biomedical engineering department periodically for electrical integrity.

The dispersive electrode (grounding pad or plate) must be properly placed and connected to avoid electrical burn to the patient. The following safeguards must be taken:

1. The dispersive electrode should be as close as possible to the site where the active electrode will be used to minimize current through the body. The patient should be in the desired position before the dispersive electrode is applied to prevent its becoming dislodged during patient positioning. Do not remove and reposition the disposable dispersive electrode because the integrity of the adhesive will be altered. A new electrode must be used each time.
2. The dispersive electrode must cover as large an area of the patient's skin as possible in an area free of hair or scar tissue, which tend to act as insulation. An area may need to be shaved. The surface area affects heat buildup and dissipation. Avoid areas where bony prominences might result in pressure points, which in turn can cause current concentration. Place the pad or plate on a clean, dry skin surface over or under as large a muscle mass area as possible. The gel conduction material on the pad is cold and sticky to the touch; a patient who is awake should be forewarned of its application.
3. The dispersive electrode should *not* be placed on skin over a metal implant, such as a hip prosthesis, because current could be diverted to the implant.

4. The dispersive electrode must be clean, free from bent edges, and adhere uniformly to skin. Some conductive lubricants will dry out and leave a high-resistance film that will prevent proper contact with skin. Inspect the integrity of the package of a disposable dispersive electrode before use. Do not use the electrode if the package is damaged or has been previously opened.
5. The metal connection between the pad or plate and the conductor cord must not touch the patient. Special care must be taken to ensure that the cord does not become dislodged. Do not put a safety belt over the electrode or cord, for example. The safest connectors are threaded or locked and also are insulated. The connector should not create a pressure point on the patient's skin.
6. The connection between the dispersive electrode and generator must be secure and made with compatible attachments. If the return circuit is faulty, the ground circuit may be completed through inadvertent contact with the metal operating table or its attachments. If the grounded area is small, current passing through an exposed area of skin contact will be relatively intense. For example, one such contact point could be the thigh touching a leg stirrup while the patient is in the lithotomy position.
7. The dispersive electrode should be positioned and connected for generators that accommodate both bipolar and monopolar mechanisms. A dispersive electrode is not used with bipolar generators.

The circulator should record on the patient's chart the location of the inactive dispersive electrode, the condition of the patient's skin before and after electrosurgery, the generator identification number, and the settings used. Some institutions also require documentation of the dispersive electrode lot number.

Safety Factors

Electrical burn through the patient's skin is the greatest hazard of electrosurgery. These burns are usually deeper than flame burns, causing widespread tissue necrosis and deep thrombosis to the extent that debridement may be required. Isolated circuits for electrosurgical units and return-electrode monitoring systems, *if used,* virtually eliminate these burns. However, nursing personnel must be aware of hazards and safeguard against injury to the patient. In addition to the precautions noted for preparing the electrosurgical unit and for positioning the dispersive electrode used with monopolar units, other precautions should be taken:

1. Alert the anesthesiologist to the anticipated use of electrosurgery. Electrosurgery should not be used in the mouth, around the head, or in the pleural cavity when high concentrations of oxygen or nitrous oxide are used. Flammable anesthetics are not used. Safety regulations for use with all inhalation anesthetic agents must be followed (see Chapter 10, pp. 152-153).
2. Electrocardiogram electrodes should be placed as far away from the surgical site as possible. Burns can occur at the site of electrocardiogram electrodes and other low impedance points from invasive monitor probes if current diverts to alternate grounds.
3. Finger rings and other jewelry should be removed. Metallic jewelry presents a potential risk of burn for the patient from diverted currents from the monopolar/unipolar unit with either an isolated or ground referenced output.
4. Flammable agents such as alcohol should not be used in skin preparation. If they are used, the skin surface must be completely dry before draping. Fumes may collect in drapes and ignite when the electrosurgical or cautery unit is used. The use of aqueous antiseptic solutions is preferred.
5. If another piece of electrical equipment is used in direct contact with the patient at the same time as the electrosurgical unit, connect it to a different source of current, such as a battery, if possible. The cutting current of the electrosurgical unit may not work if another piece of electrical equipment is on same circuit. The electrosurgical unit may interfere with operation of other equipment, such as cardiac monitors. The isolated power system of solid-state generators may prevent these problems.
6. Electrosurgery may disrupt operation of an implanted cardiac pacemaker. The patient must be continuously monitored. A defibrillator should be on standby in the OR.
7. Connection of a bipolar active electrode to a monopolar receptacle may activate current, causing a short circuit. Plugs on cords should be differentiated to prevent misconnections of active and inactive electrodes.
8. Secure the active electrode handle in an insulated holster/container when not in use. Do not immerse an active electrode in liquid.
9. To prevent fire, only moist sponges should be permitted on the sterile field while the electrosurgical unit is in use.
10. Investigate a repeated request for more current. The dispersive electrode or connecting cord may be at fault. Shock to those touching the patient may result. The patient may be burned.
11. For safety of the patient and personnel, follow instructions for use and care on the machine or in the manual provided by the manufacturer that

accompanies each electrosurgical unit. Grasp and pull only the plugs, not cords, when disconnecting attachments from the generator or the power source. Position the power cord away from the team to avoid tripping team members. Avoid rolling equipment over the power cord.

12. Any malfunctioning electrosurgical unit must be taken out of service until cleared for use by the biomedical engineering department.
13. The patient and personnel should be protected from inhaling plume (smoke) generated during electrosurgery. A suction device should be placed as close to the source of plume as possible to maximize evacuation of smoke and enhance visibility at the surgical site (see surgical plume, Chapter 10, p. 157).

Electrosurgery causes more patient injuries than any other electrical device used in the OR. Most incidents are caused by personnel error. In addition to the foregoing precautions, refer to the discussion of electrical hazards and safety in Chapter 10, pp. 148-152.

LASER SURGERY

Laser is an acronym for *light amplification by stimulated emission of radiation.* Einstein's theory, purported in 1917, explaining the difference between spontaneous and stimulated emission of light eventually led to the development of the laser. This development began in 1940 in the Soviet Union. Lasers depend on the capacity of atoms to become excited when struck by a quantum of electromagnetic energy known as a *photon.* Photons are the basic units of radiation that constitute light. When struck by a photon, the electrons of the atom move to a high energy level. On spontaneous return to a lower energy level toward normal ground state, these electrons emit another photon that will strike another atom also in the transitional *pumped up* energy state. This reaction produces a second photon of the same frequency. This sets up a chain reaction of stimulated emission of photons at high energy levels. Production of this in a sustained state, known as *population inversion,* was technically difficult. The introduction of practical lasers into scientific technology finally occurred almost simultaneously in the United States and Russia around 1960.

The laser as a surgical instrument was developed in the United States. The first surgical laser, the ruby laser, was used in ophthalmology for retinal hemorrhages. As scientists discovered that other materials could be electrically stimulated to produce lasers in a variety of wavelengths, the carbon dioxide (CO_2) and argon gas surgical lasers were developed in the mid-1960s. The argon laser replaced the ruby laser for use in ophthalmology. However, not until after Jako adapted the CO_2 laser to the operating microscope in 1972 did lasers truly become viable adjuncts to the surgical armamentarium.

Definitions

A glossary of terms necessary for an understanding of laser surgery is included in Box 15-2.

Physical Properties of Laser

The laser focuses light on atoms to stimulate them to a high point of excitation. The resulting radiation is then amplified and metamorphosed into the wavelengths of laser light. This light beam is *monochromatic,* one color, because all the electromagnetic waves are the same length, and *collimated,* parallel to each other. The light is totally concentrated and easily focused. Unlike conventional light waves, which spread and dissipate electromagnetic radiation by many different wavelengths, the *coherence* of the laser beam is sustained over space and time with wavelengths in the same frequency and energy phase.

Lasers may emit their energy in brief, repeating emissions that have a duration of only an extremely small fraction of a second. These are *pulsed laser systems.* Or, they are capable of producing continuous light beams; these are *continuous wave lasers.* All lasers have a combination of duration, level, and output wavelengths of radiation emitted when activated. Power density, the *irradiance,* is the amount of power per unit surface area during a single pulse or exposure. This is expressed as watts per centimeter squared. Regardless of beam characteristics, components of a laser system are the same (Figure 15-1). These components include the following:

1. *Medium* to produce lasing effect of stimulated emission. Gases, solid rods or crystals, liquid dyes, and free electrons are used. Each produces a different wavelength, color, and effect.
2. *Power source* to create population inversion by pumping energy into the lasing medium. This may be electrical or radio-frequency power or an optical power source such as a xenon flash lamp or another laser.
3. *Amplification mechanism* to change random directional movement of stimulated emissions to a parallel direction. This occurs within an optical resonator or laser cavity, a tube with mirrors at each end. As photons traveling the length of the resonator reflect back through the medium, they stimulate more atoms to release photons, thus amplifying the lasing effect. The power density of the beam determines the laser's capacity to cut, coagulate, or vaporize tissue.
4. *Wave guides* to aim and control the direction of the laser beam. The optical resonator has a small opening in one end that permits transmission of a small beam of laser light. The smaller the beam, the higher its power density will be. Fiberoptic

BOX 15-2

Glossary of Laser Surgery Terms

emissions Surgical lasers emit nonionizing radiation, heat, and debris.

direct laser energy Nonionizing radiation is selectively absorbed by tissues with resultant destruction at the focal point.

indirect or reflective energy Radiation can become scattered if the beam strikes a reflective surface or is unintentionally activated. Direct or indirect exposure to laser energy can burn skin and injure eyes. It can also ignite flammable materials and combustible gases.

laser plume Carbonized cell fragments, toxic hydrocarbons, viruses, and noxious fumes can be dispersed from tissues exposed to laser beam. Vaporization converts solid tissue to smoke and gas. This plume (smoke) is evacuated to maintain visibility and also to minimize hazard of inhalation by personnel.

laser Acronym for *l*ight *a*mplification by *s*timulated *e*mission of *r*adiation. Light, concentrated and focused, stimulates atoms to emit radiant energy when activated.

laser beam Light beams, either pulsed or continuous, go through a medium to produce lasing effect. The beam has three distinct characteristics as follows:

coherent Light beams are sustained over space and time because electromagnetic waves are in same frequency and energy phase with each other.

collimated Light beams are parallel.

monochromatic Light beam is one color because waves are all the same length in the electromagnetic spectrum.

power All lasers have a combination of duration, intensity, and output of radiation when wavelengths are activated.

irradiance Power density is the amount of radiant energy emitted during exposure to light beam that determines the laser's capacity to cut, coagulate, or vaporize tissue.

source Power to energize the light beam may be electrical, radio-frequency, or optical.

wavelength Electromagnetic waves transfer energy progressively from point to point through a medium. The wavelength is the distance traveled along the electromagnetic spectrum. Radiation penetration differs at different wavelengths. Each laser has a different wavelength and color, depending on the medium the light beam passes through.

color Colors vary from visible red to blue-green (near the ultraviolet end of electromagnetic spectrum) to invisible light in far-infrared range.

medium Gases, synthetic crystals, glass rods, liquid dyes, free electrons and semiconductors are used to produce lasing effect.

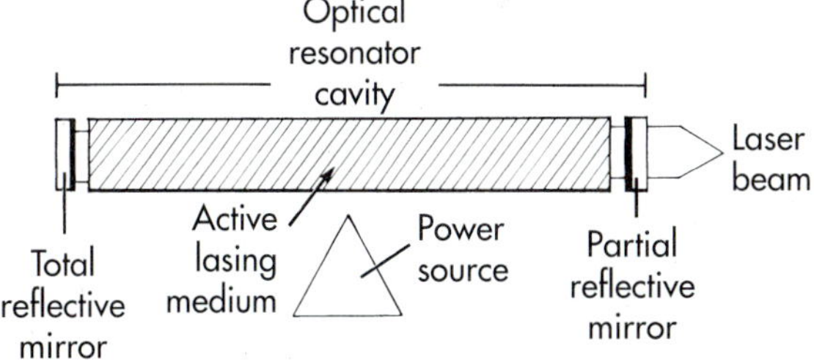

FIGURE 15-1 Basic laser components.

wave guides or a series of rhodium reflecting mirrors then direct the beam to tissue. The wave mode may be continuous, pulsed, or a Q-switched single pulse of high energy.

5. *Backstops* to stop the laser beam from penetrating beyond the expected impact site and affecting nontargeted tissue. Quartz or titanium rods will stop the beam.

Types of Lasers

Lasers use argon, carbon dioxide, holmium, krypton, neodymium, phosphate, ruby, or xenon as their active media. When delivered to tissues, laser light can be absorbed, reflected, transmitted, or scattered, depending on the characteristics of the laser and the type of tissue. Only absorbed light produces thermal effects in tissue. Thermal penetration varies according to the ratio of absorption vs. scattering. Energy absorbed at the surface will destroy superficial cells; further penetration extends cell destruction in surrounding tissues. The wavelength of the laser light, power density, rate of delivery of energy, and exposure time will vary the effects on tissue. Energy density is based on the laser's wattage, beam/spot size, and time of exposure. Spot size depends on the laser fiber size and distance of the tip from tissue; it increases and becomes defocused as fiber is moved farther from tissue. Box 15-3 lists variables in tissue reaction.

Laser beams cut, vaporize, or coagulate tissue. Coagulative effect causes collagen bonding and welding of tissue surfaces. Each laser has selective uses. Laser light

BOX 15-3

Factors Associated With Tissue Reaction to Laser Light

Type of laser (wavelength)
Intensity of laser focus
Duration of application
Depth of penetration
Type of tissue (color and composition)

colors vary from visible near ultraviolet to the invisible far infrared ranges of the electromagnetic spectrum (Figure 15-2). Wavelengths also vary, providing different radiation penetration depths. Lasers are commonly used in conjunction with the operating microscope and/or an endoscope. The surgeon selects the appropriate laser for the tissue to be incised, excised, or coagulated.

Argon Laser

Argon ion gas emits a blue-green light beam in the visible electromagnetic spectrum at wavelengths of 450 and 530 nm or 0.5 μm. This wavelength passes through water and clear fluid, such as cerebrospinal fluid, with minimal absorption. It is intensely absorbed by brown-red pigment of hemoglobin in blood or melanin in pigmented tissue and converted into heat. Thermal radiation penetrates to a depth of 1 or 2 mm in most tissue.

The argon laser operates from electrical power. A water-cooling system is often required to dissipate heat generated in the argon medium.

The argon laser beam usually is transmitted through a flexible quartz fiberoptic wave guide that is 200 to 600 μm in diameter. This can be directed to a handpiece or through an endoscope or operating microscope. Most argon laser machines deliver a nonfocused beam that vaporizes tissue poorly and scatters more radiation than other types of lasers. Irradiance may vary from less than 1 watt to 20 watts, depending on the model.

Argon lasers coagulate bleeding points or lesions involving many small superficial vessels, such as a port-wine stain. They are used primarily to destroy specific cutaneous lesions while sparing adjacent tissue and minimizing scarring. Argon lasers may be used to treat vascular lesions and remove plaque and to coagulate superficial vessels in mucosa, as in the gastrointestinal tract. They are also used in ophthalmology, otolaryngology, gynecology, urology, neurosurgery, and dermatology.

Carbon Dioxide Laser

Using a mixture of carbon dioxide, nitrogen, and helium molecular gases, the CO_2 laser emits an invisible beam from mid- to far-infrared range of the electromagnetic spectrum at wavelengths of 9600 and 10,600 nm or 10.6 μm. This wavelength is intensely absorbed by water. It raises water temperature in cells to the flash boiling point, thus vaporizing tissue. Vaporization is the conversion of solid tissue to smoke and gas. This plume should be evacuated or suctioned through a filter device from the site of lasing. The intense heat of the CO_2 laser also coagulates vessels as it cuts through them. It penetrates the surface to a depth of 0.1 to 0.2 mm per application to tissue with minimal thermal effect to surrounding tissue.

The CO_2 laser operates from electrical power. The machine has a self-contained cooling system.

The CO_2 laser beam must be delivered in a direct line of vision. It can be directed through a rigid endoscope,

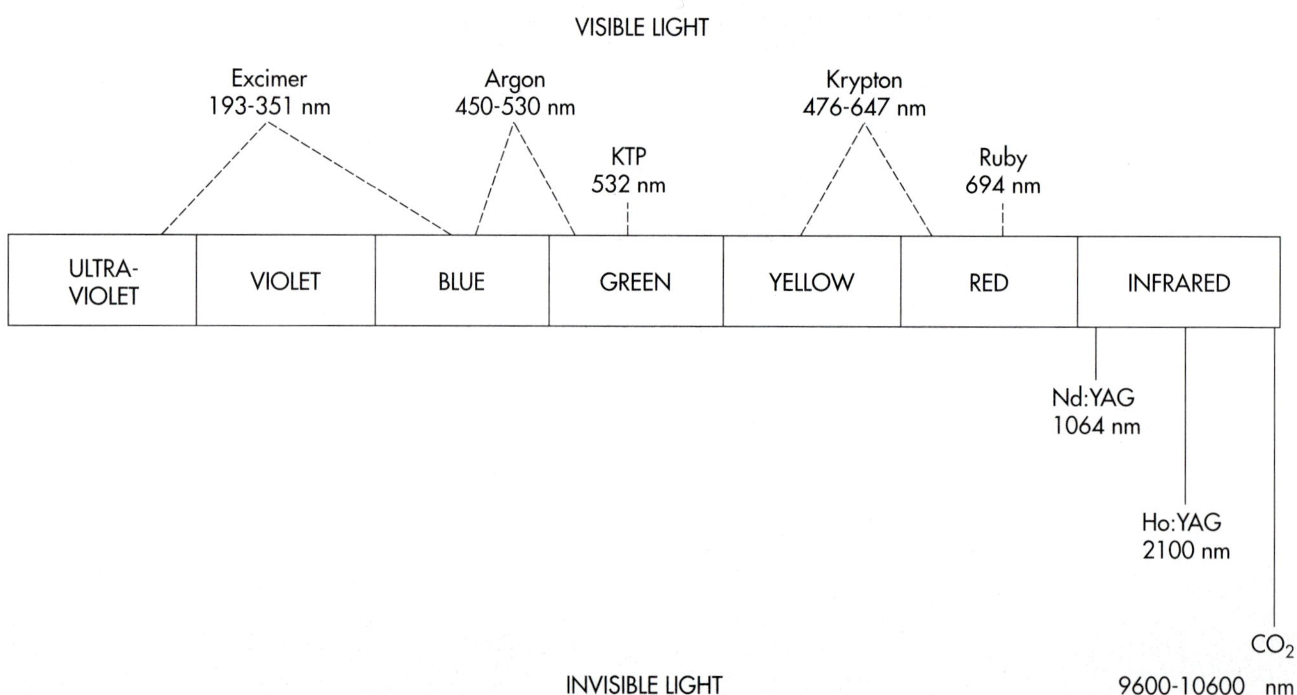

FIGURE 15-2 Electromagnetic spectrum of laser light beams at wavelengths in nanometers.

but it cannot be transmitted through a fiberoptic wave guide because its longer wavelength prevents conduction through crystal fibers. It is transmitted through an operating microscope or an articulating arm with a series of mirrors. This arm allows precise focus and direction of the beam to a pencil-like handpiece. CO_2 lasers have a helium-neon laser coaxial target beam that superimposes the invisible carbon dioxide beam to provide a visible red aiming light. The wave generated may be continuous or pulsed. Irradiance can vary from less than 1 watt up to 300 watts. A portable hand-held laser tube with a hollow needle to deliver the carbon dioxide beam is available for use in vascular surgery and microsurgery.

The vaporization and hemostatic action of the CO_2 laser is of value to the surgeon in treating soft tissue and vascular lesions. Large or small masses of tissue can be removed rapidly and efficiently. However, the CO_2 laser cannot be used in a fluid environment. A cavity, such as the peritoneal cavity or a joint, must be insufflated with gas before the beam is directed through an endoscope. This laser is used primarily in otolaryngology, gynecology, plastic surgery, dermatology, neurosurgery, orthopaedics, and cardiovascular and general surgery.

Excimer Laser

When organic molecular bonds are broken up by a photochemical reaction, a cool laser energy is emitted. Short wavelengths in the ultraviolet to visible blue-green spectrum are produced by gas used in the excimer laser combining with a halide medium. Argon fluoride produces a wavelength of 193 nm; krypton fluoride, 248 nm; xenon chloride, 308 nm; and xenon fluoride, 351 nm. These gases are extremely toxic. The beams they produce offer precision in cutting and coagulating without thermal damage to adjacent tissue. Excimer lasers have been developed for use in ophthalmology, peripheral and coronary angioplasty, orthopaedics (to cut bone), and neurosurgery.

Free Electron Laser

Free electrons, which are not bound to a specific atom, pass from a particle accelerator through a series of magnets to create a light beam. The beam can be tuned anywhere within the electromagnetic spectrum from ultraviolet to infrared. The free electron laser (FEL) produces light waves as a series of rapid superpulses of high energy and short duration, with minimal thermal damage. They can fragment calculi. The FEL can also be used for precise cutting of tissues.

Holmium:YAG Laser

A crystal that contains holmium, thulium, and chromium elements increases the wavelength of YAG laser energy to 2100 nm or 2.10 μm. This invisible beam in the mid-infrared range of the electromagnetic spectrum is absorbed by tissues containing water. Combined with high-energy pulsed delivery, it penetrates less deeply into tissue than the neodymium:YAG laser for more precise cutting and less generalized heating of tissue. It may be used percutaneously through a laser fiber threaded through a hollow needle or be delivered through a fine fiberoptic fiber. It may be used in a fluid medium. It acts on water in cells without char or extensive tissue damage. Approved for use in all joints except the spine, the holmium (Ho):YAG laser is useful in orthopaedics to cut, shape, and sculpt cartilage and bone and to ablate soft tissues.

Krypton Laser

The krypton ion gas laser emits a red-yellow light beam in visible electromagnetic spectrum at wavelengths of 476.2 to 647.1 nm or 0.6 μm. It is intensely absorbed by pigment in blood and retinal epithelium. The krypton laser resembles the argon laser in construction and use. It operates from electrical power and is water cooled. Used in ophthalmology, it is more versatile than the argon laser in selective photocoagulation of the retina (see Chapter 33, p. 696).

Neodymium:YAG Laser

Nd:YAG is the acronym for neodymium, yttrium, aluminum, and garnet comprising the solid-state crystal medium that emanates the light beam of this laser. This invisible beam in the near-infrared range of the electromagnetic spectrum has a wavelength of 1064 nm or 1.06 μm. It is poorly absorbed by hemoglobin and water but is intensely absorbed by tissue protein. The wavelength penetrates to a depth of 3 to 7 mm to denature protein by thermal coagulation and shrinkage of tissue beneath the surface.

The Nd:YAG laser operates from electric current through the optical power source of xenon flash lamps. It must have an air, carbon dioxide, or water cooling system.

The Nd:YAG laser beam can be transmitted through a flexible quartz fiber, 200 to 600 μm in diameter, which passes through a rigid endoscope. It can also be transmitted through a fiberoptic wave guide to a handpiece or a flexible endoscope or be focused through an operating microscope. An aiming light of blue xenon or red neon-helium may be used in conjunction with the Nd:YAG beam. Sapphire or ceramic tips allow direct contact with tissue for cutting and vaporizing without diffuse coagulation using less than 25 watts of power. These tips are available on hand-held scalpels or to fit on ends of fibers for endoscopic use. Many of these tips are reusable; some are disposable after a single use.

The Nd:YAG laser has the most powerful coagulating action of all the surgical lasers. Its continuous or pulsed wave penetrates deeper into tissues than other lasers, that is, up to 2 cm, and will coagulate large vessels up to 4 mm. It is used to coagulate and vaporize large volumes of tissue. This versatile laser has applications in rhinolaryngology, urology, gynecology, neurosurgery, orthopaedics, and thoracic and general surgery.

For ophthalmology the Nd:YAG laser uses a Q-switching mode to store energy in a resonator during pumping action followed by release of a single, short pulse of high energy. This does not burn tissue but disrupts it with minute shock waves.

Potassium Titanyl Phosphate Laser

The solid-state potassium titanyl phosphate (KTP) crystal emits a visible green light at a wavelength of 532 mm or 0.5 µm. This laser produces less power than CO_2 or Nd:YAG lasers but can be focused to a smaller diameter, as for precision work in the middle ear. KTP absorbs most effectively into red or black tissue for coagulation. The beam can be directed by a handpiece at or in contact with tissue or through a rigid or flexible fiberoptic fiber or micromanipulator. The beam cuts, vaporizes, or coagulates tissue with minimal lateral thermal damage and plume. Cooling gases are not necessary, but the system must be water cooled. Instruments are available that provide both KTP and Nd:YAG wavelengths selected by a button on the control panel or that pass Nd:YAG beam through the KTP crystal. Many accessories are available for specific applications in all surgical specialties. The KTP laser has good cutting properties.

Ruby Laser

The ruby solid-state crystal laser emits a visible red light at wavelengths of 694 nm or 0.6 µm. A synthetically machined crystal rod is placed in a resonator cavity with a xenon flash lamp that, when activated, creates the optical pumping to produce the ruby laser beam. Blood vessels and transparent substances do not absorb this beam. A pulsed system, the ruby laser, is capable of generating large fields of energy on impact. This shock wave effect can injure internal tissues and bone. Irradiance is 1 watt. Originally used in ophthalmology, the ruby laser currently is used primarily to eradicate port-wine stain lesions of the skin.

Tunable Dye Laser

Fluorescent liquid dyes or vapors can produce lasing energy. When exposed to intense laser light, usually an argon beam, dye absorbs light and fluoresces over a broad spectrum from ultraviolet to far-infrared. The laser may be delivered interstitially, endoscopically, externally, or retrobulbarly. A tunable prism can adjust laser wavelength from 400 to 1000 nm, in either continuous or pulsed mode, for the specific dye in use.

The argon tunable dye laser system emits a blue-green beam in a 430 to 530 nm wavelength from an argon laser that pumps a rhodamine B dye laser to produce a red laser beam of approximately 630 nm wavelength for selective destruction of malignant tumor cells. A dye laser tuned to 577 nm can be used on vascular lesions. Other wavelengths, as through copper vapor, may be used to treat skin lesions or superficial tumors, as of the bladder wall. The site can be repeatedly treated as long as cells remain photosensitive. This tunable dye laser is used most commonly for photodynamic therapy.

Photodynamic Therapy For photodynamic therapy the patient is injected 24 to 48 hours before laser therapy with a photosensitive drug that is absorbed by normal and malignant tissue. Normal tissue gradually releases the drug, but abnormal tissue retains it. The abnormal photosensitive tissue is destroyed when exposed to the laser beam. Normal adjacent tissue appears sunburned but is not permanently damaged. All dyes used with tunable lasers are potentially toxic and must be handled with caution (see Chapter 10, pp. 155-156). See Chapter 45 for a further discussion of photodynamic therapy for oncology.

Safety Factors

All surgical lasers present hazards to patients and to the OR team. This equipment must be used in accordance with established regulations, standards and recommended practices, manufacturer's recommendations, and institutional policies related to a laser program. Laser safety is based on knowledge of the specific laser to be used, its instrumentation, its mode of operation, its power densities, its action in tissues, and its risks.

Regulatory Agencies

Lasers are classified as medical devices and are subject to regulation. The Code of Federal Regulations' *Performance Standards for Light Emitting Products* provides specifications for manufacturers of medical laser systems.*

National Center for Devices and Radiological Health The National Center for Devices and Radiological Health (NCDRH) is the regulatory section of the Food and Drug Administration (FDA) in the Department of Health and Human Services (DHHS). More than 250 types of lasers are regulated by the FDA. Those intended for medical and surgical use come under the jurisdiction of medical device regulations. They are categorized as Class III, subdivision Class 4, because lasers are potentially hazardous (Box 15-4). Manufacturers must verify that their products meet all safety requirements of the federal standard. They must receive approval from NCDRH to market or test a laser for a par-

**Federal Register,* Code of Federal Regulations, Performance standards for light emitting products, Part 1040, 1982; Federal Register, Laser products; Amendments to performance standard, final rule 50(161), 1985. HHS Publication FDA 88-8035, Regulations for the administration and enforcement of the Radiation Control for Health and Safety Act of April 1988, Part 1040, sections 1040.10 and 1040.11.

BOX 15-4

Medical Device Regulations

FDA classification of medical devices
Medical devices were classified in 1976 by the FDA according to their safety factors.

Class I
Subject to general controls

Class II
Devices for which general controls are not enough

Class III
Implants and life support devices

Classification of lasers
Lasers are classified according to potential hazard of exposure.

Class 1
Enclosed system, considered safe based on current medical knowledge. No light emission escapes the enclosure.

Class 2
Limited to visible light (400-780 nm). Output power is 1 mW or less. Momentary viewing (0.25 second maximum permissible exposure) is not considered hazardous. Staring into the beam is not recommended. Protective eyewear of the correct optical density should be worn.

Class 3A
Emitted laser light viewed directly through collecting optics would cause permanent eye damage. Output power is 0.5 mW or less. Protective eyewear of the correct optical density should be worn.

Class 3B
Continuous laser light with 0.5 watt or less output can cause permanent eye damage. Exposure to the beam should be avoided. Protective eyewear of the correct optical density should be worn.

Class 4
Laser light produced is hazardous to skin and eyes. Strict control measures are enforced. Protective eyewear of the correct optical density should be worn.

ticular clinical application or use, and they must comply with labeling requirements.

American National Standards Institute The American National Standards Institute (ANSI) is a voluntary organization of experts who determine industry consensus standards in technical fields. The standard developed specifically for laser safety in health care facilities* is intended for all users. Existing federal legislation and state laser safety regulations are based on the ANSI standard. Simply stated, this standard implies that every health care facility that uses surgical lasers must establish and maintain an adequate program for control of laser hazards. This program shall include provisions for the following:

1. *Laser safety officer.* This person should have authority to suspend, restrict, or terminate operation of a laser system if hazard controls are inadequate. A laser safety committee, often a subcommittee of the OR committee, may appoint this surveillance officer.
2. *Education of users.* A safety training program must ensure that all users, including surgeons, perioperative nurses, surgical technologists, and biomedical engineers and technicians, are knowledgeable of correct operation, potential hazards, and control measures.
3. *Protective measures for patients, personnel, and the environment.*
4. *Management of accidents.* Management includes reporting accidents and developing plans of action to prevent a future occurrence.

Occupational Safety and Health Administration As elaborated in Chapter 10, the Occupational Safety and Health Administration (OSHA) is concerned primarily with the safety of health care workers. The agency can enforce ANSI standard.

State and Local Agencies State regulations and local ordinances vary. Knowledge of and compliance with any requirements must be established.

Policies and Procedures

Specific policies and procedures related to use of lasers should be written by the laser safety committee before a laser program is instituted. These policies and procedures will need to be revised or updated when new equipment is installed. Applicable policies include but are not limited to the following:

1. *Credentialing and clinical practice privileges of medical staff.* Physicians authorized to use a laser should be required to complete a postgraduate laser course in their specialties. Hands-on experience and a preceptorship with a qualified user also should be required. The physician must have training for each type and wavelength of laser. A list of approved physicians should be available to OR staff.
2. *Initial and ongoing educational programs for nursing personnel.* Nursing personnel should have thorough knowledge and understanding of laser equipment, laser physics, tissue reactions, applications, and safety precautions.
3. *Continuous quality improvement.* A program of continuous quality improvement includes appropri-

*American National Standard for the Safe Use of Lasers in Health Care Facilities, ANSI Z136.3, American National Standards Institute, Inc., New York, 1988.

ate care, use, and maintenance of equipment and prevention of laser-related accidents.

4. *Documentation.* The surgeon, procedure, type of laser used, length of use, and wattage must be recorded in the patient's medical record. This information, plus the patient's name, should also be recorded in the OR log.

Patient Safety

The surgeon must explain laser surgery and its potential complications to the patient before obtaining written consent. Some lasers are considered investigational devices by the FDA. The patient must sign a specific consent form permitting experimental use and data collection. With all lasers appropriate precautions are taken to ensure patient safety. The patient's eye, skin, and tissues surrounding the target site must be protected from thermal burns.

1. Eyes and eyelids must be adequately protected from the specific laser beam in use.
   a. Patients who are awake must wear the same type of safety glasses or goggles as those worn by the laser team (see the section in this chapter on personnel eye protection).
   b. Eyes can be taped shut on patients who are under general anesthesia.
   c. Eyepads moistened with saline solution should be taped securely in place for procedures around the head and neck, except for ophthalmic procedures and those using the Nd:YAG laser. Nonflammable material, such as aluminum foil with the reflective side down, can be taped over the eyes for Nd:YAG laser procedures. Moistened eyepads will not stop this laser beam.
   d. Protective shields should be used around eyes during ophthalmic procedures. Lead eye shields can be applied directly on an anesthetized eye to protect the cornea.
2. Antiseptic used for skin preparation should be nonflammable.
   a. Aqueous solutions are safest, but they can retain laser heat if allowed to pool on or around skin. Skin should be thoroughly dry before the laser is activated.
   b. Alcohol and tinctures are flammable and volatile when wet. Vapors must not accumulate under drapes because they can ignite.
3. Immediate area around the incision and/or tissue surrounding the target site must be protected from thermal injury. Flammable materials are avoided or safeguarded to prevent fire.
   a. Flame- or fire-resistant drapes should be used. Metallic foil and polypropylene laser-retardant and ignition-resistant drapes are available. Polypropylene and plastic incise drapes can melt if a laser beam strikes them. Woven and nonwoven fabrics can be ignited.
   b. Woven textile or cellulose-based absorbent nonwoven towels saturated with sterile normal saline solution or water should be placed over fabric drapes around the incision before the laser is used.
   c. Laser handpiece should be laid on a moistened surface. The laser tip is extremely hot and may shatter if placed in contact with a cold surface.
   d. Moistened sponges, towels, or compressed patties should be placed around target tissue except when the Nd:YAG laser is used. Sponges and other material must be removed from tissue near the target site of the Nd:YAG laser because wetting will not stop this beam and they could be ignited.
   e. Rectum should be packed with a moistened sponge to prevent methane gas, which is potentially explosive, from escaping from the intestinal tract during use of laser in the perineal area. Record placement of the sponge in the anal orifice and removal of the rectal packing.
4. Anesthetic agents must be noncombustible. Nonflammable anesthetics and oxygen mixed with nonflammable agents must be administered in a closed system.
   a. Oxygen and nitrous oxide concentrations around the head should be as low as possible during use of laser in the aerodigestive tract, that is, oral, laryngeal, bronchial, or esophageal procedures.
   b. Flexible metallic or insulated silicone endotracheal tubes are preferred for aerodigestive tract procedures. Laser-approved varieties are commercially available. If used, red rubber tubes must be wrapped with reflective aluminum or copper tape to prevent ignition. Polyvinyl chloride endotracheal tubes should *never* be used because they ignite easily. The endotracheal tube cuff should be inflated with saline solution which may be tinted with methylene blue to facilitate detection of a leak.
5. Teeth should be covered during aerodigestive procedures to protect against reflective radiation.
6. Patients who are awake may wear a protective high-filtration mask during CO_2 ablation, as of condylomata (venereal warts), to prevent inhaling airborne material into the lungs. An intubated patient is not considered at risk for respiratory contamination.
7. Postoperative instructions should include care of healing thermal skin wound.

Personnel Safety

Exposure to nonionizing laser radiation can be hazardous for personnel. Precautions must be taken to avoid eye and skin exposure to direct or scattered radiation and inhalation of plume.

Eye Protection The eye is the organ that is most susceptible to laser injury. Different laser wavelengths affect eyes differently: argon and Nd:YAG lasers will be absorbed by retina and the CO_2 laser by cornea. Therefore safety glasses or goggles of the correct optical density must be worn at all times while the laser is in use. *Optical density* is the ability of the lens to absorb a specific wavelength (Table 15-1). The color of the lens is not the protecting feature of the eyewear. Each type of wavelength requires protective eyewear of a specific optical density, as recommended by the manufacturer of the laser.

1. Protective eyewear is available outside the room near posted signs designating the specific type of laser in use. Only persons with appropriate eye protection are admitted in the room while the laser is in use.
   a. All protective eyewear (i.e., safety glasses or goggles) must shield the wearer's eyes from the top, bottom, and sides of the visual field.
   b. Goggles will fit over eyeglasses, or prescription lenses of the correct optical density can be obtained. Contact lenses do not provide eye protection.
   c. Scratches on the lens or breaks in the frame can negate eye protection.
2. Lens covers with filter caps are available for optical eyepieces of endoscopes and operating microscopes. Their use does not eliminate the need for the entire team to wear eye protection.

Skin Protection Skin sensitivities can develop from overexposure to ultraviolet radiation. Skin also can be burned from exposure to direct or reflected laser energy. These hazards are minimized if personnel are alert to precautions for environmental safety (see the section on environmental safety in this chapter). Other personnel safety precautions reduce risks.

1. Metallic jewelry should not be worn. It could absorb heat or reflect the beam.
2. Fire-resistant gowns may be worn.

TABLE 15-1

Optical Density Necessary for Protective Eyewear

Optical Density	Transmission of Light (% of Wavelength)
0	1
1	0.1
2	0.01
3	0.001
4	0.0001
5	0.00001
6	0.000001

Light transmission is measured with a spectrophotometer to calculate the optical density needed for protective eyewear.

Laser Plume Toxic substances, including carcinogens and viruses, may become airborne from vaporization of tissues, especially from CO_2 and contact Nd:YAG lasers. The smoke produced, referred to as *laser plume,* contains water, carbonized particles, mutated DNA, and intact cells. It may have a distinct odor. Laser plume should not be inhaled. Smoke evacuation from the site of lasing and high-filtration masks prevent personnel from inhaling plume. Removal of plume also enhances visibility at the target site for the surgeon. Plume can bend or refract the beam, thus inadvertently causing injury to adjacent tissues.

1. A mechanical smoke evacuator or suction with a high-efficiency filter should be turned on before or at the same time as the laser and should be run during activation and for 20 to 30 seconds after the laser is deactivated. The tip should be placed as close as possible, at least within 2 inches (5 cm), to the lasing site of tissue vaporization.
   a. Several types of mechanical smoke evacuator systems are available. Many systems have charcoal filters.
   b. Charcoal filters in most evacuators must be changed regularly. Gloves and a mask are worn when handling contaminated filters.
2. Masks should be tight fitting and should filter particles as small as 0.1 μm.

Environmental Safety

Only properly trained persons are authorized to participate in laser surgery. Others must be aware of its hazards.

1. Warning sign(s), "Laser Surgery in Progress," should be posted on the outside of all OR doors when the laser is in use. Design, symbols, and wording on the warning sign should be specific for the type of laser in use.
2. Walls and ceilings should have nonreflective surfaces. Glass, as in windows, cabinet doors, and/or the x-ray viewing box, must be covered with nonreflective material to stop beams when lasers other than CO_2 are used. CO_2 laser beams are absorbed by glass.
3. Warning labels on the machine, affixed by the manufacturer, must indicate points of danger to avoid personnel exposure to laser radiation.

4. Machine should be prepared, checked, and tested before the patient is brought into the room. A preoperative checklist is helpful. Any malfunction must be reported immediately and the equipment not used until it is in proper working order.
5. Machine should be kept on the "standby" setting with the beam terminated in a beam stop of highly absorbent, nonreflecting, fire-resistant material when not in use to avoid accidental activation. It should be turned off and locked with a key when left unattended. Only authorized personnel have access to the key.
6. Foot switch should be operated by the surgeon who delivers the laser energy to the tissue. The foot pedal can be covered when not in use so the surgeon will not inadvertently activate the laser. Foot pedals for other equipment should be moved away while the laser is in use. The laser pedal can then be removed after use.
7. Nonreflective instruments should be used in or near the beam. These instruments may be of a dull blue titanium alloy or an ebonized or anodized stainless steel. These finishes defocus and disperse the laser beam. Reflective instruments can cause burns or start fires.
8. Fire is a potential hazard that cannot be underestimated. Personnel must be aware of fire safeguards and adhere to precautions for their own and the patient's safety.
   a. Basin of sterile water or normal saline solution should be readily available at the sterile field.
   b. Halon fire extinguisher must be available.
   c. Oxygen concentration in the room should be as low as possible. Oxygen leaking from the side of a patient's face mask can be ignited by laser beam. The anesthesiologist must be knowledgeable about flash points and fire retardation when the laser is in use.
   d. Liquids should never be placed on the machine. A spill could act as a conductor and short-circuit the mechanism.
9. Electrical codes and standards must be enforced to avoid electrical hazards (see Chapter 10, pp. 148-152). An isolation transformer is recommended for a high-power laser power source to avoid dangerous overload of the existing OR power system. Electrical circuitry must provide adequate amperage for power requirements. Preferably the laser has its own dedicated circuit.
10. Manufacturer's instructions for operation, care, handling, and sterilization of the laser system must be followed. Proper care of lasers and accessory equipment is essential to patient, personnel, and environmental safety.

Laser Team

A laser team should be designated to carry out the duties that are different from those of the traditional OR team. This team may include the following personnel:

1. *Clinical laser nurse.* The responsibilities of the clinical laser nurse are different from those of the circulator. Duties include the following:
   a. Preparing and teaching the patient preoperatively, intraoperatively, and postoperatively.
   b. Bringing laser equipment to the OR and checking it. The chassis and floor around it should be inspected for water leak. Using sterile technique, the clinical laser nurse and scrub person calibrate the laser as appropriate.
   c. Covering windows, posting signs, and distributing appropriate protective eyewear.
   d. Covering patient's eyes.
   e. Positioning the laser foot pedal for the surgeon's convenience and removing it after use.
   f. Operating the key switch and monitoring activation of the laser. The wattage and exposure time are set according to surgeon's orders. These should be repeated before and after adjusting controls.
   g. Cleaning and checking laser fibers after use and preparing them for sterilization.
   h. Completing the laser log.
   i. Collaborating with the laser safety officer and biomedical engineer and/or technician to ensure safe use of laser equipment.
2. *Biomedical technician.* The biomedical technician provides preventive maintenance and handles minor problems with the laser system. A log of laser uses and maintenance is maintained.
3. *Camera operator.* Endoscopic procedures performed under video control may require an additional sterile team member to operate the camera attached to the endoscope while the surgeon controls the laser fiber.

Advantages of Laser Surgery

Surgical lasers emit nonionizing radiation. This radiation is selectively absorbed by different tissues with resultant penetration and destruction at the focal point but with differential thermal protection of surrounding tissues. Lasers offer the surgeon and the patient many advantages over other surgical techniques.

1. *Precise control for accurate incision, excision, or ablation of tissue.* The laser beam is precisely focused for localized tissue destruction. The depth of radiation penetration is precisely regulated by duration of focus, power density, and type of tissue.

2. *Access to areas inaccessible to other surgical instruments through minimally invasive techniques.* The beam can be directed through endoscopes or deflected off rhodium reflector mirrors.
3. *Unobstructed view of surgical site.* The laser beam comes in contact with tissue to be cut, coagulated, or vaporized. It can be directed through the operating microscope.
4. *Minimal handling of and trauma to tissues.* Traction on target tissue is unnecessary.
5. *Dry, bloodless surgical field.* The laser beam simultaneously cuts and coagulates blood vessels, thus providing hemostasis in vascular areas.
6. *Minimal thermal effect on surrounding tissue.* Essentially no permanent thermal necrosis of tissue occurs beyond 100 μm from the edge of the area incised. This minimizes postoperative pain.
7. *Reduced risk of contamination or infection.* The laser beam vaporizes microorganisms, thus essentially sterilizing the contact area.
8. *Prompt healing with minimal postoperative edema, sloughing of tissue, pain, and scarring.*
9. *Reduced operating time.* Because procedures can be done more quickly, both anesthesia and operating time are shorter. Many procedures can be done without general anesthesia. Many are done in ambulatory care facilities.

Disadvantages of Laser Surgery

1. *Costs to start and maintain a program.* Equipment, instrumentation, supplies, and staff education are expensive initial investments. Most aspects need frequent updates and maintenance.
2. *Decisions must be made about the use of disposable vs. reusable supplies and the impact on patient care.* Most reusables are fragile and must be replaced on a regular basis.
3. *Liability may increase as the number of users increase.* Specific credentialling and continuing education require planning and are time consuming.

ENDOSCOPY

Endoscopy is a combined form of two Greek words, *endon* (ενδον) and *skopein* (σκοπην), *endon* meaning "inside," and *skopein* meaning "to examine." *Endoscopy,* as the term is used in medicine, is a visual examination of the interior of a body cavity, hollow organ, or structure with an *endoscope,* an instrument designed for direct visual inspection.

Although physicians sought to visualize the interior of body organs, development of endoscopy was slow. It was not until the early nineteenth century that attempts were made to examine the inside of the bladder. Instruments were inadequate, however, and light was from a candle or lamp. Finally, Nitze, an Austrian, developed an instrument in 1876 that is the basis of modern endoscopy. Dr. Chevalier Jackson of Philadelphia further enhanced endoscopy by developing a laryngoscope and bronchoscope. Only after the incandescent lamp was invented and an optical system was devised could an efficient instrument be made. Improvements started about 1878, and the precise instruments of today have evolved since that time, making possible the conservative treatment of many conditions. Endoscopic inspection of the abdominal cavity, introduced in 1902, has become a common procedure since the advent of fiberoptic illumination.

An endoscope is usually inserted into a natural body orifice (i.e., the mouth, anus, or urethra). It may be inserted through a small skin incision and/or trocar puncture, as through the abdominal or vaginal wall. An endoscopic procedure is designated by the anatomic structure to be visualized. The endoscope likewise is named for the anatomic area it is designed to visualize; for example, a laryngo*scope* is used for laryngo*scopy.* From head to foot, nearly every area of the body can be visualized with an endoscope.

All endoscopic procedures are considered minimally invasive except for ophthalmoscopy, because the scope is placed into a body orifice or cavity. Many require one or more small skin incisions for insertion of the scope and accessories. Endoscopy is used for many diagnostic procedures (see Box 28-2, p. 574) and in conjunction with surgical procedures. A description of many of these is included in the chapters in Section Ten.

Design of Endoscopes

Although the sizes and shapes vary according to specific uses, all endoscopes have similar working elements (Figure 15-3).

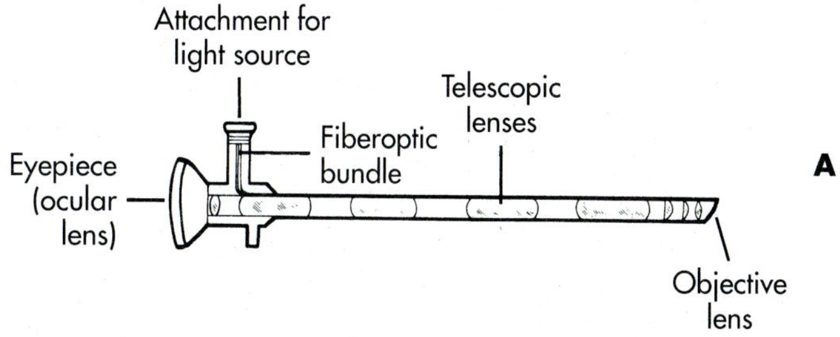

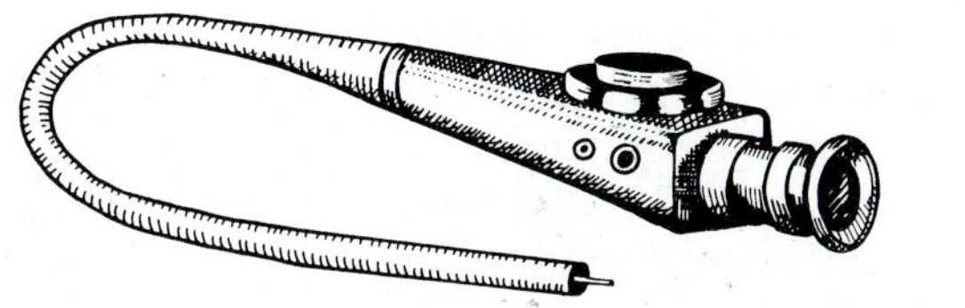

FIGURE 15-3 Schematic design of endoscopes. **A,** Rigid scope. **B,** Flexible scope.

Viewing Sheath (Scope)

The surgeon views anatomic structures through a round or oval sheath. Diameter varies from the 1.7 mm needle fetoscope to the 5 mm or less of the arthroscope to the 22 mm of an anoscope. Length must be appropriate to reach the desired structure. The scope may be rigid or flexible.

Rigid Scopes Rigid scopes are either hollow sheaths that permit viewing in a forward direction only, such as laryngoscopes, or a sheath with an eyepiece and telescopic lens system that permits viewing in a variety of directions, such as cystoscopes. Most rigid scopes are metal. Disposable plastic anoscopes and otoscope sheaths are available.

Flexible Scopes Flexible scopes have a dial adjuster that contours the lensed tip into and around anatomic curvatures to permit visualization of all surfaces of the wall of a structure, as within the hollow organs of the gastrointestinal tract viewed through a flexible gastroscope or colonoscope. The sheath of these instruments is made of plastic material.

Light Source

Illumination within the body cavity is essential for visual acuity. The light source may be through a fiberoptic bundle or from an incandescent light bulb. The light carrier may be an integral part of the viewing sheath, as in flexible scopes and rigid telescopes, or it may be a separate light carrier accessory to a hollow rigid scope.

Fiberoptic Lighting With fiberoptic lighting an intense cool light illuminates body cavities, including those that cannot be seen with other light sources. Light is conducted through a bundle of thousands of coated glass fibers encased in a plastic sheath. Each fiber is drawn from optical glass into a strand 10 to 70 μm in diameter that is coated to minimize loss of light by reflection. Light entering one end of the fiber is transmitted by refraction through its entire length. The light produced through the bundle of fibers is nonglaring and evenly distributed on the area to be visualized. Although it is of high intensity, the light is cool; however, a minimum rise of temperature in the tissues exposed to it may occur.

Bulbs Bulbs screw into the fitting either at the end of a removable light carrier or at the end of a built-in lens system. Electric current is conducted through a single-filament wire to illuminate the tiny incandescent light bulb. When changing the bulb, a bit of wax is applied to the threads of the bulb base, sealing the bulb socket from moisture to prevent short circuits. Fiberoptic lighting has replaced bulbs in most endoscopes and prevents this hazard.

Power Source

Electric current must be transmitted to the light source connected to a fiberoptic bundle or a light bulb. The electric current is entirely external to the patient with fiberoptic lighting. Current flows through a power cord attached to the endoscope inserted into the patient and through the instrument to the light bulb at the distal end of the light carrier or sheath. The power source may or may not be connected to the electrical system in the room.

Projection Lamp A quartz-halogen or mercury-arc light bulb provides an intense light source, similar to a film projector, for transmission of light through a fiberoptic bundle to the distal end of the scope. Usually a portable, compact, self-contained unit, the intensity of the light may be regulated from 400 footcandles to as much as 5200 footcandles, up to 5500° K daylight in some illuminators. The bulb must be positioned securely in its socket so output focuses on the center of the fiberoptic bundle. If it is not properly positioned, light output will not be of maximum value.

A fiberoptic power cable transmits light from the projection lamp to the endoscope. Both ends of the cable must have the correct fittings to attach to the lamp and to the scope or removable light carrier. The diameter of the cable varies from 2.0 to 5.5 mm to be compatible with the aperture for the light source. Cable lengths also vary from 6 feet (180 cm) to 9 feet (275 cm) so the projection lamp can be positioned at a distance from a sterile field. Before use, the fiberoptic cable should be checked for damage. Hold one end of the cable toward a low power light such as the overhead operating light. With a magnifying glass, focus on the opposite end. Broken fibers in the cable will appear as dark spots. The cable must be replaced if more than 20% of the area appears dark.

Battery Box One or more sets of dry-cell batteries may be used as the power source for light bulbs. The batteries may be recharged in some units, but eventually they must be replaced. A battery provides a good source of current, is safe, and can be used in conjunction with other electrical equipment.

Rheostat A rheostat is a resistor for regulating flow of current from the electrical system. Rapidly introduced high voltage may burn out the delicate filament in a light bulb. A rheostat reduces electrical potential and allows gradual increase of current to desired brightness of the light. However, safety precautions must be observed when using this power source to prevent shock to the patient and operator. Rheostats that cannot be grounded should not be used. They also cannot be used when the cutting current of the electrosurgical unit is in use. Cutting current will not work if another piece of equipment is on the same circuit.

Accessories

Accessories such as suction tubes, snares, biopsy forceps, grasping forceps, sutures, and sponge carriers are used in conjunction with endoscopes. These accessories can be passed through channels in the endoscope to remove fluid or tissue, coagulate or ligate bleeding vessels, inject fluid or gas to distend cavities, etc. Some rigid scopes have an obturator, a blunt-tipped rod placed through the lumen, to permit smooth insertion of the instrument, as into the anus. The accessories that will be needed will be determined by type of endoscope and purpose of procedure.

Carbon Dioxide Insufflator The peritoneal cavity is filled with carbon dioxide gas, creating a gas lake called *pneumoperitoneum,* before a laparoscope is inserted through the abdominal wall. The pneumoperitoneum allows for visualization of organs and structures within the peritoneal cavity. The carbon dioxide insufflator is a specially designed machine that delivers a metered flow up to 6 L per minute of carbon dioxide through disposable hydrophobic filter tubing. At the start of the procedure a small 1 to 2 mm incision is made into the abdominal wall, a special spring-loaded *Verres needle* is inserted, and the carbon dioxide is delivered into the peritoneal cavity at a rate measured by pressure predetermined by the surgeon. Initial flow is started at 6 to 7 mm Hg to establish a safe flow. It is maintained between 8 to 14 mm Hg. Once the pneumoperitoneum is established, a 10 or 12 mm trocar is inserted and the insufflation tubing is attached to a port on the side of the trocar sleeve. Occasionally a surgeon will omit using a Verres needle for initial insufflation and create the gas lake through the trocar. This procedure may be used for the patient who has many adhesions or multiple previous surgeries.

The circulator monitors the intraabdominal pressure and the amount of carbon dioxide delivered and may be asked to change the flow rate periodically throughout the procedure. The pressure should not be allowed to exceed 20 mm Hg. Problems with kinked tubing can give a false high pressure reading. High pressures are immediately reported to the surgeon.

At the conclusion of the procedure, the carbon dioxide should be evacuated through the filtered suction port on the trocar and not expelled directly into the room air. The expelled carbon dioxide gas contains blood and body fluids that cause airborne contamination.

Electrosurgical Electrodes An active electrode connected to a monopolar electrosurgical unit may be used through an endoscope, such as a laparoscope for general or gynecologic surgery or a resectoscope for urologic surgery. A variety of electrodes, both disposable and reusable, are available. They must have adequate insulation and be inspected before use for any defect. Electrical energy transfers by capacitance from the activated electrode through intact insulation into other nearby conductive materials. Unless a safe path is provided for current to return to ground, the current induced by capacitance might cause a burn on internal tissue. Direct coupling occurs when the activated electrode touches other metal instruments, particularly the laparoscope. An all-metal trocar/cannula system allows accidental contact to dissipate through the abdominal wall. The surgeon should avoid activating the electrode unless it is in contact with the tissue. A shielding and monitoring system is commercially available for monopolar endoscopic electrosurgical electrodes. Bipolar instruments, including dissectors, scissors, and graspers, eliminate the potential hazard of stray currents with monopolar electrodes.

Laser A laser beam can be focused through some endoscopes. Argon, Ho:YAG, and Nd:YAG lasers will pass through a fiberoptic system. The CO_2 laser can be directed through a rigid endoscope or the interior mirror system of a multiarticulated arm of the operating microscope (see section on laser microadaptor, p. 290). The beam is then focused through the endoscope, which is usually held in a self-retaining device. A distal smoke evacuation suction device clears fumes to maintain visibility through the scope and at the site of lasing. The endoscopes are specifically designed for adaptation to the articulated arm of the CO_2 laser, for example, the CO_2 laser laparoscope and CO_2 laser bronchoscope.

Ultrasonic Transducer A high-frequency ultrasound transducer at the end of a fiberoptic endoscope provides visualization of the heart, liver, pancreas, spleen, and kidneys. See Chapter 28, pp. 572-573, for a discussion of the use of ultrasonography for diagnosis of vascular diseases and for identifying location, size, and consistency of lesions in abdominal organs.

Operating Microscope The optical system of some endoscopes can be attached to a specially designed operating microscope such as the colpomicroscope. The illumination of the endoscope and binocular magnification of the microscope permit study of abnormal tissues and/or therapeutic procedures in areas otherwise inaccessible without an open surgical procedure.

Cameras Lensed scopes may be equipped with a still or motion picture camera so organs or lesions can be photographed during a procedure. Video cameras with recorder/player/printer equipment can be adapted for use with some endoscopes. A high-powered light source may be needed with the camera for photographic applications and video documentation. An endoscopic video camera electronically transmits images to a closed-circuit television screen. By viewing high-resolution monitor(s), the endoscopist can manipulate instruments for diagnostic examination or to perform a therapeutic procedure. Video documentation can be obtained by taping the examination or procedure. Microcomputer imaging systems with a printer reproduce these images into photographs. Fluoroscopy may be preferred to video images for certain procedures such as radioactive implantation.

Hazards of Endoscopy

Endoscopy is not without its hazards. The patient should sign a consent before an endoscopic procedure is performed in the event that a complication develops. Two major complications of endoscopy are as follows:

1. *Perforation.* Perforation is a constant cause for concern when rigid scopes are used. Flexible fiberoptic endoscopes have decreased this danger, but it remains a potential complication.
2. *Bleeding.* Bleeding can occur from a biopsy site, pedicle of a polyp, or other area where tissue has been cut.

Electrical systems used with endoscopy must conform with the standards and be subjected to routine maintenance procedures prescribed by the National Fire Protection Association code for electrical safety. Two major electrical hazards associated with endoscopy are as follows:

1. *Improperly grounded electrical equipment.* If the surgeon will use a monopolar electrosurgical unit, place the inactive dispersive electrode with adequate skin contact to allow conduction of electric current. Only solid-state generators, and preferably bipolar active electrodes, should be used to avoid variances in voltage.
2. *Unsuspected current leaks.* Corrosion or accumulation of organic material can inhibit flow of current across the screw fitting between the light carrier and bulb. Current can leak through the instrument to the patient. Ideally endoscopes should not contain electrically conductive elements or metals that can corrode. Corrosion can be caused by repeated exposure to body fluids, hard water, or chemical agents.

Microorganisms, such as *Mycobacterium tuberculosis,* can be transmitted from one patient to another via a bronchoscope. *Streptococcus pneumoniae, Pseudomonas aeruginosa, Clostridium,* and bloodborne pathogens also present potential hazards of cross contamination. Personnel are exposed to potentially infectious body fluids and blood from aerosols, splashes, and contact with contaminated instrumentation. Gloves, masks, protective eyewear, gowns, or aprons must be worn during endoscopic procedures and cleaning of equipment. Personnel should use universal precautions during endoscopic procedures and when handling and processing contaminated endoscopes and accessories.

Types of Endoscopic Procedures

Not all endoscopic procedures are performed as sterile procedures; some are *surgically clean.* An endoscope is introduced into the gastrointestinal tract through the mouth or anus. It touches only mucous membranes. However, the gastrointestinal tract normally harbors resident and transient microorganisms. Although the procedure is not considered sterile, patients and personnel must be protected from cross contamination. Endoscopes and their accessories must be thoroughly cleaned and terminally sterilized or high-level disinfected after use. Sterility is not maintained between and during patient uses. Instruments should be stored according to manufacturer's recommendations. Many endoscopic procedures are performed by gastroenterologists in an endoscopy unit, rather than in the OR.

Endoscopy is performed as a *sterile procedure* if body tissue will be incised or excised, or if a normally sterile organ or body cavity is entered such as the bladder and uterus. Ideally, the endoscope and all accessories should be sterile regardless of the point of entry. However, it may not be feasible to sterilize some heat-sensitive parts, such as a lensed telescope, between patient uses when several procedures are scheduled in succession. Control of scheduling endoscopic procedures and adequate instrumentation will help to provide sterile endoscopes for every patient. In reality, high-level disinfection may be necessary between uses. Written policies and procedures must specify accepted practices for patient care and infection control. AORN has developed recommended practices for the use and care of endoscopes to be used as a guide in establishing processing procedures. *Only sterile endoscopes and accessories should be used on patients with suppressed immune systems,* as from chemotherapy or steroid therapy and human immunodeficiency virus–related diseases.

Often described as minimally invasive surgery, *endoscopic minimal access surgery* does not require the incisions of traditional open procedures, such as for removal of the gallbladder or appendix. The procedure is performed with instruments introduced through ports established through small incisions. Routine practices should be established that reduce risks of potential patient injuries and complications. These practices include but are not limited to the following:

1. Training for and demonstrating competence in use and care of endoscopic equipment by surgeons and nursing personnel.
2. Providing complete sets of properly prepared functional instruments.
3. Monitoring the patient for changes in physiologic status. For example, development of hypercapnia

and/or hypothermia can be caused by carbon dioxide insufflation.

All patients should be prepared, that is, prepped and draped, for conversion to an open procedure when warranted by recognized or potential complications. Instrumentation and supplies for an open procedure should be readily available. The patient should be informed preoperatively of this possibility.

Care of Endoscopes

Endoscopes are delicate and expensive instruments. Avoid rough handling, jarring, or bending of parts. Never pile them on top of each other or mix them with other instruments.

All parts of endoscopes and accessories must be thoroughly mechanically cleaned and terminally sterilized or disinfected after use. The primary causes of infection transmitted endoscopically are inadequate cleaning and disinfection or sterilization of endoscopic equipment.

Cleaning

Clean all parts of the endoscope as soon as possible after use while organic debris is still moist. Mucus, blood, feces, and protein-type residue can become trapped in the channels of the scope. This is difficult to remove if it becomes dry and may render the scope useless.

Wash endoscopes in warm, never hot, water and a neutral, nonresidue liquid-detergent solution. Use a pipestem cleaner or small brush to clean inside lumen of all channels. The stopcocks on some scopes must be thoroughly cleaned, too, because dirty ones will stick. Open them to clean; never force them but loosen them with a drop of solvent or lubricant. Disassemble all removable parts.

Particular attention must be paid to cleanliness of lenses or viewing will be obstructed. Debris can be carefully removed from around the lens with a fine toothpick. Special lens paper is used on the lens itself. Lensed instruments should not be cleaned with any substance that contains alcohol since it may dissolve cement around the lens.

Rinse the endoscope thoroughly and dry well. If scopes are to be sterilized in ethylene oxide gas, they must be thoroughly dry. Gas combines with water on items that are damp to form ethylene glycol (see Chapter 13, p. 228). Use alcohol on cotton on a wire stylet or a pipestem cleaner to dry insertion tubes. Force air through channels to dry inside them. Organisms will multiply in a moist environment, so all parts must be dry during the interval before further processing or storage.

An endoscope processor is available to clean long flexible fiberoptic scopes such as a colonoscope. It has two modes of operation to process the viewing sheath and channels of the scope: wash and dry cycle; or wash, disinfectant soak with activated glutaraldehyde solution, rinse, and dry. This equipment is an automated washer/disinfector.

Accessories must be scrupulously cleaned. All debris must be removed to ensure adequate steam sterilization. Disposable single-use biopsy forceps and cytology brushes are recommended because the configurations of these accessories are particularly difficult to clean. Some trocars, scissors, and forceps have disposable or replaceable points or tips on reusable shafts or handles. These combination instruments facilitate cleaning and also ensure a sharp cutting edge with each use.

Scopes and accessories must be inspected for damage after cleaning. Preferably, all endoscopic equipment should be terminally sterilized, otherwise it must be disinfected after thorough mechanical cleaning.

Sterilization

After cleaning and drying, place each endoscope with all its parts *disassembled* in a well-padded perforated tray of convenient size. Some endoscopes, such as an arthroscope, are supplied in a perforated case lined with foam cut to fit each disassembled part. Wrap the tray or fitted case for sterilization. Instruments should be packaged immediately and sent to be sterilized by steam or ethylene oxide gas as recommended by the manufacturer.

Some parts of endoscopes can be safely steam sterilized and therefore should be. Hollow, rigid metal sheaths, such as a sigmoidoscope, can be terminally steam sterilized after use but then may be stored to keep clean rather than sterile for a surgically clean procedure. Some fiberoptic cables also can be steam sterilized. Reusable biopsy forceps must be steam sterilized.

Parts with lenses and some fiberoptic carriers, such as a colonoscope, cannot be steam sterilized. High temperature and moisture will soften the cement holding lenses or fiberoptic fibers in place. The flexible shafts of some accessory instruments may erode when steam sterilized. These parts should be sterilized in ethylene oxide gas, hydrogen peroxide plasma, or formaldehyde gas or soaked in a chemical sterilant solution if ethylene oxide or hydrogen peroxide is not available.

During ethylene oxide sterilization of a fiberoptic lighting system, the manufacturer may recommend that the pressure not exceed 5 lb. Follow manufacturer's instructions for handling, using, cleaning, and sterilizing these items. Aeration is necessary following ethylene oxide sterilization. Ethylene oxide is a vesicant if it comes in contact with skin. It also can cause eye irritation.

If endoscopes and accessories are immersed in activated glutaraldehyde, acetic acid, or formaldehyde solution, use a plastic tray without a towel in the bottom. Prolonged use of a stainless steel tray may create an electrolytic action between the metals and can cause metallic deposits on instruments. Scopes and all accessories must be well rinsed in sterile distilled water before they are used to prevent tissue irritation from solution.

Paracetic acid, another chemical sterilant in solution, is commercially available for sterilizing endoscopes for immediate patient use. The Steris system has specialized tray assemblies for endoscope processing. These assemblies are not intended for long-term storage of sterilized instruments. These chemical sterilants are discussed in Chapter 13, pp. 231-232.

High-Level Disinfection

When immediate reuse of an endoscope that cannot be steam sterilized is necessary, it should be washed in nonresidue liquid-detergent solution, rinsed, dried, and immersed in activated glutaraldehyde, acetic acid, or paracetic acid solution with parts disassembled. All channels must be filled with solution. Solution may become diluted if endoscopes are not dried before immersion.

Set a timer for a minimum of 20 minutes to kill vegetative bacteria, fungi, and hepatitis B and human immunodeficiency viruses. Time must be extended to 45 minutes for tuberculocidal activity of glutaraldehyde.

Even though high-level disinfection is not sterilization, sterile gloves are worn to remove scopes from solution. *Never handle lensed instruments with forceps.* Forceps could crush a telescope and ruin the optical system. Also, if an instrument is wet, the danger of dropping it is increased. Rinse all parts thoroughly in sterile distilled water before use.

Storage

If not immediately wrapped for sterilization and storage, endoscopes should be terminally sterilized or at least high-level disinfected before returning them to their respective storage cabinets. Store clean, *dry,* unwrapped instruments on a soft material such as plastic sheeting or foam. Towels hold a residue of laundry detergent that can cause tarnish on metal. Flexible endoscopes are stored vertically. Accessories also may be hung.

Considerations for Patient Safety

Endoscopy through a natural body orifice is usually performed on a patient who is not under general anesthesia. The following considerations should be included in the plan of care.

1. The patient must be monitored for signs and symptoms of reaction to drugs. Endoscopy is frequently performed with the use of sedatives and a topical or local anesthetic agent or with no anesthetic at all. The patient is awake during these procedures. Drugs such as midazolam (Versed) and diazepam (Valium) and narcotics such as meperidine hydrochloride (Demerol) may be administered intravenously as an adjunct to other preoperative sedation to produce relaxation and cooperation during the procedure and amnesia afterward. Respiratory depression and transient hypotension can occur. Antagonistic drugs should be available to reverse narcotic depression. Emergency resuscitation equipment should also be available.
2. A topical agent is frequently applied to nasal or oral and pharyngeal mucosa before introduction of an endoscope into the tracheobronchial tree or gastrointestinal tract. A topical agent may be instilled into the urethra before introduction of a cystoscope. See Chapter 18 for reactions to topical and local anesthetic agents.
3. Teeth, gums, and lips must be protected if the endoscope is introduced through the mouth. Dentures are removed. A mouthpiece is inserted.
4. Hydrogen and methane gases are normally present in the colon. These gases must be flushed out with carbon dioxide before laser or electrosurgery through the colonoscope to avoid the possibility of explosion within the colon.
5. Power sources and lights should be tested before each use and after cleaning. They should be kept in working order.
6. The heat generated from the projection lamp of a fiberoptic illuminator must be dissipated. It should not be enclosed in drapes because the heat could set them on fire. If the unit contains a fan for heat regulation, the direction of air flow must be away from the patient and the sterile field to minimize airborne contamination.
7. Endoscopes must be smooth, with no nicks on the surface. A scratch on the sheath could cause injury to tissue or the mucous membrane lining of an orifice. Do not handle metal endoscopes with metal lifting forceps that can scratch the sheaths. They should be handled only with hands, usually gloved.
8. Extreme care must be taken to observe patients after endoscopic procedures for effects of respiratory or circulatory distress caused by trauma or medication. Many endoscopic procedures are performed on ambulatory outpatients. They must not leave the facility until vital signs are stable and side effects have passed.

Duties of Assistant

Often only a circulator assists the surgeon with a minimally invasive procedure.

1. Set up the supplies and equipment as much as possible before the patient and surgeon arrive. Consult the procedure book. Remember that sterility must be maintained for a sterile procedure.
2. Explain the steps of the procedure to the patient as appropriate. It is important that the patient know the reasons for any discomfort that may be

experienced so that symptoms of discomfort will be recognized as normal.

3. Explain the position and need for it before positioning the patient. The position the patient must assume during the procedure is often uncomfortable.
4. Drape the patient properly to prevent unnecessary exposure.
5. Adjust room lighting. The surgeon may want the room in semidarkness. A dimmer on the room light is helpful, but if unavailable, the x-ray view boxes may be illuminated to provide indirect lighting.
6. Divert the patient's attention as much as possible during the procedure. The patient may complain of pain more than is justified as a way of expressing displeasure at the invasion of the endoscope or the position required during the procedure. The circulator should stay with the patient to offer reassurance and emotional support. Suggest that slow, deep breaths may help relaxation and lessen the discomfort. Soft music may help the patient relax. The surgeon may allow the patient to watch the procedure through a viewing attachment on the endoscope or on a video monitor.
7. Evaluate the patient's level of discomfort and inform the surgeon of unusual reactions. The circulator also monitors the patient's respiratory status, blood pressure, and pulse. Pulse oximeter and automated blood pressure devices may be used routinely. Vital signs should be documented before the procedure begins, every 15 minutes during the procedure, and again at the conclusion. Additional vital signs should be recorded when medication is given or tissue samples are excised.
8. Know how to assemble the different scopes and their accessories and how to operate them. When passing the suction tube or biopsy forceps, place the tip directly at the lumen of the scope so the surgeon can grasp the shaft and insert it without moving eyes from the scope.
9. Care must be taken not to drop endoscopic instruments; they are delicate and expensive. Fiberoptic bundles are glass; do not kink or bend them.

MICROSURGERY

Microscopy, use of a microscope, has been an essential modality in scientific investigation for centuries. Pioneers such as Anton van Leeuwenhoek, who in 1680 developed the compound microscope, which magnified objects 270 times, contributed to the adoption of the germ theory. Objects as small as bacteria could be seen only through a light microscope, as viruses can be seen only through the more recently developed electron microscope. Joseph Jackson Lister, father of the English surgeon who introduced antiseptic surgery, perfected the achromatic lens to eliminate color aberrations in the compound microscope. Ernest Abbe did further work in the nineteenth century to improve refraction and illumination through the lens. A basic system for binocular eyepieces was devised in 1902.

A microscope was first used for clinical surgery in 1921 when Nylen operated on patients with chronic otitis in Sweden. He used a monocular microscope. Subsequently, as binocular magnification, adequate illumination, and stable support were added, otolaryngology became the first surgical specialty to routinely use a microscope.

Ophthalmologists were the first to use the stereoscopic biomicroscope, commonly referred to as a *slit lamp,* in clinical examination to magnify objects in three dimensions. The principles applied to the biomicroscope led to the development of an operating microscope in 1953. Ophthalmologists quickly expanded applications and indications for ocular microsurgery. Most other specialties were slow to implement its use.

The simplest magnifying instrument consists of a single lens with relatively high magnification, for example, the magnifying glass or a jeweler's lens. Surgeons requiring lesser magnification than that provided by the microscope use an operating loupe. This simple lens magnifies approximately two times. It attaches to a headband or to the surgeon's spectacles. *Loupe surgery is not microsurgery.* It terminates where microsurgery begins. However, from loupe surgery and from refinements of the binocular microscope, microsurgery has evolved.

The first of the current operating microscopes was developed in 1960 by the Zeiss Instrument Company in collaboration with Julius Jacobson, a vascular surgeon in New York. Jacobson developed microsurgical instruments, introduced microvascular techniques, and began using the term *microsurgery.* Thus began the development of clinical applications of microsurgery in every surgical specialty.

Definitions

A glossary for microsurgery is included in Box 15-5.

Technique of Microsurgery

Performance of surgical procedures while directly viewing the surgical field under magnification affords surgeons greater visual acuity of small structures. *The microscope provides a more limited, although more readily visible, surgical field.* All things look considerably different under magnification. Tissues not otherwise visible can be manipulated. Use of microsurgical instrumentation and techniques does not simply adapt formerly learned conventional methods to use under the microscope. The techniques themselves for handling instruments, sutures, and tissues are different and infinitely more complex, precise, and time-consuming because of the meticulous skill involved. Coordination must be adapted to work with minute materials in a field of altered perception and position. Proficiency and facility in using the operating microscope entail laboratory

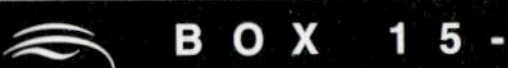

BOX 15-5

Glossary of Terms Used in Microsurgery

beam splitter Attachment to microscope that splits light; part is reflected laterally and the other part is relayed upward to the binocular tube; can be 50%/50% or 30%/70%. Greater portion may be directed to a camera or video system.
binocular Using two eyes to see in stereoscopic vision.
coaxial illumination Light path follows the same direction as visual image.
contraves stand Series of weights used to balance some microscopes.
depth of field Distance of focus.
diopter Power of the lens to assist vision by refractive correction of reflected light.
focal length Distance between the lens and the object in focus.
microscope Instrument that uses a series of lenses to magnify very small objects.
monocular Using one eye for vision. Depth of field is absent; image is two dimensional.
objective Power of the lens that determines the focal distance of vision.
ocular Eyepiece lens that multiplies the basic magnification of the microscope.
pupillary distance Measurement between pupils of eyes used to position binocular eyepieces.
stereopsis Vision with two eyes that enables objects to appear three dimensional.
working distance Physical space between objective lens of microscope and surgical field.
zoom Changing range of focus in continuous magnification; change closer or distant.

practice in movements and manipulation of instruments and suture materials under various magnifications. Mastery is achieved only by practice, repeated performance, and dedication to the task.

Divergence from tactile-manual to vision-oriented techniques requires that the surgeon and assistants pay maximum attention to detail. The most common maneuvers for placing and manipulating instruments, making an incision with a scissors, and tying sutures involve a combination of several basic movements:

1. *Compression-decompression*—to close scissors and forceps
2. *Rotation*—to insert a needle, to cut, to extract, to engage or disengage
3. *Push-pull, direct, or linear*—to incise with a razor knife

The surgeon also must be able to maintain a steady, stationary position during remote activation of equipment such as a laser beam. It is advisable that surgeons and assistants do no manual labor for at least a day before operating. Drinking coffee the morning of surgery may decrease steadiness in some individuals. Very little tremor is tolerable in microsurgery.

Advantages of Microsurgery

Microsurgery provides unique advantages in the restoration of wholeness and function of the body, such as restitution of hearing, vision, tactile sensation, circulation, and/or motion. It is used in many surgical specialties to improve precision of already established surgical procedures and to permit successful performance of procedures previously not possible. For example, blood vessels less than 3 mm in exterior diameter can be sutured. Nerves can be anastomosed. Replantation of amputated parts and some reconstructive surgery are possible only under magnification. In general, microsurgery allows the following:

1. Dissection and repair of fine structures through better visualization
2. Adaptation of surgical procedures to individual patient requirements; variation in anatomic landmarks is more distinct with magnification
3. Diminution of surgical trauma and complications because of safer dissection
4. Superior focal lighting of the surgical field, particularly in deep areas

Operating Microscope

Compound microscopes use two or more lens systems or several lenses grouped in one unit. *The operating microscope is a compound binocular instrument.* Interchangeable objective lenses combined with interchangeable eyepieces allow a wide range of magnification and working distances adjustable to the surgeon's needs. *The operating microscope uses light waves for illumination.* These waves are bent as they pass through the microscope, so the image seen by the viewer's eye is magnified.

The users must understand the parts and their functions. Basically all operating microscopes incorporate the same essential components: an optical lens system and controls for magnification and focus, an illumination system, a mounting system for stability, an electrical system, and accessories (Figure 15-4).

Optical Lens System

The ability to enlarge an image is known as *magnifying power.* This is the ratio of size of image produced on the viewer's retina by magnification to size of retinal image when the object is viewed without optical aid. To create a distinct image, adjacent images must be separated. An indistinct image remains unclear no matter

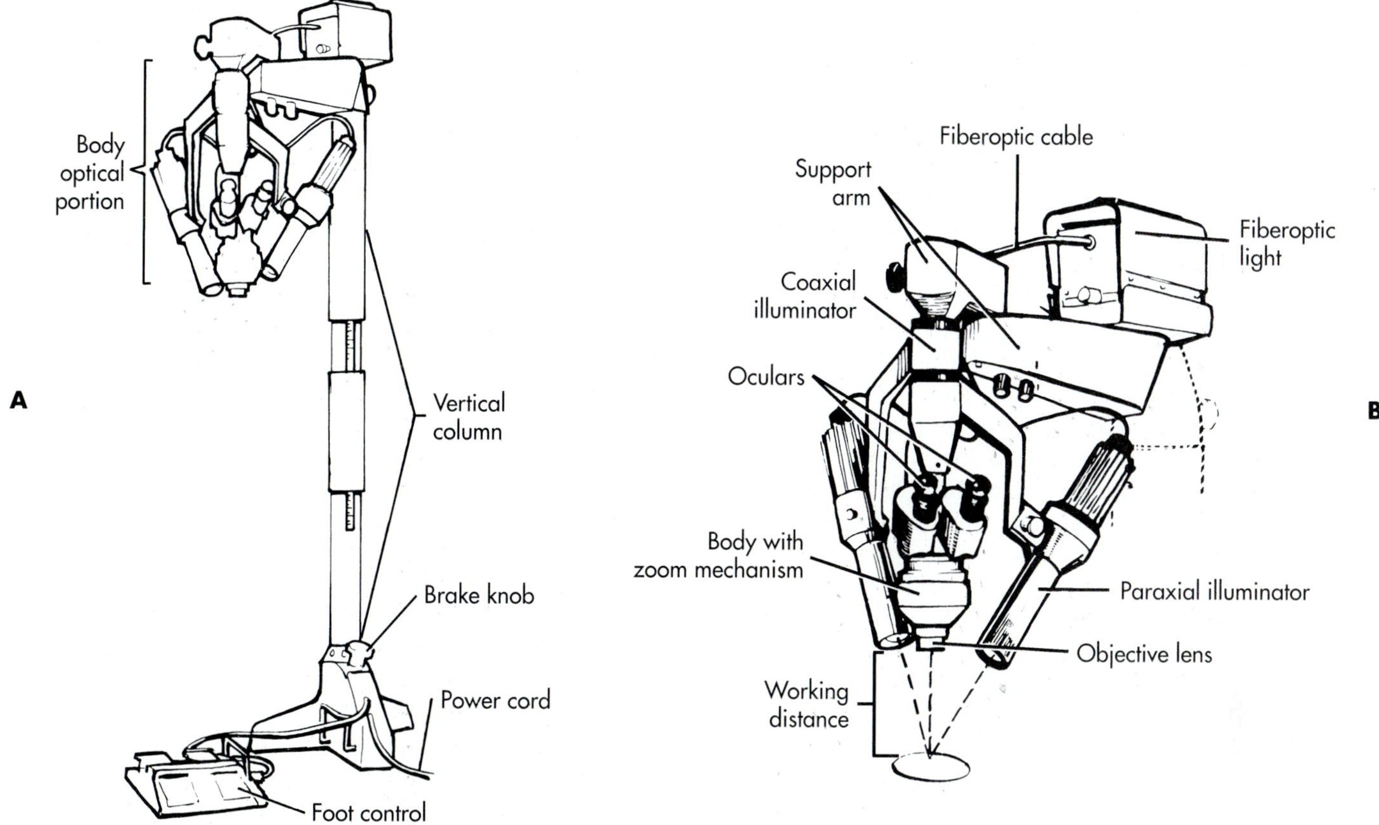

FIGURE 15-4 **A,** Floor-mounted operating microscope. **B,** Microscope body in detail.

how many times it is magnified. The ability to discern detail is known as *resolving power.*

Components The heart of the optical system is the *body,* which contains the *objective lens* (lens closest to the object). The *head* or *binocular oculars* (eyepieces) through which the surgeon looks are physically and optically attached to the body. The optical combination of the objective lens and the oculars determines the magnification of the microscope (Figure 15-4, *B*).

Objective lenses are available in various focal lengths ranging from 100 to 400 mm, with intervening increases by 25 mm increments. The 400 mm lens provides the greatest magnification. The designation of the objective lens enumerates the *working distance,* the distance from the lens to the surgical field. Distances vary from 6 to 10 inches (15 to 25 cm). For example, a 200 mm lens will be in focus at a working distance of 200 mm or approximately 8 inches (20 cm).

The oculars serve as magnifying glasses used to examine the real image formed by the objective. Most objectives are achromatic so that the true color of tissues can be viewed in sharp detail. The binocular arrangement provides stereoscopic viewing. Stereopsis is basically achieved through binocular viewing so each eye has a slightly different positional view of the object under examination. The observer's brain then combines the two dissimilar images taken from points of view a little distance apart, thus producing a perception of a single three-dimensional image. If the user is wearing corrective lenses, set the eyepieces to zero. If the user needs corrective lenses but is not wearing them, he or she should preset the eyepieces to a position of visual comfort and acuity before draping the microscope. Detachable rubber eyecups for the eyepiece are commercially available for the user's comfort.

Magnification The ability of the microscope to magnify depends on the design and quality of the parts in addition to the resolving power. The total magnification is computed by multiplying the enlarging power of the objective lens by that of the lenses of the oculars. The depth of the field, which is the vertical dimension within which objects are seen in clear focus, decreases with increase in magnification of power. Likewise, the width of the field of view narrows as the power of magnification increases. For example, at 20× magnification the field of view narrows to 10 mm, less than 1.25 cm (½ inch). Vertical viewing of the surgical field is extremely important, particularly in higher magnification ranges.

It allows the surgeon more effective use of the increasingly limited depth of field.

In more complex microscopes a third set of lenses is interposed between the oculars and the objective lens to provide additional magnification in variable degrees as desired by the surgeon. A continuously variable system of magnification for increasing or decreasing images is possible with a *zoom lens.* A faster, easier-to-handle zoom lens is preferred by most surgeons to a simpler turret magnifier that manually changes magnification by fixed increments. The zoom lens is usually operated by a foot control that permits the surgeon to change magnification without removing hands from the surgical field. The popular range of magnification in the zoom microscope is from 3.5 to 20× magnification. At 3.5× magnification, the depth of the field is 2.5 mm, or about 1⁄10 inch; at 20× magnification, the depth is 1 mm or about 1⁄25 inch. Some microscopes magnify to 40 times.

Focus Focusing is accomplished manually or by a foot-controlled motor that raises and lowers the body of the microscope to the desired distance from the object to be viewed. Some microscopes divide the focus into gross and fine. The focus of the ocular lens usually is set at zero; the surgeon adjusts the focus as desired.

Illumination System

Illumination of the operating microscope uses light waves. The shorter the wavelength, the greater the resolving power. Intensity of illumination can be varied by controls mounted on the support arm of the body. The operating microscope has two basic sources of illumination.

Paraxial Illuminators One or more light tubes, paraxial illuminators, contain tungsten or halogen bulbs and focusing lenses. The illuminators are attached to the mounting of the body of the microscope in a position to illuminate the field of view. Light is focused to coincide with the working distance of the microscope.

One of the paraxial illuminators may be equipped with a diaphragm containing a variable-width slit aperture. This device permits a narrow beam of light to be brought into focus on the objective field. This slit image assists the surgeon in defining depth perception, that is, in ascertaining the relative distance of objects within the field (which are closer, which are farther).

Coaxial Illuminators Usually fiberoptic, light is transmitted through the optical system of the microscope body. This type of illumination is called *coaxial* because it illuminates the same area in the same focus as the viewing or objective field of the microscope. The fiberoptic system provides intense, though cool, light that protects patient's tissues and the optics of the microscope from excessive heat. The light intensity ranges from 600 to 2250 footcandles without creating shadows. Reflected glare may be a problem, however. Frequent wound irrigation with a cool solution is necessary to avoid tissue damage from radiant energy during long procedures.

If a fiberoptic system is not used for coaxial illumination, a heat-absorbing filter must be interposed in the illumination system. Direct heat from a high-intensity source can damage and even burn tissues. Tungsten and halogen bulbs are used in some housings.

Another type of optical prism assembly provides a larger area of coaxial illumination with a brighter light than fiberoptic light bundles. Known as liquid light, it uses ionic, inorganic saline solution with quartz glass inserts inside a flexible aluminum spiral tube insulated with a polyvinyl chloride coating. Light is conducted throughout the cross section of the liquid, unlike a fiberoptic bundle.

Mounting Systems

Stability of the microscope is of paramount importance. The body, the optical portion, is mounted on a vertical column that may be supported by the floor, ceiling, wall, or by attachment to the operating table. The body of the microscope is attached to the column by a hinged arm and a central pivot. The mounting permits positioning as desired. It may be adjusted horizontally or vertically, rotated on its axis, and tilted at different angles. The microscope can be aimed in any direction. The objective is aimed at the principal surgical site.

Floor and ceiling mounting systems are the most popular and versatile. All microscopes must have a locking mechanism to immobilize the microscope body over the surgical field.

Floor Mount The base of the vertical support, which rests on the floor, has retractable casters for ease in moving the entire instrument. However, when lowered to working position, the base is locked into position (see Figure 15-4, *A*).

The base should be properly positioned in relation to the operating table before the anesthetic is administered or the patient is prepped. To maintain balance and control, gently push (do not pull) the microscope when moving it. The brake should be released or casters activated before moving. Arms should be folded close to the column with all attachments locked into place. Cords should be out of the way. Observation tubes should not be used as handles. Never use force in moving the microscope or in applying attachments; check the problem instead. A floor-based microscope with column support is placed to the left of a right-handed surgeon. The base should not interfere with foot controls or power cables. It must be clear of any table attachments also.

Some microscopes use a *contraves stand.* This is a counterbalanced weight system used to position the operating microscope in a suspended position over the surgical field. The weights are set and locked according to the type of attachments on the body of the microscope. The balance is set before activating the power switch.

As a safety factor the base must not be moved when the microscope is over the patient because it is top-heavy. Gross adjustments, such as height in relation to the surgical field and focus, are made with the microscope swung away from the patient. The operating table height, chair, and armrest heights are adjusted at the same time that gross adjustments are made. Fine focusing and adjustments are done after the microscope is in position for the surgical procedure. The assistant's microscope is adjusted to the same focus as that of the surgeon. During prepping and draping, the microscope is rotated out of position, then brought over the surgical field for the procedure.

Ceiling Mount A ceiling mount, either a fixed or track-mounted model, provides freer floor space. The fixed unit is suspended from a telescoping column attached directly to the ceiling. Vertical support of a track-mounted unit is suspended from a ceiling rail. It can be moved out of the way when not in use (Figure 15-5). The microscope is positioned and focused after the patient is anesthetized. A ceiling-mounted instrument is operated by a control panel on a wall (on-off switch) and by foot controls for focusing, magnifying, raising, and lowering.

A ceiling mount is generally very stable, but it is only as stable as the supporting ceiling. Mechanical devices adjacent to the OR, such as air-conditioning units, may cause vibration. The microscope *must* be vibration-free. A ceiling mount permits the same flexibility of positioning as a floor mount.

The vertical support has a memory stop mechanism that can be preset for a preselected operating table height. This setting should be checked and adjusted for each table-position change. The mechanism is a safety factor to prevent accidental lowering of the microscope at high speed too close to the patient. High-speed lowering should be done away from the patient until the memory stop is reached. As with the floor-mounted instrument, gross adjustments are never made over the patient. Fine adjustment and focusing are done after the microscope is over the surgical field.

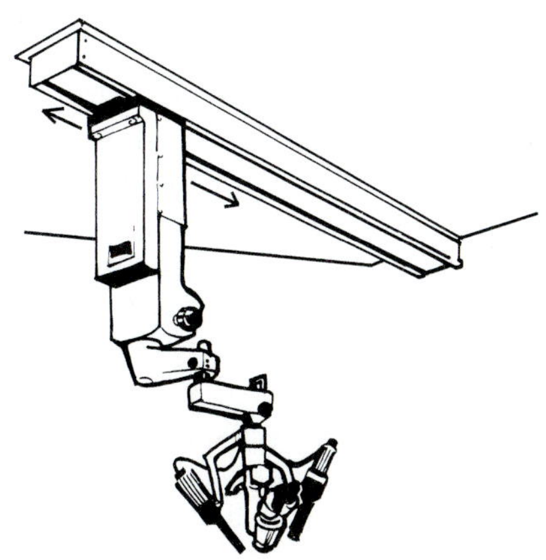

FIGURE 15-5 Ceiling track-mounted microscope.

Wall Mount The microscope is bracketed by a flexible arm to a stable wall. The swing-arm extension permits proper positioning.

Operating Table Mount Smaller microscopes may be mounted on the framework of the operating table. This system has many disadvantages and thus it is not popular.

Electrical System

The same precautions are observed with the operating microscope as with any electrical equipment in the OR. Switches and wall interlocks should be explosion-proof. Circuits must be protected from overload by breaker relays and fuses. All light controls should be in the off position when the power plug is inserted or removed from the wall outlet to avoid short-circuiting or sparking. A red pilot light illuminates on the control panel when the electric power is on.

Accessories

A number of accessories are available to enhance the versatility of microsurgery. The value of a good microscope is negated without proper ancillary equipment.

Assistant's Binoculars A separate optical body with a nonmotorized, hand-controlled zoom lens can be attached to the main microscope body for use by the assistant (Figure 15-6). This mechanism can be focused in the same plane as the surgeon's oculars. However, its field of view may not coincide exactly with that of the surgeon. This can be rectified by using a *beam splitter,* which takes the image from one of the surgeon's oculars and transmits it through an *observer tube,* thereby providing the assistant with an identical image of the surgeon's view (Figure 15-7). This is particularly important in critical areas where a difference of 1 or 2 mm is crucial.

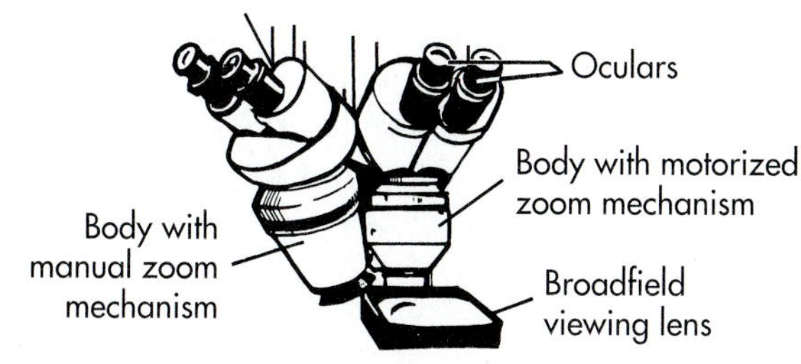

FIGURE 15-6 Surgeon's microscope on right with assistant's binoculars attached on left.

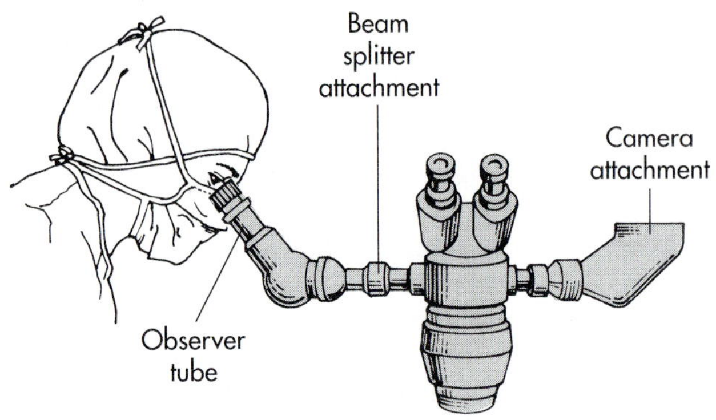

FIGURE 15-7 Microscope accessories.

Assistant's binocular co-observer tubes can be placed on the body so the assistant can work and observe from same side of table as, at a right angle to, or directly opposite the surgeon. Binocular tubes, either tiltable, straight, or inclined, can be attached on the right or left side of the body. A dual viewing bridge, the *quadroscope*, is attached when the surgeon and assistant sit opposite each other. They have exactly the same view of field with this accessory. Binoculars should be appropriately placed on the microscope body before the surgical procedure begins.

Broadfield Viewing Lens A low-power magnifying glass is used for grasping needles or for getting an overall view of the field adjacent to the objective. This lens attaches to front of the body of the surgeon's ocular (see Figure 15-6).

Couplings Couplings allow versatility in positioning the microscope for specific applications. An automated mechanism, the *X-Y attachment*, provides precision in controlling small movements of the microscope in the field of view. A coupling piece lets surgeons change the angle for side-to-side or front-to-back viewing. A universal tilt coupling can be integrated into the X-Y coupling.

Cameras Still photographic, motion picture, videotape, and television cameras may be attached to the beam splitter, permitting filming of the surgical procedure (Figure 15-7). The camera unit should be in the upright position when connected to the operating microscope. It may require the use of a stronger illumination source. Check to be sure film is in the camera by trying to rewind the film cartridge holder. Document the patient's and surgeon's names, date, and time on the film or video cartridge to prevent mixing recorded images between patients. The use of recording equipment may require special patient consent in some institutions. The recorded procedure is useful in assisting, teaching, and research.

Laser Microadaptor Laser beams can be directed through the operating microscope. The microscope and laser head couplings must be perfectly aligned in the grooves and protrusions on the metal adapters. A screw and locking pin secure the coupling. In the operating position the laser head is at approximately a 60-degree angle to the microscope. It will not fire in a horizontal or upside-down position. The microadaptor must have a compatible lens with a focal length of 200, 300, or 400 mm so the surgeon can properly adjust the focal point of the laser beam. A CO_2 laser with electronic components that delivers milliwatt energy may be used to vaporize tissues or weld tissues together. Other types of lasers are directed through fiberoptics. To protect the surgeon's eyes, filter caps over optics must be appropriate for the wavelength of laser being used. The entire team and patient must wear eye protection of the appropriate optical density when the laser is in use.

Remote Foot Controls Simple microscopes are manually operated. However, it is more convenient for the surgeon to use foot-controlled, motorized functions such as focus, zoom, and tilt. Foot controls may be activated by switches of the push-button type, heel-to-toe, or side-to-side motion. The number of switches corresponds to the number of motor-controlled functions. There may be additional foot switches for the camera or for other nonmicroscope-associated equipment such as cryosurgical, bipolar electrosurgical, or laser units. Switches may be separated by a vertical bar to prevent inadvertent contact. The bar also serves as a footrest for the surgeon. Because the surgeon and assistant usually are seated during microsurgical procedures, the height of the operating table must permit them adequate knee room to operate foot controls.

Microscope Drape The entire working mechanism and support arm of the microscope are encased in a sterile drape. Draping the entire microscope permits it to be brought into the sterile field so the surgeon can position the body and adjust the optics. Disposable drapes that are heat-resistant, lint-free, nonreflective, transparent, and quiet are available to fit the configuration of all microscopes and attachments. The scrub person slides the drape over the body, with hands protected as for draping a Mayo stand. The circulator helps guide the drape toward the vertical column and secures it. The scrub person secures the drape to the oculars. Sterile lens covers or rubber bands may be supplied with the drape for this purpose.

If not heat-resistant, a plastic drape may cause heat buildup beneath it that can damage the microscope. A heat guard may be applied over the light source or heat may be evacuated through an opening in the top of the drape.

Care of Microscope

Persons responsible for the microscope should consult the manufacturer's manual. Any malfunction should be reported to the OR manager or appropriate person who can arrange for repair service. A checklist to verify care and functioning of various parts before the surgical procedure is helpful. All persons who assist with microsurgery must know how to set up and position the microscope.

1. Microscope should be damp-dusted before use.
   a. External surfaces, *except the lenses*, are wiped with a clean cloth saturated with detergent-disinfectant solution.
   b. Casters or wheels should be clean to reduce contamination and prevent interference with mobility.
2. Lenses should be cleaned according to manufacturer's recommendations only to avoid scratching or damage to antireflective lens coating. Most manufacturers recommend sterile distilled water and lens paper. They must not be soaked in any solution.
3. Circulator should prepare the microscope.
   a. When changing oculars, care must be taken to avoid dropping and fingerprinting lenses. Avoid stripping the threads of screw mounts by seating the optics and turning in a counterclockwise direction until the threads align. Proceed by turning in a clockwise motion until secure. Take care not to overtighten. Right turns tighten, left turns loosen.
   b. Both hands should be used for attaching observation tubes, which are heavy.
   c. Extra lamp bulbs and fuses should be on hand. The circulator must know where they are stored and how to change them. It is advisable to check bulbs periodically to avoid the necessity of replacing them during a procedure. New bulbs should be inserted if a long procedure is anticipated. Bulbs should be changed with the power off.
   d. Check electrical connections for proper fit or wire fraying. Take special care of power cables to prevent accidental breakage by heavy equipment rolling over them.
   e. Check that all knobs are secured after the microscope is in operating position.
   f. Place foot controls in a convenient position so the surgeon does not have to search for them.
4. Properly store the microscope and accessories. Store away from traffic but close to areas where used.
   a. Openings into the microscope body for attachment of accessory devices, such as the observer tube, should be closed with covers provided by the manufacturer when not in use to prevent accumulation of dust.
   b. Lenses and viewing tubes should be protected.
   c. Microscope and attachments should be enclosed in an antistatic plastic cover when not in use to keep them free from dust.
   d. Power cords should be neatly coiled for storage.

Microinstrumentation

Improved results of surgical intervention utilizing microsurgical techniques are due in no small measure to the miniaturized precision instrumentation developed in association with the performance of these delicate procedures. The instruments are extremely fine, delicate, and miniature enough to handle in the very small working area. Manipulation becomes more difficult with increased size or bulk and weight. As with techniques, instruments are constantly being improved. Microsurgeons work with manufacturers to develop appropriate instruments, suture materials, and needles. Many surgeons purchase the instruments of their choice. Whether owned by the surgeon or the facility, microinstruments require exacting care to maintain desired function.

Instruments are designed to conform to hand movements under the microscope. They must permit secure grasp, ease of holding and manipulation, and fulfillment of their intended purpose. They are shaped to not obscure the limited field of view. While these factors are important criteria for any instrument, they are especially vital for microinstruments. Everyone assisting in or setting up for microsurgical procedures must know the identification and functions of these unique instruments. Design is coincident to function.

Material and Surface

Microinstruments are made of stainless steel or titanium. Titanium alloy is considerably stronger yet lighter in weight than stainless steel. Some microinstruments are malleable for desired angling. Some are disposable. All are extremely vulnerable to abuse.

Finishes of at least the portions of instruments exposed to light in the surgical field are deliberately dulled during manufacture to reduce glare, which is both annoying and tiring to the surgeon. Titanium microinstruments have a dull-blue finish.

Shape and Tips

Microinstruments are shorter than standard instruments and are often angulated for convenience of approach and avoidance of obstruction of the surgical field.

Instrument tips have minimal separation compatible with their function. Finger pressure and movement necessary to close wide tips are undesirable because they may induce tremor.

Handles

Handles are designed for secure and comfortable grasp with a diameter comparable to a pen or pencil. Minimal diameter between fingers facilitates feel and accuracy of manipulation. Double-handled instruments (scissors, needleholders) have a slightly larger diameter than single-handled ones (razor knife). The shape of the handle is also important for manipulation. For example, instruments rotated between fingers when in use, such as forceps, must be turned easily. Their handles therefore are rounded or six-sided like a pencil (Figure 15-8). Those not rotated have finger grips or are flattened. Ring-handled instruments are not practical in microsurgery.

Many instruments, particularly scissors and some needleholders, have spring handles that return tips to the open position between cutting or grasping functions (Figure 15-9). The distance from hinge to tip will vary according to function. Proper spring tension can be easily ruined by mishandling.

Handles must be long enough for comfort in the working position but must not extend beyond the working distance to contact the unsterile objective of the microscope. The maximum length of most microinstruments is about 100 mm (4 inches). Gripping surfaces should be functionally located to prevent fingers from slipping during manipulation. These surfaces serve as a guide to accurate finger positioning. The gripping area may be six-sided, round, knurled, or flat serrated.

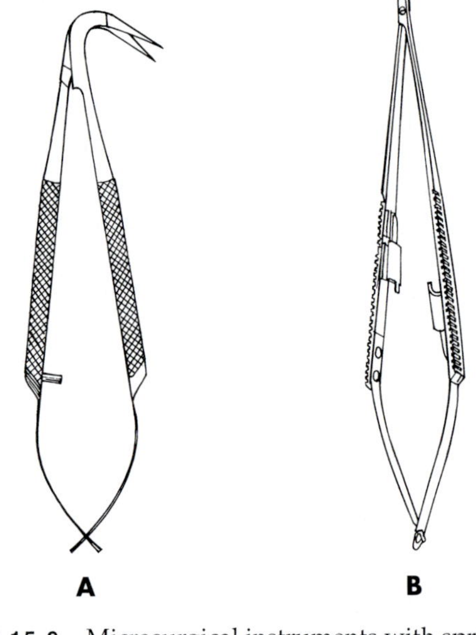

FIGURE 15-9 Microsurgical instruments with spring handles. **A,** Scissors. **B,** Needleholder.

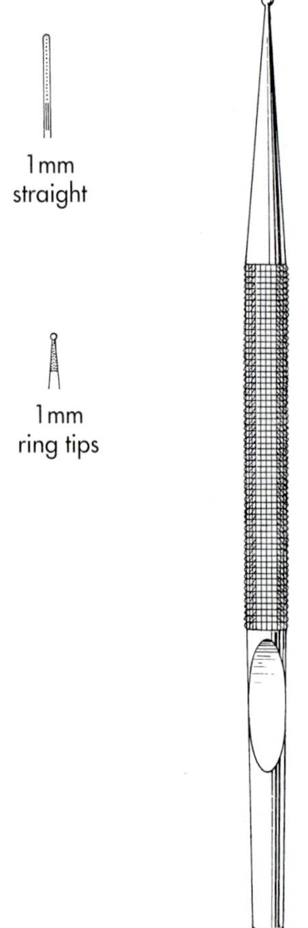

FIGURE 15-8 Microsurgical forceps.

Primary Uses

Appropriate instrumentation is used for specific types of procedures. Although all surgical instruments are structured for a definitive use, the function of microinstruments is even more restricted. Tissue can be severely injured by use of an improper or imperfect instrument. Instruments too can be damaged by use on inappropriate tissue. Primary usage includes cutting (knives, scissors, and saws), exposure (spatulas and retractors), gross and fine fixation (forceps and clamps), and suture and needle manipulation (needleholder). Instruments must not be used for manipulations other than the intended purpose.

Knives Edges of razor, diamond, and dissecting knives have different degrees of sharpness and thickness of blades appropriate to the cutting function of each, that is, to make penetrating or slicing incisions. A clean cut is desired to minimize trauma and tissue destruction.

Scissors Like knives, scissors are designed to make a specific type of incision related both to plane and to thickness. Incisions are vertical, horizontal, or of a special configuration such as curved or two-planed. Use is governed by hinging and blade relationship. Scissors are hinged to cut vertically or obliquely. Cutting is usually done by the distal part of blades for better control. Some scissors come in pairs with right and left curves. Often a part number inscribed by manufacturer on the handle will be an even number for a right-hand instrument and odd for a left-hand one. Scissor blades may be sharp or blunt, long or short, and straight or angulated. Available straight or curved, microsurgical scissors have a spring-type handle (Figure 15-9).

Powered Instruments Microsurgical air-powered drills and saws vary in sizes and shapes. They have a fingertip control; some have an optional foot control.

Spatulas and Retractors Spatulas and retractors are used to draw tissue back for better exposure or protection. Nerve hooks and elevators also are used for these purposes.

Forceps Straight and curved forceps may be toothed or smooth. They have light spring action and minimal tip separation. Teeth of some tissue forceps may be as small as 1/10 mm (1/250 inch) in diameter. Therefore many tips are barely visible to the unaided eye. Toothed forceps are used for grasping tissue but never for grasping needles or sutures. Smooth forceps are used for tying delicate ligatures and sutures. For stability of grasp and avoidance of injury to the suture strand, the tips of the forceps must be absolutely parallel and have perfect apposition of grasping surfaces. Suture must be grasped firmly but without trauma, often from a slippery surface. Other smooth forceps are used on friable tissues. Bipolar forceps are used for electrocoagulation.

Clamps Mosquito hemostats and various clamps are used for vascular occlusion and for approximation of edges of tissues such as nerves and vessels. Crushing of vessels must be avoided.

Microsutures and Needles

Microsurgical closure is unique in that the smallest sizes of sutures and needles manufactured are used. Microsuture sizes range from 8-0 (45 μm) to 11-0 (14 μm) in diameter. Because of the minute size, proportionately small needles are swaged to suture. They range from 30 to 130 μm in diameter.

Suture materials include synthetic absorbable and nonabsorbable polymers. A strand is finer than a human hair. Packets provide ready access to the needle. When in use, the needle should always be kept in view in the surgical field because the strand may easily be lost from view and difficult to pick up. The surgeon should inspect the strand for damage while passing it through tissue to be sure holding power in situ is not threatened. It is safest and easiest for the scrub person to keep these sutures in packets until the surgeon is ready to use them.

Stainless steel microsurgical needles are measured in microns of wire diameter and millimeters in length. To achieve deep placement in tissue, the needle is short and sharply curved. Less curvature is required for more superficial suturing. Straight needles may be preferred for some tissues.

To arm a needle in the needleholder, some surgeons want the scrub person to hold the open suture packet under the accessory broadfield viewing lens so they may grasp the needle themselves from foam that secures the needle. The scrub person then gently removes the packet from the strand. The surgeon grasps the needle lightly but firmly in the needleholder and takes it into the surgical field. Any readjustment of the position of the needle is done by the surgeon under the microscope.

Closure of an incision with the least trauma to produce minimal fibrosis and scarring is enhanced by placing sutures close together to yield a firm, even apposition line and anatomically secure wound. Integrity of the sutures compensates for minimal scar tissue in supporting the wound. Use of the zoom microscope facilitates tying and cutting sutures.

Needleholders Microsurgical needleholders are used only for suturing, not ligating, because the very fine suture materials would break if tied with a needleholder. They should be used to hold only minute microsurgical needles so as not to alter alignment. Handles are round to permit easy rotation between fingers. Some have spring handles. Although a lock on a needleholder may cause tips to jerk when engaged or released, some have a holding catch for use in deep wounds to prevent loss of small needles. Needleholders held closed by finger pressure, rather than a catch, firmly hold a needle shaft yet permit easy adjustment of the needle position. The tips can be curved or straight.

Sponges

Suitably small, nonfibrous sponges or lint-free patties of material such as compressed cellulose are used to accommodate the surgical field. Lint is visible under the microscope and could obstruct view.

General Considerations of Microsurgery

Patient

The patient is prepared as for a standard surgical procedure. He or she must be positioned comfortably and safely with the operating table locked in position. The surgical site is immobilized if possible.

Anesthesia

If general anesthesia is to be administered, the anesthesiologist should be informed in advance of the surgeon's intention to use the microscope. This is especially pertinent in procedures in which patient movements under light anesthesia can result in disaster. In addition, the anesthesiologist's position in relation to the patient must be considered to allow room for the microscope. The anesthesiologist should be aware that microsurgical procedures will take somewhat longer.

With local anesthesia the patient should be instructed to lie quietly and to tell the anesthesiologist or circulator of a desire to move. Many patients sleep during the procedure. A startle reflex on awakening or unexpected movement is especially hazardous in microsurgery where the surgeon's mobility and field of view are limited. If the patient jerks or turns, he or she literally may move out of the surgeon's hands and often out of view of the microsurgical field. Therefore the patient must be closely monitored.

Stability

A vital factor for successful microsurgery is stability of the surgical field, microscope, and surgeon's hands. The complete microsurgical unit consists of the operating table with the patient, the microscope, and the surgeon's chair. They must be functionally positioned in relation to each other so that major adjustments need not be made during the surgical procedure. The surgeon and circulator should check that all components are properly placed before the incision is made.

Armrests and Chair It is important that the surgeon's hands be adequately supported because a shift of even 1 mm (1/25 inch) can alter the precision of motion, particularly at high magnifications. Support of the surgeon's arm must be continuous from shoulder to hand to give stability and to minimize tremor, especially in fine finger movements. A detachable, sterile padded wrist support such as the Chan wrist rest may be affixed to the operating table.

A chair with hydraulic foot controls for raising or lowering provides the necessary forearm support by means of attached armrests. These armrests are individually draped. Mayo stand covers are convenient. Armrests can be moved independently to a variety of levels and positions. They must be secured in the desired position. The surgeon must be in a comfortable position to work.

Scrub Person Duties

Although a stabilized situation is crucial, a second fundamental necessity is for the surgeon to keep eyes on the field of view through the microscope at all times. Looking away from the field requires readjustment of vision to the field. Cooperation and coordination by the scrub person prevent the surgeon's distraction from the surgical site.

1. Set up the Mayo stand and instrument table without touching the tips of instruments. Leave protective covers on them until ready to use. Holders are available to keep tips in the air and to keep them separated. Microinstruments are handled individually. They are more susceptible to damage than standard instruments. Edges are easily dulled, and fine tips are easily bent or broken. Extreme caution is necessary not to catch tips on any object that could bend them.
2. Place instruments on the Mayo stand in anticipated order of use. Place the Mayo stand and instrument table conveniently to surgeon's hand so that he or she does not have to look around the microscope.
3. Pass instruments by placing them in the surgeon's hand in position for use and guide the hand toward the surgical field so the surgeon may keep eyes on the field.
4. Keep debris (i.e., blood, mucus, or suture ends) from the tips of instruments by wiping them *gently* on a nonfibrous sponge or lint-free gauze. Replace them in their original position on the Mayo stand, not touching each other.
5. Assist efficiently but never put hands in the surgical field unless requested to do so.
6. Understand the need for slow dissection at times. Do not let attention stray; observe the video monitor if available.

The increased time needed for use of the operating microscope can be minimized by adequate preparation and efficient assistance. Each team member should thoroughly understand the microscope and every aspect of microsurgical techniques.

Team members can be kept up to date by in-service explanation of new instruments and demonstration of the microscope. It is extremely helpful and contributory to understanding for the surgeon to show perioperative nurses and surgical technologists anatomic structures and instruments through the microscope. A comparison of microinstruments with standard instruments under the microscope is always a revelation. A television monitor is advantageous in providing the scrub person and anesthesiologist continuous observation of the surgical procedure. All members must be completely familiar with instrumentation. Not only are instruments then properly cared for, but even more important, surgical time is reduced.

ULTRASONOSURGERY

Ultrasonosurgery, also referred to as *cytoreductive debulking surgery,* is useful in removing or reducing tumors in highly vascular, delicate tissue such as the brain, liver, kidney, and spleen. The original prototypes were developed in 1967 to fragment and aspirate cataracts. An *ultrasonic aspirator,* such as the Cavitron, simultaneously fragments, irrigates, and aspirates tissue. During the fragmentation process sterile fluid passes through the handpiece to emulsify target tissue. The emulsified tissue is aspirated and collected in a closed container system.

A transducer in the handpiece converts electrical energy into mechanical motion. Ultra-high frequency sound waves produce vibrations at the tip. These vibrations are of the same physical nature as sound but with frequencies above the range of human hearing. Ultrasound has a frequency greater than 30,000 Hz. The vibrating tip of the ultrasonic aspirator fragments tissues at the cellular level. When the tip contacts tissue, vapor pockets within high-water-content cells cause cell walls to separate and collapse. The ultrasonic aspirator is used to disrupt tissues, or tracts, particularly in the central nervous system. It is also used to emulsify tumors with minimal mechanical trauma to surrounding nerves and blood vessels. A device that combines electrosurgery with ultrasonic dissection also allows coagulation during resection and aspiration of tumor mass.

An *ultrasonic probe* can be inserted through an endoscope to fragment renal or ureteral calculi, that is, kidney stones (see section on ultrasonic lithotripsy, Chapter 31, p. 640). A suction channel is incorporated into the probe to aspirate fragments as stone is pulverized by ultrasonic energy.

INTEGRATED TECHNOLOGIES

As implied in the previous discussion, several technologies may be utilized for minimally invasive surgical procedures. *Videolaseroscopy* allows the surgeon to remove organs and tumors and to ablate or repair tissues without making a major incision. An endoscope is introduced into a body cavity through a small incision. The viewing area from the telescopic lens of the scope is magnified from a video camera to a video screen. While viewing the screen, the surgeon can direct a laser beam through the endoscope to the target tissue.

Other instrumentation may be introduced through adjacent small incisions for dissection, ligation, and suturing. These instruments can be manipulated while the surgeon looks through the endoscope or at a monitoring screen. Manipulations may be observed with use of fluoroscopy or a video camera. Ultrasonic and thermal probes, electrosurgical electrodes, and laser beams can be directed through endoscopes. Laser beams can also be directed through the operating microscope.

Computers

Lasers and microscopes may be controlled by computerized systems. Computers can automatically scan tissues to select target tissue for the laser beam. Operating microscopes may contain voice-activated minicomputers that manipulate controls for fine adjustments, thus eliminating the foot and hand switches that the surgeon must operate.

THE FUTURE

A computerized, robotic surgical assistant may become one of the team members or may be already. *Robotic enhancement technology* has developed a robot that holds and moves a laparoscope into optimal position for the surgeon. The surgeon controls the position of the scope with a foot pedal or hand control connected to the robot. The robot's name is AESOP, a mnemonic for *a*utomated *e*ndoscopic *s*ystem for *o*ptimal *p*ositioning. This robot may be just the beginning of automation in the OR of the future.

Research is being done to develop virtual reality training for surgeons and operators of complex technologic equipment. *Virtual reality* is the computer science of simulating real-life motion, time, and space. Computer-generated images mimic real-life situations. The surgeon-in-training practices a procedure without touching a real patient. The surgeon dons a specialized headset/visor and sensor gloves and selects the training scenario to be practiced. The computer displays a videolike picture of human anatomy in the headset/visor. The sensor gloves signal motion, direction, and pressure to a computer and in turn create a sensation of touch for the surgeon. The entire activity looks, feels, and responds as if the surgeon were performing surgery on an actual patient. This investigative technology can allow for "practice surgery" while evaluating the skill and dexterity of the surgeon.

The possibilities for integrating advanced technologies to simplify surgery and make it less painful and safer for patients seem endless as surgeons develop and refine innovative techniques. The challenges for all members of the OR team are to learn about technologic advances and to monitor quality of patient care in their application. Engineering performance (i.e., clinical application of biotechnology) is measured by reliability, safety, maintenance, and effectiveness of equipment. Clinical performance is measured by the skills of users to achieve desired results—a successful outcome for the patient.

BIBLIOGRAPHY

Ball K: *Lasers: the perioperative challenge,* ed 2, St Louis, 1995, Mosby.

Carrington A-C: Laser safety, *Br J Theatre Nurs* 27(2):16-19, 1990.

DeKatay SM: Surgical lasers, *Surg Technol* 25(9):8-12, 1993.

Fogarty AM: Angioscopy: new developments in vascular surgery, *AORN J* 53(3):725-728, 1991.

Hladio AM: Hidden hazards: prevent the danger, *Today's OR Nurse* 12(5):42-43, 1990.

Martin MA, Reichelderfer M: APIC guideline for infection prevention and control in flexible endoscopy, *Am J Infect Control* 22(2):19-38, 1994.

Mathias JM: Minimally invasive surgery: innovative devices expanding laparoscopy; telepresence lets surgeons operate from remote site, *OR Manager* 10(6):9-11, 1994.

Mathias JM: Robotic assistant for laparoscopic surgery, *OR Manager* 10(1):1, 9-10, 1994.

Mathias JM: The future of surgery: ahead...robots, digital surgeons, and virtual reality, *OR Manager* 11(1):1, 6-7, 9, 1995.

Moak E: Electrosurgical unit safety, *AORN J* 53(3):744-752, 1991.

O'Connell WD: Video technology, *AORN J* 56(3):442-454, 1992.

Paige BA: The excimer laser: program implementation and nursing implications, *J Ophthal Nurs Technol* 11(6):251-255, 1992.

Patterson P: Endosurgery instruments: reusables vs disposables, *OR Manager* 9(1):1-8, 1993.

Patterson P: Hazards of electrosurgery in laparoscopy overlooked, *OR Manager* 9(3):1, 6-8, 1993.

Patterson P: New technology expanding endoscopic surgery market, *OR Manager* 8(12):1-9, 1992.

Pfister JI et al: Perioperative nursing care of the patient experiencing laser surgery, *Semin Periop Nurs* 1(2):96-102, 1992.

Proposed recommended practices: electrosurgery, *AORN J* 58(1):131-138, 1993. (Adopted by AORN,1994.)

Proposed recommended practices: endoscopic minimal access surgery, *AORN J* 59(2):507-514, 1994.

Proposed recommended practices: the use and care of endoscopes, *AORN J* 57(2):543-550, 1993. (Adopted by AORN, 1994.)

Rader JS et al: Ultrasonic surgical aspiration in the treatment of vulvar disease, *Obstet Gynecol* 77(4):573-576, 1991.

Recommended practices for laser safety in the practice setting, *AORN J* 58(5):1027-1031, 1993.

Reichert M: Laparoscopic instruments, *AORN J* 57(3):637-655, 1993.

Reichert M, Patterson P: Endoscopes: tough problems with their cleaning and reprocessing, *OR Manager* 6(8):1, 7-10, 1990.

Schaffner M, Martino SM: Infection control aspects for office endoscopy, *Gastroenterol Nurs* 15(5):201-204, 1993.

Stelck MJ: Proper care and handling of the flexible endoscope, *Surg Technol* 25(11):8-12, 22, 1993.

Stevens JK, Miller JI: Transrectal ultrasound, *AORN J* 53(5):1166-1178, 1991.

Tucker RD, Ferguson S: Do surgical gloves protect staff during electrosurgical procedures? *Surgery* 110(5):892-895, 1991.

Ulmer BC: Ultrasonic surgical aspiration, *AORN J* 57(4):865-869, 1993.

Verazin GT et al: Ultrasonic surgical aspirator for lung resection, *Ann Thorac Surg* 52(3):787-790, 1991.

Williams L, Gregory R: Laser surgery, *Plast Surg Nurs* 13(2):106-108, 1993.

SECTION SIX

Preoperative Patient Care

CHAPTER 16

Preoperative Preparation of the Patient

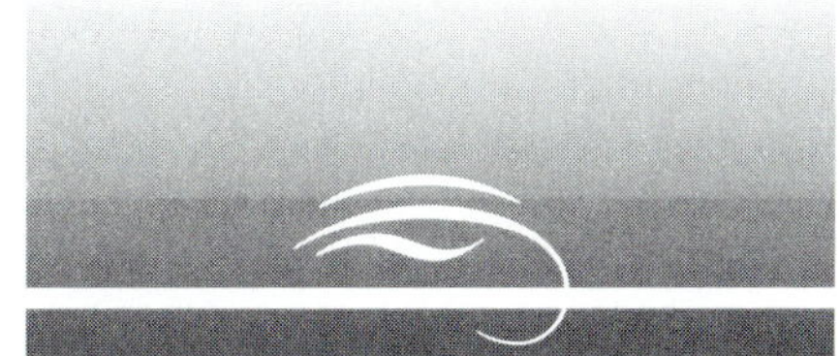

HISTORICAL BACKGROUND

For centuries before the proliferation of operating rooms (ORs) in hospitals, surgical procedures were performed on battlefields, in barber chairs, and on kitchen tables. Hospitals focused on the care of the poor, crippled, chronically ill, and insane until the eighteenth and nineteenth centuries. Even then, and on into the early twentieth century, many surgeons operated in their offices and in their patients' homes. Nurses were dispatched to homes to prepare a suitable room and to prepare the patient for the surgeons.

Achievements of surgery as a medical discipline from the late nineteenth century can be attributed to an increase in understanding of physiology, the introduction of safe anesthesia and methods of blood transfusion, the development of antimicrobials, and the management of patient before, during, and after invasive procedures. As surgeons moved into the OR arenas of hospitals, nurses became responsible for physically preparing patients for surgical procedures. Patients were admitted 4 or 5 days before the procedure in the early 1900s. By the late 1930s this time was reduced to 24 hours or less.

From around 1920, nursing leaders advocated the importance of both physiologic and psychologic preparation for surgical patients. The individual needs of patients were recognized, but they were not emphasized in nursing education until the 1940s. In the era of the 1950s, patient teaching also became a limited part of the preoperative preparation as surgeons recognized the value of early ambulation. It was not until the 1960s and 1970s, however, that nursing research studies validated a link between preoperative preparation and postoperative recovery. The risk of physiologic complications postoperatively can be reduced by teaching deep breathing, coughing, and leg exercises and by preparing the patient for early ambulation. Attention to an individual's psychosocial and spiritual needs preoperatively also has important consequences on the management of postoperative pain and the promotion of desired outcomes. Studies showed that patients who received structured preoperative teaching had a smoother postoperative recovery. During these decades OR nurses were encouraged to visit patients preoperatively to prepare them psychologically for the surgical experience by helping to alleviate their fears and anxieties and by teaching appropriate postoperative behaviors. This visit could take place at the bedside the day before a scheduled procedure.

In 1983, amendments to the Social Security Act established a prospective hospital reimbursement system for Medicare patients based on diagnosis related groups (DRGs). Historically hospitals were reimbursed for patient care on the basis of cost for room, board, and services. Under the present system inpatients are assigned to one of the DRGs for the primary diagnosis and any secondary diagnoses. The government and other third-party payers reimburse the hospital only for the care deemed necessary for the assigned DRG. Consequently, since the introduction of DRGs and prospective pricing into the health care system, the length of hospitalization of surgical inpatients has decreased both preoperatively and postoperatively. This has changed the time and place for preoperative preparation of most surgical patients who require hospital support services postoperatively. It also stimulated the development of ambulatory surgery (i.e., minimally invasive and uncomplicated procedures performed on nonhospitalized patients [see Chapter 41]). The number of surgical procedures performed in ambulatory care facilities and on patients admitted to the hospital the day of surgery increases annually.

Regardless of the physical setting in which an invasive procedure will be performed, patients must be adequately prepared so that the impact and potential risks of surgical intervention are minimized. This involves both physical and emotional preparation.

HOSPITALIZED PATIENT

The patient may be admitted to the hospital 1 or more days before a scheduled surgical procedure. Radiologic, endoscopic, or other diagnostic studies, described in Chapter 28, may be indicated to confirm the medical diagnosis. A systemic disease or chronic illness, such as diabetes or heart disease, must be under control to the extent possible. Admission criteria are established by medical staff policy. Acuity of illness or general health status and surgical procedure to be performed will influence whether the patient must be admitted to the hospital preoperatively or can arrive on the day of the surgical procedure.

Most patients who will remain in the hospital postoperatively are admitted the same day that the surgical procedure is scheduled. Often referred to as "AM admissions," these patients may be prepared for the surgical procedure in a same-day admission unit before transfer to the OR suite. Some hospitals have a preoperative check-in area within the OR suite. From the OR these patients may go to the postanesthesia care unit (PACU) to recover from anesthesia before being transferred to a surgical nursing unit. Some will be transferred directly to the intensive care unit (ICU). Magnitude of the surgical procedure and postoperative needs for complex care will determine when the patient can be discharged safely.

PREPARATION OF ALL PATIENTS FOR SURGICAL PROCEDURE

Specific procedures must be completed and documented before the patient arrives in the OR. Many of these can be done before admission to the hospital or an ambulatory care facility. Others are done after the patient arrives. For all patients preoperative physical preparation is designed to help the patient overcome the stresses of anesthesia, pain, fluid and blood loss, immobilization, and tissue trauma. Preparation often begins before the patient's hospital admission with the institution of nutritional or drug therapy. An attempt is made to bring all patients to their best possible physical status preoperatively. Appropriate consultations are sought when necessary.

Preadmission Procedures

Some of the preoperative preparation can be done in the surgeon's office. Then patients are referred to the preoperative testing center of the hospital or ambulatory care facility. Tests and records must be completed and available when the patient is admitted the day of the surgical procedure. Preoperative preparations include:

1. Medical history and physical examination. These must be done and documented by a physician.
2. Laboratory tests. Testing should be based on specific clinical indicators or risk factors that could affect surgical management or anesthesia. These include age, sex, preexisting disease, magnitude of surgical procedure, and type of anesthesia. Tests should be completed 24 hours before admission so results will be available for review.
   a. Hemoglobin, hematocrit, blood urea nitrogen (BUN), and blood glucose may be routinely tested for persons 60 years of age or older.
   b. Hematocrit is usually ordered for women of all ages before the administration of a general anesthetic.
   c. Complete blood count, SMA-6, SMA-12, SMA-18, or SMA-20 multichemistry profile may be indicated. (SMA stands for *s*equential *m*ultichannel *a*utoanalyzer.) Differential, platelet count, activated partial thromboplastin time, and prothrombin time also may be ordered.
   d. Urinalysis may be indicated by medical history and/or physical examination.
3. Blood type and crossmatch. If transfusion is anticipated, the patient's blood is typed and crossmatched. Many patients prefer to have their own blood drawn and stored for autotransfusion. They still should be typed and crossmatched, however, in the event that additional transfusions are needed.
4. Chest x-ray film. This may be required by hospital policy or medically indicated. A preoperative chest x-ray study is not routinely required for all patients. It may be medically indicated as an adjunct to clinical evaluation of patients with cardiac or pulmonary disease and for smokers, persons age 60 and older, and cancer patients.

5. Electrocardiogram. If the patient has known or suspected cardiac disease, an electrocardiogram (ECG) is mandatory. It may be routine for patients 40 years of age or older by policy.
6. Diagnostic procedures. Special diagnostic procedures are performed when specifically indicated, as for vascular surgery.
7. Written instructions. The patient must receive written instructions to follow before admission the same day as the surgical procedure. These instructions should be reviewed with the patient in the surgeon's office or in the preoperative testing center.
   a. Patient should not ingest solid foods preceding the surgical procedure to prevent regurgitation or emesis and aspiration of gastric contents. This usually is stated as "NPO after midnight." (NPO is the Latin abbreviation for *nil per os,* nothing by mouth.) Solid foods empty from the stomach after changing to a liquid state, which may take up to 12 hours. Clear fluids may be unrestricted until 2 to 3 hours before the surgical procedure but only at the discretion of the surgeon or anesthesiologist in selected patients. NPO time usually is reduced for infants, small children, diabetic patients, and elderly persons prone to dehydration.
   b. Physician may want the patient to take any essential oral medications that he or she normally takes. These can be taken with a minimal fluid intake up to 1 hour preoperatively as prescribed with 150 ml or less of water.
   c. Skin should be cleansed to prepare the surgical site. Many surgeons want patients to clean the surgical area with an antimicrobial soap for several days preoperatively. Patients who will undergo a surgical procedure on the face, ear, or neck are advised to shampoo hair before admission, since this may not be permitted for a few weeks after a surgical procedure. Male patients may be requested to have their hair cut short and to shave on the day of the surgical procedure.
   d. Nail polish and acrylic nails should be removed to permit observation of or access to the nail bed during the surgical procedure. Color of the nail bed is one indicator of oxygenation and circulation. The nail bed is a vascular area. The oxisensor of a pulse oximeter may be attached to the nail bed to monitor oxygen saturation and pulse rate. A finger cuff may be used to continuously monitor blood pressure. Nail polish or acrylic nails inhibit contact between these devices and the vascular bed. The patient should be advised that at least one fingernail should be uncovered if these devices are to be used by the anesthesiologist for monitoring.
   e. Jewelry and valuables should be left at home to ensure safekeeping. Patients should be informed that all metal jewelry, including wedding band and religious artifacts, must be removed to prevent possible burns if electrosurgery will be used.
   f. Patient should be given other special instructions about what is expected. For example, the patient must know when to arrive. An ambulatory patient must know that a responsible adult must be available to take him or her home. Family members or significant others should know where to wait and where the patient will be taken after the surgical procedure.
8. Informed consent. The patient or legal designee must give consent for the surgical procedure. After explaining the surgical procedure and its risks, the surgeon may have the patient sign the consent form. This becomes part of the patient's record and must accompany him or her to the OR. Policy and state laws dictate parameters for ascertaining an informed consent (see Chapter 3, pp. 37-39).
9. Nurse interview. A perioperative nurse should meet with the patient to make a preoperative assessment of the patient. From the assessment data and nursing diagnoses, the nurse establishes expected outcomes with the patient. The nurse develops the plan of care, which will become a part of the patient's record. Ideally an appointment with the perioperative nurse is arranged when the patient comes to the facility for preoperative tests. The nurse collects data through physiologic and psychosocial assessments for the nursing diagnoses, expected outcomes, and plan of care. The nurse reviews the written preoperative instructions and consent form with the patient to assess the patient's knowledge and understanding. The nurse also provides emotional support and teaches the patient in preparation for postoperative recovery. (See pp. 302-307 for discussion of preoperative interviewing and teaching.) Before or after the interview the patient may view a videotape to reinforce information.
10. Anesthesia assessment. An anesthesia history and physical assessment must be taken before general and regional anesthesia. The history may be taken by the surgeon, or the patient may be asked to complete a questionnaire for the anesthesiologist in the surgeon's office or in the preoperative testing center. An interview by an anesthesiologist or nurse anesthetist may be conducted before admission with patients who have complex medical histories, are high risk, or have high degrees of anxiety. All patients should understand the risks of and alternatives to the type of anesthesia to be administered. The pa-

tient should sign an anesthesia consent form after discussion with the anesthesiologist. (See information on preoperative visit by anesthesiologist on pp. 307-309.)

A preoperative phone call to the patient by a perioperative nurse a week or so in advance of the scheduled surgical procedure may prevent cancellation. The patient is reminded to have preadmission tests. The importance of preoperative preparations is reiterated, especially NPO.

Evening Before Elective Surgical Procedure

The surgeon may write specific orders for other appropriate preoperative preparations in addition to preadmission procedures previously described.

NOTE All the preadmission procedures may be done after a patient is hospitalized (i.e., admitted to a surgical unit before the surgical procedure).

1. Bowel preparation. "Enemas till clear" may be ordered when it is advantageous to have the bowel and rectum empty (e.g., gastrointestinal procedures such as bowel resection, endoscopy, and surgical procedures in the pelvic, perineal, or perianal areas). An intestinal lavage with an oral solution that induces diarrhea may be ordered to clear the intestine of feces. Solutions such as Golytely or Colyte will normally clear the bowel in 4 to 6 hours. Potassium is lost during diarrhea, so serum potassium should be checked before the surgical procedure. Elderly, underweight, and malnourished patients are prone to other electrolyte disturbances from intestinal lavage.
2. Douche. A douche to cleanse the vagina may be ordered before a vaginal or pelvic procedure.

   NOTE Patients who will be admitted the day of the surgical procedure may be instructed to self-administer enema or douche at home.

3. Hair removal. Removal of hair from the surgical site and surrounding area may be necessary (see Chapter 22, pp. 450-451).
4. Bedtime sedation for sleep.

Preoperative Visit by Perioperative Nurse

The patient's level of anxiety and fear must be assessed preoperatively. Every effort should be made through supportive measures to minimize potential hazards of adverse psychosocial distress. Ideally this assessment should take place before the day of the surgical procedure; its purpose is to alleviate anxiety and fears. Factual information and clarification of misunderstandings will be helpful in this regard, as will the opportunity for the patient to express feelings.

Although the primary area of the perioperative nurse's practice is within the OR suite, the broadened scope of perioperative nursing encompasses phases of preoperative and postoperative care that contribute to continuity of total patient care. Preoperative visits to patients are made by perioperative nurses skilled in interviewing, a technique for the development of the patient-nurse relationship. These interviews afford nurses an opportunity to learn about the patients and to establish rapport before the time they are brought to the OR.

Before the inception of preoperative visits, the perioperative nurse had only minimal time to see and get to know the unanesthetized patient. A preoperative visit to collect data at the patient's bedside, in the preoperative testing center, or home gives the perioperative nurse the time to learn about the patient, to observe patient behavior directly, and to plan appropriately before assuming responsibility for that patient's care. Knowledge about the patient and how he or she views the impending surgical procedure is a prerequisite for effective nursing intervention. The visit also fosters patient care by providing the perioperative nurse with a basis for implementing the nursing process and developing an ongoing relationship with the patient. The perioperative nurse is therefore included in all aspects of care, not just in the intraoperative phase when the patient may be medicated or under the influence of anesthesia.

Pros of Preoperative Visits

The *advantages* of preoperative visits with patients include:

1. An experienced perioperative nurse is well qualified to discuss a patient's OR experience and to orient and prepare patient and family for it and for the postoperative period.
2. The perioperative nurse can review critical data before the procedure and assess the patient before planning care.
3. Visits improve and individualize intraoperative care and efficiency and avoid needless delays in the OR.
4. Visits foster a meaningful nurse-patient relationship. Some patients are reluctant to reveal their feelings and needs to someone in a short-term relationship.
5. Visits make intraoperative observations more meaningful by establishing a baseline for measurement of patient outcomes.
6. Visits contribute to patient cooperation and involvement by facilitating communication. Mutual goals and expected outcomes are more easily developed.
7. Visits enhance the positive self-image of the perioperative nurse and contribute to job satisfaction, which in turn reduces job turnover, a bene-

fit to the hospital. Because of increased patient contact, visits make perioperative nursing more attractive to those who enjoy patient proximity and teaching.

Cons of Preoperative Visits

The *disadvantages* associated with preoperative visits include:

1. Cost-containment measures may not provide adequate staffing or allow time to visit patients.
2. Admission of patients on the day of the surgical procedure or late the day before makes timing of visits difficult.
3. Visits may produce friction among different team factions if the program is not well planned and executed.
4. Repetitious interviewing may lead to a stereotyped manner and a lack of enthusiasm and spontaneity on the part of nurse interviewers.
5. If skill is not practiced, patients may feel their privacy is being invaded.
6. Barriers to visits may arise from the perioperative nurse's inability to :
   a. Verbalize and communicate effectively
   b. Handle or accept patient's illness
   c. Handle emotionally stressed persons
   d. Understand cultural, ethnic, and value system differences
   e. Function efficiently outside of his or her customary environment
   f. Recognize how personal beliefs and biases can influence objectivity

Nurse Interviewers

Preoperative patient interviews should be performed by perioperative nurses who are experienced and possess complete knowledge of surgical procedures and preoperative and postoperative care. Ideally the circulating nurse who will be with the patient during the surgical procedure makes the visit, but this is not feasible in all situations because of staffing and time factors. Patient interviewing requires training and special skills in data collection, physical assessment, and observation. Perioperative nurses who are adept at these skills will be comfortable visiting patients.

In some hospitals a *surgical nurse liaison* or a *nurse team* sees patients who are scheduled for surgical procedures, fills out assessment forms, and prepares written individualized plans of care. The perioperative nurses review these plans before the surgical procedures and implement the plans. A team may include staff nurses, a practitioner or a perioperative nurse, and PACU nurse. The two-nurse team approach provides nurse orientation and feedback when a less experienced interviewer accompanies an experienced one. For group instruction teams of nurses representing the OR, PACU, and ICU are effective.

Interviewing Skills Interviewing, a form of verbal interaction, is a valuable tool for obtaining information. The interview can be *directive,* structured with predetermined questions in a specific, predetermined order that limits responses. An example of a directive question is: "Have you had a surgical procedure before?" A *nondirective* interview gives the patient more opportunity to respond in an open manner. An example of a nondirective question is: "Tell me about your previous surgical experience." The choice of technique depends on the information desired.

A structured form of interview is valuable in learning about an individual's health history. The unstructured type gives a portrait of the patient's emotional reactions, concerns, and personality. An effective preoperative interview usually includes questions about both facts and feelings. Informal observation of nonverbal behavior is an essential component. All questions should be relevant. The setting should be conducive to communication. The interviewer must be able to handle the situation with spontaneity, judgment, and tact. The interview must be meaningful to both the patient and the nurse.

Steps to Successful Preoperative Visits

1. Review the patient's chart and records. Focus on medical and nursing diagnoses and the surgical procedure to be performed. Collect any information relevant to planning care in the OR. If the patient is admitted to the hospital, discuss the assessment data and the plan of care with the unit nurses before visiting the patient. The nursing data include the following pertinent information:
   a. Biographic information: name, age, sex, family status, ethnic background, educational level, patterns of living, previous hospitalization and surgical procedures, religion
   b. Physical findings: vital signs, height, weight, skin integrity, allergies, presence of pain, drainage, bleeding, state of consciousness and orientation, sensory or physical deficits
   c. Special therapy: tracheostomy, inhalation therapy, hyperalimentation
   d. Emotional status: understanding, expectations, specific problems concerning comfort, safety, language barrier, and so on

   These baseline parameters are essential for accurate intraoperative and postoperative assessment.

2. Choose an optimal time and place without interruptions.

a. Patients who will be admitted on the day of the surgical procedure may be interviewed in the preoperative testing center 1 to 7 days before the surgical procedure. If this is not feasible, a telephone call to the patient may provide an alternative means of contact.
b. Patients who have been admitted to the hospital may be visited on a nursing unit the day before the surgical procedure. Early evening is usually best, after supper and before visiting hours.
c. Allow adequate time for the interview. This is usually 10 to 20 minutes unless the patient has complex problems or special needs that require more time. Give the patient time to think and respond and to ask questions.
d. If the patient is in acute physical or psychologic distress, offer support and consider rescheduling the visit. The visit may need to be canceled or conducted through a family member or significant other. An emergency surgical patient may be assessed in the preoperative holding area.
e. Do *not* conduct the interview on the morning of the procedure! Patients are not psychologically receptive to preoperative teaching at this time. Premedicated patients may be susceptible to suggestions, however, such as, "You will have minimal discomfort after the surgical procedure."

3. Greet the patient by introducing yourself and explaining the purpose of visit. Tell the patient that the visit is a routine part of nursing care, so the patient does not feel singled out because of his or her medical diagnosis. At all times demonstrate respect by addressing the patient by his or her last name, unless specifically requested to use a first name. Terms like "honey," "dear," or "sweetheart" are unacceptable. Children are usually addressed by their given first name unless the family uses a nickname.
   a. Put the patient at ease. *Sit* close so the patient can easily see and hear you.
   b. Secure the patient's attention and cooperation. Establish eye contact.
   c. Speak first with the patient alone; exceptions are small children, persons needing an interpreter, or the mentally impaired. Then, if the patient is willing, the family may be invited to participate and ask questions. This affords the patient privacy so he or she may feel free to talk. The family should be present during the preoperative teaching to learn how to assist the patient postoperatively.
   d. Allow the patient to maintain self-respect and dignity.
   e. Instill confidence in the patient by a neat appearance and positive attitude. Establish rapport by demonstrating warmth and genuine interest. Avoid an authoritative manner.
   f. Use language at the patient's level of development, understanding, and education.
4. Obtain information by asking about the patient's understanding of the surgical procedure.
   a. Assess the level of information and understanding the patient has and check its accuracy to determine whether further instruction or clarification is needed. Ask a question such as, "What has your surgeon told you about the surgical procedure?" Correct any misconceptions about the surgical procedure as appropriate within the scope of nursing.
   b. Permit the patient to talk openly. The objective is to gather data that will generate the plan of care to be implemented by the perioperative team.
   c. Direct questions must be used with caution and are not suitable for collecting all objective data. Construct open-ended questions to elicit more information than one-word answers.
   d. *Listen attentively.* To preserve self-esteem, the patient may tell you what he or she thinks you want to hear. A patient's statement that ends in a question may be either a request for more information or an expression of a feeling or attitude.
5. Orient the patient to the OR suite environment and interpret policies and routines.
   a. Tell the patient the time the surgical procedure is scheduled, approximately how long it will take, and how long the stay will probably be in the PACU. Explain the procedures to be done in the preoperative holding area before the surgical procedure, if this is the routine.
   b. Ask the patient if family members or friends will be at the facility during the surgical procedure. They should be informed how early to be there to see the patient before sedation is given. Tell the patient and family where the waiting room is located.
   c. Tell the patient that the family will be updated on the progress of the surgical procedure and informed when he or she arrives in the PACU, if this is hospital policy. Communicating the progress of the procedure, especially if it is prolonged, provides emotional support and decreases the family's anxiety.
6. Review the preoperative preparations that the patient will experience.
   a. Familiarize the patient with who and what will be seen in the OR and PACU. If you will not be in the OR, tell the patient a colleague will be there to greet him or her and provide care.

NOTE Many perioperative nurses wear OR attire and laboratory coats with name tags when they visit patients. This familiarizes patients with the way they will see personnel the next day. Attire should be changed if the nurse reenters the OR suite after the visit.

b. Use discretion as to how much the patient should know and *wants to know.* Use words that do not evoke an anxiety-inducing state of mind. Do not use words with unpleasant associations, such as knife, needle, or nausea.
c. Postoperative recovery begins with preoperative teaching but keep explanations short and simple. Excessive detail can increase patient anxiety, which itself reduces the attention span.
d. Give practical information about what the patient should expect, such as withholding fluids, drowsiness, and/or dry mouth caused by preoperative medications; transportation to the OR, the holding area, and where he or she will be taken after the surgical procedure. Instruct the patient not to hesitate to ask for assistance at any time. Give any other relevant special precautions.
e. Give basic reasons for procedures and regulations; this reduces patient anxiety. With children and the elderly the nurse may have to repeat information as a reinforcement.
f. Explain only the procedures of which the patient will be aware.
g. Inform the family as to what they will see in the ICU, such as monitors and machines, if patient will be there.

7. Tell the patient that an anesthesiologist will visit to discuss specific questions relative to anesthesia, if this is routine.
8. Answer the patient's questions about the surgical procedure in general terms. Refer specific questions to the surgeon.
   a. Be honest and responsible in communications about a proposed diagnostic or surgical procedure. Complement, but do not overlap, the surgeon's area of responsibility. Do not be unrealistic, falsify truth, or give false reassurance to the patient or the family.
   b. Be extremely cautious about spelling out specific details of treatment, procedure, and postoperative care unless you have been thoroughly briefed by the surgeon in charge. Surgeons individualize and tailor their plan of care to their own techniques and to the patient's needs. Forms of therapy may be controversial. Continual interdisciplinary communication is essential.
   c. If unable or unprepared to answer a legitimate question, tell the patient that the concern will be answered by the appropriate personnel. For example, say, "I don't know, but I'll get that information for you." Then be certain to follow up with an answer.
9. Encourage the patient and family to discuss feelings or anxieties regarding the surgical procedure and anticipated results.
   a. Motivate and assist the patient and family to gain perspective, objectivity, awareness, and insight. A skilled professional nurse will know how to discourage wishful thinking for miraculous cures while communicating understanding of their fears and wishes for an uncomplicated, fast recovery.
   b. Observe emotional reactions.
   c. As an interviewer be objective about personal feelings, emotions, pain, mutilative surgery, and death. Listen to what the patient is asking without feeling threatened. Do not superimpose personal feelings over what the patient is actually expressing. Empathy is appropriate in this environment.
   d. Acknowledge the impact of the procedure on the patient's sexuality, if appropriate. Allow the expression of the patient's personal feelings without evoking shame or guilt. Include the family or significant other as the patient desires.
   e. Try to help the patient solve his or her own problems when possible. Ask open-ended questions that help explore a subject or feelings, but do not probe to elicit specific responses. Do not destroy the patient's coping mechanism. Encourage an appropriate one. The visit is not a structured psychiatric counseling session.
   f. Listen to the anxieties of the patient, family, or significant other in a realistic time frame and get others to follow through as necessary. Do not attempt too full an agenda. Sort out what is legitimate. You cannot solve all problems in 20 minutes. For example, say, "I'll share this information with someone who can help you with this problem." Use a colleague's expertise to assist you or to make a proper referral.
   g. Comfort the patient; convey a sense of security and trust. *Touch as appropriate.* Touch has a positive effect on physiologic parameters, such as respiration and circulation. It can lower heart rate and blood pressure. Its calming effect can improve perceptual and cognitive abilities. It establishes rapport and provides reassurance. It conveys warmth, empathy, encouragement, and support. However, touch should be comfortable. A perceptive nurse can tell when a patient resents being

touched; respect his or her feelings. Patients with decreased visual acuity appreciate the assurance that touch can give, but always speak first to avoid startling the patient.

h. Reassure the patient that he or she will not be alone but will be constantly attended by competent perioperative team members. Try to increase the patient's trust and confidence in the team as a whole.

i. Allow time to deal with the patient's questions or concerns. Ask the patient, "Do you have any other concerns?" Never bring a patient's feelings into the open and then cut off the conversation. *Do not* interrupt, interrogate, or belittle an expressed fear or seemingly irrelevant topic. All questions are significant to the patient. Answer honestly and try to resolve concerns.

10. Identify special needs of the patient that will alter the plan for intraoperative care. The preoperative visit is the time for total assessment to guard against a traumatic experience for the patient.
    a. Observe physical characteristics that might affect positioning or require special setups. The plan of care will include consideration for an extra tall, obese, or left-handed patient. For example, an intravenous (IV) infusion should be started in the right arm of a left-handed person to minimize limitation of manual dexterity.
    b. Observe the patient for physical limitations such as pain on moving, an amputated extremity, paralysis, or sensory loss. This information enables the circulator to anticipate how much cooperation to expect from the patient and how much additional help may be needed. A pad of paper and pencil may be needed to communicate with a patient who is unable to speak or is deaf. In certain instances an interpreter may be needed.
    c. Ask whether the patient wears any type of prosthetic device. Explain, per accepted hospital policy, that this must be removed before the surgical procedure either at the bedside or in the OR. Also explain that jewelry must be removed.
    d. Determine how a preexisting medical condition should be managed in the OR. For example, it is important for the circulator to know about the presence of an implanted pacemaker. Monopolar electrosurgery could cause certain models to malfunction and would be contraindicated.
    e. Know the patient's special requests.
11. Offer reassurance when possible. Maintain an attitude of hope. Avoid using terminology such as, "Everything will be all right," or "You are okay." Reinforce the concept that the team will provide good care.
    a. Help both yourself and the patient turn negative feelings into positive, useful responses.
    b. Offer realistic hope but do not minimize the seriousness of the surgical procedure.
12. Use audiovisual materials to supplement the interview, if available and appropriate.
    a. Written instructions with photographs or drawings are useful for explaining procedures and equipment. These can be presented in a booklet or pamphlet that the patient can keep and share with family members or significant others.
    b. Videotapes, slide/tape programs, or films help to reinforce the preoperative teaching.

Preoperative Teaching

Teaching, a function of nursing practice, is a process of action embracing perception, thought, feeling, and performance. During the preoperative visit the perioperative nurse supplements instruction by other nursing team members and gives information unique to the patient's specific surgical procedure. The perioperative nurse teaches patients how to participate in their own postoperative recovery. Patients must have a readiness to learn, however. Preoperative teaching should take place at three levels:

1. *Information.* Explanations of procedures, patient care activities, and physical feelings that the patient may encounter during the perioperative experience help the patient identify what is happening and what to expect. They also enhance patient satisfaction with care.
2. *Psychosocial support.* Interactions enhance coping mechanisms to deal with anxiety and fears and provide emotional comfort.
3. *Skill training.* Guided practice of specific tasks to be performed by the patient in the postoperative period can decrease anxiety, hasten recovery, and help to prevent complications.

Effective Teaching Patient teaching involves emotional energy on the part of the nurse. It can produce behavioral changes in patients as they become better prepared physically and emotionally for the surgical procedure. They also learn how to use the health care system. Learning self-help has a positive effect. Discharge planning begins during preoperative teaching. The patient knows what to expect and where to go for help after discharge if needed, such as a support group.

Patient teaching may be conducted in an informal, individual manner or in a formal, group instructional setting. The nurse-instructor should first formulate, in conjunction with other team members, attainable learning objectives with the patient's input. The development of the learning objectives is based on the assessed level of the patient's emotional receptivity and mental capacity. The nurse also assesses, by observation and elicited response, the patient's acceptance of his or her problem, developmental level, sight, hearing, and so on. Before beginning an explanation, the nurse should verify what the patient already knows, needs to know, and wants to know. An understanding relationship with the patient facilitates the teaching-learning experience.

The nurse must assist family members to cope with the situation to the extent of their ability. Success or failure of treatment often depends on what happens after the patient leaves the hospital. The family's knowledge and understanding of the patient's needs, their coping skills, and their willingness to help are important factors in recovery. Teaching should be presented at the level of family members' particular resources and knowledge base. Other points to consider include the following:

1. Arrange the environment so that a teaching-learning exchange may take place; a quiet, undisturbed environment and proper timing are important.
2. Language is the fundamental tool for education. Use understandable terminology. Do not equate intelligence level with educational level. The nurse is accountable for what is taught.
3. Set priorities and teach what is significant and appropriate to the patient's particular needs.
   a. Break down instruction into manageable steps; for example, instruct the patient to deep breathe and then cough while he or she splints the site of the surgical incision with a pillow.
   b. Put content into a logical sequence of activities to facilitate learning; for example, to avoid the possibility of inappropriate dosage, instruct the patient to write down the time he or she takes medication when at home.
   c. Give reasons and benefits; for example, movement of legs and toes and ambulation postoperatively, unless contraindicated, aids circulation and prevents venous stasis.
   d. Adapt the teaching method and timing to the specific situation. The patient may reject teaching not relevant to the immediate present. For example, a patient about to have a heart valve replacement procedure may listen to instruction but may actually be concentrating on the fact that his or her heart is going to be cut open.
   e. Do not overburden the patient with a multitude of facts.
4. Recognition of the need to know, not pressure, should be the motivating factor in learning.
5. To evaluate understanding, ask the patient to repeat in his or her own words what has been explained during the instructional session and to demonstrate deep breathing and leg exercises.
6. Written information is helpful for review of verbal instruction. Go over the material with the patient. Test his or her comprehension by asking questions. A patient who is experiencing pain or anxiety or who is under the influence of medication may not fully understand verbal communication.
7. As the resource person, be consistent, concise, and organized. Repeat instructions to help the patient retain them.

Patients who receive preoperative instruction from and interact with the perioperative nurse may suffer less apprehension, tolerate the surgical procedure better, and seem more secure and comfortable postoperatively. Usually patients will remember what has been taught. They react more positively to their perioperative experience than patients who have not been given the benefit of this interaction.

At the end of the preoperative assessment and teaching session, the perioperative nurse should not depart from the patient abruptly but should briefly summarize the events that have taken place. The patient should be left with the understanding that a postoperative visit may be made after the procedure, if this is policy.

Preoperative Visit by Anesthesiologist

The anesthesiologist is knowledgeable in the pathophysiology of disease as it pertains to anesthetic agents. Participation in the patient's preoperative preparation can reduce intraoperative complications. The anesthesiologist usually assesses patients scheduled for anesthesia the evening before the surgical procedure if the patient has been admitted. Otherwise the patient may be seen before admission in the preoperative testing center, in the same-day procedures unit, or in the preoperative holding area. All patients must be evaluated before administration of anesthesia.

Judgment and skill are important in the selection of agents and administration of anesthesia, but firsthand knowledge of the patient is extremely valuable. The anesthesiologist visits the patient to seek information and to establish rapport, inspire confidence and trust, and alleviate fear. Preparation for anesthesia begins with this visit.

Before meeting the patient, the anesthesiologist reviews the patient's past and present medical records. If recent laboratory or other test reports are not in the chart, decisions and the surgical procedure are delayed until all essential information is available. Special attention is given to past surgical procedures and any disease or complicating processes, especially those involving vital organs.

After introduction to the patient, the anesthesiologist:

1. Takes a history pertinent to administration of anesthetic agents by questioning the patient about past anesthetic experiences, allergies, adverse reactions to drugs, and habitual drug usage. Tranquilizers, cortisone, reserpine, alcohol, and recreational drugs, for example, influence the course of anesthesia. Smoking habits, genetic and metabolic problems, and reactions to previous blood transfusions also influence the choice of anesthetic.
2. Evaluates the patient's physical, mental, and emotional status to determine the most appropriate type and amount of anesthetic agent(s).
   a. Examines the patient as necessary to obtain information desired, with particular interest in heart and lungs.
   b. Palpates needle insertion site and observes for skin infection if regional block anesthesia is contemplated.
   c. Assesses the patient's mental state and cognitive ability subjectively and observes for signs of anxiety.
3. Investigates patient's cardiac reserve and observes signs of dyspnea or claudication during a short exercise tolerance test, if indicated.
4. Asks about teeth. If indicated, explains that dental work may be damaged inadvertently during airway insertion.
5. Evaluates patient's physique for technical difficulties in administration of anesthesia.
   a. A short, stout neck may cause respiratory problems or difficult intubation. A stiff neck or unstable cervical spine such as from rheumatoid arthritis can make intubation difficult or dangerous, especially in an elderly patient.
   b. Active athletic and obese persons require more anesthetic than inactive persons.
   c. Accurate weight must be known because dosage of many medications is calculated from body weight. Most dosages are calculated in milligrams per kilogram.
6. Explains preference of anesthetic, pending the surgeon's approval, and informs the patient what to expect concerning anesthesia. The patient's wishes are taken into consideration, if expressed.
7. Tells patient or asks about restricted or prohibited oral intake before anesthesia and gives reasons for this. IV therapy is explained.
8. Discusses preoperative sedation in relation to the time the surgical procedure is scheduled to begin.
9. Reassures patient that constant observation will be given during the surgical procedure and in the immediate postoperative period. The methods of monitoring vital functions are also explained.
10. Explains risks of anesthesia but without causing the patient undue stress.
11. Answers patient's questions and allays fears related to anesthesia.

Following visit with the patient, the anesthesiologist:

1. Estimates the effect of the necessary position during the surgical procedure on patient's physiologic processes.
2. Records preliminary data on anesthesia chart.
3. Writes preanesthesia orders, including times for medication administration.
4. Writes a summary of the visit and the proposed anesthetic management of the patient on the physicians' progress note. This has medicolegal value if a problem subsequently develops.
5. Assigns the patient a physical *status classification* for the purpose of anesthesia, as per the taxonomy adopted by the American Society of Anesthesiologists (ASA):
   a. Class I theoretically includes relatively healthy patients with localized pathologic processes. Emergency surgical procedure, designated E, signifies additional risk. For example, a hernia that becomes incarcerated changes the patient's status to Class I-E.
   b. Class II includes patients with mild systemic disease, for example, diabetes mellitus controlled by oral hypoglycemic agents or diet.
   c. Class III includes patients with severe systemic disease that limits activity but is not totally incapacitating, for example, chronic obstructive pulmonary disease or severe hypertension.
   d. Class IV includes patients with an incapacitating disease that is a constant threat to life, for example, cardiovascular and renal diseases.
   e. Class V includes moribund patients who are not expected to survive 24 hours with or without the surgical procedure. They are operated on in an attempt to save life; the surgical procedure is a resuscitative measure, as in a massive pulmonary embolus.
   f. Class VI includes patients who have been declared brain dead but whose organs will be removed for donor purposes. Mechanical ventilation and life support systems must be maintained until organs are procured.
6. Consults with surgeon and other physicians, for example, a cardiologist, about a patient assigned a Class III, IV, or V status. Consideration is given to the critical nature of the surgical procedure in relation to the anesthesia risks.
   a. In elective situations the surgical procedure is postponed until anesthesia will be less haz-

ardous, for example, following acute respiratory infection or cardiac decompensation.

b. In emergency situations ideal practices may be altered or disregarded to meet the exigencies of the situation. For example, if a patient is hemorrhaging, there is no time to wait to restore a low red blood count. A multiple trauma victim with a full stomach may need a nasogastric tube inserted and suction applied, endotracheal intubation while awake, or spinal anesthesia as applicable, and may undergo a surgical procedure despite food ingestion.

The role of the anesthesiologist as a member of the OR team was discussed in Chapter 5. Specific functions related to the administration of anesthetic agents will be discussed in Section Seven, Chapters 17, 18, and 19. In addition to the preoperative assessment of the patient and the administration and maintenance of intraoperative anesthetic, the anesthesiologist may see the patient postoperatively. He or she has a *responsibility to inform the patient of any unfavorable reaction to a medication or agent given* so that the patient will be forewarned in the future and report these reactions to other physicians and anesthesiologists.

Before Leaving for Operating Room

The patient's physical and emotional status and vital signs should be assessed and recorded by the nurse on the surgical unit or in the same-day admission unit before the patient goes to the OR suite. Any untoward symptoms or extreme apprehension must be reported to the surgeon because they could affect the patient's intraoperative course. The following preparations are made:

1. Patient puts on a clean hospital gown.
2. Jewelry is removed for safekeeping. If a wedding ring cannot be removed, it must be taped loosely or tied securely to prevent loss. The patient may be permitted to keep a religious symbol, but the patient must understand this probably will be removed before anesthesia is induced.
3. Dentures and removable bridges are removed, unless otherwise ordered, before administration of general anesthesia to safeguard them and to prevent obstruction to respiration. Dentures may be permitted during local anesthesia, especially if the patient can breathe more easily with them in place. Some anesthesiologists prefer securely fitting dentures to be left in place to facilitate airway insertion. Dentures are necessary to retain facial contour for some plastic surgery procedures.
4. All removable prostheses, such as eye, extremity and breast, contact lenses, hearing aids, and eyeglasses are removed for safekeeping.

   NOTE
   - In some instances the patient may be permitted to wear eyeglasses or a hearing aid to the OR. The circulator must safeguard them and send them to the PACU with the patient. Contact lenses must be removed before general anesthesia because they may become dry and cause corneal abrasions.
   - The patient's personal property must be safeguarded to prevent loss or damage. Jewelry and valuables can be given to the family or sent to the hospital safe. Clothing of the patient admitted the same day as the surgical procedure can be sent to the room or unit where the patient will be admitted postoperatively.
5. Long hair may be braided. Wigs should be removed. Hairpins are removed to prevent scalp injury.
6. Antiembolic stockings or elastic bandages may be ordered for lower extremities to prevent embolic phenomena. These are applied before abdominal or pelvic procedures and for patients who have varicosities, are prone to thrombus formation, or have a history of emboli, and for some geriatric patients. They also frequently are applied for long procedures.
7. The patient voids to prevent overdistention of the bladder or incontinence during unconsciousness. This is especially important for abdominal or pelvic procedures in which a large bladder may interfere with adequate exposure of abdominal contents or may be traumatized. Time of voiding is recorded.

   NOTE Indwelling Foley catheter insertion, when indicated, is usually done in the OR after the patient is anesthetized (see Chapter 22, pp. 449-450).
8. If ordered, an antibiotic is given to increase the blood level preoperatively.
9. Preanesthesia medications are given as ordered. Their purpose is to eliminate apprehension by making the patient calm, drowsy, and comfortable. Patients receiving preanesthesia medication should be cautioned to remain in bed and not to smoke. Many of the drugs cause drowsiness, vertigo, or postural hypotension. Therefore the siderails on the bed should be raised and the call bell placed within the patient's reach.
10. The patient, bed, and chart are accurately identified, and identifications are fastened securely in place. Allergies should be prominently noted on the chart and patient's wristband.

A preoperative checklist helps ensure that the patient has been properly prepared. If preparation is inadequate, the surgical procedure may be canceled. All essential records, including the plan of care, must accompany the patient.

Emotional Preparation

By fulfilling spiritual and psychosocial needs, the nursing staff helps provide the preoperative patient with as much peace of mind as possible. Understandably, as the time for the surgical procedure approaches, the patient's tension level rises. However, the better prepared the patient is emotionally, the smoother his or her postoperative course will be.

If the patient has not seen his or her cleric or the hospital chaplain and makes such a request, the nurse should make every effort to contact that person for the patient.

Family members or significant others should be permitted to stay with the patient until he or she goes to the OR suite. Some hospitals permit parents to accompany infants and children. After leaving the patient, the family should be directed to the waiting area.

Transportation To Operating Room Suite

Patients may be taken to the OR suite about 45 minutes before scheduled procedure time. For safety they are transported via a transport stretcher (gurney). The stretcher should be pushed from the head end so the patient's feet go first. Rapid movements through corridors and around corners may cause dizziness and nausea, especially if the patient has been medicated. The attendant at the head end can observe for vomiting or respiratory distress. The patient may be more comfortable if the head end of the stretcher is raised.

Ideally elevators are designated "for OR use only." This ensures privacy and minimizes microbial contamination. The patient must be comfortable, warm, and safe during transport. Siderails are raised and restraint straps applied. The patient should be instructed to keep arms, hands, and fingers inside the siderails during transport to avoid injury going through doorways. IV solution bags hung on poles or standards during transportation must be attached securely and placed away from the patient's head to minimize danger of injury to the patient if the container should fall. Gentle handling is indicated to prevent dislodging IV needles or indwelling catheters. A unit nurse or nursing assistant should stay with the patient until relieved by a perioperative nurse or anesthesiologist, to whom the patient's chart is given. If the patient has a language barrier or is profoundly deaf, an interpreter may accompany him or her to the OR and stay until anesthesia induction.

Admission To Operating Room Suite

Exchange/Vestibular and Holding Areas

Patients are brought through the outer corridor to the holding area by outside personnel. OR personnel may transfer the patient to an OR stretcher, where he or she remains until taken into the OR. The patient goes to the PACU and from there to the unit on this stretcher. It is then brought back to a stretcher-cleaning room, where the entire stretcher, including the wheels, is decontaminated before being brought into the OR suite.

This procedure is ideal from the standpoint of contamination control. However, some conditions justify bringing patients to the OR suite in their beds. These include patients in traction, on Stryker frames, or cardiac patients who must not be moved until transferred to the operating table. A patient on a Stryker or similar frame may be operated on while on the frame. The surgeon chooses the course that best benefits the individual patient. The bed or frame can be decontaminated in the exchange area and made up with clean linen before being brought into the room after the surgical procedure.

Beds, stretchers, and frames must be stabilized by locking the wheels and by personnel when a patient is moving from one to the other. Mattresses also should be stabilized. Adequate personnel or a mechanical assist device must be available to ensure patient safety during transfer. The patient's head, arms, and legs must be protected. The patient should be instructed and assisted to prevent a fall or injury. Once transferred to a stretcher, the patient is under constant surveillance with restraining straps and siderails securely in place.

Some hospitals have individual anesthesia induction rooms where the patient waits and is administered an anesthetic before being taken into the OR.

On Admission to Holding Area

The holding area nurse greets the patient by name and introduces self. The nurse stands next to the midsection of the stretcher so the patient can see him or her comfortably. The nurse:

1. Verifies patient identification
2. Verifies surgical procedure, site, and surgeon
3. Reviews patient's chart for completeness
   a. Medical history and physical examination
   b. Laboratory reports
   c. Consent forms
4. Takes vital signs and blood pressure
5. Verifies allergies and medication history
6. Checks skin tone and integrity
7. Verifies physical limitations
8. Notes mental state

9. Puts cap on patient to protect hair (in case vomiting occurs), for purposes of asepsis, and to help prevent hypothermia
10. Puts clean gown and warm blanket on patient

The holding area nurse records pertinent findings on the perioperative nursing record. If a perioperative nursing assessment has not been done, the holding area nurse must assess the patient's needs, formulate the nursing diagnoses and expected outcomes, and prepare an individualized plan of care. If the patient has been sedated, communication may be difficult.

Preanesthesia Preparations

The following procedures may need to be completed before induction of anesthesia. Some or all of them can be performed in the holding area if adequate facilities for patient privacy are available. The patient should be informed about procedures before they are initiated by either the nurse or anesthesiologist.

1. Removal of body hair, if ordered
2. Insertion of IV infusion
3. Insertion of invasive hemodynamic monitoring lines as appropriate
4. Insertion of Foley urinary catheter, if ordered
5. Administration of preanesthesia medication and other drugs such as antibiotics, as ordered

NOTE
- The anesthesiologist may wish to talk with the patient before sedation is given.
- The patient may wish to speak to the surgeon before receiving sedation.
- Preanesthesia medication can precipitate respiratory depression and hypotension. The nurse must be alert and take prompt action if necessary. The holding area must be equipped for cardiopulmonary resuscitation.

The anesthesiologist may perform regional blocks in the holding area. All procedures done in the holding area must be documented on the patient's chart.

Despite the activities around them, patients may feel more alone in a holding area than any other location. Time passes slowly; anxiety can increase. A compassionate expression in the eyes and voice and a reassuring touch of the hand can convey concern and understanding. An anxious patient looks to the nurse for comfort, reassurance, and attention.

If the patient is drowsy, unnecessary conversation should be avoided. However, the nurse should answer questions and see to the patient's comfort. Keep the patient warm or turn down the blanket if he or she is too warm. Place an extra pillow under the patient's head or under an arthritic knee. Moisten dry lips, if appropriate. Any delay or unusual circumstances should be explained.

A quiet, restful atmosphere enables the patient to gain full advantage of premedication. Some holding areas and ORs have piped-in recorded music. Music diverts attention from the many other sounds in the environment. Music with a slow, easy rhythm and at low volume is most conducive to relaxation. Familiar music is more pleasing and relaxing because the patient can associate it with pleasant past experiences. Some facilities provide earphones or headsets so patients can listen to the music of their choice. Earphones also muffle extraneous noises and conversations. Ideally the patient should have a choice in the selection of music or no music at all; this is the advantage of individual headsets over piped-in systems.

Transfer to Operating Room

When all is in readiness for the patient, the circulator comes to the holding area for the patient. It is advantageous if this person is the perioperative nurse who made the preoperative visit. The patient appreciates seeing a familiar face. Before transporting the patient into the OR, the circulator has several important duties to fulfill.

1. Greet and check identity of the patient, stretcher or bed, and chart.
   a. Circulator should introduce himself or herself if he or she has not previously met the patient. The patient should be addressed as Mr, Mrs, or Miss, not by first name.
   b. When the patient comes to the hospital, an identifying wristband is put on in the admitting office. The unit nurse checks the band before the patient leaves for the OR. The circulator compares the information on the wristband, including identification number, with the information on the chart and with the information on the surgical schedule: name, anticipated surgical procedure, time, surgeon. The wristband may have a bar code with an identification number linked to the patient's database. The circulator uses a bar code scanner to view patient information on a computer screen or printout.
   c. Identification on the stretcher or bed ensures the patient's return to the same one following surgery, if this is the procedure. If the patient is an infant or child, the identification tag on the crib should be out of his or her reach.
   d. Verification of surgical procedure, site, and surgeon with patient provides reassurance that this is the correct patient. If the patient is heavily sedated, the surgeon may be asked to identify the patient.
2. Check siderails, restraining straps, IV infusions, and indwelling catheters.

3. Observe patient for reaction to medication.
4. Observe patient's anxiety level.
5. Check physical examination, medical history, laboratory tests, x-ray reports, and consent form in the patient's chart.
6. Review the plan of care.
   a. Pay particular attention to allergies and any previous unfavorable reactions to anesthesia or blood transfusion.
   b. Become familiar with this patient's unique and individual needs.

The patient is taken into the OR after the surgeon sees him or her and the anesthesiologist is ready to receive the patient. The main preparations for the procedure should have been completed, so the circulator can devote undivided attention to the patient. (See Chapter 21 for discussion of safety measures for transferring the patient from transport stretcher to operating table.)

Before Induction of Anesthesia

The anesthesiologist also has immediate preanesthesia duties. He or she must:

1. Check and assemble equipment before the patient enters the room. Airways, endotracheal tubes, laryngoscope, suction catheters, labeled prefilled medication syringes, and other items are arranged on a cart or table. (See Chapter 17 for discussion of anesthesia equipment.)
2. Review the preoperative physical examination, history, and laboratory reports in the chart.
3. Make certain the patient is comfortable and secure on the operating table.
4. Check for denture removal or any loose teeth. The latter may be secured with thread taped to the patient's cheek to prevent possible aspiration.
5. Check to be certain contact lenses have been removed.
6. Ask patient when he or she last took anything by mouth.
7. Check pulse, respiration, and blood pressure to obtain a baseline for subsequent assessment of vital signs while patient is anesthetized.
8. Listen to heart and lungs, then connect ECG monitor leads. Attach pulse oximeter and other monitoring devices (see Chapter 19).
9. Start IV infusion. This may be done in the holding area or an induction room. Some patients arrive with an infusion line in place.
10. Prepare for and explain induction procedure to patient. If properly premedicated, patient should be able to respond to simple instructions.

Circulator's Role During Induction

The patient's welfare and individual needs take priority over all other activities before and during induction of anesthesia. The patient is the most important person in the OR. If the circulator is more intent on equipment than on the patient, the patient may feel abandoned. At this time of stress the patient wants the physical presence of a trusted, competent, and compassionate person.

The patient expects the circulator to be cognizant of his or her problems and conditions and willing to help relieve them. The patient perceives the circulator's attitude as one of acceptance or rejection. Consequently, the behavior of the circulator affects the patient in either a positive or negative way. Positive actions include spending time with and staying close to the patient because distance may be interpreted as disapproval; paying attention to the patient's needs and discomfort; looking directly at the patient when he or she speaks; touching the patient with kindliness; and appearing poised, confident, and professional. Negative actions include frowning, ignoring the patient, and failing to respond to the patient's feelings or needs. The *way* in which something is said and done is as important as what is said and done.

Human beings react through their senses. The positive effect of *touch* is a helpful nonverbal communication in establishing nurse-patient rapport within a short time. Touch communicates caring. Gentle touch can bridge a language barrier by establishing human contact. Warmly holding a patient's hand or laying a hand on an arm during induction of anesthesia or a painful procedure can do much to alleviate anxiety and elicit trust.

A smile has been called the universal language. Even though the circulator is wearing a mask, his or her eyes can convey a smile or hope. Likewise, they can reveal anger or hostility. Physiognomy, the ancient Chinese art of discovering qualities of the mind and temperament from the expression of facial features, still has relevance. Facial expressions, eye contact, and body movements have a positive or negative effect on the patient. Warmth and solicitude can be conveyed by a pleasant manner and the expression of the eyes.

Although routine procedures for care and teaching have been established, each patient deserves personalized care in the face of a disruptive life experience. The patient must not be treated as inanimate or anonymous or categorized by disease or surgical procedure. The patient is a living, feeling person, not "Dr. Brown's hysterectomy," "the cardiac in Room 4," "the arthritic I need help to move." Jargon such as this is depersonalizing, demoralizing, offensive, and totally unacceptable. The goal of perioperative patient care is to combine *efficiency with caring*. The circulator should not become insensitive to patients because of depersonalized procedures and routines or his or her own prejudices.

Protection of modesty, dignity, and privacy whether the patient is conscious or unconscious, is essential. Unnecessary exposure must be avoided. The gown and cotton blanket protect modesty in addition to keeping the patient warm. Also, the OR door should be kept closed for privacy; this is also important in terms of aseptic technique. Surgical procedures may be viewed only by authorized persons with a definite function. All privileged information is kept confidential.

Patients are unnerved by perceptible harmful stimuli such as strange odors; disturbing sights such as a used but uncleaned operating room, soiled linen, instruments, equipment, unconscious patients, bright lights; isolation or detachment from others; the hustle and bustle of activity or a lack of preparedness; embarrassment from body exposure; and loud noises such as voices, inappropriate conversation or whistling, staff disagreements, patient's moaning, instruments clattering, and sterilizer noises.

Anxiety and preoperative sedation tend to alter the patient's ability to interpret events objectively. The patient may relate everything heard to self, although he or she may not actually be the subject of the conversation. Lack of consideration can destroy the patient's confidence in the team. An overheard thoughtless comment can create a lasting traumatic memory and fear. Negative recall can induce anxiety in similar future experiences. Think before speaking and do not converse near the patient while excluding him or her from the conversation. Sedation does not imply exclusion. The patient may be aware of conversation even if he or she appears to be asleep! Out of the patient's hearing, conversation should pertain only to the work at hand. The OR is not the place for social discourse. The patient may misinterpret or react unfavorably because hearing is the last sense lost as a person becomes unconscious. It is not known at precisely what moment a person can no longer hear and interpret what is said, but it is known that patients remain aware of their environment much longer than their seemingly unconscious state would indicate.

Time is of the essence to keep anesthesia and procedure time to a minimum, and it is a protective factor to provide as little disturbance to physiologic homeostasis as possible. However, *efficiency and safety must not be sacrificed for speed. Safety is the prime concern.* The OR suite imposes a high degree of vulnerability on patients and the entire staff. Patients lack the power to defend and protect themselves during surgical intervention. Therefore circulators are advocates and protectors. They give supportive care and safeguard patients from emotional or physical harm by constant vigilance. Circulators can minimize potential hazards by:

1. Never leaving a sedated patient unguarded. In addition to causing mental anguish from a feeling of abandonment, if left unattended, the patient may fall or be injured by equipment.
2. Correctly identifying patients, surgical sites, drugs, or medications. An incorrect surgical procedure on a patient or error in medication is usually the result of inadequate identification.
3. Creating, maintaining, and controlling an optimally therapeutic environment in the OR. This involves control of the physical environment, such as temperature, humidity, and personnel. Traffic flow in and out of the room should be kept to a minimum. The more movement and talking, the greater the room's microbial count. Once the patient is in the OR, it should be kept quiet so the effects of sedation are not counteracted. A tranquil, relaxed atmosphere is conducive to team concentration and orderly functioning so all can go well. Standards of ethical conduct should be strictly enforced.

The impact inherent in any type of surgical intervention can be reconciled when the patient has hope and confidence in caregivers. Nurses are central figures in patient care and can do much to relieve fear and provide security. Preoperative preparations can influence the outcome of the surgical procedure.

Bibliography

Allen M et al: Effectiveness of a preoperative teaching program for cataract patients, *J Adv Nurs* 17(3):303-309, 1992.

Badger JM: Calming the anxious patient, *AORN J* 94(5):46-50, 1994.

Chana CH: Documenting the nursing process: a perioperative care plan, *AORN J* 55(5):1231-1235, 1992.

DeLong DL: Preoperative holding area: personalizing patients' experiences, *AORN J* 55(2):563-566, 1992.

Drescher NI: An intergrated care plan: developing a guideline for patient care, *AORN J* 54(6):1265-1270, 1991.

Fincham JE: Perioperative implications of tobacco use, *AORN J* 56(3):531-535, 1992.

Fromm CG, Metler DJ: Preparing your older patient for surgery, *RN* 56(1):38-42, 1993.

Griffith RS: Preoperative evaluation, *Cancer* 70(5):1333-1341, 1992.

Grossman D: Enhancing your cultural competence, *Am J Nurs* 94(7):58-62, 1994.

Haines N: Same day surgery, *AORN J* 55(2):573-580, 1992.

Kratz A: Preoperative education: preparing patients for a positive experience, *J Post Anesth Nurs* 8(4):270-275, 1993.

Longinow LT, Rzeszewski LB: The holding room, *AORN J* 57(4):914-924, 1993.

Lunow K, Jung L: Practical innovations: comprehensive perioperative care—patient assessment, teaching, documentation, *AORN J* 57(5):1167-1177, 1993.

Mathias JM: NPO requirement challenged: clear liquids may be OK, *OR Manager* 10(1):1, 6, 1994.

Morrisey J: Obtaining a "reasonably accurate" health history, *Plast Surg Nurs* 14(1):27-30, 1994.

Murray S et al: How do you prep the bowel without enemas? *Am J Nurs* 92(8):66-67, 1992.

Nightingale JJ: The preoperative anaesthetic visit, *Anaesthesia* 47(9): 801-803, 1992.

Null SL: Preadmission testing, *AORN J* 59(5):1051-1060, 1994.

Oetker-Black SL: Preoperative preparation: historical development, *AORN J* 57(6):1402-1415, 1993.

Oetker-Black SL et al: Preoperative self-efficacy and postoperative behaviors, *Appl Nurs Res* 5(3):134-139, 1992.

Oetker-Black SL, Taunton RL: Evaluation of a self-efficacy scale for preoperative patients, *AORN J* 60(1):43-49, 1994.

Salzbach R: Presurgical testing improves patient care, *AORN J* 61(1):210-218, 1995.

Schmaus D: Implementing bar code technology in the OR, *AORN J* 54(2):346-351, 1991.

Schwanitz LD: Battery of routine preoperative tests no longer recommended, *OR Manager* 10(9):14-19, 1994.

Seley JJ: Patient teaching: 10 strategies for successful patient teaching, *Am J Nurs* 94(11):63-65, 1994.

Shea SI: Our patients face recovery with confidence, *RN* 55(6):17-20, 1992.

Thompson R: Preoperative visiting, *Br J Theatre Nurs* 27(4):8-9, 1990.

SECTION SEVEN

Anesthesia Concepts and Considerations

CHAPTER 17

General Anesthesia

TECHNIQUES AND AGENTS

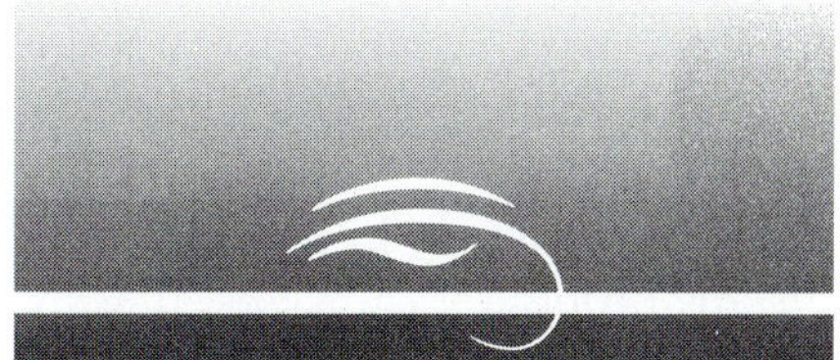

HISTORICAL BACKGROUND

Attempts to relieve pain are as old as the human race itself. Primitive people considered pain the ture of demons, which they attempted to frighten away by wearing charms and by tattooing their bodies. The medicine men used magic.

A Babylonian clay tablet, circa 2250 BC, gave a remedy for toothache. During the time of Nero, Greek and Roman surgeons gave their patients a mixture of wine and vinegar. Called a "potion of the condemned," the mixture was used to relieve anguish such as that suffered during crucifixion. These surgeons also experimented with a form of local anesthesia by placing a carbonate stone directly over the surgical site and pouring vinegar over it; they noted a numbing sensation, resulting from the formation of carbon dioxide. Sleep-producing inhalants were first used by the Egyptians and Arabians who concocted many potions from plants such as poppy and hemlock. Sponges saturated in these solutions were held to the patient's nostrils. However, death often resulted from them and from root juices used as reviving agents because dosage was unregulated and drug action unknown. The Egyptians and Assyrians produced unconsciousness by pressing on the carotid vessels in the neck, causing cerebral anoxia.

Army surgeons have always contributed to medical advancement. Ambroise Paré dulled the pain of his soldiers in the sixteenth century by compressing blood vessels and nerves near the surgical area. At this time also, half-frozen soldiers were found to have a higher pain threshold. Refrigeration anesthesia was revived in 1941 for use in amputations during World War II.

The modern concept of anesthesia was based on Joseph Priestley's experiments with oxygen and nitrous oxide. This combination and ether were first used at parties for entertainment. Traveling chemists administered these agents to induce incoherence and giddy laughter, hence the term *laughing gas*. The anesthetic properties were realized when injuries sustained during inhalation of these agents were not felt.

Dr. Crawford Long of Georgia administered the first ether anesthetic in 1842 for the painless removal of a tumor of the neck but did not publish the results of this and subsequent cases until 1849. In 1846, however, two Boston dentists, Morton and Wells, used nitrous oxide for tooth extraction. In October of that year Dr. Morton first demonstrated ether for surgical anesthesia before an astounded group of clinicians; a new era in surgery was born. Dr. Oliver Wendell Holmes devised the term *anesthesia* from the Greek words meaning "negative sensation."

Sir James Simpson, a Scottish surgeon, instituted the use of chloroform anesthesia in 1847. It was administered to Queen Victoria during childbirth by England's first anesthetist. In the late nineteenth and twentieth centuries, surgical procedures within the abdomen, thorax, and cranium evolved with administration of ether and chloroform for anesthesia. Development of the surgical specialties was concurrent with the refinement of anesthesia methods and instrumentation.

Purification of drugs such as morphine, invention of the hollow needle, and development of gas machines hastened the finding of new anesthetic techniques and agents. Endotracheal anesthesia, first used by open tracheotomy, was developed by Dr. Friedrich Trendelenburg. Dr. Chevalier Jackson's development of the laryngoscope greatly aided intubation. The importance of watching the patient's condition during anesthesia was realized ultimately and supportive measures were developed. Eminent surgeons such as Drs. George Crile and Harvey Cushing emphasized the importance of keeping accurate records of the patient's condition during the surgical procedure. In 1896 Dr. Cushing brought to the United States from Italy one of the first sphygmomanometers invented.

Special techniques such as hypothermia and extracorporeal circulation opened new vistas to surgeons, making possible advanced, complex surgical procedures that demand qualified anesthesiologists and anesthetists. Procedures lasting 6 to 24 hours are not uncommon.

Salient features of modern anesthesia include assessment of patients preoperatively; selection of appropriate agents and techniques; management of induction, maintenance, and emergence processes; and continuous monitoring of vital functions during anesthesia. The American Society of Anesthesiologists (ASA), founded in 1905, and the American Association of Nurse Anesthetists (AANA), founded in 1931, have established guidelines and standards for safely administering and monitoring anesthesia care. The ASA also developed the taxonomy for classifying patients by physical status from Class I, the lowest risk, to Class VI, the highest risk (see Chapter 16, p. 308). Historically, specialists in anesthesia have been advocates of patient safety and risk management.

With the proliferation of pain clinics anesthesiologists have essential roles in multidisciplinary teams concerned with management of acute and chronic pain. Because of their familiarity with anesthetic drugs, nerve pathways, and nerve block techniques, anesthesiologists are well qualified to assess and treat pain.

DEFINITIONS

Anesthesiology is the branch of medicine that is concerned with the administration of medication or anesthetic agents to relieve pain and support physiologic functions during a surgical procedure. It is a specialty that requires knowledge of biochemistry, clinical pharmacology, cardiology, and respiratory physiology. The American Board of Anesthesiology has defined anesthesiology as "the practice of medicine dealing with management of procedures for rendering a patient insensible to pain during surgical procedures, and with support of life functions under the stress of anesthetic and surgical manipulations." Understanding of common terms associated with these responsibilities is essential to comprehension of this complex specialty (Box 17-1).

PAIN

Pain is a perceptual phenomenon, a disturbed sensation causing suffering or distress. Physical pain is often what induces the patient to seek medical assistance. Realization of pain commences with stimulation of the nerve endings of pain fibers, which in turn produces a nerve impulse that travels to the brain. The impulse is processed and registered as an unpleasant feeling state. The quality, intensity, location, duration, and memories of pain influence one's perception and emotional response to it. Pain is undoubtedly not purely organic or strictly functional; most pain also carries a psychogenic factor. An individual's tolerance for pain, pain threshold, may be a reaction to stress, anxiety, fear, and/or external stimuli. Cultural traditions can influence expectations of pain and appropriate actions to deal with it.

Pain may be *phasic*, of short duration as a needlestick, *acute* as postoperative from tissue trauma, or *chronic* as from disease. Any patient with trauma/tissue damage from surgical procedure, ischemia from localized tissue anemia, or infarct from localized area of ischemic tissue necrosis is a candidate for pain. One must understand the anatomy and physiology of pain to assess and measure it and to attempt to relieve it. Discovery of the body's endogenous endorphins that bind to opiate receptors in the brain and spinal cord opened new horizons in understanding pain control. Methods of surgical intervention used to relieve intractable chronic pain are discussed in Chapter 37. Pain is beyond the domain of a single specialty, but in the OR, every effort is made to relieve the patient's awareness of pain. The anesthesiologist uses many drugs and agents to safely produce analgesia and amnesia (i.e., insensitivity or indifference to pain).

PREANESTHESIA PREMEDICATION

Preanesthesia medication may be given to allay preoperative anxiety, produce some analgesia and amnesia, and dull awareness of the OR environment. Elevating

BOX 17-1

Glossary of Terms Associated With Anesthesiology

amnesia Loss of memory; an indifference to pain.

analgesia Lessening of or insensibility to pain.

analgesic Drug that relieves pain by altering perception of painful stimuli without producing loss of consciousness; acts on specific receptors in nervous system.

anesthesia Loss of feeling or sensation, especially loss of the sensation of pain with loss of protective reflexes.

anesthesiologist A doctor of medicine who specializes in the field of anesthesia.

anesthetic Drug that produces local or general loss of sensibility.

anesthetist Person who has been trained to administer an anesthetic (e.g., nurse anesthetist).

anoxemia Low blood oxygen; subnormal blood-oxygen content.

anoxia Absence of oxygen.

antimuscarinic/anticholinergic Antagonist to action of parasympathetic and other cholinergic nerve fibers.

apnea Suspension or cessation of breathing.

arrhythmia Lack of rhythm designating alteration or abnormality of normal cardiac rhythm.

assisted or controlled respiration Maintenance of adequate alveolar ventilation by manual or mechanical means.

biotransformation Metabolism of anesthetic drugs. They are broken down in hepatic cells where they may accelerate their own rate of metabolism or be influenced by other drugs. Metabolic products may be inert or highly reactive chemically, possibly causing destruction of liver cells. Biotransformation is a complex process. It occurs by one or more than one of four mechanisms: oxidation, conjugation, hydrolysis, reduction. Drugs are subjected to biotransformation for inactivation and elimination.

bradycardia Slowness of heartbeat; less than 60 beats per minute.

depolarization Neutralization of polarity; reduction of differentials of ion distribution across polarized semipermeable membranes, as in nerve or muscle cells in the conduction of impulses; to make electrically negative.

drug interactions Ways in which one drug affects another.

dysrhythmia Defective rhythm, as of heart rate or brain waves; may be used interchangeably with *arrhythmia*.

emergence Return of sensation and reflexes; to regain consciousness following general anesthesia.

endotracheal Within trachea. An *endotracheal* tube may be placed in trachea to maintain a patent airway during loss of consciousness. *Intubation*, insertion of endotracheal tube. *Extubation*, removal of endotracheal tube.

epidural Space surrounding dura mater in spinal canal; injection of drugs into epidural space for relief of pain in lower abdomen and pelvis. *Epidural anesthesia* is loss of sensation below level of peridural injection without loss of consciousness.

fasciculation Incoordinate skeletal muscle contraction in which groups of muscle fibers innervated by the same neuron contract together.

general anesthesia A reversible state of unconsciousness produced by anesthetic agents in which motor, sensory, mental, and reflex functions are lost.

hemodynamics Effect of physical properties of blood and its circulation through vessels on blood flow and pressure (i.e., interrelationship of blood pressure, blood flow, vascular volumes, physical properties of blood, heart rate, and ventricular function).

hyper- or hypo- Above or below normal content (e.g., *hyperkalemia*, excess potassium level in the blood; *hypotension*, diminished or abnormally low blood pressure).

hypercapnia Excessive amount of carbon dioxide in the blood; may also be termed *hypercarbia*.

hypnosis State of altered consciousness, sleep, or trance induced artificially by means of verbal suggestion by a hypnotist or by subject's own concentration.

hypnotic Drug or verbal suggestion that induces sleep.

hypothermia State in which body temperature is lower than the physiologic normal (i.e., below 95° F [35° C]).

hypovolemia Low or decreased blood volume.

hypoxia, hypoxemia Oxygen want or deficiency; state in which an inadequate amount of oxygen is available to or utilized by tissue—inadequate tissue oxygenation.

induction Period from beginning of administration of anesthetic until patient loses consciousness and is stabilized in the desired plane of anesthesia.

laryngospasm Involuntary spasmodic reflex action that partially or completely closes the vocal cords of the larynx.

local anesthesia Loss of sensation along specific nerve pathways by blocking transmissions to receptor fibers.

lung compliance Ability of lungs to expand.

margin of safety Difference between therapeutic and lethal dosages.

narcosis State of arrested consciousness, sensation, motor activity, and reflex action produced by drugs.

narcotic Drug derived from opium or opiumlike compounds, with potent analgesic effects associated with significant alteration of mood and behavior.

neutralization Process that counterbalances or cancels the action of an agent, rendering it inert.

Continued

BOX 17-1

Glossary of Terms Associated With Anesthesiology—cont'd

P Expression for partial pressure (torr); the pressure exerted by one of the gases present in a mixture of gases. In such a mixture the partial pressures of the gases are exerted independently of each other.

Paco2 Arterial carbon dioxide tension (partial pressure of carbon dioxide in arterial blood). Normal: 35 to 45 torr.

pain threshold Individual's tolerance for pain. It may be influenced by factors such as anxiety.

Pao2 Arterial oxygen tension (partial pressure of oxygen in the arterial blood); degree of oxygen transported in the circulating blood. Normal: 80 to 100 torr.

parameter Any constant, with variable values, used as a referent for determining other variables; a constant to which a value is fixed or assigned and by which other values or functions in a given situation or system may be defined.

perfusion Introduction of fluids into tissues by their injection into blood vessels; passage of a fluid through spaces.

pH Expression for hydrogen ion concentration or acidity. In blood, alkalemia: values above 7.45; acidemia: values below 7.35; normal: 7.4.)

regional anesthesia Insensitivity of body part to pain caused by interruption of conductivity of sensory nerves supplying that area.

respiratory acidosis Reduction of carbon dioxide excretion through the lungs caused by respiratory depression or obstruction or by pulmonary disease.

sedative Drug that suppresses nervous excitement.

spinal anesthesia Intrathecal injection of drugs into subarachnoid space in spinal canal, below level of diaphragm, to produce loss of sensation without loss of consciousness.

tachycardia Excessive rapidity of heart action, heartbeat. Pulse rate is higher than 100 beats per minute.

tachypnea Abnormally rapid rate of breathing.

tension Partial pressure exerted by a component of a mixture of gases; used interchangeably with P.

tranquilizer Drug that calms, soothes, and quiets without sedating or depressing the central nervous system.

ventilation Constant supplying of oxygen through the lungs.

the pH of gastric secretions and reducing the risk of nausea and vomiting also are desirable effects. An ideal preoperative medication has quick onset, short duration of action, and minimal side effects. Some drugs decrease secretions in the respiratory tract, diminish vagal nerve effects on the heart, counteract undesirable side effects of the anesthetic, and raise the pain threshold. Preoperative medication constitutes to a greater or lesser extent a part of the overall anesthetic technique. Certain drugs may prolong the effect of the anesthetic and increase a respiratory-depressant effect.

The administration of an anesthetic actually begins with the giving of preanesthetic drugs. Discerning choice can lead to smooth, effective anesthetic management and an uncomplicated postanesthetic course as opposed to a stormy, unsatisfactory experience for all concerned.

Choice of Drugs

Selection of drugs is made by the anesthesiologist based on an assessment of the patient's physical and emotional status, age, weight, medical and medication history, laboratory tests, x-ray and electrocardiograph (ECG) findings, demands of the surgical procedure, and patient's concerns. If the patient is scheduled for local anesthesia (see Chapter 18), the surgeon may order the preoperative drugs. In choosing premedication, the anesthesiologist aims to disturb respiration and circulation as little as possible. Since more than one pharmacologic response is desired, a combination of drugs is used. Most anesthesiologists prefer to have the patient arrive in the OR awake but drowsy, free of apprehension, and fully cooperative. Drowsiness and lack of fear are not synonymous; for many patients relief from anxiety is attained only by dulling the consciousness.

Special Considerations

The patient's metabolic rate varies with age, body build, and general health. Heavy smokers, alcoholics, and patients who have problems involving hyperthyroidism, emotional instability, toxicity, or high fever have high metabolic rates and require more medication, oxygen, and anesthetic. A lower metabolic rate, as accompanies debilitating diseases and hypothyroidism, requires a smaller dosage.

Persons with drug addiction (i.e., abuse of barbiturates, narcotics, or amphetamines) present special problems concerning premedication, anesthesia, and venipuncture. These patients may have contracted human immunodeficiency virus or hepatitis. Heroin and cocaine addicts are usually given an opiate for premedication. They must be closely observed for withdrawal symptoms, especially during and after prolonged procedures.

Drugs taken simultaneously or in close sequence may act independently, may interact to reduce or increase intended effects, or may produce an undesired reaction. The anesthesiologist queries the patient about allergies, previous drug intolerance, or incidence of adverse reactions and carefully notes any medications the patient is currently taking.

Hypnosis is a valuable premedicant, especially in children, and is useful for anesthesia in selected patients (see hypoanesthesia in Chapter 18, p. 358). See Chapter 42 for other premedication agents more commonly used for pediatric patients.

In general, minimal, if any, premedication is given to ambulatory surgery patients. A sedative and antiemetic/antinauseant may be given just before surgery. Drugs associated with prolonged effects such as depression, vomiting, or a return to amnesia or a sedated state after awakening are best avoided.

Time Given

Time is calculated to maximize the effect of premedication. Peak effect is desired at the time of induction. Premedication is usually given at least 45 minutes before induction; some drugs require 60 to 90 minutes to reach peak effect.

Drugs Used

Drugs may be given orally (PO) or intramuscularly (IM), often in combination to cause drowsiness, amnesia, analgesia, and narcosis and to control vagal reflexes. Their efficacy depends on rate and extent of absorption, distribution in tissues, site of injection, degree of protein binding, and rapidity of detoxification and excretion. Drugs used for premedication are classified as sedatives and tranquilizers, narcotics, antimuscarinics/anticholinergics, and antiemetics/antinauseants.

Sedatives and Tranquilizers

Sedation reduces the effect of anxiety. Amnesia helps to provide comfort. Sedatives and tranquilizers produce a calm, hypnotic state. Many drugs are available. Each has its advantages and side effects.

Benzodiazepines Benzodiazepines produce excellent amnesia and mild sedation sufficient to reduce anxiety and fear. They cause an inhibitory effect on interneuronal transmission to sites in the central nervous system (CNS) associated with anxiety and fear. They are metabolized by the liver. Side effects are associated with overdosage. Adverse reactions are rare. The most commonly used benzodiazepines are as follows:

1. *Diazepam* (Valium), given orally for premedication. (See pp. 324 and 335 for use in induction of and emergence from general anesthesia.)
2. *Lorazepam* (Ativan), given orally for better amnesic effect than IM route. It has good antiemetic action. It acts more quickly than diazepam.
3. *Midazolam* (Versed), given IM for premedication or slow intravenous (IV) infusion for conscious sedation (see Chapter 18, p. 347). It is short acting; it metabolizes in 4 to 6 hours. It may cause respiratory depression and delayed metabolism. Dosage is highly individualized.

Barbiturates Because these drugs have a prolonged duration of action, they are seldom used for premedication on the day of the surgical procedure. They may be given orally for sleep the night before to help allay anxiety. *Secobarbital* (Seconal), *pentobarbital* (Nembutal), and *phenobarbital* have a hypnotic and sedative effect.

Antiemetics/Antinauseants Some sedatives also have antiemetic effects to minimize nausea and vomiting. They may potentiate effects of narcotics. Usually they are used in combination with other drugs. Some of the antiemetic sedatives are as follows:

1. *Promethazine hydrochloride* (Phenergan), given IM for premedication. Sedation and side effects are secondary to interactions with other drugs on CNS.
2. *Hydroxyzine hydrochloride* (Vistaril), given IM, often with a narcotic, for premedication. It causes drowsiness. This antiemetic also has antihistaminic and anticholinergic actions that cause dry mouth.
3. *Droperidol* (Inapsine), given IM for premedication. It has good sedative and antiemetic action. It may cause hypotension and tachycardia.

Narcotics

Narcotics are natural alkaloids of opium, referred to as *opiates,* or synthetics, referred to as *opioids.* They produce analgesia by acting on opiate receptors in the CNS. They effectively raise the pain threshold and lower the metabolic rate, thus moderately decreasing the amount of anesthetic needed during the surgical procedure. They also decrease alveolar ventilation and depress respiration. They should not be given to asthmatic patients and those with cardiopulmonary disease. Narcotics may cause circulatory depression and hypotension. They stimulate and constrict smooth muscles, sometimes causing nausea, vomiting, and urinary retention. Narcotics include:

1. *Morphine sulfate,* an opiate, usually is not given for premedication because of its prolonged duration of action, unless patient is in pain. (See pp. 333-334 for use as an IV anesthetic.)
2. *Meperidine hydrochloride* (Demerol), an opioid, given IM or subcutaneously for premedication. It is

short acting with fewer side effects than morphine. (See pp. 333-334 for use as an IV anesthetic.)

3. *Fentanyl* (Sublimaze), an opioid, given IM for premedication. It is short acting with good analgesia and sedation. (See pp. 333-334 for use as an IV anesthetic and p. 337 for neuroleptanalgesia.)

Antimuscarinics

Formerly known as *anticholinergics,* these drugs interfere with stimulation of the vagus nerve. They are useful in the prevention and treatment of reflex slowing of the heart, which may occur intraoperatively with stimulation of carotid sinus, intrathoracic manipulation, or traction on intraabdominal viscera or extraocular muscles. They are given preoperatively to prevent vagal mediated hypotension, cardiac dysrhythmias, and bradycardia. They increase the heart rate. Antimuscarinics are also bronchodilators and parasympathetic depressants. Because they inhibit mucus secretions, they may be given preoperatively to decrease secretions. The patient usually complains of dry mouth. The routine use of less irritating anesthetic agents has diminished their need for this purpose. Antimuscarinics are given IM. They include:

1. *Atropine sulfate* may be given preoperatively for peripheral effects. The patient will experience dry mouth and blurred vision. The preoperative dose does not provide significant vagal blocking action. Supplemental doses may be given during the surgical procedure to reduce gastric acidity.
2. *Glycopyrrolate* (Robinul) has an atropinelike effect with longer duration of action. It reduces volume and acidity of gastric secretions, thus elevating their pH. Because it does not cross the blood-brain barrier, it has less autonomic effect and causes less tachycardia than atropine.
3. *Scopolamine* decreases secretions and provides some amnesia. In combination with a narcotic, it may produce an altered state of consciousness, but it can also produce excitement, rage, and hallucinations. It is more frequently given as a supplement during the surgical procedure than as premedication for its effect on gastric secretions.

NOTE

- Nausea and vomiting may delay discharge following ambulatory surgery, especially for a patient who receives morphine during the surgical procedure. Placement of a transdermal scopolamine patch behind the ear may help relieve nausea. This can be placed up to 12 hours preoperatively and worn up to 24 hours postoperatively.
- Ephedrine and droperidol also are useful antinausea drugs. Ephedrine provides less sedation than droperidol. It may be given intramuscularly during the surgical procedure rather than preoperatively.

CHOICE OF ANESTHESIA

Selection of anesthesia is made by the anesthesiologist in consultation with the surgeon. The primary consideration with any anesthetic is that it should be associated with low morbidity and mortality. Choice of the safest agent and technique must be a personal decision predicated on thorough knowledge, sound judgment, and evaluation of each individual situation. The anesthesiologist aims to use the lowest concentration of anesthetic agents compatible with patient analgesia and relaxation. An ideal anesthetic agent or technique suitable for all patients does not exist, but the one selected should include some or all of the following:

1. Provide maximum safety for the patient
2. Provide optimum operating conditions for the surgeon
3. Provide patient comfort
4. Have a low index of toxicity
5. Provide potent, predictable analgesia extending into postoperative period
6. Produce adequate muscle relaxation
7. Provide amnesia
8. Have rapid onset and easy reversibility
9. Produce minimum side effects

Ability to tolerate stress and adverse effects of anesthesia and the surgical procedure depend on respiration; circulation; and function of liver, kidneys, and the endocrine and central nervous systems. The following factors are important:

1. Age and size/weight of patient
2. Physical, mental, and emotional status of patient
3. Presence of complicating systemic disease or concurrent drug therapy
4. Presence of infection at site of the surgical procedure
5. Previous anesthesia experience
6. Anticipated procedure
7. Position required for procedure
8. Type and expected length of procedure
9. Local or systemic toxicity of the agent
10. Expertise of the anesthesiologist
11. Preference of the patient

ANESTHETIC STATE

Both the central and the autonomic nervous systems play essential roles in clinical anesthesia.

The CNS exerts powerful control throughout the body. The effect of anesthetic drugs is one of progressive depression of the CNS beginning with the higher centers of the cerebral cortex and ending with the vital centers in the medulla. The cerebral cortex is not inactive during deep anesthesia. Afferent impulses continue to flow into the cortex along primary pathways and to excite cells in appropriate sensory areas. Also, the cerebral cortex is integrated with the reticular system. The brain represents approximately 2% of body weight but receives about 15% of cardiac output. Various factors cause alterations in cerebral blood flow and are of considerable importance in anesthesia. These factors are oxygen, carbon dioxide, temperature, arterial blood pressure, drugs, age of patient, anesthetic techniques, and neurogenic factors.

The autonomic nervous system is equally important because of its role in the physiology of the cardiovascular system, the anesthesiologist's ability to block certain autonomic pathways with local analgesic agents, specific blocking effects of certain drugs, and the sympathomimetic and parasympathomimetic effects of many anesthetic agents.

The anesthetic state involves motor, sensory, mental, and reflex functions. The anesthesiologist constantly assesses the patient's response to stimuli to evaluate specific anesthetic requirements. Specific drugs are used to achieve the desired results: *amnesia, analgesia,* and *muscle relaxation.*

Types of Anesthesia

Anesthesia may be produced in a number of ways.

1. *General anesthesia.* Pain is controlled by general insensibility. Basic elements include loss of consciousness, analgesia, interference with undesirable reflexes, and muscle relaxation.
2. *Balanced anesthesia.* The properties of general anesthesia (i.e., hypnosis, analgesia, and muscle relaxation) are produced, in varying degrees, by a combination of agents. Each agent has a specific purpose. This often is referred to as *neuroleptanesthesia* (see p. 337).
3. *Local or regional block anesthesia.* Pain is controlled without loss of consciousness. The sensory nerves in one area or region of body are anesthetized. This is sometimes called *conduction anesthesia* (see Chapter 18).
4. *Spinal or epidural anesthesia.* Sensation of pain is blocked at a level below the diaphragm without loss of consciousness. The agent is injected in the spinal canal (see Chapter 18, pp. 349-352).

Knowledge of Anesthetics

Anesthesia involves the administration of potentially lethal drugs and gases. Interactions of these with human physiology can be profound. Using discerning observation, astute deduction, and meticulous attention to the minutiae, the anesthesiologist provides skilled induction, careful maintenance of anesthesia, and prophylaxis to avoid postoperative complications. Responsible for vital functions of the patient, the anesthesiologist must know physical and chemical properties of all gases and liquids used in anesthesia. These properties determine how agents are supplied, their stability, systems used for their administration, and their uptake and distribution in the body. Important factors are diffusion, solubility in body fluids, and relationships of pressure, volume, and temperature. The synthesized general anesthetic agents are nonflammable, in contrast to the older agents.

OR and postanesthesia care unit (PACU) nurses need to be cognizant of the pharmacologic characteristics of the most commonly used anesthetics. Anesthesia and surgical trauma produce multiple systemic effects, which must be monitored (see Chapter 19).

NOTE The authors acknowledge that many anesthetics are safely administered by nurse anesthetists (CRNAs) and other qualified persons. Reference is made throughout this text to an anesthesiologist for purposes of simplicity only.

General Anesthesia

Anesthesia is produced as the CNS is affected. Association pathways are broken in the cerebral cortex to produce more or less complete lack of sensory perception and motor discharge. Unconsciousness is produced when blood circulating to the brain contains an adequate amount of the anesthetic agent. General anesthesia results in an immobile, quiet patient who does not recall the surgical procedure.

Most anesthetic agents are potentially lethal. The anesthesiologist must constantly observe the body's reflex responses to stimuli and other guides to determine the degree of CNS, respiratory, and circulatory depression during induction and the surgical procedure. No one clinical sign can be used as a reliable indication of anesthesia depth. Continuous watching and appraisal of all clinical signs, in addition to other available objective measurements, are necessary. In this way the anesthesiologist judges the level of anesthesia, referred to as *light, moderate,* or *deep,* and provides the patient with optimum care (Table 17-1).

The three methods of administering general anesthesia are *inhalation, IV injection,* or rectal instillation. The latter method is obsolete, except occasionally in pediatrics, because absorption in the colon is unpredictable. Control of each method varies.

Induction of General Anesthesia

Induction involves putting the patient safely to sleep (i.e., into a state of unconsciousness). A patent airway and adequate ventilation must be ensured. If not already running, an IV infusion is started. The anesthesiologist should wear gloves for venipuncture. A na-

TABLE 17-1

Depth of General Anesthesia

FROM	TO	PATIENT'S REACTIONS	NURSING ACTIONS
Induction and beginning of gas or drug	Loss of consciousness	Drowsy, dizzy, amnesic	Close OR doors. Keep room quiet. Stand by to assist. Initiate cricoid pressure, if requested.
Loss of consciousness	Relaxation	May be excited with irregular breathing and movements of extremities Susceptible to external stimuli (e.g., noise, touch)	Restrain patient. Remain at patient's side, quietly, but ready to assist anesthesiologist as needed.
Surgical anesthesia stage of relaxation	Loss of reflexes: depression of vital functions	Regular respiration Contracted pupils Reflexes disappear Muscles relax Auditory sensation lost	Position patient and prep skin only when anesthesiologist indicates this stage is reached and under control.
Danger stage: vital functions too depressed	Respiratory failure: possible cardiac arrest	Not breathing Little or no pulse or heartbeat	Prepare for cardiopulmonary resuscitation.

sogastric tube may be inserted to evacuate stomach contents.

Preoxygenation

The anesthesiologist may have the patient breathe pure oxygen (100%) by face mask for a few minutes. This provides a margin of safety in the event of airway obstruction or apnea during induction with resultant hypoxia.

Loss of Consciousness

Unconsciousness is induced by IV administration of a drug or by inhalation of an agent mixed with oxygen. Because the technique is rapid and simple, an IV drug usually is preferred by anesthesiologists and often is requested by patients.

Barbiturates Ultra-short-acting barbiturates given intravenously in small dosage offer a rapid, pleasant induction within 30 seconds. They provide marked sedation and amnesia. Because excessive secretions in the respiratory passage predispose the patient to coughing or laryngospasm, he or she should be asked to clear air passages as necessary before injection of the drug. Also minor laryngeal or pharyngeal stimulation of the head and neck, as during airway insertion, can precipitate coughing and laryngospasm. The most commonly used barbiturates are *thiopental sodium* (Pentothal Sodium), *methohexital sodium* (Brevital), and *sodium thiamylal* (Surital). See p. 332 for detailed description of these drugs.

Benzodiazepines Benzodiazepines are not as predictable and are slower acting than barbiturates, but they cause less hypotension, bradycardia, and respiratory depression. Their sedative effects facilitate awake intubation. The most commonly used IV benzodiazepines are *diazepam* (Valium) and *midazolam* (Versed).

Etomidate (Amidate, Hypnomidate) An ultra-short-acting IV hypnotic agent can be given for induction of general anesthesia or, in smaller amounts, for maintenance with nitrous oxide for short procedures. Like thiopental, etomidate has no analgesic activity. Its main advantage is the relative absence of cardiopulmonary effects. This drug has little or no effect on cardiac output, peripheral or pulmonary circulation, or myocardial metabolism. Pain on injection and myoclonic muscle movements can occur. But when etomidate is administered in combination with a narcotic, skeletal muscle contractions are reduced. Laryngospasm, coughing, and hiccups can occur during induction.

Etomidate is useful for patients sensitive to other induction agents because it does not seem to cause histamine release. Its use is contraindicated in children under 10 years of age and in obstetric procedures, including cesarean section.

Nitrous Oxide Usually used as an adjunct to an IV drug, nitrous oxide gas can be inhaled for a comfortable, rapid induction. It has a pleasant, fruitlike odor. The gas is administered by face mask. Relaxation is poor. Excitement and laryngospasm may occur. See p. 332 for discussion of nitrous oxide. A vaporized halogenated agent may be preferred to nitrous oxide (see pp. 329-331).

Intubation

A patent airway must be established to provide adequate oxygenation and to control breathing of the unconscious patient. The patient's tongue and secretions can obstruct respiration in absence of protective reflexes. An oropharyngeal airway, laryngeal mask, or endotracheal tube may be inserted.

Intubation is insertion of an endotracheal tube between vocal cords, usually with an oral tube by direct laryngoscopy. A nasal tube may be inserted by blind intubation or with a lightwand to aid in positioning the tube in the posterior oropharynx. These tubes are open at both ends. Most have a built-in cuff that is inflated with a measured amount of air, water, or saline after insertion to completely occlude the trachea. Tubes may be made of metal, plastic, silicone, or rubber. The anesthesiologist must be informed if a laser will be used in the mouth or throat so that a laser-resistant endotracheal tube can be inserted. The endotracheal tube must be securely fixed in place to prevent irritation of trachea and to maintain ventilation. The anesthesiologist should wear goggles or a face shield to prevent secretions from splashing in the eyes during intubation.

Neuromuscular blocking agents (see muscle relaxants, pp. 335-336) are given before intubation to relax the jaw and larynx. Intubation during induction and extubation during emergence from anesthesia are precarious times for the patient. The patient may cough, jerk, or experience laryngospasm from massive tracheal stimulation. Cardiac dysrhythmias may occur. Hypoxia is a potential complication. Aspiration is also a hazard, particularly in a patient with a full stomach or with increased intraabdominal or intracranial pressure.

Cricoid Pressure The circulator may be asked to apply pressure to cricoid cartilage to occlude the esophagus and immobilize the trachea. Referred to as Sellick's maneuver, this action prevents regurgitation and aspiration of stomach contents. The cricoid cartilage forms a complete ring around the inferior wall of the larynx below the thyroid cartilage prominence. Pressure with one or two fingers to compress the cricoid cartilage against the body of sixth cervical vertebrae obstructs the esophagus (Figure 17-1). Compression must begin with the patient awake before induction drugs are injected. It must continue until the endotracheal tube cuff is inflated.

Awake Intubation The anesthesiologist may determine that intubation must be performed before the induction of general anesthesia based on preoperative physical assessment. Acromegaly, anterior larynx, enlarged tongue, limited oral cavity, jaw fixation, short neck, or limited cervical range of motion are the most common indications for awake intubation. These conditions may inhibit visualization of the vocal cords by direct laryngoscopy and thus increase the potential risk of airway obstruction in the absence of protective reflexes, as following the induction of anesthesia. Most awake intubation is performed with a fiberoptic laryngoscope for direct visualization of vocal cords after the administration of IV sedation and application of topical

A

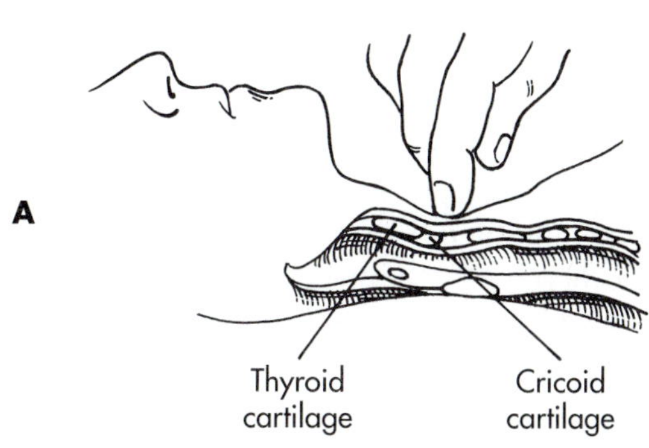

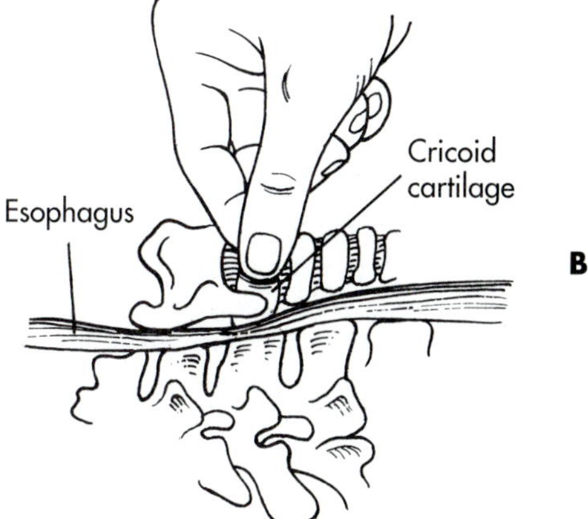

B

FIGURE 17-1 Cricoid pressure. **A,** Index finger displaces cricoid cartilage posteriorly, thus obstructing esophagus. **B,** Two-finger technique obstructs esophagus between body of sixth cervical vertebra and cricoid cartilage.

anesthetic to the posterior pharynx. The anesthesiologist may inject a local anesthetic around the laryngeal nerve to suppress the patient's gag and cough reflex. Usually two anesthesiologists work together during awake intubation. After the patient is sedated and the topical anesthetic agent is applied, one anesthesiologist inserts the endotracheal or nasotracheal tube as the second anesthesiologist gives a rapid-acting barbiturate to induce general anesthesia.

Key Points During Induction

Induction of general anesthesia is a crucial period requiring maximum attention from the OR team. The following key points are critical to the patient's welfare:

1. Circulator should remain at the patient's side to provide physical protection and emotional support and to assist anesthesiologist and closely observe monitors.
2. Although induction is quiet and uneventful for most patients, untoward occurrences are possible. Excitement, coughing, breath-holding, retching, vomiting, irregular respiratory patterns, or laryngospasm can lead to hypoxia. Secretions in air passages, from irritation by anesthetic, can cause obstruction and dysrhythmias. Induction must be gentle and not so rapid as to cause physiologic insult. To prevent these events, absolute avoidance of stimulation of the patient is mandatory. (Avoid venting steam from sterilizer in adjacent substerile room, clattering instruments, or opening paper wrappers. Do not touch patient until anesthesiologist says it is safe to do so.)
3. Precautions to be taken during induction are continuous electrocardiography, use of chest stethoscope, and readily available resuscitative equipment, including defibrillator (see Chapter 19).
4. Induction is individualized. For example, an obese patient may be induced with head raised slightly to avoid pressure of the abdominal viscera against the diaphragm. The patient is placed flat, however, if blood pressure begins to drop.
5. Small children need gentle handling. The circulator can help the anesthesiologist in making the induction period less frightening by staying close to the child. Sometimes a drop of artificial flavoring (e.g., orange, peppermint) put inside the face mask facilitates the child's acceptance of it.
6. Speed of induction depends on potency of agent, administration technique, partial pressure administered, and rate at which anesthetic is taken up by blood and tissues.

Maintenance of General Anesthesia

The anesthesiologist attempts to maintain the lightest level of anesthesia in the brain compatible with operating conditions. Five objectives must be met.

1. *Oxygenation*. Tissues, especially the brain, must be continuously perfused with oxygenated blood. Color of blood, amount and kind of bleeding, and pulse oximetry are indicators of adequacy of oxygenation. Controls on anesthesia machine and monitors of vital functions keep anesthesiologist aware of patient's condition.
2. *Unconsciousness*. The patient remains asleep and unaware of environment during the surgical procedure.
3. *Analgesia*. The patient must be free of pain during the surgical procedure.
4. *Muscle relaxation*. Muscle relaxation must be constantly assessed to provide necessary amounts of drugs that cause skeletal muscles to relax. Less tissue manipulation is required when muscles are relaxed.
5. *Control of autonomic reflexes*. Anesthetic agents affect cardiovascular and respiratory systems. Tissue manipulations and systemic reactions to them may be altered by drugs that control the autonomic nervous system.

General anesthesia is maintained by *inhalation* of gases and *IV injection* of drugs. An anesthesia machine is always used to deliver oxygen-anesthetic mixtures to the patient through a breathing system.

Anesthesia Machine

Basically the anesthesia machine includes sources of oxygen and gases with flowmeters for measuring and controlling their delivery; devices to volatize and deliver liquid anesthetics; gas-driven mechanical ventilator; devices for monitoring the ECG, blood pressure, inspired oxygen, and expired carbon dioxide; and alarm systems to signal apnea or disconnection of the breathing circuit. Breathing tubes of corrugated rubber or plastic carry gases from the machine to the face mask and breathing system. The reservoir (breathing) bag compensates for variations in respiratory demand and permits assisted or controlled ventilation by manual or mechanical compression of the bag. Sterile disposable sets containing tubing, mask, Y-connector, and reservoir bag are commercially available in conductive and nonconductive materials.

Fail-safe systems and machine design aim to eliminate delivery of a hypoxic gas mixture and to reduce the possibility of human error or mechanical failure. Reference to a checklist by the anesthesiologist before induction enhances vigilance. All anesthesia machines have the following features (Figure 17-2):

1. Sources of oxygen and compressed gases. These may come from piped-in systems, but mounted cylinders also are necessary in the event of failure of systems.
2. Means for measuring (flowmeters) and controlling (reservoir bag) delivery of gases.

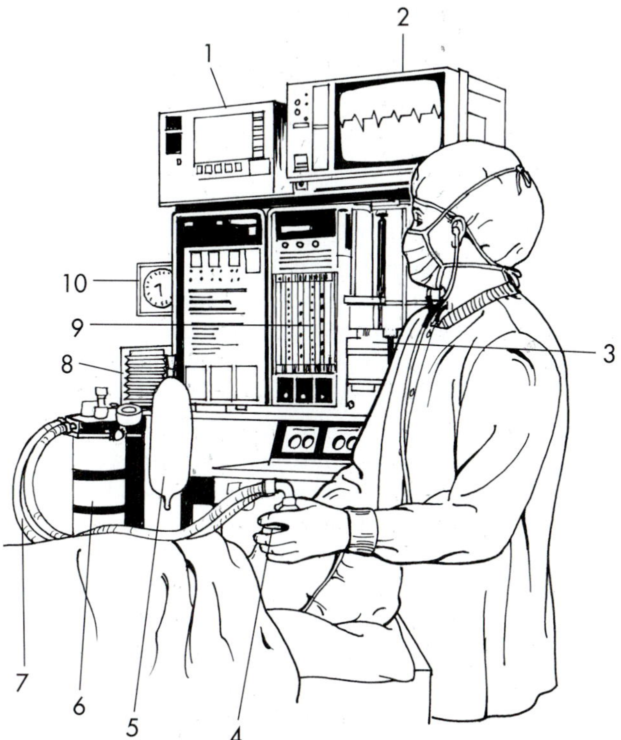

FIGURE 17-2 Anesthesia machine for maintenance of general anesthesia: *1,* anesthetic and respiratory gas monitor; *2,* physiologic monitor (channels include ECG, blood pressure, temperature, heart rate, pulse oximeter); *3,* flow-through vaporizers; *4,* face mask; *5,* reservoir "breathing" bag; *6,* carbon dioxide absorber canister; *7,* patient breathing circuit; *8,* ventilator; *9,* flowmeters for gases; *10,* sphygmomanometer for manual blood pressure.

3. Means to volatize liquid (vaporizer) and deliver (breathing tubes) anesthetic vapor or gas.
4. Device for disposal of carbon dioxide (CO_2 absorption canister).
5. Safety devices:
   a. Oxygen analyzers
   b. Oxygen pressure interlock system or equivalent to automatically shut off flow of gases in absence of oxygen pressure
   c. Pressure and disconnect alarms to notify anesthesiologist if flow of oxygen and gases becomes disproportional
   d. Pin-index safety system to release excess gases
   e. Gas scavenger system to collect exhaled gases

The elimination of waste gas, vented through an exhaust valve into a waste gas scavenger system, controls pollution of OR atmosphere. Nitrous oxide and halogenated agents can escape into room air. Substantial amounts may be an occupational health hazard to OR team members. Scavenging devices on anesthesia machine ventilator trap and remove waste gases. Breathing tubes must be checked for cracks. Valves on the machine must function properly, and connections must be secure. Room air should be monitored. This may be done by infrared spectrophotometer, for example, to monitor escape of gases from patient's exhalations and from anesthetic delivery system. Passive dosimeters may be used to monitor air in team members' personal breathing space. See Chapter 10, pp. 154-155 for further discussion of a waste gas control program for occupational safety.

Inhalation Systems

The method for administration of inhalation anesthetics through the anesthesia machine can be classified as semiclosed, closed, semiopen, or open.

1. *Semiclosed system.* The most widely used, a semiclosed system permits exhaled gases to pass into the atmosphere so they will not mix with fresh gases and be rebreathed. A chemical absorber for carbon dioxide is placed in the breathing circuit. This reduces carbon dioxide accumulation in blood. Induction is slower but with less loss of heat and water vapor than with open methods.
2. *Closed system.* A closed system allows complete rebreathing of expired gases. Exhaled carbon dioxide is absorbed by soda lime or mixture of barium and calcium hydroxide (Baralyme) in the absorber on the machine. The body's metabolic demand for oxygen is met by adding oxygen to inspired mixture of gases or vapors. This system provides maximal conservation of heat and moisture. It reduces the amount and therefore the cost of agents and reduces environmental contamination.
3. *Semiopen system.* With the semiopen system some exhaled gas can pass into surrounding air but some returns to the inspiratory part of the circuit for rebreathing. The degree of rebreathing is determined by the volume of flow of fresh gas. Expired carbon dioxide is not chemically absorbed.
4. *Open system.* In an open system valves direct expired gases into the atmosphere. The patient inhales only the anesthetic mixture delivered by the anesthesia machine. Composition of inspired mixture can be accurately determined. However, anesthetic gases are not confined to the breathing system. High flows of gases are necessary because resistance to breathing varies. Water vapor and heat are lost. Inspired gases should be humidified for respiratory mucosa to function properly, especially for children and during long surgical procedures.

Administration Techniques

Inhalation gases and vapors can be delivered from an anesthesia machine via face mask, laryngeal mask, or endotracheal tube. Respirations must be assisted or controlled.

Mask Inhalation Anesthetic gas or vapor of a volatile liquid is inhaled through a face mask attached to the anesthesia machine by breathing tubes. The mask must fit the face tightly to minimize escape of gases into room air. Significant leakage occurs around an ill-fitting mask, particularly in the area above the nose. Several sizes should be available.

Laryngeal Mask An airway can be maintained by inserting a laryngeal mask into the larynx. This flexible tube has an inflatable silicone ring and cuff. When the cuff is inflated, the mask fills the space around and behind the larynx to form a seal between the tube and trachea.

Endotracheal Administration Anesthetic vapor or gas is inhaled directly into the trachea through a nasal or oral tube inserted between the vocal cords by direct or blind laryngoscopy (see intubation, p. 325). The tube must be securely fixed in place to minimize tissue trauma. The patient is given oxygen before and after suctioning of a tracheal tube.

Advantages of endotracheal administration are that it:

1. Ensures a patent airway and control of respiration. Secretions are easily removed from the trachea by suctioning. Positive pressure can be given immediately by pressing the reservoir bag on the machine without danger of dilating the stomach.
2. Protects lungs from aspiration of blood, vomitus of gastric contents, or foreign material.
3. Preserves airway regardless of patient's position during surgical procedure.
4. Interferes minimally with surgical field during head and neck procedures.
5. Helps minimize escape of vapors or gases into room atmosphere.

Intubation, insertion of tube directly into trachea, and *extubation,* removal of tube, can cause massive tracheal stimulation. The patient may cough, jerk, or develop spasms of the larynx *(laryngospasm).* Other potential *complications* of endotracheal administration include:

1. *Trauma to teeth, pharynx, vocal cords, or trachea.* Postoperatively the patient may experience sore throat, hoarseness, laryngitis and/or tracheitis. Laryngeal edema is more common in children than in adults. Ulceration of the tracheal mucosa or vocal cords may cause granuloma.
2. *Cardiac dysrhythmias.* Cardiac dysrhythmias may occur in light anesthesia or be caused by suctioning through the endotracheal tube.
3. *Hypoxia and hypoxemia.* Hypoxia is a common complication during intubation and extubation. Endotracheal tube suctioning can cause hypoxemia.
4. *Accidental esophageal or endobronchial intubation.* The latter results in ventilation of only one lung.
5. *Aspiration of gastrointestinal contents.* This is a hazard in a patient with a full stomach or one who has increased intraabdominal or intracranial pressure. It can also occur in a patient with intestinal obstruction who is extubated before protective reflexes return.
6. *Tracheal collapse.* This may follow extubation.

Controlled Respiration Respirations may be assisted or controlled. Assistance, to improve ventilation, may easily be given by manual pressure on the reservoir (breathing) bag of the anesthesia machine. Assisted respiration implies that the patient's own respiratory effort initiates the cycle. *Controlled respiration* may be defined as the completely controlled rate and volume of respirations. The latter is best accomplished by means of a mechanical device that automatically and rhythmically inflates the lungs with intermittent positive pressure, requiring no effort by the patient. Gas moves in and out of the lungs. The combination of a volume preset ventilator with an assist mechanism maintains integrity of the respiratory center. Controlled respiration is initiated after the anesthesiologist has produced apnea by hyperventilation or administration of respiratory depressant drugs or a neuromuscular blocker.

Controlled ventilation is used in all types of surgical procedures, especially in lengthy ones. The anesthesiologist's artificial control of respiration or the patient's respiratory efforts influence the minute-to-minute level of anesthesia. Advantages of controlled respiration are that it:

1. Provides for optimum ventilation
2. Puts diaphragm at rest for thoracic procedures
3. Gives access to deep regions of thorax and upper abdomen
4. Permits deliberate production of apnea to facilitate surgical manipulation below diaphragm, ligation of deep vessels, or taking x-ray films

The patient is taken off a respirator gradually near the end of the surgical procedure and spontaneous respiration resumes. Assisted ventilation may be continued postoperatively, as in the case of an obese patient or after lengthy or open heart procedures. The endotracheal tube or laryngeal mask may remain in place until reflexes return.

Inhalation Anesthetic Agents

Inhalation is the most controllable method of administration because uptake and elimination of anesthetic agents are accomplished mainly by pulmonary ventilation. The lungs act as avenues of entrance and escape, although the agents are metabolized in the body in varying degrees. The anesthetic vapor of a volatile liquid or an anesthetic gas is inhaled and carried into the bloodstream by passing across the alveolar membrane into the general circulation and on to the tissues. Ventilation and pulmonary circulation are two critical factors involved in the process. Each can be affected by components of the anesthetic experience, such as change in body position, preanesthetic medication, alteration in body temperature, or respiratory gas tensions.

In inhalation anesthesia the aim is to establish balance between content of anesthetic vapor or gas inhaled and that of body tissues. Blood and lungs function as the transport system. Anesthesia is produced by the development of an anesthetizing concentration of anesthetic in the brain. Depth of anesthesia is related to concentration and biotransformation (see Table 17-1, p. 324).

Pulmonary blood-gas exchange is important to tissue perfusion. Defective gas exchange can cause hypoxemia and respiratory failure. It also interferes with delivery of anesthetic. Potent inhalation agents, such as myocardial depressants, affect oxygenation. Most of them induce a dose-related hypoventilation. The deeper the anesthesia, the more depressed ventilation becomes. Surgical stimulation partially corrects depression, but respiration must be controlled to keep oxygen and carbon dioxide exchange constant to prevent hypoventilation and cardiac depression.

While the respiratory system is employed for distribution of anesthetic, it also must carry on its normal function of ventilation (i.e., meeting tissue demands for adequate oxygenation and elimination of carbon dioxide and helping to maintain normal acid-base balance). The amount of anesthetic vapor inspired is influenced by the volume and rate of respirations. Gas or vapor concentration and rate of delivery are also significant. Pulmonary circulation is the vehicle for oxygen and anesthetic transport to general circulation. The large absorptive surface of the lungs and their extensive microcirculation provide a large gas-exchanging surface. In optimum gas exchange all alveoli share inspired gas and cardiac output equally (ventilation-perfusion match). Because respiratory and anesthetic gases interact with pulmonary circulation, alveolar anesthetic concentrations are rapidly reflected in circulating blood.

Alveolar concentration results from a balance between two forces: ventilation that delivers anesthetic to the alveoli and uptake that removes anesthetic from alveoli. Certain factors influence uptake of the anesthetic and therefore induction and recovery. *Uptake* has the following two phases:

1. *Transfer of anesthetic from alveoli to blood.* Rate of transfer is determined by solubility of agent in blood, rate of pulmonary blood flow (related to cardiac output), and partial pressure of anesthetic in arterial and mixed venous blood.
2. *Transfer of anesthetic from blood to tissues.* Factors influencing uptake by individual tissues are similar to those for uptake by blood. They are solubility of gas in tissues, tissue volume relative to blood flow (flow rate), and partial pressure of anesthetic in arterial blood and tissues. Tissues differ, therefore uptake of the anesthetic differs. Highly perfused tissues (heart) equilibrate more rapidly with arterial tension than poorly perfused tissue (fat), which has a slow rise to equilibrium and retains anesthetic longer.

Elimination of anesthetic is affected by the same factors that affected uptake. As an anesthetic is eliminated, its partial pressure in arterial blood drops first, followed by that in tissues.

The most important factors influencing safe administration of any anesthetic are knowledge and skills of the anesthesiologist. A perfect agent has not been found, and no agent is entirely safe. Commonly used agents are listed in Table 17-2. Advantages and disadvantages are relative.

Synthesis of potent nonflammable, halogenated, volatile liquids has replaced cyclopropane and ether, which are highly flammable agents. All inhalation agents are administered with oxygen. Volatile liquids are vaporized for inhalation by oxygen, which acts as a carrier, flowing over or bubbling through liquid in the vaporizer on the anesthesia machine. The oxygen picks up 0.25% to 5% concentration of the halogenated agent. Known sensitivity to halogenated agents or history significant for the risk of malignant hyperthermia are contraindications for their use.

Halothane (Fluothane) A widely used halogenated hydrocarbon, halothane reduces myocardial oxygen consumption more than it depresses cardiac function.

Advantages: Nonflammable, potent, versatile, chemically stable; rapid, smooth induction. High potency makes possible the use of high concentrations of oxygen for adequate ventilation; nonirritating to respiratory tract. Depth of anesthesia can be rapidly altered. Little excitement; permits early intubation because of minimal laryngeal irritation. Spontaneous ventricular dysrhythmias are rare if anoxia and respiratory acidosis are avoided. Useful for patient with bronchial asthma because it induces bronchodilatation.

Disadvantages: Potentially toxic to liver. Progressively depressant to respiration. Especially depressant to the cardiovascular system, causing hypotension, bradycardia, and, in rare cases, cardiac arrest. Sensitizes myocardial conduction system to catecholamines; avoid concomitant use of epinephrine. May cause dysrhythmias in the presence of aminophylline. Raises intracranial pressure. Limited relaxation of abdominal muscles (necessitating muscle relaxants). Has profound effect on body temperature control. May cause hypothermia. Exerts undesirable effects on rubber, some metals, and plastics. Is highly soluble in rubber and is retained in it during prolonged administration. Complete elimination of halothane takes some time.

TABLE 17-2

Most Commonly Used General Anesthetic Agents

GENERIC NAME	TRADE NAME	ADMINISTRATION	CHARACTERISTICS	USES
Nitrous oxide	—	Inhalation	Inorganic gas; slight potency; pleasant fruitlike odor; nonirritating; nonflammable but supports combustion; poor muscle relaxation	Rapid induction and recovery; short procedures when muscle relaxation unimportant; adjunct to potent agents
Halothane	Fluothane	Inhalation	Halogenated volatile liquid; potent; pleasant odor; nonirritating; cardiovascular and respiratory depressant; incomplete muscle relaxation; potentially toxic to liver	Rapid induction; wide spectrum for maintenance; depth of anesthesia easily altered; rapid reversal
Enflurane	Ethrane	Inhalation	Halogenated ether; potent; some muscle relaxation; respiratory depressant	Rapid induction and recovery; wide spectrum for maintenance
Isoflurane	Forane	Inhalation	Halogenated methyl ether; potent; muscle relaxant; profound respiratory depressant; metabolized in liver	Rapid induction and recovery with minimal aftereffects; wide spectrum for maintenance
Thiopental sodium	Pentothal Sodium	Intravenous	Barbiturate; potent; short acting with cumulative effect; rapid uptake by circulatory system; no muscle relaxation; respiratory depressant	Rapid induction and recovery; short procedures when muscle relaxation not needed; basal anesthetic
Methohexital sodium	Brevital	Intravenous	Barbiturate; potent; circulatory and respiratory depressant	Rapid induction; brief anesthesia
Propofol	Diprivan	Intravenous	Alkylphenol; potent short-acting sedative-hypnotic; cardiovascular depressant	Rapid induction and recovery; short procedures alone; prolonged anesthesia in combination with inhalation agents or opioids
Ketamine hydrochloride	Ketaject, Ketalar	Intravenous, intramuscular	Dissociative drug; profound amnesia and analgesia; may cause psychologic problems during emergence	Rapid induction; short procedures when muscle relaxation not needed; children and young adults
Fentanyl	Sublimaze	Intravenous	Opioid; potent narcotic; metabolizes slowly; respiratory depressant	High-dose narcotic anesthesia in combination with oxygen
Sufentanil citrate	Sufenta	Intravenous	Opioid; potent narcotic; respiratory depressant	Premedication; high-dose narcotic anesthesia in combination with oxygen
Fentanyl and droperidol	Innovar	Intravenous	Combination narcotic and tranquilizer; potent; long acting	Neuroleptanalgesia
Diazepam	Valium	Intravenous, intramuscular	Benzodiazepine; tranquilizer; produces amnesia, sedation, and muscle relaxation	Premedication; awake intubation; induction
Midazolam	Versed	Intravenous, intramuscular	Benzodiazepine; sedative; short-acting amnesic; central nervous system and respiratory depressant	Premedication; conscious sedation; induction in children

Use: Wide spectrum—all types of surgical procedures except routine obstetrics where uterine relaxation is not desired. It is a profound uterine relaxant. Because its metabolites have a possible effect as a hepatotoxin, some anesthesiologists avoid repeated administration within an arbitrary time, for example, a 3-month period, in adults. Recent jaundice and known or suspected liver disease (past or present) are usually contraindications to its use.

Enflurane (Ethrane) A widely used, nonflammable, stable, halogenated ether, enflurane is similar in potency and versatility to halothane.

Advantages: Rapid induction and recovery with minimal aftereffects. Pharyngeal and laryngeal reflexes are obtunded easily, salivation is not stimulated, and bronchomotor tone is not affected. Cardiac rate and rhythm remain relatively stable, although caution is advisable when used with epinephrine. Muscle relaxation is produced, but small supplementary doses of muscle relaxants may be required; nondepolarizing relaxants (see pp. 335-336) are potentiated by enflurane.

Disadvantages: Respiration and blood pressure are progressively depressed with deepening anesthesia. Although biotransformation (metabolism) of enflurane is less than occurs with other halogenated agents, small amounts of fluoride ion are released. Severe renal disease is a contraindication to use. At deeper levels an electroencephalographic pattern resembling seizures may occur. The agent is absorbed by rubber.

Use: Wide spectrum of procedures.

Isoflurane (Forane) Of the potent halogenated agents, isoflurane comes closer to ideal than other inhalation agents. Isoflurane is a nonflammable, fluorinated, halogenated methyl ether similar to halothane and enflurane yet uniquely different. It is a more potent muscle relaxant, but, unlike the others, it protects the heart against catecholamine-induced dysrhythmia. Heart rhythm is remarkably stable. Blood pressure drops with induction but returns to normal with intraoperative stimulation. A dose-related lowering of blood pressure occurs, but cardiac output is unaltered, mainly as a result of increased heart rate. Isoflurane potentiates all commonly used muscle relaxants, the most profound effect occuring with the nondepolarizing type (see pp. 335-336).

Advantages: Less cardiac depression; increased cardiac output, wide margin of cardiovascular safety; does not sensitize myocardium to effects of epinephrine. No CNS excitatory effects. Rapid induction and especially recovery with minimal aftereffects (less postoperative nausea and confusion). Innocuous to organs; low organ toxicity because of low blood solubility and minimal susceptibility to biodegradation and metabolism. Provides superb muscular relaxation. Pharyngeal and laryngeal reflexes are easily obtunded. Depresses bronchoconstriction; may be used in asthmatic patients and patients with chronic obstructive pulmonary disease.

Disadvantages: Expensive. Is a profound respiratory depressant and reduces respiratory minute volume. Respirations must be closely monitored and supported. Assisted or controlled ventilation is used to prevent respiratory acidosis. In the absence of intraoperative stimulation, blood pressure may drop as a result of peripheral vasodilation. Cerebral vascular resistance decreases, cerebral blood flow increases, and intracranial pressure rises but is reversible with hyperventilation. Secretions are weakly stimulated.

Use: Induction and maintenance for a wide spectrum of procedures except routine obstetrics. Isoflurane produces uterine relaxation. Safety to mother and fetus has not been established. The drug is metabolized in the liver, so it may be given to patients with minimal renal disease.

Desflurane (Suprane) A nonflammable, halogenated liquid with low solubility, desflurane has faster uptake by inhalation and elimination than halothane and isoflurane.

Advantages: Rapid emergence and recovery from anesthesia. Resists biotransformation (metabolism) and degradation; produces few urinary metabolites. Dosage of nondepolarizing muscle relaxants to maintain neuromuscular blockade may be reduced.

Disadvantages: Pungent odor may be irritating during induction. Increasing alveolar concentration may lower blood pressure, which may be corrected by reducing inspired concentration. Hemodynamic effects, including an elevated heart rate, preclude use alone in patient with cardiovascular disease; it may be combined with IV opioids or benzodiazepines.

Use: Induction and maintenance of anesthesia in adults. May be used for maintenance in infants and children, but it is not used for induction because of potential for coughing and laryngospasm. Because it has a high vapor pressure, desflurane is delivered only through a vaporizer specifically designed for this agent. Desflurane vaporizers require electric power to heat the liquid.

Methoxyflurane (Penthrane) A partially halogenated methyl ether, methoxyflurane is the most potent inhalation agent but is rarely used. Its high solubility makes induction slow and prolongs recovery. Its disadvantages outweigh its advantages.

Advantages: Excellent muscle relaxation and good analgesia.

Disadvantages: Depressant to cardiovascular and respiratory systems. Renal and hepatic toxicity are potential complications. Nausea and vomiting, headache, hypotension, and delirium may accompany recovery.

Use: Limited to low concentration for short duration or for analgesia in combination with nitrous oxide.

Nitrous Oxide (N_2O) An inorganic gas of slight potency, nitrous oxide supports combustion when combined with oxygen. It is the only gas still in use for anesthesia.

Advantages: Rapid uptake and elimination; few aftereffects except headache, vertigo, and drowsiness. Causes minimal physiologic change; adverse effects can be quickly reversed. Excellent analgesic for procedures not producing severe pain.

Disadvantages: No muscle relaxation. Possible excitement or laryngospasm; hypoxia a hazard; depressant effect on myocardial contractility.

Use: Because it lacks potency, nitrous oxide is rarely used alone but rather as an adjunct to barbiturates, narcotics, and other IV drugs. In combination, concentration of potent drug is reduced, thereby lessening circulatory and respiratory depressions. Because exposure can be an occupational hazard for personnel, measures are taken to minimize levels of nitrous oxide in room air (see p. 327).

Intravenous Anesthetic Agents

IV anesthesia became popular with the introduction in the 1930s of rapidly acting barbiturates. A drug that produces hypnosis, sedation, amnesia, and/or analgesia is injected directly into the circulation, usually via a peripheral vein in arm. Diluted by blood in the heart and the lungs, the drug passes in high concentration to brain, heart, liver, and kidneys, the organs of highest blood flow. Concentration in brain is rapid. With recirculation, redistribution occurs in body, decreasing cerebral concentration. Dissipation of effects depends on redistribution and biotransformation. Because removal of drug from circulation is impossible, safety in use is related to metabolism. It is advisable for the anesthesiologist to give a small test dose at induction.

Oxygen is always given during IV anesthesia. A barbiturate, dissociative agent, or narcotic may be given (see Table 17-2). Each has advantages, disadvantages, and contraindications. They may be supplemented with other drugs.

Barbiturates Thiobarbituric acid derivatives are commonly used, but they do not produce relief from pain, only marked sedation, amnesia, and hypnosis. Repeated administration has cumulative, prolonged effect. *Thiopental sodium* (Pentothal Sodium), *methohexital sodium* (Brevital), and *sodium thiamylal* (Surital) must be supplemented with other drugs to produce analgesia and relaxation during the surgical procedure. They are excellent, rapid induction agents, however.

Advantages: Nonirritating to mucous membranes of trachea or bronchi; does not stimulate salivation. Recovery is rapid, but with possible excitement; nausea and vomiting are rare.

Disadvantages: Administration of large doses can cause rapid, pronounced respiratory and circulatory depressions; small, divided doses are well tolerated with rapid uptake. Respiratory depression may be marked immediately following injection; can produce hypotension. Range of CNS depression is from mild sedation to coma or cardiac arrest.

Use: Most commonly used for induction before administration of more potent agents, such as inhalants; may be basal anesthetic for short procedures not requiring relaxation. Used for control of convulsions in patients with increased intracranial pressure; adjunct to spinal, nitrous oxide, and antimuscarinic drugs; for hypnosis during regional anesthesia.

Contraindications: Caution is necessary for patients with bronchial asthma, acute or chronic respiratory infections, or porphyria. IV barbiturates are not appropriate for patients with small superficial veins. Because solutions are highly alkaline, they are always administered via tubing of an IV infusion. Extravasation can cause thrombophlebitis, nerve injury, or tissue necrosis. Intraarterial injection is avoided.

NOTE

1. Inadvertent intraarterial injection is evidenced by sudden excruciating pain that requires immediate treatment to prevent a chemical endarteritis with tissue destruction. Arterial spasm and ischemia must be counteracted to prevent gangrene of fingers. Treatment: intraarterial injection of lidocaine (10 ml of 0.5% solution), which dilutes the barbiturate solution; local heparinization via the arterial needle to prevent arterial thrombosis; stellate ganglion block or general anesthesia with halothane to promote vasodilation.
2. For extravasation, 5 to 10 ml of 0.5% lidocaine injected into involved area dilutes barbiturate to prevent vasoconstriction.

Propofol (Diprivan) A short-acting alkylphenol, propofol is a sedative-hypnotic that produces anesthesia. It is used for rapid induction and maintenance of anesthesia for short procedures. It can also be used in combination with inhalation agents or opioids for prolonged anesthesia. Propofol is supplied in a sterile milky soybean oil–in-water emulsion. In low doses it produces sedation (i.e., drowsiness and decreased responsiveness). Continued IV administration leads to hypnosis and unconsciousness. Propofol is twice as potent as thiopental sodium.

Advantages: Rapidly distributed, metabolized, and eliminated. Emergence is very rapid with few postoperative side effects.

Disadvantages: Produces dose-related cardiorespiratory depression. Cardiovascular depressant action will decrease blood pressure. Hypotensive effect is potentiated by narcotics. Solution supports rapid growth of microorganisms if infusion pump or syringes become contaminated. Moderate to severe pain may be felt at injection site in small vein of hand or forearm; larger antecubital vein should be used or site injected with lidocaine.

Use: General anesthesia for ambulatory surgery patients; maintenance of sedation during local and regional anesthesia. Acceptable for patients allergic to barbiturates or who have porphyria.

Contraindications: Used with caution in elderly, debilitated, and hypovolemic patients. Not recommended for pediatrics, obstetrics, and some neurosurgical procedures.

Ketamine Hydrochloride (Ketalar, Ketaject) General anesthesia may be produced by a phencyclidine derivative to produce a state referred to as *dissociative anesthesia.* The drug acts by selectively interrupting associative pathways of the brain before producing sensory blockage. This permits a surgical procedure on a patient who appears to be awake (i.e., eyes are open and may move) but who is anesthetized (i.e., unaware and amnesic). Ketamine hydrochloride may be given IV or intramuscularly to yield profound analgesia. It is swiftly metabolized. Individual response varies, depending on dose, route of administration, and age. Because of a dose-response relationship, careful patient selection and dose are important. It is used alone or with nitrous oxide.

Advantages: Rapid induction. Respirations not depressed unless administered too rapidly or in too large a dose. Mild stimulant action on cardiovascular system may elevate blood pressure. Potentiated by narcotics and barbiturates.

Disadvantages: Psychologic manifestations (e.g., delirium, vivid imagery, hallucinations, and unpleasant dreams) may occur during emergence. These can be reduced by giving preanesthetic diazepam and by allowing patient to lie quietly, undisturbed during recovery except for essential procedures. Reactions more common in adults than children. IV thiopental sodium or diazepam may be given to treat emergence delirium.

Use: Mainly for children between the ages of 2 and 10 years and young adults under 30, for short procedures not requiring skeletal muscle relaxation; in plastic and eye procedures when combined with local agents; for diagnostic procedures; as induction agent before other general agents are used and to supplement nitrous oxide when adequate respiratory exchange is maintained. For longer procedures repeated doses are given that may prolong recovery time. If relaxation is needed, muscle relaxants and controlled ventilation are indicated.

Low-dose ketamine (1 mg/kg) has been recommended as an induction agent for obstetric procedures because of rapid onset, intense analgesia and amnesia, and minimal fetal effects. With its cardiovascular stimulating properties, it is useful in hypovolemic and hypotensive patients, allowing the use of high oxygen concentration, both in obstetric and trauma procedures.

Contraindications: Procedures involving tracheobronchial stimulation because pharyngeal and laryngeal reflexes are usually active. If the drug is used alone, mechanical stimulation of the pharynx should be avoided. Other contraindications include hypertension, increased intracranial pressure, intraocular procedures, and previous cerebrovascular accident because this agent increases cerebrospinal fluid and intraocular pressure.

High-Dose Narcotics Historically, natural opiates and synthetic opioids have been given to produce analgesia and sedation preoperatively and postoperatively. In addition, they are used intraoperatively as supplemental agents and/or in combination with oxygen for complete anesthesia for short procedures and in patients with little cardiovascular reserve. Cardiovascular depression must be avoided in these patients. Halogenated agents are contraindicated in patients with liver and renal disease.

The most popular narcotics for general anesthesia are the opioids *fentanyl* (Sublimaze), *sufentanil citrate* (Sufenta), *alfentanil* (Alfenta), and *meperidine hydrochloride* (Demerol), and the opiate *morphine sulfate.* (See the following discussion of these drugs.) Although they are analgesics, *to reliably achieve anesthesia, markedly larger doses of narcotics are needed,* for example, 10 to 30 times as much morphine (3 to 8 or more mg/kg body weight). High doses of fentanyl range from 50 to 100 μg/kg body weight. The drugs may be given in bolus doses or continuously via IV infusion. Surprisingly, side effects seem to occur less frequently as the potency of narcotics increases. They reduce adverse physiologic responses to the stress of the surgical procedure, such as increased work of the heart, potential dysrhythmia, sodium and water retention, and increased blood glucose. The high-dose narcotic technique for complete anesthesia reduces volatile gas pollution in the OR and PACU where patients exhale residue gases.

Narcotics produce a dose-related respiratory depression. The respiratory effects of narcotics are as follows:

1. Reduction of responsiveness of the CNS respiratory centers to carbon dioxide (less stimulation)
2. Impairment of respiratory reflexes and alteration of rhythmicity (prolonged inspiration, delayed expiration)
3. Reduction in respiratory rate before reduction in tidal volume
4. Production of bronchoconstriction (morphine, meperidine) or rigidity of chest wall (fentanyl)
5. Impairment of ciliary motion

Factors that influence narcotic respiratory actions include age, pain, sleep, urinary output, other drugs, intestinal reabsorption, and disease.

The neurophysical state obtained by use of large doses of narcotics is not the same as "the general anesthesia state" resulting from use of volatile inhalation agents such as halothane. Narcotics are more selective in action. Narcotics do *not* produce muscle relaxation. Conversely, they cause an increase in muscle tone. Neuromuscular blocking agents can block or treat this action or rigidity (see pp. 335-336).

Following high-dose narcotic anesthesia, patients are awake, pain free, with adequate though not good ventilation. *These patients need careful monitoring by a well-trained PACU staff because narcotization after large doses of narcotics can occur rapidly in an apparently awake and responsive patient.* Patient can hypoventilate, become hypoxic, and stop breathing when intraoperative stimuli cease. Vital signs, pupils, and skin color must be monitored. *Clinical signs of narcotic toxicity* are pinpoint pupils, depressed respiration, and reduced consciousness. A narcotic antagonist (see below) is given to reverse narcotic-induced hypoventilation. Potential for delayed toxicity following IM injection of narcotics, as opposed to IV administration, exists because absorption from muscle mass may be irregular.

Adjunctive Drugs

Many drugs are used to supplement nitrous oxide, halogenated inhalation agents, and IV drugs to maintain amnesia and analgesia, control hypertension, attenuate extent of postoperative respiratory depression, or other effects of general anesthesia. These drugs must be carefully controlled to avoid adverse drug interactions. For example, morphine sulfate and nitrous oxide have a synergistic action with thiopental sodium (i.e., when they are given together, each potentiates action of the other). Therefore they are given concomitantly with caution because of their combined respiratory depressant effect.

Some drugs are given preoperatively, during induction, and/or intraoperatively. Adjunctive drugs are used primarily for analgesia and amnesia or to counteract side effects of anesthesia. Some are particularly useful for ambulatory surgery patients because they are short acting.

Morphine Sulfate An opiate narcotic, morphine produces analgesia for pain relief without loss of motor, sensory, or sympathetic functions. Amnesia is incomplete (i.e., sporadic episodes of awareness may occur). Cardiovascular stability is good, but a significant dose-related vasodilatory effect can increase intraoperative blood loss. Respiratory depression is the most serious side effect; pulmonary blood volume is decreased, and pulmonary artery blood pressure is increased. Morphine may be given by IM, IV, epidural, or intrathecal injection. Duration of action varies with route of administration.

Fentanyl (Sublimaze) An opioid narcotic, fentanyl produces analgesia. It is 70 times more potent than morphine. It has minimal cardiac effects and is not associated with venodilation. Although of short duration of action, it becomes concentrated in well-perfused tissue, such as in the brain. It metabolizes slowly with possible consequent respiratory depression and chest wall rigidity. It may be given in bolus, incremental, or continuous IV infusion.

Sufentanil Citrate (Sufenta) An opioid narcotic, sufentanil produces analgesia/anesthesia and effectively reduces anxiety. It is five times more potent than fentanyl and 625 times more potent than morphine. Sufentanil does not depress the myocardium or change vascular resistance. It is short acting because onset of action is immediate, accumulation is limited, and elimination is rapid. It can cause respiratory depression and skeletal muscle rigidity. It is given IV or epidurally.

Alfentanil (Alfenta) An opioid narcotic, alfentanil is a rapid and short-acting analgesic. Respiratory depression outlasts analgesia. It is given IV by bolus or continuous infusion.

Meperidine Hydrochloride (Demerol) An opioid narcotic, meperidine produces analgesia. It causes myocardial depression and tachycardia as a result of peripheral vasodilation. It causes bronchoconstriction but has fewer undesirable side effects than morphine. Meperidine is 1000 times less potent than fentanyl and sufentanil. Commonly used for premedication and postoperative pain relief, meperidine is available in a liquid preparation that may be useful when an oral medication is preferred, as in children. It is usually given IM or IV.

Hydromorphone Hydrochloride (Dilaudid) An opioid narcotic analgesic, hydromorphone has a rapid onset and shorter duration than morphine but is 8 to 10 times more potent. It has less hypnotic quality and causes less nausea and vomiting. Hydromorphone suppresses coughing and may cause respiratory depression. It is not used in children.

Narcotic Agonists-Antagonists An *agonist* combines with receptors, such as the opiate receptors, to initiate drug actions. An antagonist neutralizes or impedes action of another drug (i.e., reverses its effects). For example, narcotics produce a dose-related respiratory depression that can be reversed by opiate antagonists. These drugs, given IV, IM, or subcutaneously, include:

1. *Naloxone hydrochloride (Narcan).* A specific narcotic antagonist, naloxone reverses respiratory depression of narcotics. It has no respiratory or circulatory action of its own in the presence or absence of a narcotic or other agonist-antagonist.
2. *Nalbuphine hydrochloride (Nubain).* A narcotic agonist-antagonist, nalbuphine is a potent analgesic. It has limited respiratory and cardiovascular effects.
3. *Butorphenol tartrate (Stadol).* A narcotic agonist-antagonist, butorphenol is an analgesic. It produces dose-related respiratory depression and some hemodynamic changes in the cardiovascular system.
4. *Pentazocine hydrochloride (Talwin).* A weak narcotic antagonist, pentazocine is a potent analgesic and mild sedative. It does not completely reverse cardiovascular and respiratory depression induced by narcotics.
5. *Buprenorphine hydrochloride (Buphrenex).* A narcotic antagonist, buprenorphine is an analgesic with a high affinity for opiate receptors. It has slight respiratory and circulatory depressant action.

Droperidol (Inapsine) A tranquilizer, droperidol produces sedation. It may be used to prevent nausea and vomiting. It is a CNS depressant. It may be given IM or IV.

Diazepam (Valium) A tranquilizer, diazepam produces amnesia, sedation, and muscle relaxation. It can lower body temperature when given preoperatively. When used for induction, it causes less hypotension and bradycardia than thiopental sodium but is slower acting. Its sedative effect facilitates awake intubation. It may extend CNS depression and somnolence during emergence, especially in elderly patients. Diazepam may be given PO, IM, or IV.

Midazolam (Versed) A sedative, midazolam is given IV or deep IM for its short-acting amnesic effect. It is a CNS and respiratory depressant. This depression can be significantly prolonged in the elderly, the obese, and patients with liver dysfunction. For pediatric surgery it may be given orally or rectally preoperatively for a smooth induction of general anesthesia and a less eventful emergence postoperatively.

Flumazenil (Mazicon) A benzodiazepine antagonist, flumazenil may be used for complete or partial reversal of sedative effects of diazepam or midazolam after anesthesia. An initial dose is given IV, followed by additional doses IV every 30 to 60 seconds until consciousness is restored. The effect peaks 6 to 10 minutes after injection.

Muscle Relaxants

Skeletal muscle relaxant drugs, referred to as *neuromuscular blockers,* facilitate muscle relaxation for smoother endotracheal intubation and working conditions during the surgical procedure. Their use has eliminated the need for deep inhalation anesthesia to produce relaxation. Administered IV in small amounts at intervals, they interfere with passage of impulses from motor nerves to skeletal muscles. They act primarily at autonomic receptor sites, the neuromuscular junction, and at prejunctional and postjunctional acetylcholine-binding sites, causing paralysis of variable duration. They also can affect transmission of impulses at preganglionic and postganglionic endings in the autonomic nervous system. Neuromuscular blockers paralyze all skeletal muscles, including the diaphragm and accessory muscles of respiration. Therefore the chief danger in their use is that they decrease pulmonary ventilation, causing respiratory depression. They also may cause circulatory disturbance. Special attention to anesthesia depth, ventilation, and electrolyte balance is required.

Neuromuscular blockers are classified as nondepolarizing and depolarizing. Although theoretically antagonistic, combinations are used. They may widen the scope of less potent anesthetics, such as nitrous oxide, or lessen the overall amount of anesthetic needed. Depolarizing and nondepolarizing drugs behave differently; depolarizers stimulate whereas nondepolarizers inhibit autonomic receptors. Duration of action should be balanced against duration of effect on ventilation.

Nondepolarizing Neuromuscular Blockers These drugs act on enzymes to prevent muscle contraction. They produce tetanic electrical impulses that gradually fade, but they do not cause muscular fasciculation on IV injection. Their effects are decreased by anticholinesterase drugs, acetylcholine, epinephrine, and depolarizing neuromuscular blockers. Action is potentiated by halogenated inhalation agents and some antibiotics. Interactions with other drugs can result in delayed recovery. For example, antibiotics may act synergistically to produce prolonged paralysis, as when peritoneal cavity is irrigated with an antibiotic solution or antibiotic is injected IV. Synergism also occurs with local and inhalation anesthetic agents. They are useful for patients on mechanical ventilators. Nondepolarizing blockers may be referred to as competitive antagonists. A peripheral nerve stimulator is useful for assessing neuromuscular transmission as a guide to dosage, degree and nature of blockade, and evidence of muscle-response recovery during and after use of nondepolarizing agents. The anesthesiologist can choose from several drugs.

1. *Tubocurarine chloride (Curare).* Obtained from plants, tubocurarine was used centuries ago by South American Indians for poison arrows. The poison caused death by suffocation from respiratory paralysis. The effects of tubocurarine on the neuromuscular junction were first described in 1856. This drug was introduced into clinical practice in 1942. Blocking transmission of nerve impulses to muscle fibers results in paralysis, predominantly of voluntary muscles. D-tubocurarine releases histamine. Autonomic blockade can cause hypotension. This neuromuscular blocker is long acting.
2. *Metocurine iodide (Metubine).* A long-acting muscle relaxant, metocurine produces less hypotension and releases less histamine than D-tubocurarine.
3. *Gallamine triethiodide (Flaxedil).* Similar in action and duration to D-tubocurarine, gallamine does not cause hypotension and bronchospasm. It may increase arterial pressure and cause tachycardia.
4. *Pancuronium bromide (Pavulon).* A long-acting synthetic muscle relaxant, pancuronium is similar in action to D-tubocurarine but about five times more potent. It has a vagolytic action that may raise pulse and heart rates.
5. *Vecuronium bromide (Norcuron).* Similar to pancuronium, vecuronium has shorter duration of action and is more potent. It does not noticeably increase heart rate or blood pressure.
6. *Atracurium besylate (Tracrium).* With intermediate action of about 30 minutes, atracurium metabolizes more quickly than the other blockers, which may be an advantage in patients with liver or renal disease. Repeated doses are not cumulative.
7. *Mivacurium chloride (Mivacron).* With this short-acting muscle relaxant, neuromuscular blockade lasts 15 to 20 minutes. It has minimal cardiovascular effect.
8. *Rocuronium bromide (Zemuron).* With rapid onset of action, rocuronium facilitates intubation. Duration of action is intermediate, about 30 minutes, with minimal overall effect on cardiovascular stability.

Depolarizing Neuromuscular Blockers These drugs have the opposite effect of the nondepolarizing drugs. They stimulate autonomic receptors. For example, they cause muscular fasciculation (i.e., involuntary muscle contractions). These contractions, the result of depolarization of nerve-muscle end plate, are seen following injection. They are followed by fatigue. Drugs may be given IM, but IV use is more common.

1. *Succinylcholine chloride (Anectine, Quelicin, Gucostrin).* An ultra-short-acting synthetic drug with onset of action in seconds, succinylcholine produces paralysis for up to 20 minutes. It is used primarily for endotracheal intubation. A dilute solution may be used to provide continuing muscle relaxation. Repeated IV administration may effect changes in heart rate and rhythm (i.e., bradycardia and ventricular dysrhythmia) until the drug is metabolized by enzymes. Muscle pain may occur after use unless fasciculation is prevented by a small preliminary dose of a nondepolarizing agent. Succinylcholine is contraindicated in patients with a known or suspected history of malignant hyperthermia episode.
2. *Decamethonium (Syncurine).* A very potent synthetic with rapid onset and short duration of action, decamethonium is not cumulative and has little effect on vital systems. It is used for deep relaxation of a short duration such as needed for endoscopy, treatment of laryngeal spasm, abdominal closure, and endotracheal intubation. It is excreted through the kidneys. Prolonged blockade may result if given to a patient in renal failure.

The anesthesiologist must constantly verify the degree of paralysis present by noting the amount of relaxation of the abdominal wall or the limpness of extremities or by using a nerve stimulator connected to the patient through needle electrodes. The use of neuromuscular blockers requires surgeon-anesthesiologist teamwork and communication. Use of these drugs always presents the hazard of overdosage, a danger alleviated by the anesthesiologist's familiarity with the surgeon's technique and requirements of the particular surgical procedure; thus the anesthesiologist can regulate dosage of anesthetic and relaxant necessary to produce the conditions required at the appropriate time. For example, a major use of neuromuscular blockers is in intraabdominal procedures. At different times during the surgical procedure, blockade may be more or less essential. Although tightness of tissues and inadequate exposure may be the result of factors other than relaxation, it is helpful to the anesthesiologist to be told before pertinent action, such as closure of the peritoneum, is taken. Inadequate muscle relaxation makes closure difficult. Controlled respiration during upper abdominal manipulation can prevent descent of the diaphragm into the surgical field.

Emergence From General Anesthesia

The anesthesiologist aims to have the patient as nearly awake as possible at the end of a surgical procedure. Pharyngeal and laryngeal reflexes must be recovered to prevent aspiration and respiratory obstruction. The degree of residual neuromuscular blockade must be determined and treated if necessary for respiratory adequacy. The action of nondepolarizing muscle relaxants may be reversed with antagonists, such as long-acting neostigmine methylsulfate (Prostigmin) or pyridostigmine bromide (Regonol), or short-acting edrophonium (Tensilon, Enlon). These *anticholinesterase drugs* must be accompanied or preceded by atropine sulfate to minimize side effects, such as excessive secretions and bradycardia.

To overcome soft tissue obstruction and to enable the patient to cough and breathe deeply, respiratory muscles must be active. A patent airway and adequate manual or mechanical ventilation are maintained until full recovery. The endotracheal tube is carefully removed when this maneuver is deemed safe. Undesirable sequelae may be associated with extubation, such as coughing and especially laryngospasm. The tube is not removed in the presence of cyanosis or inadequate respiratory exchange. Extubation is delayed until spontaneous respiration is ensured. In the absence of a means of respiratory control, as when a maxillofacial procedure endangers the airway, the endotracheal tube may be left in place.

Retching, vomiting, and restlessness may accompany emergence. Slight cyanosis, stertorous respiration, rigidity, or shivering are not uncommon as a result of a temporary disturbance of body temperature-regulating mechanisms, thus altering circulation to skin and muscles. Administering oxygen and pain medication and applying warm blankets help relieve these aftereffects. The anesthesiologist should flush the patient's lungs with oxygen to minimize exhalation of gases in the PACU.

BALANCED ANESTHESIA

Balanced anesthesia has become a widely used technique to achieve physiologic homeostasis, analgesia, amnesia, and muscle relaxation. The concept dates back to 1910, when it was noted that psychic stimuli associated with surgical procedures could be controlled by pharmacologic agents. In 1926 the concept was further developed by balancing agents and techniques to provide anesthesia. Today a combination of agents is used with many possible variations, depending on the condition of the patient and requirements of the procedure. The technique is especially useful for preventing CNS depression in older and poor-risk patients.

Induction

Induction can be accomplished with a thiobarbiturate derivative (Pentothal Sodium, Brevital), diazepam (Valium), midazolam (Versed), or other induction agent (see pp. 324-325). Oxygen is administered in physiologic quantities. Neuromuscular blockers permit control of ventilation while providing muscle relaxation during intubation.

Maintenance

Different combinations of narcotics and neuroleptic drugs (tranquilizers) are administered IV whether used alone or in combination with inhalation agents. Neuroleptics reduce motor activity and anxiety, produce a detached apathetic state, and potentiate hypnotic and analgesic effects of narcotic. Dosage can be regulated to produce desired state.

Neuroleptanalgesia

The term *neuroleptanalgesia* describes an intense analgesic and amnesic state resulting from combination of a narcotic (potent analgesic) and a neuroleptic (psychotropic tranquilizer). The analgesia, amnesia, and sedation produced are not true anesthesia. Unconsciousness may or may not occur. The dosage can be controlled so the patient can cooperate and respond to commands, if desirable, as for some diagnostic procedures. A single drug or combination of drugs may be used.

Innovar Injection Innovar injection is a combination of fentanyl and droperidol. Fentanyl, a potent, short-acting opioid narcotic, may cause respiratory depression, hypotension, and bradycardia. Therefore some anesthesiologists prefer to individualize doses separately to allow more controlled injection of fentanyl (Sublimaze). An advantage of the combination is an apparent absence of toxic effects on kidneys and liver and only slight cardiac depression. Droperidol, a potent long-acting tranquilizer, also exerts an antiemetic effect. Consciousness returns within minutes after injection, but psychotropic effects persist for 4 to 6 hours, causing drowsiness and indifference to discomfort. Respirations must be closely watched, and the patient encouraged to breathe.

Neuroleptanesthesia

When the narcotic-neuroleptic drug combination is reinforced by an anesthetic, the resulting state is referred to as *neuroleptanesthesia.* Supplementation is necessary for extensive surgical procedures. Nitrous oxide or a halogenated inhalation agent and IV narcotics provide analgesia. Neuromuscular blockers permit optimum conditions for the surgeon. An opioid agonist-antagonist may be a useful supplement. For example, nalbuphine hydrochloride (Nubain) has limited potency and toxicity. It has cardiovascular stability and limited respiratory effects.

Emergence

Residual effects of narcotics or muscle relaxants may require reversal by antagonists during and/or at the conclusion of the surgical procedure. Other precautions are taken as for any patient emerging from general anesthesia.

CONTROLLED HOMEOSTASIS

Through naturally controlled adaptive responses, the body seeks to maintain *homeostasis,* a relative steady state in its internal environment. Some functions controlled by homeostatic mechanisms include body temperature, heartbeat, blood pressure, electrolyte balance, and respiration. These parameters may be altered by anesthetic and other pharmacologic agents and by physiologic stresses during surgical manipulations. In the hands of a skilled anesthesiologist, adjunctive methods of control may be used concurrently with the administration of general anesthesia, but only when the expected outcomes will outweigh the inherent risks.

Induced Hypothermia

Hypothermia is an artificial, deliberate lowering of body temperature below the normal limits (Box 17-2). It reduces metabolic rate and oxygen needs of the tissues in conditions causing hypoxia or during a decrease or interruption of circulation. Bleeding is also decreased and less anesthetic is needed. The patient can therefore better tolerate the surgical procedure. Hypothermia may be used:

1. For direct-vision intracardiac repair of complex congenital defects in infants and in other cardiac procedures. This is the most common usage.
2. After cardiac resuscitation, to decrease oxygen requirement of vital tissues and limit further damage to brain following anoxia.
3. In treatment of hyperpyrexia and some other nonsurgical conditions, such as hypertensive crisis.
4. To increase tolerance in septic shock.
5. In neurosurgery, to decrease cerebral blood flow, brain volume, and venous and intracranial pressures.
6. To aid in transplantation of organs.

BOX 17-2

Hypothermia

Normal core temperature: 98.2° to 99.9° F or 36.8° to 37.7° C

Systemic hypothermia may be:

Light: 98.6° to 89.6° F or 37° to 32° C

Moderate: 89.6° to 78.8° F or 32° to 26° C

Deep: 78.8° to 68° F or 26° to 20° C

Profound: 68° F or below or 20° C or below

Sensorium fades at 91° to 93° F or 33° to 34° C

Attaining Hypothermia

To achieve hypothermia, heat must be lost more rapidly than it is produced. The following methods may be used.

1. *Surface-induced hypothermia.* External cooling of infants and small children weighing less than 20 lb (10 kg) may be attained by immersion in iced water, packing body in ice, or alcohol sponging. A hypothermia/hyperthermia machine with a thermal blanket or mattress is used for adults and larger children.
2. *Internal cooling.* Decrease or interruption of blood flow can be achieved by placing sterile iced saline slush packs around a specific internal organ, or by irrigation of cold fluids within a body cavity, such as intraperitoneal lavage. Cold cardioplegia technique combines cold from saline slush with drugs injected into coronary arteries for myocardial protection during heart surgery. Drugs may also be used to lower metabolism and to increase resistance to shivering during cooling.
3. *Systemic hypothermia.* The bloodstream is cooled by diverting blood through heat-exchanging devices of extracorporeal circulation (see Chapter 39, pp. 804-805) and returning it to the body by a continuous flowing circuit (e.g., core-cooling by cardiopulmonary bypass or IV administration of cold fluids). Systemic hypothermia is used in adults and larger children to 78.8° F (26° C). Oxygen consumption and metabolism of different organs vary, so uniform hypothermia is impossible. The temperature is not deliberately taken below about 84.5° F (29° C) unless arrest of the heart is desired by means of deep hypothermia (below 26° C). This is accompanied by perfusion of the rest of the body with the extracorporeal circulation method, permitting an open, motionless dry field while the blood flow is interrupted. A noncontracting heart requires very little oxygen.

The patient is progressively rewarmed at the close of the surgical procedure until temperature is 95° F (35° C) or until consciousness returns. Sometimes a degree of hypothermia is maintained for a day or two postoperatively to allow the patient to adapt more readily. Oxygen therapy and intubation, if advised, are part of postoperative care.

Complications in Use

Hypothermia carries many inherent risks. Primarily it affects the myocardium, decreasing its resistance to ventricular fibrillation and predisposing the patient to cardiac arrest. This is more likely to happen with deep hypothermia or during manipulation of the heart itself. Other dangers are heart block, effects on the vascular system, atrial fibrillation, embolism, microcirculation stasis, undesired downward drift of temperature ("overshooting"), tissue damage, metabolic acidosis, and numerous effects on other organs and systems.

Time is required for cooling and rewarming. Shivering and vasoconstriction, normal defenses of the body against cooling, can be problems during use of hypothermia. This muscle activity greatly increases oxygen needs. Shivering can be overcome by the administration of a muscle relaxant drug or IV injection of chlorpromazine or an analgesic such as meperidine.

Rewarming can be accomplished by circulating warmed blood by means of extracorporeal circulation or by using a mattress with circulating fluid and warm blankets. If external heat is applied, take care not to burn the patient. Rewarming carries potential problems such as reactive bleeding or circulatory collapse. If patient is rewarmed too rapidly, vasodilation causes a drop in blood pressure. Organ ischemia can occur from severe shivering. These superficial and systemic events impair perfusion (oxygenation) of tissues. "Rewarming shock" may be prevented by slow warming, adequate oxygenation, prevention of massive sudden vasodilation or vasoconstriction associated with shivering.

Induced Hypotension

Induced deliberate hypotension is the controlled lowering of arterial blood pressure during anesthesia as an adjunct to the surgical procedure. Hypotensive anesthesia is used to shorten operating time, reduce blood loss and need for transfusion, and facilitate dissection and visibility, especially of tumor margins in radical procedures. Visible vessels are ligated, even in the absence of active bleeding.

Adequate oxygenation of blood and tissue perfusion in vital organs (heart, liver, kidneys, lungs) and in cerebrum must be maintained to prevent damage. Degree and duration of hypotension must be carefully controlled so that the state can be rapidly terminated at any time.

Naturally, controlled hypotension is not indicated as a routine procedure. It is used only when the expected gain for a particular patient requiring a specific surgical procedure outweighs the risks. Hypotension may be specifically induced for:

1. Surgical procedure in which excessive blood loss is anticipated to decrease gross hemorrhage or vascular oozing.
2. Surgical procedure on head, face, neck, upper thorax, especially radical dissection, in which the position of the patient allows blood to pool in dependent areas and reduces venous return to the heart and cardiac output.
3. In neurosurgery when control of intracranial vessel hemorrhage may be difficult. It reduces leakage, makes an aneurysm less turgid and prone to rupture, decreases blood loss in case of rupture, and facilitates placement of ligating clips.
4. Surgical procedure in which blood transfusions should be avoided, as when compatible blood is unavailable or transfusion is against patient's religious belief.
5. Surgical procedure on spine or posterior torso. Blood loss is decreased during prone position.
6. Total hip replacement.

Precautions in Use

Potential complications of hypotensive anesthesia include cerebral or coronary ischemia or thrombosis, reactionary hemorrhage, anuria in acute renal failure, delayed awakening, or dermal ischemic lesions. *Primary contraindications* are vascular compromise to any vital organ system or the brain. Precautions include:

1. Careful selection of patient
2. Preoperative cardiac, renal, and hepatic evaluation of patient to avoid circulatory insufficiency in vital organs
3. Choice of appropriate but not arbitrary level of blood pressure
4. Administration and evaluation by expert anesthesiologists
5. Utilization for only a short time and lowering of blood pressure only enough to obtain desired result
6. Maintenance of blood volume at optimal level by continuous infusion
7. Controlled ventilation with adequate oxygenation via endotracheal tube because hypotension increases susceptibility to hypoxia
8. Extensive monitoring: ECG; core temperature; esophageal stethoscopy; urinary output, central venous pressure and arterial catheters; electrophysiologic brain monitoring

Attaining Hypotension

Several techniques will produce hypotension. Blood pressure may be lowered chemically by direct arterial or venous dilators or by ganglionic blocking drugs. Perfusion pressure drops in proportion to a decrease in vascular flow resistance, but adequate tissue blood flow exists. Fine adjustment of the desired level of hypotension can be achieved by mechanical maneuvers—namely, alterations in body position or changes in airway pressure, control of heart rate or blood volume, or addition of other vasoactive drugs in conjunction with hypotensive drugs. Properly used, these maneuvers can reduce the total dose of potentially toxic drugs needed for maintenance of hypotension.

Methods to produce hypotension include:

1. Deep general anesthesia with halothane or isoflurane, followed by a vasodilator, produce the desired minute-to-minute effect. With increased concentration halogenated agents produce hypotension as a result of myocardial and peripheral vascular depression.
2. *Sodium nitroprusside* is a potent, fast-acting vasodilator that reduces virtually all resistance in vascular smooth muscle (resistance vessels). It also reduces preload and afterload of the heart and pulmonary vascular resistance. To achieve safe arterial pressure control, administration is via calibrated drug pump. Acid-base status and blood

cyanide level are determined frequently to guard against metabolic acidosis and sodium nitroprusside–induced cyanide and thiocyanate toxicity.

3. *Nitroglycerin,* primarily a venodilator, directly dilates capacitance vessels. It reduces preload and improves myocardial perfusion during diastole, a protection against potential ischemia. Nitroglycerin for infusion (Nitrostat IV), after dilution in 5% dextrose or physiologic saline, dilates both venous and arterial beds. Arterial pressures are reduced. Nitroglycerin migrates into plastic. To avoid its absorption into plastic parenteral solution containers, dilution and storage are done in glass parenteral solution bottles. A special nonabsorbing infusion set prevents loss of nitroglycerin.
4. *Trimethaphan camsylate* (Arfonad) blocks sympathetic ganglia, which results in relaxation of resistance and capacitance vessels and reduces arterial pressure.
5. *Fentanyl* may be used as a basal anesthetic for hypotension. Blood pressure can be maintained at the desired level by addition of a small amount of a volatile agent. Fentanyl lowers arterial pressure; volatile agents reduce cardiac output.
6. Other drugs such as verapamil, nifedipine, phentolamine, tetrodotoxin, or adenosine triphosphate may be used.

Safe lower limits of arterial pressure may vary. Average is 50 mm Hg *mean,* 65 to 70 mm Hg systolic, with lower value for short periods only.

Normovolemic Hemodilution Anesthesia

Intraoperative normovolemic hemodilution has been used in cardiac surgery for several decades but more recently as an anesthetic technique in other types of major surgery when large blood loss is anticipated. It is especially useful in infants and children and in patients, such as Jehovah's Witnesses, who for religious reasons do not accept administration of blood products.

At the beginning of the surgical procedure, whole blood is withdrawn from the patient to a hematocrit of 14% to 15% and replaced with three times the volume of a balanced electrolyte solution to maintain intravascular volume. This diluted blood is transparent, giving the surgeon a clearer, almost bloodless field. This may decrease operating time. The patient is maintained under controlled hypotension with halothane anesthetic and a supplemental narcotic. Body temperature may be lowered to 89.6° F (32° C) or below for moderate hypothermia to help protect vital organs against hypoxia and hypotension.

After significant blood loss has ceased, the patient's own blood is reinfused (see section on autotransfusion in Chapter 23, pp. 485-487). Diuresis is stimulated to remove electrolyte solution. Normovolemic hemodilution can make a difficult surgical procedure easier and, in some patients, makes an otherwise impossible resection possible.

CARE OF ANESTHETIZED PATIENT

Anesthetic agents and drugs vary in potency. Therefore they differ in the amount of analgesia, amnesia, or muscle relaxation produced. Each patient's ability to detoxify anesthetic agents and to tolerate physiologic stress differs. Impairment of pulmonary function accompanies general anesthesia to some degree. General anesthesia is usually more complicated than local or regional anesthesia (see Chapter 18). Potential complications are discussed in Chapter 19.

General Considerations

The anesthesiologist keeps the surgeon informed of significant physiologic changes detected by monitoring vital functions (see Chapter 19).

1. Deficit in pulmonary and/or cardiac functions is detrimental to the patient's physiologic status. Abnormalities of pulmonary ventilation and diffusion influence the course of anesthesia and diminish tolerance to stress or the insults from the anesthetic and the procedure.
   a. Respiratory patterns vary from breath-holding and apnea to deep breathing or tachypnea.
   b. Drug action affecting respiratory stimulation or depression is related to changes in oxygen tension (PaO_2) or arterial carbon dioxide ($PaCO_2$).
   c. Hypoxia, anemia, and decreased cardiac output may produce inadequate tissue oxygenation. Subnormal cardiac reserve or oxygen-transporting ability, combined with anemia or hypoxia in an arteriosclerotic patient, for example, can be lethal.
2. Circulation is affected both centrally and peripherally. Individual agents are associated with characteristic hemodynamic patterns. Generally the agents are circulatory depressants that reduce arterial pressure, myocardial contractility, and cardiac output.
3. Liver is affected by general agents; for example, the rate of visceral blood flow. Alteration in liver function tests may follow anesthesia. Halogenated hydrocarbons have been associated with hepatotoxicity.
4. Kidney function is affected by disturbances in systemic circulation since kidneys normally receive 20% to 25% of the cardiac output. Reduced renal plasma flow and glomerular filtration rate depress renal functions related to hemodynamics and to water and electrolyte excretion. Oliguria, with re-

duced sodium and potassium excretion, accompanies induction. Postoperative fluid retention may result from a reduction in urine volume from anesthesia and intraoperative trauma and use of narcotics. In the absence of renal disease changes in renal function are usually transitory and reversible. Endocrine effects on renal function during anesthesia are important.
5. Biotransformation of agents varies with metabolites excreted by the kidneys. Urinary secretion of IV agents may be slow and unpredictable. Studies indicate that nitrous oxide may be exhaled as long as 56 hours after anesthesia, and metabolites of halothane have been recovered from patients' urine as long as 20 days after anesthesia.
6. Agents may cause nausea, emesis, or systemic complications.

General anesthesia may be contraindicated for:

1. Elective procedures on patients who are medically at high risk or severely debilitated.
2. Elective procedures during the first 5 months of pregnancy. Some anesthesiologists avoid general anesthesia because of unknown teratogenic effects of inhalation anesthetics.
3. Emergency surgical procedures on patients who have recently ingested food or fluids. Gastric suction and awake intubation are indicated if the surgical procedure cannot be delayed.

Intraoperative Awareness

The patient may be aware of conversations, noises, and even pain although seemingly anesthetized. Is it possible to imagine anything more terrifying than to feel intraoperative maneuvers but to be unable to communicate this discomfort? Intraoperative awareness varies, depending on type of procedure and depth of anesthesia.

The common use of narcotics and muscle relaxants as adjuncts has consequently decreased the amount of anesthetic used to induce and maintain unconsciousness. This is particularly true in balanced anesthesia. As a result, studies have shown evidence of *intraoperative awareness* (i.e., recall), consciously or unconsciously, of events and sounds during a state of anesthesia. Even though the patient may not consciously recall or remember the experience, unconsciously it may affect behavior and attitudes postoperatively. Subconscious memory may cause anger, generalized irritability, anxiety, repetitive nightmares, preoccupation with death, or physiologic complications.

Patient awareness of pain is rare in the hands of skilled anesthesiologists. However, hearing is the last sensation to surrender to anesthesia. Therefore OR team members must be constantly vigilant to the vulnerability of a patient to auditory stimuli, including conversations and room noise. Even potent amnesic drugs will not totally block recall of stimuli, especially disturbing ones.

Safety Factors

Team members, especially the anesthesiologist and the circulator, must be constantly aware of potential trauma to the patient since he or she is unable to produce a normal response to painful or injurious stimuli. Although safety factors are stressed throughout the text, important factors in the care of the anesthetized patient are reiterated for emphasis:

1. Patient's position must be changed *slowly and gently* to allow circulation to readjust (i.e., to compensate for physiologic changes caused by motion or position).
2. Proper positioning and padding are important to avoid pressure points, stretching of nerves, or interference with circulation to an extremity (see Chapter 21).
3. Patient's chest must be free for adequate respiratory excursions during the surgical procedure. The airway must be patent. Pressure must not be exerted on the chest. Leaning on the patient during the procedure can be devastating. Remember that the patient under the drapes is unable to complain!
4. Lungs must be adequately ventilated intraoperatively and postoperatively either by voluntary or mechanical means. Anesthetic agents are basically depressants that affect the vasomotor and respiratory centers, predisposing the patient to postoperative respiratory complications.
5. Anesthesiologist assists in transferring the patient to a stretcher or bed, safeguarding the head and neck, when it is safe to move the patient. Transfer must be made carefully and gently to avoid strain on ligaments or muscles. The relaxed, unconscious patient must be adequately supported.
6. Anesthesiologist gives the PACU nurse a verbal report, including specific problems in regard to *this* patient and completes records before the transfer of responsibility.

CARE OF ANESTHESIA EQUIPMENT

Like everyone in contact with a patient, the anesthesiologist is a potential vector in the spread of infection. He or she also may become the victim of an acquired infection from contact with a patient's body fluids or blood. Studies have found that nearly 20% of anesthesiologists and anesthetists have had hepatitis B infections.

Universal Precautions

The need for anesthesia staff to strictly adhere to universal precautions while caring for patients and equipment must be emphasized. Gloves should be worn to prevent skin contact with patient's blood and body fluids, as when starting IV infusion and when intubating and extubating the patient. Protective eyewear or a face shield should be worn for intubation and extubation to prevent splash in the eye. Hands must be washed and mask should be changed between patient contacts. Needles must be handled carefully to avoid accidental needlestick. All anesthesia equipment that has come in contact with mucous membranes, blood, or body fluids must be cleaned, disinfected, or sterilized after use to render it safe for handling and for subsequent patient use. Disposable items must be discarded in the appropriate receptacles.

Hazards of Equipment

Anesthesia techniques encompass use of drugs for parenteral administration and gases and volatile liquids for inhalation administration by means of anesthesia machines. These machines and their component parts (reservoir bags, canisters, connecting pieces, ventilators) accumulate large numbers of microorganisms during use. Consequently, the parts that come in contact with the patient's skin or respiratory tract are sources of cross contamination. Inhalation, exhalation, and the forcible expulsion of secretions create moist conditions favorable to survival and growth of a multitude of organisms (streptococci, staphylococci, coliforms, fungi, yeasts). Therefore the anesthesia circuit can become a veritable reservoir for microorganisms and a pathway for transmission of disease. When the apparatus is used on a patient with a known respiratory disease, such as tuberculosis, the risk increases.

All used accessories must be terminally cleaned and either high-level disinfected or sterilized before reuse because clinical respiratory cross infection has been traced to contaminated apparatus. Valves of the breathing circuit become contaminated from essentially healthy patients at an average rate of 35 organisms per minute. *Pseudomonas aeruginosa* has been cultured from CO_2 absorption devices. Many microorganisms accumulate in valves and air passages and in soda lime canister. Although the alkalinity of soda lime inhibits many organisms, it is not a dependable germicide or effective mechanical filter, nor is it meant to be one. Respiratory therapy equipment, mechanical ventilators, resuscitators, and suction machines and bottles present the same problems. Resistant strains of organisms, as well as opportunists, have caused nosocomial infections. Patient-to-patient infection must be eliminated. Points to remember are that:

1. Patient's respiratory tract is a portal of entry for pathogenic organisms and a source of delivering pathogens into the environment.
2. Respiratory tract loses some of its inherent defense mechanisms during anesthesia.
3. Aseptic precautions are necessary to prevent needless exposure of air passages to foreign, potentially pathogenic organisms from equipment and hands of anesthesia personnel.
4. Anesthesia machines and equipment, unless properly treated, increase danger of airborne contamination and contact transmission of pathogenic microorganisms capable of causing postoperative wound infections and systemic infections.

NOTE In the presence of tuberculosis or a virulent respiratory infection, the anesthesiologist should wear a gown and strictly adhere to universal precautions. The patient should wear a mask during transportation and until induction of anesthesia.

Disposable Equipment

Disposable equipment warrants use for reasons of safety, efficiency, and convenience. Presterilized, disposable airways, endotracheal tubes, tracheotomy tubes, breathing circuits, masks and canisters (with soda lime sealed in the plastic), and spinal trays reduce the hazard of infection. They are especially recommended for the compromised host and the bacteriologically contaminated patient. Single-use components of the anesthesia system are discarded after use. Needles must be put in puncture-resistant containers.

Care of Reusable Equipment

All parts of patient-exposed, reusable equipment must be thoroughly cleaned after *every* use to prevent pulmonary complications. Thorough cleaning to remove organic debris and drying must precede any high-level disinfection or sterilization process. *All items that can be sterilized should be sterilized.* Manufacturers strive to make the machines that cannot be sterilized more amenable to adequate terminal cleaning and freedom from microorganisms.

1. Anesthesia machine should be disinfected immediately whenever soiled by blood and secretions.
2. Surfaces of anesthesia machines, carts, or cabinets should be disinfected after *each* patient use. The specific work area used for airways, endotracheal tubes, and other items should also be cleaned. The top of a cart or tray should be draped with a disposable impervious material that is *changed between patients. All* equipment for maintenance of airway should be set up on and returned to this

drape. Disposable items should be discarded in suitable containers after use. Nondisposable equipment must be set aside after use for terminal cleaning and testing, thereby diminishing the risk of contaminating clean equipment needed for subsequent patients.

3. Monitoring equipment, including ECG and other electrodes and blood pressure cuff, should be cleaned with a detergent-disinfectant when contaminated and preferably after each use.
4. All equipment that comes in contact with mucous membranes of the patient and the inside of the breathing circuit must be terminally cleaned and sterilized preferably, or high-level disinfected.
   a. Endotracheal tubes, stylets, airways, laryngoscope blades, face masks, and suction equipment should be sterile for each patient. Suction catheters and tubing should be sterile, single-use disposable items.
   b. Interior of breathing circuits remain sterile if they stand unused in their normal position on the machine, but contamination rapidly occurs when used on patients. Parts of the circuit nearest the patient are the most heavily contaminated. Therefore corrugated hoses, breathing tubes, and reservoir bags are sterilized or high-level disinfected between each patient use.
   c. Items located farther away, such as circle systems and ventilators, are cleaned and sterilized according to a regular schedule, at least once or twice a month.
5. For cleaning, an automated process is available for decontamination. Machines wash equipment in mild detergent and hot water and rinse and dry it. Some machines incorporate a chemical disinfection cycle. If automatic equipment is not used, anesthesia and respiratory therapy equipment must be disconnected and manually cleaned before sterilization. Prompt immersion in a detergent-disinfectant solution prevents crusting of secretions. Tubing takes a long time to dry. Commercial dryers are available.
6. Sterilization methods (see Chapter 13).
   a. Steam is the preferred method for all heat-stable materials.
   b. Ethylene oxide is used for materials deteriorated by heat, such as rubber, plastics, mechanical ventilators, electronic equipment. *Thorough aeration, according to the manufacturer's recommendations, is necessary before use to remove all residual gas from the material sterilized.* Otherwise, facial burns, laryngotracheal inflammation, and obstruction or bilateral vocal cord paralysis may be caused by use of the equipment.
   c. Buffered glutaraldehyde solution does not impair conductivity of antistatic rubber. Although the least convenient method, it is preferred if ethylene oxide is not available for heat-sensitive items. Immersion for 45 minutes in Cidex solution is recommended to ensure a 100% kill of *Mycobacterium tuberculosis.* When glutaraldehyde is used, the items must be thoroughly rinsed with *sterile* water because tap water contains microorganisms and pyrogens.
7. Sterile packaged equipment should be stored in a closed, clean, and dry area. Anesthesia and respiratory therapy equipment should be kept sterile until used.
8. Policies and procedures regarding processing of equipment should be written, available, and reviewed annually.

Checking Anesthesia Equipment

Inhalation systems are tested biologically at regular intervals and checked daily for proper functioning. Preventive maintenance is essential to avoid mechanical failures, which could be fatal. Goals for quality control are to ensure that equipment is available and that it performs reliably when needed.

Bibliography

Asai T: Fiberoptic tracheal intubation through the laryngeal mask in an awake patient with cervical spine injury, *Anesth Analg* 77(2):404, 1993.

Ball K: Who's listening to whom? *AORN J* 56(5):824-827, 1992.

Beattie SJ: The laryngeal mask, *Br J Theatre Nurs* 27(2):20-23, 1990.

Beck GN et al: Comparison of intubation following propofol and alfentanil with intubation following thiopentone and suxamethonium, *Anaesthesia* 48(10):876-880, 1993.

Benumof JB, Saidman LJ: *Anesthesia and perioperative complications,* St Louis, 1992, Mosby.

Campbell LC, Weis RF: Use of anesthesia in an outpatient setting, *J Am Assoc Nurse Anesthetists* 58(3):241-247, 1990.

Cohan B: Pharmacist's corner: pharmacologic actions of commonly used preoperative medications, *AORN J* 52(3):594-598, 1990.

Curry J: Patients' memory under anesthesia: implications for the OR, *OR Manager* 9(1):14-15, 1993.

Davidson JK: *Clinical anesthesia procedures of the Massachusets General Hospital/Department of Anesthesia and Harvard Medical School,* ed 4, Boston, 1993, Little, Brown.

Edwards RM: Awake blind nasal intubation, *Anaesthesia Intensive Care* 21(2):258, 1993.

Geniton DJ: A comparison of three anesthetic agents, *AORN J* 55(6):1562-1570, 1992.

Holzman RS: Anesthesia machine, *AORN J* 52(1):69-76, 1990.

Joyce JL: Inhalation anesthetics, *AORN J* 52(1):77-83, 1990.

Mathias JM: New anesthetics have fewer side effects, *OR Manager* 11(1):16-19, 1995.

McKinney MW: Anesthetized patients may hear, understand conversations, *AORN J* 57(6):1467-1470, 1993.

Meyer C: New drugs: a faster exit from recovery, *Am J Nurs* 93(9):50-51, 1993.

Miner DG: Anesthesia: the perioperative nurse's role, *Today's OR Nurse* 12(8):24-29, 1990.

New drugs: Rocuronium (Zemuron): a safer fast muscle relaxant? *Am J Nurs* 95(3):56-57, 1995.

Patterson P: NIOSH alerts ORs to excessive nitrous oxide levels, *OR Manager* 10(7):1, 13, 1994.

Pittman SK et al: Video-assisted fiberoptic endotracheal intubation, *Anesth Analg* 78(1):197, 1994.

Propofol touted as new same-day surgery anesthesia, *Same-Day Surgery* 14(1):1-5, 1990.

Proposed recommended practices for cleaning and processing anesthesia equipment, *AORN J* 60(3):487-489, 1994.

Rogers MC: Current practice in anesthesiology, ed 2, St Louis, 1992, Mosby.

Scheller MS et al: Tracheal intubation without the use of muscle relaxants: a technique using propofol and varying doses of alfentanil, *Anesth Analg* 75(5):788-793, 1992.

Sidhu VS et al: A technique of awake fiberoptic intubation: experience in patients with cervical spine disease, *Anaesthesia* 48(10):910-913, 1993.

Vilke GM et al: Intubation techniques in the helicopter, *J Emerg Med* 12(2):217-224, 1994.

Vogelsang J: Pharmacist's corner: the treatment of postanesthesia shaking, *AORN J* 57(6):1449-1456, 1993.

Walls RM: Rapid sequence intubation in head trauma, *Ann Emerg Med* 22(6):1008-1013, 1993.

Watson DS: Pharmacist's corner: the use of the benzodiazepine antagonist flumazenil, *AORN J* 57(2):497-502, 1993.

CHAPTER 18

Local and Regional Anesthesia

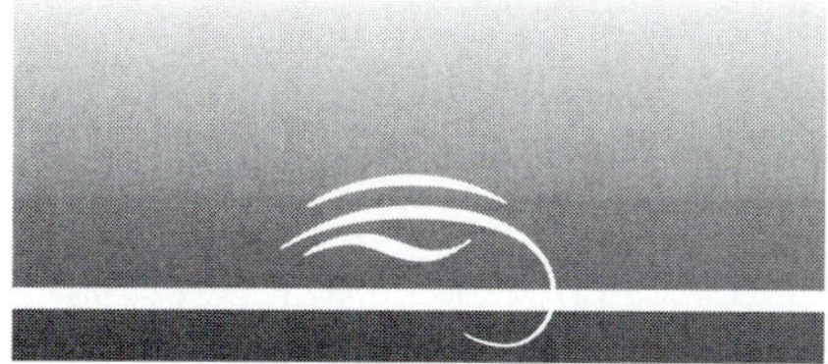

Sometimes local anesthesia is used as an adjunct to general anesthesia for decreasing intraoperative stimuli, thereby diminishing stress response to surgical trauma. Injected at the surgical site, the drug temporarily disconnects nerve impulses from the central nervous system (CNS) during manipulation of highly sensitive tissues. This reduces sensory reflexes to painful stimuli. More commonly, however, local anesthetics and regional blocks, with or without supplementary sedation, are administered as the anesthesia of choice for many diagnostic and therapeutic surgical procedures. Local anesthesia is particularly advantageous for these procedures performed in ambulatory care settings from which patients are discharged to home soon after recovery from anesthesia.

DEFINITIONS

Local anesthesia depresses sensory nerves and blocks conduction of pain impulses from their site of origin. Sensory nerves are affected first. When only an anesthetic drug is used, the patient remains conscious. Sedation may be given to relieve anxiety and to produce amnesia. This is often referred to as *conscious sedation. Regional anesthesia* may be employed, with or without conscious sedation, when general anesthesia is contraindicated or undesired. Nerve blocks, intrathecal blocks, peridural blocks, and epidural blocks are regional anesthesia techniques. These techniques block conduction of pain impulses from a specific area or region. The anesthetic drug is injected around a specific nerve or group of nerves to prevent pain of the surgical procedure. See Box 18-1 for additional terms related to local and regional anesthesia.

PREPARATION OF PATIENT

Preparation of patient who will receive a local or regional anesthetic depends on the extent of the procedure to be performed and on the anticipated technique of administration. Although it is anticipated that the patient will remain conscious, it is sometimes desirable or necessary to supplement local anesthesia with narcosis or light general anesthesia, in which case preparation for a general anesthetic is followed. Careful preoperative assessment, history taking, preanesthetic medication, and a clear explanation of what to expect (such as paresthesias) are as essential as for general anesthesia.

Assessment of the patient who is scheduled for a procedure with local or regional anesthesia, with or without intravenous (IV) conscious sedation, provides baseline data and identifies risk factors. Preoperative physiologic and psychologic assessment data that should be documented include:

1. Baseline vital signs, blood pressure, laboratory values, and results of electrocardiography and any other tests that were performed.
2. Weight, height, and age. Dosage of some drugs is calculated on the basis of body weight (i.e., mg/kg body weight). Some drugs are contraindicated for age extremes (i.e., pediatric or geriatric patients).

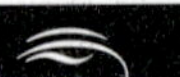

BOX 18-1

Glossary of Terms for Local and Regional Anesthesia

conduction anesthesia Loss of sensation in a region of the body produced by injecting anesthetic drug along the course of a nerve or a group of nerves to inhibit conduction of impulses to and from the area supplied by that nerve or nerves (*syn.*, block anesthesia, nerve block anesthesia).

epidural anesthesia Loss of sensation below the level of peridural injection of anesthetic drug into the epidural space in spinal canal for relief of pain in lower abdomen and pelvis without loss of consciousness.

intrathecal injection Instillation of solution, such as an anesthetic drug, into the subarachnoid space for diffusion in spinal fluid, as for spinal anesthesia.

intravenous conscious sedation Depressed level of consciousness produced by IV administration of pharmacologic agents. The patient retains ability to continuously maintain a patent airway independently and to respond to physical or verbal stimulation. Sedation may relieve anxiety and produce amnesia.

local anesthesia Loss of sensation along specific nerve pathways produced by blocking transmissions of impulses to receptor fibers. The anesthetic drug injected depresses sensory nerves and blocks conduction of pain impulses from their site of origin. The patient remains conscious, with or without IV sedation.

local infiltration Injection of anesthetic drug intracutaneously and subcutaneously into tissues to block peripheral nerve stimuli at their origin.

nerve block Loss of sensation produced by injecting the anesthetic drug around a specific nerve or nerve plexus to interrupt sensory, motor, or sympathetic transmission of impulses.

regional anesthesia Loss of sensation in a specific body part or region produced by blocking conductivity of sensory nerves supplying that area. The anesthetic drug is injected around a specific nerve or group of nerves to interrupt pain impulses. The patient remains conscious, with or without IV sedation. Regional anesthetic techniques include nerve, intrathecal, peridural, and epidural blocks.

sedative Pharmacologic agent (drug) that suppresses nervous excitement, allays anxiety, and produces a calming effect. Benzodiazepines, barbiturates, and opioids (narcotics) are the most commonly used drugs for conscious sedation.

spinal anesthesia Loss of sensation below the level of diaphragm, produced by intrathecal injection of the anesthetic drug into the subarachnoid space without loss of consciousness.

topical anesthesia Depression of sensation in superficial peripheral nerves by application of an anesthetic agent directly to mucous membrane, skin, or cornea.

3. Current medical problem(s) and past history of medical events, including history of substance abuse.
4. Current medications or drug therapy, such as insulin for diabetes or hypertensive drugs.
5. Allergies or hypersensitivities and reactions to previous anesthetics or other drugs.
6. Mental status, including emotional state and level of consciousness.
7. Communication ability. A patient with hearing impairment or language barrier may be unable to understand verbal instruction or to respond appropriately.

Preoperative orders regarding the time when the patient should cease taking anything by mouth vary with the circumstances; 8 hours before the surgical procedure is the usual cutoff time. The patient may vomit from apprehension or untoward reaction to drugs. Often a preoperative benzodiazepine is ordered before local or regional anesthesia. Medication is given as ordered. Patient is transported via stretcher if sedated.

LOCAL ANESTHESIA

The surgeon injects the anesthetic drug or applies it topically. Supplemental agents should be available for analgesia or anesthesia, if necessary, or for adverse reaction. Resuscitative equipment and oxygen must be at hand before administration of any anesthetic.

Care of Patient During Surgical Procedure

The patient must be able to respond cooperatively and to maintain respiration unassisted. However, the patient needs careful observation throughout the surgical procedure and for a period of time afterward for symptoms of delayed reaction or complications. Gentle manipulation, including concern for hearing sense, cannot be overemphasized for the patient in a conscious or semiconscious state. The care the patient will need depends on type and length of procedure, amount of sedation given, and type and amount of local anesthetic used. Psychologic support and reassurance must be given before and during the surgical procedure. The patient should be told what to expect and what is expected of him or her. The patient must be monitored for adverse effects.

Perioperative Nurse's Role

A qualified registered nurse is responsible for the patient's safety and nursing care during local anesthesia. *In the absence of an anesthesiologist or nurse anesthetist, the perioperative nurse is totally responsible for monitoring the patient* (see p. 355). *The only responsibility this nurse should have is to continually monitor and assess the patient's condi-*

tion. The perioperative nurse who assumes this responsibility should have the knowledge, skill, and ability to use and interpret data from monitoring equipment. He or she also should be able to recognize symptoms of abnormal reactions to local anesthetic drugs and to provide interventions to prevent further complications. Written institutional policies and procedures, including a format for documentation, should be in place to guide the perioperative nurse in the care of the patient receiving a local anesthetic.

Under local anesthesia, physiologic changes may require supervision of pulse, blood pressure, oxygenation, and respiration. Baseline data must be obtained preoperatively. The vital signs are monitored and compared with the patient's baseline throughout the surgical procedure. Monitoring includes blood pressure and pulse oximetry. In many instances the monitoring equipment may be more sensitive to the patient's physiologic changes than direct observation. The patient must be monitored for reaction to drugs and for behavioral and physiologic changes. Physiologic data from monitoring and direct observation must be documented frequently and at any significant event, such as the injection of medication or the removal of a specimen. Total amount of anesthetic and supplementary drugs administered must be recorded.

Intravenous Conscious Sedation

To allay the patient's anxiety and fear while allowing rapid return to ambulation, sedation may be given by IV infusion. *Intravenous conscious sedation* refers to a mild-to-moderate depressed level of consciousness that allows the patient to maintain a patent airway independently and to respond appropriately to verbal instructions or physical stimulation. A benzodiazepine, such as midazolam (Versed) or diazepam (Valium), is most commonly given either alone or in combination with a narcotic and atropine or scopolamine. Benzodiazepines provide amnesia with sedation, but they also may cause respiratory depression and fluctuations in blood pressure and heart rate and rhythm. The patient under IV conscious sedation should be monitored continuously. Optimal practice allows a registered nurse to attend and monitor the patient's physiologic state and another circulator to assist the sterile team if an anesthesiologist is not available. Written institutional policies should be in place that address the registered nurse's competency in patient monitoring and role during the use of IV conscious sedation.

All team members need to understand the goal and desired effects of IV conscious sedation. If the primary goal is to allay the patient's anxiety and fear, the therapeutic effects of the drugs given should produce relaxation and some degree of amnesia, that is, an indifference to pain, and elevate the patient's pain threshold. Because consciousness is maintained, the patient has intact protective reflexes to respond to physical stimuli. The patient also can easily be aroused from sleep to cooperate with verbal commands as necessary. In this state vital signs may fluctuate but desirably to a minimal extent. Documentation in the patient's record should reflect evidence of continuous assessment and identification of any untoward or significant reactions during administration of local anesthesia with IV conscious sedation. (Adverse reactions, monitoring, and complications are discussed later in this chapter.)

Monitored Anesthesia Care

When an anesthesiologist's presence is desired, the surgical procedure is scheduled as *monitored anesthesia care* (MAC), *attended local*, or *anesthesia standby*. Patients with particular medical problems or age-extreme patients (pediatric or geriatric) may require supervision by anesthesia personnel. Patients receiving a local anesthetic because they are too ill to undergo general anesthesia should have an anesthesiologist in attendance. Type and length of procedure also may be factors that influence the surgeon's request for an anesthesiologist to be available to give and monitor conscious sedation. The anesthesiologist may initiate and maintain a regional nerve block, such as an axillary brachial plexus block for hand surgery. Conscious sedation and regional blocks with MAC have gained in popularity with the advent of ambulatory surgery for many procedures that are not complex and do not require muscle relaxation. Many facilities require presence of an anesthesiologist or anesthetist for all patients receiving IV sedation.

Considerations in Selection of Anesthesia

A local anesthetic depresses superficial peripheral nerves and blocks conduction of pain impulses from their site of origin. Regional nerve blocks interrupt conduction of pain impulses from a specific area or region. These techniques may be employed, with or without conscious sedation, when general anesthesia is contraindicated or undesired. As with any anesthetic agent, local anesthetics offer advantages in some circumstances but have disadvantages and are contraindicated in others.

Advantages of Local Anesthesia

1. Infiltration anesthetic agents can minimize recovery period. Patient can ambulate, eat, void, and resume normal activity.
2. Local anesthesia needs minimal and simple equipment and provides economy.
3. Loss of consciousness does not occur, unless anesthesia is supplemented. Local anesthesia avoids the undesirable effects of general anesthesia.
4. It is suitable for patients who recently ingested food or fluids, as before an emergency procedure; for ambulatory patients; for minor procedures; for proce-

dures in which it is desirable to have the patient awake and cooperative.
5. Surgeon can administer the anesthetic in instances of unavailability of an anesthesiologist.

Disadvantages of Local Anesthesia

1. It is not practical for all types of procedures. For example, too much drug would be needed for some major surgical procedures; duration of anesthesia is insufficient for others.
2. There are individual variations in response to local anesthetic drugs.
3. Too rapid absorption of drug into blood, as in overdosage, can cause severe, potentially fatal reactions.
4. Apprehension may be increased by the patient's ability to see and hear. Some patients prefer to be unconscious and unaware.

Contraindications to Local Anesthesia

Local anesthesia is generally contraindicated in patients with:

1. Allergic sensitivity to the local drug.
2. Local infection or malignancy, which may be carried to and spread in adjacent tissues by injection. A bacteriologically safe injection site should be selected.
3. Septicemia. In a proximal nerve block a needle may open new lymph channels that drain through a region, thereby causing new foci and local abscess formation from the perforation of small vessels and escape of bacteria.
4. Extreme nervousness, apprehension, excitability or inability to cooperate because of mental state or age.

Techniques of Administration

Topical Application

The anesthetic is applied directly to a mucous membrane, to a serous surface, or into an open wound. A topical agent is most often applied to the respiratory passages to eliminate laryngeal reflexes and cough, for insertion of airways before induction or during light general anesthesia, or for therapeutic and diagnostic procedures such as laryngoscopy or bronchoscopy. It is also used in cystoscopy. Mucous membranes readily absorb topical agents because of their vascularity. Onset of anesthesia occurs within a minute. Volume of a topical agent in blood may equal the same level obtained by IV injection. Duration of anesthesia is 20 to 30 minutes. Ointments or solutions may be used. If a spray or atomizer is used, it should contain a visible reservoir so that quantity of drug administered is clearly observed because droplets vary in size.

Preanesthetic sedation and atropine are important before topical application within the respiratory tract. Atropine is necessary since saliva can dilute the anesthetic and prevent adequate duration of contact with mucous membranes. Also, a dry throat is necessary to prevent aspiration until the anesthetic effect has disappeared and throat reflexes have returned. Adverse reaction to topical anesthetic agents is uncommon when dosage is carefully controlled. Sudden cardiovascular collapse can occur, most frequently following topical anesthesia in respiratory tract.

Cryoanesthesia Cryoanesthesia involves blocking local nerve conduction of painful impulses by means of marked surface cooling (i.e., freezing) of a localized area. It is used in such brief procedures as the removal of warts or noninvasive papular surface lesions. Cryotherapy units are commercially available.

Simple Local Infiltration

The agent is injected intracutaneously and subcutaneously into tissues at the incisional site to block peripheral nerve stimuli at their origin. It is used to suture superficial lacerations or for excision of minor lesions.

Regional Injection

The agent is injected into or around a specific nerve or group of nerves to depress the entire sensory nervous system of a limited, localized area of the body. The injection is at a distance from the surgical site. A wider, deeper area is anesthetized than with simple infiltration. There are several types of regional blocks.

Nerve Block Anesthetizing of a selected nerve at a given point, nerve blocks are performed to interrupt sensory, motor, or sympathetic transmission. Blocks may be used intraoperatively to prevent pain of the procedure, diagnostically to ascertain cause of pain, or therapeutically to relieve chronic pain. Blocks are useful in various circulatory and neurosurgical syndromes. For prolonged pain relief, as during a long procedure or to treat chronic pain associated with disease or trauma, a continuous infusion or incremental injections through a catheter may sustain regional anesthesia. Some examples of blocks are as follows:

1. Surgical blocks
   a. Paravertebral block of cervical plexus for area between jaw and clavicle
   b. Intercostal block for relatively superficial intraabdominal procedures
   c. Brachial plexus or axillary block for arm
   d. Median, radial, or ulnar nerve block for elbow or wrist
   e. Hand and digital block for fingers; epinephrine is not added to the local agent because gangrene can result from inadequate circulation
2. Diagnostic or therapeutic blocks
   a. Sympathetic nerve ganglia block to produce desired vasodilation by paralysis of the sympa-

thetic nerve supply to the constricting smooth muscle in the artery wall

b. Stellate ganglion block to increase circulation in peripheral vascular disease in the head, neck, arm, or hand
c. Paravertebral lumbar block to increase circulation in the lower extremities
d. Celiac block for relief of abdominal pain of pancreatic origin

Bier Block A Bier block is a regional IV injection of a local anesthetic to an extremity below the level of a tourniquet. An IV catheter is introduced into a vein in the arm or leg close to the intended surgical site. Blood is drained from the extremity by compression with a tourniquet applied to the lower leg for foot surgery, arm for surgical procedure above wrist, or forearm for hand or wrist procedure. Subsequent injection of the anesthetic drug through the catheter into the vein confines the drug to infiltration into surrounding tissues. The extremity remains pain free as long as the tourniquet is in place. On release of the tourniquet at conclusion of the surgical procedure, entry of a bolus of the remaining drug into systemic circulation may cause cardiovascular or CNS symptoms of toxicity. Bier block is used most often for upper extremity procedures and for those that last an hour or less.

Field Block The surgical site is blocked off with a wall of anesthetic drug. A series of injections into proximal and surrounding tissues will provide a wide area of anesthesia, as in abdominal wall block for herniorrhaphy.

Complications

Each type of block carries unique complication potential. Examples of complications include:

1. Intercostal blocks: pneumothorax, atelectasis, total spinal anesthesia, air embolism, transverse myelitis
2. Brachial plexus blocks: pneumothorax, hemothorax, recurrent laryngeal paralysis, phrenic paralysis, subarachnoid injection, Horner's syndrome; axillary approach may be preferred to interscalene approach
3. Stellate ganglion blocks: pneumothorax
4. Celiac blocks: large vessel perforation, total spinal anesthesia

SPINAL AND EPIDURAL ANESTHESIA

Intraspinal injection of an anesthetic drug is a technique of regional anesthesia performed by a person who has been properly trained and has acquired the necessary motor skill, usually an anesthesiologist. A few states define this technique as medical practice, thereby excluding nurse anesthetists.

Intrathecal Block

Intrathecal block, commonly referred to as *spinal anesthesia,* causes desensitization of spinal ganglia and motor roots. The agent is injected into the cerebrospinal fluid (CSF) in the subarachnoid space of the meninges (the three-layered covering of the spinal cord) using a lumbar interspace in the vertebral column (Figure 18-1). The subarachnoid space is located between the pia mater (the innermost membranous layer covering the spinal cord) and the arachnoid (the thin vascular, weblike layer immediately beneath the dura mater, which is the outermost sheath covering the spinal cord). Spinal ganglia, motor nerve roots, and blood vessels pass through the meninges. The drug diffuses into the CSF around ganglia and nerves before it is absorbed into the bloodstream. Absorption into nerve fibers is rapid.

Level of anesthesia attained depends on various factors: position during and immediately after injection; CSF pressure; site and rate of injection; volume, dosage, and specific gravity (baricity) of the solution; inclusion of a vasoconstrictor, usually epinephrine; spinal curvature; interspace chosen; and coughing or straining, which can inadvertently raise the level. Spread of the anesthetic is controlled mainly by solution baricity and patient position. The period immediately following injection is decisive; the anesthetic is

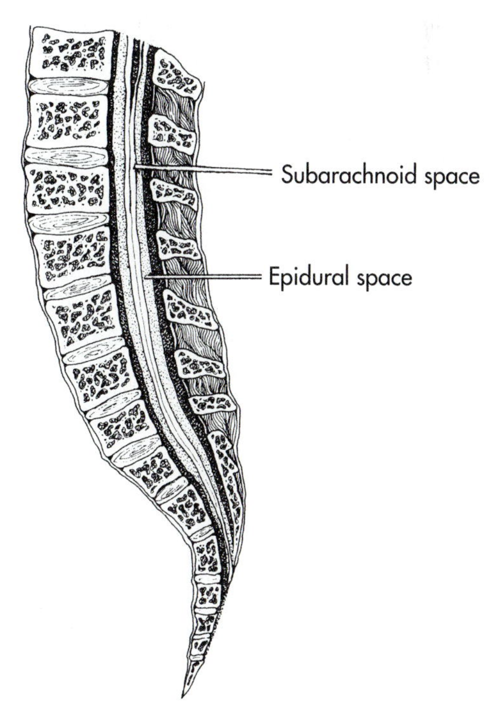

FIGURE 18-1 Agent is injected into subarachnoid space for spinal anesthesia or into epidural space for epidural anesthesia.

becoming "fixed"—that is, absorbed by the tissues and unable to travel. Further control of the anesthetic level is attained by tilting the operating table at that time. The direction of tilting depends on whether the drug is *hyperbaric* (specific gravity greater than that of spinal fluid) or *hypobaric* (lighter than spinal fluid). *Isobaric* anesthetics (same weight as spinal fluid) are made hyperbaric by the addition of 5% or 10% dextrose to the anesthetic before injection.

Immediately after injection the anesthesiologist carefully tests the level of anesthesia by pinprick, tilting the table as necessary to achieve the desired level for the surgical procedure. After anesthetic fixation and with the anesthesiologist's permission, the patient is placed in surgical position. The patient is asked to relax and let the team turn him or her. Straining or holding breath can precipitate hypotension or inadvertent rise in the level of anesthesia. The incision is never made until it is certain that anesthesia is adequate. Supplementation of spinal anesthesia is necessary if anesthesia or muscular relaxation is insufficient or the patient is unduly apprehensive. Sometimes the patient is kept in a light sleep with an IV sedative.

Choice of Agent

This depends on various factors such as duration, intensity, and level of anesthesia desired, anticipated surgical position of the patient, and the surgical procedure.

Duration of Agent

The variable duration of anesthesia depends on physiologic and metabolic factors. It is prolonged by the addition of a vasoconstrictor. Anesthesia diminishes as the agent is absorbed into systemic circulation.

Procedure

For injection, the patient is placed in the position desired by the anesthesiologist, depending on solution baricity and anesthesia to be produced.

1. *Lateral position.* The most common; the patient's back is at the edge of the operating table, parallel to it. Knees are flexed onto the abdomen and the head is flexed to the knees. Hips and shoulders are vertical to the table to prevent rotation of the spine.
2. *Sitting position.* The patient sits on the side of the operating table with feet resting on a stool. The spine is flexed, with chin lowered to sternum, arms crossed and supported on a pillow on an adjustable table or Mayo stand.
3. *Prone position.* The patient lies face downward on operating table.

The circulator or a nursing assistant supports the patient in position, observes and reassures him or her, and assists the anesthesiologist in any way possible. Attention to asepsis is extremely important. The anesthesiologist dons sterile gloves before handling sterile items. Sterile disposable spinal trays eliminate the need for cleaning and sterilizing of nondisposable equipment. They also avoid the hazards of sterilizing ampules. A *spinal tray* usually contains:

1. Fenestrated drape
2. Ampules of local anesthetic, spinal anesthetic, vasoconstrictor drug, 10% dextrose
3. Sponges, forceps, and antiseptic solution
4. Needles: 25-gauge hypodermic for infiltration of local anesthetic into the skin; 22-gauge × 2 inches (5 cm) long for intramuscular injection; blunt 18-gauge for mixing drugs; 22- or 26-gauge × 3½ inches (9 cm) long, spinal needles with stylets for intrathecal injection
5. Syringes: 5 ml for spinal anesthetic, 10 ml for hypobaric solutions, 2 ml for superficial anesthesia

Forceps and sponges are of a different type than those counted and used during the surgical procedure. The lumbar puncture site is cleansed with an antiseptic solution and draped with a fenestrated drape. Blood pressure is checked before, during, and after spinal anesthesia since hypotension is common.

Intermittent injections or continuous infusion via a plastic or silicone catheter may be used for long procedures when additional anesthesia is needed or for pain relief with a narcotic. Regional anesthesia for the latter purpose is more frequently accomplished with an epidural catheter (see pp. 351-352).

Use of Spinal Anesthesia

Spinal anesthesia is frequently used for abdominal (mainly lower) or pelvic procedures requiring relaxation, inguinal or lower extremity procedures, surgical obstetrics (cesarean section—lacks effect on fetus), and urologic procedures. It is advised for alcoholics, barbiturate addicts, very muscular patients who would need large doses of general anesthetic and muscle relaxant, and for emergency surgical procedures on patients who have eaten recently. It is also used in the presence of hepatic, renal, or metabolic disease because it causes minimal upset of body chemistry.

Advantages The patient is conscious if desired. Throat reflexes are maintained; breathing is quiet without airway problems because respiratory system is not irritated. Bowel is contracted. Muscle relaxation and anesthesia are excellent if properly executed.

Disadvantages Spinal anesthesia produces a circulatory depressant effect and stasis of blood as a result of interference with venous return from motor paralysis and arteriolar dilation in the lower extremities. Change in body position may be followed by a sudden drop in blood pressure; after fixation of anesthetic, a slight head-down position may increase venous return to the heart. The agent cannot be removed after injection. Nausea and emesis may accompany cerebral ischemia, traction on viscera, or premedication. There is possible sensitivity to the agent and danger of trauma or infection. Patient can hear. Rarely, distended bowel is perforated.

Postanesthetic Complications Transient or permanent neurologic sequelae from trauma, irritation by the agent, lack of asepsis, and loss of spinal fluid with decreased intracranial pressure syndrome are potential complications. Examples include: spinal headache; auditory and ocular disturbances such as tinnitus, diplopia; arachnoiditis, meningitis; transverse myelitis; cauda equina syndrome (failure to regain use of legs or control of urinary and bowel functions); temporary paresthesias such as numbness and tingling; cranial nerve palsies; urinary retention. Late complications include nerve root lesions, spinal cord lesions, and ruptured nucleus pulposus.

NOTE

1. True spinal headache caused by a persistent CSF leak through the needle hole in the dura usually responds to supine bed rest, copious oral or IV fluids, and systemic analgesia. Refractory postspinal headache may be treated by an epidural blood patch; 5 to 8 ml of the patient's own blood is administered at puncture site. This usually affords prompt relief.
2. If a high level of anesthesia is reached, extreme caution is essential to prevent respiratory paralysis ("total spinal"), an emergency situation requiring artificial ventilation until the level of anesthesia has receded. Respiratory arrest, although rare, is thought to be the result of medullary hypoperfusion. Apnea also can be produced by respiratory center ischemia resulting from precipitous hypotension.
3. Anesthesia machine, oxygen, and IV infusion must be in readiness before injection. Constant vigilance of respiration and circulation is mandatory. Blood pressure must be maintained.

Epidural, Peridural Block

The terms *epidural, peridural,* and *extradural* are used synonymously. The epidural space lies between the dura mater, the outermost sheath covering the spinal cord, and the walls of the vertebral column. It contains a network of blood vessels, lymphatics, fat, loose connective tissue, and spinal nerve roots. Injection is made into this space surrounding dura mater (see Figure 18-1). The drug diffuses slowly through the dura mater into CSF. Anesthesia is prolonged while the drug is absorbed from CSF into the bloodstream. Spread of anesthetic and duration of action are influenced by concentration and volume of solution injected (total drug mass) and rate of injection. The anesthetic diffuses toward the head and caudad. In contrast to spinal anesthesia, position, baricity, and gravity have little influence on anesthetic distribution. The high incidence of systemic reactions is attributed to absorption of the agent from the highly vascular peridural area and the relatively large mass of anesthetic injected. Epinephrine 1:200,000 is usually added to retard absorption. Two approaches may be used: lumbar (the more common) and caudal.

Lumbar Approach

The lumbar approach is a peridural block. Equipment is similar to that for a spinal with the addition of a 19-gauge × 3½ inches (9 cm) long, thin-walled needle with stylet with a rigid shaft and short bevel tip to minimize danger of inadvertent dural puncture. Insertion of a catheter allows repeated injections for *continuous epidural* anesthesia, requiring additional needles, stopcocks, and plastic catheter in the setup.

Caudal Approach

The caudal approach is an epidural sacral block. Epidural injection is through the caudal canal, desensitizing nerves emerging from the dural sac. Position for injection is prone with hips flexed, sacrum horizontal, and heels turned outward to expose the injection site. Sacral area is prepared and draped, with care taken to protect genitalia from irritating solution. Left lateral position is used in the pregnant patient. Care must be taken in the pregnant patient to avoid perforating the rectum or the fetal head during labor. Spread of agents in epidural anesthesia is enhanced in pregnancy, atherosclerosis, and advanced age.

The spinal tray includes the addition of 20-gauge × 1½ inches (4 cm) long spinal needle with stylet. Commercial sets are available. Skin and ligaments are infiltrated with a local anesthetic agent before the spinal needle is inserted.

Use of Epidural Anesthesia

Management and sequelae of epidural anesthesia are similar to those of spinal anesthesia. An epidural approach may be used for anorectal, vaginal, or perineal procedures. However, it is used more commonly in obstetrics as a continuous technique to control pain during labor and delivery and during and after cesarean section. The patient must be attended constantly by trained personnel once the block is initiated for obstetric analgesia. Use of an apnea monitor may be indicated. The fetal heart rate should be electronically monitored continuously because the patient is insensitive to uterine contractions.

Epidural narcotic analgesia may provide sustained postoperative relief or control of pain in patients with intractable or prolonged pain, as from muscle spasm or terminal malignancy. This may be administered by a percutaneous indwelling epidural catheter, an implanted epidural catheter with infusion port or reservoir and pump, or an implantable infusion device (see Chapter 45, p. 928). A patient may come to the OR for placement of an epidural catheter or device. A catheter for administration of a narcotic for prolonged postoperative pain relief, usually for 3 or 4 days, may be inserted before induction of general anesthesia. It may be inserted for epidural anesthesia and postoperative use. Morphine sulfate, fentanyl, sufentanil citrate, and buprenorphine hydrochloride are the drugs most commonly used for prolonged pain relief. Although probability of respiratory depression is less when the epidural route is used as compared with spinal narcotics, use of an apnea monitor is advisable. Side effects include nausea and vomiting, urinary retention, and pruritus. Epidural narcotics block pain at the level of opiate receptors in the dorsal horn of the spinal cord, not in the brain, so the patient is mentally alert and able to ambulate.

Advantages Compared with spinal anesthesia, there is a lesser degree of hypotension, headache, and potential for neurologic complications, although a higher failure rate is reported.

Disadvantages Less controllable height of anesthesia; more difficult technique; area of potential infection from anaerobic organisms with the caudal approach; unpredictable; time-consuming (i.e., longer time for complete anesthesia); larger amount of agent injected; continuous technique may slow the first stage of labor.

Complications Intravascular injection, accidental dural puncture and total spinal anesthesia, blood vessel puncture and hematoma, profound hypotension; backache, transient or permanent paralysis (paraplegia).

Spinal and Epidural Drugs

The choice of drug depends on factors such as duration, intensity, and level of anesthesia desired, anticipated surgical position of patient, and surgical procedure. Duration of action depends on physiologic and metabolic factors. The addition of a vasoconstrictor, usually epinephrine 1:200,000, prolongs duration. Diffusion of the drug into CSF is affected by solubility, molecular weight, and volume. Glucose may be added to make the drug heavier than CSF. Anesthesia diminishes as the drug is absorbed into the systemic circulation. The most commonly used anesthetic drugs for spinal and epidural anesthesia are included in Table 18-1, p. 354.

ANESTHETIC DRUGS

Local and regional anesthetic drugs interfere with initiation and transmission of nerve impulses by interacting with the membranous sheath that covers nerve fibers. By physical and biochemical mechanisms, drugs retard and stop propagation of nerve impulses, eventually blocking conduction.

Drug Interactions

Duration of action depends not only on pharmacologic properties of drugs but also on volume and concentration of solution and its systemic interactions. Drugs vary in potency, penetration, rapidity of hydrolysis or destruction, and toxicity.

Conduction Velocity

Nerve fibers vary in their susceptibility to drugs. The larger the fiber, the greater the concentration required. The least amount of lowest concentration to achieve desired effect should be administered. Conduction of a peripheral stimulus is blocked at its origin by topical application or local infiltration of the drug. Transmission of stimuli along afferent nerves from the surgical site is blocked in regional anesthesia. Conductive pathways in and around the spinal cord are blocked for spinal and epidural anesthesia.

Blocking Quality

Drugs of high potency, minimal systemic activity, prompt metabolism, and those that lack local irritation are most effective. Latency time between administration and maximum effect, duration of action, and regression time between beginning and end of pain perception determine blocking qualities of the drug. Sensory nerves are blocked initially. Motor nerves are also affected, with resultant paralysis of both voluntary and involuntary muscles. Some degree of vasodilation occurs with all anesthetic drugs except cocaine.

Absorption

Local blood flow, vasodilation, and vascularity of tissues can markedly influence local anesthetic action and systemic absorption of drugs. Fibrous tissue and fat in some injection sites act as diffusion barriers and nonspecific binding sites. Supplemental drugs can be added to anesthetic drugs to facilitate or retard absorption.

Hyaluronidase (Wydase) A soluble protein enzyme, hyaluronidase is sometimes added to a local anesthetic to facilitate its spread through subcutaneous tissues to all desired nerves. This action causes more rapid absorption of anesthetic and may reduce intensity and duration of its effect. Rapid absorption may increase possibility of a systemic reaction (see p. 356).

Epinephrine (Adrenalin) A catecholamine, epinephrine is a potent stimulant. When combined with an anesthetic drug, it causes vasoconstriction to slow circulatory uptake and absorption, thus prolonging anesthesia. It is used to counteract cardiovascular depressant effects of large doses of local anesthetic. It also decreases bleeding, which is a desired effect in many surgical procedures. Concentration of epinephrine 1:1000 (1000 mg/1000 ml = 1 mg/ml) to 1:200,000 (0.005 mg/ml) may be optimal for these purposes. Epinephrine is premixed in commercially prepared solutions. If it must be added to an anesthetic drug, it is best to do so with a calibrated syringe. Overdosage must be avoided. Epinephrine can produce an acute adrenergic response: nervousness, pallor, diaphoresis, tremor, palpitation, tachycardia, and hypertension. The patient receiving epinephrine should be well oxygenated.

Toxicity

Allergic reactions to anesthetic drugs can occur but are rare. Toxic reactions occur when the concentration of drug in the blood affects the CNS. Slurred speech, numbness of tongue, blurred vision, and tinnitus are symptoms of toxicity that can progress to drowsiness and confusion. Maximum recommended dosage for each drug should not be exceeded. Severe toxic reaction can quickly lead to cardiovascular collapse. In topical anesthesia extremely rapid systemic absorption from the mucous membranes explains the relatively high frequency of toxic reactions. In local or regional anesthesia inadvertent intravascular injection and use of fairly large quantities in highly vascular areas will contribute to local anesthetic toxicity. (See complications of local/regional anesthesia, pp. 356-358.)

Pharmacologic Agents

Many different local or regional anesthetic drugs are in use. All are direct myocardial depressants, but the CNS effects precede this depression. Detoxification occurs in the liver. They differ in structure and therefore in action. These drugs are hydrochloride salts of weak bases in solution. They are categorized by chemical structure as amino amides and amino esters (Table 18-1).

Amino Amides

Amino amides are metabolized in the liver by enzymes and are excreted by the kidneys. Patients with hepatic disease may become toxic with normal dosages because of ineffective metabolism. The *amides* include:

Lidocaine Hydrochloride (Xylocaine, Lignocaine) Probably the most widely used agent, this potent anesthetic slowly hydrolyzes in circulating plasma. It undergoes hepatic degradation. Dosage should be reduced if hepatic function or blood flow is impaired. Its major advantages are rapid onset of anesthesia and lack of local irritant effect. Allergic reactions are rare. Used extensively for surgical procedures and dentistry, it has moderate potency and duration of action. For infiltration: 0.5%; for peripheral nerves: 1% to 2%; maximum dose: 500 mg (0.5 g) or 7 mg/kg body weight. It is a good topical anesthetic, although it is not as effective as cocaine. For topical use in respiratory tract: 2% to 4%; maximum dose: 200 mg. It is commonly used topically before intubation.

Lidocaine also is used in the management of ventricular dysrhythmias during and after cardiac procedures, in resuscitation after cardiac arrest, and in treatment and prevention of irritability in patients who have experienced myocardial infarction. Clinical indications of lidocaine toxicity usually are related to the CNS. Excessive doses can produce myocardial and circulatory depression.

Mepivacaine Hydrochloride (Carbocaine) Similar to lidocaine hydrochloride, mepivacaine takes effect rapidly but produces 20% longer duration of anesthesia. It has moderate potency and duration of action. It is commonly employed for infiltration and nerve block. It produces minimal tissue irritation and few adverse reactions. Epinephrine may *not* be added to it because of its duration. For infiltration: 0.5% to 1%; for peripheral nerves: 1% to 2%; maximum dose: 500 mg.

Bupivacaine Hydrochloride (Marcaine, Sensorcaine) Four times more potent than lidocaine, bupivacaine has a high potency of long duration. Onset of anesthesia is slow, but duration is two to three times longer than that of lidocaine or mepivacaine, with toxicity approximate to that of tetracaine. Cumulation occurs with repeated injection. The drug affords prolonged pain relief following caudal block for rectal procedures. It is contraindicated for obstetric paracervical block and epidural anesthesia and for Bier block. For local infiltration or regional block, with or without epinephrine: 0.25% to 0.50%; maximum dose: 175 mg per dose without epinephrine or 225 mg with epinephrine 1:200,000 to total dose of 400 mg.

Prilocaine Hydrochloride (Citanest) With prilocaine the onset of anesthesia is slower than with lidocaine, but duration of action is longer. It is particularly useful for patients with diabetes or cardiovascular disease. It is used *without* epinephrine. For infiltration and peripheral nerves: 1% or 2%; for regional blocks: 2% or 3%; maximum dose: 600 mg.

Etidocaine Hydrochloride (Duranest) Onset of block is slower than that of lidocaine, but the block is of greater potency and toxicity and longer duration of action. For peripheral nerves: 0.5%; maximum dose: 500 mg.

Dibucaine Hydrochloride (Nupercaine, Percaine, Cinchocaine) Dibucaine is a very potent drug with a high rate of systemic toxicity. Onset is slow and

TABLE 18-1

Local and Regional Anesthetic Agents

GENERIC NAME	TRADE NAME(S)	USES	CONCEN-TRATION	DURATION OF EFFECT (HOURS)	MAXIMUM DOSAGE
Amino amides					
Bupivacaine hydrochloride	Marcaine Sensorcaine	Local infiltration* Regional block* Surgical epidural	0.25% to 0.50%	2 to 3	400 mg
Dibucaine hydrochloride	Nupercaine Percaine Cinchocaine	Local infiltration Peripheral nerves	0.05% to 0.1%	3 to 3½	30 mg
Etidocaine hydrochloride	Duranest	Peripheral nerves Epidural	0.5% to 1%	2 to 3	500 mg
Lidocaine hydrochloride	Xylocaine Lignocaine	Topical Infiltration* Peripheral nerves* Nerve block* Spinal Epidural	2% to 4% 0.5% 1% to 2%	½ to 2	200 mg 500 mg or 7 mg/kg body weight
Mepivacaine hydrochloride	Carbocaine	Infiltration Peripheral nerves Epidural	0.5% to 1.0% 1% to 2%	½ to 2	500 mg
Prilocaine hydrochloride	Citanest	Infiltration Peripheral nerves Regional block Epidural	1% to 2% 2% to 3%	½ to 2½	600 mg
Amino esters					
Chloroprocaine hydrochloride	Nesacaine	Infiltration* Peripheral nerves* Nerve block* Epidural	0.5% 2% 2% 2% to 3%	¼ to ½	1000 mg
Cocaine hydrochloride		Topical	4% or 10%	½	200 mg or 4 mg/kg body weight
Procaine hydrochloride	Novocain	Infiltration Peripheral nerves Spinal	0.5% 1% to 2%	¼ to ½	1000 mg or 14 mg/kg body weight
Tetracaine hydrochloride	Cetacaine Pontocaine	Topical Spinal	2% 1%	2 to 4	20 mg

*Epinephrine may be used.

duration of action is long. For infiltration and peripheral nerves: 0.05% to 0.1%, maximum dose: 30 mg.

Amino Esters

Amino esters are hydrolyzed in plasma by pseudocholinesterase enzymes produced by the liver. Para-aminobenzoic acid (PABA), a factor in the vitamin B complex, is a product of this metabolism. Some patients are allergic to PABA. The *esters* include:

Cocaine Hydrochloride The first local anesthetic, introduced in 1884, cocaine is a crystalline powder with a bitter taste in solution. It is the most toxic of local drugs and, in contrast to all but lidocaine hydrochloride, is a vasoconstrictor and a CNS stimulant. Cocaine reduces bleeding and shrinks congested mucous membranes. It causes temporary paralysis of sensory nerve fibers, produces exhilaration, lessens hunger and fatigue, and stimulates pulse and respiratory rates. *Administration is by topical application only* because of its high toxicity; the solution rapidly penetrates mucous membrane into highly vascular tissue. Absorption is self-limiting because of vasoconstrictive properties associated with the drug. Epinephrine should *not* be added. When applied to the throat, cocaine abolishes throat reflexes. The patient is awake and can cooperate, but disadvantages are its limited use and possible addiction. It is used topically in 4% or 10% concentration for anesthesia of the upper respiratory tract (nose, pharynx, tracheobronchial tree). Untoward reactions may occur rapidly in response to even a very small amount of the drug. Maximum dose: 200 mg or 4 mg/kg body weight. Cocaine is metabolized by the liver and excreted by the kidneys. It should be used with caution in patients with impaired liver or kidney function.

Procaine Hydrochloride (Novocain) Procaine is similar to cocaine but less toxic. Concentrations used: 0.5% for infiltration; 1% to 2% for peripheral nerves. It is injected subcutaneously, intramuscularly, or intrathecally. It has low potency, is of short duration, and is ineffectual topically. Its advantages include minimal toxicity, easy sterilization, low cost, and lack of local irritation. Newer agents are used more frequently. Maximum dose: 1000 mg (1 g) or 14 mg/kg body weight.

Chloroprocaine Hydrochloride (Nesacaine) Chloroprocaine is possibly the safest local anesthetic from the standpoint of systemic toxicity because of its fast metabolism. It has moderate potency of short duration. It is rapidly hydrolyzed in the plasma. Its action is fast, but it is not active topically. When used in obstetrics, it does not detectably alter neurobehavioral responses of newborn infants. For infiltration: 0.5%; for peripheral nerves: 2%; maximum dose: 1000 mg (1 g).

Tetracaine Hydrochloride (Cetacaine) With tetracaine the onset of analgesia is slow but duration of effect is longer than that of many other drugs. It has high potency of long duration. It is also more toxic systemically because of the slow rate of destruction in the body, but low total dosage tends to reduce the chances of reaction. It is not used for local tissue infiltration or nerve block. Tetracaine in 2% solution is used *only for topical anesthesia* on accessible mucous membranes such as the oropharynx. Maximum dose: 20 mg. Tetracaine hydrochloride is used primarily for spinal anesthesia.

MONITORING OF PATIENT RECEIVING LOCAL ANESTHETIC

Extent of monitoring, determined in consultation with the department of surgery and anesthesiology where applicable, depends on seriousness of the procedure, sedation required, and/or patient's condition. The RN assigned to monitor the patient receiving a local anesthetic, with or without IV conscious sedation, *continuously attends the patient. This nurse does not have other responsibilities* during the surgical procedure. Recommended practices of the Association of Operating Room Nurses provide guidelines for the perioperative nurse for monitoring the patient receiving a local anesthetic and the patient receiving IV conscious sedation. They may be summarized briefly as follows:

1. Patient is monitored for reaction to drugs and for behavioral and physiologic changes. The RN should recognize and report to the physician significant changes in the patient's status and be prepared to initiate appropriate interventions.
2. Nurse attending the patient should have basic knowledge of function and use of monitoring equipment, ability to interpret information, and working knowledge of resuscitation equipment.
3. Accurate reflection of perioperative care should be documented on patient's record.
4. Institutional policies and procedures in regard to patient care, including monitoring, should be written, reviewed annually, and readily available. This information should be included in orientation and in-service programs. It should include policies regarding permissible drug administration and emergency interventions by the nurse.

In addition to preoperative assessment and postoperative evaluation for continuum of care, intraoperative activities include determining and documenting the patient's baseline physiologic status before administration of sedatives, analgesics, and anesthetic drugs and monitoring the patient throughout the procedure. Parameters include, but are not limited to:

1. Blood pressure
2. Heart rate and rhythm
3. Respiratory rate
4. Oxygen saturation by pulse oximetry
5. Body temperature
6. Skin condition and color
7. Mental status and level of consciousness

Vital signs are taken before injection of a drug and at 5- to 15-minute intervals after injection. Changes in the patient's condition must be reported to the surgeon immediately. If an adverse reaction occurs, emergency measures should be instituted on request as per policy.

These may include maintaining a patent airway, starting oxygen therapy when clinically indicated, and/or administering IV therapy.

COMPLICATIONS OF LOCAL AND REGIONAL ANESTHESIA

Minor or transient complications of local and regional anesthesia are common. Serious complications, although rare, are usually permanent. They may be caused by a damaging mechanical effect of needles or a pharmacologic effect of the drug administered. As with general anesthesia, the prevention of complications requires patient assessment and preparation, knowledge of anatomy and physiology, and attention to detail. Proper choice of drug, equipment, and constant monitoring are as necessary in local and regional anesthesia as in general anesthesia. Complications of local and regional anesthesia may be summarized briefly as local effects, systemic effects, and effects unrelated to the anesthetic drug.

Local Effects

Tissue trauma, hematoma, ischemia, drug sensitivity, and infection can be minimized by use of proper drugs and equipment, sterile technique, avoidance of addition of vasoconstrictor drugs to local anesthetics in injection sites of impaired circulation (digits, penis), and avoidance of repetitive needling that promotes trauma, tissue necrosis, and infection.

Systemic Effects

Systemic effects are primarily cardiovascular, neurologic, or respiratory, for example, hypotension, convulsion, or respiratory depression. Drug interactions also are systemic. Following high blood levels, toxicity that affects more than one system may occur. Blood levels depend on the amount of drug used, its physical characteristics, presence or absence of vasoconstrictors, and the injection site. For example, because of vascularity of surrounding tissue, intercostal block produces higher anesthetic blood levels in a shorter time than axillary or epidural blocks. Absorption and blood level of drugs are related to their uptake and rate of removal from circulation. A linear relationship exists between the amount of drug administered via a given route and the resultant peak anesthetic blood level.

Predisposing Factors

True hypersensitivity that produces an allergic response can occur, but it is less frequent than reactions from overdosage of pharmacologic agents (see Chapter 19, p. 362).

1. *Immunologic sensitization.* Allergies are thought to be more common with the amino esters than the amide group of compounds. Allergy to the preservative in some solutions, such as epinephrine, also is possible. Some local anesthetics release histamine, which is the basis of an allergic response. True allergy, mediated by antigen-antibody reaction, can cause anaphylaxis, urticaria (skin wheals), dermatitis, itching, laryngeal edema, and possibly cardiovascular collapse.
2. *Overdosage.* An excessive amount of drug may enter the bloodstream if the injection exceeds maximum dose or is absorbed too rapidly. The IV route is the most dangerous route of injection because histamine is released into the systemic circulation. Injection site is also pertinent. Hazardous sites involve vascular areas of tracheobronchial mucosa, and tissues of the head, neck, and paravertebral region. The least hazardous areas are subcutaneous tissue of the extremities and trunk (abdominal wall and buttocks).

Precautions

Extraordinary precautions must be taken for a patient with history of any allergies, hypersensitivities, or reactions to previous anesthetics or other drugs. Atopic individuals, those with a hereditary tendency or with multiple allergies, may be more prone to adverse reactions to anesthetics or other drugs. Prediction of allergic reactions is unreliable. If testing for sensitivity to specific drugs is done, it is executed cautiously under well-controlled conditions.

Precautions for preventing adverse drug reactions in all patients include:

1. Assessing patient's preoperative physiologic and psychologic condition to determine potential problems and abnormal stress responses:
   a. Identify all medications patient has recently received or is currently taking, including history of substance abuse.
   b. Question patient about known or suspected previous drug reactions. Any chemically related drug is not given.
   c. Help patient cope with anxiety and fears by giving preoperative instructions and answering questions.
2. Handling drugs with care. *Before administering or placing drugs on sterile table:*
   a. Read label correctly. Check expiration date.
   b. Discard ampule or vial if label is not completely legible or has been disturbed.
   c. Observe solution for clarity and discard any suspicious ampule or vial.
3. Administering drugs selected by a physician in appropriate concentrations and dosages for anesthesia and IV conscious sedation:
   a. Give minimal effective concentration and smallest volume needed. Adjust precise amount to weight of patient as appropriate.

b. Limit total amount of drug injected or applied to prescribed safe limits. Sterile single-dose ampules and prefilled syringes are recommended.
c. Inject slowly to retard absorption and avoid overdosage. Use incremental titration of drug.
d. Pull back on syringe plunger frequently while injecting tissues to be sure solution is not entering a blood vessel inadvertently. Intravascular injection of anesthetic drug can release histamine into the systemic circulation, causing an anaphylactoid (nonimmunologic) reaction.
e. Exercise caution with drugs that depress respiratory or cardiovascular functions, such as sedatives, when upper dose limit of anesthetic drug is used.
f. Provide continuous IV access for administering drugs for IV conscious sedation or adverse reactions. An IV lifeline should be established in case of adverse reaction or inadvertent intravascular injection or bolus of anesthetic. A heparin lock device or infusion of IV fluids may be used to maintain continuous access.
g. Cease administration of drug immediately at the sign of any sensitivity.
h. Record dosage, route, time, and effects of all drugs or pharmacologic agents used.

4. Monitoring patient continuously (see section on monitoring of local anesthesia patient, p. 355):
   a. Observe patient, including facial expressions, and note responses to conversation and state of alertness.
   b. Monitor high-risk patient by electrocardiogram, in addition to blood pressure, for sudden dysrhythmia indicative of impaired cardiovascular function. Electrocardiograph should be in the room whenever IV conscious sedation is administered; it may be used routinely.
   c. Know resuscitation measures and be able to assist or initiate them as necessary, as per institutional policies and procedures.

Symptoms of Systemic Reactions

Symptoms may be those of CNS stimulation or depression or stimulation followed by depression and collapse. The cardiovascular system seems more resistant than the CNS to toxic effects of local anesthetics. The seizure threshold may differ enormously in individual patients, as may the relationship of dose to symptoms of CNS action. For example, lidocaine usually produces drowsiness before a convulsion, whereas bupivacaine may cause sudden seizure, disorientation, decreased hearing ability, paresthesias, muscle twitching, or agitation in a wide-awake patient without premonitory signs. Hypercapnia or hypoxemia from hypoventilation lowers the seizure threshold. Toxicity of local anesthetics is manifested primarily by CNS effects resulting from high blood levels.

1. *Stimulation:* talkativeness, restlessness, incoherence, excitation, tachycardia, bounding pulse, flushed face, hyperpyrexia, tremors, hyperactive reflexes, muscular twitching, focal or grand mal convulsions
2. *Depression:* drowsiness; disorientation; decreased hearing ability; stupor; syncope; rapid, thready pulse or bradycardia; apprehension; hypotension; pale or cyanotic moist skin; coma
3. *Other signs:* nausea, vomiting, dizziness, blurred vision, sudden severe headache, precordial pain, extreme pulse rate or blood pressure change, angioneurotic edema (wheeze, laryngeal edema, bronchospasm), rashes, urticaria, severe local tissue reaction

Systemic reactions or undesired effects of IV conscious sedation may include slurred speech, agitation, combativeness, unarousable sleep, hypotension, hypoventilation, airway obstruction, and apnea. Other symptoms may be related to specific drugs.

1. *Benzodiazepines and sedatives* may cause somnolence, confusion, diminished reflexes, depressed respiratory and cardiovascular function, and coma. Nystagmus (involuntary eye movements), which may be normal with large doses of diazepam (Valium), may be an abnormal reaction with other drugs.
2. *Opioids* (narcotics) may cause nausea and vomiting, hypotension, and respiratory depression.

Treatment

Treatment is aimed at preventing simultaneous respiratory and cardiac arrest. Treatment must be prompt. *Time is of the essence.* Administration of the agent thought to produce the reaction is stopped immediately (when possible) at the first indication of reaction. Therapy is generally supportive, the specifics dictated by clinical manifestations. *Treatment* consists of:

1. Maintaining oxygenation of vital organs and tissues with ventilation by manual or mechanical assistance to give 100% oxygen with positive pressure. Tracheal intubation may be indicated.
2. Reversing myocardial depression and peripheral vasodilation before cardiac arrest occurs. Patient is supine with legs elevated. IV fluid therapy is begun and a vasoconstrictor drug may be given intravenously or intramuscularly for hypotension or a weak pulse, which are signs of progressive circulatory depression. Choice of vasopressor is suggested by symptoms and the drug is used with caution. Drugs that may be used include:
   a. *Epinephrine (IV)* counteracts hypotension, bronchoconstriction, and laryngeal edema. It also stimulates beta- and alpha-adrenergic receptors

and inhibits further release of mediators. It increases arteriolar constriction and force of heartbeat. When appropriate, application of a tourniquet or subcutaneous injection of epinephrine in area of drug injection may delay absorption of toxic drug.

b. *Ephedrine* and other *vasoconstrictors* such as phenylephrine (Neo-Synephrine) or mephentermine (Wyamine) cause peripheral vasoconstriction, increased myocardial contraction, and bronchodilatation.
c. *Antihistamines* block histamine release but are not generally advocated.
d. *Steroids* enhance the effect of epinephrine and inhibit further release of histamine. Effect is not immediate, and use is directed toward late manifestations of allergic response.
e. *Isoproterenol* (Isuprel) is used predominantly in asthma and heart attack; it is a bronchodilator.

3. Giving antagonist drug in situations in which causative agent is identified.
4. Stopping muscle tremors or convulsions if they are present since they constitute hazard of further hypoxia, possibility of aspiration, bodily injury. Diazepam in 5 mg doses or a short-acting barbiturate is given intravenously to inhibit cortical irritation.

NOTE In patients in whom the adverse response is caused by hypersensitivity, the previous measures are applicable. However, aminophylline may be administered to help alleviate bronchospasm, hydrocortisone (IV) to combat shock, and sodium or potassium iodide (IV) to reduce mucosal edema.

The perioperative nurse who is monitoring the patient must know resuscitation measures and be able to assist in or initiate them when necessary. An emergency cart (see Chapter 19, pp. 402-403) with emergency resuscitative drugs and a defibrillator should be immediately available to the room where IV conscious sedation is administered. The following equipment should be *in the room* ready for use:

1. Oxygen and positive pressure breathing device (e.g., Ambu bag and mask)
2. Oral and nasopharyngeal airways and endotracheal tubes in an assortment of sizes
3. Suction

Unrelated Effects

A nerve deficit, such as pain or neuritis, that occurs in the postoperative period may be related to a preexisting condition such as multiple sclerosis. Alternatively, it may be from a cause unrelated to the anesthetic drug, such as faulty positioning; trauma from retractors; tourniquet inflated for inordinately long period, resulting in ischemia or pressure on peripheral nerves; or improperly applied cast. Less common causes involve bleeding around the nerve or reaction to epinephrine.

ALTERNATIVES TO ANESTHESIA

When local or regional anesthesia may be contraindicated but consciousness is desirable, acupuncture or hypnoanesthesia may offer alternative methods to control pain. An altered state of awareness of painful stimuli may be advantageous in selected patients.

Hypnoanesthesia

Hypnoanesthesia refers to hypnosis used as a method of anesthesia. Hypnosis produces a state of altered consciousness characterized by heightened suggestibility, selective wakefulness, reduced awareness, and restricted attentiveness. Although hypnosis has a long history of misuse, modern application by highly trained medical specialists is humane. Hypnoanesthesia, although rarely used, has been successfully employed in adult and pediatric patients. Motivation is an important factor. The method may be combined with the use of a small dose of a chemical anesthetic or muscle relaxant drug. *It must not be used indiscriminately in place of standard treatment.*

Hypnosis may be used as a therapeutic aid in *very selected* patients:

1. When chemical agents are contraindicated. The patient may be kept pain free, asleep or awake, without toxic side effects
2. When of value as an adjunct to chemical anesthesia to decrease amount of anesthesia needed
3. When it is desirable to free the patient from certain neurophysical effects of an anesthetic
4. When anxiety and fear of anesthesia are so great as to contribute to serious anesthetic risk
5. When posthypnotic suggestion may be valuable in the postoperative period
6. When it is desirable to raise the pain threshold
7. When it is desirable to have the patient respond to questions or commands

Hypnoanesthesia is advantageous for burn dressings and debridement and for patients with severe respiratory or cardiovascular disease or multiple drug allergies. The anesthesiologist must establish rapport with the patient preoperatively so the patient will listen to and obey hypnotic commands. Hypnosis is a time-consuming method and is unreliable as compared with chemical anesthesia.

Acupuncture

The ancient Chinese art of acupuncture has been practiced for more than 5000 years. Its acceptance by Western medical practitioners is fairly recent, however. *Acupuncture* is a technique of providing intense stimulation at meridian points, or planes of energy. This stimulation prompts the brain to release endorphins that can relieve pain.

Stimulation is effected by manually rotating—or applying electric current to—very fine-gauge needles inserted into meridian points. When acupuncture is used for anesthesia, a minute electric current is used to speed and enhance analgesia or anesthesia in the desired body region. The meridian point(s) generally corresponds to the area where the somatic nerve supply is located. It is a time-consuming technique. It may be used immediately after premedication is given to reduce postoperative nausea and vomiting following short procedures under general anesthesia.

Acupuncture has had limited use in surgical and dental procedures and for postoperative or intractable pain. The patient remains conscious. Procedures should be limited to use by physicians or under their direct supervision in keeping with acceptable standards of medical practice.

Bibliography

Benz JD: Injectable local anesthetics, *AORN J* 55(1):274-284, 1992.

Hinzmann CA et al: Intravenous conscious sedation use in endoscopy: does monitoring of oxygen saturation influence timing of nursing interventions? *Gastroenterol Nurs* 15(1):6-13, 1992.

Kendall F: Documenting local anesthesia patient care, *AORN J* 58(4):715-719, 1993.

Lilley LL: Epidural narcotic infusions for the management of postoperative pain, *Point of View* 27(1):4-6, 1990.

Lunow K, Jung L: Practical innovations: comprehensive perioperative care: patient assessment, teaching, documentation, *AORN J* 57(5):1167-1177, 1993.

Murphy EK: OR nursing law: monitoring IV conscious sedation, the legal scope of practice, *AORN J* 57(2):512-514, 1993.

Pasero CL, Vanderveer BL: Pain control: epidural infusions: not just for labor anymore..., *Am J Nurs* 94(12):51-52, 1994.

Patterson P: Criteria for monitoring IV sedation patients, *OR Manager* 8(1):16, 1992.

Position statement on the role of the RN in the management of analgesia by catheter techniques (epidural, intrathecal, intrapleural, or peripheral nerve catheters), *AORN J* 55(1):209-210, 1992.

Position statement on the role of the RN in the management of patients receiving IV conscious sedation for short-term therapeutic, diagnostic, or surgical procedures, *AORN J* 55(1):207-208, 1992.

Proposed recommended practices: Monitoring the patient receiving local anesthesia, *AORN J* 58(2):363-368, 1993. (Adopted in 1994.)

Recommended practices: Monitoring the patient receiving IV conscious sedation, *AORN* J 57(4):978-983, 1993.

Satterlee GB: Perioperative implications of cocaine use, abuse, *AORN J* 53(3):779-789, 1991.

Smith CJ: Preparing nurses to monitor patients receiving local anesthesia, *AORN J* 59(5):1033-1041, 1994.

Watson DS: Clinical issues: safe nursing practices involving the patient receiving local anesthesia, *AORN J* 53(4):1055-1059, 1991.

Watson DS: Pharmacist's corner: safe administration of midazolam, *AORN J* 53(1):162-165, 1991.

Watson DS, James DS: Intravenous conscious sedation, *AORN J* 51(6):1512-1522, 1990.

Wild L, Coyne C: The basics and beyond: epidural analgesia, *Am J Nurs* 92(4):26-34, 1992.

Willins JS: Giving fentanyl for pain outside the OR, *Am J Nurs* 94(2):24-28, 1994.

CHAPTER 19

Patient Monitoring and Potential Complications Related to Anesthesia

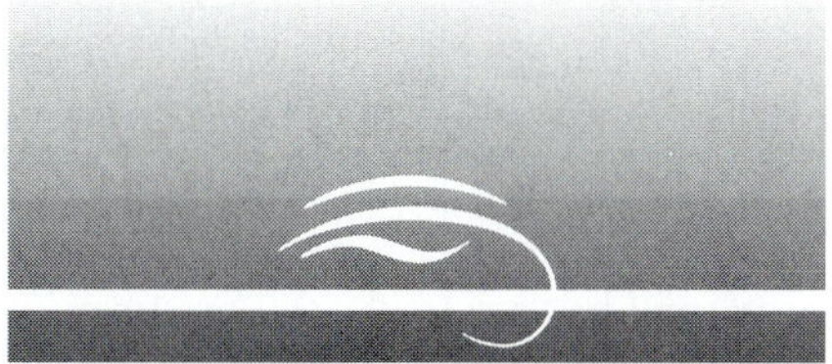

The development of successful, controllable anesthesia has made modern surgery possible. Because anesthesia is an adjunct to most surgical procedures, familiarity with various anesthetic agents, their interaction with certain drugs, and their potential hazards is a necessity. The alert, informed nurse can quietly note onset of complications and help to avert an emergency or fatality.

Working with anesthesiologists in the OR gives the learner an unparalleled opportunity to master immediate resuscitative measures and their effectiveness as well as an understanding of the care of unconscious and critically ill patients. For example, the learner daily observes tracheal intubation, ventilatory control, insertion of arterial and venous cannulae, fluid replacement, sophisticated hemodynamic monitoring, and spinal tap.

No surgical procedure is minor. Surgery and anesthesia impose upon the patient certain inescapable risks, even under supposedly ideal circumstances. Overall, however, the anesthetic-related surgical mortality rate is relatively low. Preexisting patient factors, such as age and/or medical condition, and those related to the circumstances of the surgical procedure, such as type, duration, and elective vs. emergency procedure, are more significant in determining surgical mortality. The greatest hazard of anesthesia is human error. Therefore the American Society of Anesthesiologists has established standards for basic intraoperative monitoring. Specialization in monitoring equipment and utilization of computers to record monitoring data are facets of contemporary anesthesia practice.

DRUG INTERACTIONS

Anesthesiologists and surgeons frequently administer many drugs to patients already under the influence of several different pharmacologic agents when they come to the OR. A substantial number of patients experience some form of adverse drug reaction. Some seriously ill patients may receive as many as 20 drugs concurrently. Modern balanced anesthesia may involve the use of eight or more different drugs, including those used for premedication. Spinal anesthesia, a relatively simple technique, usually involves at least five drugs. All drugs in use must be considered potential "interactors" with some other drug. A simple shift in pH can cause a significant alteration in action, effectiveness, distribution, and excretion of such common drugs as benzodiazepines and local anesthetics. Many drugs used in anesthesia are weak acids (barbiturates) and weak bases (local agents and vasopressors). Advertently or inadvertently the anesthesiologist can modify these physicochemical characteristics and thus alter the effects of drugs.

Many variables modify the action of anesthetic agents, such as dose, circulatory adaptation, ventilation management, effect of time, disease states, or concomitant surgical procedure. In selected patients, regional anesthesia or other techniques may provide better operating conditions and more safety and comfort than general anesthesia.

ADVERSE SYSTEMIC REACTIONS TO ANESTHETICS

Adverse drug reactions occurring during anesthesia and surgery are of concern to both physicians and patients. These reactions are relatively frequent, often severe, and potentially fatal. Reactions increase in ratio to the number of drugs used.

Systemic reactions manifested by symptoms referable to the central nervous system and the respiratory and cardiovascular systems are caused by absorption into the circulation of toxic amounts of local or general anesthetic drugs. The main factors then in producing these reactions are vascular uptake and circulating blood level of the anesthetic. Toxic amounts of drugs can depress peripheral vessels as well as myocardium and medullary centers. Hypoxia leads to cerebral ischemia. Hypotension, apnea, coma, respiratory and circulatory collapse, and cardiac standstill may then result.

Drugs Implicated in Reaction

Many drugs, such as the following, release histamine, which in turn is the basis of allergic response:

1. Barbiturates, used as hypnotics or anesthetics, which frequently cause skin rashes
2. Nonbarbiturates, such as ketamine, which may cause cutaneous eruptions
3. Local anesthetics, which are associated with reactions such as anaphylaxis, urticaria, and dermatitis
4. Adjuncts to anesthesia, such as tranquilizers and neuroleptics
5. Neuromuscular blockers; tubocurarine is the strongest histamine releaser
6. Other agents: nonanesthetic drugs administered during the surgical procedure such as epinephrine, antibiotics, diuretics; acrylic bone cement
7. Blood volume expanders, such as dextran

Predisposing Factors to Reaction

1. Overdosage—an excessive amount of the drug enters the bloodstream.
   a. Inattention to safe maximum dose
   b. Disregard for latent period of onset of anesthesia
   c. Too rapid injection
   d. Too rapid absorption; intravenous is most dangerous route of injection
   e. Inadvertent intravascular injection; although no antigen-antibody reaction, histamine is released to the systemic circulation
2. True hypersensitivity (immunologic sensitization) produces severe allergic responses and anaphylaxis. This can occur following very small or minimal dose. However, it is much less frequently encountered than nonimmunologic (anaphylactoid) reactions from overdosage. True allergy, mediated by antigen-antibody reaction, is accompanied by dermal reactions (such as itching, skin wheals), laryngeal edema, and possibly cardiovascular collapse.
   a. Allergic reactions are classified into four types. The response usually depends on previous exposure to the drug:
      (1) Classic anaphylactic or immediate reaction (usually mediated by immunoglobulin E antibody) with release of histamine within seconds
      (2) Cytotoxic reaction resulting in cell destruction
      (3) Immune complex hypersensitivity (e.g., serum sickness)
      (4) Delayed or cellular type hypersensitivity; at times there is a delay of 24 hours or more before onset of reaction
   b. Magnitude of allergic response is influenced by a number of factors, such as amount of antigen or antibody present and affinity of antibody for antigen. The antigen is exogenous, and the other factors are endogenous, which is the reason for extensive variation in individual susceptibility.
   c. Histamine contracts smooth muscle of bronchioles and large blood vessels, dilates venules, and increases capillary permeability.

Establishing the cause and mechanism for reaction, although difficult, is important in future management of the patient.

MONITORING OF VITAL FUNCTIONS

Concurrently, surgical and anesthesia techniques have become increasingly complex, allowing many critically ill patients, especially at age extremes, to undergo surgical procedures. The anesthesiologist keeps the surgeon instantly informed of important changes in the patient's condition, detected by precision monitoring. *Monitoring* implies keeping track of vital functions. During extensive surgery under anesthesia, the body is subjected to much stress. Bleeding, tissue trauma, potent drugs, large extravascular fluid shifts, multiple transfusions, and surgical position that may inhibit breathing and circulation all contribute to disturbed physiology. These factors can induce significant cardiac dysfunction. To continuously measure the patient's responses to these stresses, clinical evaluation by listening, observing, and feeling is augmented by the use of electronic or mechanical devices. These devices reveal physiologic trends and subtle changes, give warning of an impending dangerous state, and indicate response to therapy. Most of this equipment is expensive, constitutes electrical hazard, and takes up space in the OR. Some OR suites have permanently installed apparatus with concealed wiring and conduits in a glass-enclosed room or area adjoining the operating room. Compact, precise devices with miniaturized circuitry, better visibility, and easier maintenance are incorporated into newer anesthesia machines.

Personnel using electronic monitoring equipment must understand its function, be experienced in its use, and be able to determine equipment malfunction easily. *Instrumentation should augment, not replace, careful observation of the patient.*

Computers improve and expedite analysis of data. They are sophisticated data collection and management tools to assist in physical status assessment, diagnosis, and therapy. Clinical computers vary from single-function devices to complex multifunction, real-time systems that acquire, store, and display data, organize information, and perform calculations.

With monitoring, many aspects of respiratory, cardiovascular, and nervous system functions can be evaluated constantly. Quantitative assessment is provided by periodic specific measurements. This is desirable as anesthetic agents and surgical manipulations may initiate unwanted circulatory and respiratory reflex responses. Most anesthetics are cardiovascular and respiratory depressants. Uncorrected depression can progress to circulatory or respiratory arrest.

The spectrum of monitoring devices is broad. It ranges from noninvasive to invasive. *Noninvasive monitors* do not penetrate a body orifice. Conversely, *invasive monitors* penetrate skin or mucosa, or they enter a body cavity. Some parameters can be measured by both noninvasive and invasive methods. Nursing responsibilities may include assisting with sophisticated hemodynamic monitoring to evaluate the interrelationship of blood pressure, blood flow, vascular volumes, physical properties of blood, heart rate, and ventricular function. Detection of early changes in hemodynamics allows prompt action to maintain cardiac function and adequate cardiac output. Monitoring facilitates rapid, accurate determination of decreased perfusion. It reflects immediate response to therapeutic measures and stress.

Invasive Hemodynamic Monitoring

Hemodynamics is the study of movements of blood. Measurements of cardiac output and intracardiac pressures provide information related to functions of the heart and other major organ systems.

Invasive hemodynamic monitoring uses basic physiologic principles to detect and treat a wide variety of abnormalities. Its purpose is to avoid problems in high-risk patients and to accurately diagnose and treat patients with established life-threatening disorders. It involves direct intravascular measurements and assessments by means of indwelling catheters connected to transducers and monitors. Pressures and forces within arteries and veins are converted to electrical signals by the transducer, a device that transfers energy from one system to another. These electrical signals are then processed and amplified by the monitor into a continuous waveform displayed on an oscilloscope or monitoring screen that reproduces images received via the transducer; or the monitor may digitally display the values. These measurements yield specific information that is otherwise not usually attainable or as accurate. Although these measurements may be pertinent in guiding patient care, they present additional risks because obtaining them requires invasion of the great vessels or heart. The benefits of invasive monitoring must be balanced against the risks.

Various types of equipment, monitors, and catheters are in use. All persons caring for patients with invasive monitors must have knowledge of anatomy and physiology and understanding of the entire monitoring circuit. Every precaution must be taken to ensure patient safety. *Strict adherence to policies and procedures, manufacturer's instructions for use, and sterile techniques is absolutely essential* to minimize complications and misinterpretation of data that could lead to errors in therapy.

Indwelling arterial, venous, and intracardiac catheters permit rapid, accurate assessment of physiologic alterations in high-risk patients. Intravascular access is justified because of the high yield of information with minimal discomfort to patients. But hemodynamic monitoring techniques must not be abused. Cardiac dysrhythmias, thrombosis, embolism, and infection are serious, sometimes fatal complications of intravascular cannulation. Some facilities require the patient to sign an informed consent form before insertion of an invasive catheter.

Cannulation

Intravascular catheters usually are inserted before induction of anesthesia by a physician; a certified registered nurse anesthetist may be permitted to insert some types. They may be inserted percutaneously or by cutdown, depending on type of catheter, intended purpose(s), and location of the vessel to be cannulated. Intracardiac catheters may be placed under fluoroscopic control, or their position may be verified on a chest x-ray film after insertion. In addition to their use in hemodynamic monitoring, intravenous catheters can be used to administer blood, drugs, and nutrients. Catheters may be inserted via vena cava into the right atrium or pulmonary artery through a subclavian, jugular, brachial, or femoral vein or via an antecubital vein.

Intraarterial catheters are inserted for direct pressure measurements and to obtain blood for arterial blood gas analyses. Potential sites for cannulation include the radial, ulnar, axillary, brachial, femoral, and dorsalis pedis arteries. The radial artery is most commonly used if ulnar circulation to the hand is adequate. A Doppler ultrasonic device may be used to determine a dominant artery and to locate a weakly palpable one. When radial artery dominance exists, the ulnar, brachial, or other artery is used. As a precaution, adequacy of perfusion to the extremity below the catheter should be established before insertion, in case thrombosis or occlusion occurs. A radial artery distal to a brachial artery previously used for cardiac catheterization is avoided because of the possibility of distorted pressures or occlusion. Some physicians cannulate the femoral artery if the catheter is to remain in place for more than 24 hours. The incidence of thrombosis is lower when a large vessel is used. Thrombosis may result from irritation of the vessel wall or hypercoagulation or inadequate flushing of the catheter and line. The larger the catheter in relation to the artery lumen, the greater the incidence of thrombosis. Other complications of arterial cannulation include embolic phenomena, blood loss from a dislodged catheter or disconnected line, bruise or hematoma formation, arteriovenous fistula or aneurysm formation, systemic infection, and ischemic fingers from arterial spasm.

Catheters

Most catheters are radiopaque and have centimeter calibrations. They are flexible. They may be made of silicone, polyethylene, polyvinyl chloride, polytetrafluoroethylene (Teflon), or polyurethane. Those with soft, pliable tips are safer than stiff catheters. Shearing of a vessel with extravascular migration of the catheter has occurred from stiffness and sharpness of the catheter and movement of the patient. Soft catheters must be introduced over a guidewire or by flow-directed balloons. The catheter and related introducer, guidewire, and caps may be supplied as a prepackage sterile kit.

Many catheters have a heparin coating to prevent clot formation. Polyurethane or other uncoated catheters are available for the patient who is allergic to heparin. The catheter is kept open with a slow, continuous infusion. Routine flushing of the catheter is mandatory. Normal saline may be used if heparin is unnecessary or contraindicated. Continuous flush devices with fast-flush valves release small amounts of solution. Limited pressure diminishes the possibility of ejecting a large clot. The catheter usually is fast-flushed both hourly and after blood samples are withdrawn. Air bubbles in the line must be avoided. After flushing, check the drip rate in the drip chamber.

A catheter may have a single or multiple lumen. The catheters to be discussed are used for hemodynamic monitoring of:

1. Arterial blood gases and pressure via a single-lumen intraarterial catheter
2. Central venous pressure via a central venous, Hickman, or Broviac catheter
3. Pulmonary artery pressures via a pulmonary artery or Swan-Ganz catheter

Catheter Insertion *This is a sterile procedure.* The necessary sterile supplies should be collected before the patient arrives. Although catheters are different, the technique for insertion is basically the same for all types. Insertion is a team effort. The circulator's responsibilities may vary.

1. Explain the procedure and reassure the patient. If the patient will be awake, sedation may be ordered.
2. Document the patient's vital signs and pulse distal to the selected insertion site. If the pulse weakens after cannulation, circulation may be inadequate in an extremity and the catheter may have to be removed.
3. Position the patient as appropriate.
   a. For radial artery cannulation, affix the forearm to an armboard with the hand supinated and wrist dorsiflexed to an angle of 50 to 60 degrees over a towel. Avoid extreme dorsiflexion; this can obliterate the pulse. Tape the thumb to the armboard to stabilize the artery at the wrist.
   b. For subclavian or jugular vein insertion, place the patient in 25- to 30-degree head-down Trendelenburg's position to reduce the potential for air embolism. Elevate the scapular area with padding or a rolled towel underneath the shoulders to allow the physician to identify anatomic landmarks and locate the vein more easily. Turn the patient's head away from insertion site.
4. Prep the skin per routine procedure. Wearing sterile gloves, the physician then drapes the area. Warn the patient if his or her face will be covered.
5. Inform the patient, if awake, that he or she may have a burning sensation for a few seconds when the local anesthetic is injected before the area be-

comes numb. Explain that he or she may feel pressure, but not pain, during insertion. The skin and subcutaneous tissue are infiltrated with a local anesthetic because the skin is incised to facilitate entrance of the catheter. A cutdown to a vein may be necessary.

6. Assist the physician as appropriate. *Be familiar with and follow the manufacturer's directions for the brand of catheter and monitoring equipment being used.* (See central venous cannulation, pp. 371-372, and pulmonary artery cannulation, pp. 372-373.)
7. Make sure the connections between the catheter and infusion line are secure after the catheter has been inserted and properly placed. The catheter is sutured in place to prevent inadvertent advancement or removal and is taped to the skin. Lumens on the three-way stopcock and catheter may be capped to prevent fibrin deposits and retrograde contamination.
8. Connect the catheter line to the transducer or monitor, and take baseline pressure readings.
9. Dress the puncture site. An antibacterial ointment may be put around site. Tape must not apply pressure directly over the insertion site or catheter. Transparent dressing is preferable. The catheter beneath it must not be bent or curled.
10. Take the patient's vital signs. Using a sphygmomanometer with the blood pressure cuff on the *opposite* arm from the insertion site, check the blood pressure to compare with the monitor's pressure reading to verify the monitor's accuracy. The monitor will probably read higher systolic and lower diastolic pressures than the blood pressure cuff readings.
11. Document the procedure and initial readings. Include the insertion site; type and gauge of catheter; type of infusion solution and amount of heparin, if added; flow rate and pressure; pulse before and after insertion; tolerance of the procedure; color, sensation, and warmth of the area distal to the insertion site; time of insertion; and names of insertion team members.

Frequent checks of circuitry and calibrations are necessary to validate the recorded data. Conscientious attention to every detail is mandatory during catheter insertion and monitoring.

Drawing Blood Samples When the arterial or venous catheters are in place, the circulating nurse may be asked to collect blood samples for analysis or to take measurements, although this is not universal practice. These procedures require special training, skill, and knowledge of equipment and hazards involved.

Samples for arterial blood gas (ABG) measurements are sometimes drawn from an indwelling catheter line kept open by a continuously running infusion. The tubing incorporates a plastic three-way stopcock, usually close to the catheter insertion site. One lumen of the stopcock goes to the infusion solution, one to the cannulated vessel, and one to outside air. The latter is normally closed or covered with a sterile cap, or a sterile syringe is kept inserted in the lumen to prevent bacteria and air from entering. With a three-way stopcock, two of the three lumens are always open.

In drawing blood samples from an indwelling catheter, always *use strict sterile technique.* Blood may be drawn through a stopcock on a single-lumen catheter or from one lumen of a multilumen catheter. A sterile ABG monitoring kit with administration tubing and pressure transducers may be used for intraarterial pressure monitoring. Follow the manufacturer's instructions for turning the stopcock to draw blood samples and to flush lines. Drawing blood from a multilumen catheter is simplified when an injection port can be used. The basic procedure is similar to the following, using a stopcock. *Always wipe the stopcock or end of the catheter with alcohol before entering the system.*

1. Wear sterile gloves. Use sterile *glass* syringes if available. Pulsations can fill a glass syringe without pulling on the plunger. A *heparinized syringe* must be used to prevent the blood samples from clotting. To heparinize, draw 1 ml aqueous heparin 1:1000 into a 10 ml syringe. While rotating the barrel, pull the plunger back beyond the 7 ml calibration. With the syringe in an upright position, slowly eject the heparin and air bubbles while rotating barrel.
2. Attach a sterile 5 ml syringe to the stopcock lumen going to outside air. Turn off (close) the infusion lumen. This automatically opens the line between patient and syringe. Aspirate to clear the line of fluid and close the lumen to patient. Discard this diluted sample.
3. Quickly attach the sterile heparinized syringe to lumen to outside air, and open the lumen to the patient. This closes lumen to the infusion, permitting aspiration of undiluted blood for analysis. Arterial pressure forces blood into the syringe. Withdraw 3 to 5 ml of blood. Hold the barrel as well as the plunger of the syringe to avoid their separation. Cap the syringe for placement in properly labeled specimen bag.
4. Close lumen to the patient and flush the line and stopcock by letting the infusion solution run through them to prevent clot formation inside the catheter wall or stopcock, which could result in arterial embolization.
5. Close and recap the lumen to outside air (being careful not to contaminate the cap), thereby restarting the infusion to the patient. Regulate

the infusion rate with the clamp on the infusion tubing.

6. If air bubbles are in the syringe, remove them. Send the samples *immediately to* the laboratory. If more than 10 minutes elapse between blood drawing and analysis, the analysis cannot be considered accurate. In event of delay, the syringe with blood should be immersed in ice immediately and refrigerated at near-freezing temperature. Iced specimen bags may be used.

Parameters Monitored

Noninvasive methods can be used to monitor some cardiopulmonary and neural functions and to determine body temperature and urinary output (Box 19-1). Both noninvasive and invasive techniques are used for monitoring hemodynamic parameters to show minute-to-minute changes in physiologic variables. See Table 19-1 for normal ranges of hemodynamic parameters.

Electrocardiogram

Every heartbeat depends on the electrical process of polarization. Muscles in the heart wall are alternately stimulated and relaxed. An electrocardiogram (ECG/EKG) is a recording of electrical forces produced by the heart and translated as waveforms (Figure 19-1). It shows changes in rhythm, rate, or conduction such as dysrhythmias, appearance of premature beats, and block of impulses. An ECG does not provide an index of cardiac output. Cardiac monitoring has become standard procedure in the OR and postanesthesia care unit (PACU).

Cardiac monitoring systems generally consist of a monitor screen, a cathode-ray oscilloscope, on which the ECG is continuously visualized, and a printout system, which transcribes the rhythm strip to paper to permit comparison of tracings and provide a permanent record. The printout may be controlled or automatic. A heart-rate meter may be set to print out a rhythm strip if the rate goes below a preset figure. Lights and beepers may provide appropriate visual and audible signals of heart rate. Monitor leads or electrodes (electrically conductive discs or needles) are attached to the chest and/or extremities. These electrodes detect electrical impulses the heart generates. Connecting lead wires and cables transmit them to the cardiac monitor. A complete cardiogram includes 12 different leads, but usually only two or three electrodes are used. Careful placement of leads is important to show waves and complexes on the ECG rhythm strip. Leads to the anterior, lateral, or inferior cardiac surfaces, where ischemia most often occurs, provide myocardial ischemia monitoring. Use of multiple leads allows better definition of dysrhythmia and ischemia, the main reason for cardiac monitoring in the OR. The choice of leads is made by the anesthesiologist or by the surgeon in unattended local anesthesia.

BOX 19-1

Noninvasive Methods of Monitoring Vital Functions

Cardiopulmonary functions:

blood pressure (BP) Measurement of pressure exerted against arterial vessel walls to force blood through circulation

capnometry Measurement of end-tidal concentration of carbon dioxide by exposing expired air to infrared light

cardiac index (CI) Measurement of cardiac output in relation to body surface with ultrasound

chest x-ray study Determination of position of intravascular catheters and endotracheal or chest tubes by radiology

echocardiogram Assessment of intraventricular blood volume by observing two-dimensional color images of the beating heart produced by ultrasonic probe placed in esophagus

electrocardiogram (ECG/EKG) Recording of electrical forces produced by the heart to evaluate changes in rhythm, rate, or conduction

near-infrared reflectance Determination of amount of oxygen in hemoglobin being delivered to brain with a niroscope (NIRS)

pulse oximetry Determination of arterial hemoglobin oxygen saturation by measuring optical density of light passing through tissues

respiratory tidal volume (V_t) Measurement of volume of air moved with each respiration with a respirometer

stethoscopy Detection of cardiac rate and rhythm and pulmonary sounds by auscultation

total blood volume (TBV) Measurement of plasma and red cell volumes with an electronic device

Neural functions:

electroencephalogram (EEG) Recording of electrical activity in the brain

evoked potentials (SEP/SSEP) Recording of electrical reponses from the cerebral cortex after stimulation of a peripheral sensory organ

Temperature Measurement of core body temperature with a thermometer probe

Urinary output Measurement of urine to assess renal perfusion via indwelling catheter attached to calibrated collection device

In *placing disc electrodes,* be sure the underlying skin is clean and dry for *adequate adherence.* Shave the sites if necessary because hair can interfere with adherence. Abrade the skin slightly with a gauze pad or rough material to facilitate conduction. Peel the paper backing off the disc. As much as possible, avoid touching the adhe-

TABLE 19-1
Hemodynamic Monitoring Parameters

PARAMETER	ABBREVIATION	NORMAL RANGE FOR ADULTS
Arterial oxygen content	Cao_2	17-20 ml/dl blood
Blood pressure	BP	Systolic 90-130 mm Hg Diastolic 60-85 mm Hg
Cardiac index	CI	2.8-4.2 L/min/m^2
Cardiac output	CO	4-8 L/min
Central venous pressure	CVP	2-8 mm Hg, 3-10 cm H_2O
Cerebral perfusion pressure	CPP	80-100 mm Hg
Coronary perfusion pressure	CPP	60-80 mm Hg
Ejection fraction	EF	60%-70%
Glomerular filtration rate	GFR	80-120 ml/min
Heart rate	HR	60-100 beats/min
Intracranial pressure	ICP	0-15 mm Hg
Left ventricular end-diastolic pressure	LVEDP	8-12 mm Hg
Mean arterial pressure	MAP	70-105 mm Hg
Mean pulmonary artery pressure	MPAP	9-19 mm Hg
Oxygen saturation in arterial blood	Sao_2	95%-97.5%
Oxygen saturation in mixed venous blood	Svo_2	75%
Partial pressure of carbon dioxide in arterial blood	$Paco_2$	35-45 mm Hg (torr)
Partial pressure of oxygen in arterial blood	Pao_2	80-100 mm Hg (torr)
Partial pressure of oxygen in venous blood	Pvo_2	40 mm Hg (torr)
Pulmonary artery pressure	PAP	Systolic 15-25 mm Hg Diastolic 8-15 mm Hg
Pulmonary capillary wedge pressure	PCWP	6-12 mm Hg
Right atrial pressure	RAP	3-6 mm Hg
Right ventricular pressure	RVP	Systolic 15-25 mm Hg Diastolic 0-5 mm Hg
Stroke volume	SV	60-130 ml/beat
Systemic vascular resistance	SVR	800-1600 dyne/sec/cm
Total blood volume	TBV	8.5%-9% of body weight in kg
Venous oxygen content	Cvo_2	15 ml/dl blood

sive. Check the conductive gel within the gauze pad at the center of the disc. If it is not moist, use another disc. Place the electrode on the desired site, adhesive side down, and secure tightly by applying pressure. Begin at the center and move outward to avoid expressing gel from beneath the electrode.

One ECG tracing is taken before induction of anesthesia as a control. An ECG is especially valuable during induction and intubation when dysrhythmias are prone to occur. Early detection and rapid identification of abnormal rhythms and irregularities of the heart's actions permit treatment to be more specific. Tracings may show changes related to the anesthetic itself or to oxygenation, coronary blood flow, hypercapnia (increased $Paco_2$), or to alterations in electrolyte balance or body temperature. The ECG tracing becomes a flat line when heart action ceases, but preceding tracings may define the type of cardiac arrest, which is of value in treatment. It is beyond the scope of this text to describe normal and abnormal cardiac rhythms interpreted by ECG. However, perioperative nurses who monitor patients under local anesthesia should become familiar with them. Figure 19-2 shows example of sinus rhythms in each of 12 leads. Box 19-2 lists the characteristics of sinus rhythm.

ECG monitors should be insensitive to electrical interference. Occasionally, recording may be affected by a high-frequency electrosurgical unit. If a tracing problem occurs, check lead contacts, integrity of leads, and choice of monitoring axis.

The ECG monitor may be connected to a computer for analysis and storage of data. From the ECG readings, a device within the computer may be able to measure the amount of blood being pumped by the heart. This gives a continuous assessment of pumping capacity and cardiac output, which is useful information during open heart surgery. Impedance cardiography also provides data based on mechanical activity of the heart. This is also a noninvasive, computer-assisted measurement of cardiac output, an alternative to the thermodilution technique described on pp. 373-374.

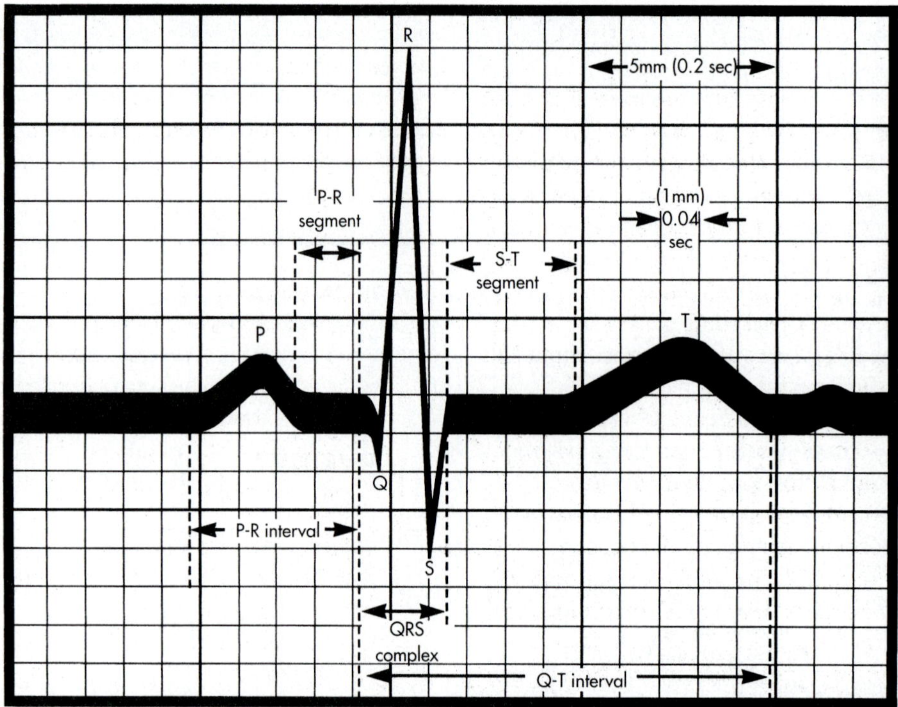

FIGURE 19-1 Electrocardiogram complex. *P wave* before each QRS complex represents atrial depolarization. *P-R interval* of sinus rhythm occurs between each P wave and R wave. *P-R segment* represents conduction of impulse through atrioventricular (A-V) node, bundle of His, bundle branches, and Purkinje's fibers. *QRS complex* following each P wave represents ventricular depolarization and occurs at regular intervals, but rate can vary. *T wave* represents ventricular repolarization.

Echocardiogram

Sound waves from a sonarlike device provide two-dimensional color images of the beating heart. An ultrasonic probe on the end of a small gastroscope is placed in the esophagus. Also referred to as *transesophageal echocardiography,* the echocardiogram can help the anesthesiologist immediately assess intraventricular blood volumes. This can be useful information for the surgeon during cardiac surgery.

Stethoscopy

Auscultation, the act of listening to the chest, detects both cardiac rate and rhythm and pulmonary sounds. A stethoscope is taped over the precordium, the region over the heart and stomach at the level of the diaphragm, or a pressure-sensitive detector may be placed within the patient's esophagus. With the trachea protected by a cuffed endotracheal tube to prevent aspiration, the stethoscope is inserted in the esophagus to the level of the heart. *Esophageal stethoscopy* is especially valuable during thoracic and abdominal procedures, when auscultatory monitoring is ineffective because of tissue manipulation or movements of the members of the operating team.

Arterial Blood Pressure

Blood pressure (BP) signifies the pressure exerted against vessel walls to force blood through the circulation. Evaluation of BP during anesthesia requires consideration of blood volume, cardiac output, and the state of the sympathetic tone of the vessels. Tissue perfusion is dependent on these factors. Arterial BP is used to assess hemodynamic and respiratory status during every surgical procedure, with very few exceptions. BP measures contraction of the heart, *systolic pressure,* and relaxation of heart between contractions, *diastolic pressure.* Blood is forced through the arteries between contractions. Pressure is higher during systole and lower during diastole. Many factors can vary BP. It is measured by millimeters (mm) of mercury (Hg). Normal range is 90 to 130 mm Hg systolic and 60 to 85 mm Hg diastolic.

The arm used for measurements should be opposite the one cannulated for intravenous fluid therapy or in-

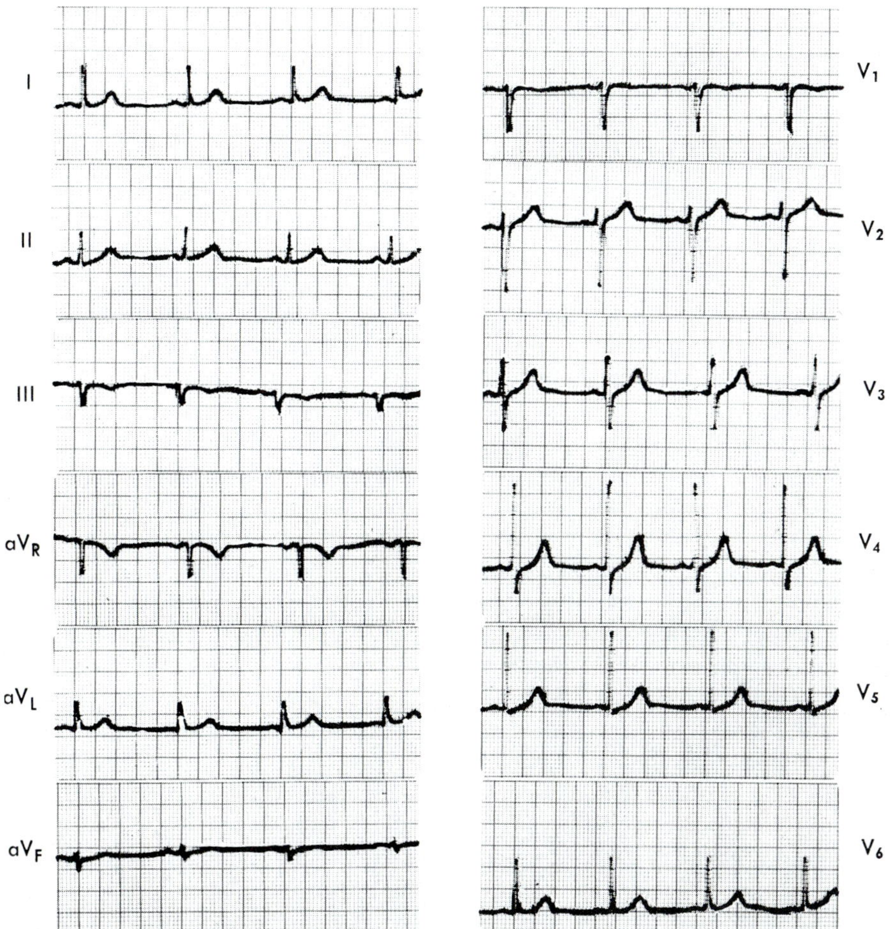

FIGURE 19-2 Example of normal sinus rhythms as they appear in each of 12 leads. (From Kinney MR et al: *Comprehensive cardiac care,* ed 8, St Louis, 1996, Mosby.)

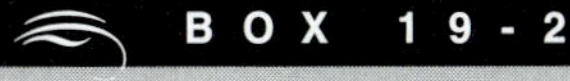

BOX 19-2

Characteristics of Sinus Rhythm

P wave is present before each QRS complex.
There is equal space between P wave and R wave (P-R interval) in each complex.
QRS complex follows each P wave (ratio 1:1).
P wave and QRS complex occur at regular intervals (rate can vary).

vasive monitoring and should be protected from contact with team members standing beside the operating table. Blood pressure can be obtained by indirect or direct methods, either intermittently or continuously.

Sphygmomanometer A pneumatic cuff is wrapped around the circumference of the upper arm. When the cuff is inflated, measurements are obtained on the sphygmomanometer as the cuff deflates. Through a stethoscope placed over an artery distal to the cuff, the systolic pressure is heard when blood begins to flow through the artery. The diastolic pressure is noted by change in sound. This is an indirect, noninvasive method for intermittent monitoring of blood pressure.

Doppler Ultrasonic Flowmeter With ultrasound, BP can be monitored automatically at preset intervals. The Doppler ultrasonic flowmeter monitor automatically inflates the cuff, takes a reading, and deflates the cuff. It can be programmed to sound an alarm if systolic pressure reaches a preset high or low level. The readings are more accurate than with sphygmomanometer pressure cuff monitoring because the ultrasonic transducer amplifies blood flow sounds. Automated, noninvasive BP monitors function well in a noisy environment. However, they do not provide continuous BP measurement nor detect extremely low pressures. Frequent inflations of the cuff can bruise skin, especially of the elderly patient.

Infrared Beams Noninvasive infrared beams (Finapres technique) may be used to indirectly monitor BP. A small cuff fits on a finger. The beams from the cuff shine through tissue. They continuously measure arterial pressure from one heartbeat to the next.

Direct Arterial Pressure From an invasive modality, beat-to-beat direct pressures are obtained through an artery, usually the radial or femoral, via an indwelling catheter inserted percutaneously. A very slow drip of slightly heparinized saline keeps the catheter open. The fluid-filled tubing from the catheter is connected to a mechanical electric transducer. The transducer is attached to an amplifier. A waveform of the amplified pulse, which represents force imposed on the transducer, is displayed. The monitor also converts waveforms into numerical measurements of systolic and diastolic rates. An alarm sounds if deviations are significant.

Mean arterial pressure (MAP), calculated by most monitors and shown on digital display, portrays perfusion pressure of the body. This is significant in evaluating myocardial perfusion. Normal MAP is between 70 and 105 mm Hg. Direct intraarterial pressure monitoring is valuable in patients with major multiple trauma or burns, inaccessibility of an extremity, unstable vital signs, or inaudible BP. Other indications are complex, extensive procedures, such as cardiopulmonary bypass with open chest; major vascular surgery with large potential fluid shifts or blood loss; total hip replacement; and major neurosurgery in the sitting position. Also included are patients in shock or with preexisting cardiac or pulmonary disease who must undergo major surgery. Direct pressure monitoring is mandatory in deliberate hypotensive anesthesia as well as in treatment of hypotensive or hypertensive crisis with continuous infusion of vasopressor or hypertensive drugs.

Blood Gases and pH

Monitoring of tissue perfusion is indispensable in evaluating pulmonary gas exchange and acid-base balance. Measurements are considered in relation to other parameters such as vital signs, venous pressure, and left atrial pressure. Oxygen and carbon dioxide in blood exert their own partial pressures (P). Measurements are expressed in mm Hg or torr. They may be differentiated as arterial (Pa) or venous (Pv). The gas being measured is identified. The partial pressure of oxygen is expressed as PO_2, or specifically in arterial blood as PaO_2 and in venous blood as PvO_2. Oxygen saturation (SO_2) in arterial blood (SaO_2) is expressed in percentage. The partial pressure of carbon dioxide is specified as $PaCO_2$, or $PvCO_2$. See Table 19-1 for normal ranges. Monitoring techniques can be either noninvasive or invasive.

Pulse Oximetry A pulse oximeter measures arterial oxyhemoglobin saturation (SaO_2). It provides a reading within seconds by measuring optical density of light passing through tissues. A sensor probe is clipped on each side of a pulsating vascular bed. Finger, toe, earlobe, and the bridge of the nose are suitable sites. The patient's skin should be clean and dry. An area with fingernail polish should be avoided or the polish removed. Skin integrity under the sensor must be intact. The sensor must be maintained flush with the skin surface and positioned so that the light source and photodetector are in direct alignment. The sensor is attached to an oximeter, which is plugged into a power source. Some power sources are battery-powered. The oximeter may have an earphone adapter and an alarm system.

Wavelengths of red and infrared light pass through tissues from the light source side of the probe. Light is picked up by receptor in the sensor on the opposite side of the tissue. The oximeter continuously calculates the amount of oxygen present in the blood by processing the ratio of red to infrared light absorbed. The presence of oxygen in hemoglobin influences this absorption. A reading below an oxygen saturation of 90% probably signifies developing hypoxia. False readings may occur in cigarette smokers because carbon monoxide can prevent red blood cells from picking up oxygen. These cells may absorb light of the oximeter, however, so the reading may be higher than actual SaO_2. Other factors may influence reliability, such as shielding of the sensor, excessive ambient light, or intravascular dyes.

Niroscope Oxygen reserves in the brain can be assessed with a near-infrared reflectance scope (NIRS), a noninvasive technique. A specific form of infrared light passes through the skull. The portion of light reflected back to sensors outside the skull is measured to determine the amount of oxygen in the hemoglobin being delivered to the brain. The niroscope provides a continuous reading of the brain's oxygen reserves.

Capnometry Changes in exhaled carbon dioxide reflect changes in respiration, circulation, or metabolism. Capnometry measures end-tidal concentration of carbon dioxide. Normal concentration is 38 torr (5%). Carbon dioxide production is in direct relationship to cellular metabolism. Monitoring carbon dioxide can detect onset of inadvertent hypothermia (see pp. 382-383) or malignant hyperthermia (see pp. 383-386). Capnometry, a noninvasive technique, also can detect anesthesia equipment problems, inadvertent esophageal intubation, inadequate neuromuscular blockage, air embolus, or ventilation-perfusion problem.

A mainstream or sidestream adapter is placed in the breathing circuit as close to the face mask as possible so that expired carbon dioxide will approximate alveolar concentration. The analyzer, attached to the adapter, exposes expired air to infrared light. The amount of light absorbed by carbon dioxide determines the end-tidal concentration. A sidestream analyzer can be used to monitor patients receiving local or regional anesthesia by placement of the sampling end of tubing in the patient's nostril or mouth.

A capnographic waveform printout provides data to evaluate respiratory rate and rhythm. Some gas monitors continuously measure carbon dioxide, oxygen, and nitrous oxide parameters of the patient's airway. Digital values are displayed on the monitor.

Optode An optode is an optical fiber inserted through an 18- or 20-gauge radial artery cannula. The tip contains chemicals that react to oxygen, carbon dioxide, and acidity of the blood. The optode is connected to a monitor that generates light through the fiber. The chemicals produce luminosities that vary in intensities for oxygen and carbon dioxide. These are measured. Readings are instantaneously and continuously shown on a digital display. Precautions must be taken to maintain sterile technique with this equipment as for other methods of percutaneous radial artery cannulation.

Direct Arterial Blood Analysis Blood samples may be drawn intermittently, as described on pp. 365-366, from arterial or venous indwelling catheters. Arterial blood gas (ABG) determinations of $Pa{O_2}$, $P{CO_2}$, and $S{O_2}$ monitor adequacy of oxygenation and carbon dioxide elimination. This is especially important in patients requiring mechanical ventilation. Tidal volume, respiratory rate, and concentration of oxygen can be appropriately adjusted. ABG monitoring also permits laboratory analyses of pH, base excess, bicarbonate, and electrolytes to evaluate metabolic processes and acid-base status. Differentiation of respiratory or metabolic acidosis or alkalosis is a guide to appropriate treatment. Samples may be taken also for other analyses, for example, glucose or coagulation factors.

Hypoventilation, uneven ventilation in relation to blood flow, impairment of diffusion, and venous-to-arterial shunting lead to anoxemia unless oxygen in inspired air is increased. Hypoventilation of the whole lung or a major portion leads to retention of carbon dioxide and predisposes the patient to cardiac dysrhythmias. Disturbances of acid-base balance have many serious consequences in many organs. They must be corrected to achieve normal physiologic functioning.

Central Venous Pressure

Because it accurately measures right atrial blood pressure, which in turn images right ventricular blood pressure, central venous pressure (CVP) assesses function of the heart's right side. It measures the pressure under which blood returns to the right atrium. It reflects pressure in the major veins as blood returns to the heart. In other words, CVP represents the amount of venous return and filling pressure of the right ventricle. This information helps determine the patient's circulatory status.

CVP also aids in evaluating blood volume and the relationship between circulating blood volume and the pumping action of the heart, that is, adequacy of volume presented to the heart for pumping. Therefore CVP is a useful guide in blood or fluid administration to avoid circulatory overload in patients having limited cardiopulmonary reserve. Too great or too rapid replacement can cause pulmonary edema. Generally a low CVP indicates that additional fluid can be given safely. CVP may be used during shock or hypotension to judge adequacy of blood replacement. However, CVP is not a measure of blood volume per se or of cardiac output.

Some indications for CVP monitoring are major surgical procedures in patients with preexisting cardiovascular disease; surgical procedures in which large volume shifts are anticipated (e.g., open heart surgery); critically ill patients (e.g., massive trauma); surgical procedures in which venous air emboli are a risk (e.g., craniotomy in sitting position); and rapid administration of blood or fluid.

Although CVP monitoring provides valuable data for assessing adequacy of vascular volume, it only indirectly reflects the function of the left side of the heart. There is no direct relationship between right and left ventricular filling pressures. Because of the distensibility (compliancy) of the pulmonary blood vessels, the lungs can accept a marked increase in blood flow before significant congestion appears. Backup of blood caused by impaired function of the left ventricle and subsequent increase in pulmonary vascular resistance (PVR) may occur before this increased pressure affects the right side of the heart, as exhibited by CVP values. Thus CVP does not correlate with left-sided heart performance in patients with left ventricular dysfunction or pulmonary congestion.

Central Venous Cannulation CVP may be monitored with a single-lumen or multilumen radiopaque catheter. A double- or triple-lumen Hickman or Broviac catheter is used most commonly. The right atrial lumen of a Swan-Ganz pulmonary artery catheter also can be used to obtain CVP readings. The lumens are labeled and color-coded on multilumen catheters.

The catheter is inserted (see pp. 364-365) preferably percutaneously through a subclavian vein. A brachial, external or internal jugular, or femoral vein may be used or, by cutdown, the antecubital vein. If the patient is awake, he or she is asked to bear down (Valsalva maneuver) as the vein is punctured. This increases intrathoracic pressure and counteracts negative pressure from the vein, thus reducing the possibility of air embolism.

The catheter is threaded through the vein and advanced into the superior vena cava or right atrium. This may be done under fluoroscopy, or a chest x-ray film may be taken to verify accurate placement of the catheter tip.

The catheter may be attached to a transducer and monitor. Pressure readings are expressed in millimeters of mercury (mm Hg). The catheter can be attached to a fluid-filled manometer that measures pressure in centimeters of water (cm H_2O). To set up this line, connect the intravenous (IV) solution bag to the tubing; insert the manometer into the line by attaching it to the stopcock between the IV tubing and the extension tubing; run air out of the line and clamp it; and secure the manometer upright to an IV pole. The hub of the catheter lumen is connected to the stopcock. Connections to the three-way stopcock should be taped to prevent inadvertent disconnection and air leaks. Cyclic variations in intracaval venous pressure occur; pressure becomes negative during atrial filling and respiratory inspiration. Sucking of air into the system during negative venous pressure can result in air embolus.

Baseline measurement is taken as soon as the catheter is in place and attached to the monitor. This is also a presumptive check for proper placement of the cannula tip. Because expansion of the lungs increases intrathoracic pressure and deflation decreases it, fluid in the manometer should fluctuate with each breath. To take a CVP reading on the manometer, zero scale must be level with the patient's right atrium. Shut off the lumen of the stopcock to the catheter, allowing the IV fluid to run into the manometer to desired level. Shut off the infusion, and open the catheter. After obtaining the reading, open the infusion lumen to the catheter to keep the line open.

Electronic transducer systems provide continuous monitoring of venous pressure. Continuous monitoring supplies good measurement of the right side of the heart and portrays the trend of heart function that is more valuable than are isolated readings obtained with a manometer. CVP values may vary somewhat, but normal readings range from 2 to 8 mm Hg, or 3 to 10 cm H_2O.

Multilumen central venous catheters provide access for administration of drugs, blood, fluids, and hyperalimentation. Blood can be removed for blood gas analyses or autotransfusion. These catheters also provide access for removal of air embolism.

Pulmonary Artery Pressures

Because a pulmonary artery (PA) catheter measures function of both the right and left sides of the heart, it provides faster, more accurate indication of impending left ventricular failure than does CVP alone. Pressures of the left side of the heart are reflected in pulmonary artery and pulmonary capillary wedge pressures, measured by the PA catheter. This is more sensitive to rapid changes in the cardiovascular system than CVP and more sensitive to the ability of the heart to accommodate fluid loads. Measurement of pulmonary pressures enables precise, rapid assessment of the left ventricle's ability to eject an adequate cardiac output. Continuous evaluation of left ventricular function is extremely important in patients whose left-sided heart dysfunction has a greater direct effect on cardiac output, circulating volume, and respiratory function than impaired right-sided heart function. Data procured include pulmonary artery pressure (PAP), pulmonary capillary wedge pressure (PCWP), right atrial pressure (RAP), and cardiac output (CO) computation. These pressures reveal the hemodynamic status of cardiovascular and pulmonary functions. They also serve as guidelines for administration of fluids, diuretics, or cardiotonic drugs to obtain optimal cardiac output.

Indications for pulmonary artery (PA) monitoring include preexisting cardiac or pulmonary disease in a patient undergoing a major vascular, intraabdominal, or neurosurgical procedure, and a potential risk of development of cardiopulmonary instability from the stress of the surgical procedure. Other conditions may include shock, burns with large fluid shifts, renal failure with low cardiac output, or pulmonary embolism. PA catheters may be used in patients who require long-term monitoring. Some multipurpose catheters may be used with ventricular and atrial pacing wires in patients with heart block or severe bradycardia. These catheters may be used to measure CO in patients with intracardiac shunts or during titrated drug administration.

Contraindications to invasive pulmonary catheter monitoring are abnormal cardiac anatomy in the patient, as well as inadequate monitors or lack of personnel trained in their use.

Pulmonary Artery Cannulation Various PA catheters are available. The number of lumens vary from two to five, depending on the range of functions desired. These catheters are used with transducers for monitoring. The type of transducer varies according to the balloon flotation device in the catheter.

To set up the monitoring system, the manufacturer's instructions must be followed explicitly. Check all equipment, including the oscilloscope. Attach the stopcocks and flush devices in the lines to the transducer head(s). Preassembled tubing systems and disposable transducer domes are commercially available. If the patient also will have a peripheral arterial line, two transducers and a triple stopcock manifold are needed. Simultaneous monitoring of PA and RAPs is thus possible. Backflush the transducer dome. The monitor should be balanced and calibrated according to the manufacturer's directions. *Be sure no air bubbles remain in the lines or system.*

Before insertion, the physician inspects the catheter for defects and tests the balloon for leakage by inflating it, submerging it in sterile saline solution, and watching for air bubbles. The balloon must then be deflated. Moistening the catheter tip with saline solution or lidocaine reduces possibility of venospasm at insertion.

Vital signs are taken before insertion of the catheter. An ECG oscilloscope should be monitored for dysrhythmias during insertion. With the introducer set, the catheter is inserted and advanced rapidly to prevent kinking or knotting. It is advanced through the vein into the inferior or superior vena cava and on into the right atrium. Continued manipulation irritates or damages vessel walls. Watching the increment markings on the side helps determine how far the catheter has advanced. It is possible to keep pushing the catheter while it is not going into the right place. It can coil up and knot in the ventricle.

When the catheter tip reaches the *right atrium* (RA) and an RA waveform appears on the oscilloscope screen or readout strip, the balloon is inflated slowly with air with a tuberculin syringe to enable it to float with the flow of blood. *The balloon is never inflated without a visible oscilloscope trace.* If the patient is awake, a voluntary cough confirms the position of the catheter in the thoracic cavity if the RA wave fluctuates. *The amount of air is specified by the manufacturer* (usually about 1.3 to 1.5 ml). Overinflation could rupture the balloon. Carbon dioxide is used for balloon inflation in patients with intracardiac shunts. If balloon ruptures in arterial criculation, carbon dioxide is more soluble than ambient (room) air in blood. A feeling of resistance should accompany inflation. Absence of resistance is a sign of a ruptured balloon; inflation should be stopped immediately. Fluid is *never* used for inflation because it would prevent proper catheter flotation and complete deflation.

Passing through the tricuspid valve, the catheter enters the *right ventricle* (RV). A typical RV waveform should appear. If dysrhythmia develops or is persistent, a bolus of lidocaine may be injected. Then after the catheter floats through the pulmonary semilunar valve into the *pulmonary artery,* a PA tracing should appear on the monitor. This waveform has a steep upstroke at the beginning from right ventricle ejection and opening of the pulmonic valve, followed by a dicrotic notch on the downstroke at closing of the pulmonic valve. PA blood flow carries the balloon into one of the artery's smaller branches. When the vessel diameter becomes too narrow for it to pass, the balloon wedges in the vessel and occludes it. A PCWP waveform should appear. After recording of this wedge pressure, the physician permits the balloon to deflate passively; air is not aspirated with the syringe. The catheter will then slip back into the main branch of the PA. A PAP waveform should reappear on the monitor. Thus the physician depends on these sequential characteristic pressure waveforms to reveal the catheter tip's location *at all times.* The circulator records pressure at each location. *The catheter remains in the pulmonary artery with the balloon deflated, continuously recording PA pressures, except when PCWP reading is desired.* If a PAP waveform persists and a PCWP is unobtainable or if resistance is not felt at an attempt to inflate the balloon, it may be that the balloon is ruptured. An x-ray film is taken to confirm the catheter position. In case of rupture, the catheter may be left in place to record PAP, provided that it has not slipped back to the right ventricle. The physician may also elect to remove it. *The balloon is always inflated during catheter advancement and deflated during catheter withdrawal.*

To prevent an air embolus after catheter insertion, the catheter must not be attached to the monitoring system until all air has been expelled. Check all lines and transducers for secure connections and patency. Each transducer's balancing port must be leveled with the patient's right atrium. Right atrial, pulmonary artery, pulmonary capillary wedge pressures and waveforms, as well as the patient's response to the procedure, must be documented.

Swan-Ganz Thermodilution Catheter The No. 7 Swan-Ganz thermodilution catheter has four separate lumens or passages within its outside wall. It is versatile and widely used. It is 110 cm (43¼ inches) long, with 10 cm increments marked on the side to permit observation of how far the catheter has advanced during insertion. Like all PA catheters, it is a balloon-tipped flotation catheter that is inserted into a major vein and advanced to the inferior or superior vena cava. When inflated, the thin latex balloon at the tip permits the catheter to float with the flow of blood through the right atrium, tricuspid valve, right ventricle, pulmonary semilunar valve, and pulmonary artery, and to wedge in a small PA branch (arteriole) for recording PCWP during occlusion of the vessel. When the balloon is not inflated, the catheter lies in the pulmonary artery to record PA pressures. It is essential to achieve proper catheter placement to minimize the risk of vessel damage and complications as well as to validate pressure readings.

The end of the catheter inserted in the patient is referred to as the distal end; the opposite one is the proximal end. The latter comprises the lumen ports or external openings. The PA port is used for monitoring PAP and PCWP. A syringe is connected to the balloon port for the desired balloon inflation. The thermistor port is used for cardiac output calculation. The right atrial port is used for measuring right atrial pressure. This port also can be used to administer fluids or can be connected to a flush system for maintenance of catheter patency. For cardiac output measurement (see pp. 375-376), normal saline or dextrose solution is injected into the cardiovascular system via the proximal lumen. The pulmonary artery and right atrial ports should be labeled.

The catheter has four separate lumens or passages. The *pulmonary artery lumen,* the largest and most distal, terminates in the opening at the catheter's tip. With proper catheter positioning, this opening lies in the pulmonary artery. In this position with the balloon deflated, PA systolic, diastolic, and mean pressures are recorded on the monitor. These are indicative of pulmonary function. When the balloon is inflated and the catheter migrates to a PA branch to wedge, PCWP is recorded. PCWP is sometimes referred to as PAWP (pulmonary artery wedge pressure) or PAOP (pulmonary artery occlusion pressure). Occlusion of a PA branch creates a no-flow system, thereby blocking blood flow from the right side of the heart to the lungs and permitting pressure equilibration in the pulmonary vascular bed distal to the catheter. Occlusion of an arteriole and low resistance of the pulmonary systems give a pressure measurement equal to the left atrial pressure, which in turn is equal to left ventricular end-diastolic pressure. *To prevent pulmonary infarction, ischemia, or hemorrhage from prolonged wedging, the balloon is always deflated immediately after a reading is taken.* The catheter will float back into the main pulmonary artery. The PA lumen can provide blood samples for blood gas measurements and mixed venous blood, which is also of value in judging cardiac function.

The *balloon lumen* opening, permitting inflation and deflation, is about 1 cm from the catheter tip. When inflated, the balloon surrounds but does not cover the opening in this tip.

The *thermistor lumen* opening is about 4 cm from the catheter tip. This lumen contains temperature-sensitive wires that run its length and transmit the temperature of blood flowing over them from the thermistor to the computer used to determine cardiac output by the thermodilution technique (see pp. 375-376).

The proximal *right atrial lumen* opening is about 30 cm from the catheter's tip. This opening lies in the right atrium to monitor right atrial pressure when the catheter is in place.

Interpretation of Pressures The range of normal pressure values may vary slightly from one authority to another. Characteristic waveforms appear on the oscilloscope or screen, depending on the location of the catheter tip during insertion and continuous monitoring. *These waveforms must be watched carefully to ascertain that the catheter is in the desired position.* The catheter enters the right atrium via the vena cava.

RIGHT ATRIAL PRESSURE (RAP) Normal RAP is 3 to 6 mm Hg. RAP reflects right atrial filling diastolic pressure, equivalent to central venous pressure and right ventricular end-diastolic pressure (RVEDP), pressure at the end of filling just before contraction. Rise in the right atrial pressure may indicate right or left ventricular failure, volume overload (hypovolemia), or air embolism. Fall in RAP may indicate vasodilation, hypovolemia, or peripheral blood pooling.

RIGHT VENTRICULAR PRESSURE (RVP) Normal RVP is 15 to 25 mm Hg systolic, 0 to 5 mm Hg diastolic. Rise in the right ventricular pressure may indicate mitral insufficiency, congestive heart failure, hypoxemia, or left ventricular failure.

PULMONARY ARTERY PRESSURE (PAP) Normal PAP is 15 to 25 mm Hg systolic, 8 to 15 mm Hg diastolic; the mean is 9 to 19 mm Hg. These pressures estimate venous pressure in the lungs as well as mean filling pressure of the left atrium and left ventricle. They reflect right ventricular function unless the patient has pulmonary stenosis, because commonly the PA systolic pressure approximates the right ventricular systolic pressure. Changes in PA systolic and mean pressures indicate changes in pulmonary vascular resistance. Alterations in pulmonary vascular resistance (PVR) occur in hypoxemia, respiratory insufficiency, pulmonary edema, pulmonary embolism, shock, or sepsis. Thus these pressures are indices of pulmonary function. Rise in PAP may indicate left ventricular failure, increased pulmonary arteriolar resistance as present in pulmonary hypertension and hypoxia, or fluid overload.

PULMONARY CAPILLARY WEDGE PRESSURE (PCWP, PAWP, PAOP) Normal pressure is 6 to 12 mm Hg. PA diastolic pressure and PCWP are prime determinants of function of the left side of the heart because they reflect end-diastolic pressures in the left ventricle just before it contracts (LVEDP), except in patients with mitral valve impairment.

Normally, when the mitral valve between the right atrium and right ventricle is open (ventricular diastole), flow of blood from the pulmonary artery to the pulmonary veins and left side of the heart is unimpeded. Then pressures throughout the pulmonary circulation and left side of the heart are comparable. Because PCWP usually approximates left atrial pressure, an indicator of left heart function, it is an important determinant of left ventricle preload. Intraoperative monitoring PCWP usually can give early disclosure of left ventricular dysfunction. Rise in PCWP may indicate left ventricular failure, mitral insufficiency, pulmonary hypertension, fluid overload, or pulmonary congestion. A rise also may occur during anesthesia induction. A fall in PCWP may indicate a reduction in LVEDP and cardiac output, or hypovolemia.

Complications of Pulmonary Artery Catheter Monitoring Invasion of the great vessels and heart carries many inherent perils. Probably the most common one during insertion is cardiac dysrhythmia, especially premature contractions. Other problems include local or systemic infection (septicemia, endocarditis), thrombus formation, pulmonary embolism, pulmonary infarction, pneumothorax, hemothorax, major vessel or heart chamber perforation, kinking or knotting of the catheter, balloon rupture, postoperative bleeding, or erroneous diagnosis from misinterpretation of data.

Although rare, PA perforation is very serious. Predisposing factors are pulmonary hypertension, anticoagulation, hyperthermia, or an overinflated balloon or catheter. Hemoptysis and sudden hypotension are symptoms of PA rupture. Equipment for endobronchial intubation, chest tube insertion, and surgical intervention must be available.

Complications that are potentially life-threatening increase markedly after 48 to 72 hours of indwelling catheterization. The physician must be notified of any change in patient status. *Catheter withdrawal* is performed by and at the discretion of a physician. To prevent injury to the heart valves, the balloon is slightly inflated until the catheter is withdrawn to the right atrium. Then the balloon is completely deflated for withdrawal. Dysrhythmias may occur. Pressure is applied to the insertion site to prevent bleeding. Pulse and BP are checked before and after withdrawal. A postwithdrawal dressing is applied. The patient is monitored for at least 24 hours.

In addition to patient problems, *monitoring problems* may arise. Each requires a specific intervention. A major problem is a damped pressure or PAP waveform. This means decreased amplitude in pressure tracings or loss of sharpness in the image that suggests a defect in the circuit. Common causes are air in the system or blood in the transducer; loose connections; a kinked, overwedged or malpositioned catheter; falling systolic pressure in the patient; or a clot in the monitor system. If the latter is suspected, gently try to aspirate blood. If no blood can be aspirated, do *not* flush. Flushing could dislodge a clot. Notify the physician, who may withdraw the catheter.

Another problem involves sudden change in configuration of a pressure tracing. Potential causes include transducer not at the RA level, transducer in need of calibration, transducer connection to the catheter not secure, catheter no longer in proper position, or loss of pressure in the pressure bag. If a PCWP waveform persists after a reading, the balloon may not be completely deflated or the catheter tip may be caught in the wedge position, requiring immediate attention. Circulators must be familiar with the appropriate interventions in both patient problems and monitoring problems, in addition to being knowledgeable about the causes and preventive measures. Only in this way can patient safety be maximized in invasive monitoring.

Cardiac Output

Cardiac output (CO) is measured by the *thermodilution technique* to determine liters per minute of blood pumped by the left ventricle into the aorta. Normal resting value is 4 to 8 L per minute. A known amount of fluid at a known temperature is injected into a lumen of an arterial catheter, and a temperature gradient at a point downstream is measured via a second lumen. Iced cold or room-temperature physiologic saline solution or 5% dextrose in water (10 ml) usually is used. Blood flow supplies the thermal dilution; for example, saline mixes with blood in the superior vena cava or right atrium, depending on catheter location, reducing the temperature of blood in the heart. The cooled blood flows past a transistorized intravascular thermistor in the thermodilution catheter that detects changes in blood temperatures that are then used to compute CO. When the solution is injected via the proximal RA lumen of a PA Swan-Ganz catheter, a digital display of CO is seen within 4 to 5 seconds.

Cardiac output reflects the mechanical activity of the heart and represents total blood flow to all tissues and vascular shunts. It depends on rate of heartbeat, contractile strength of heart muscle (myocardial contractility), peripheral resistance of vessels, and venous return. Inotropic agents such as digitalis or epinephrine increase contractility and CO except in patients with loss of functioning ventricular muscle, for example, after myocardial infarction or an aneurysm of the left ventricle. Agents such as beta blockers decrease the work of the heart by reducing contractility and CO. Calculation of the *left ventricular stroke work index* reflects pumping ability. During systole the ventricle does not totally eject the blood received during diastole. The amount of blood ejected with each contraction is referred to as the *stroke volume (SV)*. Normal resting SV is 60 to 130 ml/beat. Determinants of stroke volume are left atrial pressure, afterload, contractile state of the myocardium, and left ventricular end-diastolic pressure. *Ejection fraction (EF)*, a commonly used indicator of ventricular function, is the percentage value of stroke volume. Normal EF is 60% to 70%. Major stroke volume determinants of cardiac output are preload, contractility, and afterload. Only in limited circumstances does adjustment of heart rate therapeutically enhance cardiac output.

Preload, the amount of blood in the ventricle at the end of diastole, may be referred to as *left ventricular end-diastolic volume (LVEDV) or filling pressure (LVEDP)*. Assessment of changes in volume by measurement of changes in filling pressure helps to describe cardiac function. The Starling principle concerns the relationship between volume, stretch, and contractility. It relates myocardial fiber length to the force of the contraction. The greater the preload and stretch of myocardial fibers, the greater the subsequent contraction, thereby increasing stroke volume until at some point ventricular failure commences. Fiber overstretch weakens contractions. As the pumping ability decreases, the left ventricle is unable to empty completely. Residual blood, combined during diastole with incoming oxygenated blood from the pulmonary veins and left atrium, increases workload and elevates the left ventricular volume and pressure. As ventricular efficiency declines, cardiac output falls. Unpumped blood in the left ventricle backs up into the left atrium and pulmonary circulation, increasing these pressures. Pulmonary edema and respiratory insufficiency result as fluid is impelled into the alveoli. The CVP catheter measures the right-sided heart preload; the PA catheter measures left atrial and left ventricle end-diastolic pressures.

Cardiac function may be classified as normal, compromised, or failing. In normal hearts, maximum ventricular performance seems to be achieved at 8 to 12 mm Hg filling pressure. In compromised hearts this pressure is higher.

A reduced cardiac output results in decreased perfusion of the capillary circulation. During hemorrhage, when circulating blood volume is reduced, the resulting diminished venous return and preload lead to a lowered cardiac output. Atrial fibrillation also can modify the filling of the ventricles. Venous dilation contributes to pooling of blood, with subsequent decreased venous return to the heart. Low CO states result from reduced preload, as in hypovolemia, venous dilation, or cardiac tamponade; reduced contractility, as from anesthetic drugs, ischemia, infarction, or cardiac decompensation; dysrhythmias; or increased afterload, as in hypertension, pulmonary embolism, or elevated or diminished heart rate. Body position can influence circulation, as can age, body surface area, oxygen consumption, body temperature, basal metabolic rate, and activity. Thus many factors can affect cardiac output.

Afterload indicates the resistance the heart must overcome to eject blood into the systemic circulation. This impedance to flow is called *systemic vascular resistance* (SVR). Left ventricular pressure must exceed pressure in the aorta to open the aortic valve and force blood from the heart into the circulation. Afterload, not a direct measure, is deduced by calculating the SVR. Elevated afterload can produce increased left ventricle wall tension in an attempt to generate adequate intracavitary ventricular pressure to overcome resistance and permit systolic ejection. The subsequent increase in myocardial oxygen demand must be met or ventricular function deteriorates. Diminution of afterload reduces wall tension, thereby improving ventricular contraction. Improving cardiac function involves cost in myocardial oxygen consumption. Augmenting the cardiac output by increasing the heart rate and contractility increases myocardial oxygen consumption. Improving the cardiac output by augmenting preload or by reducing afterload results in relatively little oxygen cost to the myocardium.

A comprehensive view of cardiac function can be obtained by measurements of filling pressure, cardiac output, and calculation of peripheral resistance. Repeated measurements offer evaluation of treatment.

Cardiac Index The cardiac index (CI) assesses the heart's ability to provide the body's need for oxygen and other nutrients. With noninvasive ultrasound, CI measures cardiac output in relation to body surface. A CI less than 2 L of blood per minute per square meter of body surface identifies high risk for untoward cardiovascular events during or following anesthesia. The blood pressure may drop; irregular heartbeats may develop. If anticipated, these adverse events can be prevented or treated.

Total Blood Volume

Blood volume is useful in determining the total amount of blood replacement required. An accurate method of total blood volume (TBV) measurement involves measuring plasma and red cell volumes separately, then adding the results together. To measure red cell volume, cells are tagged with detectable, nontoxic, radioactive chromium, subsequently injected intravenously, and counted after an appropriate mixing time. Or radioactive iodinated human serum albumin, in standard-dose packages, can be injected, mixed, and counted. Counting may be done rapidly by an electronic device. This technique may be used in place of estimation of blood loss, as described in Chapter 23, pp. 480-481.

Respiratory Tidal Volume (V_t)

The volume of air moved with each respiration may be measured with a respirometer placed on the expiratory limb of the anesthesia machine or mechanical ventilator. Alarms may be incorporated to signal disconnection, failure to cycle, or excessive pressure.

Body Temperature

The body continuously produces heat through metabolic activities and loses heat through convection, evaporation, conduction, and radiation. When rate of production is equal to rate of loss, a heat balance of constant core body temperature is maintained. *Core temperature* is that of the interior of body as opposed to the body surface temperature. Normal core temperature ranges from 98.2° to 99.9° F (36.8° to 37.7° C). Under anesthesia, the average adult loses 0.9° to 2.7° F (0.5° to 1.5° C); the greatest loss occurs during the first hour through convection from exposure to the environment, through evaporation via respiration, through conduction from contact with cool surfaces, and through radiation from tissues. Intraoperative *hypothermia,* core temperature below 96° F (35° C), is a common complication of surgery under general anesthesia, especially in pediatric and elderly patients. Some anesthetic agents inhibit heat production; halogenated agents cause vasodilation that contributes to surface cooling; muscle relaxants prevent shivering, which is a thermoregulatory protective reflex. Other factors can change core temperature. *Hyperther-*

mia, retention of heat, may be caused by premedication, drapes, closed anesthesia breathing circuit, or fever from sepsis. (See also malignant hyperthermia, pp. 383-386.) Physical reactions are not seen in the anesthetized patient. Therefore the body temperature should be continuously monitored for metabolic changes.

Electronic telethermometers with dial or digital readouts measure body and surface temperatures with thermistor or thermocouple probes. A core temperature probe can be inserted into a body orifice (i.e., nasopharynx, esophagus, bladder, or rectum). An esophageal probe measures body temperature at the level of the right side of the heart and is responsive to changes in body heat. A rectal probe responds slowly to changes in body temperature. These probes are available in various sizes and have flexible tips; some are disposable. The sensor of a bladder probe is in the tip of a sterile Foley catheter. A sterile catheter-probe may also be inserted into the pulmonary artery. A probe can be placed on the tympanic membrane via the external auditory canal of an ear. This measures temperature closest to the hypothalamus, which is the thermoregulatory center in the brain.

Skin surface probes have either small tips or discs that are attached to the skin, often on an extremity, with an adhesive-backed foam pad. Cutaneous liquid crystal thermography, with temperature-sensitive chemicals laminated within an adhesive plastic strip, may be used for surface monitoring. The strip is usually applied to the forehead; its chemicals visibly change color with a temperature variation. Proximity to major arteries, insulation from the external environment, and the location of an inflammatory process and the surgical site are considerations in choice of the temperature monitoring site.

Urinary Output

Urinary output can be measured by an indwelling Foley catheter attached to a calibrated collection bag. The sterile disposable collection system must be below the level of the bladder to prevent distention and allow flow without reflux. Output is valuable in assessing effective blood volume and fluid administration, except when a diuretic is given. Volume, electrolytes, osmolarity, and pH are important.

A reduction in urinary volume may indicate reduced renal perfusion. Oliguria can result from stress of the surgical procedure, antidiuresis from the anesthetic agent, impending renal failure, or reduced volume of circulating blood. Output above 30 to 60 ml/hr usually shows adequate intravascular volume.

The collecting system should be able to accurately measure half-hour output between 1 and 200 ml and provide observation of the urine. Hemoglobinuria can be a manifestation of transfusion of incompatible blood. An electronic monitoring system is available with digital display of data that can be fed into a computer. The system records output in milliliters for both the present and the immediately past hours. It also shows the number of minutes elapsed in the current hour. Early warning of possible cardiovascular or renal problems is facilitated by visual alert signals if urine flow falls below 15 ml/hr or ceases.

Chest X-Ray Film

A chest x-ray film is essential for checking the position of the PA (Swan-Ganz) catheter, CVP line, endotracheal tube, and chest tube and for observing changes in lung and heart during therapy.

Electroencephalogram

Electrical activity of the nervous system reflects neurologic function. Therefore electrophysiologic monitoring provides information about the functional integrity of the central nervous system during anesthesia and is especially valuable in patients undergoing high-risk neurosurgical, cardiac, vascular, or orthopaedic procedures. Electrodes placed on the scalp transmit the electrical signals, alpha rhythms, from brain activity. Alpha rhythms normally occur at a rate of 8 to 13 waves per second. On the electroencephalogram (EEG), these wave patterns vary among individuals in response to anesthetics, drugs, and pathologic and physiologic changes. They reveal the presence of organic brain damage, abnormal physiologic alterations, and actions of drugs.

Regional cerebral blood flow correlates well with EEG activity. Computer analysis offers visual recognition of cerebral hypoperfusion or ischemia. The EEG is used particularly in surgical procedures involving expected localized brain ischemia caused by intentional surgical occlusion. An EEG also is a means of determining cessation of circulation, an index of expected prognosis, and brain vitality.

Scalp electrodes (cups or discs of silver/silver chloride, gold, or tin) are fixed in place with paste or collodion. Or subdermal platinum electrodes can be used. Electrodes are placed over areas of cerebral cortex according to a system that uses measurements of head circumference, distance between the ears, and distance from the nasion (point where the sagittal plane intersects the frontonasal suture) to the inion (external protuberance of the occipital bone). The small neurophysiologic signals recorded are amplified for analysis and display. Multiple channels are necessary to detect regional vs. global alterations in function. As many as 8 to 32 channels may be recorded simultaneously. Paper records or strip-charting provides comparisons of EEG activity during crucial periods with the activity seen before anesthesia induction or surgical manipulation. Methods of EEG analysis that permit automated pattern recognition and alarm generation enhance monitoring in the OR or ICU. Devices are available that process EEG signals to simplify and facilitate the complex EEG analysis.

Cerebral Function Monitor The cerebral function monitor provides trend recording of amplitude and amplitude variability for a single channel of EEG and is mainly useful for detecting marked global alterations in EEG activity during cardiopulmonary bypass, induced hypotension, or metabolic coma. During carotid endarterectomy, paired monitors can detect EEG asymmetries. Although they simplify monitoring, they may be less sensitive to ischemia than the 16-channel strip-chart recording.

Compressed Spectral Array Compressed spectral array (CSA) programs may give a time-compressed "mountain-and-valley" representation of brain activity. The mountains move to the left with slower brain activity and to the right with faster activity. CSA helps determine if the brain is ischemic because of a lack of contralateral circulation during vascular surgery, such as carotid endarterectomy. This type of computerized EEG can be run on general-purpose minicomputers or microcomputers.

Neurometrics Monitor A neurometrics monitor is also a single-channel device for displaying processed EEG signals. From 4 to 32 minutes of EEG can be seen at one time, but trends are less easily seen.

Evoked Potentials

Sensory information (sight, sound, smell, taste, and touch) evokes an electrical response when it reaches the brain. Evoked potentials are those electrical responses recorded from the cerebral cortex after stimulation of a peripheral sensory organ. A computer is programmed to average the brain's repetitive responses to the stimuli. The computer displays these as waves on a video screen or prints them on a plotter.

Auditory Evoked Potentials A clicking sound is delivered in the ear to stimulate the auditory nerve. Brain waves are recorded by the evoked potential computer. The evoked potentials can be used to assess function of the auditory nerve, as during removal of acoustic neuroma. Because the auditory nerve enters the brainstem, evoked responses provide an indirect assessment of brainstem activity.

Somatosensory Evoked Potentials Intraoperative monitoring of somatosensory evoked potentials is used to continuously assess spinal cord function and to protect the cord from injury during orthopaedic or neurosurgical procedures on the spine or spinal cord. Because hypotension increases the insult of direct pressure on the cord and heightens damage to cord function, the spinal cord is monitored when induced hypotension is employed for spinal surgery. Impulses generated below the site of the surgical procedure travel over lateral afferent neural pathways and through the operative spinal area and are recorded by electrodes at brain level. Abnormal brain responses are marked by changes in arrival time of electrical impulses or amplitude of the waves on a graph. Change in latency and amplitude of the recorded signal, which normally averages 30 to 50 evoked responses, alerts the team to the danger of spinal cord compression or ischemia. Corrective measures taken immediately can prevent serious sequelae. Evoked responses then return to normal.

COMPLICATIONS OF SURGICAL PROCEDURE WITH PATIENT UNDER ANESTHESIA

The anesthesiologist must be constantly aware of the surgeon's actions. He or she must do everything possible to ensure the safety of the patient and reduce the stress of surgery. Continuous appraisal of the patient's overall condition helps prevent complications. Some complications may occur as a direct result of anesthesia; others may have additional contributing factors. Some conditions may occur during the procedure; others may appear in the postoperative period. Tragically, catastrophic emergencies may sometimes arise when least expected. Minutes can make the difference in life and death for the patient. Anticipation and preparedness may spell that difference.

Injuries

Injuries are many and varied. The anesthesiologist may inadvertently loosen teeth or damage dental work during endotracheal intubation. Nerves can be injured from faulty positioning, such as hyperabduction or extension of the arm. Careless handling of an anesthetized patient can result in paralysis, fractures, or postoperative pain.

Eyes can be injured from irritating anesthetics, face masks, or from drying of the cornea if the eyelids are not closed. The latter occurs most often in patients with loss of normal lubrication by eye movement, protruding eyes, faces covered by drapes, or those in prone positions. Use of an ocular lubricant protects the cornea from drying.

Extravasation, thrombophlebitis, or air emboli are associated with intravenous infusions. Keep intravenous needles visible and not entirely hidden beneath drapes; check infusions frequently; fill the tubing with solution before connecting it to a needle or catheter. *Precaution is the best prevention of injuries.*

Chemical Dependency/Withdrawal

The anesthesiologist must address the special needs of chemically dependent patients to prevent potential risks of postoperative complications. Patients who are actively addicted have a physiologic dependence on alcohol and/or drugs. A person, either active or in recovery, may be addicted to alcohol, narcotics, benzodiazepines, barbiturates, amphetamines, other mind-altering drugs, or a combination of these. Chemically dependent patients are likely to have an altered response, that is, either increased or decreased effectiveness following administration of anesthetic agents, narcotics, and/or sedatives. These drugs may trigger active addiction in a patient in recovery. Patients with a history of chemical dependency, including alcoholism, must be monitored for the effects of drug interactions and symptoms of withdrawal.

Hypotension during anesthesia may be a manifestation of withdrawal from narcotics. Some anesthetic agents will potentiate depressive effects of barbiturates and opiates, with resultant postoperative respiratory depression that can be fatal.

Patients who consume large amounts of alcohol regularly (i.e., more than 4 oz daily) require larger doses of thiopental sodium to produce anesthesia. These doses may cause significant cardiopulmonary depression.

A declining blood alcohol level can alter electrolyte balance and lower blood glucose. Cardiac dysrhythmias or central nervous system dysfunction can lead to vasomotor or respiratory collapse. The chronic alcoholic is likely to have hallucinations, disorientation, and convulsions within 48 hours following withdrawal.

Many chemically dependent patients have coexisting malnutrition, hepatitis, hepatic dysfunction, cardiopulmonary disturbances, and/or renal disease. These patients frequently come to the OR as a result of trauma. An addict should not be withdrawn from the drug of choice until the acute problem is under control.

Fluid and Electrolyte Imbalances

Fluid and electrolyte imbalances may be caused by many different factors and may be manifested by numerous symptoms. Maintenance of correct balance, which greatly influences outcome of surgical intervention, is a very relevant aspect of intraoperative and postoperative care.

Fluid loss is replaced by intravenous (IV) infusion. Usually normal saline or dextrose (5% or 10% in water or saline) solution is started initially. Electrolytes may be added to the solution as needed. Two other IV solutions are used frequently to maintain balance.

1. *Mannitol,* an osmotic diuretic agent, has an effect on renal vascular resistance. Depending on the percentage of drug in solution, it can either increase or decrease renal blood flow. It may be given prophylactically to prevent renal failure. It also is used to decrease intracranial and intraocular pressure. It is rapidly excreted by the kidneys.
2. *Ringer's lactate solution,* a physiologic salt solution, may be infused when the body's supply of sodium, calcium, and potassium has been depleted or for improvement of circulation and stimulation of renal activity. Its electrolyte content is similar to that of plasma.

Blood volume expanders, such as dextran, and blood replacement are discussed in Chapter 23, p. 481 and pp. 484-487. Nutritional supplements, often initiated preoperatively, are discussed in Chapter 8, pp. 110-112.

Changes in fluid and electrolyte balance affect renal function, cellular metabolism, and oxygen concentration in the circulation.

Acid-Base Balance

For enzyme systems to function, a normal balance must be maintained between acidity and alkalinity of body fluids located within intracellular and extracellular compartments. The symbol *pH* represents the hydrogen ion concentration that determines acidity or alkalinity of a solution; neutral pH is 7.0, below 7 is acid, and above 7 is alkaline. Urine is usually acid, within pH range down to 4.6. Normal serum pH is 7.40, within a range of 7.35 to 7.45.

Hydrogen ions do not exist as separate electrolytes in body fluids but are maintained in balance with other electrolytes to ensure neutrality. Because most metabolic processes produce acids, chemical buffers interact with hydrogen ions. Carbonic acid and a hydrogen ion form bicarbonate (HCO_3), the most important buffer. The kidneys and lungs regulate this system by excreting or retaining needed ions in body fluids. Abnormal acid-base balance results from:

1. *Respiratory* malfunction in handling CO_2 produced from carbonic acid
   a. *Acidosis,* pH less than 7.35 with CO_2 above 45 torr
   b. *Alkalosis,* pH more than 7.45 with CO_2 below 35 torr
2. *Metabolic* abnormality in balance between hydrogen and serum HCO_3
   a. *Acidosis,* pH less than 7.35 with HCO_3 less than 22 mEq/L
   b. *Alkalosis,* pH more than 7.45 with HCO_3 more than 26 mEq/L

Electrolytes

Compounds that separate into ions, which are charged particles capable of conducting electric impulses, are essential in maintaining fluid and acid-base balance and in regulating cell functions. The primary electrolytes (see Table 19-2 for normal values) in the body are:

1. *Sodium.* A key regulator in water balance, sodium is necessary to the normal function of muscles and nerves. Large amounts are in extracellular fluid in concentrations of 136 to 145 mEq/L; intracellular concentration is 10 mEq/L. This balance is necessary for normal metabolism.
   a. *Hyponatremia,* insufficient serum sodium, usually accompanies excessive fluid loss or adrenal insufficiency. Muscle twitching, hypovolemia, hypotension, and tachycardia may be symptoms.
   b. *Hypernatremia,* elevated serum sodium, may be caused by hyperglycemia or administration of mannitol. Diaphoresis (sweating) may be the only obvious symptom. Convulsions can occur.
2. *Chloride.* Essential to electrochemical reactions for acid-base regulation, chloride is in extracellular fluids in large amounts. Chlorides are retained or excreted by the kidneys to offset HCO_3 excretion. Sodium tends to carry chloride with it.
   a. *Hypochloremia,* loss of chloride, may occur from vomiting, suctioning, sweating, and diuresis. It produces symptoms of metabolic alkalosis: slow, shallow respirations and muscular tightening.
   b. *Hyperchloremia,* excessive chloride, can result in renal failure. Acidosis develops and breathing becomes labored.
3. *Potassium.* One of the main constituents of cell protoplasm, potassium is primarily (98%) in intracellular fluid. It is essential for elctrochemical reactions for cellular functions.
   a. *Hypokalemia,* a shift of potassium from the blood to the cells or depletion of potassium from the body, can be associated with metabolic alkalosis. Cardiac dysrhythmias can occur when the serum potassium level falls.
   b. *Hyperkalemia,* an increase in serum potassium, may be caused by renal failure and may lead to respiratory and/or cardiac arrest. Metabolic or respiratory acidosis can occur.
4. *Calcium.* Essential to normal muscle physiology, calcium also is an integral part of the blood-clotting mechanism.
   a. *Hypocalcemia,* decreased calcium intake or absorption, may be the result of increased excretion. This can cause cardiac dysrhythmias.
   b. *Hypercalcemia,* increased serum calcium, may be the result of a shift of calcium from the bones to plasma, decreased excretion, or increased uptake and absorption. It causes neuromuscular depression and cardiac dysrhythmias.
5. *Magnesium.* Essential to electrochemical reactions for normal body functions, magnesium is primarily in intracellular fluid. An imbalance may be accompanied by calcium and/or potassium imbalances.
   a. *Hypomagnesemia,* low magnesium level, usually is associated with hypokalemia. This may be the most undiagnosed electrolyte deficiency in geriatric patients or in patients who have illnesses associated with malabsorption in the intestine or kidneys. It may cause cardiac dysrhythmias and nervous system and muscular irritabilities, and it may exaggerate drug toxicities.
   b. *Hypermagnesemia,* elevated serum magnesium, can inhibit nerve and muscle responses. It may lead to respiratory depression and cardiac arrest.
6. *Phosphate.* Normally in intracellular fluid, phosphate allows electrochemical reactions for metabolic functions. Phosphate and calcium vary inversely, so phosphate will buffer acidosis from rising calcium.
   a. *Hypophosphatemia,* low serum phosphate level, may produce tissue hypoxia.
   b. *Hyperphosphatemia,* increase in phosphate, usually occurs in renal failure. It is associated with hypocalcemia.

TABLE 19-2

Normal Blood Chemistry Laboratory Values

PARAMETER	NORMAL VALUES FOR ADULT
Base excess of blood	0 ± 2 mmol/L
Bicarbonate (HCO_3)	22-26 mEq/L
Bilirubin (total)	0.1-1.0 mg/dl
Blood urea nitrogen (BUN)	5-20 mg/dl
Calcium (Ca)	9.0-10.5 mg/dl
Carbon dioxide (CO_2) in serum	23-30 mEq/L
Chloride (Cl)	90-110 mEq/L
Creatinine	0.7-1.5 mg/dl
Creatinine phosphokinase (CPK)	12-80 U/L
Glucose	70-115 mg/dl
Magnesium (Mg)	1.6-3.0 mEq/L
pH of serum	7.35-7.45
Phosphate (P)	2.5-4.5 mg/dl
Potassium (K)	3.5-5.0 mEq/L
Sodium (Na)	136-145 mEq/L
Serum glutamic oxaloacetic transaminase (SGOT)	5-40 IU/L
Serum glutamic pyruvic transaminase (SGPT)	5-35 IU/L

Disturbances in fluid and electrolyte balance can result from:

1. Acid-base imbalances associated with chronic disease or organ dysfunction; acidosis increases serum chloride, potassium, and calcium; alkalosis decreases chloride, potassium, calcium, and phosphate.
2. Cell destruction leading to hyperkalemia; cellular potassium is depleted, with serum potassium increase.
3. Shift of potassium from blood into cells causing hypokalemia; it may be caused by the effects of epinephrine, insulin, bicarbonate, hypothermia, or cardiopulmonary bypass.
4. Changes in blood lipids; calcium and magnesium are depleted by poor absorption.
5. Fever increases metabolic rate; water and electrolytes are lost.
6. Stress; glucose tolerance is diminished and blood sugar and serum potassium levels are increased.
7. Gastric drainage; sodium and chlorides are lost.
8. Fluid loss from drainage tubes, diaphoresis, vomiting, or diarrhea; sodium, chloride, and potassium are lost.
9. Maxillofacial injury; oral intake is inhibited.
10. Radiation enteritis; magnesium and potassium are diminished.
11. Disease of bowel, liver, or biliary tract, intestinal tract obstruction, or gastrointestinal fistula; calcium and phosphate are poorly absorbed.
12. Loss of muscle mass as result of preoperative malnutrition; nitrogen loss is increased.
13. Drugs can adversely affect metabolic balance; losses of potassium, magnesium and chloride from diuretics are examples.
14. Inadequate oxygen/carbon dioxide exchange; acid-base balance is disrupted.

Hypovolemia

Hypovolemia is a decreased circulating blood volume from loss of blood and plasma or a deficit of extracellular fluid volume commonly referred to as *dehydration.* When excessive fluid loss is greater than absorption of interstitial fluid into circulation, the patient may go into *hypovolemic shock.*

Etiology

Etiologic factors include reduced fluid intake; hemorrhage; plasma loss, as through extensive burns and wound drainage; and dehydration from loss of gastrointestinal fluids as by vomiting, from diaphoresis as from fever, or from diuresis. Impaired renal function and metabolic acidosis are predisposing factors. Prolonged cardiopulmonary bypass can cause hypovolemic shock.

Symptoms

Symptoms include dry skin and mucous membranes, depressed blood pressure, elevated pulse, oliguria, decreasing central venous pressure and blood volume determinations, and deep rapid respirations.

Treatment

Hypovolemic shock resulting from hemorrhage or underestimated blood loss is most often seen in the OR. This is usually reversed by prompt restoration of circulating blood volume (see blood replacement, Chapter 23, pp. 484-487). The extent of hypovolemia will determine treatment.

1. *Fluid volume replacement.* Whole blood, plasma expander, or infusion of Ringer's lactate or other intravenous fluid is indicated to increase blood volume. Hypervolemia must be avoided in replacement.
2. *Position.* Elevation of the legs may aid venous return and cardiac output except in severe oligemia (low total blood volume).
3. *Temperature.* Keep the patient warm, but not overheated. Perspiration increases fluid loss. Shivering can cause hypothermia.
4. *Oxygen.* Oxygen is administered when Po_2 is low because the circulation is not delivering enough oxygen to tissues.
5. *Drugs.* Drugs are administered as needed to maintain blood pressure, correct acidosis, or protect kidneys from failure. (See listing of cardiovascular drugs, pp. 395-399.)

Prevention

Decreased blood volume, if present preoperatively, increases surgical risk and morbidity. It should be treated and the electrolyte imbalance should be corrected. Fluids, blood gases, and blood loss must be monitored intraoperatively.

Hypervolemia

Hypervolemia is an excess of extracellular fluid in the blood, commonly referred to as *edema.* Intravenous infusions given too rapidly or in excessive amounts, especially isotonic saline solution, can cause hypervolemia. Prolonged administration of adrenocorticosteroids is also a predisposing factor. Hypervolemia may progress to pulmonary edema (see p. 389).

Dyspnea, moist crackles (rales), elevated pulse and respiration, and diminished urine output are symptomatic of hypervolemia. Increasing central venous pressure may indicate fluid overload with venous distention. Diuretics and fluid restriction ameliorate hypervolemia and prevent pulmonary edema.

Convulsions

Convulsions occur most often in patients with a hyperactive metabolic rate, especially in dehydrated or hyperpyretic children. Anoxia and death can occur.

Etiology

Etiologic factors include severe hypoxia and carbon dioxide retention, hypernatremia, hyperthermia, overdose of regional anesthetic drugs, air embolism, and epilepsy.

Symptoms

Symptoms include muscular twitching, dilated pupils, rapid snorting respirations, rapid pulse, grimacing, and cyanosis.

Treatment

Administer oxygen to maintain respiration and diazepam, rapid-acting barbiturate, or neuromuscular blocker to stop muscular activity. Mechanical ventilation may be needed for apnea or to support circulation.

Prevention

Maintain normal body temperature and fluid and electrolyte balance.

Inadvertent Hypothermia

A decrease in the patient's core body temperature to below 96° F (35° C) can affect vasoconstriction and vasodilation, cardiac output, and renal function. Depending on degrees of body heat loss, *hypothermia* is categorized as mild (down to 90° F [32° C]), moderate (down to 85° F [30° C]), and deep (down to 80° F [27° C]). Below 68° F (20° C), brain activity ceases. Patients can emerge from anesthesia with a body temperature below normal. *Inadvertent hypothermia* occurs spontaneously intraoperatively; it not to be confused with induced hypothermia (see Chapter 17, pp. 338-339). Age-extreme, thin, and debilitated patients are most susceptible, as are patients undergoing neurosurgical, cardiovascular, thoracic, and abdominal procedures.

Etiology

Anesthesia inhibits the protective reflexes that generate body heat (i.e., shivering). It also depresses the thermoregulating center in the hypothalamus, decreases basal metabolic rate, and increases vasodilation for heat loss by radiation and conduction. Core body heat is lost by exposure to a cool external environment, as during skin preparation, and through the surgical incision. Other factors include preoperative sedation, general vs. regional anesthesia, adjunctive drugs, length of the surgical procedure, blood and fluid loss and replacement, room temperature, and evaporative loss through the respiratory tract.

Symptoms

Hypothermia can cause adverse cardiovascular, hematologic, immunologic, metabolic, and neurologic effects. Cardiac dysrhythmias, hypoxia, metabolic acidosis, hyperglycemia, and dilated pupils may be the result. A depressed central nervous system, which can lead to coma, may not be evident until the postoperative period. Shivering, impaired speech, muscle rigidity, cyanosis, weak pulse, falling blood pressure, and dysrhythmias seen in the PACU may be symptoms of hypothermia.

Treatment

The hypothermic patient must be rewarmed as soon as possible. However, postanesthesia shivering during the rewarming process can by hazardous. Shivering is an involuntary rhythmic contraction of muscle groups with irregular and intermittent relaxation. This physiologic response to cold is activated when the hypothalamus senses that the core temperature has dropped. Some postanesthesia shivering is caused by anesthetic agents. Untreated shivering leads to increased oxygen consumption as a result of muscular activity and to increased cardiac stress as a result of hypoxia. In the PACU, a forced-air skin surface warmer (Bair Hugger) or an ultraviolet or infrared heat lamp directed at lightly covered patient are effective means for raising body temperature. A temperature-regulating hypothermia/hyperthermia machine, set at 104° to 107° F (40° to 42° C), may be used with a heated blanket beneath the patient. If warmers are not available, warm blankets placed over and underneath the patient should be changed at 15-minute intervals. Blankets can be heated to 105° F (40.5° C) for an adult or 100° F (38° C) for a small child or infant. Keep a cap on the patient. Warmed humidified oxygen and IV fluid should be administered. Clonidine, an alpha-2 adrenergic agonist, or analgesics such as meperidine or morphine derivative may suppress shivering.

Prevention

Prevention of hypothermia is the best treatment. Preparations can begin before the patient arrives in the OR.

1. Place a hypothermia/hyperthermia mattress or reflective blanket on the operating table. A radiant heat source can be placed over an infant.
2. Check the room temperature and humidity.
3. Apply warmed blankets as soon as patient arrives in the OR and immediately after drapes are removed. Warm blanket can be put on the stretcher under the patient.
4. Limit skin exposure during positioning and skin preparation (i.e., keep the patient covered as much as possible).
5. Minimize the time of exposure between skin antisepsis and draping.

6. Keep the sheet under and the drapes over the patient and around the surgical site dry to provide insulation, prevent heat loss, and maintain asepsis. Dry the area following skin prep.
7. Warm antiseptic, irrigating, and intravenous solutions before administration, including blood. Anesthetic gases (including oxygen) can be warmed also.
8. Monitor body temperature (see pp. 376-377).
9. Leave a cap on the patient; a plastic head covering retains more heat than other materials.

Malignant Hyperthermia/ Hyperpyrexia

Malignant hyperthermia (MH) is a fulminant hypermetabolic crisis in susceptible persons, which is triggered by potent halogenated anesthetic agents and depolarizing skeletal muscle relaxants. MH, a potentially fatal complication of anesthesia, is characterized by uncontrolled acceleration of muscle metabolism accompanied by tremendous oxygen consumption and heat and carbon dioxide production. The body temperature can rapidly rise at a rate of 1.8° F (1° C) every 5 minutes if untreated. A temperature as high as 117° F (47° C) has been recorded, but 111.2° F (44° C) is probably highest with survival. The survival rate with appropriate treatment is between 80% and 90%. The mortality rate without appropriate treatment is around 10%; thus MH is of significant concern.

Etiology

The exact cause of MH is unknown. It is understood that certain patients are susceptible, and some anesthetic agents may trigger this crisis.

Susceptible Patients A familial genetic transmission exists as an autosomal dominant trait with variable multifactorial inheritance patterns. The genetic defect manifests by increasing calcium levels in skeletal muscles. The crisis results from a hereditary inability of the sarcoplasmic reticulum, a skeletal muscle cell membrane, to control intramyoplasmic levels of calcium. Skeletal muscle undergoes contraction as a result of releases of calcium ions in response to drugs or stress. Rapid increase of calcium in muscle fiber leads to generalized catabolism. As biochemical reactions occur, the body produces heat and carbon dioxide.

Susceptible patients also include those with any type of myopathy or acquired muscle disease, such as ptosis, strabismus, hernia, area of muscle weakness or hypertrophy, or muscular dystrophy. The incidence of MH is higher in children than adults. Patients, especially children, with rheumatoid arthritis are particularly susceptible to MH.

Some patients have a history of temperature instability with minor illness such as a sore throat. A majority will have an unexplained preoperative elevation of creatinine phosphokinase (CPK) above 280 U/L, although other conditions can produce levels above normal range.

MH may occur in a patient's first exposure to anesthesia or in a later one; one third of reported cases of MH have occurred in a second or subsequent anesthesia.

Triggers Several agents may trigger this abnormal hypermetabolic response in susceptible individuals. However, succinylcholine, halothane, enflurane, desflurane, and isoflurane are the main triggers of MH.

Symptoms

Clinical signs and symptoms occur according to swiftness of onset. Onset may develop rapidly immediately after induction or develop after several hours of general anesthesia, or even in the postoperative recovery period.

Spasm of the jaw muscles with rigidity of the masseter muscles or severe fasciculations following succinylcholine administration should suggest development of MH to the anesthesiologist.

The most common presenting sign of MH is unexplained *ventricular dysrhythmia,* mainly tachycardia or premature ventricular contractions. This is associated with an unexplained increase in end-tidal carbon dioxide tachypnea, cyanosis, skin mottling, and unstable blood pressure. Blood in the surgical field may appear dark as a result of central venous desaturation.

When a sudden, generalized hypermetabolic state is produced, the temperature rises rapidly as more heat is produced than the body can eliminate. *Elevated temperature may be a late sign or absent in MH syndrome.* Fever, hot skin or tissues, and diaphoresis are symptoms of heat buildup. A favorable prognosis decreases when excessive heat in the tissues is noted through the surgeon's gloves or when the anesthesiologist senses heat in the reservoir bag or soda lime canister on the anesthesia machine. The body tries to adjust by vasodilation and increased cardiac output. If rapidly increasing tissue demands are not met, hypoxia, central venous hypercapnia, and severe respiratory and metabolic acidosis occur, progressing to cardiovascular collapse. Blood tests will reveal increased serum levels of potassium, magnesium, CPK, and myoglobin. Excessive myoglobin release caused by rapid muscle destruction, rhabdomyolysis, can cause renal failure and lead to anuria.

Late clinical findings include hyperkalemia, acute renal failure, left-sided heart failure, disseminated intravascular coagulopathy, skeletal muscle swelling or necrosis from hypoxia and acidosis, pulmonary edema, neurologic sequelae including paraplegia and decerebration, and coma from ischemia secondary to hypoxia. Recurrence of MH crisis can occur 24 to 72 hours postoperatively.

Monitoring Parameters to be monitored routinely in patients at risk for MH who undergo general anesthesia are ECG, blood pressure, core temperature by esophageal probe, pulse oximetry, capnometry, nerve stimulation to measure the level of muscle relaxation, and precordial stethoscopy. Rise in temperature greater than one-half degree per hour should raise suspicion of MH.

Treatment

Success is contingent on complete preparedness (preplanned action, written protocol, immediate equipment supply), early diagnosis, and vigorous therapy. The following treatment outline is the suggested protocol established by the Malignant Hyperthermia Association of the United States (MHAUS). Institutional policies and procedures should be in place to guide the perioperative team in caring for a patient in MH crisis.

1. *Discontinue anesthesia and stop the surgical procedure immediately.* The anesthesiologist immediately institutes *hyperventilation with 100% oxygen* at a high flow rate of at least 10 L/min. Research has shown that the breathing circuit and anesthesia delivery machine need not be changed because the high concentration of oxygen delivery clears the machine of anesthetic gases very rapidly. If the surgical procedure cannot be interrupted, safe agents may be employed to maintain anesthesia during the stabilization period.
2. Immediately start drug therapy. Administer:
   a. *Dantrolene sodium (Dantrium IV)* 2 to 3 mg/kg in an initial IV bolus, and repeat every 5 to 10 minutes until the maximum dose of 10 mg/kg is given or the MH episode is controlled. Patients generally respond to the drug quickly. The onset of action is usually 2 to 3 minutes. Occasionally doses higher than 10 to 20 mg/kg are needed.

      Dantrolene is a specific drug for treatment of MH. It directly blocks accumulation of calcium within the muscles by preventing its release from the sarcoplasmic reticulum and by uncoupling excitation-contraction, thus relaxing skeletal muscle. It has no effect on cardiovascular or respiratory functions. Calcium channel blockers may not be given with dantrolene because they may cause hyperkalemia, myocardial depression, and cardiovascular collapse.

      Given intravenously, dantrolene is supplied in 70-ml vials as a sterile, lyophilized powder that contains 20 mg of dantrolene and 3 g of mannitol. Each vial must be reconstituted before use with 60 ml of sterile water for injection *without* a preservative agent. The large quantities of sterile water that are needed would contain the preservative agent in toxic amounts. A semiautomatic fluid-dispensing syringe expedites mixing. If this is not available, additional personnel should help with the reconstitution process because large quantities of the diluted drug will be needed and each vial will require vigorous shaking to mix. The solution will be yellow-orange when mixed. In *extreme* circumstances, the drug may be given through a filter to remove particulates from the solution. Once reconstituted, dantrolene must be used within 6 hours and must be protected from exposure to light.

      If other IV solutions have been running, the line should be flushed with sterile water before dantrolene is injected; this will prevent precipitation. Do not use Ringer's lactate solution because it will increase the level of acidosis. An additional IV site should be established to infuse iced normal saline solution at the rate of 15 ml/kg every 15 minutes for at least 45 minutes.

      Dantrolene is continued postoperatively at a minimum of 1 mg/kg every 6 hours for 24 to 72 hours postepisode. After the initial 48 hours, 1 mg/kg every 6 hours may be given orally for 24 hours. No serious side effects have been reported with short-term use, but muscle weakness may be evident for 24 to 48 hours after administration. Few isolated reports of nausea, vomiting, and fatigue have been documented. Prolonged administration may lead to hepatotoxicity.

   b. *Procainamide (Pronestyl)* 15 mg/kg diluted in 500 ml physiologic saline solution IV over 60 minutes. Procainamide treats cardiac dysrhythmia if required.
   c. *Sodium bicarbonate* 1 to 2 mEq/kg IV stat and repeated as guided by blood gas analysis. An alkali, sodium bicarbonate raises pH temporarily. It combats acidosis and antagonizes hyperkalemia by lowering the plasma potassium level. It can cause rebound acidosis. Monitoring of arterial pH and P_{CO_2} is necessary to determine subsequent doses.
   d. *Regular insulin* 10 units in 50 ml 50% dextrose in water IV. Insulin offsets the high glucose metabolic demands and improves the glucose uptake. It shifts potassium back into the cells to help treat hyperkalemia. Blood glucose and potassium levels must be monitored.
   e. *Calcium chloride* 2.5 mg/kg to treat severe cardiac toxicity caused by hyperkalemia.
   f. *Mannitol* 0.25 g/kg IV and *furosemide (Lasix)* 1 mg/kg IV, up to four doses each. These drugs dislodge myoglobin from the renal tubules and sustain urinary flow. Urine output greater than

2 ml/kg/hr must be maintained to prevent renal failure. The dose is calculated in consideration of the mannitol contained in the dantrolene solution.

3. *Begin active cooling.* Administer refrigerated or iced normal saline intravenously. Lavage the stomach and rectum. Avoid irrigating the bladder, because accurate measurement of urine output is important. It the peritoneal or thoracic cavity is open, cool sterile saline may be poured into the opening. Cool the body surface by placing the patient in a plastic sheet and applying ice bags and ice water, or use a hypothermia blanket. If readily available, use extracorporeal perfusion apparatus for partial (femoral to femoral) cardiopulmonary bypass to cool the viscera. Body temperature must be carefully monitored to avoid accidental cooling to dysrhythmic levels. Medication may be given to limit shivering, normally a heat-retaining mechanism that also increases oxygen consumption. Surface cooling is considered more effective in children because of their high ratio of surface area to body volume. Too vigorous cooling can result in inadvertent hypothermia and cardiac arrest. To avoid hypothermia, cooling should be discontinued when the core temperature reaches 100° F (38° C).
4. Correct the electrolyte imbalance on the basis of blood sampling of electrolytes, pH, and blood gases. After the presumed onset of MH, an arterial line must be established if one is not already in place. Blood samples are taken at 10-minute intervals for pH, P_{CO_2}, P_{O_2}, sodium, potassium, chlorides, calcium, magnesium, and phosphate. Hypocalcemia and hyperkalemia followed by hypokalemia may be expected.

   Also measured are CPK, serum glutamic oxaloacetic transaminase, alkaline phosphatase, and lactate dehydrogenase for indication of muscle destruction. Blood urea nitrogen for kidney function, bilirubin for liver function, coagulation studies, blood lactate and pyruvate, and serum thyroxine levels may be ordered.
5. Central venous pressure should be monitored. A CVP line may need to be inserted if one is not already in place.
6. Urinary output is monitored via an indwelling Foley catheter. In addition to the measurement of volume, urine is sampled for hemoglobin and myoglobin. The urine will be brown as the amount of hemoglobin and myoglobin increases.

Supplies for Malignant Hyperthermia Supplies should be kept in a specific location and must be immediately available for both adult and pediatric patients. A cart marked for use in MH is convenient. Supplies that may be needed include:

1. Monitors: ECG, electronic temperature probes and recorder
2. IV equipment: blood administration sets and pumps; CVP line setup; IV solutions—12 bags, 1000 ml each, of physiologic saline kept in refrigerator
3. Arterial line setup
4. Intubation equipment
5. Ice chips and plastic bags; hypothermia blankets
6. Gastric lavage set; three-way indwelling catheter for insertion into the rectum; 50 ml syringes
7. Blood sampling and arterial blood gas equipment
8. Indwelling Foley catheter and urimeter bag
9. Drugs:
   a. 36 vials, 20 mg each, of dantrolene sodium (quantity needed to treat and stabilize a 70 kg adult)
   b. 36 vials, 60 ml each, of sterile water without preservative agent to reconstitute dantrolene (quantity needed for 70 kg adult is 2100 ml)
   c. Five 100 ml prefilled syringes of sodium bicarbonate 5%
   d. Six 1 g ampules of procainamide
   e. Ten 50 ml vials of 20% mannitol
   f. Four 2 ml (20 mg) prefilled syringes of furosemide
   g. One 100-unit vial of regular insulin
   h. Two 50 ml vials of 50% dextrose in water
   i. Three 1000-unit vials of heparin
   j. Ten 250 mg vials of hydrocortisone sodium succinate (Solu-Cortef)
10. Associated needles and syringes
11. Extracorporeal perfusion apparatus, if available
12. Defibrillator machine and electrodes

Prevention

Identification of susceptible patients is the best prevention. *Preoperative history* should routinely include questions about the patient's previous anesthesia experiences, unexplained incidents or death of family members who underwent anesthesia, and known muscular abnormalities or episodes of heat stroke of the patient and relatives. Hereditary predisposition has been detected in three generations; however, family history frequently is not known. *The most prominent clue to identification of a patient susceptible to MH is a family history of unexplained death under general anesthesia.* Genetic counseling of the patient and family is advised. Although the crisis usually occurs under general anesthesia, it can occur during periods of emotional or physical stress. Susceptible persons should wear a medical-alert bracelet or tag.

Diagnosis of susceptibility to MH can be accomplished by *preoperative muscle biopsy.* A 1 g specimen of skeletal muscle is excised from the thigh under local anesthesia. The specimen is removed from the muscle as a strip and outstretched between the prongs of a double-tipped clamp. Evaluation of the muscle response to caffeine-induced contracture during exposure to halothane reveals sensitivity. Although local anesthetic is used to obtain the muscle biopsy, dantrolene should be readily available in the unlikely event of an episode of MH.

The blood CPK level may be elevated in susceptible patients, but it also can be influenced by alcohol consumption or strenuous exercise. A normal CPK level does not ensure absence of the MH trait. Phosphorus nuclear magnetic resonance imaging also may detect susceptibility, but it is not always a reliable indicator.

Prophylaxis Dantrolene may be given preoperatively to susceptible patients. The suggested dose is 1 mg/kg increments every 4 to 6 hours orally up to a 4 mg/kg total dose, followed by 2.5 mg/kg IV 30 minutes before induction of general anesthesia. Intraoperative monitoring is mandatory. When nontriggering anesthetic agents are used, prophylactic dantrolene therapy may be unnecessary. Each patient should be evaluated individually. Some indications for dantrolene prophylaxis may include:

1. Previous history of suspected MH episode
2. Family history of MH (actual or suspected)
3. Known MH susceptibility
4. Prolonged procedure anticipated in MH-susceptible patient
5. Underlying disease or physiology causing suspicion of MH susceptibility

Nontriggering anesthetic agents should be administered to MH-susceptible individuals. Barbiturates, benzodiazepines, and narcotics are considered safe. Nitrous oxide by inhalation or intravenous propofol or ketamine hydrochloride can be administered for general anesthesia. Most of the synthetic nondepolarizing neuromuscular blockers are safe muscle relaxants. Amino amide and ester agents can be used safely for local anesthesia.

Postoperatively, the patient should be continuously monitored in the PACU for 4 to 6 hours. If the vital signs remain stable during this time, the patient may be discharged.

Pulmonary Complications

One of the primary areas of postoperative complications is the respiratory tract. Potential for developing pulmonary problems depends on several factors. Any preexisting lung disease such as emphysema, infection, or asthma predisposes the patient. Heavy smokers have the highest risk of succumbing to postoperative pulmonary problems caused by chronic irritation of the respiratory tract with consequent production of excess mucus. Chest wall deformities, obesity, and extremes of age are other pertinent preoperative influences. *Intraoperative factors* include:

1. Type of preoperative medications
2. Type and duration of anesthesia
3. Type and duration of assisted ventilation
4. Position of the patient during the surgical procedure
5. Extent of the surgical procedure

Postoperatively, one of the most critical factors is the patient's ability to mobilize secretions by deep breathing, coughing, and ambulation. Patients undergoing chest and abdominal surgery are likely to breathe shallowly because of pain and therefore may not adequately raise accumulated secretions. Development of one pulmonary complication frequently predisposes the patient to development of another.

Pulmonary embolism (see Chapter 23, pp. 488-489) is a major cause of death during a surgical procedure and in the immediate postoperative period. Some intraoperative problems may extend into postoperative recovery. *Adult respiratory distress syndrome,* also known as *progressive pulmonary insufficiency* or *shock lung,* may develop in the first 24 to 48 hours following a traumatic injury.

Aspiration

Aspiration of gastric contents into the lungs may occur during abolition of throat reflexes when the patient is unconscious or is conscious with the throat anesthetized, as for bronchoscopy. Residual effects impede lung function and blood-gas exchange. A chemical pneumonitis results from aspiration of highly acidic gastric juices. Edema forms, alveoli collapse, ventilation-perfusion mismatch occurs, and hypoxemia results. Aspiration of solids in emesis results in edema, severe hypoxia, and respiratory obstruction. Bronchospasm and atelectasis may be followed by pneumonitis or bronchopneumonia. Most aspiration is irritative, but it can be infectious if nasopharyngeal flora are aspirated. Pneumonia or lung abscess may result with necrosis of the pulmonary parenchyma.

Etiology Every patient who has food in the stomach is a poor risk for anesthesia (e.g., a patient with traumatic injuries who requires immediate surgical intervention). Increased intragastric pressure is an aspiration hazard and may result from conditions such as pylorospasm, diaphragmatic hernia, gastrointestinal bleeding, intestinal obstruction, or gas forced into the stomach by application of positive-pressure ventilation without use of a cuffed endotracheal tube.

Symptoms Symptoms include cyanosis, dyspnea, and tachycardia, followed by cardiac embarrassment, lung collapse, and consolidation.

Treatment Most effective treatment occurs during the first minutes after aspiration. The strategy is to remove as much aspirate as possible and limit the spread of what is left in the lung. Lower the head of the table with a right lateral tilt for postural drainage; right mainstem bronchus bifurcates slightly higher than left bronchus. Suction the oropharynx and tracheobronchial tree. If the patient has aspirated particulate matter that causes obstruction of airways, bronchoscopy must be performed to remove it. Suctioning must be interrupted every 10 to 15 seconds to give oxygen. Oxygenation and carbon dioxide removal are high priorities. Aspiration of acid gastric content injures the alveolar capillary interface, resulting in intrapulmonary shunting and pulmonary edema. Intensive pulmonary care is aimed at improving ventilation-perfusion ratios and decreasing abnormal gas exchange. This may require tracheal intubation for mechanical ventilation with continuous positive pressure. Most severe hypoxemia is expected to occur rapidly within the first 30 to 60 minutes after aspiration. Careful cardiovascular monitoring and frequent blood-gas and acid-base determinations guide therapeutic measures to maintain intravascular volume. Prophylactic antibiotics may be given for aspiration of bowel-contaminated fluid to prevent infection, and a bronchodilator may be used to treat spasm. Most permanent injury or death results from the initial hypoxemia.

Prevention Prevention involves adequate preoperative preparation (withholding oral intake 8 to 10 hours before induction) and careful administration of anesthetic agents. The anesthetic is decreased near the end of the surgical procedure, hastening the return of throat reflexes. All trauma and obstetric patients receiving general anesthesia should be treated as if they have full stomachs. Gastric evacuation is delayed during labor and by analgesic medications. A nasogastric tube may be inserted preoperatively or intraoperatively.

Laryngospasm and Bronchospasm

Laryngospasm is a partial or complete closure of the vocal cords as an involuntary reflex action. *Bronchospasm* is contraction of smooth muscle in the walls of bronchi and bronchioles, causing narrowing of the lumina. These spasms or abnormal narrowings are produced by a marked increase in smooth muscle tone of the airway walls. Marked elevation of airway resistance profoundly alters gas flow into and out of the lungs. Accompanying changes result in a decreased ventilation-perfusion ratio, with subsequent reduction in PaO_2 and rise in $PaCO_2$. Many factors can precipitate spasm.

Etiology Etiologic factors include mechanical airway obstruction, certain anesthetics and drugs, allergic conditions such as asthma, vagal reflex, stimulation of the pharynx and larynx under light anesthesia, traction on the peritoneum, foreign material in the tracheobronchial tree, movement of the head or neck or traction on the carotid sinus, and painful peripheral stimuli. Degree of spasm varies from mild to severe.

Symptoms Symptoms include wheezing respirations or stridor, reduced compliance, cyanosis, and respiratory obstruction.

Treatment Treatment depends on the precipitating factor. Methods generally used include positive-pressure oxygen, tracheal intubation, and neuromuscular blockers for relaxation. Bronchodilator drugs such as aminophylline, isoetharine, and metaproterenol sulfate are given with caution because they act as cardiac stimulators and, in the presence of hypoxia, they may contribute to cardiac dysrhythmia and cardiac arrest. Patients may be refractory (unresponsive) to bronchodilators because of acid-base abnormalities. Correction can reduce the side effects and augment the beneficial effects of bronchodilators. If the etiologic factor is an allergy, steroids and antihistamines may be given. Vagal reflexes are inhibited by atropine. If reflex is the cause, anesthesia is deepened. Drying agents are given for excessive secretions. Immediate effective treatment is mandatory to counteract hypoxia and prevent cardiac arrest.

Prevention Prevention involves maintenance of a patent airway, appropriate premedication such as atropine, avoidance of factors stimulating the vagal reflex, and treatment of predisposing pulmonary condition.

Airway and Respiratory Obstruction

An airway is maintained with an oral airway or endotracheal tube. However, airway obstruction is the most frequent cause of respiratory difficulty in the immediate postoperative period. The patient may exhibit paradoxical respiration (i.e., downward movement of the diaphragm occurring with contraction rather than expansion of the chest) resulting in hypoxia and carbon dioxide retention. As the condition worsens, the patient becomes restless, diaphoretic, cyanotic, and finally unconscious. If not relieved in seconds, this serious complication may lead to cardiac arrest.

Etiology Etiologic factors include blocking of the airway by the tongue, soft tissue, excessive secretions, or a foreign body; laryngospasm or bronchospasm; or positioning of the head with the chin down.

Symptoms Symptoms include increased respiratory effort with inadequate respiratory exchange, visible use of accessory muscles, and respiratory motion of the chest and abdomen without audible air movement at the airway. If the airway is totally obstructed, breath sounds will be absent; if it is partially obstructed, a snoring sound will be elicited. Pulse is rapid and thready. Pallor and cyanosis rapidly follow hypoxia, which develops more slowly if the patient has been breathing a high concentration of oxygen.

Treatment Eliminate the cause of obstruction by suctioning blood, mucus, or emesis; gently hyperextend the neck and elevate the chin. Administer oxygen by positive pressure; a nasal airway or endotracheal intubation may be necessary.

Hypoventilation

The ability to oxygenate depends on hemoglobin concentration, cardiac output, and oxygen saturation. Inadequate or reduced alveolar ventilation can cause a deficit in oxygenation. This can lead to *hypoxia*, decreased level of oxygen in arterial blood and tissues, *hypoxemia*, decreased level of oxygen in arterial blood, and *hypercapnia* (hypercarbia), an elevated level of carbon dioxide in arterial blood. The body compensates for mild hypoxia with increased heart and respiratory rates, bringing more oxygen to the blood and tissues. If hypoxia progresses, this compensation is inadequate. If it is prolonged, cardiac dysrhythmia or irreversible brain, liver, kidney, and heart damage results from hypoxia. Retention of carbon dioxide also leads to acidosis.

Etiology Pain, a faulty position, a short, thick neck, or a full bladder are contributing factors to hypoventilation. Inadequate pulmonary ventilation from depression of the respiratory center by narcotics or anesthetics, reduced cardiac output, severe blood loss, obstruction to the respiratory passages, or abnormality of ventilation-perfusion ratio also can contribute to hypoxia and hypercapnia.

Symptoms Symptoms include increased pulse rate; pallor or cyanosis from hypoxia or flushed or reddened appearance from hypercapnia; decreased volume of respirations; stertorous or labored respirations; and dark blood in the surgical field. The acid-base balance can be affected.

Treatment Immediate adequate oxygen intake stimulates the medullary centers to prevent respiratory system failure. An endotracheal tube may be left in place postoperatively to support assisted ventilation.

NOTE

1. Oxygen is a medication requiring proper dosage. Patients with chronic obstructive pulmonary disease (COPD) cannot tolerate high concentrations. To prevent cardiac arrest, a 2 to 3 L flow is recommended postoperatively.
2. The patient is encouraged to cough and breathe deeply postoperatively. If the patient received naloxone hydrochloride (Narcan) to reverse the respiratory depressant effect of a narcotic, the patient may awaken rapidly and cough, inadvertently causing extubation. The patient must be watched closely during recovery.

Prevention A patent airway, adequate oxygenation, and proper positioning help prevent hypoventilation. Intraoperative measurements of arterial pH, PCO_2, and PO_2 enable the anesthesiologist to evaluate oxygenation and carbon dioxide removal. To prevent hypoventilation and hypoxia patients may be given oxygen and assisted ventilation during transport to the recovery area.

Pneumothorax

Although it is rare, insertion of a needle into the thoracic cage can occur during a nerve block or subclavian catheter insertion. The prime symptom is shortness of breath. Confirmation is made by x-ray study. If the pneumothorax is extensive and the lung fails to reexpand, a chest tube with an underwater seal is required.

Intercostal Muscle Spasm

"Rigid chest" may occur after large doses of intravenous fentanyl or on emergence from general anesthesia. It may reverse itself, or neuromuscular blockers may be needed.

Atelectasis or Pulmonary Collapse

Partial collapse of a lung is one of the most common postoperative problems. If mucus obstructs a bronchus, air in the alveoli distal to the obstruction is resorbed. That segment of lung then collapses and consolidates. Retained mucus, although initially sterile, becomes contaminated by inhaled bacteria; the patient may develop bronchopneumonia.

Etiology Factors that promote increased production of mucus, such as certain irritating anesthetics, and decreased mobilization of mucus, such as from a tight abdominal dressing, predispose to pulmonary collapse. Furthermore, normal respiration includes a deep sigh several times an hour to help keep lungs expanded. This natural sigh is inhibited by anesthetics, narcotics, and sedatives. Oxygen and carbon dioxide are absorbed into the pulmonary blood flow, and the alveoli collapse. Low tidal volume intensifies the problem. High concentrations of oxygen remove nitrogen from lungs, leaving oxygen, carbon dioxide, and water in alveoli.

Symptoms Atelectasis increases temperature, pulse, and respiratory rate. The patient may appear cyanotic and uncomfortable, with shallow respirations and pain on coughing. Breath sounds are diminished, with fine crackles. Chest x-ray study reveals collapsed areas of lung as patch opacities, generally involving the lung bases.

Treatment and Prevention Measures to help prevent or treat atelectasis are abstention from smoking, a regimen of coughing and deep breathing, and early ambulation. An upright position allows for better lung expansion. Medication for pain, when appropriate, before breathing exercises or ambulation, improves ability to breathe deeply and cough effectively. Splinting the thoracic or abdominal incision with a pillow also helps decrease the pain of coughing. Repeated vigorous coughing is contraindicated in some patients, for example, following cataract extraction, craniotomy, or herniorrhaphy.

Pulmonary Edema

Pulmonary edema may be defined as an abnormal accumulation of water in extravascular portions of the lungs, including both alveolar and interstitial spaces. In surgical patients, the cause is most probably increased microvascular pulmonary capillary permeability or capillary endothelial injury. Blood stagnates in the pulmonary circulation. Fluid exudes from capillaries into the alveoli and interstitial spaces. Reduction of capillary membrane perfusion leads to hypoxia. Symptoms, usually seen postoperatively in the PACU or ICU, may include a bounding rapid pulse, crackles, dyspnea, and engorged peripheral veins.

Cardiovascular Complications

The emotional and physical stresses to which a surgical patient is subjected may lead to cardiovascular complications. The patient who fears dying while under anesthesia runs a greater risk of cardiac arrest on the operating table than patients with known cardiac disease. Psychologic stress can have physiologic manifestations (see discussion of anxiety in Chapter 7, p. 101). Extreme preoperative anxiety predisposes the patient to a difficult induction and intraoperative period and to postoperative discomfort. Patients with a history of cardiovascular problems are prone to develop complications. These may include dysrhythmias, hypotension, thromboembolism and/or thrombophlebitis, myocardial infarction, or congestive heart failure. Cerebral thrombosis or embolism may result in prolonged coma. Patients must be closely monitored for symptoms of cardiovascular complications. Those related to hemorrhage and coagulation are discussed in Chapter 23, pp. 487-488. Anoxia, the complete or almost total absence of oxygen from inspired gases, arterial blood, or tissues, is a precursor to cardiovascular collapse. Cardiac arrest can result in death in the OR.

Hypotension

Reduced blood pressure, with resultant inadequate circulation, may accompany depression of the myocardium, depression of the vasomotor center in the brain, decline in cardiac output, or dilation of the peripheral vessels. Hypotension may occur also when positive pressure is applied to the airway. Progressive deepening of general anesthesia usually produces peripheral vasodilation and diminished myocardial contractility. Adequate blood flow to the brain and heart, the two most vulnerable vascular beds because of their high metabolic demand, must be maintained. If arterial hypotension is uncontrolled, it may cause cerebral vascular accident, myocardial infarction, or death.

Etiology Overdosage of general anesthetic or rapid vascular absorption of local agents may result from an amount of the agent exceeding the patient's tolerance. Tendency to overdosage occurs during prolonged anesthesia with large amounts of drugs absorbed, in age-extreme patients, or with unrecognized hypothermia during lengthy abdominal or thoracic procedures. Circulatory effects of spinal or epidural anesthesia, such as diminished cardiac output or reduced peripheral resistance, also produce hypotension.

Other causes are hemorrhage, loss of whole blood, or loss of plasma into tissues during extensive surgical procedures; circulatory abnormalities such as cardiac tamponade, heart failure, hypovolemia, cerebral or pulmonary embolism (fat embolism from fracture sites, amniotic fluid emboli during delivery, or air emboli from introduction of air into the circulation during an infusion or procedure); myocardial ischemia or infarction; changes in position, especially if executed rapidly or roughly; excessive preanesthetic medication (postural hypotension may follow narcotic administration); potent therapeutic drugs (tranquilizers, adrenal steroids, antihypertensives) given before anesthetic; or hypoxia.

Surgical manipulation may induce hypotension mechanically by obstructing venous return to the heart with packs, retractors, or body rests. Or hypotension may result from a vagal-induced reflex precipitated by intraperitoneal traction, manipulation in the chest or neck areas, rapid release of either increased intraabdominal pressure or overdistention of the bladder, anorectal stimulation, or stimulation of the periosteum or joint cavities. Other causes are transfusion reaction (suggested by accompanying cyanosis and oozing at surgical site), septic shock, severe hyperthermia, and anaphylactic reaction.

Symptoms Early reversible shock is accompanied by unstable blood pressure, vasoconstriction, elevated serum pH, and elevated catecholamine levels. Late manifestations are pallor or cyanosis, clammy skin, dilated pupils, decreased urinary output, tachycardia, decreased bleeding in the surgical field, or pallor of organs caused by compensatory vasoconstriction, nausea, vomiting, sighing respirations, or air hunger in conscious patients.

Diagnosis Determination of arterial blood pressure and pulse rate and estimation of pulse volume are indicative of the volume of cardiac ejection. Arbitrary figures of measured blood pressure are not as important as individual circulatory status. A specific measurement in a healthy adult may be relatively insignificant, whereas the same figure in an aged patient could be hazardous. In critically ill patients, direct arterial pressure, central venous pressure, and urine output are monitored.

Treatment Treatment must be prompt to avoid circulatory collapse. The aim is to increase perfusion of the vital organs and to treat any specific cause while giving general supportive therapy. Supportive measures include oxygen by mask with assisted respiration; elevation of the legs to increase blood pressure by draining pooled blood, especially after sympathetic blockade; and rapid intravenous fluid therapy to increase blood volume. Because the volume of fluid is more vital than its composition, various solutions are applicable for early treatment in an emergency. If whole blood is not available, crystalloid solutions (e.g., Ringer's lactate), 5% dextrose in water, physiologic saline solution, plasma or serum albumin, or 6% dextran (plasma expander) may be given. Rapid infusion under pressure may be necessary. Vasoactive drugs are given as necessary; these are usually vasopressors (see pp. 398-399) to constrict arterioles and veins while increasing the myocardial contractile force. Blood gases should be monitored.

Prevention The causes must be reversed or avoided. Therefore, observe the patient constantly throughout anesthesia; in suspected individuals, test the cardiovascular response to the desired surgical position before induction; avoid overdosage of premedications and anesthetic drugs; change position slowly; manipulate tissue gently; and replace blood and fluid loss promptly. The anesthesiologist administers a minimal amount of the anesthetic and takes adequate time to induce and deepen anesthesia so as not to raise the blood level of the anesthetic too rapidly. Positive pressure is applied to the airway prudently.

Some narcotics and anesthetic agents, surgical trauma, anoxia, and blood loss can lead to postoperative hypotension. When combined, these factors interfere with the complex physiologic mechanisms that support blood pressure. Peripheral vessels dilate. A degree of cardiovascular collapse ensues. Vasoconstriction reduces renal blood flow, causing decrease or failure of kidney function. Patients must be monitored postoperatively for sudden drops in blood pressure or other signs of shock. Vasoactive drugs and oxygen may be administered. Fluid management is critical during the recovery phase of renal function following restoration of systemic blood pressure to avoid hypertension.

Hypertension

Abnormal elevation of blood pressure may occur, especially in a hypertensive or arteriosclerotic patient. Even mildly hypertensive patients are prone to myocardial ischemia (inadequate blood flow to heart) during induction of and emergence from anesthesia. Intubation stimulates the sympathetic nervous system. Other predisposing factors include pain, shivering, hypoxia, hypercapnia, effects of vasopressor drugs, or hypervolemia from overreplacement of fluid losses. Treatment consists of administration of oxygen, diuretics, and antihypertensive beta-blocker drugs as indicated. If not controlled, hypertension may precipitate a cerebrovascular accident or myocardial infarction. It may cause bleeding from the surgical site or may threaten the integrity of a vascular bypass.

Circulatory Shock

Shock is a complex phenomenon, a life-threatening condition in which circulation fails for one or several reasons. Loss of circulating blood volume, loss of pumping power of the heart, or loss of peripheral resistance can result in insufficient flow of blood for adequate tissue perfusion or oxygenation. If prolonged, inadequate organ blood flow with deficient microcirculation profoundly depresses vital processes. Because the objective of circulation is achieved in the capillaries, defective cellular metabolism derived from shock interferes further with the body's inherent defenses and metabolic acidosis occurs. Normal defense mechanisms are reflex vasoconstriction and increased pulse rate, which tend to redistribute the flow of blood to the heart and brain at the expense of the other vital organs. If shock is promptly recognized, treated, and reversed, permanent damage is avoided. If it progresses to irreversibility, death ensues from cellular dysfunction and organ hypoperfusion.

Multiple kinds and causes of shock present problems in relationships among the heart, circulatory system, and blood volume. Circulatory inadequacy may originate from a marked decrease in cardiac output, venous return to the heart, or peripheral vascular resistance. All forms of shock carry high mortality rates. The best treatment is prevention. Shock is classified by cause of inadequate tissue perfusion.

Hypovolemic Shock Fluid loss is greater than compensatory absorption of interstitial fluid into the circulation (see hypovolemia, p. 381).

Hemorrhagic Shock Shock results from hemorrhage or inadequate blood volume replacement (see Chapter 23, p. 487).

Cardiogenic Shock The pumping action of the left ventricle is insufficient to pump enough blood to vital organs. Cardiogenic shock may be precipitated by congestive heart failure, myocardial contusion or infarction, coronary air embolism, mechanical venous obstruction, or hypothermia. In addition to drugs, various mechanical devices may be used, such as an auxiliary ventricle or counterpulsation with the intraaortic balloon to temporarily increase left ventricular function.

Neurogenic Shock Loss of vasomotor tone in peripheral blood vessels leads to sudden vasodilation and pooling of blood. Vasodilation produces hypotension. Peripheral resistance is too great for compensation by increased cardiac output, increasing the risk for congestive heart failure and pulmonary edema. Causes may be brain damage, deep anesthesia, emotional trauma, vagal reflex from pain or surgical manipulation, or spinal cord injury.

Traumatic Shock Damage to the capillaries caused by soft tissue trauma increases capillary permeability, with loss of blood volume into the tissues. This state is aggravated by pain, which inhibits the vasomotor center, leading to vasodilation and hypovolemia. Toxic factors associated with intravascular coagulation lead to pulmonary, renal, and/or multiple organ failure. (See disseminated intravascular coagulation [DIC], Chapter 23, p. 488.)

Vasogenic Shock Anaphylaxis (see p. 395) and septic shock (see Chapter 25, p. 534) are the most common types of vasogenic shock.

Venospasm

If caused by cold IV fluid infusion, venospasm may manifest as very slow flow. It may result from pressure infusion or extravasation. Intravenous procaine relieves spasm. Thrombophlebitis may follow venospasm.

Coronary Thrombosis

Coronary thrombosis can occur from severe hypoxia and lack of oxygen to coronary vessels. Sometimes its occurrence is the reason for a patient's never regaining consciousness following a surgical procedure.

Air Embolism

Air embolism may occur intraoperatively with the patient in a sitting position for craniotomy or posterior cervical operation. Cerebral diploic veins are noncollapsible; venous sinuses in the skull remain open. Air entering a vein is carried rapidly to the right side of the heart and pulmonary circulation, obstructing ventricular flow. Cardiac dysrhythmias and unexplained hypotension are prime symptoms. Characteristic heart murmur may be audible by precordial stethoscope or Doppler device. Air embolism may also occur during cardiopulmonary bypass, thyroidectomy, or laparoscopy.

Preoperative placement of a central venous catheter (see pp. 371-372) allows immediate aspiration of air. To relieve ventricular obstruction if no catheter is in place, the patient is placed in steep head-down position with right side up. If cardiac arrest occurs, cardiopulmonary resuscitation is begun. Closed heart massage may move an embolus obstructing the coronary artery.

Cardiac Dysrhythmias

An alteration of normal cardiac rhythm may decrease cardiac output, exhaust the myocardium, and lead to ventricular fibrillation or cardiac arrest. *Bradycardia* is the slowing of the heart or pulse rate. *Tachycardia* is an excessive rapidity of the heart's action. Ventricular tachycardia and ventricular fibrillation are dysrhythmias of most serious consequence and thus most feared.

Etiology Etiologic factors include hypoxia; hypercapnia; acidosis; electrolyte imbalance; coronary disease; myocardial infarction; vagal reflexes; anesthetic agents; toxic doses of digitalis, epinephrine or other drugs; and laryngospasm and coughing initiated by the presence of secretions in the airway following induction. Other causes may be hypotension, hemorrhage, hypovolemia, pneumothorax, and mechanical injuries.

Ventricular Dysrhythmias An impulse originating in the ventricles must travel to the rest of the myocardium from one ventricle, proceeding then to the other ventricle. Because the impulse does not travel via the rapid, specialized conduction system, depolarization of both ventricles takes longer and is not simultaneous. The complexes of dysrhythmias have an abnormal appearance on ECG compared to normally initiated and conducted impulses.

PREMATURE VENTRICULAR CONTRACTIONS An ectopic focus in the ventricles stimulates the heart to contract or beat prematurely before the regularly scheduled sinoatrial impulse arrives (Figure 19-3). Main precipitating factors are electrolyte or acid-base imbalance, myocardial infarction, digitalis toxicity, and caffeine. The premature ventricular contraction (PVC) must be distinguished from a premature atrial contraction (PAC). Isolated PVCs may not require treatment, but those occurring in clusters of two or more or over five or six a minute require therapy. The aim is to quiet the irritable myocardium and restore adequate cardiac output.

Treatment consists of a lidocaine bolus followed by a continuous drip by infusion; correction of the cause

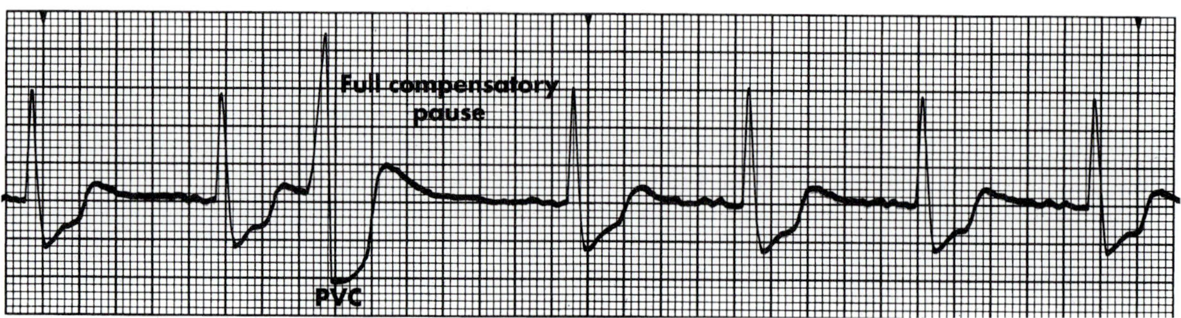

FIGURE 19-3 Premature ventricular contractions. (From Huszar RJ: *Basic dysrhythmias: interpretation and management*, ed 2, St Louis, 1994, Mosby.)

(e.g., hypoxia): and other antiarrhythmic drugs if indicated (e.g., procainamide or quinidine). Temporary pacing may be used for severe bradycardia. Paired PVCs pose an increased danger of ventricular tachycardia.

VENTRICULAR TACHYCARDIA Rapid heart rate (100 to 220 beats per minute) may be caused by ventricular ischemia or irritability, anoxia, or digitalis intoxication. The heart rate does not give time for ventricular filling (Figure 19-4). The resultant reduced cardiac output predisposes the patient to ventricular fibrillation or cardiac failure. It is treated by prompt intravenous administration of lidocaine, procainamide, or intramuscular quinidine.

Synchronized cardioversion of 10 to 200 joules may be used if the blood pressure is palpable. This is the application of high-intensity, short-duration electric shock to the chest wall over the heart to produce total cardiac depolarization. This countershock is timed to interrupt an abnormal rhythm in the cardiac cycle, thereby permitting resumption of a normal one. Cardioversion is usually applied in instances of nonarrest for a nevertheless dangerous ventricular tachycardia. It may be an elective or emergency treatment. Asynchronous cardioversion is used if the patient is pulseless. Treatment includes correction of underlying cause.

VENTRICULAR FLUTTER Often called *fine ventricular fibrillation,* the flutter appears as a transient state between ventricular tachycardia and ventricular fibrillation. The patient will show signs of poor cardiac output.

VENTRICULAR FIBRILLATION The most serious of all dysrhythmias, fibrillation is characterized by total disorganization of ventricular activity (Figure 19-5). There are rapid and irregular, uncoordinated random contractions of the small myocardial groups without effective ventricular contraction and cardiac output. Circulation ceases. The patient in fibrillation is unconscious and possibly convulsing from cerebral hypoxia.

Treatment of Ventricular Fibrillation Because respiratory and cardiac arrest quickly follow, ventricular fibrillation is rapidly fatal unless successful *defibrillation* is effected.

1. *Precordial thump.* In a *monitored* patient, a fast, sharp, single blow to the midportion of the sternum (using the nipple line as a landmark) may be delivered with the bottom fleshy part of a closed fist struck from 8 to 12 inches (20 to 30 cm) above the chest. The blow generates a small electrical stimulus in a heart that is reactive. It may be effective in restoring a beat in cases of asystole or recent onset of dysrhythmia.
2. *Asynchronous cardioversion.* Prompt defibrillation by short-duration electric shock to the heart produces simultaneous depolarization of all muscle fiber bundles, after which spontaneous beating (conversion to spontaneous normal sinus rhythm) may resume if the myocardium is oxygenated and not acidotic. Defibrillation of an anoxic myocardium is difficult. *The time fibrillation is started should be noted.* The electric shock is coordinated with controlled ventilation and cardiac compression. Cardiopulmonary resuscitation (see CPR, pp. 399-404) begins as soon as fibrillation is identified. Many variables may affect defibrillation, such as body weight, paddle position, electrical waveform, and resistance to electric current flow. Procedures follow an established protocol.
3. *Adjunct drug therapy.* Drugs are given as necessary: vasopressor, cardiotonic, and myocardial stimulant drugs to maintain a useful heartbeat; vasodilator or antiarrhythmic drugs to prevent recurrence; and sodium bicarbonate to combat acidosis (see pp. 396-399). Continuous monitoring of the heart and laboratory analysis of arterial blood gases are essential.

Defibrillation: Equipment and Technique Necessary equipment for defibrillation includes a defibrillator machine and two paddle electrodes. Defibrillators use direct electric current. Most have integrated monitors; monitor and defibrillator switches may be separated or combined. An operational monitor does not always indicate that fibrillation power is on. Many monitor-defibrillator units can monitor the ECG from

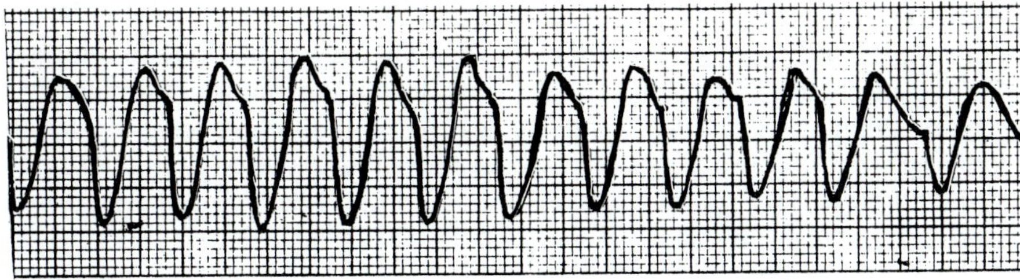

FIGURE 19-4 Ventricular tachycardia. (From Phipps WJ et al: *Medical-surgical nursing: concepts and clinical practice,* ed 5, St Louis, 1995, Mosby.)

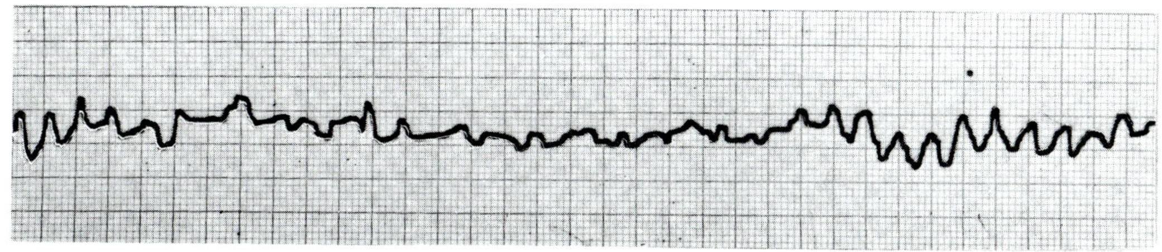

FIGURE 19-5 Ventricular fibrillation. (From Phipps WJ et al: *Medical-surgical nursing: concepts and clinical practice,* ed 5, St Louis, 1995, Mosby.)

the paddle electrodes as well as from separate patient leads. These paddles and patient leads cannot operate simultaneously, however. Depending on the type of defibrillator, the electrical cord must be plugged in or batteries charged. All defibrillators should be checked regularly with suitable test equipment. Paddles must be cleaned immediately and prepared for reuse. This is emergency equipment and must be available at all times.

EXTERNAL DEFIBRILLATION External defibrillation of the heart is used unless the chest is already open, as for intrathoracic surgery. Standard electrode paste or jelly or saline-soaked 4 × 4 gauze pads reduce the resistance of the skin to passage of the electric current. If paste is used on paddles, it should not extend beyond the electrodes or onto any part of the handles. Gel pads between the paddles and the patient's skin provide the advantage that if external cardiac compression is resumed after defibrillation, hands will not slip on the chest. The large diameter of the paddles increases the area of skin contact, thus reducing the possibility of skin burns by spreading of the current. The paddles must be held flat against the skin and more than 2 inches (5 cm) apart to prevent electrical arcing. They must be kept scrupulously clean because foreign material reduces the uniformity of the shock. The electrodes must be pressed firmly against the chest wall for good contact. One of two *external paddle positions* may be used:

1. *Standard position.* One electrode is placed just to the right of the upper sternum below the clavicle. The other is positioned to the left of the cardiac apex (i.e., left of the nipple at the fifth intercostal space along the left midaxillary line). The delivered current flows through the long axis of the heart.
2. *Anterior-posterior position.* One electrode is placed anteriorly over the precordium between the left nipple and sternum. The other is positioned posteriorly behind the heart immediately below the left scapula, avoiding the spinal column. This allows for more energy passage through the heart, but placement is more difficult.

INTERNAL DEFIBRILLATION For internal defibrillation, sterile electrodes are placed on the myocardium, one over the right atrium, the other over the left ventricle. If these electrodes are gauze-covered, they are dipped in sterile saline solution before use. Minimal current is needed when paddles are placed directly on the heart.

Team members must understand the functioning of the defibrillator for the patient's safety and their own. The person holding the electrode paddles delivers the electric charge by pressing a switch on the handle or a foot switch. The safest method is to activate both paddles simultaneously for discharge of electric energy. The operator should have dry hands and stand on dry floor. *To avoid possible self-electrocution when using a defibrillator, neither the person holding the electrodes nor anyone else should touch the metal operating table or the patient while the current is applied. No part of the operator's body should touch the paste or the uninsulated electrodes. Loud verbal warning is given before discharge.* Countershock is repeated at intervals if fibrillation persists. Transthoracic impedance falls with repetitive closely spaced electric discharges. After each countershock, reassess the ECG and pulse.

Myocardial damage resulting from defibrillatory efforts is in direct proportion to the energy used; therefore maximal settings, when not required, may increasingly impair an already damaged myocardium. The energy level delivered through a specific ohm load should be indicated on the front panel of the defibrillator. Delivery-output ranges vary with machines. Strength of the countershock is expressed in energy as joules or watt-seconds, the product of power and duration. If the patient's chest muscles do not contract, no current has reached the patient. Check the defibrillator's connection to the electrical source and "off" button to the synchronizer circuit. If the machine is battery operated, the battery must be charged enough to energize the capacitor. *Be familiar with and follow operating instructions for the defibrillator in use.*

Prevention Appropriate preoperative sedation and skillfully administered anesthesia help to prevent hazardous cardiovascular reflexes. As premature ventricular contractions are precursors to fibrillation, in itself a precursor to cardiac arrest, any cardiopulmonary emergency in a prearrest phase requires:

1. *Monitoring of heart rhythm and rate.* Ability to recognize the rhythms that precede arrest permits intervention that may prevent arrest. If the cardiac status is not under constant monitoring, hypoxia and acidosis may be present and require correction before other therapeutic modalities can be used effectively.
2. *Establishment of an intravenous lifeline.* Venous cannulation provides access to peripheral and central venous circulation for administering drugs and fluids, obtaining venous blood specimens for laboratory analysis, and inserting catheters into the right side of the heart and pulmonary arteries for physiologic monitoring and electrical pacing. If cardiac arrest appears imminent or has occurred, cannulation of a peripheral or femoral vein should be attempted first so as not to interrupt cardiopulmonary resuscitation. To keep the infusion open, the rate should be kept low. The usual complications to all intravenous techniques should be guarded against.

Cardiac Arrest (Circulatory Arrest)

In cardiac arrest, there is cessation of cardiocirculatory action; the pumping mechanism of the heart ceases. Cardiac standstill represents total absence of electrical cardiac activity, asystole, reflected as a straight line on an ECG rhythm strip. It may occur as primary cardiac failure or secondary to failure of pulmonary ventilation. The types of circulatory arrest are profound cardiovascular collapse, electromechanical dissociation, ventricular fibrillation, and ventricular asystole or standstill. Cardiac arrest may precede or follow failure of the respiratory system because the systems are interrelated.

Incidence Arrest may occur during induction of anesthesia, intraoperatively, or postoperatively. Occurrence during cardiac surgery or following massive hemorrhage is not uncommon. Patients more prone to arrest include those at age extremes and those with previously diagnosed paroxysmal dysrhythmias, primary cardiovascular abnormalities, myocarditis, heartblock, or digitalis toxicity. Unexpected arrest is one that happens in a patient of general good health who is undergoing a low-risk or relatively routine procedure. These arrests are associated with major morbidity and mortality.

Etiology A single factor or combination of factors may precipitate arrest, but the general cause is inadequate coronary arterial blood flow. Defective respiratory function produces systemic hypoxemia, causing myocardial hypoxia and depression. It also increases myocardial irritability and the heart's susceptibility to vagal reflexes. Some of the specific precipitating factors are dysrhythmias, emboli, extreme hypotension or hypovolemia, respiratory obstruction, aspiration, effects of drugs, anesthetic overdosage, excessively rapid or unsmooth induction, sepsis, pharyngeal stimulation, metabolic abnormalities (acidosis, toxemia, electrolyte imbalance), poor cardiac filling caused by positioning, manipulation of the heart, central nervous system trauma, anaphylaxis, and electric shock from ungrounded or faulty electrical equipment.

Symptoms Symptoms include loss of heartbeat and blood pressure, sudden fixed dilated pupils, sudden pallor or cyanosis, cold clammy skin, absence of reflexes, unconsciousness or convulsions in a previously conscious patient, respiratory standstill, and dark blood or absence of bleeding in the surgical field.

Diagnosis Arrest is readily detected by the ECG monitor during anesthesia, with absence of blood pressure and precordial heart sounds and the lack of a palpable carotid pulse. Onset of pupillary dilatation is within 45 seconds after cerebral anoxia; full dilatation is reached about 90 to 110 seconds after cessation of cerebral circulation.

Treatment Cardiopulmonary resuscitation (see pp. 399-404) is initiated *immediately* to restore oxygenation to vital organs. Defibrillation may be needed for ventricular fibrillation (see pp. 392-394). Intravenous drugs usually are used (see following discussion) to improve cardiopulmonary status.

Prevention Optimal psychologic preoperative assessment to identify the level of anxiety and testing for abnormalities and sensitivities are important preoperative preparations. Intraoperative precautions include use of ECG and temperature monitoring; no stimulation during induction; maintenance of an adequate airway, oxygenation, and arterial blood pressure; proper timing and use of medications; proper positioning and slow position changes under anesthesia; no weight on the patient; gentle handling of tissues, with minimal traction and manipulation, especially of the heart and great vessels; and skillful anesthetic administration.

INTRAVENOUS CARDIOVASCULAR DRUGS

An important factor in optimal anesthesia management is prompt recognition of causes of hypotension, shock, and other complications that could lead to cardiac arrest. Prompt correction of reversible precipitants is critical. Many intravenous drugs are used to correct hypoxia, correct metabolic acidosis, manipulate cardiovascular variables, or treat pulmonary edema.

Pharmacodynamics

Uptake, movement, binding, and interactions of drugs vary at the tissue site of their biochemical and physiologic actions. Drug action is determined by how the drug interacts in body. Some drugs alter body fluids; others, such as anesthetics (see Chapter 17), interact with cell membranes; most act through receptor mechanisms.

Receptor Mechanisms

Most drugs mimic naturally occurring compounds and interact with specific biologic molecules to produce biologic responses. For example, cardiovascular drugs are *sympathomimetics.* They evoke physiologic responses similar to those produced by the sympathetic nervous system. A receptor is a structural protein molecule on a cell surface or within cytoplasm that binds with a drug to produce a biologic response. Three types of receptors are noteworthy in understanding the drugs used to counteract complications that may occur during anesthesia.

Adrenergic Receptors These are innervated by sympathetic nerve fibers and activated by epinephrine or norepinephrine secreted at the postganglionic nerve endings. These receptors are classified as *alpha, beta$_1$,* or *beta$_2$* depending on their sensitivity to specific adrenergic activating and blocking drugs. Alpha receptors are located primarily in peripheral and renal arteriolar muscles; beta$_1$ receptors predominate in the heart; beta$_2$ receptors are primarily in smooth muscle of the lungs and blood vessels.

Cholinergic Receptors These are sites where acetylcholine exerts action to transmit nerve impulses through the parasympathetic nervous system to regulate heart rate and respirations.

Opiate Receptors These are regions in the brain capable of binding morphine in areas related to pain.

Drug Interactions

No drug has a single action. Each modifies existing functions within the body by interactions to stimulate or inhibit responses. The desired action may be accompanied by side effects or an exaggerated response. An *allergic reaction* may occur immediately after exposure or may be delayed.

Anaphylaxis is a life-threatening, acute allergic reaction in which cells release histamine or a histamine-like substance. Anaphylaxis, a form of vasogenic shock, causes vasodilation, hypotension, and bronchiolar constriction. Within seconds, the patient will exhibit edema, wheezing, cyanosis, and dyspnea. Treatment includes epinephrine and antihistamines to control bronchospasm. Isoproterenol, vasopressors (see pp. 398-399), corticosteroids, and aminophylline may also be administered.

In combination with local, regional, or general anesthetics, drugs must be carefully administered and monitored. The action of one drug may counteract another. Patients who do not respond to one drug (e.g., a catecholamine) may respond to another. Physicians do not always agree on the use of potent drugs. For example, a vasoconstrictor used to treat hypotension may possibly cause ischemic damage to organs. *Follow the physician's orders for all drugs.*

Intravenous Administration

Speed of administration and dosage will depend on the drug and its intended action. Dosages given in this text vary according to individual patient circumstances. Technique of intravenous administration also varies.

Continuous Intravenous Drip The drug is diluted in a volume of dextrose or normal saline solution. The rate of administration is regulated by adjusting the number of drips per minute from the solution container into the IV tubing. A drug that might be absorbed by plastic should *not* be added to solution in a plastic infusion bag.

Bolus A bolus is a single rapid injection of the full dosage of a drug that cannot be diluted. It is usually given through an existing IV line. It may be injected directly into a vein or an intrathecal catheter. Some drugs can be given via an endotracheal tube for absorption through the alveoli. The drug quickly reaches peak level in the bloodstream.

Intravenous Push A drug may be injected slowly into an IV line or through an intermittent infusion pump over a period of minutes. The total dose may be diluted and given in repeated doses over hours. An infusion pump may be used to control rate of delivery precisely.

Titration Dosage is calculated on the basis of body surface area (BSA) and hemodynamic parameters. Cardiac output is evaluated in terms of BSA. This may be determined by the ratio of the patient's height and weight on the BSA scale or by thermodilution (see p. 375). The patient's physiologic responses also will determine total dosage.

NOTE

1. Some drugs are inactivated by others. The IV tubing should be flushed or changed to avoid precipitation, as can occur with sodium bicarbonate.
2. Many potent drugs should be infused through an IV catheter, which is safer than a needle to prevent extravasation. If a drug extravasates at the site of injection, the area must be promptly infiltrated with phentolamine (Regitine) to prevent necrosis.

Drugs by Classification

Pharmacokinetics includes mechanisms of absorption, distribution, and metabolism of drugs in the body and elimination from the body. Nurses must have knowledge of drug actions and of how to prepare and administer drugs. The following drugs are classified by their pharmacodynamics to counteract adverse cardiovascular and pulmonary status.

Sympathomimetics are most often used to:

1. Increase force (inotropic effect), maintain contractility (noninotropic effect), or decrease stroke volume of myocardial contractions
2. Increase pulse rate
3. Increase or decrease arterial blood pressure
4. Correct dysrhythmias
5. Increase renal blood flow
6. Stimulate the central nervous system
7. Treat bronchospasm
8. Prolong effect of local anesthetics
9. Manage life-threatening emergencies

Patients receiving any of the following drugs must be carefully monitored.

Antiarrhythmics/Antidysrhythmics

These drugs control heart rate and rhythm. They may induce a decreased rate and cardiac output. They may reduce cardiac conduction and increase dilation of peripheral vessels.

Lidocaine Hydrochloride (Xylocaine) Lidocaine increases the threshold for ventricular irritability by exerting a focal anesthetic effect on the myocardial cell membrane. It is used for ventricular tachycardia and fibrillation, especially if resistance to defibrillation effort occurs. It can be given intravenously, intrathecally, or by endotracheal tube. *Dosage:* 1 mg/kg or 75 to 100 mg IV push over 30 to 60 seconds, followed by half the initial dose every 8 to 10 minutes to a total of 3 mg/kg, if ectopic heartbeats continue. After conversion, a maintenance dose of 2 to 4 mg/min can be given by IV drip. Half these dosages are used to treat shock or pulmonary edema.

Bretylium Tosylate (Bretylol) Bretylium lowers the defibrillation threshold, permitting otherwise refractory rhythms to be electrically converted. It is indicated for ventricular tachycardia and fibrillation unresponsive to other therapy. *Dosage:* 5 mg/kg by rapid IV bolus, followed by defibrillation. If fibrillation continues, dose can by doubled and repeated as necessary. For ventricular fibrillation, 300 to 600 mg may be required. The drug may be diluted for continuous IV drip at a dosage of 1 to 2 mg/min for ventricular tachycardia and to prevent fibrillation. Some degree of hypotension may occur.

Procainamide Hydrochloride (Pronestyl) Procainamide suppresses ventricular premature contractions and recurrent tachycardia. This drug may be used if lidocaine is contraindicated or has not controlled ventricular tachycardia. *Dosage:* 100 mg IV push every 5 minutes until dysrhythmia ceases, or to a total of 1 g. Maintenance IV drip is 1 to 4 mg/min. Marked hypotension may occur if infusion is too rapid.

Adenosine Triphosphate (Adenocard) Adenosine slows atrioventricular (AV) node conduction. This action converts supraventricular tachycardia to normal sinus rhythm. *Dosage:* 6 to 12 mg by IV bolus followed immediately by a saline bolus. If given via a central venous catheter, 3 mg may be therapeutic. Incremental doses of 0.05 mg/kg can be given as necessary. This drug is contraindicated for asthmatics.

Verapamil Hydrochloride (Isoptin, Calan) A calcium channel blocker, verapamil inhibits calcium ions to slow myocardial contractility, heart rate, and demand for oxygen. It is used as an antiarrhythmic to treat paroxysmal supraventricular tachycardia, acute atrial flutter, and atrial fibrillation. *Dosage:* 5 to 10 mg (0.075-0.15 mg/kg adult body weight) by slow IV push over 2 minutes; may be repeated after 30 minutes. This drug is *not* given to patients with severe hypotension or cardiogenic shock, nor is it given concurrently with an intravenous beta-adrenergic blocker, such as propranolol.

Propranolol Hydrochloride (Inderal) A beta-adrenergic receptor blocking agent, propranolol is used to control supraventricular dysrhythmias and to treat hypertension. It reduces myocardial oxygen consumption by blocking catecholamine-induced increases in heart rate, blood pressure, and cardiac contractions. It may be used if control of ventricular fibrillation is not achieved with lidocaine or other drugs. *Dosage:* 1 to 3 mg IV push, not to exceed 1 mg/min, titrated for heart rate and rhythm. This drug is contraindicated for asthmatics and patients with bronchospasm or cardiac depression.

Isoproterenol Hydrochloride (Isuprel) A beta-adrenergic receptor stimulant, isoproterenol stimulates sympathetic tone, rate, and strength of myocardial contractions and cardiac output. It increases myocardial demand for oxygen. It may be used for ventricular dysrhythmias, but it may produce tachycardia or dysrhythmia. It is indicated to control hemodynamically significant bradycardia in a patient who has a pulse but who is unresponsive to atropine. It is a vasodilator and bronchodilator. *Dosage:* IV drip of 1 mg to 500 ml of dextrose or saline solution at rate of 1.25 ml/min, titrated according to heart rate and rhythm.

Antimuscarinics/Anticholinergics

These drugs block passage of impulses through the parasympathetic nerves to the heart and smooth muscles. When both the sympathetic and parasympathetic components of the autonomic nervous system are stimulated, the parasympathetic dominates to slow heartbeat and respirations. An anticholinergic allows desired sympathetic action.

Atropine Sulfate Atropine reduces cardiac vagal tone, enhances atrioventricular conduction, and increases cardiac output. It accelerates cardiac rate in sinus bradycardia with severe hypotension or in bradycardia associated with hypoxia and reduced cardiac output. It may restore cardiac rhythm in atrioventricular block or ventricular asystole. It is a primary drug used in cardiopulmonary arrest. Atropine may be given intravenously, intrathecally, or via an endotracheal tube. *Dosage:* 1 mg IV bolus for asystole, 0.5 mg for bradycardia, at 5-minute intervals until desired rate is achieved or to a total dose of 2 mg. Full vagal blockage could result from overdosage.

Vasodilators

These noninotropic drugs relax smooth muscle in the capillaries and cause peripheral dilation. They dilate arteries and veins almost equally without increasing myocardial contractility. This reduces venous return to heart. They are used to alter blood flow and lower blood pressure in patients with severely reduced cardiac output or in hypertensive crisis.

Sodium Nitroprusside (Nipride, Nitropress) Sodium nitroprusside acts rapidly as a direct peripheral vasodilator to increase cardiac output and redistribute cardiac work in patients with pump failure. It increases tissue perfusion without reflex tachycardia. *Dosage:* IV drip not to exceed 10 µg/kg/min of 50 mg dissolved in 2 to 3 ml of dextrose added to 250 to 1000 ml of dextrose in water for infusion. An infusion pump or microdrip-regulating system ensures a precise flow rate. The solution deteriorates in light, so it must be protected by opaque material such as aluminum foil. No other drug should be injected into the IV line while sodium nitroprusside is running.

Nitroglycerin (Nitrostat IV, Nitrol IV, Tridil) Nitroglycerin decreases venous return to the heart and reduces preload and afterload, thus lowering myocardial oxygen demands. It is used for control of blood pressure in hypertension associated with cardiovascular procedures or endotracheal intubation, or in the immediate postoperative period. *Dosage:* up to 50 µg/min by IV push. Titrate to increase dose and adjust time intervals between infusions, depending on lowering of the blood pressure. This potent drug must be diluted in dextrose or saline solution. It is absorbed by polyvinyl chloride (PVC) plastic, so glass solution bottles and tubing that is not made of PVC should be used. The drug is also light-sensitive.

Trimethaphan Camsylate (Arfonad) A ganglionic blocking agent, trimethaphan camsylate is used to produce controlled hypotension during surgical procedure and to lower blood pressure in patient with hypertension or in an acute hypertensive crisis. *Dosage:* 500 mg diluted in 500 ml of 5% dextrose in water (1 mg/1 ml) IV drip. Initially drug is infused slowly at rate of 1 to 2 mg/min and increased gradually to an average dose range of 3 to 6 mg/min.

Cardiotonics

These drugs combine inotropic effect on the contractility of muscle with vasodilation of blood vessels. They stimulate myocardial function. Vasodilation reduces cardiac afterload, thereby improving cardiac performance and correcting peripheral vascular compensations.

Amrinone (Inocor) Amrinone possesses significant vasodilator activity to improve tissue perfusion, especially to the kidneys, and to improve cardiac output. It is used for short-term effect in patients with ischemic heart disease and severe heart failure. Blood pressure and heart rate remain unchanged, while peripheral arteriolar resistance falls. *Dosage:* 0.5 to 3.5 mg/kg IV bolus followed by IV drip of 5 to 10 µg/kg/min. Titrated to hemodynamic response, a second bolus can be given after 30 minutes.

Dobutamine Hydrochloride (Dobutrex) A synthetic derivative of dopamine, dobutamine increases myocardial contractility while producing little systemic arterial constriction. It is used for short-term treatment of refractory heart failure, cardiogenic shock, and hemodynamically significant hypotension. *Dosage:* 2.5 to 10 µg/kg/min IV drip. Tachycardia or dysrhythmia may result from a larger dose. It is incompatible with alkaline solutions and drugs such as sodium bicarbonate.

Catecholamines

These drugs are vasoconstrictors that improve tissue perfusion by maintaining perfusion pressure, preventing or diminishing blood loss, decreasing tissue vascularity, and improving coronary blood flow. Among indications for their use are anesthesia overdose, hypotension associated with blood loss, and adrenergic insufficiency. They raise blood pressure. They are antispasmodic.

Epinephrine Hydrochloride (Adrenalin) An endogenous catecholamine and alpha-adrenergic receptor stimulant, epinephrine plays an essential role in restoration of spontaneous circulation in asystole; therefore it is the first drug administered in cardiac arrest. By increasing systemic vascular resistance, it improves coronary perfusion pressure and cardiac output produced by cardiac compression during CPR. It improves myocardial contractility and tone and causes vasoconstriction of arteries. It may be given intravenously, intrathecally, or via endotracheal tube or intracardiac injection. *Dosage:* 0.5 to 1.0 mg IV bolus, repeated every 5 minutes as necessary. It is available in preprepared syringes of 1:10,000 dilution (1 mg/10 ml). It may be added to an IV infusion of 250 ml of 5% dextrose in water. It is inactivated by alkaline solutions. Continuous infusion may increase heart rate, blood pressure, and cardiac output. Side effects include myocardial oxygen demand and possible premature ventricular contractions or ventricular fibrillation.

Norepinephrine Bitartrate (Levophed) An endogenous catecholamine, norepinephrine restores and maintains blood pressure. It may be given following peripheral vascular collapse as a result of severe hypotension or cardiogenic shock. It constricts renal and mesenteric vessels and may cause severe peripheral vasoconstriction. *Dosage:* 16 mg/L (16 µg/ml) IV drip in 5% dextrose in water, titrated to desired blood pressure; average dose range is 2 to 4 µg/min. Drug is toxic if extravasation occurs. Hypotension from hypovolemia is a contraindication.

Diuretics

These drugs increase the amount of urine excreted. Potent diuretics are used to treat pulmonary edema and postarrest cerebral edema. They inhibit reabsorption of sodium. They are used with caution, as they may have a direct venodilating effect or may lead to fluid and electrolyte depletion. The most commonly used diuretics are:

1. *Furosemide (Lasix),* 0.5 to 2.0 mg/kg injected slowly over 1 to 2 minutes by IV push; dose can be repeated in 2 hours.
2. *Ethacrynate sodium (Sodium Edecrin),* 40 to 50 mg or 0.5 to 1.0 mg/kg injected slowly by IV push.

Vasopressors

These vasoactive drugs exert an inotropic vasoconstriction action on arterioles and veins through stimulation of alpha-adrenergic receptors, and they increase myocardial contractility, blood pressure, and heart rate by activation of beta-adrenergic receptors. These drugs cause vasomotor depression of the peripheral circulation but increase coronary flow. They may increase ventricular contractile force, alter sinoatrial nodal activity, constrict smooth muscles, and dilate renal and mesenteric blood vessels. They may produce ventricular dysrhythmia, which can be intensified by hypoxia or hypercapnia. Drug effectiveness is reduced in the presence of respiratory or metabolic acidosis.

Dopamine Hydrochloride (Intropin) In high dosage (greater than 10 µg/kg/min IV drip), dopamine causes peripheral vasoconstriction to increase blood pressure and cardiac output. It may be used during cardiogenic shock, severe hypotension, and asystole and then be titrated to the desired blood pressure. Discontinuance should be gradual. A low dose, 1 to 2 µg/kg/min IV drip, dilates renal and mesenteric blood vessels to maintain urinary output but may not increase heart rate or blood pressure. Rate may be increased until organ perfusion is evidenced by blood pressure and urinary output. Tachydysrhythmias are an indication for reduction in dose or discontinuation. Dopamine is inactivated in alkaline solution and by sodium bicarbonate. It is caustic if it extravasates. It should be diluted immediately before use.

Metaraminol Bitartrate (Aramine) Metaraminol produces marked vasoconstriction and increases cardiac output and blood pressure, which may be useful to treat severe hypotension. It may be given IV or via endotracheal tube. *Dosage:* 0.4 mg/min IV drip in 5% dextrose in water.

Other Vasopressors These drugs have various actions. Selection will depend on action needed. Drugs that may be used include:

1. Isoproterenol hydrochloride (Isuprel)
2. Methoxamine hydrochloride (Vasoxyl)
3. Mephentermine sulfate (Wyamine)
4. Norepinephrine bitartrate (Levophed)
5. Phenylephrine hydrochloride (Neo-Synephrine)

Other Drugs

The foregoing list is not intended to be all-inclusive. Other drugs are used for specific problems. Life-threatening acid-base or electrolyte imbalances associated with cardiovascular or pulmonary complications may need to be corrected, as following cardiopulmonary resuscitation. Two drugs may be used *with caution;* they are *not recommended for routine administration at onset of cardiopulmonary resuscitation.*

Calcium Salts Calcium should be avoided unless the patient has hyperkalemia, hypocalcemia, or calcium channel blocker toxicity. It may be administered by IV bolus as *calcium chloride,* 2 ml of 10% (1 g/10 ml) solution repeated as necessary at 10-minute intervals; *calcium gluconate,* 5 to 8 ml; *calcium gluceptate,* 5 to 7 ml.

Sodium Bicarbonate Metabolic acidosis secondary to accumulation of lactic acid produced by respiratory metabolism may need to be corrected. Bicarbonate binds with hydrogen ion from lactic acid to produce carbonic acid that breaks down into carbon dioxide and water. Sodium bicarbonate may be given after other resuscitation measures to reverse acidosis. *Dosage:* 1 mEq/kg by IV bolus initially, titrated according to blood gas analyses for subsequent doses, usually no more than 0.5 mEq/kg at 10- to 15-minute intervals. An excessive dose can produce metabolic alkalosis. Sodium bicarbonate should not be mixed in an IV line with any other drug; it will precipitate calcium salts and inactivate catecholamines.

CARDIOPULMONARY RESUSCITATION

Cardiopulmonary resuscitation (CPR) is aimed at rapidly restoring oxygen delivery to vital organs to reverse the processes that lead to death. CPR is as emergency procedure requiring special training to recognize cardiac or respiratory arrest and to perform artificial ventilation and circulation. To prevent irreversible brain damage, resuscitative measures must be instituted immediately, within 3 to 5 minutes after the arrest. The combination of anoxia and acidosis can make restoration of normal function impossible. Resuscitation is not a one-person job. *The team must be completely familiar with the preplanned routine before the necessity for its use arises.* Success depends on prompt diagnosis and immediate effective treatment. Outcome is directly related to the rapidity with which a functional, spontaneous heart rhythm can be restored. Patients who experience arrest in an operating room may be on monitors with an intravenous line already in place and resuscitation equipment on hand. These arrests are referred to as *witnessed arrests. Note time of onset of arrest and start the time-elapsed clock.* Basic life support is instituted *at once* to reestablish oxygenation and restore the heartbeat.

Basic Life Support

Basic life support (BLS) is that particular phase of emergency cardiac care that either prevents circulatory or respiratory arrest or insufficiency through prompt recognition and intervention or externally supports circulation and respiration of a victim of cardiac or respiratory arrest through CPR. BLS can and should be initiated by any person present when cardiac arrest occurs.

The ABCs of resuscitation are:

A *Airway:* patent and free of secretions or foreign body for effective pulmonary ventilation
B *Breathing:* prompt restoration and maintenance of oxygenation through artificial ventilation
C *Circulation:* provision of oxygen to vital tissues by means of cardiac compression (artificial circulation)

These steps should be started immediately and performed in the order given except when the patient is already intubated. A precordial thump, advanced life support, or both procedures should be instituted without delay to restore circulation. Resuscitation must continue until the patient can resume normal, spontaneous respiration and circulation or until its discontinuation is warranted by cardiac or central nervous system biologic death.

When the arrested patient is in the operating room, anesthesiologists and other team members are present. In a witnessed arrest, the carotid pulse is palpated. The carotid artery is located in the groove between the trachea and muscles of the side of the neck. Palpation of the femoral artery is an acceptable option. If the patient has respiratory arrest, four quick, full lung inflations are given without allowing for full lung deflation between breaths. Maintenance of positive pressure in the lungs more effectively fills, ventilates, and prevents collapse of alveoli. If pulse and breathing are not immediately restored, CPR is begun.

If the patient is being monitored by ECG at the time of arrest, a fast precordial thump may be given and the monitor checked for cardiac rhythm while the carotid pulse is checked. If ventricular fibrillation or tachycardia without a pulse is evident, countershock is delivered as soon as possible (DC 200 to 300 joules delivered energy in adult, 2 joules/kg or 1 joule per pound in infant or child). If this is unsuccessful, additional countershocks and medications are given as ordered or per written protocol. In open heart defibrillation, between 5 and 40 joules are delivered. Begin with lower energy levels.

In infants and small children, a hand is placed over the precordium to feel the apical beat or the brachial pulse is checked in lieu of a carotid pulse. The brachial pulse is on the inside of upper arm midway between the elbow and shoulder. Use index and middle fingers. *Do not give a precordial thump to an infant or child.* In infants and children, bradydysrhythmias and heart block lead to cardiac arrest more commonly than ventricular fibrillation.

Artificial Ventilation (Pulmonary Resuscitation)

Immediate opening of the airway is mandatory to combat respiratory failure. If respiratory obstruction is present, it must be cleared. During general anesthesia, either an oropharyngeal or nasopharyngeal airway or endotracheal tube is in place to maintain a patent air passage. Oxygen (100%) can be delivered at once under positive pressure by manual ventilation. If not, ventilation by other means, such as an esophageal obturator airway or expired-air technique, should be initiated to sustain oxygenation, followed by tracheal intubation as soon as possible. A cuffed endotracheal tube permits continual delivery of high-oxygen concentration without the hazard of stomach distention or aspiration. It facilitates adequate ventilation since, with its use, interposed breaths are not necessary, thereby permitting a faster, uninterrupted cardiac compression rate of 80 per minute. When a tube or airway is lacking, the most rapid means of reestablishing oxygenation is by an *expired-air technique or mouth-to-mouth or mouth-to-nose artificial ventilation.* When artificial ventilation is combined with cardiac compression, tissues receive oxygen.

In the OR the anesthesiologist manages artificial ventilation.

NOTE

1. If attempts to ventilate are unsuccessful despite proper opening of airway, further attempts to remove obstruction should be made. Laryngoscopy, cricothyrotomy, or tracheotomy may be indicated.
2. Tracheal suctioning should last no longer than 5 seconds at a time without ventilation to prevent hypoxia.
3. If spinal injury is suspected or present, extension of the neck is avoided and modified jaw thrust technique is employed. Head, neck, and chest are kept aligned.
4. Ventilation is assessed by seeing the chest rise and fall and hearing and feeling air escape during the patient's exhalation.

Artificial Circulation (Cardiovascular Resuscitation)

Cardiac compression must accompany ventilation in a pulseless patient to maintain adequate blood pressure and circulation, thereby keeping tissues viable, preserving cardiac tone and reflexes, and preventing intravascular clotting. This may be accomplished by *external closed-chest cardiac compression,* the rhythmic application of pressure over the lower half of the sternum above the xiphoid process (Figures 19-6 and 19-7). Because the heart occupies most of the space between the sternum and the thoracic spine, intermittent depression of the sternum raises intrathoracic pressure and produces car-

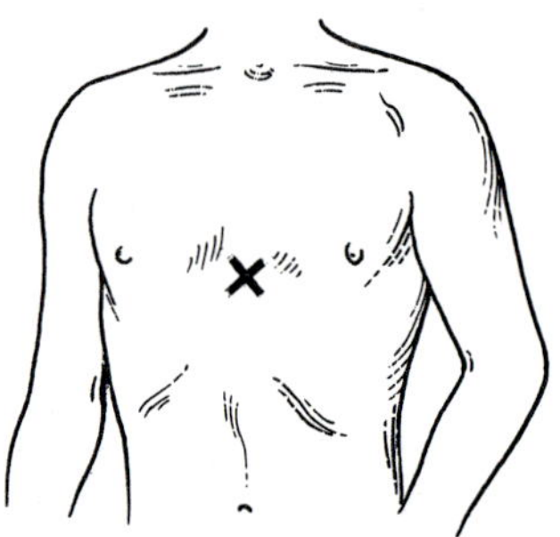

FIGURE 19-6 Cross indicates correct spot to place hands for performing closed-chest cardiac compression: over lower half of sternum and above xiphoid process.

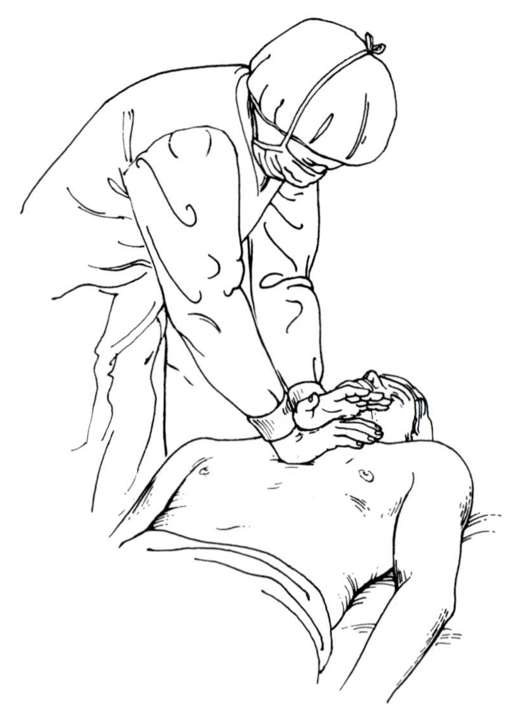

FIGURE 19-7 Closed-chest cardiac compression. Patient is supine on hard flat surface. Resuscitator places heel of one hand over lower half of sternum with heel of other hand on top. Fingers are arched upward to avoid exerting force on ribs. Elbows are straight and locked with shoulders straight over hands.

diac output (Figure 19-8). Blood is forced from the heart into the pulmonary artery and aorta. During relaxation of pressure, negative intrathoracic pressure causes venous blood to flow back into the heart from the pulmonary and systemic circulatory systems (Figure 19-9). Blood moves in the arterial direction through the heart valves. Carotid artery blood flow from this technique usually is only one quarter to one third of normal (mean BP 40 mm Hg), although systolic blood pressure is raised. It may peak to 100 mm Hg, but the diastolic pressure is low. Artificial ventilation is *always* required when external cardiac compression is employed because oxygenation of the circulating blood is inadequate. The brain and myocardium must be perfused effectively for survival. External cardiac compression must be instituted immediately on cessation of circulation. Any interruption in compression causes cessation of blood flow and drop in blood pressure.

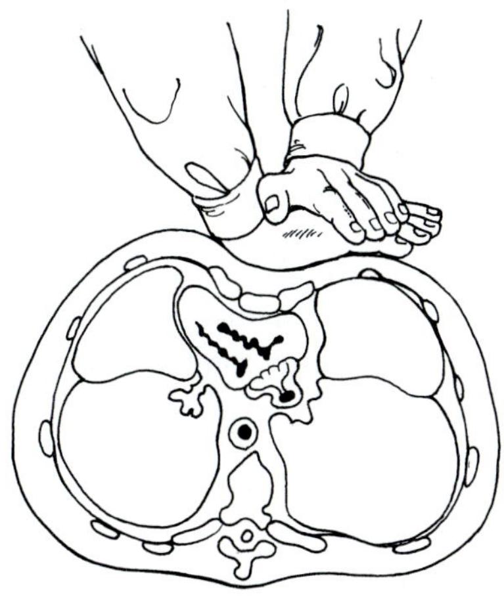

FIGURE 19-8 Manual depression of sternum raises intrathoracic pressure and produces cardiac output. Blood is sent from heart into pulmonary artery and aorta.

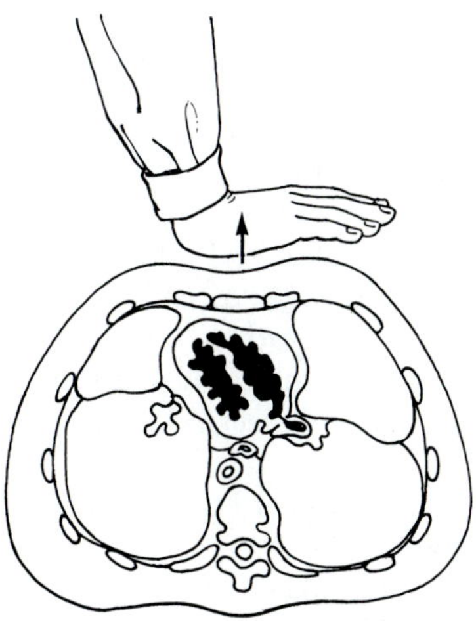

FIGURE 19-9 Releasing pressure on sternum allows heart to fill with venous blood.

Cardiac compression must be performed with knowledge and care. All physicians and nursing personnel must be trained and certified in CPR. Basic principles are the same for infants and children. Differences in technique are related to the position of the heart in the chest, small chest size, and faster heart rate.

Basic life support should not be interrupted for more than 5 seconds at a time except for endotracheal intubation. If intubation is difficult, the patient must be ventilated between short attempts. CPR is never suspended for more than 30 seconds. Preferably, the patient should not be moved until stabilized and ready for transport or until arrangements are made for uninterrupted CPR during movement.

Elevation of the legs to a 60-degree angle with the trunk aids venous return and augments artificial circulation. Cardiac compression is successful only if the heart fills with blood between compressions and the resuscitator can move an adequate volume of oxygenated blood. The carotid or femoral pulse is checked every few minutes to indicate compression effectiveness or return of spontaneous effective heartbeat.

Manual external cardiac compression causes fatigue leading to variation in cardiac output; therefore it is advisable to have additional relief personnel available. Commercially available, manually operated mechanical chest compressors or automatic compressor-ventilators that provide simultaneous compression and ventilation eliminate this problem. When such devices are used, *compression must always be started with the manual method first*. Compressor-ventilators should be used only with a cuffed endotracheal tube, esophageal obturator airway or mask, and only by experienced operators. Use should be limited to adult patients.

Complications of external compression are minimized by careful attention to detail. Compression must be performed with extreme caution to prevent injuries such as rib or sternal fracture, costochondral separation, fat embolism, laceration of the liver, lung contusion, pneumothorax, and hemothorax. *To prevent fractures, never compress the xiphoid process at the tip of the sternum or exert pressure on the ribs.*

Internal Cardiac Compression This is instituted if the patient's chest is already open, as during a cardiothoracic procedure. Thoracotomy may be performed and internal compression administered in instances where external compression may be ineffective, for example, internal thoracic injuries such as penetrating wounds of the heart, flail chest, pericardial tamponade caused by hemorrhage, and chest or spinal deformities. The advantages of internal compression are more complete ventricular emptying with greater outflow of blood into the circulation and rapid diastolic filling for a faster stroke rate than with external compression. Less blood flows in a retrograde manner. The disadvantages are delay in compression, potential trauma to the lungs and myocardium, and possible infection.

If the chest is not open, the incision is made through the left fifth or sixth intercostal space. The pericardial sac is opened for direct manual compression of the myocardium. A rib spreader is placed to avoid strangulation of the operator's hands. By cradling heart in both hands, the operator compresses the ventricles between the thumb and fingers of one hand or fingers of both hands 80 times a minute. Venous filling is necessary for adequate ventricular stroke volume.

Checking Effectiveness of Cardiopulmonary Resuscitation

Signs suggestive of effective compression are constricted reactive pupils, palpable peripheral pulse, audible heartbeat, and improvement in color of mucous membranes, skin, and blood. Additional signs indicative of potential recovery are prompt return of spontaneous respiration and consciousness. Continuous compression is stopped when arterial blood pressure remains above 70 to 90 mm Hg and a strong spontaneous pulse is resumed. CPR may be performed intermittently as necessary to assist the restored heart.

Persistent dilatation of the pupils and lack of reaction to light are ominous signs usually indicative of brain damage. Cell destruction is also manifested by convulsions, hyperpyrexia, and persistent coma. Survival in relation to these symptoms is usually accompanied by tragic consequences such as decerebration or paralysis.

If oxygenation and sternal compression (basic life support) do not promptly produce spontaneous cardiac action, additional supportive therapy is also used (advanced life support).

Advanced Cardiac Life Support

Advanced cardiac life support (ACLS) consists of *definitive therapy* intended to reinstitute spontaneous oxygenation. It includes BLS; use of adjunctive equipment and special techniques for establishing and maintaining effective ventilation and circulation; cardiac and supplemental monitoring; recognition and control of dysrhythmias; defibrillation; establishing and maintaining an IV infusion route; drug administration; and postresuscitative care. It requires the supervision and direction of a physician. It should be initiated within 8 minutes of arrest to improve long-term functional survival. Subsequent insertion of an arterial line supplies access for direct pressure monitoring and arterial blood gases.

Intravenous Drugs

Compression is usually accompanied or followed by judicious use of drugs, administered intravenously to manipulate cardiovascular variables, such as hypoxia and acidosis. (See listing of drugs on pp. 396-399.) These drugs may improve the patient's cardiopulmonary status by increasing the perfusion pressure during cardiac compression, stimulating spontaneous or more forceful myocardial contractions, accelerating the cardiac rate, and suppressing abnormal ventricular activity.

Oxygen, epinephrine, and atropine are the mainstays of pharmacologic management in CPR. Used in combination with basic life support, lidocaine, and defibrillation (see pp. 392-394), they correct most CPR oxygen delivery problems. Each additional drug serves as a vital adjunct in definitive therapy and postresuscitative care.

Emergency Arrest/Crash Cart

An *emergency arrest cart* should be available at all times in all critical care areas (i.e., OR, ED, PACU, and ICU). Specific drugs and equipment vary depending on how well equipped the anesthesiologist is for emergencies. Equipment on a portable cart usually includes:

1. Oxygen and resuscitation equipment: oxygen cylinder, tubing, mask, Ambu bag or bag-valve-mask
2. Laryngoscope tray, blades; endotracheal equipment and tubes; assorted airways—oral and nasal, stylet, padded tongue blades
3. Tracheotomy tray
4. Sterile gloves, sterile gauze sponges, prep swabs or spray, adhesive tape, tourniquets, sutures, armboard, drapes
5. Suction machine and catheters
6. IV infusion solutions and sets, IV needles and catheters (14 and 16 gauge), tubing stopcocks, infusion pump, additive labels
7. Cutdown tray; venous cannulas, wire-guided catheters
8. Assorted sterile syringes: 3, 5, 10, 20, and 50 ml
9. Assorted sterile needles: 25 gauge × ⅝ inches, 20 gauge × 1½ inches, 18 gauge × 1½ inches, 20 gauge × 3 inches (intracardiac) and spinal needles
10. Arterial blood sampling kit with needles, heparinized syringes; arterial line tray
11. Disposable scalpels, hemostats
12. Emergency thoracotomy set: scalpel with No. 20 blade, rib retractor, self-retaining retractor
13. ECG monitor, leads, recording sheets
14. Cardiac arrest board
15. Defibrillator with paddles (adult, pediatric, external, internal), electrode jelly or paste, saline pads
16. Cardiac arrest record for treatment documentation/flow sheets
17. Cardiac pacemaker
18. Drugs: mainly vasoconstrictors, cardiotonics, vasopressors, cardiac depressants, anticholinergics,

cerebral dehydrating agents, pulmonary dehydrating agents. (Many frequently used emergency drugs are available in sterile commercially prefilled syringes to avoid delay in preparation. They must be routinely checked for expiration dates.)

19. CVP manometer
20. Nasogastric tube and bulb syringe
21. Flashlight

Personnel Responsibilities

During cardiopulmonary resuscitation, team members must *remain calm* but react quickly and act efficiently.

1. *Director:* One person, the most knowledgeable, *usually the anesthesiologist,* commands resuscitation efforts. He or she is assisted by surgeons, nurses, surgical technologists, and other available personnel. A cardiologist is usually summoned. Resuscitation teams are multidisciplinary. The person in charge directs lifesaving interventions that entail minute-to-minute decisions such as medications and defibrillation. To avoid confusion, the director issues orders for others to follow. Every circulator should be prepared to be a team captain.
2. *Circulator*
   a. Start the time-elapsed clock (if available) and record the time of arrest.
   b. Activate the emergency alarm to alert the OR manager and summon assistance.
   c. Help reposition the patient as necessary into supine position for CPR. Lower the operating table and provide the resuscitator with a standing platform to facilitate cardiac compression. The circulator must be able to perform chest compressions if an additional resuscitator is not immediately available.
   d. Obtain and prepare necessary equipment, such as medications, the defibrillator, and the ECG if it is not already in use.
   e. Help with and observe intravenous and monitoring lines, such as an arterial line. Assist in collection of blood samples.
   f. Maintain accuracy of sponge, needle, and instrument counts and sterility to best of ability if wound closure progresses (but sterility is secondary to resuscitation efforts).
   g. Supervise termination of the procedure as necessary.
   h. Delegate duties to assisting personnel.
   i. Control traffic. Exclude unauthorized personnel from the room. Provide an optimum environment for successful resuscitation.
   j. Document all medications given, time and amount, and the sequence of procedures performed. Documentation is important in guiding therapy and providing legal protection.
   k. Assist where needed most.
   l. In unsuccessful resuscitation, follow protocol regarding notification of family, care of the deceased, specimens to be saved, and forms to be filled out after a death in the OR.
3. *Scrub person*
   a. Remain sterile and keep the tables sterile if possible. If arrest occurs during the surgical procedure, when chest is not open, the wound is packed with saline-soaked sponges, covered with sterile drape, and the patient is repositioned as necessary for CPR. If the wound can be closed rapidly during resuscitation, this may be done.
   b. Keep track of sponges, needles, and instruments. Counts are completed and the wound is closed as soon as possible despite the outcome. Follow the written institutional policy and procedure for counts during emergency situations.
   c. Give attention to the field and the surgeon's needs. If the patient is hemorrhaging, keep suction tubing clear and tapes available.
   d. If the circulator is performing chest compressions, obtain the emergency cart and assist as required.
4. *OR manager/head nurse*
   a. Assign professional and assistive support personnel to augment the team, for example, an extra circulator, medication nurse, personnel to obtain supplies or handle laboratory samples.
   b. Notify the attending physician, if not present, and appropriate administrative personnel.
   c. Have the patient placed on the critical list. Alert the ICU of a potential patient admission.
   d. Reassign subsequent patients' scheduling.
   e. Keep track of resuscitation progress.
   f. Evaluate the arrest procedure and emergency equipment; verify the documentation.
   g. Support the team as necessary. Keep the surgical suite running smoothly during the emergency.

Duration of Cardiopulmonary Resuscitation

CPR may be done as long as necessary to restore cardiocirculatory function if adequate ventilation and a good peripheral pulse have been restored. It is not uncommon for a second arrest to occur following successful resuscitation. The time frame for survival is shortened drastically if the arrest is unwitnessed. When the patient's condition is adequately stabilized and the wound is closed, he or she is transferred to the ICU.

The decision to discontinue resuscitative efforts in the OR is made by a physician. However the resuscitation team is included in this decision. The decision is based on assessment of cerebral and cardiovascular status. The end point of cardiovascular unresponsiveness is suggested as the most reliable basis for this decision.

Appropriate administrative personnel and services, such as the nursing unit, ICU, and clergy, as well as the patient's family, are notified of the cardiac arrest as required. In case of death, the surgeon notifies the family.

Postresuscitation Care

Postarrest supportive therapy depends on the cause and duration of arrest. Care centers on cardiac and cerebral preservation, maintenance of circulation and ventilation, and minimizing of sequelae such as cerebral edema. The patient must be carefully monitored and closely observed for 48 to 72 hours postarrest. In select patients, hypothermia may be used to reduce oxygen needs. Vital signs, acid-base and electrolyte balances, and urinary output are closely watched. Seizures should be controlled to prevent further anoxia. The patient is observed for signs of embolism, pulmonary edema, fractured ribs, or hemopericardium. A chest x-ray film is taken as soon as feasible after the arrest. An IV fluid lifeline must be left in place. If there is evident cerebral damage, the prognosis is guarded.

Staff Education

Practice sessions of a cardiac arrest emergency and CPR with subsequent evaluation and revision are valuable to review the protocol and prepare the OR staff before need for implementation. Current CPR/BLS certification is required of all OR personnel. Many ORs require yearly BLS review with recertification every 2 years. ICU personnel are required to be ACLS certified.

Today's research is tomorrow's practice. The search for new anesthetic drugs tailored to affect only selected cells continues. Research also continues in the development and refinement of processes and monitors for automatic assessment of many vital functions. Nursing staff should be informed when new agents and technology are introduced and be instructed in their use as appropriate.

Bibliography

Anderson S: Six easy steps to interpreting blood gases, *Am J Nurs* 90(8):42-45, 1990.

Beck CF: Malignant hyperthermia: are you prepared? *AORN J* 59(2):367-390, 1994.

Benumof JL, Saidman LJ: *Anesthesia and perioperative complications,* St Louis, 1992, Mosby.

Bohony J: 9 common IV problems and what to do about them, *Am J Nurs* 93(10):45-49, 1993

Braun AE: Emergency cardiac care, *RN* 56(9):50-56, 1993.

Brody GM, Elberger ST: Hypothermia and the heart, *Emerg Med* 23(2):80-89, 1991.

Chabot RJ, Gugino VD: Quantitative electroencephalographic monitoring during cardiopulmonary bypass, *Anesthesiology* 78(1):209-211, 1993.

Chernow B: Blood conservation in critical care—the evidence accumulates, *Crit Care Med* 21(4):481-482, 1993.

Cicek S et al: Intraoperative echocardiography: techniques and current applications, *J Cardiac Surg* 8(6):678-692, 1993.

Clark DJ et al: Measurement technique for the determination of blood oxygen saturation, *J Biomedical Engineering* 14(2):168-172, 1992.

DeAngelis R, Lessig ML: Hyperkalemia, *Crit Care Nurs* 12(3):55-59, 1992.

Dennison RD: Making sense of hemodynamic monitoring, *Am J Nurs* 94(8):24-31, 1994.

Donnelly AJ: Part I. Antiarrhythmic agents use in the surgical patient, *AORN J* 53(5):1261-1266, 1991; Part II. Pharmacodynamics of parenteral antiarrhythmic agents, *AORN J* 54(1):121-130, 1991.

Donnelly AJ: Malignant hyperthermia: epidemiology, pathophysiology, treatment, *AORN J* 59(2):393-405, 1994.

Eichorn JH: Effect of monitoring standards on anesthesia outcome, *Int Anesthesiol Clin* 31(3):181-196, 1993.

Erwin CW, Erwin AC: Up and down the spinal cord: intraoperative monitoring of sensory and motor spinal cord pathways, *J Clin Neurophysiol* 10(4):425-436, 1993

Gangloff LB: Practical innovations: sterile defibrillator test probe checks circuits, cords, *AORN J* 58(3):573-574, 1993.

Grauer K: *Practical guide to ECG interpretation,* St Louis, 1992, Mosby.

Hayden RA: Trend-spotting with an Svo_2, *Am J Nurs* 93(1):26-33, 1993.

Hayden RA: What keeps oxygenation on track? *Am J Nurs* 92(12):32-40, 1992.

Hess D et al: Resistance to flow through the valves of mouth-to-mask ventilation devices, *Respir Care* 38(2):183-188, 1993.

Hurray JM, Saver CL: Arterial blood gas interpretation, *AORN J* 55(1):180-185, 1992.

Johannsen JM: Update: guidelines for treating hypertension, *Am J Nurs* 93(3):42-49, 1993.

Kudzma EC: Drug response: all bodies are not created equal, *Am J Nurs* 92(12):48-50, 1992

Mackowiak PA et al: A critical appraisal of 98.6° F, the upper limit of the normal body temperature, and other legacies of Carl Reinhold August Wunderlich, *JAMA* 268(12):1578-1580, 1992.

Malignant Hyperthermia Association of the United States: *Understanding malignant hyperthermia,* Westport, Conn, 1992, The Association.

Malignant Hyperthermia Association of the United States: *Managing malignant hyperthermia: drugs and equipment,* Westport, Conn, 1993, The Association.

Metheny NM: Why worry about IV fluids? *Am J Nurs* 90(6)50-55, 1990.

Morgan PD: Intraoperative evoked potentials: an overview, *Semin Periop Nurs* 2(1):13-19, 1993.

Murphy TG: Adenosine: slow down and take a look, *Am J Nurs* 92(11):22-24, 1992.

Murphy TG, Bennett EJ: Low-tech, high-touch perfusion assessment, *Am J Nurs* 92(5)36-46, 1992.

Murray EW: Probing the safety of central venous catheters, *Am J Nurs* 93(4):72-76, 1993.

Nash CA, Jensen PL: When your surgical patient has hypertension, *Am J Nurs* 94(12):38-44, 1994.

Nobel JJ: Carbon dioxide monitors: exhaled gas, *Pediatr Emerg Care* 9(4):244-246, 1993.

O'Neal PV: How to spot early signs of cardiogenic shock, *Am J Nurs* 94(5):36-40, 1994.

Owens MW: Keeping an eye on magnesium, *Am J Nurs* 93(2):66-67, 1993.

Pasero C, McCaffery M: Avoiding opioid-induced respiratory depression, *Am J Nurs* 94(4):24-30, 1994.

Pearlman RC, Schneider PL: Intraoperative neural monitoring, *AORN J* 59(4):841-849, 1994.

Penn F, Mancini J: Hemodynamic effects of vasoactive infusions, *AORN J* 54(3):613-621, 1991.

Puterbaugh S: Hypothermia related to exposure and surgical intervention, *Today's OR Nurse* 13(7):32-33, 1991.

Roberts I et al: Estimation of cerebral blood flow with near infrared spectroscopy and indocyanine green, *Lancet* 342(8884):1425, 1993.

Saul L: Arrhythmia mimics, Part I, *Am J Nurs* 91(3):40-43,1991; Part II, *Am J Nurs* 91(5):41-45, 1991.

Saver CL: Decoding the ACLS algorithms, *Am J Nurs* 94(1):27-35, 1994.

Saver CL: Your guide to first- and second-line code drugs, *Am J Nurse* 94(2):15, 1994.

Saver CL, Hurray JM: Electrocardiogram monitoring: interpreting normal cardiac rhythms, *AORN J* 52(2):264-271, 1990; interpreting abnormal cardiac rhythms, *AORN J* 52(2):273-283, 1990.

Shafer AL: Cardiopulmonary resuscitation drug therapy, *AORN J* 54(5):1070-1081, 1991.

Smith EA, Kilpatrick ES: Intraoperative glucose measurements: the effect of hematocrit on glucose monitoring strips, *Anaesthesia* 49(2):129-132, 1994.

Smith ML et al: In-line measurement of electrolytes, glucose, and blood gases, *Int Anesthesiol Clin* 31(3):159-180, 1993.

Spry CC: Opinion: Perioperative nurses should keep monitoring their specialty, *AORN J* 51(4):1071-1072, 1990.

Stein E: *Rapid analysis of electrocardiograms: a self-study program,* ed 2, Malvern, Penn, 1992, Lea & Febiger.

Stringfield YN: Acidosis, alkalosis, and ABGs, *Am J Nurs* 93(11):43-44, 1993.

Vaska PL: Fluid and electrolyte imbalances after cardiac surgery, *AACN Clin Issues Crit Care Nurs* 3(3):664-671, 1992.

Vogelsang J: The treatment of postanesthesia shaking, *AORN J* 57(6):1449-1456, 1993.

Vos HR: Making headway with intracranial hypertension, *Am J Nurs* 93(2):28-35, 1993.

Willens JS: Strengthen your life-support skills, *Nursing* 23(4):54-58, 1993.

Wilson BA et al: *Nurse's drug guide,* Norwalk, Conn, 1994, Appleton & Lange.

Yelderman M: Continuous cardiac output by thermodilution, *Int Anesthesiol Clin* 31(3):127-140, 1993

Zbar RI: Liver laceration after cardiopulmonary resuscitation: a case report, *Heart Lung* 22(5):463, 1993.

SECTION EIGHT

Intraoperative Patient Care

CHAPTER 20

Coordinated Roles of Scrub Person and Circulator

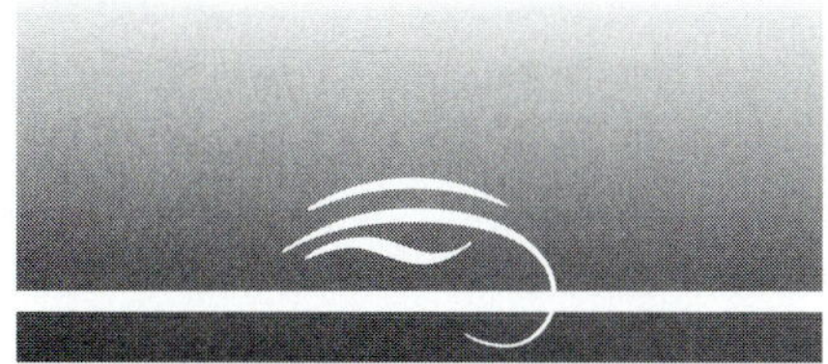

The duties of the scrub person and circulator are many and varied. They are responsible for the cleanliness of the environment so that microorganisms are kept to a minimum. They must prepare and maintain the sterile field. This chapter outlines the preparation of the operating room (OR) for the patient and the division of duties immediately before and during a surgical procedure. Special detailed discussion is devoted to responsibility and accountability for sponges, sharps, and instruments because of their overall importance to the success of the surgical procedure. Perioperative nurses and surgical technologists should be prepared to handle all situations.

PRELIMINARY PREPARATIONS

Preliminary preparations are completed by the circulator and scrub person before each patient enters the OR. Sometimes assistance is provided by a nursing assistant or housekeeping personnel. It is a cooperative effort. Clean surroundings are part of the skill and care that are the patient's rights. Cleaning the room is part of total patient care. (The cleanup procedure following each surgical procedure is detailed in Chapter 27.)

Before First Surgical Procedure of Day

The following housekeeping duties should be done at least 1 hour before scheduled incision time:

1. Remove unnecessary tables and equipment from the room.
2. Damp-dust overhead operating light, furniture, flat surfaces, and all portable or mounted equipment with a disinfectant solution.
3. Damp-dust tops and rims of sterilizer and/or washer-sterilizer and countertops in substerile room adjacent to the OR.
4. Wet-vacuum floors with detergent-disinfectant (see Chapter 27, p. 552, for technique).

Before Each Surgical Procedure

After the room is clean and all surfaces are dry:

1. Place a clean sheet, lift sheet, armboard covers, and restraining strap(s) on the operating table. Put a thermal blanket or pressure mattress on the table if needed to induce hypothermia or hyperthermia or to relieve pressure during a long procedure (see Chapters 17 and 21).

2. Position the operating table under the overhead operating light fixture.
3. Turn on the operating light to check focus and intensity, and preposition it as much as possible. The light should be positioned in relationship to the location of surgeon at the operating table and to that part of the patient's anatomy that will be encountered during the surgical procedure.
4. Connect and check suction between the receptacle and the wall outlet to be certain suction functions at maximum vacuum.
5. Place a waterproof laundry bag or antistatic plastic bag for disposal of reusable woven items in the laundry hamper frame.
6. Place appropriately marked receptacles in the room for disposal of biohazardous items, such as sharps, disposable drapes, or other biologically contaminated materials.
7. Line each kick bucket and wastebasket with an impervious liner with a cuff turned over the edge. Plastic waste disposal bags are nonconductors on which electrostatic charges may accumulate. Use care in handling them. Antistatic bags are safest.
8. Arrange furniture with those pieces that will be draped to become part of the sterile field at least 18 inches (45 cm) away from walls or cabinets. They should be kept side by side, away from the laundry hamper, anesthesia equipment, doors, and paths of traffic.
9. Put sterile drape pack on the instrument table in place so that when opened the wrapper will adequately drape the table and the drapes will be in their proper place (see Figure 20-1). Sterile drape packs may contain reusable woven fabric or disposable nonwoven drapes. Types of drapes and contents of the pack vary. Some sterile drape packs will be specifically packaged according to surgical specialty. Sterile drape packs may contain:
   a. Reusable woven fabric drapes assembled, packaged, and sterilized within the facility. These may be generic or designated for a particular specialty.
   b. Combination of reusable woven fabric and disposable supplies assembled, packaged, and sterilized by a commercial processing company. These may be specific to a particular specialty.
   c. Disposable nonwoven drapes assembled, packaged, and sterilized by the manufacturer. These may be specific to a particular specialty.
   d. Disposable nonwoven drapes, disposable supplies, sutures, blades, and other specialty items. These are commonly referred to as *custom packs*. Custom packs are assembled, packaged, and sterilized by a custom pack supplier or manufacturer according to the request of the facility.

   NOTE Although the term *linen pack* is frequently used, many packs contain disposable drapes. (See Chapter 22, pp. 458-460, for discussion of draping materials.)

10. Put a sterile basin set into the ring stand.
11. Obtain an appropriate set of sterile instruments, or if a sterile instrument set is unavailable, place a tray of unsterile instruments in the steam sterilizer in the substerile room and sterilize them.
12. Select the correct size gloves for each member of the sterile team.
13. Collect additional instruments and supplies, according to the procedure book and the surgeon's preference card, from cabinets in the room or other supply area within the OR suite.

    NOTE If a case cart system is used, all or most of the needed supplies will be on the cart. These should be checked to ascertain that everything is there.

14. Obtain special equipment, such as table appliances, pillows, or padding, needed to position and protect the patient.
15. Obtain appropriate patient monitoring equipment.
16. Obtain any specialized equipment that will be needed, such as electrosurgical unit, pneumatic tourniquet, or operating microscope, and check/test for proper function.

Individual Patient Setups

Each patient has a right to individual supplies prepared just for him or her. Sterile supplies should not be opened until they are ready to be used. Tables should *not* be prepared and covered for use at a later time. The scrub person, working with an efficient circulator, should have time to set up the instrument table immediately before each surgical procedure.

The practice of covering sterile setups is *not* in the best interest of the patient. Unless it is under constant surveillance, sterility of any setup cannot be guaranteed. Uncovering a sterile table is difficult and may compromise sterility. However, should a scheduled surgical procedure be delayed and a sterile setup *not* be contaminated by the patient's presence in the room, the setup may remain open, under surveillance, by someone in the room with doors closed. The setup should be used as close to the time of preparation as possible. Sterility is mainly event-related, not time-dependent.

If a patient is taken into the OR and for some reason the surgical procedure is canceled, the tables should be torn down and the room cleaned as if the surgical procedure had taken place.

Opening Sterile Supplies

Before any sterile supplies are opened, the integrity of each package must be checked for tears and watermarks. If either is present, the package is unsafe to use. Also check the process monitor. To open packages:

1. Remove tape from packages wrapped in woven wrappers. The tape should be opened by breaking the seal on paper or nonwoven material. Removing tape strips from paper-wrapped items increases the risk of tearing the wrapper and exposing the contents to contamination. Check the chemical indicator to be certain the item has been exposed to a sterilization process.
2. Open drape pack, instrument set, gown pack, and basin set so the inside of each inner wrapper becomes the sterile table cover. With hands on outside of the wrapper in a folded cuff, lift the wrapper toward yourself to avoid contaminating contents of the pack. The area touched falls below table level, and the inside of the wrapper remains sterile. Do not reach over the inside of the sterile table cover or contents of the pack. Always lift the wrapper toward yourself (Figure 20-1).

   NOTE If packs or sets have sequential double wrappers, both layers are opened by the person opening supplies. The outer wrapper is considered the dust cover, and the inner wrapper the microbial barrier.

3. Open other packages, such as sponges, gloves, and sutures, maintaining a sterile transfer to the appropriate sterile table. Touch only the outside of the outer wrapper. Avoid reaching over sterile contents and sterile table. Enclose hand in wrapper to the extent possible.

   NOTE
   - If small packages are sequentially double-wrapped (i.e., a package inside a package), only the outer wrapper may be removed. Consideration must be given, however, to the type of packaging material and the conditions and duration of storage. Remember shelf life is event-related.
   - If a sterile package is dropped, the item may be considered safe for immediate use only if it is enclosed in an impervious material and the integrity of the package is maintained. Dropped items wrapped in woven materials should not be transferred to the sterile table.

4. Open the gown and gloves for the scrub person on the Mayo stand or small table.

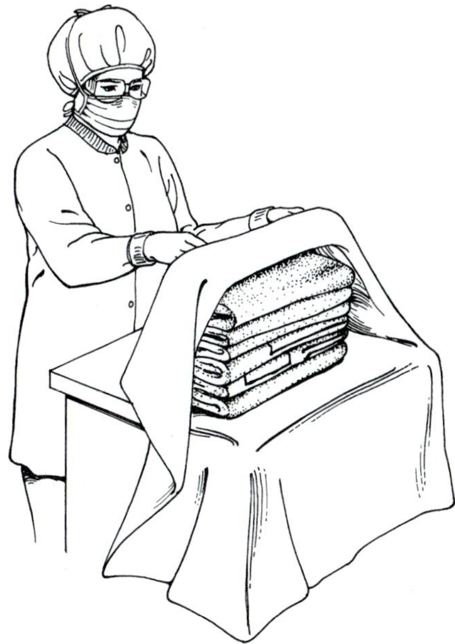

FIGURE 20-1 Opening sterile drape pack. Wrapper is lifted back while keeping hands on the outside. Hands are in folded cuff to avoid contaminating contents of pack. Area touched falls below unsterile table level; sterile inside of wrapper (now table cover) remains sterile.

DIVISION OF DUTIES

The circulator and scrub person should plan their duties so that, through coordination of their efforts, the sterile and nonsterile parts of the surgical procedure move along *simultaneously*. From the time the scrub person starts the surgical scrub until the surgical procedure is completed and dressings are applied, an invisible demarcation line separates the scrub and circulating duties that neither person may cross. The duties of the two positions are listed separately, but a spirit of mutual cooperation is essential to move the schedule of surgical procedures efficiently and to serve the patients' best interests.

Scrub Person Duties

When all is in readiness for arrival of the patient, the scrub person prepares for arrival of the surgeon.

Before Surgeon Arrives

1. Do a complete scrub according to the institutional procedure (see Chapter 11).
2. Gown and glove from a surface separate from the intended sterile field. Wipe the powder off gloves before handling drapes, instruments, and other sterile items.
3. Drape tables as necessary according to the institutional procedure.
   a. A second instrument table may be needed for extensive surgical procedures or special types of instrumentation.
   b. The scrub person may drape and set a small table for the patient's skin preparation. More

commonly, the circulator opens and prepares a disposable or prepackaged prep tray (see Chapter 22).

c. The surgeon and assistant(s) may gown and glove themselves from a separate small table or may be gowned and gloved by the sterile scrub person.

NOTE In draping a nonsterile table, always cuff the drape over your gloved hands in preparation for opening it. Lift the table drape toward yourself to cover the nonsterile front edge of the table first and to minimize the possibility of contaminating the front of your gown. Then place the drape over back of the table. Avoid leaning over the table. After the ends of the drape are unfolded over the sides of the table, be careful not to lift them to table level again while opening the crosswise folds (review Figures 12-3 through 12-6).

4. Move the remaining contents of the drape pack to a corner of the instrument table if they are not preset on the table drape in a convenient place. Before being wrapped for sterilization, contents of the pack can be stacked in sequence of use and set on the table drape in the spot where they should be on the table. Then when the pack is opened, the contents do not need to be handled or moved. The pack contains, from top to bottom, at least:
   a. One Mayo stand cover
   b. Six to eight towels
   c. One fenestrated sheet (The types of fenestrated sheets are discussed in Chapter 22.)
5. Drape the Mayo stand. Both the frame and the tray are draped unless the tray is wrapped and sterilized separately.

   The Mayo stand cover is like a long pillowcase. It is fanfolded with a wide cuff to protect gloved hands. With hands in the cuff, folds of the drape are supported on the arms, in the bend of the elbows, to prevent its falling below waist level. While sliding the cover on, place a foot on base of stand to stabilize it (Figures 20-2 and 20-3).

   A snugly wrapped sterile tray may be placed on top of the draped Mayo frame. Or a waterproof barrier, such as a nonabsorbent disposable towel or antistatic plastic film, is placed over the cover on the tray and tucked in along the edges.
6. Leave large solution basin in ring stand and take remainder of the basins to the instrument table. The wrapper on the basin set serves as the cover for the ring stand with the large basin. The surgeon and assistants may need to wash their gloves during the surgical procedure. Sterile normal saline or water is usually used in this "splash" basin. *Splash basins are not used in many ORs.* Instead this basin may be used to collect used instruments. Only demineralized sterile water should be used for this purpose.

   One basin is left on the instrument table until needed for the specimen. A round basin will be used for moistening sponges. Place an absorbent towel on the instrument table under it.

NOTE In addition to these basins, the basin set may also contain solution cups for the skin preparation table and a basin specifically intended for trash disposal. Attaching a trash bag to the side of the table compromises the sterility of the field by hanging lower than the sterile table surface.

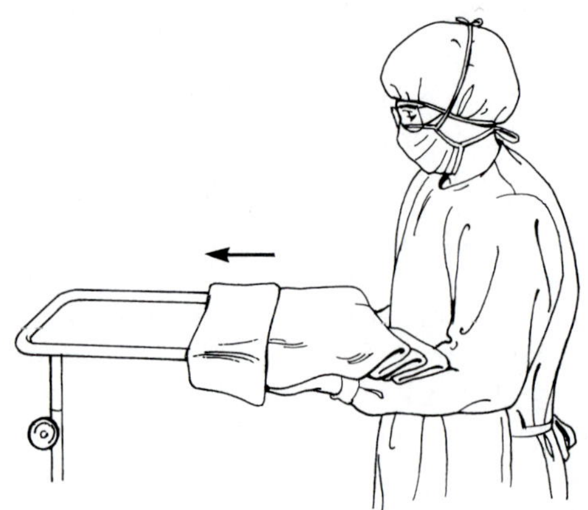

FIGURE 20-2 Starting to drape Mayo stand. Scrub person's hands are protected in cuff of drape. Folds of drape are supported on arms, in bend of elbows, to prevent their falling below waist level. Foot on base of stand stabilizes it.

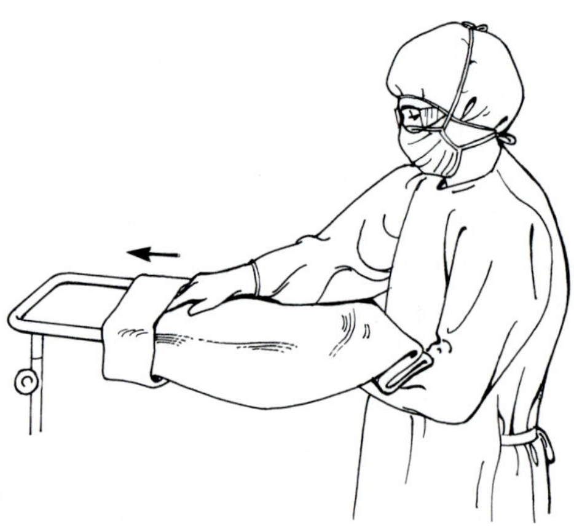

FIGURE 20-3 Completing draping of Mayo stand. Hands are protected in cuffs.

7. Count sponges, surgical needles and other sharps, and instruments with the circulator according to established institutional policy and procedure. These items and counting procedures are discussed on pp. 425-429 later in this chapter.
8. Arrange instruments and accessory items on the Mayo stand for making and opening the initial incision. Arrange other instruments and items on instrument table.

   Instruments for each surgical procedure should be selected according to standard basic sets and the preferences of the surgeon. For each step of the surgical procedure, instruments of suitable size, shape, strength, and function are needed. The styles and numbers of instruments will be dictated by type of surgical procedure. Instruments are classified as:

   a. Cutting or dissecting—knives and scissors
   b. Grasping and holding—tissue forceps
   c. Clamping and occluding—hemostatic forceps and clamps
   d. Exposing—retractors
   e. Suturing—needleholders

   Instruments are described in detail in Chapter 14; see pp. 252-253 for setting up instrument table.

   A few of each classification of instruments, plus sutures, surgical needles, and sponges, are put on Mayo stand initially. If a local anesthetic will be used, a syringe and injection needle will be needed also (see p. 414, point 13).

   Do not overload the Mayo stand initially (Figure 20-4). Additional instruments and supplies can be added as necessary as the surgical procedure progresses. Long-handled forceps and clamps and deep retractors can be substituted for those used on superficial structures. The Mayo stand should be kept neat throughout the surgical procedure, with instruments organized by classifications.
9. Put blades on knife handles. To avoid injury, always use an instrument; never use fingers alone. Holding the cutting edge down and away from eyes, grasp the blade at its widest, strongest part with a needleholder and slip the blade into groove on knife handle. A click indicates that the blade is in place. To prevent damage to the blade, the instrument should not touch the cutting edge (Figure 20-5).
10. Prepare sutures in the sequence in which the surgeon will use them. The surgeon *ligates* (ties off) blood vessels shortly after the incision is made, unless electrosurgery is preferred to seal vessels. Prepare *ligatures* (free hand ties) first if they will be used.

    Tear suture packets at notch in the hermetically sealed edge. Remove suture material from the packet unless packet is designed for single-strand dispensing. Work over the instrument table and hold onto the ends to prevent strands from dropping over the edge of the table and thus becoming contaminated.

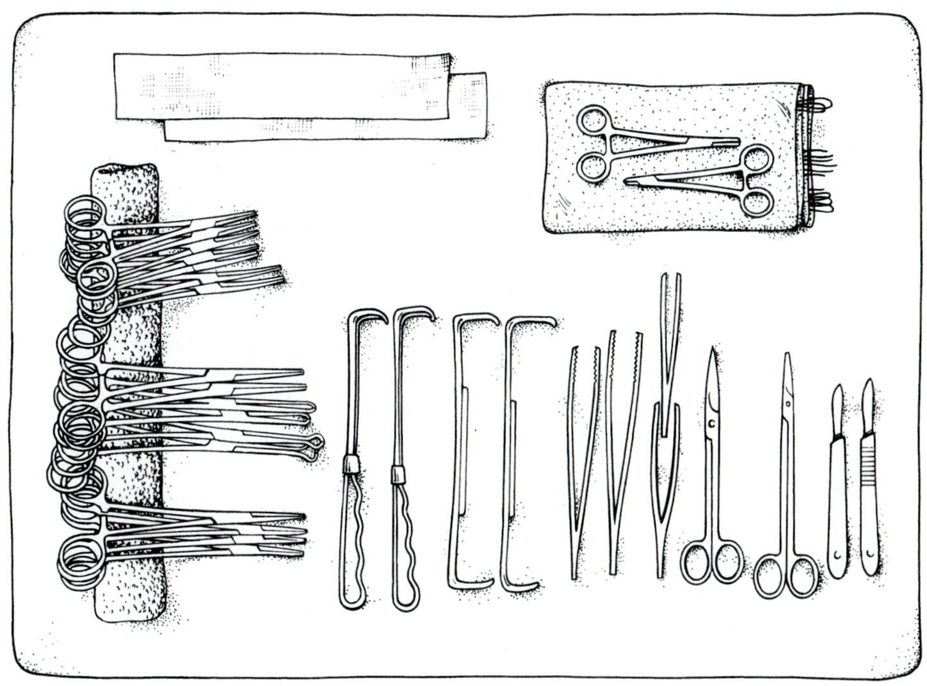

FIGURE 20-4 Contents of Mayo stand, in preparation for surgical procedure.

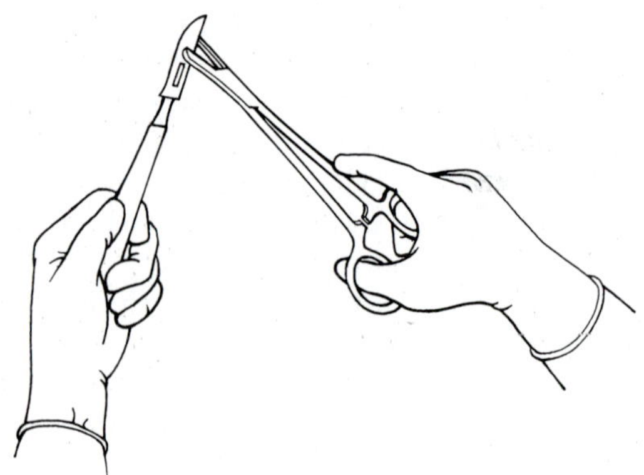

FIGURE 20-5 Putting scalpel blade on knife handle. To avoid injury, always use an instrument; never use your fingers alone. Holding it down and away from your eyes, with strong needleholder (not a hemostat), grasp blade at its widest, strongest part and slip it into groove on handle. To prevent damage to blade, needleholder must not touch cutting edge.

Place dispensing packets or strands of ligating material in a *suture book,* a fanfolded towel, with the ends extended far enough for rapid extraction. Place the largest size in the bottom layer along the fold that will be farthest away when placed on the Mayo stand. The next smaller size is placed in the next layer so that the ends are not overriding those below; if three sizes are prepared, the medium size can be placed midway between the other two. The smallest size will be along the closest fold. The suture book may be placed on the Mayo stand with the ends on it, *not over the edges,* and toward the sterile field. Strands are pulled out toward the surgical field, *never away from it,* to prevent possible contamination.

After ligatures are prepared, a *few* packets may be opened and prepared for *suturing* (sewing or stitching). Seldom is it necessary to prepare large amounts of suture material in advance. Suture materials, preparation, and handling are discussed in detail in Chapter 24.

11. Secure surgical needles and all other sharps, including knife blades, after completing the count with the circulator. Refer to the methods of accounting for sharps on pp. 428-429. *Surgical needles and sharps should never be loose on Mayo stand.*

    Surgical needles are discussed in detail in Chapter 24. If eyed reusable needles are used, each needle must be inspected before threading for cleanliness, burrs, and integrity of the eye.
12. Place a few appropriate-size sponges for the initial incision on the Mayo stand after completing the count with the circulator. These may be opened to their full length. Fix two or three sponges on sponge forceps, if these will be used, but leave the forceps on the instrument table. Put x-ray–detectable rings on tapes, if used. Many different kinds of sponges are available. These are described on pp. 426-427. Also refer to methods of guarding sponges on p. 427.
13. Fill a syringe with the correct agent if a local infiltration anesthetic is to be used. Attach an appropriate-size needle and put it on the Mayo stand. This will be the first thing the surgeon will use after the patient is draped. State the kind and percentage of the solution when handing syringe to the surgeon. The solution label should be checked by a registered nurse when it is poured and verified when it is given. Sterile labels and marking pens are commercially available to label the containers for medications, radiopaque dyes, and other solutions used in the sterile field. Labeling should include the name and strength of the solution. An appropriate label should be placed on syringes, basins, and medicine cups to prevent inadvertent use of the wrong solution in the wrong manner.
14. Syringes with needles are used for injection and aspiration, and syringes without needles are used for irrigation. Most hospitals use sterile disposable syringes and needles. Glass syringes and reusable needles in the same models and sizes are occasionally used.
    a. Syringes commonly used for injection or aspiration are:
        (1) *Luer-Lok tip.* This has a tip that locks over the needle hub. It is used whenever pressure is exerted to inject or aspirate fluid. Sizes are available from 2 to 100 ml.
        (2) *Ring control.* This has a Luer-Lok tip. The barrel has one fingerhold and a thumbhold, which give the surgeon a secure grip when injecting with only one hand. Sizes range from 3 to 10 ml.
        (3) *Luer slip tip.* This has a plain tip that may not give a secure connection on a needle hub. It is necessary when using some catheter adapters or a rubber connection for aspiration. Sizes vary from 1 to 100 ml.

    NOTE When using a sterile syringe, be very careful not to touch the plunger except at the end, even with gloves on. Contamination of the plunger contaminates the inner wall of the barrel and thus the solution that is drawn into it. Glove powder can act as a contaminant.

    b. Syringes used for irrigation are:
        (1) *Bulb with barrel.* A plastic or rubber bulb is attached to the neck of the barrel. The barrel has a tapered or blunt end. This is used with a one-hand control for irrigation during many types of surgical procedures. It

is commonly referred to by the trade name Asepto syringe. Sizes have a solution capacity of ¼ to 4 oz (7.6 to 118 ml).

(2) *Bulb without barrel.* This is a one-piece bulb that tapers to a blunt end. It is used to irrigate small structures. This type may be used for suctioning nasal and oral fluids from neonates during cesarean section deliveries. This variety is usually disposable because it is not possible to clean the interior of the bulb after use.

NOTE To fill the barrel or bulb, depress bulb, submerge the end in solution, and release. The bulb will reinflate, thus drawing solution into it. Warm, not hot, solution is usually used for irrigation, so check the temperature before giving the syringe to the surgeon. Irrigating solution may be stored in a warmer maintained at a temperature ranging from 99° to 122° F (37° to 50° C). For use, solution usually should not exceed body temperature.

c. Needles for injection or aspiration: The size of needles with a lumen is designated by length and gauge. *Gauge* is the outside diameter of needle. The gauge gets smaller as the number gets larger (i.e., a 30-gauge needle is smaller than a 20-gauge needle). Although numerous sizes of needles are available, only a few representative sizes and their uses are mentioned.
   (1) ½ inch (12.7 mm) × 30 gauge, for local anesthetic in plastic surgery
   (2) ¾ inch (19 mm) × 24 or 25 gauge, the usual needle for any subcutaneous injection
   (3) 1½ inches (3.8 cm) × 22 gauge, for subcutaneous or intramuscular injection
   (4) 2 inches (5 cm) × 18 or 20 gauge, for aspiration or transfusion of blood products
   (5) 4 inches (10 cm) × 20 or 22 gauge, for deep injections of local anesthetic or for intracardiac injections

After Surgeon and Assistant(s) Scrub

1. Gown and glove surgeon and assistant(s) as soon after they enter the room as possible, if this is routine procedure. This should take precedence over other activities of setup. However, *do not interrupt a count* to do so. Such interruptions lead to incorrect counts. The surgeon and assistant(s) may take gowns and gloves from a separate table set up for this purpose. (See Chapter 11, pp. 177 and 179, for discussion on gowning and gloving other team members.)
2. Assist in draping the patient according to the routine procedure (see Chapter 22).
   a. Some surgeons use self-adhering plastic sheeting as the first drape. Stand on the opposite side of operating table from the surgeon to apply this drape.
   b. Some surgeons use towels and clips with or instead of a plastic drape. To prevent reaching over the nonsterile operating table, go to the same side of table as the surgeon to hand towels and clips. Skin towels may be held in place with sutures or staples rather than clips.

NOTE Once a perforating towel clip has been fastened through a drape, do not remove it; points are contaminated. If it is necessary to remove one, discard it from the field and cover the area with another sterile drape or towel. Nonperforating ball-tip towel clips are preferred for securing drapes. Because of risk of contamination, drapes, once positioned, should not be moved.

3. Bring the Mayo stand into position over the patient after draping is completed. Be sure that it does not rest on the patient. Position the instrument table at a right angle to the operating table (see Figure 20-8, p. 420).
4. Lay a towel or magnetic pad for instruments below the fenestration (opening) in the drape. Lay two sponges on this.
5. Attach suction tubing and electrosurgical cord, if either or both are to be used, to drapes with a nonperforating clamp. Allow ample length to reach both the incision area and the equipment. Drop the ends off the side of the table nearest the unit to which the circulator will attach them.
6. Attach a container (holder/holster) to the drape with a nonperforating clip for containment of the active electrosurgical electrode handpiece when not in use.

During Surgical Procedure

1. Pass the skin knife to the surgeon and a hemostat to the assistant. Some surgeons do not want the knife handed to them. Lay the knife on an instrument towel, magnetic pad, or tray for them to pick up.

NOTE When passing a knife, always hold the handle with blade down, with the tip angled away from yourself and the surgeon. Hold hand pronated with thumb apposed against tip of index finger and flex the wrist.

Because skin cannot be sterilized, the skin knife may be considered contaminated whether or not the surgeon has cut through an adhering plastic drape. The skin incision exposes deep skin flora of hair follicles and sebaceous gland ducts. This probably will not bring microbes from skin into deep tissues, however.

2. Hand up sterile towels or lap sponges if requested for covering skin at the incision edges. Rearrange the instrument towel to make a smooth field.
3. Watch the field and try to anticipate the surgeon's and the assistant's needs. Keep one step ahead of

them in passing instruments, sutures, and sponges and handing up the specimen basin. Notify the circulator if additional supplies are needed or if the surgeon asks for something not on the table. Ask quietly for supplies to avoid distracting the surgeon.

4. Pass instruments in a decisive and positive manner. When instruments are passed properly, surgeons know they have them; their eyes do not have to leave surgical site. When the surgeon extends his or her hand, the instrument should be placed firmly into the palm in proper position for use (see Figure 14-11, p. 254).

   Some surgeons use hand signals to indicate the type of instrument needed. These signals eliminate the need for talking, but such signs should be clearly understood. An understanding of what is taking place at the surgical site makes the signals meaningful. When bleeding is obvious, the surgeon needs a hemostatic forceps. When a suture needs cutting, the need is for scissors.

   Keep instruments as clean as possible. Wipe blood and organic debris from them with a moist sponge. Remove debris from electrosurgical tips. Flush suction with saline or sterile water periodically to keep the tip and tubing patent. Keep track of the amount of solution used to clear the line. The volume of fluid in the suction canister may be confused with blood loss.

   Return instruments to the Mayo stand or instrument table promptly after use. Their weight or sharp tip could injure the patient.

5. Place a ligature in the surgeon's hand. The surgeon keeps both eyes on the field and does not reach for a ligature except to hold a hand out to receive it. Draw a strand out of the suture book, toward the sterile field, grasp both ends, and place securely in surgeon's outstretched hand. The end of a ligature may be placed in a forceps, referred to as a "tie on a passer." When handing a tie on a passer, place the forceps in the surgeon's hand in the same manner used to pass any hemostatic forceps. Trail the end of the ligature until it is taken by the assistant during the tying procedure.

   Have ready, at all times during the surgical procedure, a fine and a heavy suture on needles placed in needleholders. After handing a suture to the surgeon, hand the suture scissors to the assistant and prepare another suture just like it at once. The needle or suture may break. *Account for each needle in its entirety as the surgeon finishes with it.* Check its integrity. Tell the surgeon immediately if a needle is broken so that both pieces can be retrieved.

   Repeat the size of a suture or ligature when handing it to surgeon. Obviously, if the surgeon is using a long series of interrupted sutures or many ligatures in rapid succession, this repetition is not necessary. Use good judgment.

   Be logical in selecting instruments used for suturing. Give the surgeon long needleholders to work deep in a cavity. Short ones may be used for surface work. Give the assistant a needleholder to pull the needle through tissue for the surgeon. Then have scissors ready when the knot is tied. Hemostatic forceps are sometimes used to secure the ends of multiple interrupted sutures placed in rapid succession. Many times the knot tying and cutting take place after all sutures are in position.

   Remove waste ends of suture material from the field, Mayo stand, and instrument table. Place them in the trash disposal container. Put used needles on a magnet, needle rack, or into the suture book or other container for this purpose until the needle count is completed. Follow established institutional policy and procedure for securing sharps during the surgical procedure.

6. Keep two clean lap sponges or tapes on the field. Put up clean ones before removing soiled ones on an exchange basis. Discard soiled sponges into a kick bucket. Soiled sponges should not accumulate in the sterile field.

   Count all sponges or tapes added during the surgical procedure with the circulator before moistening or using them. Do not mix types of sponges and tapes, either on the table or in a basin of solution. Because it is isotonic, normal saline solution, warmed to at least body temperature, is usually used to moisten sponges and tapes. Special irrigating solutions may be requested by the surgeon.

7. Save and care for all tissue specimens according to policy and procedure. Some states require that all tissue, including exudates, removed from a patient should be sent for pathologic examination. Therefore it is advisable to send all tissue to the laboratory even though it may appear to be of no value for examination or diagnostic purposes.

   Specimens are put in a specimen basin or another container. Never put a large clamp on a small specimen; this may crush cells, making tissue identification difficult. Some specimens have borders or margins the surgeon will mark with specific sutures as tags for the pathologist's identification of and attention to certain areas. Disposable glove wrappers, marked *right* and *left*, can be used for holding bilateral specimens (e.g., right and left breast biopsies). Hand the specimen from the field in a basin or wrapper or on a towel; *never place it on a sponge.* Keep the specimen basin on the field until all tissue has been removed or all contaminated items are in it. Tell the circulator exactly what the specimen is and if there are any identifying notations for the pathologist. If there are any doubts about the specimen's identification or markers, ask the surgeon to clarify.

8. Maintain sterile technique. Watch for any breaks. Observe the following points:
   a. Step away from sterile field if contaminated. Ask circulator for another glove, gown, or sleeve—whatever is needed to reestablish sterile conditions for yourself or another sterile team member. If the lower arm of the gown becomes contaminated, a sterile gown sleeve can be drawn over it to cover the site of contamination if the area is not saturated with blood or biohazardous material. A saturated gown can be a potential site of contamination to the wearer's skin and should be changed.
   b. Change glove at once and discard the needle or instrument if a glove is pricked by a needle or snagged (i.e., torn) by an instrument even if the skin has not been broken. (See discussion of penetrating injuries in Chapter 10, p. 157.)
   c. Without touching the contaminated part, discard a piece of suture material, tubing, or a sponge that falls over the edge of the sterile field.
   d. Keep hands at table level when at rest.
   e. Keep contact with sterile field to a minimum. No one should lean on or against the operating table, Mayo stand, or instrument table, and especially not on the patient. Remember that the patient under the drapes is unable to complain!
   f. Leave a wide margin of safety in moving about the room. Gowns balloon out, requiring more space than usual attire. In passing nonsterile objects, turn your back to them.
   g. Do not turn back to the sterile field or to members of the sterile team. Face sterile areas to pass them.
   h. Do not reach behind a member of sterile team; go around. Pass another member of sterile team back to back (see Figure 12-7, p. 204).
   i. Keep the table and sterile field as dry as possible. Spread extra towels as needed. Keep loops and rings on tapes in the basin, not dangling over the side of it and dripping on the instrument table.
   j. Discard soiled sponges from the sterile field. Do not allow them to accumulate.
   k. Keep talking to a minimum. Avoid coughing and sneezing.
   l. Drape nonsterile equipment, such as a microscope, endoscopic camera, or articulating laser arm, before it is brought over the sterile field.

During Closure

1. Count sponges, sharps, and instruments with the circulator when the surgeon begins closure of the wound, in accordance with established count procedures (see third and fourth counts, pp. 425-426).
2. Clear off the Mayo stand, as time permits, leaving a knife handle with blade, tissue forceps, suture scissors, four hemostats, and two Allis's forceps.

   NOTE Policy usually requires that the setup and the Mayo stand remain sterile until the patient has left the room. Cardiac arrest, tracheal collapse, hemorrhage, or other emergency can occur in the immediate postoperative-postanesthesia period. Even though sterile instrument sets are nearby, valuable time can be lost in opening sterile supplies when every second counts in an emergency situation. Sterile instruments on the Mayo stand, regardless of their previous use, can be used for emergency intervention. These can be lifesaving until other ones become available.

3. Have a clean, saline-moistened sponge ready to wash blood from the area surrounding the incision as soon as skin closure is completed.
4. Have dressings ready. (See discussion of dressings and drains in Chapter 25, pp. 527-532.)

Circulator Duties

Circulators should wash their hands and arms as required by institutional policy and procedure at the beginning of the day before entering the OR, but they do not don sterile gowns and gloves. Persons who wear sterile attire touch only sterile items; persons who are not sterile touch only unsterile items. Therefore the circulator should assist the sterile scrub person by providing the sterile supplies needed to prepare for arrival of surgeon.

After Scrub Person Scrubs

1. Fasten the back of the scrub person's gown.
2. If the tray of instruments is in the sterilizer in the substerile room, several methods may be employed to transfer the sterile tray to the field if the scrub person is unable to retrieve it. (See discussion of transfer of sterile tray to the sterile field in Chapter 14, p. 252). Do not reach over sterile instruments or a sterile surface when placing the tray. The tray may be set on the sterile basin in a ring stand or on a separate sterile surface to avoid the danger of contaminating the instrument table with moisture.
3. Open packages of sterile supplies, such as syringes, suction tubing, sutures, sponges, and gloves. Many of these items are prepackaged, presterilized, disposable products. Others are wrapped and sterilized by on-site personnel. Care must be taken in opening all sterile packages to avoid contamination of the contents. Many items

do not transfer easily. Use an appropriate method of sterile transfer.

a. Place the item on the edge of the sterile instrument table with the inside of the wrapper everted over hand. *Never reach over the sterile field and shake an item from package.*
b. Expose the contents for the scrub person to remove the item from the wrapper or package with a forceps or to grasp the item (Figure 20-6). The scrub person avoids touching the unsterile outside. Remember that the sterile boundary of a peel-open package is the inner edge.
c. Flip only *rigid* items from a package designed for this purpose, but with caution (Figure 20-7). Flipping an item from a package may result in missing the intended sterile surface, thus landing on the floor. Do not reach over a sterile surface to drop an item from a package. Flipping creates air turbulence and thus is the least preferred method of sterile transfer.

NOTE

- If a sterile package wrapped in porous material drops to the floor, discard it. Compression resulting from the fall can cause air and dust to enter the package. The enclosed item should not be considered safe for use on the sterile field.
- *The routine use of transfer forceps is obsolete.* Should a need arise, such as for removing a single instrument from a flash sterilizer, a sterile transfer forceps may be used. At this time a sterile package containing a forceps is opened and used for a single transfer.

4. Check the list of suture materials and sizes on the surgeon's preference card, but verify with the surgeon before opening packets. Avoid opening suture packets that will not be used. The surgical procedure might be canceled and then the sutures would be wasted. If the surgeon's need for sutures cannot be anticipated and further instructions

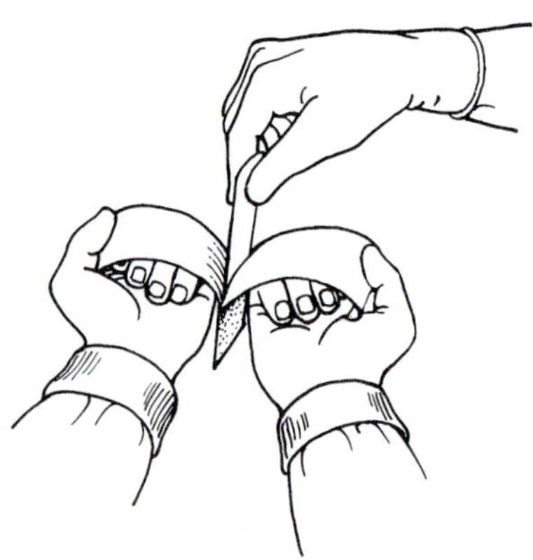

FIGURE 20-6 Scrub person taking contents from suture packet opened and held by circulator. Scrub person avoids touching unsterile outer wrapper.

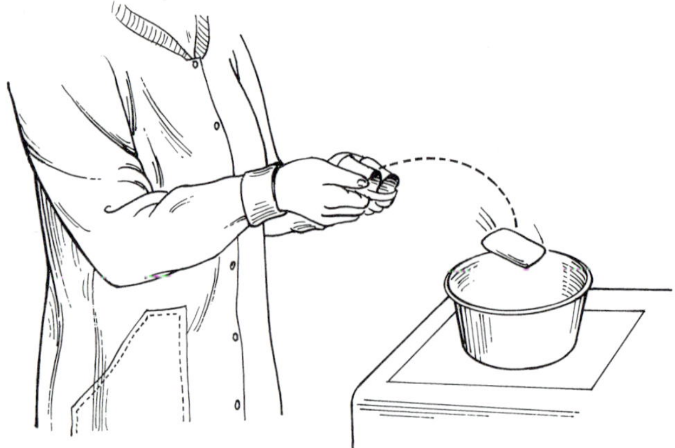

FIGURE 20-7 Circulator flipping sterile suture packet from overwrap into basin on scrub person's sterile instrument table.

have not been given, keep a packet or two ahead of actual need during the surgical procedure. Once the surgical procedure is started, more suture can be added to the field to prevent waste.

5. Pour solution (usually normal saline) into the round basin for sponges on the instrument table and into the splash basin in the ring stand if this will be needed. Pour a small amount of antiseptic agent for skin preparation in solution cups to be used for this purpose.
6. Count sponges, sharps, and instruments with the scrub person as required by institutional policy and procedure. Record immediately (see section on second count later in this chapter, p. 425).

After Patient Arrives

While the scrub person continues to prepare for the arrival of the surgeon, the circulator attends to the patient.

1. Greet and identify the patient. Introduce yourself to the patient if you have not made the preoperative assessment. Check the wristband for identification by name and number. Verify any allergies or chemical sensitivities the patient may have. These may be identified by an additional wristband and/or by a special notation on patient's chart.
2. Check the plan of care and the patient's chart for pertinent information, including consent.
3. Be sure the patient's hair is covered with a cap to prevent dissemination of microorganisms, to protect it from being soiled, and to prevent a static spark near the anesthesia machine. Loosen the neck ties on the patient's gown and untuck the blanket from the foot of the transport stretcher.
4. Assist the patient to move onto the operating table, taking care that the patient's gown, blanket, intravenous (IV) infusion tubing, or catheter drainage

tubing is not caught between the stretcher and the operating table. Use good body mechanics to prevent injury to yourself. An additional person should be on the opposite side of the transport stretcher during the move from one surface to another. The patient could fall if assistance or stabilization of the stretcher and table are inadequate. The wheels of the transport stretcher and the operating table must be locked during the transfer.

5. Apply a restraint strap over the thighs and secure the arms. The restraints should not impair circulation to the extremities. Keep the patient covered with a blanket to protect modesty and to provide warmth. The restraint strap should be placed over the blanket and should be visible.
   a. Patient's legs must not be crossed.
   b. Place the left arm of a right-handed patient (or vice versa) on the armboard if an IV infusion will be started. Remove arm from sleeve of the gown before securing it to the armboard.
   c. The angle of abduction of the arm on the armboard should *never* be greater than 90 degrees, a right angle with body. The brachial nerve plexus can be damaged by lengthy, severe abduction of the arm.
6. Help the anesthesiologist, as needed, to apply and connect monitoring devices.
7. Assist anesthesiologist, surgeon, or assistant as necessary if an IV infusion will be started. Obtain the following equipment before the patient arrives:
   a. Nonsterile gloves for the person who will do a percutaneous venipuncture. Sterile gloves are required for a venous cutdown or insertion of arterial monitoring lines.
   b. Tourniquet to help expose the vein for percutaneous insertion.
   c. Sponges saturated with antiseptic solution for skin preparation. Thorough skin antisepsis is imperative.
   d. IV administration set of sterile tubing with air filter and needle, cannula, or catheter. A cutdown tray may be needed.

NOTE
- 1½ inch (3.8 cm) × 20- or 21-gauge needles usually are used for IV fluids when blood transfusion is not anticipated; 1½ inch (3.8 cm) × 18-gauge or 2 inch (5 cm) × 20-gauge needles are used when blood transfusion is anticipated.
- When prolonged postoperative fluid therapy or hyperalimentation is anticipated, an inert, nontoxic, radiopaque plastic catheter is inserted through either a venipuncture through the skin (percutaneous insertion) or a cutdown through a skin incision to expose the vein. A venous cutdown is done in other selected situations: for central venous pressure monitoring, thrombosed superficial veins, or superficially collapsed veins caused by shock or prolonged preoperative IV therapy. The cutdown site is an open wound. Catheter insertion should be considered a minor surgical procedure. Sterile gloves, drapes, and tray of sterile instruments and sutures are needed. Have assorted sizes of IV catheters available so the surgeon can choose the size best suited to the vein. A soft, pliant catheter takes the contour of the anatomy and is not easily dislodged by movement of the patient.

   e. Parenteral infusion solution. IV solutions usually started initially in the OR include:
      (1) Normal saline
      (2) Dextrose, 5% or 10%, in water
      (3) Dextrose in 0.25% saline
      (4) Ringer's lactate solution
      (5) Dextrose in Ringer's lactate solution

NOTE Gently squeeze the plastic bag to detect leaks; check glass for cracks. Check the solution for clarity or discoloration. A cloudy solution is contaminated. If the circulator hangs the solution, a registered nurse or physician must check the label on the container before it is administered. All solutions given are charted and monitored to see that they are running at the proper speed. Usually this is the responsibility of anesthesiologist.

   f. Adhesive tape strips to firmly secure the needle or catheter and tubing to the patient's skin to prevent motion that may cause entry of microorganisms into the skin wound or traumatize the vein. If the patient is sensitive to adhesives, paper tape may be used.
   g. Stopcock to regulate or stop flow of solution through the tubing into the vein. Ports should remain covered until needed to prevent microbial migration into the system.

During Induction of General Anesthesia

1. Stay in the room and near the patient to comfort him or her and assist the anesthesiologist in the event that excitement or any emergency situation occurs. The patient must be guarded during induction to prevent possible injury or fall from the operating table. Further restrain or hold the patient if necessary.
2. Maintain a quiet environment. Excitement may occur during induction from tactile or auditory stimulation. It occurs more commonly in substance abusers. A strong startle reaction to sound can provoke life-threatening cardiac dysrhythmias in any patient, however. Hearing is the last sense lost. Any stimulation while the patient is under light anesthesia is highly dangerous and must be avoided. A quiet, undisturbed induction makes for a much safer and easier maintenance of and recovery from anesthesia.

After Patient Is Anesthetized

1. Reposition the patient only after the anesthesiologist says the patient is anesthetized to the extent that he or she will not be disturbed by being moved or touched. (Positioning of patient is discussed in Chapter 21.)
2. Attach anesthesia screen and other table attachments as needed. These always are placed after the patient is anesthetized and positioned to prevent injury to the patient.
3. Note the patient's position to be certain all measures for his or her safety have been observed.
4. Place the inactive electrosurgical dispersive electrode pad or plate in contact with patient's skin if the electrosurgical unit is to be used. Avoid scar tissue and hairy or bony areas. (See Chapter 15 , pp. 266-270 for discussion of electrosurgical units.)
5. Expose the appropriate area for skin preparation. Turn the blanket downward and the gown upward neatly to make a smooth area around surgical site.
6. Turn on overhead spotlight over the site of the incision. Bright light should not be focused on the patient before he or she is asleep or the eyes are covered. Preoperative medication affects the protective pupillary reflex. Dim light is restful and not irritating.
7. Arrange the sterile prep tray and pour solutions if this has not already been done. Don sterile gloves and prepare the surgical site. (Patient skin preparation is discussed in Chapter 22.)

   NOTE The first assistant may be the person who preps the patient. This person first scrubs his or her own hands and arms, then puts on sterile gloves.

8. Cover or bag the prep tray immediately after use. The preparation sponges are not included in the sponge count so they should not be discarded in the kick bucket. A disposable tray may be bagged for disposal with trash after the surgical procedure is completed.

After Surgeon and Assistant(s) Scrub

1. Assist with gowning. Reach inside the gown to the shoulder seam. If closed-glove technique is used, pull the gown sleeves only so far that the hands remain covered. If open technique is used, pull each sleeve over the hands so the gown cuffs are at the wrists. Fasten the back of the gown.

   NOTE After gloving, the surgeon and assistant(s) should wipe their gloves with a sterile damp towel to remove glove powder. If the surgeon rinses gloves in a splash basin, this basin should be removed from the sterile field immediately after use for this purpose to avoid carrying powder into the surgical wound if the gloves are rinsed of blood and debris during the surgical procedure.

2. Observe for any breaks in technique during draping (see Chapter 22). Stand near the head end of the operating table to assist the anesthesiologist in fastening the drape over the anesthesia screen or around an IV standard next to the armboard.
3. Assist the scrub person in moving the Mayo stand and instrument table into position, being careful not to touch the drapes (Figure 20-8).
4. Focus the overhead operating light on the site of incision unless sterile handles will be used. The beam of light should pass the surgeon's right ear and center at the tip of his or her right index finger (or left for left-handed surgeon).
5. Place steps or platforms for team members who need them, or place stools in position for surgeon who prefers to operate seated. If the surgeon is seated, the entire team should be seated to protect the level of the sterile field.
6. Position kick buckets on each side of the operating table and splash basin, if used, near the surgeon (Figure 20-8).
7. Connect suction if necessary. Suction caps are designed so the inlet for fluid is below the outlet for vacuum. These connections must not be reversed. If they are, contents of the container are picked up and carried into the vacuum system, clogging it and making it nonoperational. Disposable suction collection units facilitate disposal.

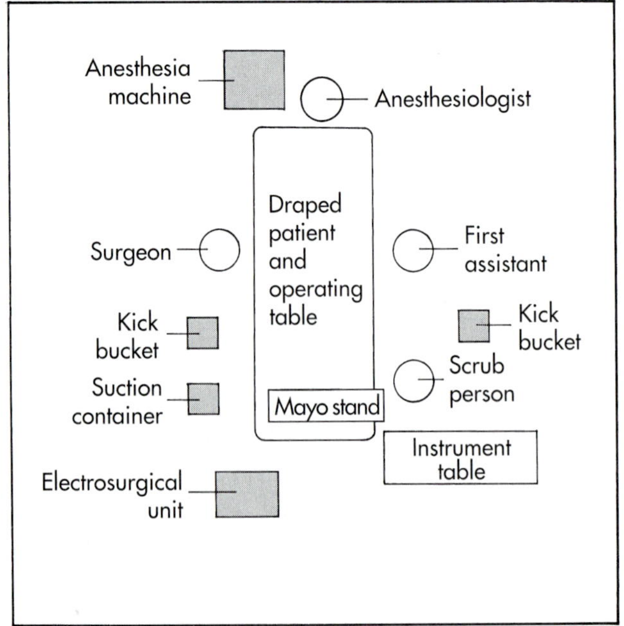

FIGURE 20-8 Arrangement of sterile field, team members, and unsterile equipment *(shaded)*.

8. Connect electrosurgical electrode cord or any other powered equipment to be used. Place footpedals within easy reach of the surgeon's foot. Tell the surgeon which footpedal is placed by which foot and confirm the desired settings on all machines.

During Surgical Procedure

1. Be alert to anticipate needs of the sterile team such as adjusting the operating light, removing perspiration from brows, and keeping the scrub person supplied with sponges, sutures, warm saline, etc. Ideally the circulator watches the surgical procedure closely enough to see when routine supplies are needed and gives them to the scrub person without him or her having to ask for them. The circulator should know how to use and care for all supplies, instruments, and equipment and be able to get them quickly. This is particularly important in emergency situations such as cardiac arrest.
2. Stay in the room. *Inform the scrub person if you must leave.* Be available to answer questions, obtain supplies, and assist team members.
3. Keep discarded sponges carefully collected, separated by sizes, and counted. Sponge forceps or gloves, *never bare hands,* are used to handle and count sponges. Soiled sponges should be placed away from traffic, cabinets, and doors but in full view of the scrub person and anesthesiologist. They must be kept at a level well below the sterile field in a leakproof container. Lint, dust, and trapped organisms will be dispersed into the air as sponges dry and are handled for counting. Gathering them directly into containers, such as clear plastic bags that can be closed, eliminates hazards. The method used depends on provision made for care of soiled sponges. (Refer to suggested methods of guarding sponges on pp. 427-428 of this chapter.)
4. Assist in monitoring blood loss. Weigh sponges if requested by the anesthesiologist or surgeon. Estimate blood volume in the suction container by subtracting irrigation and body fluids from the total volume in the container. Total blood volume monitoring determinations may be used for estimation of the surgical blood loss (see Chapter 19, p. 376). Refer to discussion of blood loss and procedure for weighing sponges in Chapter 23, p. 481.
5. Obtain blood products for transfusion as necessary from the refrigerator, or send nursing assistant to the blood bank. If the patient's own blood will be recovered for intraoperative autotransfusion, obtain the necessary equipment. Refer to the discussion of blood transfusion (pp. 484-485) and autotransfusion (pp. 485-486) in Chapter 23.
6. Know the condition of the patient at all times. Inform the OR manager of any marked changes, unanticipated procedure, or delays. In a busy department it may be necessary to rearrange the schedule. Communicate periodically with the patient's family or significant other(s) to inform them of the progress of the procedure as appropriate.
7. Prepare and label specimens for transportation to the laboratory. An error in labeling a tissue specimen or culture could cause an inaccurate diagnosis, improper therapy, or reoperation. Each container is labeled with the patient's name and identification number. A requisition specifying the laboratory test the surgeon desires accompanies the specimen. This includes date, name of surgeon, preoperative and postoperative diagnoses, surgical procedure, desired testing to be performed, and tissue to be examined, including its source.

   Containers for storing specimens may be plastic containers, waxed cardboard cartons, or glass jars with preservative solution. The closed, labeled container is placed into a plastic bag or additional container for transport to the laboratory. Handling of specimens should be held to a minimum and *never done with bare hands;* wear gloves. If instruments are used for handling, be careful not to tear or damage tissue. The routine for each type of tissue specimen may vary as follows:

   a. Pathologic specimens should not be allowed to dry out. A solution of aqueous formaldehyde most often is used as the fixative until the specimen is processed further in laboratory. Some pathology labs prefer moistening the specimen with sterile normal saline. Check for the preference of the laboratory examining the specimen.
   b. Cultures should be refrigerated or sent to the laboratory immediately. When placed immediately into media, they can be stored in an incubator indefinitely.

      Cultures are obtained under sterile conditions. Tips of swabs must not be contaminated by any other source. The circulator may hold the tube with gloved hands; however, swabs are handled only by sterile team members. OR and laboratory personnel must be protected from contamination. The circulator, wearing gloves, can hold open a small paper or plastic bag for the scrub person to drop the tube into if it is handled on the sterile field.

      Cultures for suspected anaerobic pathogens require immediate attention. Exposure to room air may kill anaerobes in a few minutes. Most laboratories provide special transport devices or media for their survival. If these are not available, purulent material can be aspirated into a sterile disposable syringe with a disposable needle attached. The needle is removed and placed with counted sharps on the instrument table. Air is expelled away from the field, and the syringe is capped with the syringe tip supplied with the syringe and sent immediately to the laboratory. The syringe should not be sent to the laboratory with the needle attached. The needle should not be recapped by hand because of the potential for a needlestick injury.

c. Smears and fluids should be taken to the laboratory as soon as possible. These may be placed on glass slides or drawn into evacuation tubes.
d. Stones are placed in a dry container so they will not dissolve.
e. Foreign bodies should be disposed of according to policy and a record kept for legal purposes. A description of the object is recorded. A foreign body may be given to the police, surgeon, or patient, depending on legal implications, policy, or surgeon's wishes.
f. Amputated extremities are wrapped before sending them to a refrigerator, which is usually in the morgue. To comply with a religious mandate that his or her body be buried in its entirety, the patient may request that an extremity be sent to a mortuary. This must be noted on the requisition sent to the laboratory. Refer to institutional policy and procedure for the care of amputated limbs.

Use care to avoid contaminating the outside of a specimen container. If contaminated, wipe with a tuberculocidal disinfectant. Always wash hands thoroughly after removing gloves worn to handle specimens.

8. Complete the patient's chart, permanent OR records, and requisitions for laboratory tests or chargeable items, as required.
   a. Documentation in patient's chart of direct intraoperative care should include:
      (1) Disposition of sensory aids or prosthetic devices accompanying the patient on arrival in OR
      (2) Position, supports, and/or restraints used during the surgical procedure
      (3) Placement of monitoring and electrosurgical electrodes, tourniquets, and other special equipment and identification of units or machines used, as applicable
      (4) Skin preparation area and antiseptic agent
      (5) Medications administered by RN
      (6) Contact with the patient's family or significant other(s)
   b. Circulator documents other activities that may affect patient outcomes of surgical intervention. These may include:
      (1) Type, size, and manufacturer's identifying information of prosthetic implants or type, source, and location of tissue transplants or inserted radioactive materials
      (2) Disposition of tissue specimens and cultures
      (3) Placement of drains, catheters, and packing
   c. Requisitions are made out as a record of:
      (1) Charges to patients for supplies, according to hospital routine.
      (2) Piece of equipment sent from OR with patient to unit (e.g., an instrument such as an intestinal clamp left on patient following a colostomy, a tracheotomy set that accompanies patient following thyroidectomy, wire scissors if patient has had teeth wired together). These items are to be returned. The requisition usually is made out in duplicate; the copy accompanies the item, and original is filed by the lender until the item is returned.
9. Be alert to any breaks in sterile technique.
   a. Do not touch or reach over the sterile field. When placing sterile items, transfer should be made to the edge of the instrument table to avoid exposing it to contamination with microorganisms in dust or lint shed from a sleeve or wrapper.
   b. Face sterile areas when passing. Just as no unsterile equipment should be placed between two sterile surfaces, no unsterile person should pass between two sterile surfaces or two sterile team members. All unsterile personnel should face and remain at least 1 foot (30 cm) from any sterile surface.
   c. Do not touch unwrapped sterilized items to the nonsterile rim or door when removing them from the sterilizer.
   d. Do not touch the edge of a cap or the lid to the lip of the container before or after pouring sterile solution. The outside of a cap is not sterile.
   e. Wash hands vigorously after each patient contact or handling contaminated items and after removing gloves. Wash hands frequently with an antiseptic agent. Work up a good lather and use friction. Be sure to clean under fingernails; microorganisms can grow under them. Turn faucet handles off with a paper towel if a knee or foot control is not available.
   f. Keep conversation to a minimum. Do not handle mask and cap unnecessarily. Keep hair covered and the mask in place.

g. Decontaminate the floor and walls promptly during the surgical procedure if contaminated by organic debris such as blood, body and irrigation fluids, and sputum. A broad-spectrum tuberculocidal detergent-disinfectant can be applied from a squeeze bottle to the soilage. Wear gloves to wipe it up. This prompt decontamination helps prevent microorganisms from drying and becoming airborne.
h. Do not wear gloves when handling charts, x-ray films, requisitions, etc. Gloves should be worn only for direct contacts with the patient and inanimate items contaminated by blood, blood products, and body fluids. Do not handle sterile packages or touch items in cabinets while wearing contaminated gloves.

During Closure

1. Count sponges, sharps, and instruments with the scrub person. Report counts as correct or incorrect to the surgeon (refer to count procedures, pp. 425-426). Complete the count records. Collect used sponges for disposal in appropriately marked receptacles.
2. If another patient is scheduled to follow (TF):
   a. Phone or ask clerk-receptionist to call the unit where the next patient is waiting at least 45 minutes before the scheduled time of the surgical procedure to request that preoperative medication be given if ordered. This usually is not necessary for the first scheduled patient of the day but is important for subsequent patients when the exact time of the surgical procedure is uncertain. For these patients the anesthesiologist usually orders medication "on call."
   b. Send a nursing assistant for the patient or notify the unit to transport the patient. The patient should be in the OR suite 30 minutes before the time of anticipated incision. If a holding area is included in the OR suite, the patient may arrive earlier to receive preoperative medication there.
   c. Check the surgeon's preference card and procedure book. Collect supplies that will be needed; get them organized to the extent possible. These can be assembled in the substerile room or left in a cabinet. They cannot be put on furniture in the room until it is cleaned after this surgical procedure is completed. Advance preparation is not necessary if a case cart system is used.
3. Prepare for room cleanup so that minimal time will be expended between surgical procedures.
   a. Remove x-ray films from the viewbox, place them in an envelope, and take them to the designated area to be returned to the x-ray department.
   b. Return blood not needed for transfusion to the refrigerator or have it taken to the blood bank by a nursing assistant.
   c. Obtain the washer-sterilizer tray, instrument tray, and other items necessary for the cleanup procedure.
4. Send for a postanesthesia care unit (PACU) stretcher, intensive care unit (ICU) bed, or prepare the patient's stretcher or bed with a clean sheet, whatever is the institutional procedure. Also alert nursing assistants and housekeeping personnel that the surgical procedure is nearing completion so that they can be ready to assist as needed. This helps shorten time between surgical procedures.
5. Obtain a transfer monitor and oxygen tank with tubing if needed.

After Surgical Procedure Is Completed

1. Open the neck and back closures of gowns of the surgeon and assistants so they can remove them without contaminating themselves.
2. Assist with dressing the surgical wound. Refer to discussion of dressings in Chapter 25, pp. 530-532. The scrub person should roll the drapes off the patient before the outer layer of dressing is applied.
3. Connect all drainage systems as indicated. Refer to the discussion of drains in Chapter 25, pp. 527-530.
4. See that the patient is clean. Wash off blood, feces, or plaster. Put on a clean warm gown and blanket.
5. Have a nursing assistant bring in a clean PACU stretcher or ICU bed. Check the patient's name on the stretcher or bed if procedure is to return patient to same one used for transport to the OR suite.
6. Help move the patient to the stretcher or bed. Lock the wheels. Remove arm and leg restraints and table appliances. A lifting frame or patient roller is a great help in moving unconscious and obese patients. The Davis patient roller consists of a series of rollers, mounted in a frame long enough to accommodate an adult patient. The edge of the roller is placed under the lift sheet and the patient's side. With the patient's head and feet supported, pull on the lift sheet and roll the patient onto the stretcher or bed. The following precautions should be taken in lifting or rolling an unconscious patient:
   a. Splint the arm if an IV line is running, thus protecting the needle.
   b. Support the arms at the sides with the lift sheet so they do not dangle.
   c. The anesthesiologist guards the head and neck from injury.

d. Lift or roll the patient gently and slowly to avoid circulatory depression. At least four people are needed; one to lift the head, one to lift the feet, one beside the stretcher or bed to pull, and one beside the patient to lift him or her from the operating table. The action of all should be synchronized. The count of three is called by the anesthesiologist.
e. Remove the lift sheet from under the patient by rolling the patient gently from side to side. Brush burns result if the fabric is pulled from under the patient.
f. Place the patient in a comfortable position most conducive to maintenance of respiration and circulation. This may vary with the type of surgical procedure; usually the patient should:
   (1) Be supine following laparotomy, with the head of the stretcher elevated 15 degrees
   (2) Be semiprone following tonsillectomy, for drainage
   (3) Be lateral, on the affected side, following transthoracic surgical procedures, thus splinting the side
   (4) Have the affected extremity supported on a pillow
g. Raise the siderails before the patient is transported out of the OR.

7. Secure IV solution bags on a standard, attached preferably near the foot end of the stretcher or bed, where there is less danger of injury to the patient if it should fall or break.
8. Be sure the chart and proper records accompany the patient. Send extra units of blood as needed. Send other supplies as indicated. Final completion of the patient's chart by the circulator should include documentation of:
   a. Time of arrival in OR and start of procedure
   b. Method of anesthesia and by whom; the type and amount of local infiltrate used
   c. Participants in the procedure (i.e., surgeon, assistants, scrub person, and circulator)
   d. Presence of students or other authorized personnel
   e. Vital sign trends throughout a procedure performed under local anesthesia
   f. Assessment of patient's skin condition before and at completion of the surgical procedure (i.e., skin discoloration, rashes, pressure sores, burns)
   g. Fluid intake, urinary output, and estimated blood loss, if measurement during the surgical procedure was appropriate
   h. All types and amounts of intraoperative medications administered
   i. Results of all counts and personnel performing the counts as defined by institutional policy and procedure
   j. Type of dressing, placement of drains, and/or packing
   k. Time of discharge from OR and method of transport
9. Have the nursing assistant help transport patient to the PACU, ICU, or nursing unit.

Transfer from Operating Room

The patient should be constantly observed during transport by someone familiar with his or her condition. The circulator may accompany a patient who has had local anesthesia. An anesthesiologist or anesthetist should accompany an anesthetized patient. The circulator may go with the anesthesiologist to give a nursing report, including review of the plan of care, to the nurse receiving the patient in the PACU, ICU, or nursing unit. A report is imperative for continuity of care and recovery of the patient. A concise verbal report from the anesthesiologist and/or circulator includes:

1. Name and age of patient
2. Type of surgical procedure and surgeon
3. Type of anesthesia and anesthesiologist
4. Vital signs, preoperative and intraoperative, including current body temperature
5. Types and locations of drains, packing, and dressings
6. Level of consciousness preoperatively and current status
7. Medications given preoperatively and intraoperatively, and those regularly taken by prescription or self-medicated
8. Medical history, including previous surgical procedures
9. Allergies and responses to allergens, substance sensitivity
10. Positioning on the operating table and devices attached to the skin
11. Complications during the surgical procedure
12. Intake and output, including IV fluids and blood
13. Location of the waiting family or significant other(s)
14. Special considerations
    a. Sensory and/or physical impairments

       NOTE Eyeglasses, hearing aid, dentures, or other personal property brought to the OR with the patient is returned to the patient when the level of consciousness is appropriate.

    b. Language barrier
    c. Use of tobacco, alcohol, and/or addictive drugs

d. Orders such as "no code" or "do not resuscitate" or "do not attempt resuscitation"

SPONGES, SHARPS, AND INSTRUMENT COUNTS

The foregoing outline repeatedly mentions counting of sponges, needles and other sharps, and instruments. These supplies are crucial to the surgical procedure. They must be accounted for throughout every procedure.

A sponge left in the wound after closure is a possible cause for a lawsuit following a surgical procedure. A piece of a broken needle or a whole needle and occasionally an instrument may be left in a patient. A foreign body unintentionally left in a patient can cause unnecessary physical injury and can be the source of wound infection or disruption. Foreign bodies inadvertently left in the wound must be retrieved. Therefore, to ensure adequate patient protection, items are counted before and after use. The kinds and numbers of sponges, needles and other sharps, and instruments vary for each surgical procedure.

Counts are also performed for infection control and inventory control purposes. A contaminated sponge or needle, unaccounted for at the close of procedure, could inadvertently come in contact with the personnel who clean the room. Blood or body fluids are sources of pathogens such as human immunodeficiency virus (HIV) or hepatitis B virus (HBV). Inventory control is monitored by accounting for the instrument set in its entirety. Counting ensures that expensive instruments such as towel clips and scissors are not accidentally thrown away or discarded with the drapes. Surgical instruments can cause major damage to equipment in the laundry services. Injury to the laundry and housekeeping/environmental services personnel by contaminated sharp edges of surgical instruments, blades, and needles is a potential risk.

Counting Procedures

A *counting procedure* is a method of accounting for items put on the sterile table for use during the surgical procedure. Sponges, sharps, and instruments should be counted on all procedures.

First Count

The person who wraps items for sterilization counts them in standardized multiple units. If commercially prepackaged sterile items are used, such as sponges, this count is done by the manufacturer.

Second Count

The scrub person and the circulator together count all items before the surgical procedure begins and as each additional package is opened and added to the sterile field during the surgical procedure. These initial counts provide the baseline for subsequent counts. A useful method for counting is as follows:

1. As the scrub person touches each item, he or she and the circulator number each one aloud until all items are counted.
2. The circulator immediately records the count for each type of item on the count record. Preprinted forms are helpful for this purpose.
3. Count additional packages away from counted items already on table in case it is necessary to repeat the count or discard an item.
4. Counting should not be interrupted. If uncertain about the count because of interruption, fumbling, or any other reason, repeat it.

NOTE If either the scrub person or circulator is permanently relieved by another person during the surgical procedure, the incoming person should verify all counts before the person being relieved leaves the room. Persons who perform final counts are held accountable for the entire count.

Third Count

Counts are taken in three areas before the surgeon starts the closure of a body cavity or a deep or large incision.

1. *Field count.* Either the surgeon or the assistant assists the scrub person with the surgical field count. This area may be counted first. Counting this area last could delay closure of the patient's wound and prolong anesthesia.
2. *Table count.* The scrub person and the circulator together count all items on the instrument table and Mayo stand. The surgeon and assistant may be closing the wound while this count is in process.
3. *Floor count.* The circulator counts sponges and any other items that have been recovered from the floor or passed off the sterile field. These counts should be verified by the scrub person.

The circulator totals field, table, and floor counts. If the second and third counts match, the circulator tells the surgeon the counts are correct.

NOTE By written policy and procedure, final counts may be deleted if all items are easily accounted for in their entirety. This exclusion usually applies only to instruments used for superficial incisions or minimally invasive procedures.

Fourth or Final Count

A fourth count is performed to verify any counts and/or if institutional policy and procedure stipulates additional counts before any part of a cavity or a cavity within a cavity is closed. A final count may be taken during subcuticular or skin closure. A count should be reported to the surgeon as correct only after a physical count by number actually has been completed.

The circulator documents on the patient's record what was counted, how many counts were performed and by whom, and if the counts were correct. A registered nurse should participate to verify that all counts are correct. However, the personnel actually performing the counts are responsible for the accuracy of the counts. The counting procedure, outcome, and participating personnel should be documented according to institutional policy and procedure.

Omitted counts because of extreme patient emergency should be recorded on the patient's record, and the event should be documented according to institutional policy and procedure. If a sponge or sponges are intentionally retained for packing or an instrument remains with the patient, these also should be documented on the patient's record. Any time a count is omitted, refused by a surgeon, or aborted, the reason should be fully documented.

Records can be subpoenaed and admitted as evidence in court. The accountability for all items used during the surgical procedure is placed on the scrub person and the circulator who jointly perform the counting procedures as defined by institutional policy and procedure.

Incorrect Count

If any count is incorrect, a specific policy and procedure should be defined by each institution including, but not limited to:

1. Informing the surgeon immediately.
2. Repeating the entire count.
3. Circulator searches trash receptacles, under furniture, on floor, in laundry hamper, and throughout room.
4. Scrub person searches drapes and under items on the table and Mayo stand.
5. Surgeon searches surgical field and wound.
6. Circulator should call the immediate supervisor to check the count and assist with the search.
7. After exhausting all search options, policy should stipulate that an *x-ray film be taken before the patient leaves the OR* whenever a sponge, sharp, or instrument count is incorrect. The surgeon may wish an x-ray film taken at once, with a portable machine, to determine whether the item is in the wound. Because of the patient's condition or reasonable assurance, based on wound exploration, that the item is not in the patient, the surgeon may prefer to complete the closure first.
8. Circulator should write an incident report, indicating all efforts and actions to locate the missing item even if item is located on an x-ray film. This report has legal significance to verify that an appropriate attempt was made to find the missing item. If the item is not found on the x-ray film, the report brings to the attention of personnel the need for more careful counting and control of sponges, sharps, and instruments.

Sponges

Sponges are used for absorbing blood and fluids, protecting tissues, applying pressure or traction, and dissecting tissue. Many different kinds of sponges are available. Those placed on the sterile table and field should be *x-ray detectable.* A radiopaque thread or marker is incorporated into commercially manufactured sponges.

Types of Sponges

The following are representative of the types of sponges used:

1. *Gauze sponges,* called "swabs" in some countries, are supplied folded.
   a. 3 × 3 inch (7.6 × 7.6 cm) sponges may be used in small incisions.
   b. 4 × 4 inch (10 × 10 cm) sponges, the most common size, are usually used dry. They are usually opened to their full length for swabbing superficial tissues. They may be folded into a 2 × 2 inch (5 × 5 cm) square and used on sponge forceps deep in body cavities.
   c. 4 × 8 inch (10 × 20 cm) sponges may be used for sponging or as a moist pack in a large exposed area.

   NOTE Do not open gauze sponges out to a single ply. Fibers along raw edges would become foreign bodies in the wound, as could the radiopaque marker if it became dislodged.
2. *Tapes,* also called *lap pads* or *packs,* are used for walling off the viscera and keeping them moist and warm. Either square or oblong, they may have a loop of twilled tape sewed on one corner over which a metal or plastic radiopaque ring, about 1½ inches (3.8 cm) in diameter, can be fastened. If rings are used, they remain outside the edges of incision while the tape is inside. Normal saline is usually used to moisten tapes because it is an isotonic solution.
3. Dissecting sponges:
   a. *Peanut sponges* are very small gauze sponges used for blunt dissection or to absorb fluid in delicate procedures. They are clamped into the tip of a forceps during use.
   b. *Kitner dissectors* are small rolls of heavy cotton tape. They are held in a forceps for use.
   c. *Tonsil sponges* are cotton-filled gauze with a cotton thread attached. They are held in a forceps for use.

4. *Compressed absorbent patties (cottonoids),* made of compressed rayon or cotton, are used moist on delicate structures such as nerves, brain, and spinal cord. Smaller pieces have a thread attached so they can be located in the wound. Patties are very absorbent. Press them out flat after moistening before handing them to the surgeon. The surgeon will pick up the patty with a forceps and apply it to the area of intended use.
5. *Pledgets,* made of polymeric felt, are used as a buttress under sutures in friable tissues. Usually prethreaded onto suture, pledgets may be supplied separately in multiple units.

Counting Sponges

Radiopaque, x-ray–detectable gauze sponges, tapes, dissecting sponges, and cottonoid patties are counted in multiples of 5 or 6 (i.e., 10 or 12, 20 or 24 per package). Types of sponges and number of different sizes should be kept to a minimum. To count them, the scrub person:

1. Holds the entire pack of sponges, of whatever type including tapes, in one hand. The thumb should be over the edges of folded sponges.
2. Shakes pack gently to separate the sponges.
3. Picks each sponge separately from pack with the other hand and numbers it aloud while placing it in a pile on the table.

If a pack contains an incorrect number of sponges, the scrub person should hand the pack to circulator. Attempts should not be made to correct errors or compensate for discrepancies. The pack should be isolated and not used.

Methods of Guarding Sponges

Regardless of types and numbers of sponges counted, various methods may be used to help ensure that one is not left in the patient or misplaced.

By Scrub Person

1. Keep sponges, tapes, peanuts, etc., separated on the instrument table and far away from each other and away from draping material, especially towels.
2. Keep sponges far away from small items such as needles and clips that might be dragged into the wound by them.
3. Do not give the surgeon or assistant a sponge to wipe powder off gloves. It may end up in laundry hamper or trash.
4. Do not cut sponges or tapes.
5. Do not remove the radiopaque thread or marker.
6. Never mix sponges and tapes in a solution basin at same time, to avoid the danger of dragging a small sponge unknowingly into the wound along with a tape.
7. Do not give the pathologist a specimen on a sponge to take from the room; put it on a towel instead.
8. Discard all soiled sponges into the kick bucket, leaving two clean ones on field. If the surgeon needs more, keep a mental count of the number of sponges or tapes on the field at any given time. Put up clean ones before removing soiled ones on an exchange basis.
9. Do not be wasteful of sponges. Besides the economy factor, the more sponges that are used, the more there are to count and the greater the chance for error.
10. Once the peritoneum is opened or the incision extends deep into a body cavity where a sponge could be lost, three alternative precautions can be taken:
    a. Remove all small sponges from the field and use only tapes. Rings, if used, hang over wound edges.
    b. Use 4 × 4 inch (10 × 10 cm) sponges on sponge forceps only.
    c. Give sponges to the surgeon one at a time on an exchange basis.
11. Count sponges and tapes added during the surgical procedure with the circulator before moistening or using them.
12. *Do not add or remove sponges from the surgical field during a sponge count until count is verified as completed and correct.* Before beginning the final count, place one or two tapes or sponges on the field for use while the count is taken.

By Circulator

1. To prevent the possibility of a sponge being taken into the OR and causing confusion in the count, different types and sizes should be used on trays, such as spinal, shave, or prep trays, and should be contained before the incision is made. A tray, including the used sponges, may be bagged in plastic and stored temporarily. Sponges from these trays should never be put in a kick bucket or trash receptacle until after the final count is completed.
2. Unfold each discarded sponge and shake tapes to be sure no sponges are on them. To avoid transmission of bloodborne pathogenic organisms, *soiled sponges are never touched with bare hands.* Use sponge forceps or gloves to separate sponges for counting and stacking.
3. Count sponges into multiple or submultiples of the total number in a package as recorded on sponge count record; count and stack them into separate units for each type of sponge.

NOTE The kick bucket should be lined with a bag made of antistatic plastic or other impervious material.

Sponges may be hung over the rim of the bucket until the count unit is complete, or they may be transferred into compartmentalized containers. Several types are available; some facilitate blood loss estimation by visualizing or weighing. When the number needed to complete a unit is obtained, the sponges should be enclosed in an impervious bag or container to minimize airborne contamination. The scrub person should verify the count with the circulator before the unit is closed. The number of sponges in each unit and the number of units are recorded so that when it is time for the final count the circulator has a record of the number bagged or in containers. The units can be placed on an impervious surface, such as a waterproof sheet on the floor, within sight of the anesthesiologist and scrub person. Hanging sponges on a rack or laying moist sponges on a wrapper on the floor is a potential source of environmental contamination.

4. Give additional sponges or tapes to the scrub person when it is convenient for him or her to count them. Count and record them immediately.
5. Collect all soiled sponges into a plastic or other moisture-proof bag, usually the kick bucket liner, after the final count. Wear gloves or use sponge forceps to handle soiled sponges. Discard the gloves with the sponges and wash hands immediately.
6. Give the scrub person dressings after the final sponge count. Radiopaque sponges are not used for dressings because they could distort a postoperative x-ray film of the site.
7. Do not remove sponges from the room before the surgical procedure is completed.

Sharps

Sharps include surgical needles, hypodermic needles, knife blades, electrosurgical needles and blades, and safety pins. Each item must be accounted for. Surgical needles are the most difficult to keep track of and are used in the largest quantity. All surgical needles and other sharps are counted as they are added to the sterile table and/or separated from other instruments in the instrument tray.

Surgical Needles

Surgical needles are used for suturing (i.e., bringing tissues together). The types and methods for handling them are discussed in detail in Chapter 24, pp. 498-502. However, the type will determine the method of transfer to the sterile table.

1. Reusable eyed needles put in a needle rack or a suture book are uniformly counted into sets in multiples of two or three of each type and size the surgeon will need. These needles usually are sterilized in the instrument set.
2. Disposable eyed or eyeless (swaged) needles are precounted by the manufacturer. The label specifies whether the sterile packet contains a single or multiple needles.

Counting Sharps

Each sharp, or packet containing them, is separated for counting individually. Suture packets containing swaged needles can remain unopened. The count is taken according to the label on each packet. The scrub person must verify this count when the packet is opened. Some packets contain multiple needles, as described in Chapter 24, p. 505.

Methods of Accounting for Sharps

If a needle has broken, both the scrub person and the circulator must make sure all pieces are recovered or accounted for if the surgeon decides not to retrieve a piece. Sometimes the risk of retrieving a piece of a needle is more hazardous than letting it encapsulate in tissue.

By Scrub Person Needles, knife blades, safety pins, and other small sharps *should never be loose on the Mayo stand* because they could be dragged into the incision or knocked onto the floor.

1. Leave needles swaged to suture material in their inner folder or dispenser packet until the surgeon is ready to use them. These folders or packets can be placed in a fold of the suture book or secured on the Mayo stand. Suture packets can remain sealed until the scrub person anticipates their use, thus minimizing the number of loose unused needles on the sterile table.
2. Give needles to surgeon on an exchange basis; that is, one is returned before another is passed. Account for each needle as the surgeon finishes with it. Never let a needle lie loose on the field or Mayo stand. Keep them away from sponges and tapes.
3. Use needles and needleholders as a unit. A good rule is: *no needle on the Mayo stand without a needleholder and no needleholder without a needle.*
4. Secure used needles and sharps until after the final count. Many methods for efficient handling are available.
   a. Sterile adhesive pads with or without magnets facilitate counting and safe disposal. Separate pads can be used for needles that may be used again and for those that will not be. When a large number of swaged needles will be used, the scrub person and circulator may determine the number of needles a pad will hold and work out a unit system. When the maximum number is reached and counted by them, the pad is closed. This method eliminates the hazard of handling loose needles on the Mayo stand or instrument table.

b. Swaged needles can be inserted through or into their original packet. An empty packet indicates an unaccounted-for needle at the time of the final count.
c. Used eyed needles can be returned to the needle rack or threaded into top layer of the suture book.
d. Accumulation of used needles in a medicine cup or other container is the least desirable method because each must be handled individually to count them. This not only potentially contaminates gloves but may puncture them as well.

By Circulator

1. Open only the number of packets of sutures with swaged needles that will be needed. Overstocking the table not only is wasteful but also complicates needle count.
2. Counted sharps should not be taken from the OR during the surgical procedure. If a scalpel with a counted knife blade is given to pathologist to open a specimen, it must remain in the room after gross examination; it must not be taken to the laboratory with the specimen.
3. A sharp is passed off the sterile field if it punctures, cuts, or tears the glove of a sterile team member. These sharps must be retained and added to the table and field counts to reconcile the final sharp count.
4. A magnetic roller may be used to locate a surgical needle that has dropped on the floor.

Instruments

Surgical tools and devices are designed to perform specific functions that include cutting or dissecting, grasping and holding, clamping and occluding, exposing, or suturing. For each basic maneuver, an instrument of suitable size, shape, strength, and function is needed. Variation in style and number of instruments will be dictated by type of surgical procedure and, to some extent, by personal preferences of the surgeon. See Chapter 14 for detailed discussion of surgical instruments.

Counting Instruments

Instrument counts are recommended for all surgical procedures. Specific written policies and procedures must be followed without deviation. To count instruments, the scrub person:

1. Removes the top rack of instruments from the instrument tray or container and places it on a rolled towel or over the lip of a tray or container. Instruments are counted as they are assembled in standardized sets. Groups of even numbers of each of the basic clamps facilitate handling and counting.
2. Exposes all instruments left in tray for counting. Removes knife handles, towel clips, tissue forceps, and other small instruments from the tray and places them on the instrument table. Do not put instruments on the Mayo stand until they are counted or as they are being counted.
3. Accounts for all detachable and disassembled parts. These must be counted or accounted for during assembly.
4. Recovers and retains all pieces of an instrument that breaks during use. A replacement instrument must be added to the count.
5. Counts any instruments added to the table after the initial count is taken, with one exception. If the circulator decontaminates and sterilizes an instrument that has dropped to the floor or has been passed off table, an adjustment in the count is unnecessary. Instruments recovered from the floor or passed off that are not sterilized are retained by the circulator and added to the designated counts.

Simplifying Instrument Counts

Reducing the number and types of instruments and streamlining standardized sets makes counting easier. Inform the OR manager if unused, unnecessary instruments are routinely included in basic sets. Keep the surgeon's preference cards up-to-date. Instruments peculiar to specific surgical procedures or surgeons can be wrapped separately and added to the basic set only when needed.

Standard count sheets for each basic instrument set will facilitate the process. The person who prepares the set verifies the initial count as listed. The sheet accompanies the set. The circulator can check the items as they are counted with the scrub person.

OTHER NURSING CONSIDERATIONS

Accounting for sponges, sharps, and instruments throughout every surgical procedure guards against the potential for leaving a foreign object in the wound. The insertion of drains to evacuate fluids and air from the surgical site and the application of sterile dressings also are important aspects of wound management. Both the scrub person and the circulator assist in these final stages of the surgical procedure (see Chapter 25, pp. 529-532).

The outcome of surgical intervention is always expected to be favorable. However, in reality this does not always occur. Patients can die on the operating table. Team members must deal psychologically with the death of a patient (see Chapter 4, pp. 64-65). The perioperative nurses and surgical technologists also must care for the body.

Regardless of the outcome, the sterile field must be dismantled and the OR cleaned in preparation for the next patient (see Chapter 27).

A discussion of the duties of the scrub person and the circulator would not be complete without consideration of efficiency, productivity, and work habits.

Efficiency of Operating Room Team

The scrub person and circulator working together coordinate their efforts to accomplish the tasks necessary to achieve a common goal in the OR. This common goal is to provide for the safety and welfare of every patient. Efficiency, therefore, depends primarily on individual effort and the working relationship among team members.

Appropriate Behaviors

Pride in one's own work and in that of other team members leads to satisfaction. Unethical discussions, unprofessional conduct, lapses in sterile technique, carelessness in handling expensive equipment, preventable breakage, and forgetfulness make negative impressions on patients and coworkers. They may carry these impressions to others outside the hospital. Constant vigilance is necessary.

Behavioral Objectives

To enhance efficiency, the scrub person and circulator need to develop personal attributes that foster teamwork. Behavioral objectives include the following:

1. Demonstrate initiative and energy.
2. Develop a spirit of cooperation. A responsive and pleasing personality will make any situation tolerable. It never hurts to say "please" and "thank you."
3. Display positive regard and respect for coworkers. Individuals from different backgrounds and a divergence of lifestyles contribute new ideas and approaches to the workplace. Compassion and understanding of individual differences promote trust and respect from others.
4. Maintain a tasteful sense of humor. Situations encountered in the OR are often difficult. Humor relieves stress and tension.
5. Keep an open mind and be flexible. Changes in work schedules and procedures are made when a need for change accommodates or improves patient care. Adaptability eases the difficulty frequently associated with unexpected change.
6. Accept and benefit from constructive criticism. Keep a balanced perspective. Many times it is not the incident itself but one's reaction to it that can be devastating. Constructive criticism should be given and received tactfully and kindly.
7. Maintain personal integrity by not discussing patients, surgeons, surgical procedures, and the multitude of incidents involving them outside the OR suite. To seek advice or to resolve a problem, discuss work-related questions or situations with your immediate supervisor.
8. Seek proper instruction in the use and care of equipment and supplies before assuming responsibility for them.
9. Review departmental policies and procedures and follow them.
10. Strive to work smoothly and efficiently as a team member. Team members anticipate the needs of the group as a whole and function as an integral part in the attainment of common goals.
11. Support an atmosphere in which the surgeon and team members work well together. Usually a calm, serious atmosphere with intense concentration without excessive tension is best. The surgeon should not feel rushed. Respect the surgeon's mood and temperament, which may vary with the progress of the surgical procedure.
12. Maintain a stable temperament. The surgeon may vent frustration if the patient's condition deteriorates. Verbal outbursts are a release of tension and are not intended as a personal affront. Be tolerant and forgiving; have patience. Learn to compromise and negotiate without antagonism. Avoid being defensive. Verbal abuse is not acceptable and should not be tolerated. The immediate supervisor should be consulted if this situation occurs.
13. Communicate and collaborate with team members in the best interests of the patient. Seek and share pertinent data. Keep others informed. This may necessitate telling the surgeon or another team member that a break in technique has taken place, which must be promptly corrected.
14. Admit an error, and then take steps to rectify the situation. Be accountable and responsible for yourself. Provide the rationale for your actions without becoming defensive. Perform within the appropriate scope of practice and qualifications, and seek help with new or unfamiliar duties. A team member has the right to refuse inappropriate work assignments.
15. Evaluate sterile processing monitors for reasonable assurance of sterility. Know if an item was sterilized commercially, in the OR suite, or in the sterile processing department. Know how supplies are packaged and sterilized to open them correctly, to supervise their use by others, or to evaluate their level of quality and safety for the patient.
16. Be responsible for all work assignments. Look for ways to help others until all work is finished. Be willing to help others, to learn, and to do any task required within the limitations of the job description. The department as a whole will benefit.

17. *Be dependable, ethical, honest, and trustworthy.* Team members should have confidence in each other.

Productivity

Productivity and efficiency go hand in hand. Literally, productivity is directly related to what a person does and how he or she does it. But it is also the quantity and quality of work *(output)* in relation to the costs in terms of labor and time *(input)*. Labor costs can amount to as much as 60% of the OR budget. To be productive, perioperative nurses and surgical technologists should develop psychomotor skills, competencies, and mental capacities. This requires an accurate perception of the factors and conditions that affect the patient, surgeon, and other team members. Described as *situational awareness,* this concept means staying in touch with the environment and thinking ahead in preparing for and participating in the surgical procedure. Productivity is enhanced by ability to:

1. Organize work efficiently and effectively. Efficiency is important to keep to a minimum the length of time that a patient is anesthetized and that the anxious family is waiting.
2. Work rapidly with precision and dexterity. Learn to follow directions quickly and accurately, with attention to the smallest detail. Carelessness is unacceptable.
3. Adapt to changes or unexpected situations quickly, calmly, and efficiently. A change in diagnosis during the surgical procedure may require an altogether different setup and a different surgical approach from the one anticipated. Emergencies will arise. You should know *what* to do, but also *why* you should do it. Exercise good judgment, prioritize actions, and function competently under pressure.
4. Anticipate the needs of the surgeon and the team, and keep one step ahead. The surgeon becomes distracted if handed the wrong instrument or is made to wait for supplies. Be alert and try to read the surgeon's mind logically.
5. Maintain physical and emotional stamina. Situational awareness can be compromised by fatigue, poor physical health, and emotional distress. Be sensitive to the health and well-being of other team members.

Time and Motion Economy

Time is money; do not waste it. Know the policies and procedures, and efficiently follow them. Learn to do things right the first time and continue to do them that way; time is wasted in correcting errors. Motions should be productive.

Time Is Costly

Time is an important element in the OR. If time is wasted between surgical procedures, for example, the day's schedule is slowed down and later surgical procedures are delayed. Surgeons' time is wasted and they tend to come late, anticipating delays. The patients become anxious waiting for their surgical procedures and more uncomfortable during the prolonged period without fluids.

Poor managers of time tend to become less efficient and thus drift into poor work habits. *Common sense* is a great ally. Take time to stop and think. Is there a quicker, easier, or more efficient way of doing the job? Most work habits can be improved. Analyze them in a methodical manner.

Recognition that a problem exists is the first step toward solving a problem. Gather facts needed to support the desirability of adopting alternatives. Seek to develop more efficient and economical work methods.

Associations

Each patient, surgeon, and surgical procedure is unique, but all have commonalities. A logical thought process will simplify preparations of the OR for the patient and the surgeon. Supplies and equipment must be in readiness before they arrive. Developing a mental checklist can help you to make associations quickly of the requirements for a specific procedure according to surgical specialty and surgeon and for the individualized needs of the patient (Box 20-1).

Association is a great aid to memory and organization of work. The mention of one article brings to mind the others used with it. For instance, the scrub person knows a suture calls for a tissue forceps to the surgeon, needleholder to the assistant, then scissors.

Think of the order in which instruments and supplies are going to be needed, and *do first things first* (e.g., prepare sutures for closing deep tissue layers before skin sutures).

To be proficient, know the organization of work and the relative importance of factors in accomplishing it. For example, if, as the patient is being prepped, the surgeon requests stainless steel retention sutures for closure instead of the usual sutures, the circulator should realize there is plenty of time to get them after other duties are completed. He or she must tie the gowns, supervise the draping, adjust the Mayo stand and instrument table, focus the light, etc., to start the surgical procedure before getting the closing sutures. When getting steel sutures, association tells the circulator to also get wire scissors and bumpers or bridges.

Watch for and try to establish associations to increase efficiency. If surgeons must devote time and attention to details that the perioperative nurses and surgical technologists should know, they are distracted from their

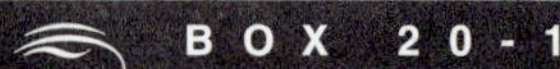

BOX 20-1

Basic Associations Facilitate Preparations for Each Surgical Procedure

All surgical procedures
Housekeeping: room cleaned
Furniture: present and arranged
Suction: connected and functional
Operating light and table: prepositioned and functional

Specific to scheduled procedure
Basic instrument set
Basic drape pack
Basin set
Skin preparation setup
Sterile supplies

Specific to surgical specialty
Electrosurgical unit
Laser
Microscope
Tourniquet
Endoscope
Drapes
Instruments
Sterile supplies
Fluoroscopy or x-ray control

Specific to surgeon
Gloves
Instruments
Sutures
Personal preferences/preference card

Specific to patient
Age
Body build
Allergies
Physical limitations/impairments
Autotransfusion/blood transfusion
X-ray films
Special considerations/plan of care

primary concerns. Time is wasted for all involved, including the patient.

Motion Economy

Wasted motion is not only time-consuming but also adds to physical fatigue. Fatigue is the result of body movement. Ten principles of motion economy can reduce fatigue from physical activity and improve your level of efficiency.

1. *Motions should be productive.* Once the steps in a procedure are learned, work to increase speed and psychomotor skill to perform them. Avoid rushed or disorganized motions. Make each movement purposeful. Work quietly and quickly. Work as fast as possible without sacrificing accuracy and technique for speed.

   The corollary to this principle is *a place for everything and everything in its place.* Keep an orderly work area to avoid fumbling and rehandling items. Arrange them properly and leave them there. This corollary is justification for standardization of procedures, such as a standardized instrument table setup and stocking of supplies in cabinets or on carts. If everything has a place and is in its place, supplies will be easily obtained by instinct when needed. A neat and orderly work area is one of the first requirements for productive motions. Consider the work flow so that minimal motions can be made to accomplish productive work.
2. *Motions should be simple.* Body movements should be confined to the lowest classification with which it is possible to perform work properly. Movements of the upper extremity are classified in five levels:
   a. Class 1 involves the fingers. The knuckle provides the pivot for motion for such tasks as fingering through a card file, turning a set screw on an instrument, and using a pair of scissors.
   b. Class 2 involves both the hand and fingers. The wrist is the pivot for motion as in passing instruments, counting sponges, and picking up or writing on an intraoperative record.
   c. Class 3 includes the forearm. Using the elbow as a pivot, more effort and time are expended in the third and succeeding classifications because the movements of any one class involve movements of all classes preceding it. It takes longer and more effort to turn the pages of a procedure book or a patient's chart than to thumb through a file of surgeon's preference cards. The elbow pivots to open a peel-down package, unfold drapes, and unwrap small supplies.
   d. Class 4 includes the upper arm. The shoulder pivot is used when opening a door, setting up the Mayo stand, and prepping a patient.
   e. Class 5 adds the torso. The trunk bends or stretches to lift a patient, take supplies from a low shelf or drawer, hang an IV bag, or count the sponges in a kick bucket.

   Upper extremity work should be arranged to reduce work to the lowest possible classification. Finger motion is the least fatiguing; shoulder motion is the most fatiguing. The scrub person should be positioned at the operating table so that elbow, wrist, and finger motions can be used. He or she should be positioned opposite the surgeon so that both can work with their elbows at their sides. This avoids prolonged shoulder motion for both of them.

It is quicker for the circulator to stretch to hang an IV bag than to take time to use finger action to loosen the set screw on an IV standard, lower it with shoulder movement, hang the bag with elbow action, and repeat the sequence in reverse. However, stretching is more fatiguing. Increasing fatigue causes slower motion as the day progresses. Maybe 30 seconds was saved with the first patient of the day, but what happens to the last patient of the day? Time is lost because energy wanes.

3. *Motions should be curved.* Motions should go along curved rather than straight paths whenever possible. A circular motion to clean the flat surfaces of furniture is less fatiguing than straight push-and-pull strokes.
4. *Motions should be symmetrical.* Motions should be rhythmic and smooth flowing, and, when possible, both hands should be used symmetrically. Damp cloths in both hands, going in opposing circles, will get flat surfaces cleaned faster and easier.
5. *Work should be within grasp range.* All work materials should be arranged so they are within grasp range to avoid changes in body position. Grasp range is within the radius from the pivot point of the elbow or shoulder, either horizontally or vertically. The minimum grasp range is within the radius of the arcs formed with only forearms extended, using the elbows as pivot points on the horizontal plane (Figure 20-9).

The optimum grasp range is within the area where the left-hand and the right-hand arcs overlap. This is the area in which two-handed work, such as putting a needle in a needleholder, can be done most conveniently.

The maximum grasp range is within the arcs formed from the shoulder pivots. The overlapping of these arcs is the maximum extent at which two-handed work can be done within reach without changing body position.

The Mayo stand should be placed over the operating table at a height and in a position within the minimum and optimum grasp range of the scrub person. It must not rest on the patient, but it can be lowered to an inch or two above. The instrument table should be positioned as close to the horizontal plane within maximum grasp range as possible. Instruments or supplies requiring two-handed work should be placed on the Mayo stand and the instrument table as close to the optimum grasp range as possible.

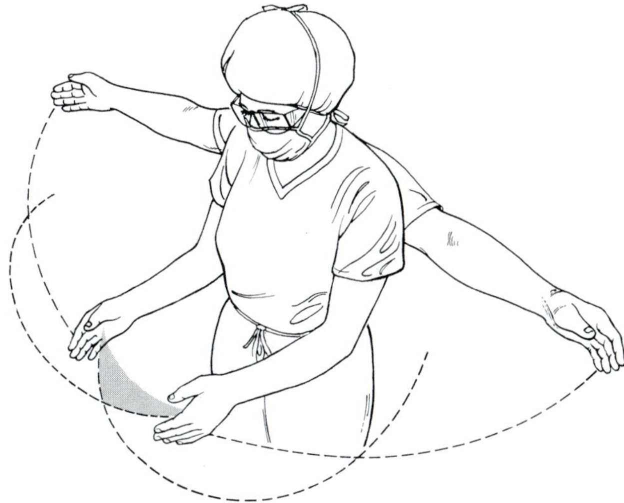

FIGURE 20-9 Grasp ranges. Minimum range is within radius of arcs formed with only forearms extended, using elbows as pivotal points. Optimum range is within area where arcs of hands overlap. Maximum range is within the arcs formed from shoulder pivots.

6. *Hands should be relieved of work.* Hands should be relieved of any work that can be done more advantageously by other parts of the body. Many electrical instruments have foot pedals to facilitate operation.
7. *Work materials should be prepositioned.* Supplies can be arranged for convenient use and minimal handling. Drapes are packaged in order of use so they do not need to be handled by the scrub person, except to move the stack to a corner of the instrument table, until ready to use. Instruments can be arranged in containers so that all of them do not need to be removed until needed.

Economize time and effort by placing items on the instrument table and Mayo stand in the order in which they will be used, and put them in their proper places without rearranging them. Arrange instruments on the Mayo stand in position to hand to the surgeon or assistant. In passing an instrument, place it in the surgeon's hand in the position in which it will be used so that readjustments will not be necessary (see Figure 14-11, p. 254). Grasp it with the thumb and the first two fingers, far enough away from the handle so that the surgeon can grasp it. Hand a needle in the needleholder the same way, supporting the suture so it does not drag, and with the needle pointing in direction in which the surgeon will start to use it. Hand thumb forceps so that the surgeon can grasp the handle; do the same with retractors.

8. *Gravity should be used.* Scrub sponges or brush dispensers operate on the principle that gravity should be used whenever possible. Cabinets for smaller packages in the sterile supply room can be vertical and divided into appropriate-size slots. These can be filled from the top and dispensed from the bottom of each slot. This is convenient, saves space, and ensures that older items are used first. Shelves for large, heavy packs can be made of rollers and slanted slightly to facilitate handling. Gravity-feed and drop-delivery installations eliminate or reduce motions. The quickest way to dispose of an object is to drop it. This may be the quickest way to break or contaminate it too, so the application of this principle requires good judgment.
9. *Supplies should be combined.* Items should serve two or more purposes whenever possible. Sterilizer indicator tape, for example, serves a dual purpose: to hold the package closed and to tell you if it has been exposed to a sterilization process. And only inches, not a yard, of tape accomplish the job.

   Disposable kits and trays are purchased, or sets are made up of reusable items so that all the supplies and materials needed for a procedure are combined into a single unit. This eliminates opening many separate packages.

   Some knife blade packets can be sterilized in the instrument tray with the knife handle. This eliminates a sterile transfer to the instrument table.

   Put instruments that are sterilized in sets of various sizes, such as expensive prostheses, on a small sterile table or at one side of the instrument table. When the surgeon decides which size is needed, remove it from the set without contaminating the others, thus making their cleanup and reprocessing easier.
10. *Worker should be at ease.* Tiring body motions or awkward or strained body posture should be avoided. A pleasant, quiet environment is less fatiguing, with fewer psychologic and physiologic adverse effects on team members, and enhances greater efficiency. See discussion of body mechanics and other factors that contribute to a comfortable working environment in Chapter 10, pp. 143-144.

Economical Use of Supplies and Equipment

As the cost of supplies increases, circulators and scrub persons should be conscious of ways to eliminate wasteful practices. For example, throw away disposable items only. Avoid throwing away reusable ones.

The OR suite is one of the most expensive departments of a hospital. Adequate instruments and supplies are necessary for patient care. Cost is not always the primary consideration. Beyond the point of safety, economy becomes a hazard. But supplies do not need to be used lavishly just because they are available. Remember the following principles.

"Just Enough Is Enough"

Varieties and numbers of instruments and supplies needed for each surgical procedure can be kept to a minimum. If the procedure book and surgeon's preference cards are kept up-to-date, articles no longer used are eliminated. Items to "have available" are not opened unnecessarily.

1. Pour just enough antiseptic solution for skin preparation according to the manufacturer's recommendation; it takes only a small amount. Do not unnecessarily open a bottle for a small amount if you know the remainder will not be used.
2. Follow procedures for draping to provide an adequate sterile field without wasting disposable draping material or opening launderable woven textiles unnecessarily.
3. Do not open another packet of sutures for that last stitch. Usually a few leftover pieces are long enough to complete the closure.
4. Suction tubing, syringes, hypodermic needles, drains, catheters, extra drapes, etc., are kept sterile. Supplies should be opened only as needed, not routinely "just in case" they may be needed.
5. Do not soak too much plaster when helping with cast applications. Keep just ahead of the surgeon. Watch to see when it appears the cast is almost finished. Ask if more is needed before soaking an extra one or two rolls of plaster.
6. Turn off lights when they are not needed.

Use Supplies and Equipment for Intended Use

1. Use operating table appliances according to manufacturer's instructions for positioning and stabilizing patients.
2. Nonsterile gloves are available for nonsterile procedures in which the use of gloves is for hand protection. Open sterile gloves for sterile procedures only.
3. Use fabrics only as needed and for their intended purpose. If water runs over onto the floor, do not soak it up with good material; use the wet-vacuum pickup or mop. But do not let it run over!
4. Do not use hemostats to clamp drapes or tubing; that ruins both the hemostat and the tubing. Use a

stopcock or special tubing clamp. Use a nonpiercing towel clip to secure drapes.

5. Give the assistant a needleholder for pulling needles through tissue for the surgeon. A hemostat can be ruined by using it for this purpose. A needle can be damaged.
6. Use wire scissors for wire, tissue scissors for tissue, dressing scissors for drains and dressings, and suture scissors to cut sutures.

Avoid Damage

Handle all supplies and equipment carefully to avoid damage and breakage.

1. Slip the patient's gown sleeve off before the IV transfusion is started preoperatively to avoid having to cut off a wet, soiled gown after the surgical procedure is completed.
2. Rotate sterile and older supplies so that items will not deteriorate or integrity of packaging will not be compromised.
3. Take special care to preserve the edges of sharp instruments.
4. Follow established procedures for the proper sterilization and care of instruments, electrical equipment, etc. If you are uncertain how to sterilize or care for any equipment, find out; do not ruin items by guessing. Items for ethylene oxide gas sterilization should be plainly tagged "for gas" to help avoid possibility of inadvertently putting them into the steam sterilizer.
5. Remove all tape from packages wrapped in woven fabrics. It will clog the washers in the laundry.
6. Do not handle adhesive with rubber gloves; it sticks to the gloves and tears them.
7. Check drapes to be certain instruments are not discarded in disposable drapes or sent to the laundry. At end of the surgical procedure, the scrub person should look for instruments, needles, and equipment before discarding drapes.
8. Take defective instruments and equipment out of use immediately. Report the defect or malfunction promptly for corrective action. Also report a surgeon's complaints about the function or quality of an instrument or equipment.
9. Adhere to routine preventive maintenance schedule for equipment.

Carelessness Can Cause Infection

Careless and accident-prone personnel are hazardous in the OR.

1. Avoid banging furniture against walls and doors. Chipped walls or doors can harbor microorganisms and interfere with effectiveness of housekeeping.
2. Avoid contamination of sterile supplies when opening sterile packages and transferring items to sterile field. If in doubt about sterility, discard the item.
3. Thoroughly clean and properly sterilize instruments. Dirty instruments corrode, do not function smoothly, and are a source of infection for the patient.
4. Thoroughly clean all reusable items before sterilizing. The risk of infection associated with reusable items is directly related to cleaning, processing, and handling them. If carelessness exists, many avenues for potential infection become a threat to everyone's welfare.
5. Dispose of sharps safely so that housekeeping personnel or other staff members do not accidentally stick themselves or get cut. Hepatitis and HIV can be contracted from a penetrating injury with contaminated needle or knife blade.

The circulator and scrub person coordinate their efforts to achieve a favorable outcome so that the patient will be free of infection following surgical intervention.

Bibliography

Abbott CA: Intraoperative nursing activities performed by surgical technologists, *AORN J* 60(3):382-393, 1994.

Allen GJ: Reducing waste and costs in the operating room, *Surg Technol* 26(12):15-17, 25, 1994.

Cowlard DM: Practical innovations: annotated tray lists save time, decrease errors, *AORN J* 55(1):286-292, 1992.

Fox V: Clinical issues: passing surgical instruments, sharps without injury, *AORN J* 55(1):264-266, 1992.

Meeker MH, Rothrock JC: *Alexander's care of the patient in surgery*, ed 10, St Louis, 1995, Mosby.

Murphy EK: OR nursing law: counts, documentation revisited, *AORN J* 54(4):875-878, 1991.

Murphy EK: OR nursing law: documentation, counts cause concern, *AORN J* 53(2):491-494, 1991.

Murphy EK: OR nursing law: documenting potential for injury; malpractice; absent anesthesia providers; retained sponges; first assistant liability for counts, *AORN J* 58(5):1037-1039, 1993.

Murphy EK: OR nursing law: nurses' liability for inaccurate counts, *AORN J* 51(4):1067-1069, 1990.

Murphy EK: OR nursing law: technician starting lines; counts when a patient dies; count documentation, *AORN J* 56(4):747-748, 1992.

O'Neale M: Clinical issues: sterile processing; instrument safety; instrument counts; aseptic technique, *AORN J* 53(1):146-149, 1991.

O'Neale M: Clinical issues: used sponge exposure; processing peel packages; flash sterilization; protective arm attire; beverages in the OR, *AORN J* 59(2):503-506, 1994.

Phippen ML, Applegeet C: Clinical issues: unlicensed assistive personnel in the perioperative setting, *AORN J* 60(3):455-458, 1994.

Ponder KS: The RN circulator, *AORN J* 60(3):459-462, 1994.

Proposed recommended practices for sponge, sharp, and instrument counts, *AORN J* 61(2):404-411, 1995.

Rappaport W, Haynes K: The retained surgical sponge following intra-abdominal surgery, *Arch Surg* 125(3):405-407, 1990.

Recommended practices: aseptic technique, *AORN J* 54(4):819-824, 1991.

Recommended practices: sanitation in the surgical practice setting, *AORN J* 56(6):1089-1095, 1992.

Schram CA: Forensic medicine, *AORN J* 53(3):669-692, 1991.

Smith CD: Clinical issues: instrument use; contaminated glove removal; used sponge display; foot pedal operation; instrument disassembly for processing, *AORN J* 59(3):687-690, 1994.

Zuffoletto JM: OR nursing law: nurses' vs surgeons' responsibility for sponge counts, *AORN J*, 57(6):1457-1458, 1993.

CHAPTER 21

Positioning the Patient

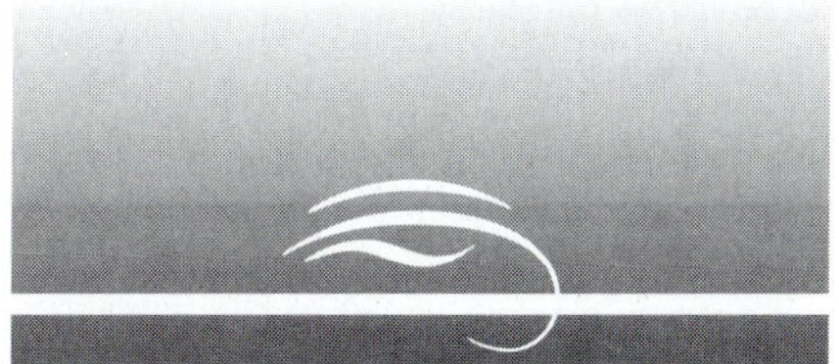

PRELIMINARY CONSIDERATIONS

Proper positioning for a surgical procedure is a facet of patient care that is as important to patient outcome as adequate preoperative preparation and safe anesthesia. It requires knowledge of anatomy and *application of physiologic principles,* as well as familiarity with the necessary equipment. Safety is a prime consideration.

Patient position is determined by the procedure to be performed, with consideration of the surgeon's choice of surgical approach and of anesthetic administration technique. Factors such as age, height, weight, cardiopulmonary status, and preexisting diseases (e.g., arthritis) also influence position and should be incorporated into the plan of care. Preoperatively, the patient should be assessed for alteration in skin integrity, joint mobility, and presence of joint or vascular prosthesis. Expected outcome is that the patient will not be harmed by positioning for surgical procedure. See Chapter 42 for positioning and restraining pediatric patients.

Responsibility

Choice of position for surgical procedure is made by the surgeon in consultation with the anesthesiologist, and adjustments are made as necessary for anesthesia. Responsibility for placing the patient in surgical position may be that of the circulator, with guidance, approval, and sometimes assistance of the anesthesiologist and the surgeon. In essence, it is a shared responsibility among all team members. In cases of complex positioning or obese, heavy patients, the plan of care will include the need for additional help in lifting and/or positioning the patient.

Time

The patient is usually supine, on his or her back face up, after transfer from the stretcher to the operating table. The patient may be anesthetized in this position and then positioned for the surgical procedure or may be positioned and then anesthetized. Factors influencing the time at which the patient is positioned are site of surgical procedure, age and size of patient, anesthetic administration technique, and pain on moving if the patient is conscious. The patient is not positioned or moved until the anesthesiologist indicates it is safe to do so.

Preparations for Positioning

Before the patient is brought into the operating room (OR), the circulator should:

1. Review the proposed position by referring to the procedure book and the surgeon's preference card.
2. Ask for assistance if unsure how to position the patient.
3. Consult the surgeon as soon as he or she arrives if not sure which position is to be used.
4. Check the working parts of the operating table before bringing the patient into the room.

5. Assemble all attachments and protective pads anticipated for the surgical procedure.
6. Test positioning devices for patient safety. Check for cleanliness.
7. Review plan of care for unique needs of patient.

Safety Measures

Safety measures must be observed while transferring, moving, and positioning patients. These include:

1. Patient must be properly identified before transfer to the operating table and the surgical site affirmed.
2. Operating table and transport vehicle must be securely locked in position, with the mattress stabilized during transfer to and from table.
3. Two persons should assist an awake patient with the transfer by positioning themselves on each side of the patient's transfer path. The person on the side of the transport stretcher assists the patient to move toward the operating table. The person on the opposite side prevents the patient from falling over the edge of the table. Take care not to allow the patient's gown or blanket to become lodged between the two surfaces.
4. Adequate assistance in *lifting* unconscious, obese, or weak patients is necessary to prevent injury. A minimum of four persons is recommended. Transfer devices and lifters may be used. The patient is moved on the count of three. The anesthesiologist gives the signal. Sliding or pulling the patient may cause dermal abrasion or injury to soft tissues.
5. Anesthesiologist guards the anesthetized patient's head at all times and supports it during movement. The head should be kept in neutral axis and turned as little as possible to maintain airway and cerebral circulation.
6. Physician assumes responsibility for protecting an unsplinted fracture during movement.
7. Anesthetized patient is not moved without permission of the anesthesiologist.
8. Anesthetized patient must be moved *slowly* and gently to allow the circulatory system to adjust and to control body during movement.
9. No body part should extend beyond the edges of the table or contact metal parts or unpadded surfaces.
10. Body exposure should be minimal to prevent hypothermia and to preserve dignity.
11. Movement and position should not obstruct or dislodge catheters, intravenous (IV) infusion tubing, and monitors.
12. Armboard must be guarded to avoid hyperextending the arm or dislodging the infusion needle.
13. When the patient is supine (on the back), ankles and legs must not be crossed. This would create occlusive pressure on blood vessels and nerves.
14. When the patient is prone (on the abdomen), the thorax must be relieved of pressure to facilitate chest expansion with respiration.
15. When patient is lateral (lies on side), a pillow must be placed lengthwise between legs to prevent pressure on bony prominences, blood vessels, and nerves.
16. Patient must be protected from crush injury at flex points during articulation of the table.
17. When the operating table is elevated, feet and protuberant parts must be protected from compression by overbed tables, Mayo stands, and frames. Adequate clearance of 2 to 3 inches is maintained.

ANATOMIC AND PHYSIOLOGIC CONSIDERATIONS

Tolerance of the stresses of the surgical procedure depends greatly on the normality of functioning of vital systems. The patient's physical condition must be considered. Proper body alignment is important. Criteria must be met for physiologic positioning to prevent injury from pressure, obstruction, or stretching.

Respiratory Considerations

Unhindered diaphragmatic movement and a patent airway are essential to maintain respiratory function, to prevent hypoxia, and to facilitate induction by inhalation. Chest excursion is a concern because respiration expands the chest anteriorly. Some positions limit the amount of mechanical motion of the chest for respiration. Some hypoxia is always present in a horizontal position. Tidal volume, the functional residual capacity of air moved by a single breath, is reduced by as much as a third when patient lies down. Therefore there should be no constriction about the neck or chest. Patients' arms should be at their sides, on armboards, or otherwise supported, not crossed on the chest. Patients who are obese, who smoke, or have pulmonary disease have additional respiratory compromise.

Circulatory Considerations

Adequate circulation is necessary to maintain blood pressure, to perfuse tissues with oxygen, to facilitate venous return and prevent thrombus formation, and to prevent circulatory disturbances. Occlusion and pressure on peripheral blood vessels must be avoided. Body support and restraining straps must not be fastened too tightly. Anesthetic agents alter normal body circulatory mechanisms. Some drugs cause constriction or dilation of blood vessels, which is further complicated by positioning.

Peripheral Nerve Considerations

Prolonged pressure on or stretching of peripheral nerves can result in injuries ranging from sensory and motor loss to paralysis. Extremities, as well as the body, must be well supported at all times. Appliances, restraints, and equipment in contact with skin must be well padded. Most frequent sites of injury are divisions of the brachial plexus and the ulnar, radial, peroneal, and facial nerves. Axons may be stretched or disrupted. Extremes of position of the head and arm easily cause injury to the brachial plexus. The ulnar, radial, and peroneal nerves may be compressed against bone, stirrups, or operating table if the patient is improperly positioned. Femoral nerve injury may be caused by retractors during pelvic procedures. Sciatic nerve injury may be caused by tissue retraction or manipulation during hip surgery. Facial nerve injury may result from too vigorous a manual effort to elevate the mandible to maintain airway or from too tight a head strap.

Musculoskeletal Considerations

Strain on muscles results in injury and/or needless postoperative discomfort. An anesthetized patient lacks protective muscle tone. If the head is extended for a prolonged time, the patient may suffer more pain from a resulting stiff neck than from the surgical wound. Proper body alignment must be maintained.

Soft Tissue Considerations

Body weight is distributed unevenly when the patient lies on the operating table. Weight concentrated over bony prominences can cause skin pressure ulcers. These areas must be protected from constant external pressure against hard surfaces, particularly in thin or underweight patients. Also, tissue subjected to prolonged mechanical pressure, such as a fold in skin under an obese patient, will not be perfused adequately. Debilitated, poorly nourished, and diabetic patients are at high risk for decubitus ulcers. Wrinkled sheets and edges of a positioning or other device under the patient can cause pressure on the skin. Pressure injuries are more common after surgical procedures that last 2 hours or longer. Reposition the head and other body parts, if possible, during lengthy procedures.

Accessibility of Surgical Site

Surgical procedure determines the position in which the patient is placed. The surgeon must have adequate exposure to minimize trauma and operating time.

Accessibility for Anesthetic Administration

The anesthesiologist must be able to attach monitoring electrodes, administer anesthesia, observe its effects, and maintain IV access.

Individual Positioning Considerations

If a patient is extremely obese (e.g., with torso occupying the table width), his or her arms may be placed on armboards. Patients with arthritis deformans may need special individualized care because of limited range of motion in their joints. A cardiac patient may experience dyspnea when lying flat.

EQUIPMENT FOR POSITIONING

Operating Table

Many different tables with suitable attachments are in use. Practice is necessary to master adjustments. Tables are versatile and adaptable to a number of diversified positions for all surgical specialties. However, orthopaedic, urologic, and fluoroscopic tables are used frequently for specialized procedures. Consult the manufacturer's recommendations for operation of each model of table.

Most tables consist of a rectangular metal top that rests on an electric or hydraulic lift base. Some models have interchangeable tops for the various specialties. The table top is divided into three or more hinged sections. Basically, these are the head, body, and leg sections. Each can be manipulated, flexed, or extended to the desired position. This procedure is called *breaking the table.* The joints are referred to as *breaks.* Some tables have a metal crossbar or body elevator between the two upper sections that may be raised to elevate a gallbladder or kidney. The head section is removable, permitting insertion of special headrests for cranial procedures. An extension may be inserted at the foot of the table to accommodate an exceptionally tall patient. An x-ray penetrable tunnel top extending the length of the table permits the insertion of an x-ray cassette holder at any area. A self-adhering, sectional, conductive rubber mattress covers the table top. The mattress is at least 3 inches (8 cm) thick.

Standard operating tables have posturing controls for manipulating the table into desired positions. Some tables are electrically controlled, either by remote hand or foot control switches or a lever-operated electrohydraulic system; movement of others is manual. By setting the selector control on *back, side, foot,* or *flex,* the desired section(s) of the table top can be articulated. By activating other selector controls, the table top may be tilted laterally from side to side and raised or lowered in its entirety. A tiltometer indicates the degree of tilt between horizontal and vertical. All operating tables have a brake or floor lock for stabilization in all positions.

Special Equipment and Table Attachments

Equipment used in positioning is designed to stabilize the patient in the desired position, thus permitting optimal exposure of the surgical site. All devices must be clean, free of sharp edges, and padded to prevent trauma or abrasion. Each operating table has attachments for specific purposes. Many positioning devices to protect pressure points and joints are commercially available. If reusable, they must be washable; some may be sterilized between uses.

Safety Belt (Knee Strap)

A sturdy, *wide* strap of durable material, such as nylon webbing or conductive rubber, is placed over the thighs, above the knees, and around the table top and fastened to restrain leg movement. Some straps are attached at each side of the table and fastened together at the center. This belt must be secure but not so tight as to impair circulation. The circulator should be able to pass a finger between the strap and the patient. It is used during the surgical procedure except for certain positions (e.g., lithotomy). Placement depends on body position. Padding, such as a folded blanket, should be placed between the skin and the belt to prevent injury to underlying tissue. The strap should be placed over, not under, the blanket on the patient for easy visualization.

Anesthesia Screen

A metal bar attaches to the head of the table and holds the drapes from the patient's face, separating the nonsterile from the sterile area at the head end of the operating table. It is adjustable, allowing rotation or angling. It is placed after induction and positioning of patient.

Lift Sheet (Draw Sheet)

A double-layer sheet of broad, heavy fabric, stitched vertically through the middle, is placed horizontally across the top of a clean sheet on the operating table. A smooth, folded bedsheet also may be used for this purpose. After the patient is transferred, the arms are enclosed in lower flaps with the hands placed palms down with fingers extended on the mattress or turned inward toward the body. Upper flaps are brought down over the arms and tucked under the patient's sides. Avoid tucking the sheet under the sides of the mattress because the combined weight of the mattress and the patient's torso may impair circulation. The full lengths of the arms are supported at the patient's side, protected from injury, and secured. The patient should be told this is to support the arms when he or she is asleep and relaxed. The word "restraint" is avoided. At the end of the surgical procedure, this may be used to lift the patient from the operating table.

Armboard

An armboard is used to support arm(s) when IV fluids are infused; arm or hand is the site of the surgical procedure; arm at the side would interfere with access to the surgical area; space is inadequate for the arm on the table beside the body, as with an obese patient; or the arm requires support, as in lateral position. The armboard is padded to a height level with the operating table. The patient's arm is placed palm up, except when patient is in prone position, to prevent ulnar nerve pressure and abnormal shoulder rotation. The armboard has adjustable angles, but *the arm is never abducted beyond an angle of 90 degrees from shoulder.* A self-locking type of armboard is safest to prevent displacement.

Double Armboard Both arms are supported with one directly above the other in lateral position. This is sometimes called an *airplane support* or *overbed arm support.* Both levels must be padded.

Wrist or Arm Strap

Narrow straps, at least 1½ inches (3.8 cm) wide, placed around the wrists, secure hands and arms to the armboard or to the table at the patient's side. The hands must never be placed under the body because compression results. They must be secured, but without pressure or tourniquet effect from the strap.

Upper Extremity Table

For a surgical procedure on an arm or hand, an adjustable extremity table may be used in lieu of an armboard. Sometimes this attachment is referred to as a *hand table.* It is slipped under the mattress at one end. The other end is supported by a metal leg. Some models attach directly to the operating table and require no additional floor support. A solution drain pan may fit into some tables. After skin preparation or irrigation, the pan is removed and the top panel is reinserted. A firm foam rubber pad is placed on the table and covered to receive the arm, which is then draped. The table provides a large firm surface for the surgical procedure. The surgeon and sterile team usually sit around the table.

Shoulder Bridge (Thyroid Elevator)

A metal bar is slipped onto the table under the mattress between the head and body sections by temporarily removing the head section. This bridge can be raised to hyperextend the shoulder or thyroid area for surgical accessibility.

Shoulder Braces or Supports

Adjustable, well-padded concave metal supports are used to prevent the patient from slipping when the head of table is tilted down, as in Trendelenburg's position. Braces should be placed equidistant from the head of the table, with a ½ inch (13 mm) space between shoulders and braces to eliminate pressure against the shoulders. The braces are placed over the acromion processes, not over muscles and soft tissues near the neck. To avoid nerve compression a shoulder brace is not used when the arm is extended on an armboard. Ankle straps may be used instead to stabilize the patient.

Body Rests or Braces

A metal brace with a foam rubber pad covered with conductive rubber is placed in metal clamps on the side of the table and slipped in from the table edge against the body at various points to stabilize it in lateral position.

Kidney Rests

Concave metal pieces with grooved notches at the base are placed under the mattress on the body elevator part of the table. They are slipped in from the table edge snugly against the body for stability in the kidney position. Be careful that the upper edge of the rest does not press too tightly against the body, even though padded. Some tables have kidney rests built in. They are raised and lowered electrically or by a hand crank.

Body (Hip) Restraint Strap

A wide belt with center portion padded to protect the skin is placed over the patient's hips and secured by hooks to the sides of the table. This strap helps hold the patient securely in the lateral position.

Hemorrhoid Strap

Made of a piece of 3-inch (7.5 cm) adhesive 6 inches (15 cm) in length with a buckle and canvas strap on one end, a hemorrhoid strap is placed on each buttock, 4 inches (10 cm) lateral to the surgical site, to separate the buttocks for anal procedures. Each strap is fastened to the table frame at the side with the patient in Kraske position.

Adjustable Arch Bar

The adjustable arch bar consists of two padded rolls mounted on a frame. The rolls extend from shoulders to knees. The patient is placed on the abdomen on this arch. The degree of flexion desired for thoracic or lumbar vertebral procedures is achieved by adjusting the height of the arch by means of a lever. Other types of frames are available.

Stirrups

Metal stirrup posts are placed in holders, one on each side of the table to support the legs and feet in lithotomy position. The feet are supported by canvas or fabric loops, thus suspending the legs at a right angle to the feet. These are sometimes called *candy cane* or *sling stirrups.*

During extensive surgery, special leg holders supporting the lower legs and feet may be used. Metal or high-impact plastic knee-crutch stirrups with adjustments for knee flexion and extension are available. Even if well-padded, these stirrups may create some pressure on the back of the knees and lower extremity, jeopardizing the popliteal vessel and nerve.

Metal Footboard

The footboard can be left flat as a horizontal extension of the table or raised perpendicular to the table to support the feet, with the soles resting securely against it. It must be padded for reverse Trendelenburg's position.

Headrests

Padded headrests attach to the table to support and expose the occiput and cervical vertebrae. They are used with supine, prone, sitting, or lateral positions. The head must be held securely but without pressure that could cause blindness, for example.

Accessories

Various sizes and shapes of pads, pillows, and bead bags (often called bean bags) that fit anatomic structures are used to protect, support, or immobilize body parts. Foam rubber, polymer pads, silicone gel pads, bead bags, and any other accessories are covered with washable materials unless they are designed for single-patient use.

Donut, a ring-shaped foam rubber or silicone gel pad, or a bead bag, may be used for procedures on the head or face to keep the surgical area in a horizontal plane. Donuts also are used to protect pressure points, such as the ear, knee, or elbow.

Protectors made of foam rubber, polymers, silicone gel, or other material may be used to protect joints from pressure. A hard plastic shell with a soft liner (sometimes referred to as a sled or toboggan) is commercially available for the elbow, for example. Many other types of protectors are available.

Bolsters are used to elevate a specific part of the body (e.g., to hyperextend the spine for laminectomy). Solid rolls of cloth or firm foam under each side of the patient's chest raise it off the table to facilitate respiration. These are called *chest rolls.* Commercially available bolsters and elevating pads are commonly used. Check the manufacturer's literature for latex content. The patient may have a latex sensitivity.

Pressure Mattress

To minimize pressure on bony prominences, peripheral blood vessels, and nerves during prolonged surgical procedures (more than 2 hours), an alternating pressure mattress is put over the mattress on the operating table before the patient arrives. This may be a positive-pressure air mattress, a circulating water thermal mattress, a foam rubber mattress with indentations similar in configuration to an egg crate, a gel pad, or a dry polymer pad. Unless designed to be placed next to patient's skin, thermal blankets used to induce hypothermia or hyperthermia and pressure mattresses should be covered with an absorbent sheet or thin pad. Folds and creases in covering should be avoided to prevent pressure indentations in the skin. Follow manufacturer's instructions for use of these devices.

Surgical Positioning System

A convenient, efficient, comfortable means of patient positioning is available that eliminates sandbags, bolsters, and adhesive tape. Soft pads filled with tiny plastic beads are placed under or around the body part to be supported. Suction is attached to the pad and, as air is withdrawn, the pad becomes firm. During air evacuation, the circulator and assistant mold the pad to the body area with their hands. The suction is disconnected. With a vacuum inside pad, the surrounding atmospheric pressure presses the beads together and friction between them prevents their moving, creating a solid mass that keeps its molded shape. Various sizes and shapes of pads provide firm, yet pressure-point relieving support. To change the patient's position during the surgical procedure, the valve on the pad is squeezed until the pad is slightly soft. The patient is repositioned, and suction is applied to remold the pad.

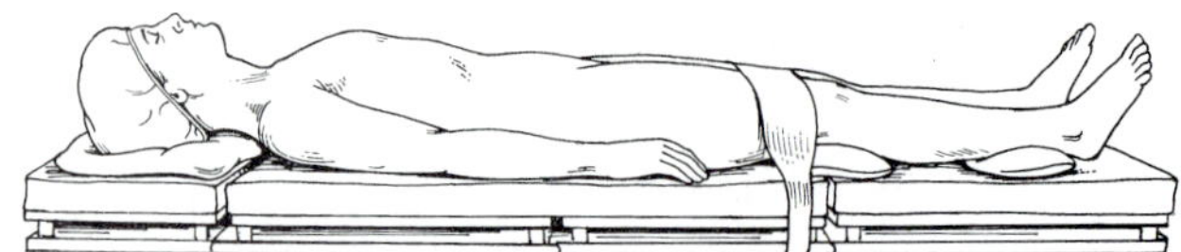

FIGURE 21-1 Supine position. Patient lies straight on back, face upward, with arms at sides, legs extended parallel and uncrossed, feet slightly separated. Strap is placed above knees. Head is in line with spine. Note small pillow under ankles to protect heels from pressure.

SURGICAL POSITIONS

Many positions are used for surgical procedures. Only the most commonly employed ones are discussed here. If IV fluids will be infused in the arm during the surgical procedure, the arm will be on an armboard. This fact is assumed in the following discussion because IV fluids are usually given. If electrosurgery will be used, the inactive dispersive electrode should be placed after the patient is in position for the surgical procedure.

Supine (Dorsal) Position

Figure 21-1 shows the patient in the supine position. This is the most natural position for the body at rest. The patient lies flat on the back with the arms secured at the sides with the lift sheet or wrist strap, palms down or along side of body. The elbows may be protected with plastic shells. The legs are straight and parallel, in line with the head and spine. The hips are parallel with the spine. The safety belt is placed across the thighs 2 inches above the knees. Small pillows may be placed under the head and lumbar curvature. The heels must be protected from pressure on the table by a pillow, ankle roll, or donut. The feet must not be in prolonged plantar flexion. The soles may be supported by a pillow or padded footboard to prevent footdrop. This position is used for procedures on the anterior surface of the body such as abdominal, abdominothoracic, and some lower extremity procedures. Modifications of supine position are used for specific body areas:

1. For procedures on *face* or *neck.* The neck may be slightly hyperextended by lowering the head section of the table or by placing a narrow pad between the scapulae. With the patient in supine position, the head may be supported in a headrest or donut and/or turned toward the unaffected side. The eyes must be protected from injury or irritating solutions. They should be kept closed with eye pads taped in place during skin preparation and surgical procedure. They should be inspected at the end of the surgical procedure.
2. For *shoulder* or *anterolateral* procedures. With the patient in supine position, a small sandbag, roll, or pad is placed under the affected side to elevate the shoulder off the table for exposure. The length of body must be stabilized to prevent rolling or twisting of the spine. Hips and shoulders should be kept in a plane. The operating table can also be tilted laterally to elevate the part.
3. *Dorsal recumbent.* For some *vaginal* or *perineal* procedures, the patient is in supine position except that the knees are flexed and thighs externally rotated. Soles of the feet rest on the table. Pillows may be placed under the knees if needed for support.
4. *Modified recumbent (frog legged).* For some surgical procedures in region of the *groin* or *lower extremity,* the patient is in supine position except that the knees are *slightly* flexed with a pillow beneath each (Figure 21-2). The thighs are externally rotated.
5. *Arm extension.* For *breast, axillary, upper extremity,* or *hand* surgery, the patient is in supine position with arm on the affected side on an armboard or upper extremity table extension that locks into position at right angle to the body. The affected side of body must be close to the table edge for access to the surgical area. If the axilla is involved, the arm is even with the lower edge of the armboard for accessibility. Hyperextension of the arm must be avoided to prevent neural or vascular injury, such as brachial plexus injury or occlusion of the axillary artery. The armboard must be well padded.

Trendelenburg's Position

The patient lies on the back in supine position with knees over the lower break of the table (Figure 21-3).

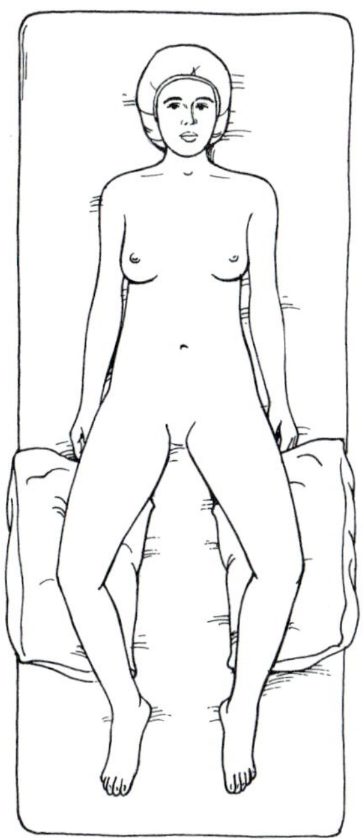

FIGURE 21-2 Modified recumbent position. Patient lies on back with arms at sides. Knees are slightly flexed, with pillow under each. Thighs are externally rotated.

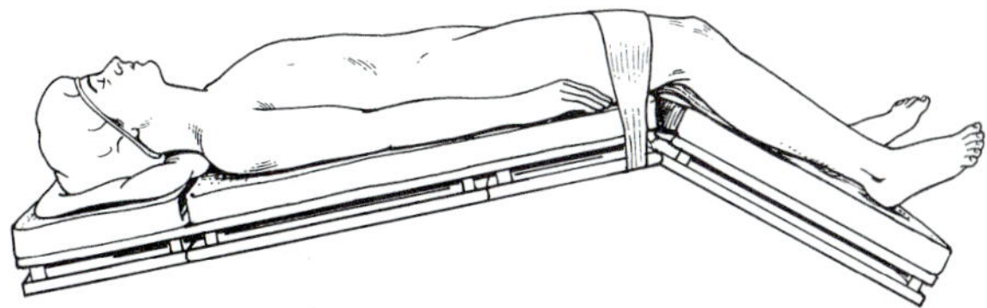

FIGURE 21-3 Trendelenburg's position. Note knees are over lower break in table, knee strap is above knees.

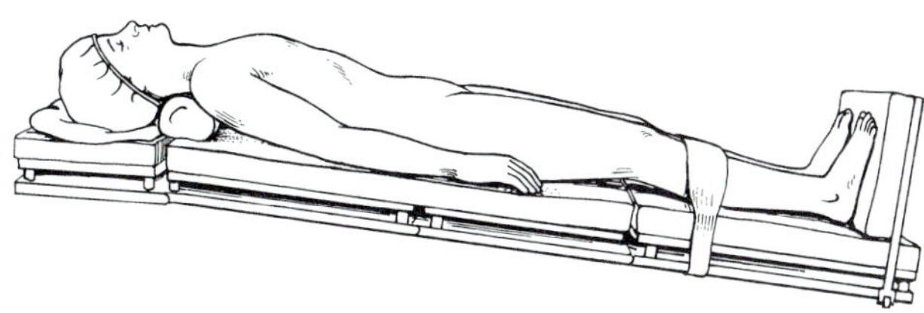

FIGURE 21-4 Reverse Trendelenburg's position. Patient lies on back. Footboard is padded and raised. Entire table is tilted so head is higher than feet. Strap is below knees.

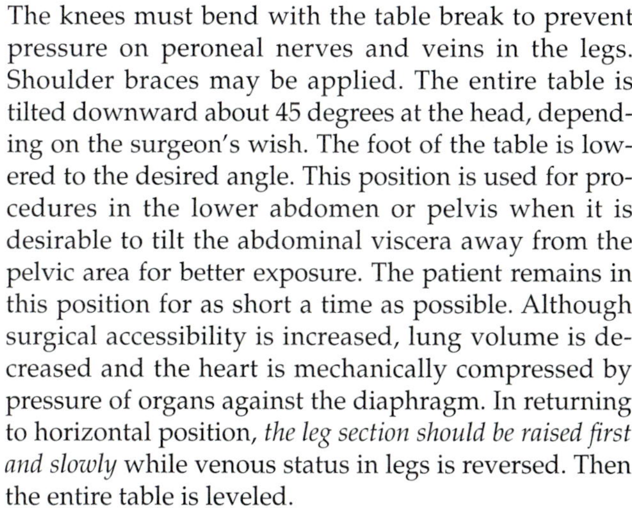

The knees must bend with the table break to prevent pressure on peroneal nerves and veins in the legs. Shoulder braces may be applied. The entire table is tilted downward about 45 degrees at the head, depending on the surgeon's wish. The foot of the table is lowered to the desired angle. This position is used for procedures in the lower abdomen or pelvis when it is desirable to tilt the abdominal viscera away from the pelvic area for better exposure. The patient remains in this position for as short a time as possible. Although surgical accessibility is increased, lung volume is decreased and the heart is mechanically compressed by pressure of organs against the diaphragm. In returning to horizontal position, *the leg section should be raised first and slowly* while venous status in legs is reversed. Then the entire table is leveled.

A modification of position may be used for patients in hypovolemic shock. Many anesthesiologists prefer to keep the trunk level and to elevate the legs by raising the lower part of the table at the break under the hips. Others prefer to tilt the entire table head-downward. Either position reduces venous stasis in the lower extremities.

Reverse Trendelenburg's Position

The patient lies on the back in supine position (Figure 21-4). The mattress is adjusted so the surgical area is over the elevator bridge on the table. The entire table is tilted so the head is higher than the feet. A padded footboard is used to prevent sliding toward the tilt. The position is used for thyroidectomy to facilitate breathing and to decrease blood supply to surgical site (blood will pool caudally). It is used also for gallbladder or biliary tract procedures to allow abdominal viscera to fall away from the epigastrium, giving access to upper abdomen. Small pillows may be placed under the knees and the lumbar curvature. A small pillow or donut may stabilize the head. If the elevator bridge is not used, the surgical area may be hyperextended by a pad.

Fowler's Position

The patient lies on the back with the buttocks at the flex in the table and knees over the lower break. The foot of the table is lowered slightly, flexing the knees. The body section is raised 45 degrees, thereby becoming the back rest. Arms may rest on armboards parallel to table or on a large soft pillow on the lap. The safety belt is secured 2 inches above the knees. The entire table is tilted slightly head-end downward to prevent the patient slipping caudad. Feet should rest on the padded footboard to prevent footdrop. For cranial procedures, the head is supported in a headrest. The table looks like a modified armchair in this position. This may be used for shoulder, nasopharyngeal, facial, and breast reconstruction procedures.

Sitting Position

The patient is placed in Fowler's position except that the torso is in an upright position. Shoulders and torso should be supported with body straps but not so tightly as to impede respiration and circulation. Pressure points must be padded, especially ischial tuberosities, to reduce risk of sciatic nerve damage. The flexed arms rest on a large pillow on the lap or on a pillow on an adjustable table in front of the patient. The head is seated forward in a cranial headrest for neurosurgical procedures. Air embolism is a potential complication. Antiembolic stockings or pneumatic counterpressure devices are used to counteract postural hypotension (see Chapter 23, pp. 473-474). This position is used for some otorhinologic and neurosurgical procedures.

Lithotomy Position

Nonsterile cotton boots or leggings may be put on the patient's legs before transfer to the operating table for perineal, vaginal, endourologic, or rectal procedures. Patient's buttocks rest along the break between the body and leg sections of the table. So that the patient's legs do not extend over the foot of the table, a padded metal footboard is used as a table extension. Stirrups are secured in holders on each side of the table at the level of the patient's upper thighs. They must be adjusted at equal height on both sides and at appropriate height for the length of the patient's legs to maintain symmetry when the patient is positioned (Figure 21-5). After the patient is anesthetized, *the legs are raised simultaneously by two persons.* Each grasps the sole of a foot in one hand and supports the calf at the knee area with the other. Knees are flexed and legs are *inside* the posts of the stirrups. The feet are then placed in canvas slings of the stirrups at a 90-degree angle to the abdomen. One loop of canvas encircles the sole; the other loop goes around the ankle. Simultaneous movement is essential as knees are flexed to avoid straining the lower back. If the legs are properly placed, undue abduction and external rotation are avoided. The lower leg or ankle must not touch the metal stirrup. Padding is placed as necessary. If the legs are put in stirrups before induction, the patient can identify discomfort and pressure on the back and/or legs.

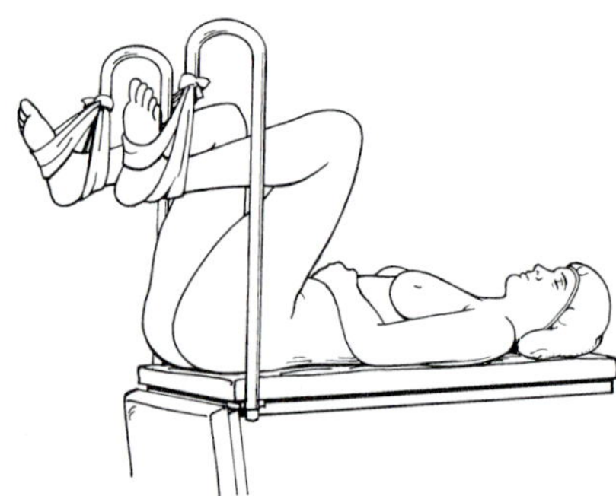

FIGURE 21-5 Lithotomy position. Patient is on back with foot section of table lowered to right angle with body on table. Knees are flexed and legs are on inside of metal posts with feet supported by canvas straps. Note that buttocks are even with table edge.

The lower section of mattress is removed and the leg section of the table lowered. The mattress is pulled down on the table, as necessary, until *the buttocks are even with the table edge.* They must not extend beyond the edge, causing strain on lumbosacral muscles and ligaments as body weight rests on the sacrum.

Arms may be placed on armboards or loosely cradled over the lower abdomen and secured by the lower end of the blanket. Arms must not rest on the chest and impede respiration. Lung compliance is decreased by pressure of the thighs on the abdomen, which hinders descent of the diaphragm. The hands should *not* extend along the table where they could be injured in the break during manipulation of the table or movement of the patient. Hands have been crushed in the break as the leg section of table was raised at the conclusion of a surgical procedure.

Antiembolic stockings may be worn or legs may be wrapped in elastic bandages before the surgical procedure to prevent formation of thrombi or emboli. Blood pools in the lumbar region of the torso, especially during prolonged surgical procedures. Distal pulses, skin color, and evidence of edema in legs should be checked during long procedures. Nerve damage or compartment syndrome can occur in the lithotomy position from direct pressure and/or ischemia of muscles that compromises viability of tissues.

At the conclusion of the surgical procedure, raise the leg section of the table and replace the lower section of mattress. Legs must be removed *simultaneously* from the stirrups and lowered *slowly* to prevent hypotension as blood reenters the legs and leaves the torso. As they are lifted from stirrups, the legs are fully extended and brought together to prevent wide abduction of the thighs. The safety belt should be reapplied over the thighs during the patient's emergence from anesthesia.

Prone Position

The patient is anesthetized and intubated in the supine position, usually on the transport stretcher. When the anesthesiologist gives permission, the patient is slowly and cautiously turned onto the abdomen on the operating table by a team of at least four persons to maintain the patient's body alignment. The body is rotated like rolling a log. Prone position is used for all procedures with a dorsal or posterior approach (Figure 21-6).

Chest rolls or bolsters under the axillae and along the sides of the chest from clavicles to iliac crests raise the weight of the body from the abdomen and thorax. Weight of the abdomen will fall away from the diaphragm and keep pressure off the vena cava and abdominal aorta. This facilitates respiration, although the position reduces vital capacity and cardiac index. To ensure cardiac filling and to reduce hypotension, venous return from the femoral veins and inferior vena cava

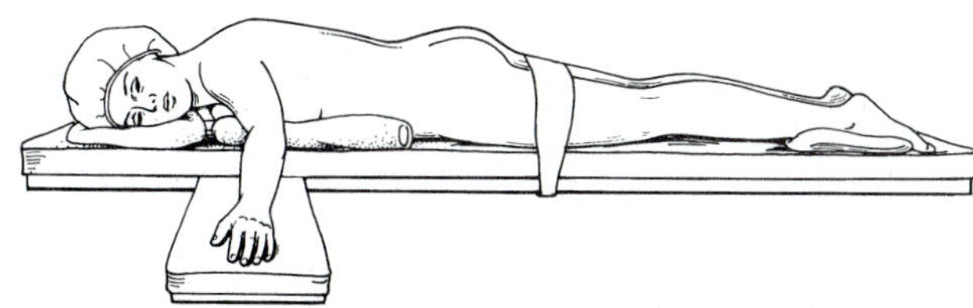

FIGURE 21-6 Prone position. Patient lies on abdomen. Chest rolls under axillae and sides of chest to iliac crests raise body weight from chest to facilitate respiration; pillow under feet protects toes. Patient is anesthetized in supine position before being turned into prone position.

must be uninterrupted. Female breasts should be moved laterally to reduce pressure on them. Male genitalia must be free from pressure.

The arms may lie supported along the sides of the body, with palms up or inward toward the body. This position places more pressure on female breasts. The arms may be placed on angled armboards by lowering them toward the floor and rotating them upward in natural range of motion. Elbows are slightly flexed to prevent overextension, and padded. The palms are down. The arms may extend beyond the head. The head is turned to one side, resting on a padded donut to prevent pressure on ear, eye, and face.

A pillow or padding under ankles and dorsa of feet prevents pressure on the toes and elevates the feet to aid venous return. Donuts under the knees prevent pressure on the patellae. The safety belt is placed above the knees.

Modified Prone Positions

For surgical procedures on the spine, the mattress is adjusted on the table so the hips are over the break between body and leg sections. A large soft pillow is placed under the abdomen. The upper break of the table is flexed and the table tilted so the surgical area is horizontal. Some surgeons prefer a special assembly for the orthopaedic table, an adjustable arch, and a Hastings or an Andrews frame for spinal surgery. The patient must be carefully lifted and properly positioned on special tables or frames. The patient may be placed in a prone sitting or kneeling position with the torso at a right angle to the thighs. The lower legs, at right angles at the knees, rest on the foot extension, which is at 90-degree angle. The midsection of the abdomen is allowed to hang free. This allows the anesthesiologist to use hypotensive anesthetic technique for hemostasis.

For neurosurgical procedures, the head rests in a cranial headrest exposing the occiput and cervical vertebrae. Eyes must be protected. Ophthalmic ointment is applied to protect the corneas and to keep the lids closed before turning the patient onto the headrest. Ears must be protected with foam support. When the patient is face down on a headrest, the head should be raised periodically to prevent pressure necrosis of cheeks and forehead.

Kraske (Jackknife) Position

The patient is supine until anesthetized, then turned onto the abdomen into the prone position by rotation. The hips must be over the center break of the table between body and leg sections. Chest rolls or bolsters are placed to raise the chest if the patient is under general anesthesia. Arms are extended on angled armboards with elbows flexed and palms down. The head is to side, supported on a donut or pillow. The dorsa of the feet and toes rest on a pillow. The safety belt is placed below the knees. The leg section of the table is lowered the desired amount, usually about 90 degrees, and the entire table is tilted head downward so that the hips are elevated above the rest of the body. The patient must be well balanced on the table (Figure 21-7). For procedures in the rectal area such as pilonidal sinus or hemorrhoidectomy, buttocks are retracted with hemorrhoid straps or wide tape strips. Because of the dependent position, venous pooling occurs cephalad (toward head) and caudad (toward feet). It is very important to return the patient slowly to horizontal from this unnatural position.

Knee-Chest Position

An extension is attached to the foot section. The table is flexed at the center break. The lower section is broken until it is at a right angle to the table. The patient kneels on the lower section and the entire table is tilted cephalad to elevate the pelvis. The knees are thus flexed at a right angle to the body. The upper portion of the table may be raised slightly to support the head, which is turned to the side. The arms are placed around the head with elbows flexed, with a large soft pillow beneath. The chest rests on the table. The safety belt is above the knees. The table is tilted head downward so the hips are

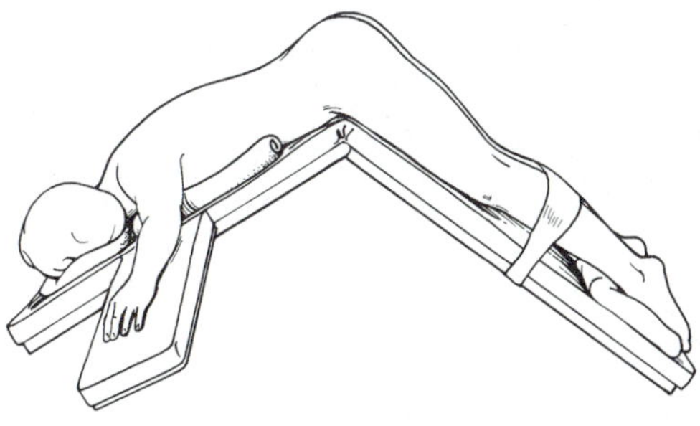

FIGURE 21-7 Kraske position. Hips are over central break in table and knee strap is below knees. Note chest rolls in place and pillow under feet.

at highest point—modified jackknife. This position is used for sigmoidoscopy or culdoscopy.

Lateral Position

The patient is anesthetized and intubated in the supine position, then turned to the unaffected side. The table remains flat. In the *right lateral position,* the patient lies on the right side with the left side up for a left-sided procedure; *left lateral position* exposes the right side (Figure 21-8). Referred to synonymously as *lateral, lateral decubitus,* or *lateral recumbent,* these positions are used for access to the hemithorax, kidney, or retroperitoneal space. The position contributes to physiologic alterations. Respiration is affected by differing gas exchange ratios in the lungs. Because of gravity, the lower lung receives more blood from the right side of the heart and so has increased perfusion but less residual air because of mediastinal compression and weight of abdominal contents on the diaphragm. Positive pressure to both lungs helps control respiratory changes. Circulation is also compromised by pressure on abdominal vessels. In the right lateral position, compression of the vena cava impairs venous return.

The patient is turned by no fewer than four people to maintain body alignment and achieve stability. The patient's back is drawn to the edge of the table. The knee of the lower leg is flexed to prevent rolling and to aid in stabilization. The knee may need to be padded to prevent pressure. The upper leg remains straight. A large soft pillow is placed lengthwise between the legs. This prevents pressure on the peroneal nerve, as well as circulatory complications, by taking pressure off the lower leg. The ankle and foot of the upper leg should be supported to prevent footdrop. Bony prominences are padded. A safety belt or 3-inch (7.5 cm) wide tape is placed over the hip for additional stability.

Arms may be placed on a padded double armboard, the lower arm with palm up, the upper arm slightly flexed with the palm down. Blood pressure should be taken from the lower arm. A small roll or pad under the axilla relieves pressure and protects neurovascular structures. Shoulders should be in alignment.

The head must be in cervical alignment with the spine. It should be supported on a small pillow between the shoulder and neck to prevent stretching the neck and brachial plexus and to maintain a patent airway.

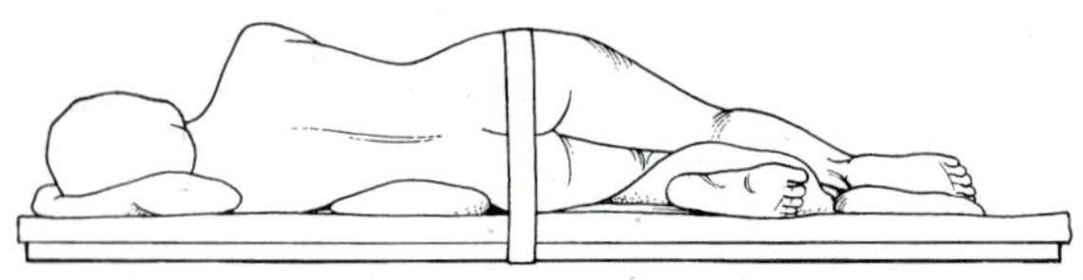

FIGURE 21-8 Left lateral position. Note strap across hip to stabilize body. Pillow between legs relieves pressure on lower leg.

Kidney Position

When the patient is turned onto the unaffected side, the flank region must be over the kidney elevator on the table (Figure 21-9). The short kidney rest is attached to the elevator at the patient's back. The longer rest is placed in front at a level beneath the iliac crest to minimize pressure on abdominal organs. Both rests must be well padded. In an obese patient, folds of abdominal tissue may extend over the end of the anterior rest and be bruised if caution is not taken. The table is flexed slightly at level of the iliac crest so the kidney elevator can be raised as desired to increase space between the lower ribs and iliac crest. Table flexion combined with use of the kidney elevator may cause cardiovascular responses. Blood tends to pool in the lower arm and leg. Circulation is further compromised by increased pressure on abdominal vessels when the kidney elevator is raised. Used for procedures on the kidney and ureter, this position is not well tolerated.

A body strap or tape is placed over the hip to stabilize the patient *after* the table is flexed and the elevator is raised. Skin and underlying tissue could be damaged by excessive pressure during flexion. The entire table is tilted slightly downward toward the head until the surgical area is horizontal. The upper shoulder and hip should be in a straight line. A pillow may be used to support the chest and protect the breasts. A chest roll may be placed to take body weight off the deltoid muscle in the shoulder. Before closure, the table is straightened for better approximation of tissues.

Lateral Jackknife Position

After the patient is placed in lateral position, the table is flexed at the level of the patient's flank or lower ribs. The table is tilted so the torso is level. This drops the legs into a dependent position. Blood tends to pool in the legs. Extreme table flexion into a lateral jackknife position may occlude the inferior vena cava, causing venous obstruction. Pulmonary compliance is reduced, making

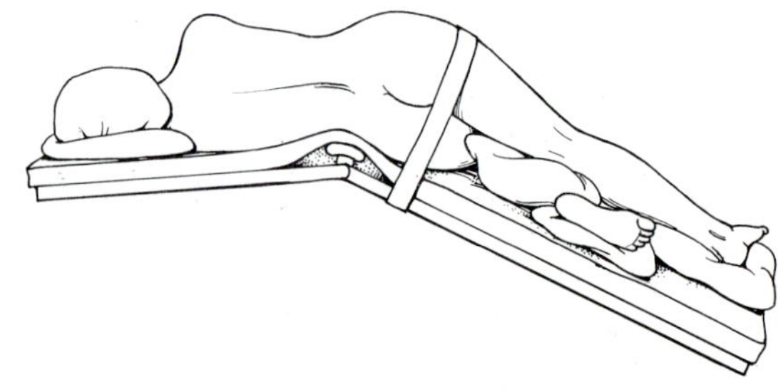

FIGURE 21-9 Right kidney position. Patient is in lateral position with kidney region over table break. Note kidney strap across hip to stabilize body, raised kidney elevator for hyperextending surgical site, and pillow between legs. Patient's side is horizontal from shoulder to hip.

ventilation difficult. Similar to the kidney position already described, this position is not well tolerated.

Lateral Chest Position

Modifications of lateral position are used for unilateral transthoracic procedures with the lateral approach. After the patient is turned onto the unaffected side and positioned as described, a second strap may be placed over the shoulder for stability unless it interferes with skin preparation. The arms may be extended on a double armboard, or the lower arm is extended on an armboard with the palm up while the upper arm is brought forward and down over a pad to draw the scapula from the surgical area. Position depends on site and length of chest incision. A small firm pillow or pad under the axilla and surgical area relieves pressure on the lower arm and assists in spreading the intercostal space for better exposure.

One body rest is placed at the lumbar area to facilitate respiratory movements and provide support. Another body rest is placed along the chest at axillary level. This must be well padded to avoid bruising the breasts. Bead bags or bolsters may be used instead of body rests. Shoulders and hips should be level. Lowering the head of the table slightly assists postural drainage during the surgical procedure. This position is restricting to the cardiopulmonary system, especially if prolonged.

Anterior Chest Position

For thoracoabdominal procedures with anterior approach, the position is more supine than the lateral chest position. After the patient is anesthetized, a small firm pillow is placed under the shoulder and another under the buttocks on the affected side. The knee on the affected side is flexed slightly, with a large soft pillow beneath it to relieve strain on the abdominal muscles. The table can be tilted laterally to raise the incisional site. The safety belt is above the knees. The arm on the unaffected side is supported at the side. The arm on the affected side is padded well and bandaged loosely to the anesthesia screen. To avoid injury to the brachial plexus the arm must not be hyperextended. The head of the table is lowered slightly for postural drainage.

Sims' Recumbent Position

In Sims' recumbent position, a modified left lateral recumbent position, the patient lies on the left side with the upper leg flexed at the hip and knees. The lower leg is straight. The lower arm is extended along the patient's back with weight of the chest on the table. The upper arm rests in a flexed position on the table. This position may be preferred for endoscopic examination performed via the anus in obese or geriatric patients.

MODIFICATIONS FOR INDIVIDUAL PATIENT NEEDS

The patient's individual needs must be met in positioning as in everything else. Anomalies and physical defects are accommodated. Avoidance of unnecessary exposure, whether the patient is unconscious or conscious, is an essential consideration for all patients. Objectively observe the patient's position before skin preparation and draping to see that it adheres to physiologic principles. Reassess protective devices, positioning aids, and padded areas before draping, because the placement could have shifted during insertion of an indwelling urinary catheter or skin preparation procedure. Careful observation of patient protection and positioning facilitates expected outcome.

The circulator should document in the patient's record any limitations in range of motion preoperatively, the condition of the skin before and after the surgical procedure, and the position in which the patient was positioned during the surgical procedure, including special equipment used.

BIBLIOGRAPHY

Biddle C, Cannady MJ: Surgical positions, *AORN J* 52(2):350-359, 1990.

Fogg DM: Clinical issues: lateral positioning techniques, *AORN J* 57(2):495-496, 1993.

Fogg DM: Clinical issues: patient positioning, *AORN J* 56(3):553-554, 1992.

Fogg DM: Clinical issues: patient positioning, *AORN J* 58(6):1192, 1993.

Graling PR, Colvin DB: The lithotomy position in colon surgery: postoperative complications, *AORN J* 55(4):1029-1039, 1992.

Insinger J, Bailes BK: Care of the patient undergoing spinal surgery, *AORN J* 58(3):511-526, 1993.

Kemp MG et al: Factors that contribute to pressure sores in surgical patients, *Res Nurs Health* 13(10):293-301, 1990.

Martin JT: *Positioning in anesthesia and surgery,* ed 2, Philadelphia, 1987, Saunders.

O'Neale M: Clinical issues: positioning aids, *AORN J* 54(5):1063, 1991.

Paschal CR, Strzelecki LR: Lithotomy positioning devices: factors that contribute to patient injury, *AORN J* 55(4):1011-1022, 1992.

Proposed recommended practices for positioning the patient in the perioperative practice setting, *AORN J* 61(2):414-417, 1995.

Scott SM et al: Pressure ulcer development in the OR, *AORN J* 56(2):242-250, 1992.

Smith KA: Positioning principles, *AORN J* 52(6):1196-1208, 1990.

CHAPTER 22

Skin Preparation and Draping of the Surgical Site

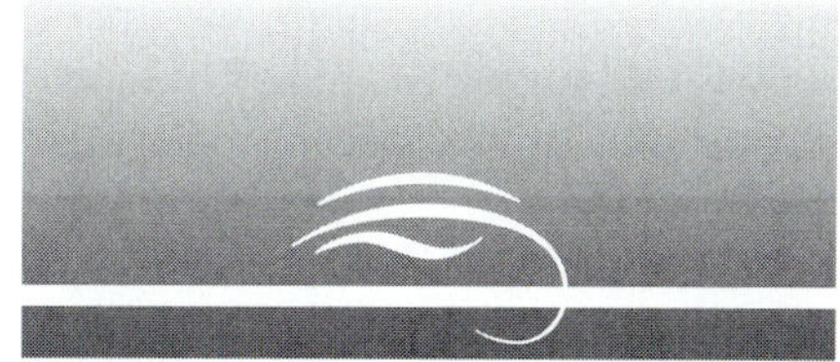

PHYSICAL PREPARATION OF PATIENT

The type of surgical procedure to be performed, age and condition of the patient, and preferences of the surgeon will determine specific procedures to be carried out before the incision is made. Consideration must be given to control of urinary drainage, to skin antisepsis, and to establishment of a sterile field around the surgical site.

URINARY TRACT CATHETERIZATION

The patient should void to empty the urinary bladder just before transfer to the operating room (OR) suite, unless an indwelling Foley catheter is in place. If the patient's bladder is not empty or the surgeon wishes to prevent bladder distention during a long procedure or following the surgical procedure, catheterization may be necessary after the patient is anesthetized. An indwelling Foley catheter may be inserted. This maintains bladder decompression to avoid trauma during a lower abdominal or pelvic procedure, to permit accurate measurement of output during or following the surgical procedure, or to facilitate output and healing after a surgical procedure on genitourinary tract structures. Catheterization is performed before the patient is positioned, except for a patient who will remain in lithotomy position.

Urinary tract infection can occur following catheterization from contamination or trauma to structures. Sterile technique must be maintained during catheterization. A sterile, disposable catheterization tray is used, unless the patient is being prepared for a surgical procedure in the perineal or genital area. For these latter procedures, a sterile catheter and lubricant may be added to the skin preparation setup. For other surgical procedures, the perineal area should be scrubbed (sterile gloves are worn) with an antiseptic agent to reduce normal microbial flora and to remove gross contaminants before the catheterization procedure.

Urinary catheterization is an invasive procedure requiring sterile technique. Sterile gloves are worn to handle the sterile catheter. Catheter size should be small enough to minimize trauma to the urethra and prevent necrosis of the meatus; usually a size 16 or 14 French catheter is inserted in an adult female, a 16 or 18 French in an adult male.

If an indwelling Foley catheter is to be inserted, check the integrity of the balloon by inflating it with the correct amount of sterile water or air before insertion. Balloon size may be 5 or 30 ml (5 ml is used most frequently); 10 ml of sterile water is needed to properly inflate a 5 ml balloon to compensate for volume required by the inflation channel. Most Foley catheters have a rubber valve over the lumen to the inflation channel that can be penetrated by a plain Luer slip tip syringe. Some require a needle on the syringe to penetrate the rubber cover. Solution or air must be evacuated before insertion of the catheter into the urethra.

The hand used to spread the labia or stabilize the penis is considered contaminated and should not be used to handle the catheter. Sponges used to cleanse the labia minora or glans penis should be handled to avoid contaminating the gloved hand used to insert the catheter. To facilitate insertion and minimize trauma, lubricate the tip of the catheter with a sterile, water-soluble, antimicrobial lubricant. Urine will start to flow when the catheter has passed into the bladder. Drain the bladder. Inflate the balloon of a Foley catheter.

Attach the catheter to a sterile closed-drainage system. Secure the tubing to the patient's leg with enough slack in it to prevent tension or pull on the penis or urethra. Drainage tubing should be positioned to enhance downward flow but must not fall below the level of the collection container. Attention must be paid to the catheter and tubing during positioning of the patient for the surgical procedure to prevent compression or kinking. If the container must be raised above the level of the bladder during positioning, clamp or kink the tubing until the container can be lowered and secured under the operating table to avoid contamination by retrograde, backward flow of urine.

SKIN PREPARATION OF PATIENT

Skin preparation begins before the patient arrives in the OR.

Purpose of Patient's Skin Preparation

The purpose of skin preparation (usually called *skin prep*) is to render the surgical site as free as possible from transient and resident microorganisms, dirt, and skin oil so the incision can be made through the skin with minimal danger of infection from this source.

Preliminary Preparation of Patient's Skin

Mechanical Cleansing

Bathing removes many microorganisms from the skin. This action can be enhanced to progressively reduce the resident microbial population with daily use of a skin-cleansing agent containing chlorhexidine gluconate or iodophor or an antimicrobial bar soap. Bacteriostatic action takes place in the cumulative deposits of fatty acids in the skin. Many surgeons advise their patients to use such a product at home for several days before an elective surgical procedure.

All patients should shower, preferably, or bathe the evening before and morning of a surgical procedure with an antimicrobial agent, preferably chlorhexidine because of its residual activity. Patients whose surgical procedures will be through the scalp or on the face, eye, ear, or neck are advised to shampoo their hair. This may not be permitted for days or weeks postoperatively.

Skin should be free of gross dirt and debris. The surgical site and surrounding area should be thoroughly cleansed with a rapid-acting, skin-degerming, antiseptic agent. *History of allergies must be obtained before applying any chemical agent to a patient's skin.* Usually the surgeon is responsible for designating in the patient's preoperative orders the limits of the skin area and how it is to be prepared. The procedure book specifies anatomic areas that must be mechanically cleansed and corresponding areas for hair removal, *if ordered,* for each type of surgical procedure (see Figures 22-1 through 22-6).

The patient's general skin condition must be observed. Abnormal skin irritation, infection, or abrasion on or near the surgical site might be a contraindication to the surgical procedure and must be reported to the surgeon.

Hair Removal

Hair removal can injure skin. Breaks in skin surface afford an opportunity for entry and colonization of microorganisms and are a potential source of infection. However, hair surrounding the surgical site may be so thick that removal is necessary. Hair may interfere with exposure, closure, or dressing. Hair may also prevent adequate skin contact with electrodes.

Hair removal is carried out per the surgeon's order, either on the preoperative unit or in the OR suite as close to scheduled time for the surgical procedure as possible. The procedure can be done in a preoperative holding area only if privacy is assured. Skin preparation can be an embarrassing procedure for the patient. Drape the patient to expose the area to be prepared, but avoid unnecessary exposure.

Most patients, especially women and children, do not require any form of hair removal. If necessary, hair may be removed with clippers, by applying a depilatory cream, or by shaving with a razor.

Clippers Electric clippers with fine teeth cut hair close to the skin. The short stubble, usually about a millimeter in length, that remains does not interfere with antisepsis or exposure of the surgical site. Clipping can be done immediately before the surgical procedure or up to 24 hours preoperatively using short strokes against the direction of hair growth. The blade lies flat against the skin surface. After use, the blade assembly must be disassembled, cleaned, and sterilized if a disposable clipper blade assembly is not used. The clipper handle is cleaned and disinfected. Cordless handles with rechargeable batteries are available.

Depilatory Cream Hair can be removed by chemical depilation before the patient comes to the OR suite. A preliminary skin patch is tested on a forearm before general application. If the patient is not sensitive, a thick layer of cream is applied over the hair to be removed. Depilatories should not be used around the eyes or genitalia. After the cream has remained on the skin for the required time, usually about 20 minutes, it is washed off. The hair comes off in the cream. The skin is intact and free from cuts, but any evidence of irritation should be documented.

Razor Shaving should be performed as near the time of incision as possible if this method must be used. Avoid making nicks and cuts in the skin. Nicks made immediately before the surgical procedure (i.e., up to 30 minutes) are considered clean wounds. However, nicks and abrasions made several hours before may present as infected wounds at the time of surgical incision. Notify the surgeon if the skin is not intact at the surgical site. This may be cause for cancellation of the surgical procedure. Time lapse between the preoperative shave and the surgical procedure may increase risk of postoperative infection.

Wear gloves to prevent cross contamination even though this is a surgically clean procedure. Wet shaving is preferable. Soaking hair in lather allows keratin to absorb water, making hair softer and easier to remove. Use a sharp, clean razor blade. Hold the skin taut and shave by stroking in the direction of hair growth. Blades are either discarded (in sharps disposal container) after use or terminally sterilized. If disposable razors are not used, razors must be terminally sterilized between uses.

Skin Degreasing

The skin surface is composed of cornified epithelium with a coating of secretions that include perspiration, oils, and desquamated epithelium. These surface sebaceous lubricants are insoluble in water. Therefore a skin degreaser, or fat solvent, may be used to enhance adhesion of electrocardiogram (ECG) electrodes. It also may be used before a skin prep to improve adhesion of self-adhering drapes (p. 458) or to prevent smudging of skin markings (p. 458). Isopropyl alcohol and acetone are effective fat solvents. A fat-solvent emollient is incorporated into some antiseptic agents. Some solvents are flammable.

PATIENT'S SKIN PREP ON OPERATING TABLE

After the patient is anesthetized and/or positioned on the operating table, the skin at the surgical site and an extensive area surrounding it is mechanically cleansed again with an antiseptic agent immediately before draping.

Setup

Prewarmed solutions, *if composition will not be changed by warming,* may help reduce the patient's heat loss during the skin preparation procedure. Prep trays and/or solutions may be placed in a solution warmer or in an open steam sterilizer for a few minutes to warm them. Solutions should not be warmed beyond 104° F (40° C).

Some disposable sterile skin prep trays include applicators and/or containers of a premeasured amount of antiseptic solution. The solution of choice must be added to other trays. If prepackaged trays are not used, a sterile table must be prepared with the following sterile items:

1. Two towels to define upper and lower limits of area to be prepared. Two absorbent towels are used to prevent pooling under body parts along sides of area.
2. Small basins for solutions—usually at least two. One or two ounces of solution usually is sufficient.
3. Sponges—may be 4 × 8 inches (10 × 20 cm) for large areas; 4 × 4 (10 × 10 cm) or 3 × 3 (7.5 × 7.5 cm) for small areas. *These should not be counted sponges from the instrument table.* Textured foam sponges may be preferred.
4. Cotton applicators as necessary.

Sterile gloves must be worn and a sterile setup must be used to prep skin around an open wound or to include urinary catheterization as part of the procedure. A clean but unsterile setup may be used for intact skin. Skin cannot be sterilized; it is mechanically cleansed and chemically decontaminated to reduce skin flora.

Antiseptic Solutions

The infection control committee usually determines the chemical agent(s) to be used in the OR for skin antisepsis. Maximum concentration of a germicidal chemical that can be used on skin and mucous membranes is limited by its toxicity for these tissues. The agent should have the following qualities:

1. It has broad-spectrum antimicrobial action and rapidly decreases microbial count.
2. It can be quickly applied and remains effective against microorganisms.
3. It can be safely used without skin irritation or sensitization. It must be nontoxic.
4. It effectively remains active in presence of alcohol, organic matter, soap, or detergent.
5. It should be nonflammable for use with laser, electrosurgery, or other high-energy devices.

Chlorhexidine Gluconate

A tincture of 0.5% chlorhexidine gluconate in 70% isopropyl alcohol (Hibitane Tincture) is a broad-spectrum, rapid-acting, nontoxic, antimicrobial agent. It binds to negative charges on microbial cell walls to produce irreversible damage and death. Activity is adversely affected by traces of soap and is reduced in the presence of organic matter. This agent is not absorbed through intact skin. It significantly reduces and maintains a reduction of microbial flora for at least 4 hours. Its activity increases at elevated temperature. It is available either tinted for color demarcation of skin area being prepped or nontinted to prevent skin staining if the surgeon needs to observe skin color. Because it is an irritant to the eyes, it is contraindicated for facial antisepsis.

Iodine and Iodophors

A solution of 1% or 2% iodine in water or in 70% alcohol is an excellent antiseptic. However, potential hazards of skin irritations and burns led to decline in its use. If used, iodine should dry and then be rinsed off with 70% alcohol to neutralize the burning effect.

Iodophors are iodine complexes combined with detergents. Povidone-iodine has a surfactant, a wetting and dispersive agent, in an aqueous solution such as Betadine surgical scrub, a commonly used iodophor. Iodophor in 70% alcohol also is available. These are excellent cleansing agents that remove debris from skin surfaces while slowly releasing iodine. Iodophors are broad-spectrum antimicrobial agents and have some sporicidal activity. They are relatively nontoxic and virtually nonirritating to skin or mucous membranes.

The brown film left on the skin clearly defines the area of application. This should *not* be wiped off because microbial activity is sustained by release of free iodine as the agent dries and color fades from skin. It should remain on skin for at least 2 minutes. To hasten drying of skin, alcohol may be painted on the area without friction before a self-adhering drape is applied (see p. 458).

NOTE

1. Iodophors should *not* be used to prep the skin of patients allergic to iodine or sea food. Shellfish, for example, contains iodine.
2. Type of preparation, concentration of iodine, and presence of surfactants affect microbial activity of products. Povidone-iodine complexes are available in solution, spray, or gel forms. Tinctures are in solution. Manufacturer's instructions must be strictly followed for product in use.
3. Concentration of povidone-iodine may be altered by evaporation if solution is warmed. Patient may be burned by an increase in iodine concentration. Follow manufacturer's recommendation.

Alcohols

Isopropyl and ethyl alcohols are broad-spectrum agents that denature proteins in cells. A 70% concentration with *continuous contact* for several minutes is satisfactory for skin antisepsis if the surgeon prefers a colorless solution that permits observation of true skin color. Because alcohol coagulates protein, it is not applied to mucous membranes or used on an open wound. Isopropyl alcohol is a more effective fat solvent than ethyl alcohol. Both are volatile and flammable. They must not pool around or under the patient, especially if an electrosurgical unit or laser will be used.

Triclosan

A solution of 1% triclosan is a broad-spectrum antimicrobial agent. It is blended with oils and lanolin in a mild detergent. Cumulative suppressive action develops slowly only with prolonged routine use. It is safe for use on the face around eyes.

Basic Prep Procedure for Clean Areas

Skin preparation requires coordination of hands, eyes, and body movements of the person doing the prep. Mechanical friction with an antiseptic agent is the basis for effective skin antisepsis.

1. Expose only the skin area to be prepared by folding back the cotton blanket and gown to 2 inches (5 cm) beyond limits of the prep area. Double-check the surgical procedure.

   NOTE If the surgical procedure is unilateral, be sure which side is affected. Consult the chart and x-ray films. Before amputation of an extremity, expose the opposite one also for comparison. Check with surgeon.

2. Don gloves.
3. Place towels above and below the area to be cleansed to mark the limit of the area and also to protect gloved hands from touching the blanket or gown. Also place absorbent towels along each side of the area to act as an absorber of runoff solution. These two towels are removed after the prep is completed.
4. Wet the sponge with antiseptic agent, but squeeze out excess solution.

   NOTE Solution should not run off the skin area onto the operating table to pool under patient. A patient lying in solution may develop skin irritation even though the solution itself is nonirritating. Waterproof pads or additional absorbent towels may be placed under the patient during prep and then removed. Flammable solutions, such as alcohol or tinctures and solvents, must evaporate before drapes are applied to prevent accumulation of fumes under them.

5. Scrub the skin, starting at the site of incision, with a *circular motion* in ever-widening circles to the periphery. Use enough pressure and friction to remove dirt and microorganisms from the skin and pores. Effective skin antisepsis is achieved through mechanical and chemical action. (See Figure 22-1 for abdominal prep and Figure 29-3, p. 583, for abdominal incisions.)

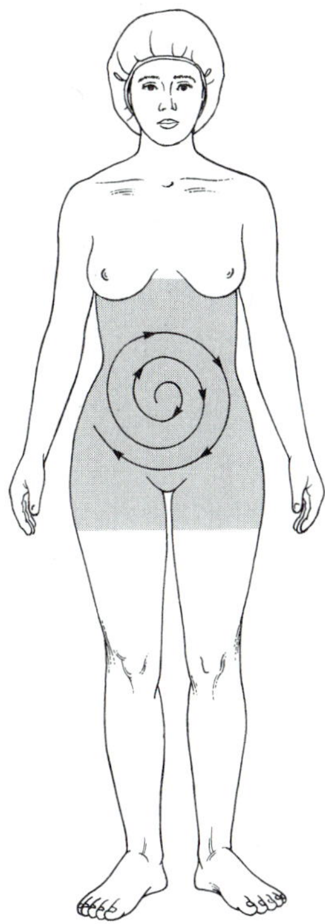

FIGURE 22-1 Abdominal preparation. Area includes breast line to upper third of thighs, from table line to table line, with patient in supine position. *Shaded area* shows anatomic area to be prepared. *Arrows* within area show direction of motion for skin preparation on operating table.

NOTE

- Some surgeons prefer to have the antiseptic agent applied over cancerous areas by painting rather than scrubbing. During vigorous scrubbing, cancer cells may be freed, picked up by blood and lymph streams, and carried to other parts of the body. To paint, secure a folded sponge in a sponge forceps, dip in the solution, squeeze out excess solution, and apply to the skin in circular motions from incision site to periphery.
- No-touch technique may be used (i.e., an applicator device or sponge forceps rather than hands is used to apply the solution and scrub the skin).
- Scrub brushes with bristles should not be used. Bristles might fall out and remain on the skin to become foreign bodies in the surgical wound. Bristles can be abrasive to the skin. Sponges or commercially prepared foam applicators should be used.

6. Discard the sponge after reaching the periphery. *Never* bring the sponge back toward the center of the area.
7. Repeat the scrub with a separate sponge for each round.

Apply antiseptic agent and scrub for the time recommended by the manufacturer of the agent(s) used. Recommended minimum time may be 2 to 5 minutes, but consideration should be given to the extent of the area being prepped. The prepped area needs to be large enough to provide a wide margin around the full length of the anticipated incision and to accommodate potential drain sites and opening in draping material.

Contaminated Areas Within Surgical Field

Umbilicus

The umbilicus is considered a contaminated area in relation to the surface surrounding it because it may harbor microorganisms in the detritus that often accumulates there. Solution may be squeezed into the umbilicus to soften detritus while the remainder of the abdomen is scrubbed. Or the umbilicus may be cleansed first with separate sponges and applicators to avoid runoff of dirty solution over cleansed skin area. Then the abdominal prep begins with new sponges at the line of incision, moving with circular motions to the periphery and including the umbilicus again each round as it is approached within the area. The umbilicus is thoroughly cleansed with cotton applicators as the final step of the abdominal prep.

Stoma

The external stoma (orifice) of a colostomy, ileostomy, etc., may be sealed off from the surgical site with a self-adhering towel drape. If this is not possible, follow the same rule for use of sponges as for the umbilicus; come back to that area last, or use a separate sponge each round for the contaminated area only. The opening of the stoma may be packed with a sponge while surrounding area is scrubbed.

Other Contaminated Areas

Draining sinuses, skin ulcers, vagina, anus, etc., are considered contaminated areas also. In all these, follow the general rule of scrubbing the most contaminated area last or with separate sponges.

Foreign Substances

Adhesive, grease, tar, and similar foreign materials must be removed from skin before the area is mechanically cleansed with an antiseptic agent. A nonirritating solvent should be used to cleanse the skin. The solvent must be nonflammable and nontoxic. However, do not allow the solution to collect underneath the patient.

Traumatic Wounds

In the preparation of an area in which the skin is not intact because of a traumatic injury, wound irrigation may be part of the skin preparation procedure. The wound may be packed or covered with sterile gauze while the area around it is thoroughly scrubbed and shaved if necessary. Extent and type of injury will determine the appropriate procedure.

Solutions irritating to a denuded area must not be used. Small areas may be irrigated with warm sterile solution, usually normal saline, in a bulb syringe. When a bulb syringe is used, care must be taken not to force debris and microorganisms deeper into the wound. The wound is irrigated gently to dislodge debris and flush it out.

Copious amounts of warm sterile solutions may be needed to flush out a large wound. A container of warm sterile normal saline or Ringer's lactate solution attached to intravenous tubing can be hung on IV pole near the area to be copiously irrigated. If the area is on an extremity, a sterile irrigating pan with a wire screen fitted over the top is placed under the extremity. During irrigation, solution runs from the wound into the pan. A piece of tubing connected to an outlet on the pan carries the irrigating solution into a kick bucket on the floor near the table.

It may be necessary to place dry towels or sheets under the patient if the area has not been protected during irrigation. A moistureproof pad placed under the wound before irrigation will help channel solutions into a drainage pan.

Debridement of the wound (excision of all devitalized tissue) usually follows irrigation. The surgeon may wish to have sterile tissue forceps and scissors on the preparation table for removal of nonviable tissue.

Areas Prepared for Grafts

Separate setups are necessary for skin preparation of recipient and donor sites before skin, bone, or vascular grafting procedures. The donor site is usually scrubbed first.

The donor site for a skin graft should be scrubbed with a colorless antiseptic agent so surgeon can properly evaluate vascularity of the graft postoperatively. The recipient site for skin grafts is usually more or less contaminated (e.g., following a burn or other traumatic injury). Items used in preparation of the recipient site must not be permitted to contaminate the donor site. Also, microorganisms on the skin of the donor site must not be transferred to a denuded recipient site.

Special Considerations in Specific Anatomic Areas

Eye

1. Eyebrows are never shaved or removed unless the surgeon deems this essential. Eyebrows do not grow back completely.
2. Eyelashes may be trimmed, if ordered by the surgeon, with fine scissors coated with sterile petrolatum or water-soluble lubricant to catch the lashes.
3. Eyelids and periorbital areas are cleansed with a nonirritating antiseptic agent, commonly triclosan detergent, then rinsed with warm sterile water. The prep starts centrally and works to the periphery (i.e., from center of the lid to brow and cheek).
4. Conjunctival sac is flushed with a nontoxic agent, such as sterile normal saline, with a bulb syringe. The patient's head is turned slightly to the affected side. The solution is contained with sponges or an absorbent towel. *Care must be taken to prevent prep solution from entering the patient's eyes or ears.*

NOTE Chlorhexidine gluconate and iodophors can cause corneal damage if accidentally introduced into the eyes. Chlorhexidine also may cause sensorineural deafness if it enters the inner ear, as through a perforated tympanic membrane. Chlorhexidine is contraindicated for facial preps. Iodophors must be used with caution around the eyes.

Ears, Face, or Nose

1. Usually it is not possible to define the area with towels.
2. Protect the eyes with a piece of sterile plastic sheeting. If the patient is awake, ask that eyes be kept closed during the prep.
3. As much of the surrounding area is included as is feasible and consistent with aseptic technique. Skin surfaces should be cleansed at least to the hair line.
4. Cotton applicators are used for cleansing the nostrils and external ear canals.

Neck

1. One sterile towel is folded under the edge of the blanket and gown, which are turned down almost to the nipple line.
2. Area includes the neck laterally to the table line and up to the mandible, tops of shoulders, and chest almost to the nipple line.
3. For combined head and neck surgical procedures, include the face to the eyes, shaved areas of the head, ears, posterior neck, and the area over the shoulders.

Lateral Thoracoabdominal

1. Gown is removed. The blanket is turned down well below the lower limit of the area to be prepared. A towel is folded under the edge of the blanket.
2. Arm is held up during preparation.
3. Beginning at the site of incision, the area may include axilla, chest, and abdomen from the neck to crest of the ilium. For surgical procedure in the region of the kidney, it extends up to the axilla and down to the pubis. The area also extends beyond midlines, anteriorly and posteriorly and may include the arm to the elbow (Figure 22-2).

Chest and Breast

1. Anesthesiologist turns the patient's face toward the unaffected side.
2. One towel is folded under the blanket edge, just above the pubis. Another is placed on the table under the shoulder and side.
3. Arm on the affected side is held up by grasping the hand and raising the shoulder and axilla slightly from the table.
4. Area includes the shoulder, upper arm down to the elbow, axilla, and chest wall to the table line and beyond the sternum to the opposite shoulder (Figure 22-3).

Shoulder

1. Anesthesiologist turns the patient's face toward the opposite side.
2. Towel is placed under the shoulder and axilla.
3. Arm is held up by grasping the hand and elevating the shoulder slightly from the table.
4. Area includes the circumference of the upper arm to below the elbow, from the base of the neck over the shoulder, scapula, and chest to the midline.

Upper Arm

1. Towel is placed under the shoulder and axilla.
2. Arm is held up by grasping hand and elevating the shoulder slightly from table.
3. Area includes the entire circumference of the arm to the wrist, axilla, and over the shoulder and scapula.

Elbow and Forearm

1. Towel is placed under the shoulder and axilla.
2. Arm is held up by grasping the hand.
3. Area includes the entire arm from the shoulder and axilla to and including the hand.

Hand

1. Towels are omitted. The anatomy of the hand furnishes sufficient landmarks to define the area, and towels are apt to slip over the scrubbed area.
2. Arm must be held up by supporting it above the elbow so that the entire circumference can be scrubbed.
3. Area includes the hand and arm to 3 inches (7.5 cm) above the elbow.

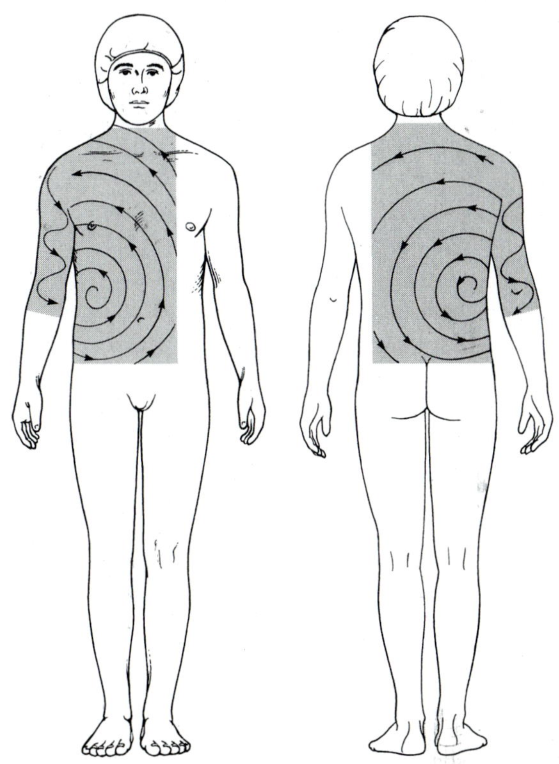

FIGURE 22-2 Lateral thoracoabdominal preparation. Area includes axilla, chest, and abdomen from neck to crest of ilium. Area extends beyond midline, anteriorly and posteriorly. Patient is in lateral position on operating table.

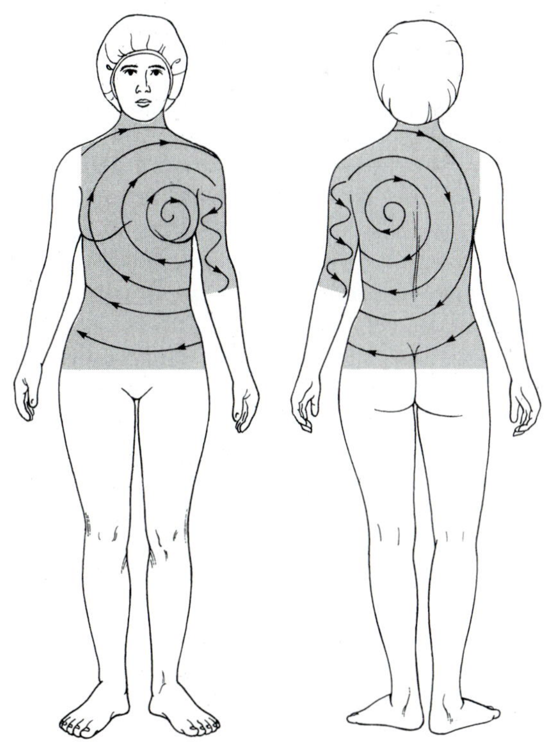

FIGURE 22-3 Chest and breast preparation. Area includes shoulder, upper arm down to elbow, axilla, and chest wall to table line and beyond sternum to opposite shoulder. If patient is in lateral position, back is prepped also.

Rectoperineal

1. One towel is folded under the edge of the blanket above the pubis. Another towel is placed under the buttocks.
2. Area includes the pubis, external genitalia, perineum and anus, and inner aspects of the thighs (Figure 22-4).
3. Begin the scrub over the pubic area, scrubbing downward over the genitalia and perineum. Discard the sponge after going over the anus.
4. Inner aspects of the upper third of both thighs are scrubbed with separate sponges.
5. Rectoperineal area is prepped first, with the patient in lithotomy position, followed by an abdominal prep, with the patient in supine position, for a combined abdominoperineal procedure. Two separate prep trays are used.

Vagina

1. Sponge forceps should be included on the preparation table for a vaginal prep because a portion of the prep is done internally. A disposable vaginal prep tray, with sponge sticks included, is available.
2. With the patient in lithotomy position, a moistureproof pad is placed under the buttocks and extends to the kick bucket that receives solutions and discarded sponges.
3. Towel is folded under the edge of the blanket above the pubis.
4. Area includes the pubis, vulva, labia, perineum, anus, and adjacent area, including inner aspects of the upper third of the thighs (Figure 22-4). *The vagina is prepped last.*
5. Begin over the pubic area, scrubbing downward over the vulva and perineum. Discard each sponge after going over the anus.
6. Inner aspects of the thighs are scrubbed with separate sponges from the labia majora outward.
7. Vagina and cervix are cleansed with sponges on sponge forceps or disposable sponge sticks after external surrounding areas are scrubbed. The cleansing agent should be applied generously in the vagina because vaginal mucosa has many folds and crevices that are not easily cleansed.
8. After thoroughly cleansing the vagina, wipe it out with a dry sponge to prevent possibility of the fluid entering the peritoneal cavity during the surgical procedure on pelvic organs.
9. Catheterize, if indicated.

Hip

1. One towel is placed under the thigh on the table. Another towel is placed on the abdomen and folded under the edge of the gown, just above the umbilicus.
2. Leg on the affected side is held up by supporting it just below the knee.
3. Area includes the abdomen on the affected side, thigh to the knee, buttocks to table line, groin, and pubis (Figure 22-5).

Thigh

1. One towel is placed under the thigh on the table. Another towel is placed on the abdomen and folded under the edge of the gown, just below the umbilicus.

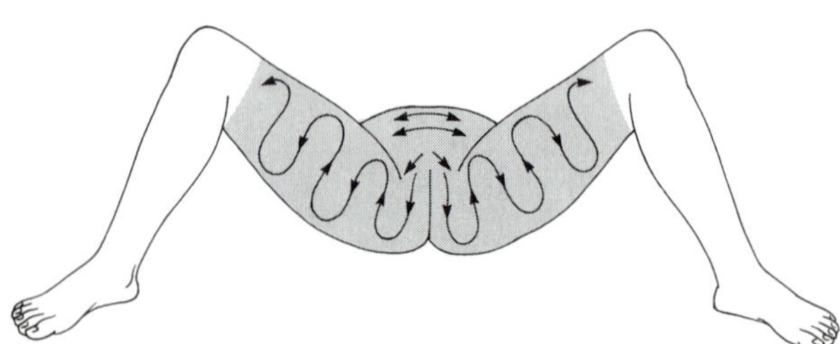

FIGURE 22-4 Rectoperineal and vaginal preparation. Area includes pubis, vulva, labia, perineum, anus, and adjacent area, including inner aspects of upper third of thighs.

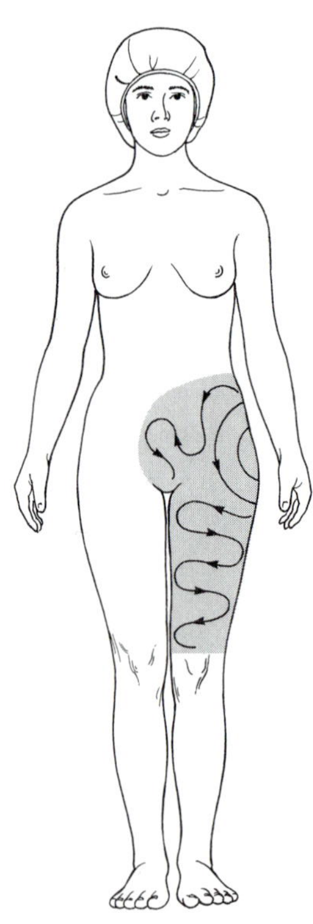

FIGURE 22-5 Hip preparation. Area includes abdomen on affected side, thigh to knee, buttock to table line, groin, and pubis.

2. Leg is held up by supporting the foot and ankle.
3. Area includes the entire circumference of thigh and leg to the ankle, over the hip and buttocks to the table line, groin, and pubis.

Knee and Lower Leg

1. Towel is placed over the groin.
2. Leg is held up by supporting it at the foot.
3. Area includes the entire circumference of the leg and extends from the foot to the upper part of the thigh (Figure 22-6).

Ankle and Foot

1. Towels are omitted.
2. Foot is held up by supporting the leg at the knee. A leg-holder device is useful.
3. Area includes the foot and entire circumference of the lower leg to the knee.

NOTE

- A moistureproof pad should be placed on the operating table under a lower extremity to retain drops of solution. This is removed after the prep so table will be dry.
- An extremity remains supported and elevated until sterile drapes are applied under and around the prepped area.
- A full extremity prep may be done in two stages to provide adequate support to joints and to ensure that all areas are scrubbed. It may include the foot for hip, thigh, knee, and lower leg procedures.
- Caution must be taken to prevent solution from pooling under a tourniquet. If a pneumatic tourniquet is used (see Chapter 23, pp. 474-476), it is positioned before the prep. A towel tucked under the tourniquet cuff absorbs excess solution. This is removed before the tourniquet is inflated.

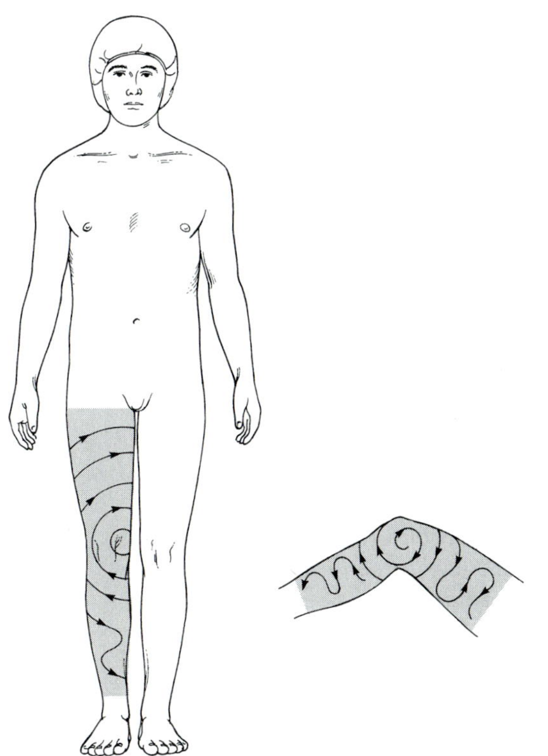

FIGURE 22-6 Knee and lower leg preparation. Area includes entire circumference of affected leg and extends from foot to upper part of thigh.

Skin Marking

Some surgeons use a staining solution to mark the incision lines on the skin. This may be done before the patient is prepped. If so, the stain must withstand scrubbing without washing off. If the skin is marked after prep, a sterile dye solution and applicator or a sterile marking pen must be used. Methylene blue or alcoholic gentian violet are used for this purpose.

Documentation

Details of preoperative skin condition and preparation should be documented in the patient's intraoperative record. These should include but are not limited to:

1. Condition of skin around surgical site
2. Hair removal, if done, including method and location, areas for attachment of monitors or electrodes, and time of removal
3. Antiseptic solutions, fat solvents, irrigating solutions, and any other agents used
4. Skin area prepared and skin reaction, if any
5. Name of person who did prep

DRAPING

Draping is the procedure of covering the patient and surrounding areas with a sterile barrier to create and maintain an adequate sterile field. An effective barrier eliminates or minimizes passage of microorganisms between nonsterile and sterile areas. Criteria to be met in establishing an effective barrier are:

1. Blood- and fluid-resistant to keep drapes dry and prevent migration of microorganisms. Material should be impermeable to moist microbial penetration (i.e., resistant to strike-through).
2. Resistant to tear, puncture, or abrasion that causes fiber breakdown and thus permits microbial penetration.
3. Lint free to reduce airborne contaminants and shedding into the surgical site. Cellulose and cotton fibers can cause granulomatous peritonitis or embolize arteries.

4. Antistatic to eliminate risk of a spark from static electricity. Material must meet standards of National Fire Protection Association.
5. Sufficiently porous to eliminate heat buildup so as to maintain an isothermic environment appropriate for patient's body temperature.
6. Drapable to fit around contours of patient, furniture, and equipment.
7. Dull, nonglaring to minimize color distortion from reflected light.
8. Free of toxic ingredients, such as laundry residues, and nonfast dyes.
9. Flame-resistant to self-extinguish rapidly on removal of an ignition source. This is a concern with use of lasers, electrosurgical units, and other high-energy devices, which provide an ignition source at the sterile field. Drapes become fuel for a fire. Some materials are more flammable than others; some are fire-retardant.

Draping Materials

Self-Adhering Plastic Sheeting

Sterile, waterproof, antistatic, and transparent or translucent plastic sheeting may be applied to dry skin.

Incise Drape The entire drape has an adhesive backing that is applied to skin. This may be applied separately or the sheeting may be incorporated into the drape sheet. The skin incision is made through the plastic.

Antimicrobial incise drapes have an antimicrobial agent impregnated in the adhesive or the polymeric film. A film coated with an iodophor-containing adhesive, for example, slowly releases active iodine during the surgical procedure to effectively inhibit proliferation of organisms from patient's skin. The antimicrobial may be triclosan or another agent that does not contain iodine. The skin is usually prepped with alcohol and allowed to dry before the drape is applied. Time is a factor in microbial accumulation from resident bacteria. Antimicrobial incise drapes are used, particularly for procedures lasting more than 3 hours, to sustain suppression.

Towel Drape The plastic sheeting has a band of adhesive along one edge. Used as a draping towel, it will remain fixed on skin without towel clips. This is advantageous when clips might obscure the view of a part exposed to x-rays during the surgical procedure. It also is used to wall off a contaminated area, such as a stoma, from the clean skin area to prevent spilling contents and causing infection or chemical irritation.

Aperture Drape Adhesive surrounds a fenestration (opening) in the plastic sheeting. This secures the drape to the skin around the surgical site, such as an eye or ear.

NOTE Caution must be used in applying this type of drape around the face of patient who is awake. Be sure the patient has breathing space. Some patients experience claustrophobia. Fabric towels may not feel as confining.

Advantages of a self-adhering plastic drape are:

1. Resident microbial flora from skin pores, sebaceous glands, and hair follicles cannot migrate laterally to the incision.
2. Microorganisms do not penetrate through the impermeable material.
3. Landmarks and skin tones are visible through the transparent plastic.
4. Inert adhesive holds drapes securely, eliminating the need for towel clips and possible puncture of the patient's skin.
5. Plastic sheeting conforms to body contours and has elasticity to stretch without breaking adhesion to skin.

Some self-adhering drapes have sufficient moisture-vapor permeability to reduce excessive moisture buildup that could macerate the skin and/or loosen adhesive. A nonporous material should not cover more than 10% of body surface as it may interfere with the patient's thermal regulatory mechanism of perspiration evaporation. The heat-retaining property of plastic causes the patient to perspire excessively, but its nonporous nature prevents evaporation.

This material is used in the following manner:

1. Usual skin preparation is done.
2. Scrubbed area must be dried. It may dry by evaporation, or excess solution may be blotted or wiped off with a sterile sponge or towel.

   NOTE Alcohol may be applied after an iodophor scrub to hasten drying by evaporation. Ether, a highly flammable agent, is *not* recommended for skin preparation. A combination of alcohol and Freon can produce chemical irritation on skin.

1. Transparent plastic material is applied firmly to the skin with initial contact along the proposed line of incision. Smooth the drape away from the incision area.
2. Regular fabric drapes are applied over the plastic sheeting unless plastic is incorporated into the fenestrated area of the drape.

Nonwoven Fabric Drapes

Most nonwoven disposable materials are compressed layers of synthetic fibers (i.e., rayon, nylon, or polyester) combined with cellulose (wood pulp) and bonded together chemically or mechanically without knitting, tufting, or weaving. This material may be either nonabsorbent or absorbent. Polypropylene and foil also are used. Those fabrics that comply with criteria for establishing an effective barrier have the following *advantages as disposable drapes:*

1. Moisture repellancy retards blood and aqueous fluid moisture strike-through to prevent contamination

NOTE Not all nonwoven fabrics have this characteristic: only nonabsorbent materials or those laminated with plastic are impermeable to moisture.

2. Lightweight, yet strong enough to resist tears
3. Lint free, unless cellulose fibers are torn or cut
4. Contaminants are disposed of along with drapes
5. Antistatic and flame-retardant for OR use
6. Prepackaged and sterilized by manufacturer, which eliminates washing, mending, folding, and sterilizing processes

Some drapes have a reinforced area of multiple layers surrounding the fenestration. The outer layer absorbs fluids, but the underneath layer is impermeable to strike-through. An antimicrobial may be incorporated into this reinforced area. Other drapes have an impermeable layer around the fenestration. Drapes that are completely laminated with a plastic layer may be used for an extremity or for instrument table covers. They are not used over the entire body of the patient because of their heat-retention property.

Many nonwoven drapes have pouches or troughs incorporated close to the fenestration or along the sides of the drape to collect fluids. The pouch may have drainage ports, or fluid may be suctioned out. Some drapes also have pockets, skid-resistant instrument pads, and/or devices for holding cords incorporated in them (see Figure 22-7).

NOTE If blood is collected for autotransfusion from a pouch or trough, the plastic must be FDA-approved for blood recovery.

Laser-Resistant Drapes Nonwoven drapes that contain cellulose ignite and burn easily. Polypropylene drapes will not ignite, but they can melt. An aluminum-coated drape may be safest for use with lasers, especially around the oxygen-enriched environment of the head and neck area.

Thermal Drape An aluminum-coated plastic body cover reflects radiant body heat back to the patient to reduce intraoperative heat loss. (See section on inadvertent hypothermia in Chapter 19, pp. 382-383.) A sterile, nonconductive, radiolucent thermal drape may be used as the final drape. The patient may be wrapped in nonsterile reflective covers (Thermadrape) in the preoperative holding area. These may remain in place through the surgical procedure under standard sterile drapes and during postoperative recovery in the postanesthesia care unit (PACU). A reflective blanket or thermal drape is recommended when more than 60% of body surface can be covered and when surgical procedure will last more than 2 hours.

Nonwoven, disposable drapes are supplied prepackaged and presterilized by the manufacturer. A sterile package may contain a single drape, or it may have all the drapes needed for a procedure, including towels, Mayo stand and instrument table covers, and gowns. Unused disposable drapes and gowns should *not* be resterilized unless the manufacturer provides written instructions for reprocessing.

Woven Textile Fabrics

Thread count and finish of woven natural fibers determine the integrity and porosity of reusable fabrics. Tightly woven textile fabrics may inhibit migration of microorganisms. Cotton fibers swell when they become wet. This swelling action closes pores or interstices so that liquid cannot diffuse through tightly woven fibers. The fabric can be treated to further repel fluids (i.e., be impermeable to moisture strike-through). Reusable drapes may be made of 270- or 280-thread count pima cotton with a Quarpel finish. This fluorochemical finish combined with phenozopyridine or a melanin hydrophobe produces a durable water-resistant fabric. However, this fabric has essentially the same heat-retaining qualities as plastic lamination, so it cannot be used for complete patient draping. This treated material can be used as reinforcement around fenestrations in otherwise untreated drapes.

Tightly woven 100% polyester reusable fabrics are hydrophobic, repel water droplets, but allow vapor permeation. Other reusable fabrics with different construction but similar barrier properties may be used.

Points about reusable woven textile drapes to consider:

1. Material must be steam penetrable and must withstand multiple sterilization cycles.
2. When packaged for sterilization, drapes must be properly folded and arranged in sequence of use. Drapes may be fanfolded or rolled.
3. Material must be free from holes and tears. The person who folds the drape is responsible for inspecting it for holes. Those detected may be covered with heat-seal patches. Tears or punctures, as from towel clips or sharp instruments, compromise barrier qualities of drape.
4. Drapes should be sufficiently impermeable to prevent moisture from soaking through them. Moisture has a wicking action that can cause migration of microorganisms.

5. Reusable fabrics must maintain barrier qualities through multiple launderings. Densely woven treated cotton will become moisture permeable after about 75 washings, untreated cotton in as few as 30 washings. Repeated drying, ironing, and steam sterilizing also alters fabric structure. Number of uses, washings, and sterilizing cycles should be recorded, and drapes that are no longer effective as barriers should be taken out of use.

Style/Type of Drapes

Towels

Towels may be used to outline the surgical site. The folded edge of each towel is placed toward the line of incision. When reusable fabric is packaged, four towels intended for this purpose can be placed together with the folded edges graduated. Nonabsorbent disposable towels are used for this technique. Towels usually are secured with towel clips but may be sutured or stapled to skin.

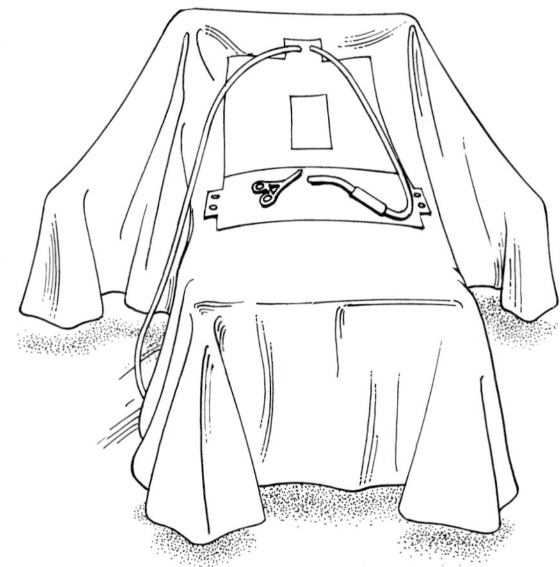

FIGURE 22-7 Fenestrated laparotomy drape sheet with reinforcement around fenestration.

Fenestrated Sheets

The drape sheet has an opening (fenestration) that is placed to expose the anatomic area where the incision will be made. Many styles of disposable nonwoven or reusable woven fabrics are available for specific uses. The size, direction, and shape of the fenestration vary to give adequate exposure of the surgical site. The sheet is long enough to cover the anesthesia screen at the head and extend down over the foot of table. Fenestrated sheets are usually marked to indicate the direction in which they should be unfolded. This may be an arrow or label designating *top* or *head, bottom* or *foot*. It is wide enough to cover one or two armboards.

Reinforcement around the fenestration (Figure 22-7) for both nonwoven and woven fabrics provides an extra thickness to minimize the passage of microorganisms from nonsterile area under the drape to the sterile field. The reinforced area is usually 24 inches (60 cm) wide.

Drapes described are basic styles of fenestrated sheets.

Laparotomy Sheet The laparotomy sheet is often called a *lap sheet;* the longitudinal fenestration is placed over the surgical site on the abdomen, back, or a comparable area (Figure 22-7). The opening, about 40 inches (102 cm) from the top in the center of the sheet, is 9 × 4 inches (23 × 10 cm), which is large enough to give adequate exposure in the usual laparotomy. The sheet is at least 108 × 72 inches (274 × 183 cm). It is unfolded toward the feet first (see Figure 22-9).

Thyroid Sheet The thyroid sheet is the same size as a laparotomy sheet. The fenestration is transverse and closer to top of the sheet.

Breast Sheet The breast sheet is the same as a laparotomy sheet except that the fenestration is 11 × 11 inches (28 × 28 cm), which provides for a larger exposure. Besides its use for breast procedures, it is used for surgical procedures within chest cavity.

Kidney Sheet The kidney sheet is the same size as a laparotomy sheet. The fenestration is transverse to accommodate a transverse kidney incision.

Hip Sheet The hip sheet is the same as a laparotomy sheet except that it is somewhat longer to completely cover the orthopaedic fracture table.

Perineal Sheet The perineal sheet is of adequate size to create a sterile field with the patient in the lithotomy position. It has large boots incorporated into it to cover the legs in stirrups. It has an opening 6½ to 7 inches (17 cm) in diameter with a 10-inch (25 cm) reinforcement around it.

Combined Sheet A combined sheet is a combination laparotomy and perineal sheet. It is used for combined abdominoperineal resection of the rectum when the entire procedure is done with the patient in lithotomy position. It has two fenestrations.

Separate Sheets

Although fenestrated sheets are used for most surgical procedures, they are not always practical. The openings may be much too large for small incisions, such as taking specimens for biopsies, procedures on hands or feet, etc. Smaller, separate sheets may be used for these purposes, leaving exposed only the small surgical area, or for providing additional drapes on the surgical field.

Split Sheet The split sheet is the same size as a laparotomy sheet. Rather than being fenestrated, one end is cut longitudinally up the middle at least one third the length of sheet to form two free ends (tails). The upper end of this split may be U-shaped. Bands may be sewn on each tail approximately 8 inches (20 cm) from the end of the split to snug sheet around an extremity or head.

Minor Sheet The minor sheet is 36 × 45 inches (91 × 114 cm). It has many uses. Wrapped around an extremity, it permits the extremity to remain on the sterile field for manipulation during the surgical procedure. It is used under an arm to cover an armboard for shoulder, axillary, arm, or hand procedures.

Medium Sheet The medium sheet is about 36 × 72 inches (91 × 183 cm). It is used to drape under legs, as an added protection above or below the surgical area, or for draping areas in which a fenestrated sheet cannot be used.

Single Sheet The single sheet is 108 × 72 inches (274 × 183 cm). Folded lengthwise, it is placed above the sterile field to shield off the anesthesiologist and anesthesia machine or other equipment near the patient's head or operating table. A single sheet also is used to cover the patient and operating table below the surgical area around the face.

Leg-Pocket Drapes Leg-pocket drapes are supplied in pairs to cover the legs of a patient in the lithotomy position. A rectangle, approximately 36 × 72 inches (91 × 183 cm), is closed on two sides to form a tentlike pocket. One open edge is folded into a cuff to protect gloves from contamination during application.

Stockinette

Stockinette is used to cover an extremity. This seamless tubing of stretchable material contours snugly to the skin. The material is very porous and absorbent, so it is not a microbial barrier. Therefore it may be covered with a layer of plastic. A two-ply tubular disposable drape is available that has an inner layer of stockinette and an outer layer of vinyl. An opening is cut through the material over the line of incision. Edges may be secured with a plastic incise drape before the incision is made, or it may be clipped to the wound edges after the incision.

Techniques to Remember in Draping

Because draping is a very important step in the preparation of the patient for a surgical procedure, it must be done correctly. The entire team should be familiar with the draping procedure. The scrub person must know it perfectly and be ready to assist with it. Check beforehand to see that necessary articles are arranged in proper sequence on the instrument table.

The person responsible for draping the patient may vary, as do materials and styles of drapes used to create a sterile field. The surgeon or assistant usually places the self-adhering drape and/or towels and towel clips to outline the surgical site. The scrub person assists with placing the remainder of drapes.

During any draping procedure, the circulator should stand by to direct the scrub person as necessary and to watch carefully for breaks in technique. A contaminated drape or exposure of a nonsterile area is a potential source of infection for the patient.

1. Place drapes on a dry area. The area around or under the patient may become damp from solutions used for skin preparation. The circulator must remove damp items or cover the area to provide a dry field on which to lay sterile drapes.
2. Allow sufficient time to permit careful application.
3. Allow sufficient space to observe sterile technique.
4. Handle drapes as little as possible.
5. Never reach across the operating table to drape the opposite side; go around the table.
6. Take towels and towel clips, if used, to the side of the table from which the surgeon is going to apply them before handing them to him or her.
7. Carry *folded drapes* to the operating table. Watch the front of the sterile gown; it may bulge and touch the nonsterile table or blanket on the patient. Stand well back from the nonsterile table.
8. Hold drapes high enough to avoid touching nonsterile areas, but avoid touching the overhead operating light.
9. Hold drape high until it is directly over proper area, then lay it down where it is to remain. Once a sheet is placed, do not adjust it. Be careful not to slide the sheet out of place when opening the folds. If a drape is incorrectly placed, discard it. The circulator peels it from table without contaminating other drapes or the prepped area.
10. Protect gloved hands by cuffing the end of the sheet over them. Do not let gloved hands touch the skin of the patient.
11. In unfolding a sheet from the prepped area toward the foot or head of the table, protect the gloved hand by enclosing it in a turned-back cuff of sheet provided for this purpose. Keep hands at table level.
12. If a drape becomes contaminated, do not handle it further. Discard it without contaminating gloves or other items.

13. If the end of a sheet falls below waist level, do not handle it further. Drop it and use another.
14. If in doubt as to its sterility, consider a drape contaminated.
15. A towel clip that has been fastened through a drape has its points contaminated. Remove it only if absolutely necessary, then discard it from sterile setup without touching points. Cover the area from which it was removed with another piece of sterile draping material.
16. If a hole is found in a drape after it is laid down, the hole must be covered with another piece of draping material or the entire drape discarded.
17. A hair found on a drape must be removed and the area covered immediately. Although hair can be sterilized, the source of a hair is usually unknown when it is found on a sterile drape. It would cause a foreign-body tissue reaction in a patient if it got into the wound. Remove the hair with a hemostat and hand instrument off sterile field; cover the area with a towel or another piece of draping material.

Procedures for Draping Patient

Draping procedures establish the sterile field. Standardized methods of application should be practiced using adequate draping materials. The most common procedures are discussed here merely to elaborate the principles. *The following details procedures using only absorbent woven draping materials* because it is more complex to establish a microbial barrier with them. The draping procedure is simplified when single-thickness, impermeable materials are used. Consult the procedure book for specific draping procedures.

Laparotomy

The term *laparotomy* refers to an incision through the abdominal wall into the abdominal cavity. All flat, smooth areas are draped in the same manner as the abdomen. These areas include the neck, chest, flank, and back.

1. Hand up four towels and towel clips. With practice these can be held in the hands at the same time and separated one by one as the surgeon takes them. Go to the side of the table on which the surgeon is draping to avoid reaching over the nonsterile table. The surgeon places these towels within the prepped area, leaving only the surgical area exposed.
2. Hand one end of a fanfolded medium sheet across the table to the assistant, supporting the folds, keeping it high, and holding it taut until it is opened; then lay it down. Place this medium sheet below the surgical site with the edge of it at the skin edge, covering the draping towel. This sheet provides an extra thickness of material under the area from the Mayo stand to the incision, where instruments and sponges are placed, and closes some of the opening in the laparotomy sheet if necessary. This sheet may be eliminated if a self-adhering incise drape or impermeable drapes are used.
3. Place a laparotomy sheet with the opening directly over the prepped area outlined by the towels in the direction indicated for the foot or head of the table. Drop the folds over the sides of the table. However, if an armboard is in place, hold the folds at table level until the sheet is opened all the way. Open it downward over the patient's feet and upward over anesthesia screen (Figures 22-8 and 22-9).

   NOTE Sheets with appropriate fenestrations are used to expose the surgical site.
   - For the neck, use a thyroid sheet.
   - For the chest, with patient in either supine or lateral position, use a breast sheet.
   - For the flank, with patient in kidney position for transverse incision, use a kidney sheet.
   - For the back, use a laparotomy sheet the same as for the abdomen.
4. Place a large single sheet crosswise on the table above the fenestrated site. This sheet provides an extra thickness above the area and closes some of the opening in the laparotomy sheet if necessary. It also covers the armboard if one is in use. A single sheet may be needed for this latter purpose even if an impermeable lap sheet is used.

Head

An overhead instrument table may be positioned over the patient. The table drape is extended down over the patient's shoulders to create a continuous sterile field between the instrument table and surgical site.

1. Surgeon places four towels around the head and secures them with towel clips or affixes them in place with sutures or skin staples. Towel clips and staples are not used if x-ray films will be taken during the surgical procedure.
2. Hand one end of a fanfolded medium sheet to the assistant. Holding it taut, unfold and secure it over head end of the operating table below the surgical site at the skin edge of the draping towel.
3. Place a fenestrated sheet with the opening over the exposed skin area of the head. Unfold the sheet across front edge of the overhead table and secure it before allowing the remainder of the drape to drop over head of operating table toward the floor.

NOTE If a split sheet is used, the tails are placed toward the head end of the operating table, draped around the patient's head, and secured with towel clips.

Face

Even if the surgical site is unilateral, the surgeon may want the entire face exposed for comparison of skin lines.

1. Surgeon places a drape under the head while the circulator holds up the head. This drape consists of a towel placed on a medium sheet. The center of the towel edge is 2 inches (5 cm) in from the center of the sheet edge. The towel is drawn up on each side of the face, over the forehead or at hairline, and fastened with a clip. This leaves the desired amount of the face exposed.
2. Hand up three more towels and four towel clips. These four towels surround the surgical site.
3. Place a medium sheet just below the site. This sheet must overlap the one under the head.
4. A fenestrated drape may be placed to complete draping.
5. Cover the remainder of the foot of the table, as necessary, with a single sheet.

NOTE

- If the patient is receiving inhalation anesthesia, use a minor sheet instead of a towel on a medium sheet for the first drape under head. A minor sheet is large enough to draw up on each side of the face and to enclose breathing tubes from the anesthesia machine for a considerable distance, thus keeping them from contaminating the sterile field.
- If the surgical procedure on the face is unilateral, the anesthesiologist may sit along the unaffected side, near the patient's head, with the anesthesia screen placed on this side of the table.
- Wide skin staples may be used to affix towels around the contours of the face and neck. Each staple overlaps the skin and edge of drape.

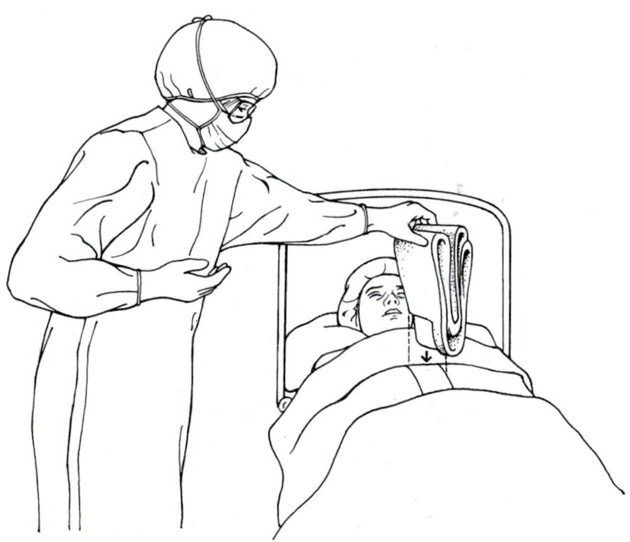

FIGURE 22-8 Draping with sterile laparotomy sheet. Scrub person carries folded sheet to table. Standing far back from table, with one hand scrub person lays sheet on patient so opening in sheet is directly over prepared skin area.

Eye

After the skin prep, protect the unaffected eye by covering it with a sterile eye pad before draping the patient.

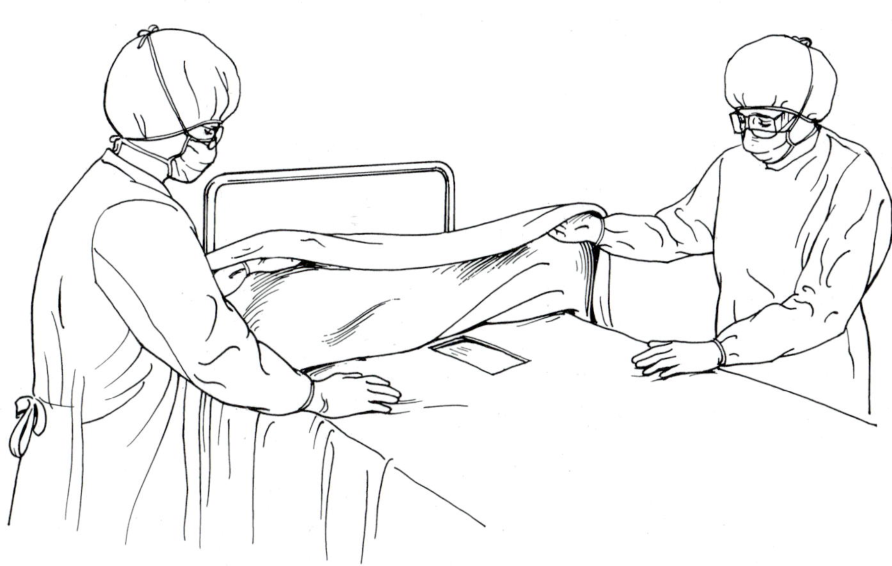

FIGURE 22-9 Unfolding upper end of laparotomy sheet over anesthesia screen. Note that hands approaching unsterile area are protected in cuff of drape and sheet is stabilized with other hands.

1. Surgeon places two towels and a medium sheet under the head while the circulator holds the head up, as described for face drape. One towel is drawn up around the head, exposing only the eyebrow and affected eye, and fastened with a clip without pressure on the eyes.
2. Hand up four towels and towel clips to isolate the affected eye. Some surgeons prefer a self-adhering aperture drape.
3. Cover the patient and remainder of the table below the surgical area with a single sheet.

NOTE

- If local anesthetic will be administered, the drapes must be raised off the patient's nose and mouth to permit free breathing. A Mayo stand or anesthesia screen positioned over the lower face before the draping will elevate the drapes. Oxygen, 6 to 8 L/min, can be supplied under the drapes by tube or nasal cannula.
- For a microsurgical procedure, a sterile U-shaped steel wrist rest for the surgeon and assistant is fastened to the head of the table after towels are put around the patient's head, before the rest of draping is completed.
- If irrigation will be used, a plastic fenestrated drape is placed over the four towels to keep them dry if an aperture drape is not preferred.

Ear

Basic draping procedure is the same as for draping a face or eye, except that only the affected ear is exposed. The head will be turned toward the unaffected side. Oxygen can be supplied under the drapes, as previously described.

Chest and Breast

While the arm is still being held up following skin preparation:

1. Place a minor sheet on armboard, under the patient's arm, extending the sheet under the side of the chest and shoulder. The person who has been holding the arm lays it on the armboard and fastens it with a wrist strap. The distal portion of the arm may be encased in sterile stockinette so that the arm can be manipulated during the surgical procedure.
2. Hand up towels and towel clips; five or six are required.
3. Apply a breast sheet so axilla is exposed for anticipated axillary dissection.

Shoulder

While the arm is still being held up following skin preparation:

1. Place a medium sheet over the chest and under the arm.
2. Place a minor sheet under the shoulder and side of chest.
3. Surgeon outlines the surgical site with towels and secures them with clips.
4. Place a minor sheet over the patient's chest, covering the neck. Keep this sheet even with edge of the towel that limits the surgical site laterally.
5. Wrap the arm in a minor sheet or encase it in sterile stockinette and secure it with a sterile gauze bandage. At this point, a sterile team member relieves unsterile person who has been holding the arm.
6. Place a medium sheet above the area and secure these sheets together with towel clips.
7. Laparotomy or breast sheet may be used. Pull the arm through the opening. Or a single sheet may be placed above the area and the foot of the table covered with a medium sheet.

Elbow

While the arm is still being held up following skin preparation:

1. Place a medium sheet across the chest and under the arm, up to axilla.
2. Surgeon defines the surgical area on the upper arm by placing a towel around the arm and securing it with a clip.
3. Wrap the hand and lower arm in a minor sheet or a double thickness of towel and secure it with a sterile bandage. At this point, a sterile team member relieves unsterile person who has been holding the arm.
4. Draw stockinette over the exposed surgical site.
5. Place a medium sheet across the chest, on top of the arm, even with the towel on the upper arm and covering it. Secure this sheet around the arm with a towel clip.
6. Lay a laparotomy sheet over the hand and pull the arm through it, opening the sheet across the patient. Cover foot of the table with a medium sheet.

Hand

While arm and hand are still being held up following skin preparation:

1. Place an impervious minor sheet, folded in half, on the armboard or extremity table.
2. Surgeon places a towel around the lower arm, limiting the exposed area to the affected hand, and secures it with a towel clip.
3. Pull stockinette over the hand. At this stage in draping, the unsterile person is relieved of holding the arm. The arm is laid on the armboard.

4. Place a minor sheet across the armboard just above the surgical site.
5. Place a laparotomy sheet on the hand with foot end toward the patient. Do not drop folds *below* the level of the armboard. Open lap sheet across the patient's body.
6. Place a medium sheet below the laparotomy sheet to finish covering the patient.
7. Place a single sheet over the anesthesia screen.

Perineum

With the patient in lithotomy position for a genital, vaginal, or rectal procedure:

1. Place a medium sheet under the buttocks. The circulator can grasp the under sides and assist in placement. With the patient's legs elevated in stirrups, this drape hangs below the level of the table and covers the lowered section of the operating table.
2. Slide leg-pocket drape over each leg, protecting gloved hands in the folded cuffs, if this type of leg cover is used.
3. Hand up three towels and four towel clips for the surgeon to square off the perineum. The anus is covered if not part of the surgical site. An adhesive towel drape may be used for this purpose.
4. Place a medium sheet across the abdomen, from the level of the pubis, extending over the anesthesia screen.

NOTE A fenestrated perineal sheet may be used rather than a pair of leg-pocket drapes. After towels are placed, hand one end of sheet to the assistant, opening out folds, and draw the boots over the feet and legs simultaneously. Hands are kept on the outside of the sheet to avoid contaminating gloves and gowns.

Hip

If the leg will be manipulated during the surgical procedure, while the leg is still being held up following skin preparation:

1. Place a medium sheet on the table under the leg, up to the buttock.
2. Place another medium sheet on the table, overlapping the first one, to cover the unaffected leg.
3. Surgeon wraps a towel around the thigh, just below the surgical site, and clips or sews it in place if x-ray films will be taken.
4. Hand up additional towels to surround the surgical area, with towel clips to secure them.
5. Surgeon wraps the foot and leg, including a towel around the thigh, in a minor sheet and bandages it on. Some surgeons prefer to use stockinette. The leg, held up to this point, is laid on the table.
6. Place a minor sheet lengthwise of the table on each side of the exposed area, even with the skin. The sheets under the leg and above the site do not overlap.

NOTE Some surgeons prefer to omit step 6 and draw the leg through the opening of a hip sheet or place a split sheet under the leg with the tails crossed over it toward the patient's head.

7. Place a medium sheet above the exposed area. Secure these last three sheets with towel clips.
8. Place a single sheet above the surgical area and over the anesthesia screen.

If manipulation of the leg is not necessary during the surgical procedure, drape the same as for a laparotomy, using a hip sheet instead of a laparotomy sheet.

Knee

While the leg is still being held up following skin preparation:

1. Place a medium sheet lengthwise on the table, under the leg, up to the buttock.
2. Place another medium sheet on the table overlapping the first sheet to cover the unaffected leg.
3. Surgeon limits the sterile field above the knee by placing a towel around the leg and securing it with a towel clip.
4. Lay a minor sheet on the sterile sheets under the leg. The person who has been holding the leg lays it on this minor sheet. The surgeon wraps the leg in the minor sheet and secures it with a sterile bandage. Stockinette may be preferred for this step.
5. Place a medium sheet above exposed area, at skin edge, over the draping towel, and fasten it with a towel clip.
6. Place a laparotomy sheet, with the opening on foot and the longer part of the sheet toward the table head. Open it and draw the leg through the opening. A split sheet may be used.

Lower Leg and Ankle

While the leg is still being held up following skin preparation:

1. Place a medium sheet under the leg and over the unaffected leg to above the knees.
2. Surgeon limits the sterile field by placing a towel around the leg above the area of the intended surgical site and securing it with a towel clip.
3. Put stockinette over the foot and draw it up over the leg to above the skin edge of the towel. The person who has been holding the leg is relieved, and the leg is held by a sterile team member.
4. Place a medium sheet above the surgical area, and secure around the leg with a towel clip.

5. Place a laparotomy sheet or split sheet with the leg drawn through the opening.
6. Cover the remainder of the table over the anesthesia screen with a single sheet as necessary.

Foot

The general method of draping a foot is the same as that for hand. While the foot is still being held up following skin preparation:

1. Place a medium sheet on table under foot.
2. Surgeon limits exposed area to the foot by placing a towel around the ankle and securing it with a towel clip.
3. Enclose the foot in stockinette. A sterile team member relieves unsterile person who has been holding the leg.
4. Place a medium sheet above the foot, and secure it around the ankle with a towel clip.
5. Place a laparotomy sheet with the opening over the foot and longer part of the sheet toward the head of the table.

Draping of Equipment

A pneumatic tourniquet (see Chapter 23, pp. 474-476) frequently is used to control bleeding during surgical procedures on the upper and lower extremities. The tourniquet cuff is placed around the extremity before skin preparation. It is enclosed within (i.e., covered by) the draping material. The towel that delineates the upper limit of the surgical area is placed around the extremity below the tourniquet cuff.

Equipment that is brought into the sterile field but cannot be sterilized must be draped before it is handled by sterile team members.

1. Tailored disposable drapes are available to cover equipment, such as the operating microscope, so it can be manipulated in the sterile field by surgeon.
2. If x-ray films are to be taken during the surgical procedure, a cassette holder may be placed on the operating table, under the patient, before the patient is positioned, prepped, and draped. The circulator raises the drape for the radiology technician to place and remove the cassette. The holder and/or cassette may be covered with a sterile Mayo stand cover or specially designed disposable cover and placed on sterile drapes when a lateral view is needed.
3. Cords, attachments, or tubings that are not sterile must be inserted into sterile coverings before they are placed on the sterile field.

Nonsterile equipment that must stand near the sterile field must be excluded from the sterile area by a drape shield. IV poles frequently are used to attach drapes to shield off power-generating sources of mechanical and electrical equipment, such as electrosurgical and cryosurgical units, fiberoptic lighting units, and air-powered or electrical instruments. The drape over the patient or a separate single sheet is extended from the operating table upward in front of or over the nonsterile equipment. The circulator fastens the drape to IV poles on each side of the equipment that stands above level of the sterile field or near it.

NOTE Heat-generating equipment must have adequate ventilation to dissipate heat. Impermeable, heat-retaining materials cannot completely encase these units.

Some nonsterile equipment, of necessity, will be moved over the sterile field. The sterile field must be protected.

1. Sterile disposable drapes are available to cover x-ray equipment, image intensifiers, etc.
2. When ready to move an x-ray tube or image intensifier over the sterile field, cover the field with a minor sheet. Discard this sheet after use.
3. Photographic equipment and video cameras should be draped as much as feasible when used over the sterile field.

PLASTIC ISOLATOR

A plastic isolator (a shield around the patient's bed or the operating table) may be used to exclude microorganisms from the environment immediately surrounding the patient. It may isolate a patient who is highly susceptible to infection, such as a burned or immunosuppressed patient, or it may isolate a patient with a gross infection and provide protection for others. In the OR, plastic isolators are used to isolate the sterile field from both room air and OR team and thus exclude microorganisms normally in the OR environment.

The portable, lightweight, optically transparent surgical isolator forms a bubble over the patient when inflated. This *surgical isolation bubble system (SIBS)* has two elements: a filter/blower unit and a prepackaged sterile, disposable bubble. Its floor provides a sterile drape that adheres to prepared skin around incision site. Built into the sides are ports (armholes) through which the team works and a port for passing sterile supplies from the circulator.

A patient isolation drape may be used that is a modification of the total isolator. It isolates the sterile field from equipment, such as the C-arm image intensifier used for hip procedures. The drape is suspended from a steel frame but does not enclose the patient. The incise portion of the drape may be impregnated with a time-release iodophor. Storage and irrigation pouches are incorporated into the side.

Bibliography

Belkin NL: Barrier materials, *AORN J* 55(6):1521-1528, 1992.

Chevalier J, Cremieux A: Comparative study on the antimicrobial effects of hexamedine and Betadine on the human skin flora, *J Appl Bacteriol* 73(4):342-348, 1992.

Gauthier DK et al: Clean vs sterile surgical skin preparation kits, *AORN J* 58(3):486-495, 1993.

Hedin G, Hambraeus A: Daily scrub with chlorhexidine reduces skin colonization by antibiotic-resistant *Staphylococcus epidermis, J Hosp Infect* 24(1):47-51, 1993.

Howard RJ: Comparison of a 10-minute aqueous iodophor and a 2-minute water-insoluble iodophor in alcohol preoperative skin preparation, *Complications Surg* 10(7):43-45, 1991.

Jepsen OB, Bruttomesso KA: The effectiveness of preoperative skin preparations, *AORN J* 58(3):477-484, 1993.

Kovach T: Nip it in the bud: controlling wound infection with preoperative shaving, *Today's OR Nurse* 12(9):23-26, 1990.

Kutarski PW, Grundy HC: To dry or not to dry: an assessment of the possible degradation in efficacy of preoperative skin preparation caused by wiping skin dry, *Ann R Coll Surg Engl* 75(3):181-185, 1993.

Mathias JM: Do surgical prep sets need to be sterile? *OR Manager* 7(6):1, 13, 1991.

Murphy L: Cost/benefit study of reusable and disposable OR draping materials, *J Healthcare Material Manage* 11(4):44-48, 1993.

Murphy L: Preoperative skin preparation of patients, *Plast Surg Nurs* 13(2):101, 1993.

O'Neal M: Clinical issues: preoperative shaves,..., *AORN J* 54(3):604-606, 1991.

Patterson P: An examination of three draping questions, *OR Manager* 6(8):14-15, 1990.

Patterson P: Draping: what's necessary, what's proven, *OR Manager* 6(7):1, 15-16, 1990.

Patterson P: Hair clipping superior to preoperative shave, *OR Manager* 6(2):6-7, 1990.

Patterson P: Reusable textiles with a new look make OR comeback, *OR Manager* 10(3):1, 6-9, 1994.

Recommended practices: Protective barrier materials for surgical gowns and drapes, *AORN J* 55(3):832-835, 1992.

Recommended practices: Skin preparation of patients, *AORN J* 56(5):937-941, 1992.

Smith CD: Clinical issues: combined vaginal/abdominal preps; seated personnel, *AORN J* 59(6):1313-1318, 1994.

Solitz TJ: Using an abdominal pouch drape to control fluid spills during liver transplantations, *AORN J* 52(5):1071-1075, 1990.

Welch T: Advances in surgical draping: weaving a non-linen future, *Br J Theatre Nurs* 27(3):26-27, 1990.

CHAPTER 23

Hemostasis and Blood Loss Replacement

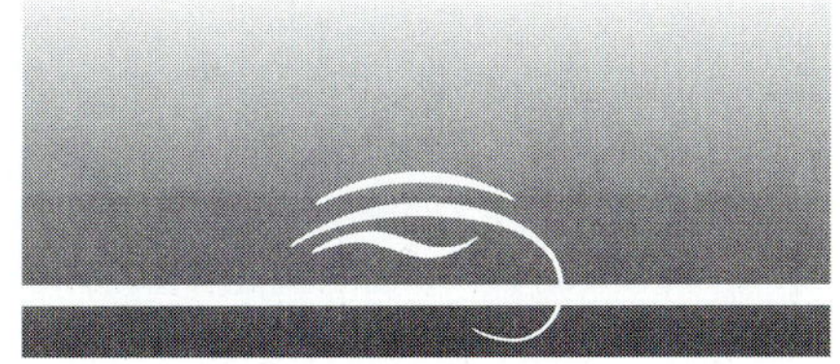

HISTORICAL BACKGROUND

From Egyptian artifacts and writings, historians believe that surgery dates back to 6000 BC. The first surgical procedures probably were performed to control hemorrhage and to close war injuries. Tourniquets were used to control bleeding. Mummies that have been exhumed reveal wounds that were sewn together with sutures.

Around 1000 BC, Homer described the Greek method of caring for battle wounds. They were cleansed, hemorrhages were controlled with crushed roots and leaves, and then the wounds were covered with compresses.

Hippocrates (460-377 BC) noted the analgesic action of temperature as a therapeutic entity. He used ice and snow to control bleeding. Although the effects of cold as well as ligatures were known to him, Hippocrates recommended hot irons to stop hemorrhage. This custom persisted for more than 2000 years.

Even in early times, it was known that loss of blood meant loss of life. However, the circulation of blood was not understood. The writings of Aristotle (384-322 BC) reveal that veins were thought to contain all or most of the blood. Arteries were thought to contain air, with only a small amount of blood. This doctrine continued until the physiologist Galen (130-200 AD) demonstrated in the second century that arteries, like veins, contain blood, which he believed just ebbed and flowed. This theory held for about 1500 years, until William Harvey (1578-1657), an English anatomist, realized that blood circulated and could flow only in one direction. His prediction that it passed from arteries to veins through capillaries was proved under the microscope in 1661 by Marcello Malpighi (1628-1694), an Italian anatomist.

Galen emphasized the importance of avoiding further injury to arteries, muscles, and nerves during the treatment of war wounds. To stop the flow of blood from a vein, he suggested grasping it with a hook and twisting it moderately. If bleeding was from an artery, he said a ligature of linen should be applied.

Hemostasis, as practiced by early surgeons, combined styptics with pressure, bandages, and elevation of the part. Surgeons used materials at hand to cover the wound to create a framework for a blood clot. Hare's fur, shredded bark of trees, egg yolk, dust, or cobwebs were bandaged onto a bleeding part. The early lithotomists who cut into the bladder to remove stones controlled bleeding by assigning an assistant to compress the ends of vessels between his fingers until bleeding stopped.

Through the Middle Ages, gangrene was thought to be the natural result of wounds. The accepted treatment for bleeding and infection was boiling oil and hot irons. One day in the sixteenth century Ambroise Paré (1509-1590), a French army barber-surgeon, found that his supply of oil was inadequate to treat the many wounded on the battlefield. He hastily concocted poultices of egg yolk, oil of roses, and turpentine. He observed that these men had less pain and their wounds healed better than those treated with boiling oil. The difference so impressed him that he never used oil again. Paré became best known, however, for the use of ligatures to control bleeding from amputations. He also was the first to grasp blood vessels with a pinching instrument.

The progress of surgery was so slow through the Renaissance era that for another 200 years after Paré's time surgeons still used the inhumane, destructive irons and boiling oil. With the advent of gunpowder in warfare, surgeons cleansed and cauterized the wounds with hot oil, believing that gunpowder poisoned wounds.

Mention is made of ligatures and sutures in writings of the early eighteenth century, as is the use of pressure on bleeding points to control bleeding. The process of coagulation was recognized also during this century, but it was believed to be the result rather than the cause of hemostasis.

In the early nineteenth century, the pus and infection present in wounds were thought to be caused by sutures because the long ends of silk or flax left hanging from wounds sloughed out. Secondary hemorrhage from abscess formation and ulceration of ligatures through vessels was common.

Before the advent of anesthesia in 1846, surgical skill was based on speed. Most surgical procedures were done for major injuries or life-threatening conditions, such as gangrene or infection in an extremity. Amputations were swift, guillotine style. Blood dripped onto the floor or into a box of sawdust.

By the end of the nineteenth century, anesthesia and asepsis made surgery a viable branch of medicine. But many technical difficulties faced the surgeon. Loss of blood was one of the most dangerous complications of surgery.

The first attempt to transfuse blood occurred in 1818 when James Blundell of London salvaged vaginal blood from a postpartum hemorrhage. By syringe he reinfused the blood into the patient. Later in the century, in 1886, John Duncan transfused blood directly from the surgical field into a trauma patient by femoral injection. Continuing into the twentieth century patients were transfused with their own (autologous) blood salvaged from body cavities. Then in 1901 Karl Landsteiner (1868-1943), an Austrian-American pathologist, discovered the blood groups A, B, and O. This led to the feasibility of donor (homologous) blood transfusions. Plasma was first used during World War I to combat shock.

The development of blood banking superseded previous attempts at autotransfusion. The first blood bank was established in 1936 at the Mayo Clinic in Rochester, Minnesota. Interest in homologous blood prospered during World War II because a large donor pool collected by the Red Cross, along with improved methods of typing and crossmatching, made banked blood easier to obtain and safer to use. Resurgence of interest in autologous blood occurred, however, during the Vietnam War with direct salvage devices. The first technically safe commercial autologous blood recovery equipment was marketed in 1971.

Transfusion of blood products, homologous or autologous, is not a substitute for blood conservation measures. Meticulous hemostasis and the use of blood volume expanders, normovolemic hemodilution, and pharmacologic agents can decrease surgical blood loss.

MECHANISM OF HEMOSTASIS

Hemostasis is essential to successful wound management. Literally, *hemostasis* is the arrest of a flow of blood or hemorrhage. The mechanism is *coagulation*, formation of a blood clot. The clotting of blood takes place in several stages by enzyme reaction.

When severed by incision or traumatic injury, a blood vessel constricts and the ends contract somewhat. Platelets rapidly clump and adhere to connective tissue at the cut end of a constricted vessel. Interaction with collagen fibers causes platelets to liberate adenosine diphosphate (ADP), epinephrine, and serotonin from their secretory granules. In turn, ADP causes other platelets to clump to the initial layer and to each other, forming a platelet plug. This may be sufficient in small vessels to provide primary hemostasis.

The reaction of plasma from vessels with connective tissue cells at the site of injury activates clotting factors and causes a series of other reactions. *Prothrombin*, normally present in blood, reacts with *thromboplastin*, which is released when tissues are injured. Prothrombin and thromboplastin, along with calcium ions in the blood, form *thrombin*. This requires several minutes. Thrombin unites with *fibrinogen*, a blood protein, to form *fibrin*, which is the basic structural material of blood clots. This last reaction is very rapid.

The fibrin strands reinforce the platelet plug to form a resilient hemostatic plug capable of withstanding arterial pressure when the constricted vessel relaxes. Massive thrombosis within the vessels would occur once coagulation is initiated, if it continued. However, fibrin is digested during the process. The products of this digestion, as well as antithrombins normally present in blood, act as anticoagulants. The coagulation mechanism rapidly and efficiently inhibits excessive blood loss so that excessive coagulation does not occur (Figure 23-1).

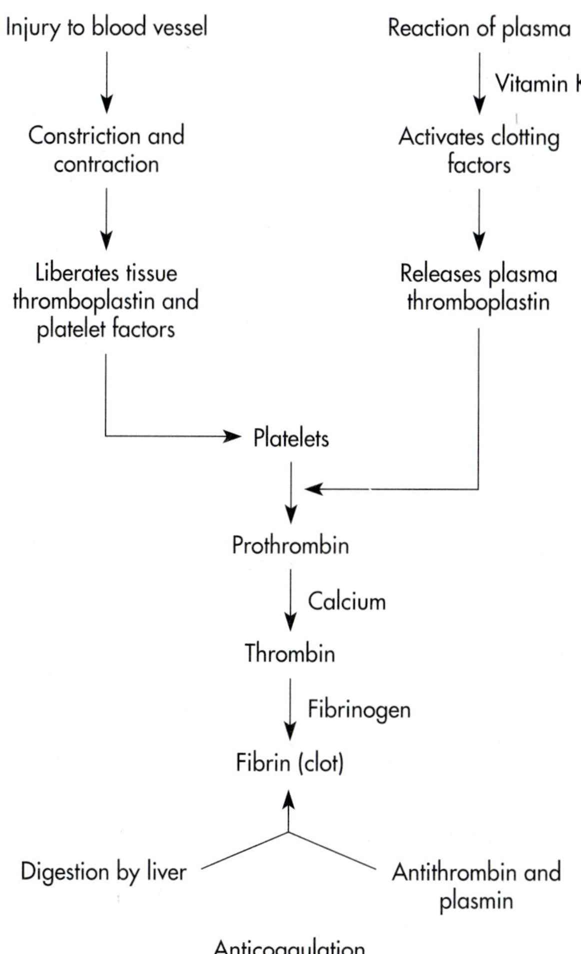

FIGURE 23-1 Mechanism of hemostasis.

METHODS OF HEMOSTASIS

Basically two types of bleeding occur during surgical procedures: gross bleeding from transected or penetrated vessels and diffuse oozing from denuded or cut surfaces. Although the need to control gross bleeding is obvious, insidious but continuous loss of blood from small vessels and capillaries can become significant if oozing is uncontrolled. Complete hemostasis, gentle tissue handling, elimination of dead space, precise wound closure, and protective wound dressing are essential to minimize trauma to tissue and to enhance healing without complication. Incomplete hemostasis may cause the formation of a hematoma. *Hematoma* is a collection of extravasated blood in a body cavity, space, or tissue caused by uncontrolled bleeding or oozing. It may be painful and firm to the touch. Some hematomas require evacuation to prevent infection; others reabsorb with time.

Numerous agents, devices, and sophisticated pieces of equipment are used to achieve hemostasis and wound closure. These various methods can be classified as chemical, mechanical, and thermal.

Chemical Methods

Absorbable Gelatin

Available in either powder or compressed-pad form, gelatin (Gelfoam) is an absorbable hemostatic agent made from purified gelatin solution that has been beaten to a foamy consistency, dried, and sterilized by dry heat. As a pad, it is available in an assortment of sizes that can be cut as desired without crumbling. When it is placed on an area of capillary bleeding, fibrin is deposited in the interstices and the sponge swells, forming a substantial clot. The sponge is not soluble; it absorbs 45 times its own weight in blood. It is denatured to retard absorption, which takes place in 20 to 40 days. It is frequently soaked in thrombin or epinephrine solution, although it may be used alone. Before a gelatin sponge is handed to the surgeon, it is dipped into warm saline, if used without thrombin or epinephrine, and pressed between the fingers or against the sides of the basin to remove air from it. The same procedure is used with thrombin or epinephrine solution, but then the sponge is dropped back into the solution and allowed to absorb solution back to its original size.

In powder form, gelatin is mixed with sterile saline to make a paste for application to cancellous bone to control bleeding or to denuded areas of skin or muscles to stimulate growth of granulation tissue.

Absorbable Collagen

Hemostatic sponges (Collastat, Superstat, Helistat) or felt (Lyostypt) of collagen origin are applied *dry* to oozing or bleeding sites. The collagen activates the coagulation mechanism, especially the aggregation of platelets, to accelerate clot formation. The material dissolves as hemostasis occurs. Any residual will absorb in the wound. Because of an affinity for wet surfaces, it must be kept dry and should be applied with dry gloves or instruments. Absorbable collagen is contraindicated in the presence of infection or in areas where blood or other fluids have pooled. It is applied directly to bleeding surface as supplied from the sterile package.

Microfibrillar Collagen

Available in compacted nonwoven web form or in loose fibrous form, microfibrillar collagen (Avitene, Instat) is an absorbable topical hemostatic agent. It is produced from a hydrochloric acid salt of purified bovine corium collagen. It is applied *dry*. When it is placed in contact with a bleeding surface, hemostasis is achieved by adhesion of platelets and prompt fibrin deposition within the interstices of the collagen. Tissue cohesion is an inherent property of the collagen itself. It functions as a hemostatic agent only when it is applied directly to the source of bleeding from raw, oozing surfaces including bone and friable tissues or directly to active bleeding from irregular contours, crevices, and around suture lines. Firm pressure must be applied quickly with a dry gauze sponge, which is held either by the fingers in accessible areas or a sponge forceps in less accessible areas. It is important that the material be compressed firmly against the bleeding surface before excessive wetting with blood can occur. Effective application is evidenced by a firm adherent coagulum with no break-through bleeding from either surface or edges. Excess material should be removed from around the site without recreating bleeding. The remaining coagulum absorbs during wound healing.

Oxidized Cellulose

Absorbable oxidation products of cellulose are available in the form of a pad of oxidized cellulose (Oxycel) similar to absorbent cotton or oxidized regenerated cellulose in a knitted fabric strip that is of low density (Surgicel) or high density (Surgical Nu-Knit). These products may be sutured to, wrapped around, or held firmly against a bleeding site or laid dry on an oozing surface until hemostasis is obtained. When oxidized cellulose comes into contact with whole blood, a clot forms rapidly. As it reacts with blood, it increases in size to form a gel and stops bleeding in areas in which bleeding is difficult to control by other means of hemostasis. Except in situations in which packing is required as a lifesaving measure, only the minimal amount required to control capillary or venous bleeding is used. If left on oozing surfaces, it will absorb with minimal tissue reaction. It is not recommended for use on bone unless it is removed after hemostasis because it may interfere with bone regeneration. Oxidized regenerated cellulose has some bactericidal properties, but it is not a substitute for antimicrobial agents.

Oxytocin

Oxytocin is a hormone produced by the pituitary gland. It can be prepared synthetically for therapeutic injection. This is sometimes used to induce labor. It also causes contraction of the uterus after delivery of the placenta. It is a systemic agent used to control hemorrhage from the uterus, rather than a hemostatic agent per se.

Phenol and Alcohol

Some surgeons use 95% phenol to cauterize tissue when cutting across the lumen of the appendix or gastrointestinal tract. Phenol coagulates proteins and in high concentration is so caustic that it can cause severe burns. Therefore it must be neutralized with 95% alcohol as soon as the surgeon has used it; burning action continues until the phenol is neutralized with alcohol.

Styptics

A styptic is an agent that checks hemorrhage by causing *vasoconstriction,* contraction of blood vessels. Styptics have the disadvantage of being rapidly carried away by the bloodstream.

Epinephrine A hormone of the adrenal gland, epinephrine (Adrenalin) is prepared synthetically for use as a vasoconstrictor to prolong the action of local anesthetic agents or to decrease bleeding. Used in some local anesthetic agents to constrict the vessels locally, epinephrine keeps the anesthetic concentrated within the area injected and reduces the amount of bleeding when the incision is made. However, it is rapidly dispersed, leaving little local effect. Within the incision, gelatin sponges soaked in 1:1000 epinephrine may be applied to bleeding surfaces. These are especially useful in ear and microsurgical procedures in which localized hemostasis is critical.

Silver Nitrate Crystals of silver nitrate in solution or mixed with silver chloride and molded into applicator sticks are applied topically. Both an astringent and an antimicrobial, silver nitrate is most commonly used in the treatment of burns. It may be used to seal areas of previous surgical incisions that fail to heal with time.

Tannic Acid A powder made from an astringent plant, tannic acid is used occasionally on mucous membranes of the nose and throat to help stop capillary bleeding.

Thrombin

An enzyme extracted from bovine blood is used therapeutically as a topical hemostatic agent. Thrombin accelerates coagulation of blood and controls capillary bleeding. It unites rapidly with fibrinogen to form a clot. Topically it may be used as a dry powder to sprinkle on an oozing surface or as a solution, alone or to saturate a gelatin sponge. Topical thrombin may be sprayed on areas of capillary bleeding that do not lend themselves to other means of hemostasis, such as sealing a skin graft onto a denuded area. Do not allow it to enter large vessels.

Thrombin is used for topical application only. *It is never injected.* When a thrombin solution is on the instrument table, it must be kept separated from any other solutions. Place a sterile label on the container with the name of the drug and the concentration. It is recommended that thrombin be mixed just before use because it loses potency after several hours. Refer to the manufacturer's instructions for mixing solution. Thrombin is contraindicated if the patient is allergic to beef products.

Sclerotherapy

A caustic sclerosing solution may be injected into veins, as in the mucosal lining of the esophagus or anus to stop or prevent bleeding. The solution may be sodium morrhuate or a mixture of equal parts of dehydrated alcohol, bacteriostatic saline, and sodium tetradecyl. Other sclerosants are mixtures of absolute ethanol or ethanolamine.

Hyperbaric Oxygenation

Although technically not a method of hemostasis because it does not arrest the flow of blood, *hyperbaric oxygen (HBO) therapy* is used for specific types of wounds and conditions to enhance healing. Pure oxygen is administered under pressure that is several times greater than atmospheric pressure. Under this pressure, plasma saturates with oxygen. This raises oxygen tension in tissues to normal or above-normal levels. The increased oxygenation physiologically effects intense vasoconstriction, vascular proliferation, bone formation and resorption, and bone marrow suppression. It also has a bacteriostatic or bactericidal action. These effects may be used selectively.

HBO therapy is administered in specially designed chambers. The patient may be enclosed in a monoplace, single-patient chamber or in a multiplace chamber with other patients and/or caregivers. The patient breathes 100% oxygen via a mask. Some of the surgical conditions for which HBO is used include crush injuries, severed extremities, central nervous system injuries, burns, acute traumatic ischemia, acute blood loss anemia, venous stasis, radiation necrosis, osteomyelitis, diabetic skin ulcers, and gas gangrene. HBO increases the vascularity of soft tissues and bone. It is adjunctive to surgical debridement, but it may help preserve the viability of tissues or sustain life until definitive treatment can be carried out.

HBO chambers are not in common use, primarily because of their cost. Hospitals that have them will accept patients from other hospitals if the treatments will be beneficial.

Mechanical Methods

Mechanical hemostasis is achieved by occluding severed vessels until normal forces of blood have time to form a clot. During the surgical procedure, the surgeon uses many mechanical devices to apply pressure or to create a mechanical barrier to the flow of blood. Pressure also is used prophylactically preoperatively and postoperatively.

External Pressure Devices

Mechanical devices are applied externally either before the patient arrives in the operating room (OR) or after the patient is transferred to the operating table. The intended purpose may be prophylactic to prevent venous stasis, deep vein thrombosis, or pulmonary embolus intraoperatively and postoperatively. Or the function may be therapeutic to control internal hemorrhage preoperatively or hematoma postoperatively. A bloodless surgical field also can be created by external pressure devices.

Antiembolic Stockings Elastic stockings or bandage (Ace bandage) may be applied to the lower extremities to prevent thromboembolic phenomena. Static compression on the legs helps prevent venous stasis. Stockings are available in knee- or groin-length sizes. To apply, the circulator rolls the stocking from top to toe. After being placed over the patient's toes, the stocking is gently unrolled over the leg from foot to ankle to calf, etc. An elastic bandage also is applied from the foot upward to allow venous return of blood flow as vessels are compressed.

Sequential Pneumatic Compression Device Inflatable, double-walled vinyl or woven fabric leg wraps use alternating compression and relaxation to reduce the risk of deep vein clotting in the legs of high-risk patients undergoing general anesthesia. The leg wraps may be used over antiembolic stockings on each leg. The circulator should measure the patient's thigh or calf for correct size selection (i.e., small, medium, large, or extra-large) for either full-leg (thigh-high) or knee-high leg wraps. The foot is not encased within wrap. Proper selection and application are essential for effective compression. Disposable leg wraps are commercially available. A motorized pump, attached by tubing to each wrap, sequentially inflates leg wraps at the ankles, then at the calves, and then at the thighs for full-leg compression. The pressure of this wavelike action is greatest at the ankles. The leg wraps are divided into chambers so that pressure can be regulated by preset or adjustable gauges. Pressure between 40 and 50 mm Hg applied for 12 seconds and then released for 48 seconds, for example, empties blood from deep leg veins. The action prevents venous stasis and accumulation of clotting factors in deep veins. The pumping action must be started before induction of anesthesia because general anesthesia reduces venous return and causes vasodilation.

The circulator should check operation of the pump regularly and periodically inspect the leg wraps and tubing. The type of device, time started, pressure and cycle settings, and time discontinued must be documented on the intraoperative record. If the surgeon wants leg wraps to remain on the patient postoperatively, the device is transported to the postanesthesia care unit (PACU) or intensive care unit (ICU) with the patient. Frequently, sequential compression is continued for 24 hours postoperatively or until the patient is fully ambulatory following an abdominal, hip, or neurosurgical procedure.

Pneumatic Counterpressure Device Although the concept dates back to 1903, external counterpressure was not a popular medical device until the Vietnam

War. There it was used to control hemorrhagic shock until definitive hemostasis became available to casualties. Circumferential pneumatic compression counteracts postural hypotension, maintains venous pressure, and controls hemorrhage. Several types of *pneumatic antishock garments* (PASG) are used, primarily to treat hypovolemic shock. The acronym MAST can refer to *medical antishock trousers, military antishock trousers,* or *military antigravity suit.* An inflatable, waterproof garment is fastened around the patient from ankles to rib cage. The trouser chambers are inflated first to prevent venous stasis in the legs. The entire suit or only specific chambers of it can be inflated from the feet up. Each chamber is inflated separately with a foot pump. By increasing pressure on vessel walls of the legs and abdomen, systemic vascular resistance of peripheral vessels increases blood flow to the heart, lungs, and brain. Compression of torn vessel walls reduces the size of the laceration and diminishes blood loss.

The PASG device may be in place when the trauma patient arrives in the OR. Deflation begins after induction of anesthesia, beginning with the abdominal chamber. Leg chambers may remain inflated for counterpressure if blood pressure remains unstable. *Deflation must be slow and gradual.* Rapid deflation reduces cerebral and cardiopulmonary circulation, with resultant shock. Blood pressure must be monitored; it should not drop more than 5 mm Hg.

Pneumatic counterpressure devices may be used to prevent air embolism during some head and neck procedures performed with the patient in a sitting position. The increased venous filling produced decreases the possibility of an air embolus. Also, these devices may be used postoperatively to reduce bleeding or to stabilize the patient following massive blood loss during the surgical procedure.

Tourniquet A tourniquet is a device used to constrict the flow of blood by compression of the blood vessels. It is frequently used on an extremity to keep the surgical site free of blood. A bloodless field makes dissection easier and less traumatic to tissues and reduces operating time. However, the tourniquet is not a form of hemostasis per se; bleeding must be controlled before pressure is released.

Precautions for tourniquet application and use must be observed. A tourniquet should never be used when circulation in distal part of an extremity is impaired or when an arteriovenous access fistula for dialysis is present. A tourniquet can cause tissue, nerve, and vascular injury. Paralysis may result from excessive pressure on nerves. Prolonged ischemia can cause gangrene and loss of the extremity. Tourniquet time should be kept to a minimum. Metabolic changes may be irreversible after 1 to 1½ hours of tourniquet ischemia.

A tourniquet is dangerous to apply, to leave on, and to remove. A tourniquet may be applied by the surgeon or by an assistant or the circulator on the surgeon's orders. A pneumatic tourniquet is used most frequently to produce a bloodless field (see next discussion). *Other types of tourniquets include:*

1. *Blood pressure cuff.* The cuff is inflated with ambient air. The surgeon determines the amount of pressure to be sustained. The regulator valve is tightened. The pressure gauge or sphygmomanometer must be monitored for pressure deviations.
2. *Rubber band.* This may be used as a tourniquet for a finger or toe. The surgeon will put a sterile rubber band on the digit after draping.
3. *Rubber bandage (Esmarch's bandage).* Friedrich von Esmarch, a German military surgeon, introduced an elastic bandage for the control of hemorrhage on the battlefield in 1869. Known today as Esmarch's bandage, a 3-inch (7.5 cm) latex rubber roller bandage is used to compress superficial vessels to force blood out of an extremity. An Esmarch's bandage is not used, however, to empty vessels of blood preoperatively in a patient who has sustained traumatic injury or if the patient has been in a cast. Danger exists that thrombi might be present in vessels because of injury or stasis of blood. These could become dislodged and result in emboli. An extremity with active infection or malignant tumor also is not wrapped with an Esmarch's bandage.

   Starting at the distal end of the extremity, the surgeon wraps a sterile Esmarch's bandage tightly, overlapping it spirally, to the level of the blood pressure cuff or a pneumatic tourniquet. (An elastic Ace bandage may be used.) The circulator tightens the tourniquet. Then the rubber bandage is removed. Or, starting from the distal end of the extremity, the rubber bandage can be partially removed, leaving the last three rounds, which constitute a tourniquet.

   After terminal cleaning of a reusable Esmarch's bandage, a layer of gauze bandage is rolled between layers of the rubber bandage to ensure sterilization of all surfaces. The gauze must be removed and the bandage rerolled before use.
4. *Rubber tubing.* When an intravenous (IV) infusion is started, a small length of rubber tubing is tied around the extremity, usually an arm, while needle is being inserted. This stops venous return and makes the vein more visible for venipuncture.

Pneumatic Tourniquet Similar to a blood pressure cuff, although heavier and more secure, the pneumatic cuff consists of a rubber bladder shielded by a plastic insert inside a fabric cover with a hook and loop (Velcro) closure. Many different types of cuffs are available; some are straight and cylindrical in shape, others are contoured. A cuff of appropriate length and width must be used; various sizes are available. Cuffs are inflated automatically with compressed gas (air, oxygen, or Freon) by means of tubing interconnected between the cuff and a pressure cartridge, piped-in system, or battery-powered unit. The desired pressure is uniformly maintained by a pressure valve and registered on a pressure gauge. The tourniquet console, a pressure regulator with a gauge, may be contained in a unit mounted on a portable stand or hung on an IV pole. An automated tourniquet with a computerized microprocessor control signals both audible alarms and visual indicators for deviations from preset pressure and for elapsed time of inflation.

Correct pressure is the minimum amount required to produce a bloodless field. The calculation of tourniquet cuff pressure is according to the systolic blood pressure. An exact pressure to which the cuff should be inflated has not been determined. In a healthy adult, upper extremity pressure 30 to 70 mm Hg higher than the systolic value of the blood pressure may be sufficient to suppress arterial circulation. Tourniquet pressure on an average adult arm usually ranges from 250 to 300 mm Hg (up to 6 lb). In the lower extremity, cuff pressure should be higher than the systolic pressure by one half the value. This may require 350 mm Hg on the thigh. Thin adults and children require less pressure; muscular and obese extremities may require more. Inflation time should also be kept to a minimum. If needed for more than 1 hour on an arm or 1½ hours on a leg, the tourniquet is deflated at intervals periodically at the discretion of the surgeon.

A pneumatic tourniquet should be used and maintained according to the manufacturer's written instructions. These and institutional policies and procedures should be available to users of this complex equipment. The cuff, tubing, connectors, gauges, and pressure source should be maintained in working order. *Precautions* to be taken when using a pneumatic tourniquet include the following, in addition to those listed on p. 474 for all tourniquets.

1. Inspect and test pneumatic tourniquet equipment before each use.
   a. Inspect inflatable cuff, connectors, and tubing for cleanliness, integrity, and function.
   b. Ensure that cuff and tubing are intact and connectors are securely fastened to the tourniquet pressure source.
   c. Check pressure gauge for accuracy. An aneroid pressure gauge can be checked by comparing it with a mercury manometer. Pressure drifts can be detected by wrapping cuff around a rigid cylinder, inflating it to 300 mm Hg, and observing for pressure variations.
2. Protect patient's skin under the tourniquet cuff.
   a. Place wrinkle-free padding around extremity. A length of stockinette or lint-free cotton sheet wadding may be used. Disposable padded covers are commercially available.
   b. Keep padding and cuff dry. Antiseptic solutions and other fluids should not contact or accumulate under the cuff. Skin maceration or burns could result. Placing an impervious drape around the cuff prevents the pooling of fluids.
3. Position cuff at point of *maximum circumference* of the extremity.
   a. Avoid vulnerable neurovascular structures. Nerves and blood vessels may be compressed against bone when the cuff is inflated. Soft tissue provides padding for underlying structures. The cuff should be placed on upper arm or proximal third of thigh.
   b. Select cuff of appropriate width for size and shape of extremity. A wide cuff occludes blood flow at a lower pressure than a narrow cuff.
   c. Select cuff with adequate length to overlap at least 3 inches (7.5 cm) but not more than 6 inches (15 cm).
   d. Apply cuff smoothly and snugly over padding, if used, before prepping extremity.
   e. Apply sterile cuff, if used, after prepping and draping. A sterile cuff may be used for an immunocompromised patient.
4. Preset pressure gauges. The surgeon determines pressure setting according to the patient's age, limb size, and systolic blood pressure and the width of cuff to be used.
5. Exsanguinate extremity after prepping and draping, but before cuff inflation, to prolong tourniquet time.
   a. Wrap rubber bandage around extremity to compress superficial vessels. An Esmarch's bandage may be applied unless contraindicated as previously noted on p. 474.
   b. Elevate arm or leg for 2 minutes to encourage venous drainage by gravity if a rubber bandage is contraindicated.
   c. Deflate cuff completely and exsanguinate again if cuff inflates either excessively or insufficiently. Reinflation over blood-filled vessels may cause intravascular thrombosis.
6. Inflate cuff *rapidly* to occlude arteries and veins simultaneously to predetermined minimum pressure.
7. Monitor safety parameters during use of the pneumatic tourniquet.

a. Monitor pressure gauge to detect pressure fluctuations within the bladder of the cuff.
b. Monitor duration of inflation. Inform the surgeon when cuff has been inflated for 1 hour and every 15 minutes thereafter. In some ORs the circulator posts tourniquet time on a tally board in view of the surgeon.

8. Document use of a tourniquet on the intraoperative record.
   a. Record times tourniquet is applied, inflated, deflated, and removed. The anesthesiologist also records inflation time on the anesthesia sheet when a tourniquet is used with a Bier block for regional anesthesia (see Chapter 18, p. 349).
   b. Record location of cuff and the pressure setting.
   c. Record model and serial number of the tourniquet used.
   d. Document assessment of skin condition of the extremity preoperatively and evaluation of skin and tissue integrity after removal of the cuff.
9. Clean and inspect the pneumatic tourniquet after each patient use.
   a. Wash reusable cuff and bladder according to the manufacturer's instructions. An enzymatic detergent should be used if blood or body fluid came in contact with the cuff. A disposable cuff cover facilitates cleaning.
   b. Rinse and dry cuff and bladder. Water droplets inside the bladder can damage the pressure mechanism if forced backward during subsequent deflation. Care should be taken to prevent water getting into the bladder during washing.
   c. Wipe connecting tubing with a disinfectant.
   d. Test cuff, tubing, connectors, and gauges before storage between uses. A malfunctioning device must be removed from service until repaired and tested by appropriate personnel.

Pressure Dressings Pressure on the wound in the immediate postoperative period can minimize the accumulation of intercellular fluid and can decrease bleeding. Pressure dressings are used on some extensive wounds to eliminate dead space and to prevent capillary bleeding, thus decreasing edema and potential hematoma formation. They may be used as an adjunct to wound drainage to distribute pressure evenly over the wound. (See Chapter 25, p. 531, for a description of materials used.)

Packing Packing is used with or without pressure to achieve hemostasis and to eliminate dead space in an area where mucosal tissues need support, such as the vagina, rectum, or nose. Packing impregnated with an antiseptic agent, such as iodoform gauze, may be used to ensure closure of an incision from the wound base toward the outside (i.e., healing by second intention) as in a large abscess cavity. The surgeon inserts sterile packing as the final stage of the surgical procedure. It is usually removed in 24 to 48 hours. The intraoperative record and patient's chart must reflect type and location of packing.

Internal Mechanical Methods

Meticulous hemostasis during the surgical procedure is essential to control bleeding and to minimize blood loss. The surgeon uses many mechanical tools to achieve hemostasis.

Hemostatic Clamps Clamps for occluding vessels are used to compress blood vessels and to grasp or hold a small amount of tissue. The *hemostat* is the most frequently used surgical instrument and the most commonly used method of hemostasis. This instrument has either straight or curved jaws that narrow to a fine point. Often the pressure of clamping an instrument is sufficient to constrict and seal a vessel with minimal trauma or adjacent tissue necrosis. A wide variety of hemostatic clamps are used for vessel occlusion, including noncrushing vascular clamps that do not damage large vessels. (See Chapter 14 for a description of surgical instruments.)

Ligating Clips When placed on a blood vessel and pinched shut, clips occlude the lumen and stop the vessel from bleeding. Metallic clips are small pieces of thin, serrated wire, bent in the center to an oblique angle. Absorbable polymer clips are similar in configuration. Clips are most frequently used on large vessels or those in anatomic locations difficult to ligate by other means. *A specific forceps is required for the application of each type available.* Single clips may be mounted in a sterile plastic cartridge that can be secured in a heavy stainless steel base to facilitate loading the applier forceps. Disposable appliers preloaded with multiple clips also are available.

Ligating clips were devised in 1917 by Dr. Harvey Cushing for use in brain surgery. Cushing clips are made of silver. Stainless steel, tantalum, and titanium clips are more common today. The serrations across the wire prevent their slipping off the vessels. Polymeric clips have a locking device to secure them on vessels. Many surgeons use clips for ligating vessels, nerves, and other small structures.

Metallic clips also may be used to mark a biopsy site or other areas to permit x-ray visualization and thus detect postoperative complications. For example, migration of a marker clip could indicate the presence of a hematoma in the wound. The artifacts (i.e., distortion) caused by clips may be a disadvantage, however, in future radiologic studies or magnetic resonance imaging (MRI). Titanium and absorbable polymeric clips are used to eliminate or decrease image distortion of computerized tomography and MRI.

Ligature A ligature, commonly called a *tie,* is a strand of material that is tied around a blood vessel to occlude the lumen and prevent bleeding. Frequently the ligature is tied around a hemostat and slipped off the point onto the vessel and pulled taut to effect hemostasis. Vessels are ligated with the smallest-size strand possible and include the smallest amount of surrounding tissue possible. Ends are cut as near the knot as possible.

Large and pulsating vessels may require a *transfixion suture.* A ligature on a needle is placed through a "bite" of tissue and brought around end of vessel. This eliminates any possibility of its slipping off the vessel. All bleeding points should be ligated before the next layer of tissue is incised.

Pledgets Small pieces of Teflon felt are used as a buttress under sutures when bleeding might occur through the needle hole in a major vessel or when friable tissue might tear. Placed over an arteriotomy site, they exert pressure to seal off bleeding. Pledgets are used most frequently in cardiovascular surgery.

Packs Packs are used to sustain pressure on raw wound surfaces. The application of sponges or laparotomy tapes effectively controls capillary ooze by occluding the capillaries. The surgeon usually wants these moistened, often with cold but sometimes with hot normal saline solution. Hot packs promote hemostasis by accelerating the coagulation mechanism.

Compressed Absorbent Patties Compressed absorbent radiopaque patties (cottonoids) are used for hemostasis when placed on the surface of brain tissue and to absorb blood and fluids around the spinal cord or nerves. These patties are available in an assortment of sizes. Before use, the scrub person moistens them with normal saline solution, presses out excess solution, and keeps them flat.

Bone Wax Composed of a sterile mixture of beeswax and a softening agent, bone wax provides a mechanical barrier to stop oozing from cut bone surfaces. The packet should be opened just before use to minimize the drying of wax. The scrub person can warm wax to the desired consistency by manipulating it with the fingers or by immersing the unopened packet in warm solution. Small pieces can be rolled into balls and placed around the rim of a medicine cup. When needed, the cup can be presented to the surgeon. Bone wax is used in some orthopaedic and neurosurgical procedures and when the sternum is split (sternotomy) for cardiothoracic procedures. Bone wax should be used sparingly and excess should be removed from the surgical site because it is minimally resorbed.

Digital Compression When digital pressure is applied to an artery proximal to the area of bleeding, such as in traumatic injury, hemorrhage is controlled. The main disadvantage of digital pressure is that it cannot be applied permanently. Firm pressure is applied on the skin on both sides as the skin incision is made to help control subcutaneous bleeding until vessels can be clamped, ligated, or cauterized. Pressure is applied while the surgical area is sponged to locate a bleeding vessel.

Suction Suction is the application of pressure less than atmospheric either continuously or intermittently. It is used during surgical procedures for removal of blood and tissue fluids from the surgical field, primarily to enhance visibility. An appropriate style tip for locating bleeding is attached to sterile disposable suction tubing. (See Chapter 14, p. 251, for description of suction tips; many are disposable.) The scrub person hands end of the tubing to the circulator, who attaches it to a suction collection container.

A powered suction/irrigation system may be used to simultaneously irrigate wound and evacuate solution. The irrigation may be pulsed (i.e., intermittent to remove debris and clots) or continuous with gravity flow. The surgeon adjusts flow of irrigation and suction with controls on the disposable tip assembly.

Drains Postoperatively, drains aid in removal of blood, fluid, and air from the surgical site to obliterate dead spaces and to enhance opposition of tissues, thus preventing hematoma formation and edema. Drains usually are placed through a stab wound in the skin adjacent to the primary incision. (See Chapter 25, pp. 527-530, for discussion of drains and drainage systems.)

Thermal Methods

Hemostasis may be achieved or enhanced by application of either cold or heat to body tissues.

Cryosurgery

Cryosurgery is performed with the aid of special instruments for local freezing of diseased tissue without harm to normal adjacent structures. Extreme cold causes intracapillary thrombosis and tissue necrosis in the frozen area. Frozen tissue may be removed without significant bleeding during or after the surgical procedure. Cryosurgery is also used to alter cell function without removing tissue. It tends to be hemostatic and lymphostatic, particularly in highly vascular areas.

Extreme cold is delivered to extract heat from a small volume of tissue in a rapid manner. Liquid nitrogen is the most commonly used refrigerant; however, Freon or carbon dioxide gas may be used. The liquid or gas is in a vacuum container and comes through an insulated vacuum tube to a probe. All but the tip of the probe is insulated. Freezing of tissue at this tip is result of the liquid nitrogen at the lowest temperature of −320° F (−196° C) becoming gaseous. In the process, heat is removed from the tissue. A ball of frozen tissue gradually forms around the uninsulated tip. The extent of tissue destruction is controlled by raising or lowering temperature of cells surrounding the lesion to −46° to −40° F (−20° to −40° C).

The machines vary in range of temperatures obtained according to their design and type of refrigerant used. Some are nonelectric with foot-switch–operated probes. Special miniature, presterilized, disposable models for single-patient use are particularly suitable for ophthalmic applications.

Because the process is rapid, involves less trauma to destroy or remove tissue, controls bleeding, and minimizes local pain, cryosurgery is used to alter the function of nerve cells and to destroy otherwise unapproachable brain tumors. Other techniques for which it is used include removal of superficial tumors in the nasopharynx and the skin, destruction of the prostate gland, removal of highly vascular tumors and some otherwise nonresectable liver tumors, removal of lesions from the cervix and anus, cataract extraction, and retinal detachment. The amount of tissue destroyed is influenced by the size of the tip of the probe, temperature used, duration of use, kind of tissue and its vascularity, and skill of the surgeon.

Hypothermia

Cooling of body tissues to a temperature as low as 78.8° F (26° C) in adults and large children and 68° F (20° C) in infants and small children, well below normal limits, decreases cellular metabolism and thereby decreases need for oxygen by tissues. The decreased requirement for oxygen decreases bleeding. Hypothermia lowers blood pressure to slow the circulation and increases the viscosity of blood. This process results in hemoconcentration, which contributes to capillary sludging and microcirculatory stasis to provide an essentially dry field for the surgeon. Hypothermia may be localized or generalized (systemic). See Chapter 17, pp. 338-339, for a detailed description of the methods of local and systemic hypothermia by both internal and external body cooling. Hypothermia is used as an adjunct to anesthesia, particularly during heart, brain, or liver procedures.

Diathermy

Oscillating, high-frequency electric current generates enough heat to coagulate and destroy body tissues. Heat is generated by resistance of tissues to passage of alternating electric current. A short-wave diathermy machine produces a high frequency of 10 to 100 million cycles per second. The machine should not be activated until the surgeon is ready to deliver this current. Diathermy is useful in stopping bleeding from small blood vessels. It is used primarily to repair detached retina and to cauterize small warts, polyps, and other small superficial lesions.

Electrocautery

A small loop heated by a steady, direct electric current to red heat will coagulate or destroy tissue on contact. Heat is transferred to tissue from the preheated wire. The hemostatic effect is a result of searing or sealing the tissues. A variety of sterile, disposable, battery-powered models are available. The hot point of the cautery must be at least 24 inches (60 cm) from the anesthesia machine and face mask, with a protecting screen between the tip and the patient's head. Cautery should not be used in the mouth, around the head, or in the pleural cavity. *Cautery must not be used when any flammable agent is present.* To prevent fire, only *moist* sponges should be permitted on the field while cautery is in use.

Electrosurgery

High-frequency electric current provided from an electrosurgical unit frequently is used to cut tissue and to coagulate bleeding points. The concentration and flow of current generates heat as it meets resistance in passage through tissue. Because air has low electrical conductivity, an active electrode tip delivering radio-frequency energy must be in direct contact with tissue. Both cutting and coagulating currents are used in many open and minimally invasive surgical procedures. Some surgeons prefer electrosurgery to other methods of cutting and ligating vessels. Coagulated tissue produces foreign-body reaction, however, which must be absorbed by the body during healing. If a large amount of coagulated tissue is present, sloughing may result so wound may not heal by first intention. Because the high-frequency electric current goes through tissues, patient must be grounded and safety precautions taken to avoid accidental injury. See the discussion of electrosurgery in Chapter 15, pp. 265-270.

Fulguration

Sparks of high-voltage electric current char the surface of tissue, producing a thin coagulated crust (eschar) without damaging underlying tissues. Fulguration uses higher-frequency currents than does electrocoagulation. The cutting current from a spark-gap generator is used for fulguration. This high-voltage arcing, described as spray coagulation, is used primarily for transurethral bladder and prostate procedures.

Argon Beam Coagulator

Argon gas effectively delivers radio-frequency energy to tissue in a directional noncontact white light beam for the purpose of rapid hemostasis by coagulation. The argon beam coagulator directs a gentle flow of ionized argon gas from a generator to a pencil-shaped handpiece. The gas flow over tissues clears blood and fluid from the target site and allows creation of a superficial eschar directly on tissue. Less necrotic tissue is produced than with the high current density of electrocoagulation because the temperature never exceeds 230° F (110° C), and penetration is approximately half the depth, which minimizes tissue destruction. The depth of penetration depends on power, duration of application, and electrical characteristics of tissue. Coagulation occurs through the arcing effect of electrical energy, not through the action of argon gas. The coaxial flow of gas delivers monopolar current that coagulates the surface with practically no smoke or odor. The patient must be grounded with a dispersive pad, however, to complete the electrical circuit. The pad is placed in an area that allows good skin contact.

The argon beam coagulator is used to control hemorrhage from vascular structures, surface bleeding, and diffuse oozing and to achieve hemostasis of bone marrow. Handpieces and electrodes are available for use through endoscopes, but they are not used in fluid environments such as joints.

Hemostatic Scalpel

The sharp steel blade of the hemostatic scalpel seals blood vessels as it cuts through tissue. The disposable blade, size No. 10 or 15, has a heating and sensing microcircuitry between the steel and a layer of copper coated with electrical insulation and a nonstick surface. The blade fits into a reusable handle that contains control switches. The scrub person hands the end of the electrical cord attached to the handle to the circulator, who plugs it into the controller unit. When the surgeon activates it, the blade transfers thermal energy to tissues as the sharp edge cuts through them. The temperature can be controlled between 230° and 518° F (110° and 270° C). The surgeon can raise or lower the temperature in increments of 50° F (10° C). The blade also can be used cold, like any other scalpel.

The hemostatic scalpel can be used to incise skin, soft tissues, and muscle. This is particularly advantageous in vascular areas, such as scalp, head and neck, and breast. This scalpel may be used to debride burns. Blood flow into the incised area is minimal, providing the surgeon with a clear, dry field, thus shortening surgical time. The rapid hemostasis with minimal tissue damage promotes wound healing and may eliminate a need for blood replacement. Because electric current from the microcircuitry does not pass through tissue, a grounding pad is not required. This also prevents muscle contractions.

Thermal Probe

A thermal probe generates heat at the tip. By direct contact at the point of bleeding, it coagulates vessels. No electric current is released into tissues.

Laser

Laser beams are used for control of bleeding or for ablation and excision of tissues in organs that can be exposed or are accessible. The laser furnishes an intense and concentrated light beam of a single wavelength from a monochromatic source of nonionizing radiation. Thermal energy of this beam may simultaneously cut, coagulate, and/or vaporize tissue. The laser wound is characterized by minimal bleeding and no visible postoperative edema. The amount of tissue destruction is predictable by adjusting width and focus of the beam. Different lasers have selective uses. See Chapter 15, pp. 270-279, for a detailed discussion of laser surgery.

Photocoagulation

The photocoagulator uses an intense multiwavelength light furnished by a xenon tube to coagulate tissue. Because its use is limited to ophthalmology, see Chapter 33, p. 696.

Plasma Scalpel

The plasma scalpel vaporizes tissues and stops bleeding as it simultaneously cuts and coagulates tissue. Within the instrument, which looks like a large ballpoint pen, argon or helium gas passes through an electric arc that ionizes it into a high thermal state. These gases are inert and noncombustible. As the instrument moves over tissue, the gas that flows from the tip is visible so the surgeon can see depth and extent of the incision. Tissue damage, with resultant inflammatory response during wound healing, is greater than that caused by a steel knife blade but less than that caused by other electrosurgical instruments and lasers. Because it will coagulate blood vessels up to 3 mm in diameter, the plasma scalpel is useful in highly vascular areas.

Ultrasonic Scalpel

The titanium blade of the scalpel moves by a rapid ultrasonic motion that cuts and coagulates tissue simultaneously. The portable generator, a microprocessor with piezoelectric disks, converts electrical energy into mechanical energy. This energy is transmitted through a handpiece to a single-use blade. All three parts of the system lock into a frequency of 55,500 movements per second. When this happens, the system is said to be in harmony, thus the name *Harmonic Scalpel.* The scalpel can be used for sharp or blunt dissection without damage to adjacent tissues. Vibrations from the blade denature protein molecules as it cuts through tissue, producing a coagulum that seals bleeding vessels. The continuous vibration of the denatured protein generates heat within the tissue to cause deeper coagulation. This action does not raise tissue temperature above 176° F (80° C) so that char or smoke is not produced. A fatty particulate mist may be generated. The vibrating blade also produces a cavitational effect as it cuts through tissue with high water content that disrupts cell walls and separates tissue, which aids in dissection.

The ultrasonic scalpel is used primarily for laparoscopic and thoracoscopic procedures. Blades and accessories for open procedures will make this technology available to all surgical specialties. Because electricity is not required for effects on tissue, a grounding pad is not necessary.

BLOOD LOSS

Some blood loss is inevitable whenever tissues are severed by intent or traumatic injury. Blood loss is computed as a percentage of total blood volume (TBV). TBV averages from 6% to 8% of total body weight. In the average healthy adult male this equals about 75 ml/kg and in the female 60 to 70 ml/kg. Calculation of TBV depends on venous hematocrit value. Normal *hematocrit,* the volume of red cells expressed as a percentage of volume of whole blood, is 42% to 52% in males and 37% to 47% in females. An infant reaches these blood volume levels at about 3 months of age. An increase in hematocrit indicates a decrease in plasma volume, normally by dehydration and loss of sodium. A decrease in hematocrit indicates a decrease in number of red cells, but this does not necessarily reflect blood loss; it may be caused by overhydration. Fluid and electrolyte balance is important for maintenance of blood volume. Inadequate fluid replacement can lead to decrease in cardiac output and cardiovascular collapse.

A decrease in red blood cells (erythrocytes) and in hemoglobin, the chief oxygen-carrying component of these cells, causes hypoxia if values fall below normal (Table 23-1). Therefore determination of operative blood loss may be critical to physiologic functions. The extent of blood loss will depend on the location and magnitude of the surgical procedure. Blood loss can be categorized as:

1. *Minor:* loss of 500 to 700 ml is about 15% of TBV.
2. *Moderate:* loss of 750 to 1500 ml is about 15% to 30% of TBV. A resultant decrease in pulse pressure and slight tachycardia (rapid heart rate) may progress to tachycardia, tachypnea (rapid breathing), and postural hypotension (reduced blood pressure).
3. *Major:* loss of 1500 to 2250 ml is about 30% to 45% of TBV. Blood pressure drops, skin becomes cold and clammy, and urinary output decreases.
4. *Catastrophic:* loss over 2250 ml is greater than 45% of TBV. Hypoxia (decrease in oxygen level) develops from loss of hemoglobin (red blood cells). Prolonged hypoxia leads to irreversible heart, brain, liver, and kidney damage.

Estimation of Blood Loss

An accurate determination of total blood volume involves measuring plasma and red cell volumes separately, and adding these values together. This may be done rapidly by an electronic counting device (see Chapter 19, p. 376). In lieu of this, blood loss is estimated in all surgical procedures in which a major loss is anticipated. This can be done by:

1. Visual inspection of blood on drapes and floor by the anesthesiologist.
2. Estimation of blood in suction container. Allowance must be made for presence of other body fluids and irrigating solution, if used. The scrub person must estimate the amount of solution suc-

TABLE 23-1

Normal Values of Blood*

	MALES	FEMALES	CHILDREN
Red cells (RBC)	4.7-6.1 million/mm^3	4.2-5.4 million/mm^3	3.8-5.5 million/mm^3
Hemoglobin (Hgb)	14-18 g/dl	12-16 g/dl	11-16 g/dl
Hematocrit (Hct)	42%-52%	37%-47%	31%-43%
Prothrombin time (PT)	11.0-12.5 sec	Same	Same
Platelets	150,000-400,000/mm^3	Same	Same after 1 wk of age
Partial thromboplastin time (PTT)	30-40 sec	Same	25-35 sec

*Values vary depending on calibration of testing equipment in laboratory that services the health care facility.

tioned into the container through irrigation of wound and/or tubing. This can be done by knowing capacity of the irrigation syringe in use and keeping track of number of times it is used. The circulator subtracts these amounts to estimate volume of blood in the container.
3. Visual inspection of blood in sponges by the anesthesiologist.
4. Measurement of blood in sponges by weighing them. Sponges are weighed after use as they are discarded from the surgical field.

Weighing Sponges

Some anesthesiologists and surgeons prefer to have sponges weighed for blood loss rather than visually estimating it. A scale calibrated in grams is used. The dry and wet weights of each type of sponge (see Chapter 20, p. 426) must be known. Wet weight is that of sponge soaked in normal saline solution and wrung out until almost dry. A chart of these weights should be available; often it is attached to the scale. The number of sponges being weighed is multiplied by the appropriate dry or wet weight. Each type must be weighed separately, with the dry separated from the wet. To allow for (i.e., by subtracting) dry or wet weights and weight of a moisture-proof cover on the scale platform or a container, adjust scale to register at zero. When blood-soaked sponges are weighed, the reading on the scale equals the blood loss; 1 g equals 1 ml. The scale must be checked at each use for readjustment to zero. Some scales are controlled by a microprocessor that automatically makes calculations.

The circulator must weigh sponges *before they dry out.* Blood loss is recorded each time sponges are weighed, adding new weight to previous ones to keep a current total. A tally board for this purpose may be mounted on the wall where the anesthesiologist and surgeon can read it. The estimated blood in the suction container can be recorded here also.

Reduction of Blood Loss

When significant bleeding can be anticipated, several techniques are used to reduce red blood cell loss during the surgical procedure or to eliminate blood transfusion requirements.

Hemodilution

Acute normovolemic or isovolemic hemodilution reduces red cells in blood but maintains normal or equal blood volume. After induction of anesthesia, a physician, usually the anesthesiologist, withdraws blood through an arterial or venous catheter. The blood is drawn into bags containing anticoagulant, usually citrate. Citrate metabolizes rapidly, thus minimizing risk of systemic anticoagulation when blood is reinfused. The amount withdrawn depends on anticipated blood loss and the patient's estimated TBV and hematocrit. A plasma volume expander is infused intravenously while blood is removed to restore blood volume. This hemodilution technique reduces red blood cell loss during the surgical procedure because the hematocrit has been lowered. The surgical procedure begins when the hematocrit is between 27% and 30%. Adequate intravascular volume and oxygenation are maintained. Urinary output must be measured.

Each bag of blood must be labeled with patient's name and identifying number and the time of withdrawal. Blood may be stored at room temperature for 6 hours or in a refrigerator for 24 hours. At the conclusion of the surgical procedure, or sooner if indicated, the blood is reinfused intravenously to raise the hematocrit back to the preoperative level. Units are reinfused in reverse order of withdrawal (i.e., last one first) so that the unit with the highest concentration of red cells and coagulation factors is infused last.

Blood Volume Expanders

Artificial nonblood crystalloid or colloid solutions are administered intravenously for fluid replacement and plasma volume expansion. They are not sole replacements for blood loss. They must be used with caution. The most commonly used plasma volume expanders are:

1. *Dextran.* This crystalloid polymer of glucose acts by drawing fluid from tissues to decrease blood viscosity. It remains in circulation for several hours. It interferes with the crossmatching of blood: thus a blood sample for this purpose must be drawn before dextran is infused. It may be used until blood or blood products are available or for hemodilution. As a 6% or 10% solution, it may be mixed in water with glucose or sodium chloride.
2. *Ringer's lactate solution.* This crystalloid physiologic salt solution is infused for the improvement of circulation and stimulation of renal activity and in patients in whom the body's supply of sodium, calcium, and potassium has been depleted.
3. *Hetastarch* (Hespan). This colloid polymer expands plasma volume slightly in excess of the volume infused. It approximates the action of serum albumin. Large volumes may alter coagulation factors. It can be used for hemodilution.

Pharmacologic Agents

The action of specific pharmacologic agents either stimulates or retards the coagulation mechanism. This action may reduce blood loss and help to provide hemostasis in patients with hematologic disorders (see pp. 482-484). Some of these disorders are associated with cardiovascular disease or end-stage renal disease. Others are congenital or acquired coagulopathies. Three types of agents affect bleeding.

Desmopressin Acetate Desmopressin promotes hemostasis in patients with von Willebrand's disease and shortens bleeding time in patients with uremia. When given prophylactically, this synthetic vasopressin analogue can decrease surgical blood loss in patients undergoing spinal surgery and reduce blood loss after cardiac surgery.

Vasodilators Vasodilators lower systemic blood pressure, thus decreasing bleeding. Sodium nitroprusside, nitroglycerin, and trimethaphan camsylate are most commonly used (see Chapter 19, p. 397).

Anticoagulants Anticoagulants minimize the tendency of blood to clot yet do not lead to excessive bleeding during or following the surgical procedure. These agents provide adequate anticoagulation with a minimum of hemorrhagic complications. They help prevent venous stasis to reduce the incidence of deep vein thrombus and pulmonary embolus. They may be given orally, subcutaneously, or intravenously beginning preoperatively, especially in patients who have a history of thromboembolic disease. The action of each anticoagulant is different.

1. *Heparin* acts to inhibit conversion of prothrombin to thrombin. This prolongs clotting time. It may be administered subcutaneously to keep activated partial thromboplastin time in the high normal range between 30 and 40 seconds. Given intravenously, heparin is effective immediately. It may be used as a flush to keep IV lines open or to flush the lumen of a blood vessel (1 ml heparin in 100-ml normal saline solution). Heparin does not dissolve a thrombus, but it will prevent a clot from becoming larger.
2. *Coumarin derivatives* depress blood prothrombin and decrease tendency of blood platelets to cling together, thus decreasing normal tendency of blood to clot. They also interfere with action of vitamin K to prevent the synthesis of prothrombin and fibrinogen. *Warfarin sodium* is the most commonly used coumarin derivative.
3. *Low molecular weight dextran* reduces platelet adhesiveness and aggregation to prevent sludge from forming in the bloodstream. It coats blood platelets to keep them from massing together.
4. *Aspirin* diminishes clumping of platelets by inhibiting release reaction of platelet factors and action of vitamin K.

Vitamin K enables the liver to produce clotting factors in blood, including prothrombin. To reduce the possibility of intraoperative hemorrhage, patients who have been on anticoagulant therapy and those who have faulty metabolism or absorption of vitamin K are given it preoperatively. It also is given to elderly or debilitated patients before intraocular surgery, to newborns preoperatively, and to mothers just before delivery. The latter helps prevent postdelivery hemorrhage and ensures that the baby has an adequate prothrombin level until a sufficient amount is produced by the liver.

Hypotensive Anesthesia

In selected situations when excessive blood loss is anticipated or encountered, arterial blood pressure may be deliberately lowered to produce an essentially bloodless field. When induced, hypotension is carefully controlled by the anesthesiologist (see Chapter 17, pp. 339-340).

Hematologic Disorders

Some hemolytic and hemorrhagic disorders require special consideration during perioperative care to minimize risks of surgical intervention. Concern is for the maintenance of adequate tissue perfusion and oxygenation and for hemostasis and coagulation in patients at risk. Patients at risk for intraoperative bleeding or who have a known hematologic disorder should have a complete blood count, SMA-18 (sequential multichannel autoanalyzer) test, and urinalysis done preoperatively. Hemoglobin, hematocrit, and red blood cell counts are critical determinants for blood replacement requirements preoperatively and intraoperatively. Precautions can be taken to minimize the risks of surgical intervention with adequate blood replacement.

Anemia

Anemia is a symptom of a deficiency in either the quantity or quality of red blood cells (erythrocytes). *Hemoglobin,* the chief component of these cells, delivers oxygen to tissues. Normal hemoglobin values are 14 to 18 g/dl of blood in males, 12 to 16 g/dl in females, and 11 to 16 g/dl in children. These values are lower in anemic patients. Thus anemia may result in tissue hypoxia. The various types of this disorder may be caused by:

1. Blood loss from massive bleeding, as from a traumatic injury, or chronic blood loss, as from a gastric or intestinal ulcer. This blood loss can be replaced by transfusion of blood products.
2. Dietary deficiency of sufficient iron, protein, vitamins, and minerals to form red blood cells or produce hemoglobin. Dietary supplements are given to correct the deficiency.
3. Diseases or drugs that inhibit the bone marrow from producing blood cells, such as tumors or chronic renal disease. The cause must be diagnosed and treated.
4. Destruction of red blood cells by an overactive reticuloendothelial system in the spleen or liver. A splenectomy may be indicated for hypersplenism or hereditary spherocytosis, for example.

5. Destruction of red blood cells by foreign substances entering the circulatory system, such as an incompatible blood transfusion. Neonatal anemia may necessitate an exchange transfusion.
6. Abnormal blood cells produced by the bone marrow, usually by genetic or hereditary factors.

The average normal life span of red blood cells is 120 days. In patients with any one of the many forms of *hemolytic anemia,* red blood cells have a shortened life span. Hemolytic anemias may be acquired or inherited. All must be adequately assessed preoperatively.

Sickle Cell Hemoglobinopathies A severe chronic inherited hemolytic disorder, *sickle cell anemia* is most prevalent among blacks of African descent. It may be found in other ethnic groups, particularly people of Mediterranean descent. Pairing of identical abnormal recessive genes causes substitution of a single amino acid for glutamic acid in the polypeptide chain, which alters the hemoglobin. These abnormal cells, known as *hemoglobin S,* become distorted in shape when exposed to low oxygen tension in the venous circulation. Dehydration, cold, infection, and physical or emotional stress may precipitate crisis periods that vary in duration and intensity when sickling occurs. A crisis also may occur spontaneously without apparent cause. The resultant sickle-shaped red blood cells occlude the microcirculation through the capillaries, arterioles, and venules. Occlusion results in blood stasis, hypoxia, vasospasm, ischemia, and necrosis, which causes pain and ultimately permanent damage to tissues and organs. Stasis ulcers and biliary tract disease are common complications that may require surgical intervention. Elective surgical procedures are performed when the patient is not in crisis, but these patients are always at risk of crisis.

Sickle cell trait is present when one abnormal gene is inherited. The red blood cells have both hemoglobin A (normal) and hemoglobin S (sickle cell). Persons with this trait usually are asymptomatic and tolerate routine anesthesia and surgical intervention well. But when stressed by hypothermia, acidosis, or hypoxemia, local or regional sickling can occur during the surgical procedure.

Sickle cells have a life span of 15 to 30 days. The severity of the hemolytic process is proportional to the amount of hemoglobin S in the blood. Hemoglobin in patients with sickle cell anemia usually ranges from 6 to 9 g with a hematocrit of 25% to 30%. Patients of African descent and other susceptible persons should be tested preoperatively. Electrophoresis is the standard laboratory test for hemoglobin S. Consideration then must be given to the following in the perioperative management of patients with sickle cell anemia or sickle cell trait:

1. Transfusion of whole blood, packed cells, or low molecular weight dextran may be administered preoperatively, especially if the patient's hemoglobin is 5 g or less.
2. Urea may be given orally or intravenously prophylactically to prevent a sickle cell crisis. It may also be used to reverse a crisis.
3. Systemic antibiotics are initiated preoperatively because these patients are susceptible to postoperative infection.
4. Normal body temperature must be maintained. Any lowering increases oxygen requirement. The patient must be kept warm to avoid hypothermia.
   a. Add extra blankets during transport to the OR suite.
   b. Avoid drafts from the air-conditioning system in the holding area, OR, and PACU.
   c. Cover patient's head for warmth.
   d. Raise temperature in the OR to 80° to 85° F (27° to 29° C).
   e. Place patient on a hyperthermia blanket on the operating table.
   f. Monitor patient's temperature intraoperatively with an electronic probe.
   g. Place warm blankets over the patient before transfer to the PACU.
5. Oxygen is administered during induction of anesthesia, intraoperatively, and following extubation to prevent deoxygenation of the sickle cells and subsequent ischemic infarction in tissues.
6. Blood gases are monitored to avoid hypoxia, acidosis, hypotension, and hypovolemia. Fluid and blood replacement intraoperatively reduces the risk of crisis from dehydration.
7. Scheduling an elective surgical procedure early in the morning minimizes dehydration following a period of nothing by mouth (NPO).

Hemorrhagic Disorders

Patients with a disorder in the mechanism of blood coagulation have abnormal bleeding tendencies. These may be related to:

1. Hemorrhagic diseases, such as a type of *purpura* in which spontaneous bleeding occurs under the skin, through mucous membranes, or in the gastrointestinal tract, that is idiopathic (cause unknown) or secondary to a systemic or an infectious disease or to exposure to chemical agents
2. Platelet deficiency in the blood, such as *thrombocytopenia* as a result of decreased production of platelets by bone marrow or excessive destruction of platelets in the peripheral circulation
3. Abnormal blood clotting factors, such as in *hemophilia* and *von Willebrand's disease,* which are inherited genetic disorders

A baseline of blood values should be established preoperatively. The baseline consists of a complete blood count, including platelets, plasma clotting time, bleeding time, prothrombin time, and partial thromboplastin time. Adequate blood replacement of the deficient factors must be available during the surgical procedure and postoperatively.

Hemophilia The term *hemophilia* refers to a group of genetic bleeding disorders characterized by abnormal blood clotting factors.

Hemophilia A, the classic disorder, is caused by a deficiency of functional factor VIII, the antihemophilic globulin in plasma. *Hemophilia B,* also known as Christmas disease, is caused by a lack of functional factor IX, the plasma thromboplastic cofactor. A carrier mother transmits to her son this sex-linked recessive trait of the specific clotting factor. Hemophilia occurs most commonly in males of Russian-Jewish descent.

Severity of the disorder depends on the percentage of functional vs. nonfunctional factor in the blood. Partial thromboplastin times or thromboplastin generation times are the standard tests for this determination. These patients have normal vasculature and platelets (150,000 to 400,000/mm^3 of blood); thus bleeding time (1 to 3 minutes by the Duke method) and prothrombin time (11 to 12.5 seconds) test results are normal.

Severely affected hemophiliacs have spontaneous bleeding episodes into the skin, muscles, and joints, most commonly the ankles, knees, wrists, and elbows. If untreated, joint deformities can result. Bleeding will be excessive from even a minor wound such as a bruise or cut.

For hemostasis during a severe bleeding episode, replacement therapy must be initiated to raise the clotting factor to between 60% and 100% (normal individuals have clotting factor levels of 60% to 120%). In hemophiliacs fibrin clots do not form and bleeding continues. The missing clotting factor must be raised temporarily to control hemorrhage. This is started preoperatively for elective surgery. Concentrates available for replacement therapy include:

1. Factor VIII for hemophilia A
   a. Lyophilized concentrate products, such as Hemofil M and Koāte-HP reconstituted with sterile water
   b. Cryoprecipitate
   c. Fresh frozen plasma or concentrate
2. Factor IX for hemophilia B
   a. Lyophilized concentrate products, such as Konȳne and Profilnine reconstituted with sterile water
   b. Fresh frozen plasma
3. Lyophilized concentrate with inhibitors to neutralize the antibody that prevents clotting

Lyophilized concentrates are made from pooled normal human plasma obtained by plasmapheresis, a process of separating red cells by centrifugation. The circulator should obtain factor concentrate from the blood bank and must be familiar with how to prepare it. The dosage for factor deficiency is calculated on the basis of plasma volume, half-life of the factor, and percentage of the deficit. It is given by IV infusion intraoperatively and postoperatively.

NOTE

1. Because they may have received many blood transfusions and/or infusions of clotting factor concentrates, many hemophiliacs are HIV-seropositive and carriers of hepatitis B and may have had hepatitis C. (See Chapter 12 for discussion of hepatitis and human immunodeficiency virus [HIV].)
2. Blood and blood products should be prepared and administered by a registered nurse or physician.

BLOOD REPLACEMENT

Despite meticulous hemostasis and methods to reduce blood loss, blood replacement is necessary during many extensive surgical procedures, particularly cardiovascular, orthopaedic, organ transplantation, and trauma surgery. Surgeons limit use of transfused blood whenever possible. However, to compensate for blood loss of more than 1200 ml or hematocrit below 30% and to prevent shock, transfusions of whole blood, fresh frozen plasma, packed red cells, platelets, serum albumin, or blood substitutes must be carried out according to policy. Transfusions may be of homologous, autologous, or artificial blood.

Homologous Blood

Homologous blood is that drawn from one individual for transfusion into another. It must be compatible, that is, not cause a reaction. Therefore blood typing and crossmatching are essential to determine compatibility between donor and recipient. The four main blood types are A, B, O, and AB. In addition, many subgroups of antigens exist in red blood cells. Also, agglutinogens, known as Rh factor positive, may be present. If these are not present in red cells, the blood is Rh negative. A recipient must receive donor blood of the same type and Rh factor. In extreme emergency situations, O negative blood, referred to as universal donor blood, may be given until the patient's blood can be typed and crossmatched or until compatible blood can be obtained.

A transfusion of the wrong blood type can be fatal. Transmission of hepatitis B or C, HIV, and other viruses and infections is a potential danger even with current testing of all donor blood. Consequently, many patients prefer "directed donors." When blood replacement is anticipated before a surgical procedure, a family member or friend with a compatible blood type can be asked to donate blood to be held in the blood bank for the patient. Directed donations are not necessarily safer than nondirected voluntary donations supplied from the blood bank, however. When multiple units of blood must be transfused, packed cells, fresh frozen plasma, and platelets usually are given to supplement units of whole blood. These components are not part of whole blood replacement.

Basic rules apply to the transfusion of all homologous blood products. All established measures must be strictly observed for the patient's safety.

1. Blood products are obtained from the blood bank by a person responsible for signing them out to a specific patient. Usually a nursing assistant from the OR staff can do this.
2. To have blood nearby, a refrigerator with controlled temperature may be installed in the OR suite. Blood products for transfusion are kept at a constant temperature between 34° and 43° F (1° and 6° C), verified by a recording thermometer on the outside and a standard one inside. Both audible and visible alarms are activated if a dangerous temperature is reached. Fluctuations in temperature cause red blood cells to deteriorate. Microorganisms can multiply in unrefrigerated blood. If blood is brought into the OR and not needed, it should be returned to the refrigerator in the suite or blood bank immediately. Do not allow whole blood or its derivatives to stand unrefrigerated in the OR.
3. Blood products are administered by a physician or nurse after a careful comparison of label on the bag with identity of the patient. A second professional person confirms the data. The label stays on the container while blood product is being transfused.
4. Cold, refrigerated blood may induce hypothermia. Blood should be warmed as it is transfused by immersion of administration tubing in a controlled water bath or through coils in a temperature-modifying device. The temperature must be maintained between 89° and 105° F (32° and 41° C). Hemolysis may occur if the temperature exceeds 110° F (43° C).
5. Another solution may be infused immediately before a blood product is administered. In changing to the blood product, avoid the possibility of air entering tubing. A blood filter must be used for transfusion. The filter should be changed after the second or third unit of whole blood because the filter can become clogged with microaggregates.
6. Anesthesiologist records on the anesthesia record the following information for each unit transfused:
   a. Name of person who started transfusion
   b. Type and amount of product transfused (i.e., whole blood, plasma, packed cells, platelets, or albumin)
   c. Time started and drops per minute
   d. Information on label, including blood group, Rh factor, and number
7. Patient is observed closely for any type of reaction. This probability increases in direct proportion to the number of units transfused. The most common type of reaction is *allergic; febrile* is almost as common, and *hemolytic* reactions are possible. Transfusion reactions under anesthesia may be accompanied by profound hypotension, temperature change, blood in urine, and/or skin rash. However, the common physical reactions and chills are not seen in an anesthetized patient. If any suspicious reactions occur:
   a. Stop transfusion. Keep IV line patent with IV solution as directed by physician.
   b. Return unused blood to the blood bank along with a sample of the patient's blood.
   c. Send a urine sample to the laboratory as soon as possible.
   d. Take vital signs every 5 to 10 minutes until stable.
   e. Have emergency medications available.
   f. Document on patient's chart the type of reaction, action taken, patient's response, and other documentation as required by the institution.

Autologous Blood

Autologous blood is that recovered from the patient and reinfused. Referred to as *autotransfusion,* this process is the preferable method of replacement for either elective or emergency procedures. The patient's own blood is the safest form of transfusion; it eliminates concerns about compatibility/reactions and transmission of exogenous organisms. Autologous blood is equal or superior in quality to homologous blood. It may be obtained preoperatively from patients and returned to them intraoperatively or postoperatively as needed.

NOTE Some patients who, because of religious beliefs, will not accept homologous blood may accept autotransfusion. Jehovah's Witnesses, for example, believe that receiving blood or blood products violates a biblical prohibition against consumption of blood. They have the right to refuse transfusion. Written informed consent should be obtained from all patients for whom autotransfusion is contemplated.

Preoperative Blood Donation

One or more units of whole blood or blood components can be obtained by phlebotomy from the patient preoperatively and stored in the blood bank. Blood may be donated as often as every fourth day, if hemoglobin remains at least 11 g/dl or hematocrit is 33%, with the final unit donated no less than 72 hours before the scheduled surgical procedure. If two or more units are donated, an oral or intramuscular iron supplement may be prescribed.

Autologous blood is usually stored in a liquid state as whole blood or packed red cells. Whole blood, with anticoagulant, can be stored for 35 days and red cells, with preservative, for 42 days. Red cells and plasma can be frozen for prolonged storage. The same protocol is used in the OR for reinfusing autologous blood as described (p. 485) for homologous transfusions. If the patient does not need reinfusion, the blood is discarded. It is not given to another patient.

Intraoperative Autotransfusion

Recovery of blood as it is lost requires sterile equipment that suctions blood from the surgical site, filters and anticoagulates it, and contains it for reinfusion intravenously to the patient with minimal damage to cells. Blood can be suctioned directly from a body cavity or the wound, or it may be collected from drapes and sponges. Disposable drapes with plastic pouches to contain blood and fluid are available. (Any plastic devices, including suction tubing and pouches, used for blood recovery must be approved by the Food and Drug Administration [FDA].) Red blood cells can be salvaged from bloody sponges by rinsing them in a basin of normal saline solution used only for this purpose. The scrub person *gently* squeezes out sponges, then suctions the solution into an autotransfusion unit with a cell processor.

Blood is *not* salvaged if microfibrillar collagen has been used for hemostasis. This may not wash out when red cells are processed and can predispose the patient to disseminated intravascular coagulation or adult respiratory distress syndrome. Also, blood contaminated with enteric organisms or amniotic fluid is not salvaged. If a malignant tumor can be resected intact, autotransfusion may benefit the patient with cancer. Most cancer cells will filter out of processed blood. Autologous blood is not collected from patients with known systemic infections or from open traumatic wounds. Other patients, of all ages, are candidates for autotransfusion.

The autotransfusion unit must be easily and quickly assembled as it may be lifesaving for a trauma patient in an emergency situation. All fluid paths should be disposable and must be sterile. Three basic systems are used for intraoperative autotransfusion.

Automated Cell Salvage Processor Blood is suctioned through double-lumen tubing. An anticoagulant solution of heparinized saline or citrated dextrose mixes with blood at the tip end of the tubing. The aspirate passes through a 140-μm filter before entering the collection reservoir. This filter removes fat and debris. When a sufficient quantity to be processed has accumulated, the blood is pumped into a centrifuge bowl. The centrifugal force separates red cells from plasma, platelets, white cells, and other debris including anticoagulant. These red blood cells are washed with normal saline solution. A suspension of red cells in saline solution is pumped into a reinfusion bag. Each bag contains about 250 ml of washed packed red cells with a hematocrit of 50% to 55% ready for IV reinfusion. The entire cycle takes 3 to 7 minutes. Some autotransfusion units have automatic, programmed cycles, including process air and foam detectors; others operate manually. Platelet-rich plasma suitable for autotransfusion can be sequestered from some units.

Canister Collection Method Blood is suctioned and anticoagulated as described for the cell processor. From the tubing, the blood collects in a reservoir with a disposable liner. When the reservoir becomes full, or at the end of the surgical procedure, the liner is removed. The contents are washed in a standard red cell washer before being reinfused. This equipment may be located in the blood bank. The liner must be labeled with patient's name and identifying number if it leaves the OR for washing. Autologous blood obtained using this technique has a high hematocrit level and is almost free of protein, anticoagulant, and debris.

Salvage Collection Bag An anticoagulant, usually citrate, is added to blood collected directly into a single-use, self-contained transfusion bag. The blood is not washed. It is reinfused through a blood filter. This simple method is most appropriate when profuse bleeding occurs in areas that form pools that can be easily suctioned, such as the abdominal or chest cavities.

All three methods are safe when used according to the manufacturer's instructions. The automated cell salvage devices are the most sophisticated and complex. Only properly trained personnel should operate them. OR personnel may be trained to set up the sterile suction and containers.

Postoperative Autotransfusion

Autologous blood may be collected, processed, and bagged during a surgical procedure for reinfusion postoperatively. Bags must be labeled with name and identifying number of the patient and time processed. Autologous blood also can be salvaged postoperatively from a drainage tube placed into the surgical wound, most commonly a chest tube. The tube may be connected to a cell washer in a portable unit that attaches to wall suction in the PACU or ICU. Another method collects wound drainage by suctioning it directly into a filtered collection bag. With both of these methods blood is anticoagulated. It may be collected for a maximum of 6 hours. The concentrated red cells, either washed or unwashed, are reinfused intravenously. Unwashed blood can be kept at room temperature for 4 hours and washed blood for 6 hours at room temperature or refrigerated for 24 hours at 39.2° F (4° C), whether obtained intraoperatively or postoperatively.

Blood Substitutes

Oxygen-carrying blood substitutes offer another alternative to transport oxygen to the brain and throughout the body when the patient's blood volume or hemoglobin level is decreased because of blood loss. Fluosol-DA, an emulsion of perfluorochemicals, is an artificial blood substitute. Other infusions are prepared from a diluted stroma-free human hemoglobin solution or pure cattle hemoglobin in a saline solution. These substitutes may be used in anemic patients, for persons who refuse blood or blood products for religious reasons, or when compatible homologous blood is not available.

COMPLICATIONS

The patient must be constantly monitored (see Chapter 19) to detect any complications that might be developing as a result of blood loss or replacement or as a compromise of the cardiovascular system. Hemorrhage, shock, and disseminated intravascular coagulation (DIC) can have serious consequences on the outcome of surgical intervention. They may be the reason for or the result of a surgical procedure. Other complications associated with the vascular system can have serious cardiovascular, pulmonary, and renal sequelae.

Hemorrhage

Severe bleeding into or from a wound is a major contributing factor to intraoperative and postoperative morbidity and mortality. If uncontrolled, exsanguination can occur. Massive hemorrhage may cause hypovolemic shock, ventricular fibrillation, or death as a result of marked decrease in cardiac output. Common symptoms are arterial hypotension, pale or cyanotic moist skin, oliguria, bradycardia from hypoxia, or tachycardia after moderate to marked blood loss, restlessness, and thirst in the conscious patient.

In the OR, hemorrhage is readily visible. Meticulous hemostasis during every step of the surgical procedure and good nutritional status of the patient preoperatively are crucial to prevention. Preoperative evaluation of clotting time and history of bleeding (personal and familial), type and crossmatch of blood, and insertion of an IV line before incision are necessary precautions.

In treating hemorrhage, the surgeon locates the source of bleeding and applies digital compression to severed or traumatized blood vessels until noncrushing vascular clamps can be placed to occlude the vessel proximally and distally to the site of bleeding. The vessel is then ligated, electrocoagulated, or sutured. Circulating blood volume must be restored promptly. If homologous blood is transfused, it must be fresh and warmed to limit electrolytic changes. Sodium bicarbonate may be given intravenously to reduce acidosis. Multiple IV infusion routes can be used, by cutdown if necessary, to infuse blood under pressure. Ringer's lactate solution or other plasma expanders are used when blood is contraindicated (e.g., for religious reasons). Oxygen is administered to combat hypoxia. Accurate measurement of blood and fluid losses intraoperatively, followed by adequate replacement, will help prevent hypovolemic shock. Autotransfusion may be feasible.

Hemorrhage can be detected postoperatively by observation of blood-soaked dressings. The patient must be checked frequently for both observable and nonobservable symptoms of hemorrhage. Internal bleeding can be caused by slipping or sloughing of a ligature or by the blowout of clots from ligated or coagulated vessels.

Shock

Shock is a state of inadequate blood perfusion to parts of the body. If untreated, it will become irreversible and result in death. All forms of shock carry high mortality. See Chapter 19, pp. 390-391, for discussion of the six main classifications of circulatory shock.

Hemorrhagic shock results from a decrease in circulating blood volume caused by loss of blood, plasma, or extracellular fluid. Fluid loss is excessive when it is greater than compensatory absorption of interstitial fluid into circulation. Shock resulting from hemorrhage or inadequate blood volume replacement, as seen in the OR and PACU, usually is reversed by prompt restoration of circulating blood volume. (See Chapter 19, p. 381, for discussion of hypovolemic shock.)

Venous Stasis

Venous return of blood from the lower extremities can be slowed by the effects of general or spinal anesthesia and by the position of legs during prolonged surgical procedures. The venous stasis that develops in most patients during a surgical procedure can be effectively counteracted. To prevent thrombophlebitis and thrombosis in patients with thromboembolic disease, anticoagulants may be administered. Antiembolic stockings, with or without a sequential pneumatic compression device, augment venous flow from the legs. Elevation of legs as little as 15% above horizontal can assist in venous return.

Postoperatively, the patient may be placed in Trendelenburg's position with legs elevated. Flexion and extension of legs and feet, frequent turning, and early ambulation, unless contraindicated, aid circulation.

Deep Vein Thrombosis

Venous stasis, changes in clotting factors in the blood, and damage to vessel walls are the primary causes of deep vein thrombosis (DVT) in the lower extremities. Age, obesity, immobility, and a history of thromboembolic or other cardiovascular disease are predisposing factors. The type, location, and extent of the surgical procedure can contribute also. Preoperative prophylactic interventions, including anticoagulants and compression stockings, can reduce the risk of postoperative pulmonary embolism, which is a life-threatening complication of DVT.

Disseminated Intravascular Coagulation

Although a rare event, DIC is a life-threatening syndrome. It is a complex derangement of clotting factors. The hemostatic process involves vasoconstriction with platelet aggregation and clotting. In DIC, the normal clotting mechanisms do not function. Instead, a repetitive, overactive cycle of clot formation and simultaneous clot breakdown (fibrinolysis) occurs. This leads to consumption of platelets and coagulation factors and release of fibrin degradation products that act as potent anticoagulants. DIC can follow hemorrhage, thrombi, emboli, infection, or allergic reaction to an incompatible blood transfusion. It may be precipitated by septic shock, abruptio placentae during pregnancy, or massive soft tissue damage of extensive trauma or burns. As blood becomes depleted of platelets and major clotting factors, coagulation is initiated throughout the bloodstream, especially in microcirculation. Prolonged bleeding may be noted; hematomas and cutaneous petechiae may appear. Massive hemorrhage and ischemia of vital organs may ensue. Bleeding may be noted from various sites, such as through the nasogastric tube. The patient may have hypotension and oliguria. Postoperatively the patient may have nausea and vomiting, severe muscular pain, and convulsions and may lapse into a coma. Diagnosis is based on laboratory blood studies. Treatment begins with control of the primary condition. Blood, plasma, and dextran can be administered intravenously. Heparin and clotting factors, if given early, may prevent hemorrhage.

Pulmonary Embolism

Pulmonary embolism is an obstruction of the pulmonary artery or one of its branches by an embolus, most often a blood clot. The most important factor leading to *pulmonary emboli* is stasis of blood, particularly in deep veins of the legs and pelvis where the majority of thrombi arise. These become detached and are carried to the lungs. Changes in vessel walls and coagulative changes in blood are also important factors. A prolonged period on the operating table may decrease blood flow to the lower extremities by more than 50%. Blood flow is impaired further if the knees are raised on a pillow, putting pressure on the vessels. Venous stasis also is correlated with obesity, congestive heart failure, and atrial fibrillation. Local trauma to a vein or venous disease enhances the chance of thrombus formation. Hypercoagulability may coexist with conditions such as pregnancy, fever, myocardial infarction, and some malignancies and after abrupt cessation of anticoagulant therapy. Prevention consists of a regimen of prophylactic anticoagulants or antiplatelets for high-risk patients and routine measures to prevent venous stasis, such as intermittent compression or antiembolic stockings.

Because of the origin of thrombi in deep veins, it is important to observe the patient postoperatively for thrombophlebitis, evidenced by heat, edema, redness, pain in the calf, or a positive Homans' sign, which is pain in the calf upon forceful dorsiflexion of foot. Nonspecific symptoms depend on whether the embolism is mild or massive. The patient may have dyspnea, pleural pain, hemoptysis, tachypnea, crackles, tachycardia, mild fever, or persistent cough. Patients with massive emboli have air hunger, hypotension, shock, and cyanosis. Treatment of pulmonary emboli consists of bed rest, oxygen therapy, anticoagulant therapy, thrombolytic agents, and sometimes a surgical procedure to remove the emboli or prevent their recurrence.

Fat embolism occurs primarily following fracture of a long bone, pelvis, and ribs. However, it sometimes occurs after a blood transfusion, cardiopulmonary bypass, or renal transplant. Fat globules enter the bloodstream. Symptoms develop when globules block pulmonary capillaries, causing interstitial edema and hemorrhage. Frequently, *adult respiratory distress syndrome* (ARDS) ensues 24 to 48 hours after injury, with hypoxia and decreased surfactant production, resulting in collapse of the alveolar membrane and microatelectasis. The syndrome develops most frequently in patients older than 10 years of age, especially those who have traveled long distances with an immobilized fracture. Symptoms include disorientation, increased pulse and temperature, tachypnea, dyspnea, crackles, and pleuritic chest pain. Other significant signs are fat in the sputum and urine and a petechial rash on the anterior chest. Treatment is supportive. Mortality is high.

Air embolism may follow injection of air into a body cavity or a bolus of air in an IV or intraarterial infusion. Another portal of entry is transection of large veins with the patient in a sitting position (see Chapter 21, pp. 443-444). The pull of gravity on the blood column exerts a significant negative pressure that sucks air down the veins and into the heart. This can be a complication in handling central venous catheters and using syringes to obtain blood for gas analysis.

Intrauterine fetal death or placenta previa may precipitate an *embolism of amniotic fluid*. Also, tumors may cause emboli from primary or metastatic sites.

Overriding Concerns

The physical stresses to which a surgical patient is subjected may lead to cardiovascular complications, including thromboembolism and/or thrombophlebitis, hypotension, various dysrhythmias, and congestive heart failure. Pulmonary edema may result from congestive heart failure or fluid overload. Renal function also is a major concern. Control of blood loss and blood replacement are essential aspects of surgical intervention. Meticulous hemostasis and wound closure are basic surgical techniques.

Bibliography

Allen GJL: Intraoperative autotransfusion: an old idea comes of age, *Surg Technol* 24(1):8-12, 1992.

Assalia A, Schein M: Resuscitation for haemorrhagic shock, *Br J Surg* 80(2):213, 1993.

Bailes BK: Disseminated intravascular coagulation, *AORN J* 55(2):517-529, 1992.

Bickwell WH: Are the victims of injury sometimes victimized by attempts at fluid resuscitation? *Ann Emerg Med* 22(2):225-226, 1993.

Bright LD, Georgi S: How to protect your patient from DVT, *Am J Nurs* 94(12):28-32, 1994.

Campbell AD: Pneumatic compression stockings: preventing deep vein thrombosis and pulmonary embolus, *Today's OR Nurse* 12(7):4-9, 1990.

Carstens VL, Earnshaw PH: Postoperative orthopedic autotransfusion, *AORN J* 56(2):272-280, 1992.

Curry J: Bloodless surgery meets patient needs for alternatives, *OR Manager* 9(1):12-13, 1993.

Domsky MF, Wison RF: Hemodynamic resuscitation, *Crit Care Clin* 9(4):715-726, 1993.

Donner C: Detecting venous thrombosis, *Am J Nurs* 93(6):48, 1993.

Drago SS: Banking on your own blood, *Am J Nurs* 92(3):61-64, 1992.

Falk JL et al: Fluid resuscitation in traumatic hemorrhagic shock, *Crit Care Clin* 8(2):323-340, 1992.

Ferguson KJ et al: Physician recommendation as the key factor in patients' decisions to participate in preoperative autologous blood donation programs, *Am J Surg* 168(1):2-5, 1994.

Flynn JC: Perioperative autotransfusion: avoiding donated risks, *Today's OR Nurse* 12(7):20-23, 1990.

Gruen GS et al: The acute management of hemodynamically unstable multiple trauma patients with pelvic ring fractures, *J Trauma* 36(5):706-711, 1994.

Hennessy B et al: Venous air embolism: keeping your patient out of danger, *Am J Nurs* 93(11):54-56, 1993.

Huston CJ: Disseminated intravascular coagulation, *Am J Nurs* 94(8):51, 1994.

Johnson GN, Bowman RJ: Autologous blood transfusion, *AORN J* 56(2):282-292, 1992.

Martinelli AM: Sickle cell disease, *AORN J* 53(3):716-724, 1991.

Mathews K: Argon beam coagulation, *AORN J* 56(5):885-896, 1992.

Mathias JM: No-heat surgical device uses ultrasonic motion for cutting, *OR Manager* 10(2):16-17, 1994.

Miller SR, Waxman K: Advances in the management of hemorrhagic shock, *West J Med* 155(4):404-405, 1991.

National Blood Resource Education Program's Nursing Education Working Group: Tranfusion nursing: trends and practices for the '90s, *Am J Nurs* 91(6):42-52, 1991.

Phillips GR et al: Massive blood loss in trauma patients: the benefits and dangers of transfusion therapy, *Postgrad Med* 95(4):61-72, 1994.

Proposed recommended practices: use of the pneumatic tourniquet, *AORN J* 59(3):693-704, 1994.

Puri VK: Colloid versus crystalloid war—a time for truce, *Crit Care Med* 18(4):457-458, 1990.

Usuba A et al: Oxygen transport capacity and hemodynamic effect of newly developed artificial blood "Neo Red Cells (NRC)," *Int J Artif Organs* 16(7):551-556, 1993.

Wicker P: Electrosurgery: Part I: the history of diathermy, *Br J Theatre Nurs* 27(8):6-7, 1990.

CHAPTER 24

Wound Closure Materials

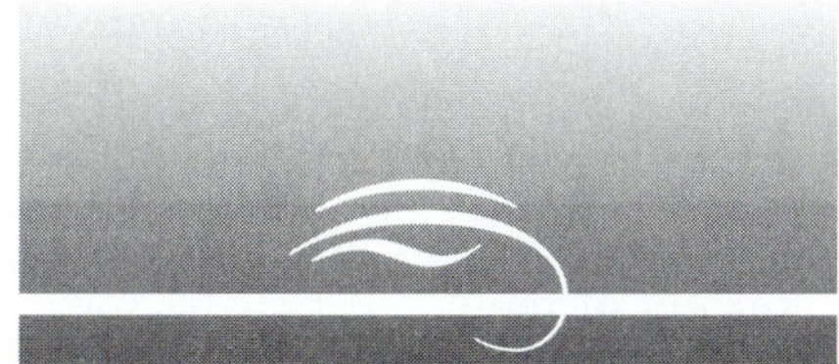

HISTORICAL BACKGROUND

As a distinct discipline of medicine, surgery is based on techniques to control bleeding and close wounds. The story of sutures, in some measure, is the story of surgery itself. Many kinds of materials were used in the past, and many are used today, to close or cover wounds.

The first written description of sutures, which were probably made of linen, to approximate wound edges is in the Edwin Smith papyrus from the sixteenth century BC. The *Shusruta Samhita,* an ancient Indian classic written between 600 and 1000 BC, refers to plaited horsehair, cotton, strips of leather, and fibers from tree bark for use as sutures. These and other writings dating back to 2000 BC refer to strings and animal tendons for ligating and suturing. In 30 AD Celsus referred to the use of twisted sutures.

Galen (130-220 AD) mentioned the use of animal gut sutures for the primary closure of wounds in Roman gladiators, although he recommended silk when it could be obtained. Previous knowledge of ligatures seems to have been lost until Galen wrote of using them to stop bleeding after trying all other methods known at the time.

Muhammadan religious laws required caravan leaders to carry sutures and needles to care for injuries. Sometimes camel hair was used for sutures. Arabian surgeons used harp strings. Rhazes (circa 854-930 AD) of Persia is credited with first employing *kitstrings* to suture abdominal wounds. In Arabic, a kit is a fiddle. The fiddle strings were made from sheep intestines, which were twisted and dried in the sun. They were called *kitgut.* However, a young cat also is a kit. The term *catgut* is believed to have evolved from its origin as kitgut. Suture material is still made from sheep or beef intestine but is more accurately called *surgical gut* today.

Sutures fell into disuse during the Middle Ages, accompanying a general regression in surgical technique. Their use was revived by Ambroise Pare´ (1510-1590), a French army surgeon. He ligated arteries to stop the bleeding following amputations.

Early in the nineteenth century Dr. Philip Syng Physick (1768-1837) found that the body absorbs sutures made from animal tissue. Probably the first surgeon to realize this, Physick was the first American to use catgut extensively. He also fashioned a curved needle for circumventing an artery.

Catgut sutures were used in the early nineteenth century by English surgeons. But Joseph Lister (1827-1912) is credited with sterilizing and chromicizing them. Only since Lister's time have wound closure techniques been brought to an advanced state of development.

Many materials have been used as ligatures and sutures through the centuries, including gold, silver, and tantalum wire, silk, silkworm gut, horsehair, kangaroo tendon, cotton, and linen. The synthetic polymers developed in the twentieth century resulted in the demise of many of these materials for use as surgical sutures. Polymer chemistry has revolutionized the manufacture of sutures, although silk and surgical gut continue to be widely used.

Needles are used to place suture through tissues. Needles were used by primitive man to sew hides together for clothing. Eyed needles made of bone date back to the Upper Paleolithic period between 20,000 and 35,000 years ago and were used until the Renaissance, which began in the fourteenth century. By the nineteenth century steel needles, either straight like those used by dressmakers or curved, were employed. They were manipulated by the fingers of the operator, however. Succeeding generations of surgeons have fashioned hundreds of modifications of needles. Needles were first *swaged* (i.e., permanently attached to the suture material) in 1928. Today more than a hundred shapes, sizes, and types of surgical needles are swaged to the suture materials that are in common use.

Although surgical stapling is considered to be an innovation of the twentieth century, the concept of mechanically holding tissues together dates back to antiquity. The *Shusruta Samhita* describes the use of termites to hold wound edges in apposition. The termite would bite through the skin at wound site and, with subsequent beheading, would hold the wound edges together with its pincers. Ancient Egyptians and some modern South American tribes used ant jaws. East Africans closed wounds with acacia thorns. These insects and plants were forerunners of the skin staplers used today.

The first internal stapler was introduced in Budapest by Professor Hamer Hültl in 1908 for closing the stomach. This was followed in 1924, also in Hungary, by a mechanical device for gastrointestinal anastomosis developed by Aladar von Petz. Although cumbersome and heavy, weighing over 7 lb (5 kg), the von Petz clamp received worldwide acceptance. The Russians subsequently became the leaders in the field of stapling tissue with their refinements in instrumentation during the 1950s. Most of the reusable staplers currently in use are available through patents licensed from the former Soviet Union. A disposable skin stapler was introduced in 1978, and disposable internal staplers have been available since 1980.

Halsted Suture Technique

The education a physician receives during postgraduate surgical training exerts a lasting influence on his or her surgical techniques. The classic example of the influence of a professor on his students is that of Dr. William Stewart Halsted (1852-1922). Dr. Halsted, a professor of surgery at Johns Hopkins Hospital in Baltimore from 1893 to 1922, is acknowledged to have been one of the greatest surgeons of all times. He perfected and brought into use the fine-pointed hemostat for occluding vessels, the Penrose drain, and rubber gloves. However, he is best known for his principles of gentle tissue handling. In addition to his surgical techniques, he inspired his assistants with his high ideals—as near perfection as possible in all surgical procedures. The silk suture technique he initiated in 1883, or a modification of it, is in use today. Its features are as follows:

1. Interrupted sutures are used for greater strength. Each stitch is taken and tied separately. If one knot slips, all the others hold. Halsted also believed that interrupted sutures were a barrier to infection, for he thought that if one area of a wound became infected, the microorganisms traveled along a continuous suture to infect the entire wound. A continuous suture is a running stitch tied only at the ends of the incision.
2. Sutures are as fine as is consistent with security. A suture stronger than the tissue it holds is not necessary.
3. Sutures are cut close to the knots. Long ends cause irritation.
4. A separate needle is used for each skin stitch.
5. Dead space in the wound is eliminated. *Dead space* is that space caused by separation of wound edges that have not been closely approximated by sutures. Serum or blood clots may collect in a dead space and prevent healing by keeping the cut edges of tissue separated.
6. Two fine sutures are used in situations usually requiring one large one.
7. Silk is not used in the presence of infection.
8. Tension is not placed on tissue. Halsted warned against bringing tissue together under tension and thus endangering the blood supply.

Halsted's principles are, in general, still highly regarded. However, they were based on use of the only suture materials available to him, silk and surgical gut. With the advent of less reactive synthetic materials, wound closure may be safely and more quickly performed with different techniques and without complications.

SUTURES

Common Terms

Suture is an all-inclusive term for any strand of material used for ligating or approximating tissue.

Tie

If the material is tied around a blood vessel to occlude the lumen, it is called a *ligature* or *tie*. A *free tie* is a single strand of material handed to the surgeon or assistant to ligate a vessel. A strand attached to a needle before use is referred to as a *stick tie* or *suture/ligature*.

The needle is used to anchor the strand in tissue before occluding a deep or large vessel.

Suture

The verb *to suture* denotes the act of sewing by bringing tissues together and holding them until healing has taken place. The noun *suture* is the strand of material used for this purpose.

Specifications for Suture Material

1. It must be *sterile* when placed in tissue. Sterile techniques must be rigidly followed in handling suture material. For example, if the end of a strand drops over the side of any sterile surface, discard the strand. *Almost all postoperative wound infections are initiated along or adjacent to suture lines.* Affinity for bacterial contamination varies with the physical characteristics of the material.
2. It must be predictably uniform in tensile strength by size and material. *Tensile strength* is the measured pounds of tension or pull that a strand will withstand before it breaks when knotted. Minimum knot-pull strengths are specified for each basic raw material and for each size of that material by the *United States Pharmacopeia* (USP). Tensile strength decreases as the diameter of the strand decreases.
3. It must be as small in diameter as is safe to use on each type of tissue. The strength of the suture usually need be no greater than the strength of the tissue on which it is used. Smaller sizes are less traumatic during placement in tissue and leave less suture mass to cause tissue reaction. The surgeon ties small-diameter sutures more gently and thus is less apt to strangulate tissue. A small-diameter suture is flexible, easy to manipulate, and leaves minimal scar on skin.
4. Sizes range from heavy 7 to very fine 11-0; ranges vary with materials. Taking size 1 as a starting point, sizes increase with each number above 1 and decrease with each 0 added. Thus size 7 is the largest and 11-0 is the smallest. The more 0s in the number, the smaller the size of the strand. As the number of 0s increases, the size of the strand decreases. In addition to this system of size designation, the manufacturer's labels on boxes and packets also may include metric measures for suture diameters. These metric equivalents vary slightly by types of materials.
5. It must have knot security, remain tied, and give support to tissue during the healing process. However, sutures in the skin are always removed 3 to 10 days postoperatively, depending on the site of incision and cosmetic result desired. Because they are exposed to the external environment, skin sutures can be a source of microbial contamination of the wound that inhibits healing by first intention.
6. It must cause as little foreign-body tissue reaction as possible. All suture materials are foreign bodies, but some are more inert, less reactive, than others.

Choice of Suture Material

Surgical sutures as defined by the USP* are divided into two classifications: absorbable and nonabsorbable.

1. *Absorbable sutures* are sterile strands prepared from collagen derived from healthy mammals or from a synthetic polymer. They are capable of being absorbed by living mammalian tissue but may be treated to modify resistance to absorption. They may be colored by a color additive approved by the Federal Food and Drug Administration (FDA).
2. *Nonabsorbable sutures* are strands of natural or synthetic material that effectively resist enzymatic digestion or absorption in living tissue. During the healing process, suture mass becomes encapsulated and may remain for years in tissues without producing any ill effects. They may be colored by a color additive approved by the FDA. They may be modified with respect to body, texture, or capillarity. *Capillarity* refers to a characteristic of nonabsorbable sutures that allows the passage of tissue fluids along the strand, permitting infection, if present, to be drawn along the suture line. These suture materials may be untreated or may be treated to reduce capillarity. *Noncapillarity* is the characteristic of some nonabsorbable sutures in which the nature of the raw material or specific processing meets USP tests that establish them as resistant to "wicking" transfer of body fluids.

The two classifications of suture materials are subdivided into monofilament and multifilament strands.

1. *Monofilament* suture is a strand consisting of a single threadlike structure that is noncapillary.
2. *Multifilament* suture is a strand made of more than one threadlike structure held together by braiding or twisting. This strand is capillary unless treated to resist capillarity or is absorbable.

The surgeon selects the type of suture material best suited to promote healing. Factors that influence choice include:

1. Biologic characteristics of the material in tissue, for example, absorbable vs. nonabsorbable, capillary vs. noncapillary, inertness.

**United States Pharmacopeia*, ed 22, Rockville, Md, 1990, US Pharmacopeial Convention.

2. Healing characteristics of tissue. Tissues that normally heal slowly such as skin, fascia, and tendons usually are closed with nonabsorbable sutures. Absorbable suture placed through the skin may cause a stitch abscess to develop because it is inclined to act as a culture medium for microorganisms in the pores of the skin. Tissues that heal rapidly such as stomach, colon, and bladder may be closed with absorbable sutures.
3. Location and length of the incision. Cosmetic results desired may be an influencing factor.
4. Presence or absence of infection, contamination, and/or drainage. If infection is present, sutures may be the origin of granuloma formation with subsequent discharge of suture and sinus formation. Foreign bodies in potentially contaminated tissues may convert contamination to infection. Foreign bodies in the presence of some body fluids may cause stone formation, as in the urinary or biliary tract.
5. Patient problems such as obesity, debility, advanced age, and diseases, which influence rate of healing and time desired for wound support.
6. Physical characteristics of the material such as ease of passage through tissue, knot tying, and other personal preferences of the surgeon.

Absorbable Sutures

Surgical Gut

Often still referred to as catgut, *surgical gut* is collagen derived from the submucosa of sheep intestine or serosa of beef intestine. The intestines from these freshly slaughtered animals are sent to processing plants. There they undergo many elaborate mechanical and chemical cleaning processes before intestinal ribbons of collagen are spun into strands of various sizes, ranging from the heaviest size 3 to the finest size 7-0. Although the larger sizes are made from two or more ribbons, the behavior of surgical gut is that of a monofilament suture.

Surgical gut is digested by body enzymes and absorbed by tissue so that no permanent foreign body remains. The rate of absorption is influenced by:

1. *Type of tissue.* Surgical gut is absorbed much more rapidly in serous or mucous membrane. It is absorbed slowly in subcutaneous fat.
2. *Condition of tissue.* Surgical gut can be used in the presence of infection; even knots are absorbed. However, absorption takes place much more rapidly in the presence of infection.
3. *General health status of patient.* Surgical gut may be absorbed more rapidly in undernourished or diseased tissue, but in elderly or debilitated patients it may remain for a long time.
4. *Type of surgical gut.* Plain gut is untreated, but chromic gut is treated to provide greater resistance to absorption. Surgical gut may be made pliable to enhance its handling characteristics, but the process significantly reduces tensile strength.

Plain Surgical Gut Plain surgical gut loses tensile strength relatively quickly, usually in 5 to 10 days, and is digested within 70 days because collagen strands are not treated to resist absorption. Plain surgical gut is used to ligate small vessels and to suture subcutaneous fat. It is not used to suture any layers of tissue likely to be subjected to tension during healing. It is available in sizes 3 through 6-0. Usually used in its natural yellow-tan color, it may be dyed blue or black.

Fast absorbing plain surgical gut is specially treated to speed absorption and tensile strength loss. It may be used for epidermal suturing where sutures are needed for no more than a week. These sutures are used only externally on skin, not internally, particularly for facial cosmetic surgery.

Chromic Surgical Gut Chromic surgical gut is treated in a chromium salt solution to resist absorption by tissues for varying lengths of time depending on the strength of the solution and duration and method of the process. The chromicizing process either bathes each ribbon of collagen before it is spun into strands or applies solution to the finished strand. This treatment changes the color from the yellowish-tan shade of plain surgical gut to a dark shade of brown. Chromic surgical gut is used for ligation of larger vessels and for suture of tissues in which nonabsorbable materials are not usually recommended because they may act as a nidus for stone formation, as in the urinary or biliary tracts. In closure of muscle or fascia it has the disadvantage of rapidly declining tensile strength. If the absorption rate is normal, chromic surgical gut will support the wound for about 14 days, with some strength up to 21 days, and will be completely absorbed within 90 days. Sizes range from 3 through 7-0. Chromic surgical gut may be dyed blue or black.

Collagen Sutures

Collagen sutures are extruded from a homogeneous dispersion of pure collagen fibrils from the flexor tendons of beef. Both plain and chromic types are similar in appearance to surgical gut and may be dyed blue. Sizes range from 4-0 through 8-0. These sutures are used primarily in ophthalmic surgery.

Handling Characteristics of Surgical Gut and Collagen

1. Most surgical gut and collagen sutures are sealed in packets that contain fluid to keep the material pliable. This fluid is chiefly alcohol and water *but may be irritating to ophthalmic tissues.* Hold packet over a basin, and open carefully to avoid spilling

fluid on the sterile field or splashing it into your own eyes. Rinsing is necessary *only* for surgical gut or collagen sutures to be implanted into the eye.

2. Surgical gut and collagen sutures should be used immediately after removal from their packets. When the material is removed and not used at once, the alcohol evaporates and the strand loses pliability. Many surgeons prefer that the scrub person quickly dip the strand into water or normal saline solution to soften it slightly. *Do not soak.* Excessive exposure to water will reduce the tensile strength. Before unwinding, the strand can be dipped momentarily in water or normal saline solution at room temperature; heat will coagulate the protein.
3. Unwind the strand carefully. Handle it as little as possible. Never jerk or stretch surgical gut; this weakens it. Do not straighten suture by running fingers down length of strand; excessive handling with rubber gloves can cause fraying. Grasp the ends and tug gently to straighten.

Synthetic Absorbable Polymers

Polymers, either dyed or undyed, are extruded into absorbable suture strands. These synthetic sutures are absorbed by a slow hydrolysis process in the presence of tissue fluids. They are used for ligating or suturing except when extended approximation of tissues under stress is required. They are inert, nonantigenic, and nonpyrogenic and produce only a mild tissue reaction during absorption. They may be monofilament or multifilament, coated or uncoated.

Polydioxanone (PDS Suture) Monofilaments extruded from polyester poly (p-dioxanone), PDS and PDS II sutures are particularly useful in tissues in which slow healing is anticipated, as in the fascia, or where extended wound support is desirable, as in the elderly, but an absorbable suture is preferable. They may be used in the presence of infection; they will not harbor bacterial growth because of their chemical and monofilament construction. PDS II sutures are more pliable than PDS sutures. Absorption is minimal for about 90 days, then complete within 6 months. Approximately 50% of the tensile strength is retained for 4 weeks and 25% for 6 weeks. PDS suture retains its breaking strength longer than any other synthetic absorbable suture. Violet PDS suture is available in sizes 2 through 9-0, blue in sizes 7-0 through 10-0 for ophthalmic tissues, and clear in sizes 1 through 7-0.

Poliglecaprone 25 (Monocryl Suture) Prepared from a copolymer of glycolide and epsilon-caprolactone, Monocryl suture is the most pliable of the monofilament synthetic sutures. It retains approximately 50% to 60% of its tensile strength in tissue for 7 days, retains approximately 20% to 30% at 14 days, and loses all tensile strength by 21 days. Absorption is essentially complete between 91 and 119 days. Because of its strength retention and absorption profiles, it is indicated for use in all types of soft tissue approximation and/or ligation, especially in general, gynecologic, urologic, and plastic surgery, but it is not indicated for use in cardiovascular, neural, or ophthalmic tissues. Undyed natural golden in color, it is available in sizes 2 through 6-0.

Polyglyconate (Maxon Suture) A monofilament is prepared from a copolymer of glycolic acid and trimethylene carbonate. It is indicated for approximation of soft tissue except in cardiovascular, neural, and ophthalmic tissues. Absorption is minimal for about 60 days, then is complete within 6 months. Approximately 70% of tensile strength remains at 2 weeks, 55% at 3 weeks. Clear or dyed green, this suture is available in sizes 2 through 7-0. Maxon CV monofilament absorbable suture is available for pediatric cardiovascular and peripheral vascular procedures.

Polyglactin 910 (Vicryl Suture) The precisely controlled combination of glycolide and lactide results in a copolymer with a molecular structure that maintains tensile strength longer than surgical gut, but not as long as polydioxanone. Approximately 30% of original strength is retained at 3 weeks. Absorption is minimal for about 40 days; then it absorbs rapidly within 90 days. The acids of both glycolide and lactide exist naturally in the body and are readily excreted in urine. Polyglactin 910 sutures are available in two forms: uncoated monofilament and coated multifilament.

1. *Uncoated monofilament polyglactin 910 (Vicryl suture)* is available dyed violet in sizes 9-0 and 10-0 for ophthalmic procedures.
2. *Coated multifilament polyglactin 910 (Coated Vicryl suture)* is a braided strand coated with a mixture of equal parts of a copolymer of glycolide and lactide (polyglactin 370) and calcium stearate. The coating provides a nonflaking lubricant for smooth passage through tissue and precise knot placement. This absorbable coating does not affect the absorption rate or tensile strength of the suture. It absorbs with the suture. Coated Vicryl suture is available dyed violet in sizes 2 through 9-0 and undyed in sizes 1 through 8-0.

Polyglycolic Acid (Dexon Suture) The homopolymer of glycolic acid loses tensile strength more rapidly and absorbs significantly more slowly than polyglactin 910. Strands are smaller in diameter than surgical gut of equivalent tensile strength. Polyglycolic acid suture loses approximately 45% of its tensile strength by 14 days and absorbs significantly by 30 days. It is a braided suture material available in two forms: uncoated and coated.

1. *Uncoated polyglycolic acid (Dexon S suture)* is available dyed green in sizes 2 through 8-0, and undyed natural beige in sizes 2 through 7-0. (A 9-0 monofilament suture, dyed green, is also available.)
2. *Coated polyglycolic acid (Dexon Plus suture)* has a surfactant, poloxamer 188, on the surface that becomes slick in contact with body fluids for smooth passage through tissue. This suture requires two or three extra throws in knot tying, and the ends must be cut longer than for uncoated material. The coating virtually disappears from the suture site within a few hours, which may strengthen knot security. Sutures are available in the same sizes as uncoated polyglycolic acid sutures.

Handling Characteristics of Synthetic Absorbable Polymers

1. Synthetic absorbable sutures have an expiration date on the package. Therefore, rotate stock. *First in, first out* is a good rule to follow.
2. Sutures are packaged and used dry. Do not soak or dip in water or normal saline solution. The material hydrolizes in water so that excessive exposure to moisture will reduce the tensile strength. It is smooth, soft, and will retain its pliability.

Nonabsorbable Sutures

Surgical Silk

Surgical silk is an animal product made from the fiber spun by silkworm larvae in making their cocoons. From the raw state, each fiber is processed to remove natural waxes and gums. Fibers are braided or twisted together to form a multifilament suture strand. The braided type is used more frequently because surgeons prefer its high tensile strength and better handling qualities. Surgical silk is treated to render it noncapillary. It also is dyed, most commonly black, but also is available in white. Sizes range from 5 through 9-0.

Silk is not a true nonabsorbable material. It loses much of its tensile strength after about 1 year and usually disappears within 2 years. It gives good support to wounds during early ambulation and generally promotes rapid healing. It causes less tissue reaction than surgical gut, but it is not as inert as most of the other nonabsorbable materials. It is used frequently in the serosa of the gastrointestinal tract and to close fascia in the absence of infection.

Virgin Silk Virgin silk suture consists of several natural silk filaments drawn together and twisted to form 8-0 and 9-0 strands for tissue approximation of delicate structures, primarily in ophthalmic surgery. It is white or dyed black.

Dermal Silk Dermal suture is a strand of twisted silk fibers encased in a nonabsorbing coating of tanned gelatin or other protein substance. This coating prevents ingrowth of tissue cells and facilitates removal after use as a skin suture. Because of its unusual strength, it is used for suturing skin, particularly in areas of tension. It is black in sizes 0 through 5-0.

Handling Characteristics of Silk Sutures

1. Silk sutures are used dry. They lose tensile strength if wet. Therefore, do not moisten before use.
2. If it is necessary to sterilize silk suture, do so at 250° F (121° C) for 15 minutes. Silk shrinks during steam sterilization. Therefore, if supplied nonsterile, it must never be sterilized on a spool. Some tensile strength is lost during sterilization.

Surgical Cotton

Cotton is a natural cellulose fiber. Suture is made from individual, long-staple cotton fibers that are cleaned, combed, aligned, and twisted into a smooth multifilament strand. Sizes range from 1 through 5-0. Usually white, it may be dyed blue or pink.

Cotton is one of the weakest of the nonabsorbable materials; however, it gains tensile strength when wet. Moisten before handing to the surgeon. Tensile strength is increased 10% by moisture. Also, moisture prevents clinging to the surgeon's gloves. Like silk, cotton suture may be used in most body tissues for ligating and suturing, but it offers no advantages over silk.

Linen

Surgical linen is spun from long-staple flax fibers, then twisted into tight strands and treated for smooth passage through tissue. Tensile strength is inferior to all other nonabsorbable materials. Linen suture, available in sizes 0 and 2-0, is used almost exclusively in gastrointestinal surgery.

Surgical Stainless Steel

Stainless steel sutures are drawn from 316L-SS (L for low carbon) iron alloy wire. This is the same metal formula used in the manufacture of surgical stainless steel implants and prostheses.

NOTE *Two different kinds of metal must not be embedded in the tissues simultaneously.* Such a combination creates an unfavorable electrolytic reaction. Some implants and prostheses are made of Vitallium, titanium, or tantalum. Suture material in the wound must be compatible with these metals.

Before the availability of surgical stainless steel from suture manufacturers, commercial steel was purchased by weight, using the Brown & Sharpe (B&S) scale for diameter variations. Many surgeons still refer to surgical stainless steel size by the B&S gauge from 18, the largest diameter, to 40, the smallest. One manufacturer labels surgical stainless steel with both B&S gauge and equivalent USP diameter classifications from 7 through 6-0. Both monofilament and twisted multifilament stainless steel strands are available.

Surgical stainless steel is inert in tissue and has high tensile strength. It gives the greatest strength of any suture material to a wound before healing begins and supports a wound indefinitely. Some surgeons use stainless steel for abdominal wall or sternal closure or for retention sutures to reduce the danger of wound disruption in the presence of contributing factors. It may be used in the presence of infection or in patients in whom slow healing is expected. It is used for secondary repair or resuture following evisceration.

Unlike most other suture materials, steel lacks elasticity. A suture tied too tightly may act as a knife and cut through tissue. Stainless steel sutures are harder to handle than any other suture material. A painstaking knot-tying technique is required. For most surgeons this disadvantage more than outweighs the advantages for routine use. However, in selected situations it fills an important need. It is used in the respiratory tract, in tendon repair, in orthopaedics and neurosurgery, and for general wound closure.

Handling Characteristics of Stainless Steel

1. Surgical stainless steel strands are malleable and kink rather easily. Kinks in the strand can make it practically useless. Therefore care must be taken in handling to keep the strand straight.
2. Use wire scissors for cutting stainless steel sutures. Barbs on the end of a strand can tear gloves, thus breaking sterile technique, or traumatize tissue.
3. If surgical stainless steel must be threaded to a needle, some surgeons prefer one or two twists of the end around the strand just below the eye of the needle to prevent unthreading during suturing.

Synthetic Nonabsorbable Polymers

Although silk is the most frequently used nonabsorbable suture material, synthetic nonabsorbable materials are used because they offer unique advantages in many situations. They have higher tensile strength and elicit less tissue reaction than silk. They retain their strength in tissue. Knot tying with most of these materials is more difficult than with silk. Additional throws are required to secure the knot. The surgeon may sacrifice some handling characteristics and ease of knot tying for strength, durability, and nonreactivity of the synthetics. These advantages may outweigh the disadvantages.

Surgical Nylon Nylon is a polyamide polymer derived by chemical synthesis from coal, air, and water. It produces minimal tissue reaction. Nylon has high tensile strength, but it degrades by hydrolysis in tissue at a rate of about 15% to 20% per year. It may be used in all tissues where a nonabsorbable suture is acceptable, except when long-term support is critical. It is available in three forms: monofilament, uncoated multifilament, and coated multifilament.

1. *Monofilament nylon (Ethilon suture and Dermalon suture)* is a smooth single strand of noncapillary material, clear or dyed black, blue, or green. The smaller the diameter becomes, the stronger the strand becomes proportionately. Sizes range from 2 through 11-0; the latter is the smallest of all sutures manufactured for use in microsurgery. Monofilament nylon is also used frequently in ophthalmic surgery because it has a desirable degree of elasticity. Larger sizes are used for skin closure, particularly in plastic surgery where cosmetic results are important, and for retention sutures. Wet or damp monofilament nylon is more pliable and easier to handle than dry nylon. A limited line of sutures is supplied in a moisturized state; most are supplied dry.
2. *Uncoated multifilament nylon (Nurolon suture)* is very tightly braided and treated to prevent capillary action. Usually used dyed black, but also available in white, nylon looks, feels, and handles similarly to silk, but it is stronger and elicits less tissue reaction. Sizes range from 1 through 7-0. It may be used in all tissues in which a multifilament nonabsorbable suture is acceptable.
3. *Coated multifilament nylon (Surgilon suture)* is a braided strand of nylon treated with silicone to enhance its passage through tissue. Otherwise its characteristics are similar to silk and uncoated multifilament nylon.

Polyester Fiber A polymer of terephthalic acid and polyethylene, Dacron polyester fiber is braided into a multifilament suture strand available in two forms: uncoated and coated fibers.

1. *Uncoated polyester fiber suture (Mersilene suture and Dacron)* is closely braided to provide a flexible, pliable strand that is relatively easy to handle. However, uncoated braided polyester fiber suture has a tendency to "drag" and exert a sawing or tearing effect when passed through tissue. It may be used in all tissues in which a multifilament nonabsorbable suture is indicated. It is especially useful in the respiratory tract and for some cardiovascular procedures. Available white or dyed green or blue, sizes range from 2 through 11-0.
2. *Coated polyester fiber suture* has a lubricated surface for smooth passage through tissue. It is widely used in cardiovascular surgery for vessel

anastomosis and placement of prosthetic materials because it retains its strength indefinitely in tissues. Sutures are available with different coating materials:

a. *Polybutilate* is the only coating developed specifically as a surgical lubricant. This polyester material adheres strongly to the braided polyester fiber. Polyester fiber coated with polybutilate *(Ethibond suture)* provides a strand superior to any other braided material, coated or uncoated, in decreasing drag through tissue. Colored green or white, sizes range from 5 through 7-0.
b. *Polytetrafluoroethylene,* a commercial product of DuPont trade named Teflon, is used as a coating bonded to the surface *(Polydek suture)* or impregnated into spaces in the braid of the polyester fiber strand *(Tevdek suture).* Minute particles of this coating can flake off the strand. Because these particles are insoluble and resistant to enzymes, foreign-body granulomas may be produced. Sutures with this material on them are white or dyed green and are available in sizes 5 through 10-0.
c. *Silicone,* a commercial lubricant, provides a slippery coating but does not bond well to polyester fiber. It can become dislodged in tissues as the strand is tied. Sutures with this coating *(Ti-Cron sutures)* are available white or dyed blue in sizes 5 through 7-0.

Polybutester (Novafil Suture) A copolymer of poly (glycol) terephthalate and poly (butylene) terephthalate is extruded into a monofilament strand. It is more flexible and elastic than other synthetic polymers, which may be a physiologic advantage in limited circumstances for apposing wound edges. It is available clear or dyed blue in sizes 2 through 10-0.

Polyethylene (Dermalene Suture) A long-chain polyethylene polymer is extruded into a monofilament strand. It is available dyed blue in sizes 0 through 6-0 for use in some situations in which a monofilament material is desirable.

Polypropylene (Prolene Suture and Surgilene Suture) A polymerized propylene is extruded into a monofilament strand. It is the most inert of the synthetic materials and almost as inert as stainless steel. Polypropylene is an acceptable substitute for stainless steel in situations in which strength and nonreactivity are required, and it is easier to handle. The suture may be left in place for prolonged healing. It can be used in the presence of infection. It has become the material of choice for many plastic surgery and cardiovascular procedures because of its smooth passage through tissues as well as its strength and inertness. It is frequently used for continuous abdominal fascia closure, as a subcuticular pull-out suture, and for retention sutures. It is available pigmented with blue dye in sizes 2 through 10-0 and clear in sizes 4-0 through 6-0.

Handling Characteristics of Synthetic Nonabsorbable Polymers

1. Physical damage to suture materials can occur from the time the suture is removed from a packet if the strand is mishandled. Handle all sutures and needles as little as possible. Avoid pulling or stretching. Sutures should be handled without using instruments except when grasping the free end during an instrument tie. Clamping instruments, especially needleholders and forceps with serrations, on strands can crush, cut, and weaken them.
2. All synthetic materials require a specific knot-tying technique. Knot security requires additional flat and square ties. Multifilament materials are generally easier to tie than monofilament sutures.

SURGICAL NEEDLES

Except for simple ligating with free ties, surgical needles are needed to safely carry suture material through tissue with the least amount of trauma. The best surgical needles are made of high-quality tempered steel that:

1. Is strong enough so it does not break easily
2. Is rigid enough to prevent excessive bending, yet flexible enough to prevent breaking after bending
3. Is sharp enough to penetrate tissue with minimal resistance, yet need not be stronger than the tissue it penetrates
4. Is approximately the same diameter as the suture material it carries to minimize trauma in passage through tissue
5. Is appropriate in shape and size for the type, condition, and accessibility of the tissue to be sutured
6. Is free from corrosion and burrs to prevent infection and tissue trauma

NOTE Because needles are made of steel, they are theoretically detectable by x-ray if inadvertently lost in tissue. However, the location in tissue may preclude the needle from appearing on an x-ray film. For example, the angle of the needle or its position behind bone may obstruct detection. The smaller the size of the needle, the more likely the image is to be obstructed. All needles must be accounted for so they do not become foreign bodies in tissue.

Many shapes and sizes of surgical needles are available. Names vary from one manufacturer to another; general classification only, not nomenclature, is standardized. They may be straight like a sewing needle or curved. All surgical needles have three basic components: the point, the body or shaft, and the eye. They are classified according to these three components.

Point of Needle

Points of surgical needles are honed to the configuration and sharpness desired for specific types of tissue. The basic shapes are cutting, tapered, or blunt (Figure 24-1).

Cutting Point

A razor-sharp honed cutting point may be preferred when tissue is difficult to penetrate, such as skin, tendon, and tough tissues in the eye. These make a slight cut in tissue as they penetrate. The location and degree of sharpness of cutting edges vary.

Conventional Cutting Needles Two opposing cutting edges form a triangular configuration with a third edge on the body of the needle. Cutting edges are on the inside curvature of a curved needle. Cutting edges may be honed to precision sharpness to ensure smooth passage through tissue and a minute needle path that heals quickly.

Reverse Cutting Needles A triangular configuration extends along the body of the needle. The edges near the point are sharpened or honed to precision points. The two opposing cutting edges are on the outer curvature of a curved needle.

Side Cutting Needles Relatively flat on top and bottom, angulated cutting edges are on the sides. Used primarily in ophthalmic surgery, they will not penetrate underlying tissues. They split through layers of tissue.

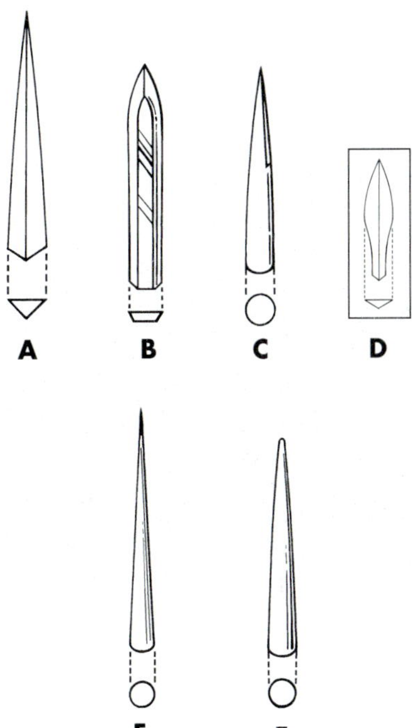

FIGURE 24-1 Configurations of needle points. **A,** Conventional cutting and reverse cutting. **B,** Side cutting. **C,** Cutting edge at end of tapered body with, **D,** trocar point. **E,** Taper. **F,** Blunt.

Trocar Points Sharp cutting tips are at the points of tapered needles. All three edges of the tip are sharpened to provide cutting action with the smallest possible hole in tissue as it penetrates.

Taper Point

These needles are used in soft tissues, such as intestine and peritoneum, which offer a small amount of resistance to the needle as it passes through. They tend to push the tissue aside as they go through rather than cut it. The body tapers to a sharp point at the tip.

Blunt Point

These tapered needles are designed with a rounded blunt point at the tip. They are used primarily for suturing friable tissue, such as liver and kidney. Because the blunt point will not cut through tissue, it is less apt to puncture a vessel in these organs than is a sharp-pointed needle. Blunt needles may also be used in some tissues to reduce the potential for needlestick injuries, especially in general and gynecologic surgery.

Body of Needle

The body, or shaft, varies in wire gauge, length, shape, and finish. Nature and location of tissue to be sutured influence selection of needles with these variable features.

1. Tough or fibrosed tissue requires a heavier gauge needle than the fine-gauge wire needed in microsurgery.
2. Depth of "bite" (placement) through tissue determines the appropriate needle length.
3. Body may be round, oval, flat, or triangular. The point determines the shape: round or oval bodies have trocar, taper, or blunt points; flat or triangular bodies have cutting edges. The shape also may be straight or curved (Figure 24-2).
   a. Straight needles are used in readily accessible tissue. They have cutting points for use in skin, which is their most frequent use, or tapered points for use in intestinal tissue.
   b. Curved needles are used to approximate most tissues because quick needle turnout is an advantage. The curvature may be ¼, ⅜, ½, ⅝ circle, half-curved with only the tip curved, or compound curved. *Curved needles always are armed in a needleholder before being handed to the surgeon.*
4. Curved needles that have longitudinal ribbed depressions or grooves along the body on inside and outside curvature can be cross-locked in the needleholder. This feature virtually eliminates twisting or turning of the needle in any position in the needleholder.
5. Body of all needles must have a smooth finish. Many needles have a surface coating of microthin plastic or silicone to enhance smooth passage

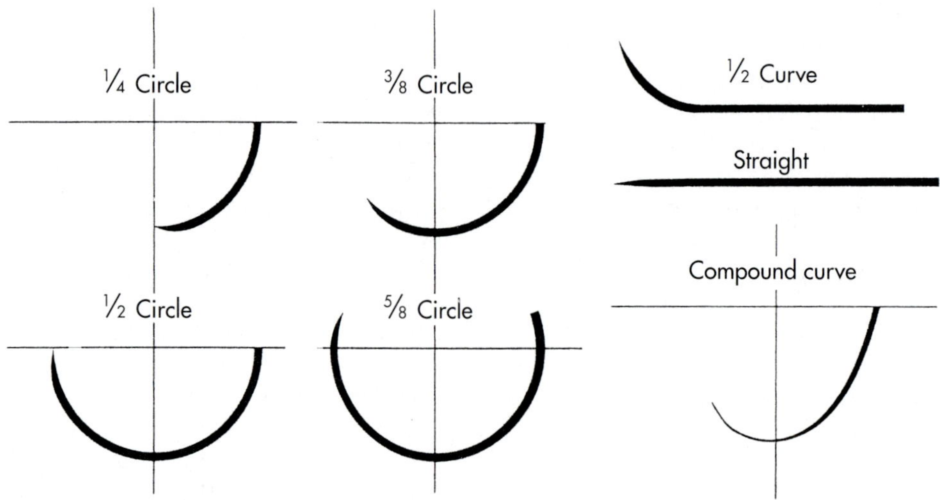

FIGURE 24-2 Shapes of needle bodies.

through tissue. Others have a black surface finish to enhance visibility at the surgical site.

Eye of Needle

The eye is the segment of needle where the suture strand is attached. Surgical needles are classified as eyed, French eye, or eyeless (Figure 24-3).

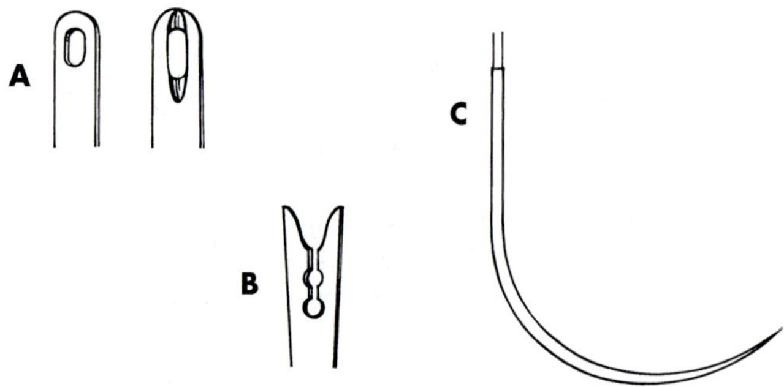

FIGURE 24-3 Eyes of needles. **A,** Oblong eyes. **B,** French eye. **C,** Eyeless (swaged).

Eyed Needle

The closed eye of an eyed surgical needle is like that of any household sewing needle. Shape of the enclosed eye may be round, oblong, or square. The end of the suture strand is pulled 2 to 4 inches (5 to 10 cm) through the eye so the short end is about one sixth the length of the long end.

French Eye Needle

Sometimes referred to as *spring eye* or *split eye,* a French eye needle has a slit from inside of the eye to end of the needle through which the suture strand is drawn. To thread a French eye after arming needle in a needleholder, secure 2 to 3 inches (5 to 7.5 cm) of the strand between fingers holding the needleholder. Pull the strand taut across center of V-shaped area above the eye, and draw down through slit into the eye (Figure 24-4). French eye needles as a general rule are used with pliable braided materials, primarily silk and cotton, of medium or fine size. These needles are not practical for surgical gut; the strand may fray or the eye may break because the diameter is usually too large for the slit.

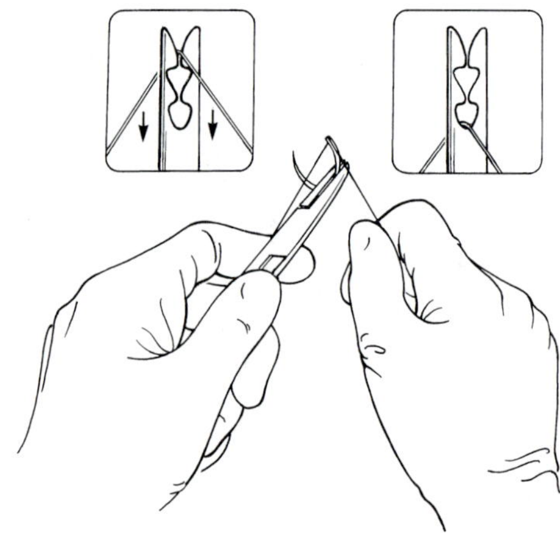

FIGURE 24-4 To thread French eye needle, pull strand taut across center of V-shaped area and draw down through slit into eye.

Handling of Eyed and French Eye Needles

Eyed and French eye needles have disadvantages for scrub person, surgeon, and patient.

1. Each needle must be carefully inspected by scrub person before and after use for dull or burred points, corrosion, and defects in the eye.
2. Care must be taken to avoid puncturing gloves with the needle point when threading.
3. If the scrub person must choose an appropriate needle to thread, needle should be same approximate diameter as the suture size requested by the surgeon.
4. Needles can unthread prematurely. This is an annoyance to the surgeon and prolongs operating time for the patient. To avoid this, the surgeon may prefer the suture strand threaded double with both ends pulled the same length through the eye; ends may be tied together in a knot, if desired. Or the scrub person may lock suture strand by threading the short end through the eye twice in the same direction.
5. Two strands of suture material are pulled through tissue when threaded needles are used. The bulk of the double strand through the eye creates a larger hole than the size of needle or suture material with additional trauma to tissue.

Eyeless Needle

An eyeless needle is a continuous unit with the suture strand. The needle is swaged onto end of strand in the manufacturing process. This eliminates threading at the operating table and minimizes tissue trauma because a single strand of material is drawn through tissue. Diameter of the needle matches size of the strand as closely as possible. The surgeon uses a new sharp needle with every suture strand. Usually referred to as *swaged needles,* four types of eyeless needle-suture attachments are available.

Single-Armed Attachment One needle is swaged to a suture strand.

Double-Armed Attachment A needle is swaged to each end of the suture strand. The two needles are not necessarily the same size and shape. These are used when the surgeon wishes to place a suture and then continue to approximate surrounding tissue on both sides from a midpoint in the strand.

Permanently Swaged Needle Attachment This attachment is secure so needle will not separate from suture strand under normal use. The needle is separated by cutting it from the strand.

Controlled-Release Needle Attachment This attachment is secure so suture strand does not separate from needle inadvertently, but it does release rapidly when pulled off intentionally. The surgeon grasps the suture strand just below the needle, pulling strand taut, and releases the needle with a straight tug of the needleholder on the needle. This facilitates fast separation of needle from suture when desired.

Placement of Needle in Needleholder

Needleholders have specially designed jaws to securely grasp surgical needles without damage if used correctly. The scrub person should observe the following principles in handling needles and needleholders:

1. Select a needleholder with appropriate size jaws for size of needle to be used. An extremely small needle requires a needleholder with very fine-tipped jaws. As wire gauge of the needle increases, jaws of the needleholder selected should be proportionately wider and heavier. Curved jaws or angulated handles may be needed for placement of needle in tissues.
2. Select an appropriate length needleholder for area of tissue to be sutured. When the surgeon works deep inside the abdomen, chest, or pelvic cavity, a longer needleholder will be needed than in superficial areas.
3. Clamp body of needle in an area one fourth to one half of the distance from the eye to the point (Figure 24-5). *Never clamp the needleholder over the swaged area.* This is the weakest area of an eyeless needle because it is hollow before the suture strand is attached. Pressure on or near needle-suture juncture may break the needle.
4. Place needle securely in the tip of the needleholder jaws, and close it in the first or second ratchet. If the needle is held too tightly in the jaws or the needleholder is defective, the needle may be damaged or notched in such a manner that it will have a tendency to bend or break on successive passes through tissue.
5. Pass needleholder with the needle point up and directed toward the surgeon's thumb when grasped so it is ready for use without readjustment. If a hand-free technique is preferred, place needleholder on a tray or magnetic mat with the needle point down.

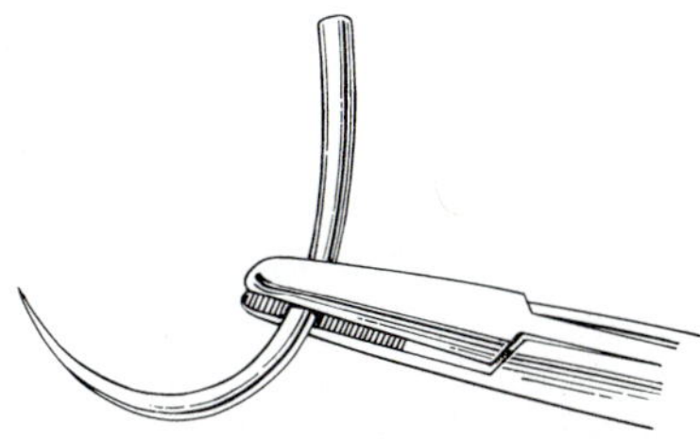

FIGURE 24-5 Correct position of curved needle in needleholder, about one third down from swage or eye.

6. Hand needleholder to the surgeon so the suture strand is free and not entangled with the needleholder. Hold free end of suture in one hand while passing needleholder with the other hand. Protect the end of the suture material from dragging across the sterile field. The assistant may take hold of free end to keep the strand straight for the surgeon and to keep it from falling over side of the sterile field.
7. Hand a needleholder to assistant to pull the needle out through tissue. A hemostat or other tissue forceps is *not* used for this purpose because the instrument may be damaged or may damage the needle. The needle should be grasped as far back as possible to avoid damage to taper point or cutting edges.

COMMON SUTURING TECHNIQUES

Primary Suture Line

The *primary suture line* refers to those sutures that hold wound edges in approximation during healing by first intention (see Chapter 25, pp. 522-523). This line may have one continuous strand of suture material or a series of suture strands. A variety of techniques are used to place sutures in tissues. The most common terms for these techniques are described.

Continuous Suture

A series of stitches is taken with one strand of material tied only at the ends of the suture line. This may be referred to as a *running stitch.* Closure is rapid, and less suture mass remains in the tissue. It distributes tension evenly across the suture line. A continuous suture is used to close peritoneum and vessels because it also provides a leakproof suture line. The configuration of the stitches varies with tissue and desired cosmetic result.

Interrupted Suture

Each stitch is taken and tied separately. This is the technique recommended by Dr. Halsted for two reasons: if an interrupted suture breaks or loosens, the remaining sutures may still hold the wound together; in the presence of infection, microorganisms are less likely to follow the primary suture line. It has the disadvantage of isolating tension to each stitch. The technique is time consuming.

Buried Suture

A suture placed under the skin, buried, may be either continuous or interrupted.

Purse-String Suture

A continuous suture is placed around a lumen and tightened, drawstring fashion, to close the lumen. This is used when inverting the stump of the appendix, for example.

Subcuticular Suture

A continuous suture is placed beneath the epithelial layer of the skin in short lateral stitches. The suture comes through upper layer of skin at each end of the incision only. A perforated lead shot may be crushed tightly on each suture end. The suture is drawn tight enough to hold skin edges in approximation. It is easily removed by cutting off the shot at one end, grasping the other shot, and pulling the entire strand through the length of the incision. It leaves a minimal scar. This technique was first used by Dr. Halsted.

Endoscopic Suture

Sutures are available as ligatures and preknotted loops or with curved or straight permanently swaged needles for use through an endoscope. The ligatures are fashioned into loosely knotted loops before being passed through the endoscope to tie off vessels and tissue pedicles. After the loop is placed around the target site, the knot is slid into position and tightened. The ends are cut with endoscopic scissors and removed through the endoscope. Suture with a permanently swaged needle is placed through either a 3 mm suture introducer for a straight needle or an 8 mm suture introducer for a curved needle. Used to suture vessels, reconstruct organs, approximate opposing tissue surfaces, and anastomose tubular structures, the technique varies according to the method used for knot tying. The methods of endoscopic knot tying are:

1. *Extracorporeal.* The swaged needle and both ends of the suture are brought outside the body through the trocar. The needle is cut off, and the knot is loosely fashioned. The knot is reintroduced into the body through the trocar by means of a knot-sliding cannula. It is snugged into position and tightened against the tissue. The ends of the suture are cut close to the knot with endoscopic scissors. Excess suture ends are removed through the endoscope.
2. *Intracorporeal.* The needle and suture are passed through the tissue with an endoscopic needleholder. Endoscopic instruments are used to tie the knot and cut the suture inside the body.

Secondary Suture Line

The *secondary suture line* refers to those sutures that reinforce and support the primary suture line, obliterate dead space, and prevent fluid accumulation in the wound during healing by first intention. These sutures exert tension lateral to the primary suture line, which contributes to the tensile strength of the wound. Sutures used for this purpose are referred to as *retention, stay,* or *tension sutures.*

Retention Sutures

Interrupted nonabsorbable sutures are placed through tissue on each side of the primary suture line, a short distance from it, to relieve tension on it. Heavy strands are used in sizes ranging from 0 through 5. The tissue through which retention sutures are passed includes skin, subcutaneous tissue, and fascia and may include rectus muscle and peritoneum of an abdominal incision. Following abdominal surgical procedures, retention sutures are used frequently in patients in whom slow healing is expected because of malnutrition, obesity, carcinoma, or infection; in the elderly; for patients receiving cortisone; or patients with respiratory problems. Retention sutures may be used as a precautionary measure to prevent wound disruption when postoperative stress on the primary suture line from distention, vomiting, or coughing is anticipated. Retention sutures should be removed as soon as the danger of sudden increases in intraabdominal pressure is over, usually on the fourth or fifth postoperative day. Retention sutures are also used to support wounds for healing by second intention and for secondary closure following wound disruption for healing by third intention (see Chapter 25, p. 523).

Retention Bridges, Bolsters, and Bumpers

To prevent heavy retention suture from cutting into skin, several different kinds of bridges, bolsters, or bumpers are used.

1. *Bridges* are plastic devices placed on the skin to span the incision. The retention suture is brought through the skin on both sides of the incision and through holes on each side of the bridge and is fastened over the bridge. One type allows adjustment of tension on the suture during the postoperative healing period.
2. *Bolsters* and *bumpers*—the names are used interchangeably—are segments of plastic or rubber tubing. One end of suture is threaded through the tubing before the suture is tied. It covers all of the retention suture strand that is on the skin surface (see Figure 29-4, p. 584). Compression bolsters are made from polyethylene foam held in place with malleable aluminum buttons to secure and distribute tension of retention sutures.
3. *Buttons and beads* are used as bolsters and bumpers to prevent the suture from retracting or cutting into skin or friable tissue. The suture is pulled through holes and tied over a button (e.g., with pull-out tendon sutures). Beads, usually lead shot, may be crushed on ends of pull-out subcuticular skin suture. The devices are used most frequently in plastic and orthopaedic surgery.

Traction Suture

A *traction suture* may be used to retract tissue to the side or out of the way, such as the tongue in a surgical procedure in the mouth. Usually a nonabsorbable suture is placed through the part. Other materials may be used to retract or ligate vessels.

1. *Umbilical tape.* Aside from its original use for tying the umbilical cord on a newborn, umbilical tape may be used as a heavy tie or as a traction suture. It may be placed around a portion of bowel or a great vessel to retract it.
2. *Vessel loop.* A length of flat silicone can be placed around a vessel, nerve, or other tubular structure for retraction. It can be tightened around a blood vessel for temporary vascular occlusion.
3. *Aneurysm needle.* An aneurysm needle is an instrument with a blunt needle on the end. The eye is on the distal end of the needle. The needle forms a right or oblique angle to the handle, which is one continuous unit with the needle. The needles are made in symmetric pairs—right and left. The surgeon uses them to place a ligature around a deep, large vessel, such as in a thyroidectomy or in thoracic surgery.

SURGEON'S CHOICE

The surgeon chooses from available types and sizes of sutures and needles the ones that best suit each purpose. In general, fine sizes are used for plastic, ophthalmic, pediatric, and vascular surgery; medium sizes for all other kinds of surgery; heavy sizes are used for retention and for anchoring bone. In general, cutting needles are used in tough tissue such as skin, fascia, tendon, and mucous membranes, including the cervix, tonsil, palate, tongue, and nose. Medium tissue calls for round taper point or cutting needles. Round taper point needles usually are used for nerve, peritoneum, muscle, and other soft tissue, such as lung and intestine, subcutaneous tissue, and dura.

It is almost impossible to learn the needle-tissue-suture-surgeon combinations by memory alone because of the unlimited number of combinations. Learning the general classification of needles, sutures, and tissues is the first step; practical experience is necessary to remember the combinations. Do not feel discouraged when you cannot anticipate the surgeon's wishes, and do not hesitate to ask when you are uncertain of the proper combination at the proper time.

The preference card usually lists the surgeon's usual suture and needle routine by tissue layer. Some cards list swaged sutures by code number. Others list sutures by size and materials and needles by size and shape. Remember, suture and needle sizes are as variable as patient sizes. Therefore the surgeon may unexpectedly request a smaller or larger size out of routine for a particular patient's situation.

SUTURES AND NEEDLES: PACKAGING AND PREPARING

Most suture material is individually packaged and supplied sterile by the manufacturer. It is sterilized by cobalt 60 irradiation or ethylene oxide gas. A few materials can be steam sterilized, but most cannot. Protein in absorbable materials derived from animals will coagulate; synthetic absorbable materials are affected by moisture and heat. Only stainless steel can be repeatedly steam sterilized. Nylon, polyester fiber, and polypropylene can be steam sterilized a maximum of three times without loss of tensile strength. Follow the manufacturer's recommendations for sterilization of *nonsterile* suture materials.

Swaged needles come in sterile packets with the suture material. They eliminate labor and expense of cleaning, packaging, and sterilizing needles. Disposable eyed and French eye needles are packaged and sterilized by the manufacturer. Needles are counted when dispensed to the sterile field (see needle counts, Chapter 20, p. 428).

Preparation of Reusable Needles

Standard sets of reusable eyed and French eye needles may be prepared for each surgical procedure. This necessitates preparing many more needles in a set than any one surgeon uses if each surgeon's preferences are to be accommodated. An alternative may be to choose needles for each procedure on the surgical schedule according to each surgeon's preferences as listed on the preference card.

Eyed needles can be loaded on a metal rack with a spring to hold them. The rack can be steam sterilized with the instruments for that surgical procedure, or it may be wrapped, labeled, and sterilized separately. Needles are counted before and after use.

Packaging of Suture Materials

A strand of sterile suture material is supplied with as many as four coverings.

Box

Each box contains one, two, or three dozen packets of sterile suture material. The label on the box may be color-coded by suture material, for example, light blue for silk, yellow for plain surgical gut. Most boxes fit into a suture cabinet rack.

Overwrap

Each packet has a hermetically sealed outer overwrap. This is coated Tyvek on one side and clear plastic film on the other. The overwrap is peeled back to expose the inner primary packet for sterile transfer to the sterile table. The circulator must not contaminate the sterile inner primary packet as the overwrap is peeled apart and the packet is flipped onto the sterile table or presented to the scrub person (see Figures 20-6 and 20-7, p. 418).

Primary Packet

Suture material, with or without swaged needles, is hermetically sealed in a primary packet that is opened by the scrub person. The primary packet may be made of foil, paper, plastic, or combinations of these. Labels may be color-coded by material, the same as the box. If a swaged needle is enclosed, a silhouette of the needle is included on the label, along with the size and type of suture material. A single strand of material or multiple strands may be in the primary packet. The packet may be designed for dispensing individual strands from a multiple suture packet.

NOTE

1. Suture packets, both overwrap and primary, should be opened only as needed to minimize waste.
2. Custom kits with multiple suture packets within a single package facilitate dispensing sutures to and organizing them on the sterile table. The kit may have appropriate sutures, with or without swaged needles, to meet the requirements of a particular surgeon or procedure. The packets are organized in order of use. The contents are listed on cover of package to facilitate counts.
3. Sterile suture packets are labeled "Do Not Resterilize." Component layers of the packaging materials cannot withstand exposure to the heat of steam sterilization without potential physical damage to contents and packets. The manufacturer will not guarantee product stability or sterility for packets sterilized in the hospital or for strands removed from packets and sterilized.
4. Some suture materials have an expiration date stamped on box and primary packet to indicate known shelf life of the material. Oldest sutures should be used first.

Inner Dispenser

Suture material is contained within the primary packet in a manner that facilitates removing or dispensing. This may be a folder, reel, organizer, or tube that may or may not be removed with the suture strands.

Preparation of Suture Material

The length of each strand of suture material within the primary packet varies; the shortest is 5 inches (approximately 13 cm) and the longest is 60 inches (150 cm). The most commonly used lengths range from 18 to 30 inches (45 to 75 cm). The length the surgeon prefers should be noted on the preference card. The scrub person may have to cut the strands to the desired length, depending on the lengths available.

Standard Length

The term *standard length* refers to a 60-inch (150 cm) strand of nonabsorbable or a 54-inch (135 cm) strand of absorbable material without a swaged needle. It is never handed to the surgeon in this length. The scrub person may cut it into a half-length, third-length, or fourth-length for use as a free tie or thread it for a stick tie or suture as shown in Figures 24-6 and 24-7.

Ligating Reels

Twelve feet (approximately 4 m) of nonabsorbable or 54 inches (135 cm) of absorbable suture are wound on disklike plastic reels. These reels are color-coded by material and have size identification. The surgeon keeps the reel in palm of hand for a series of free ties. The reel is radiopaque in case it is inadvertently dropped in a body cavity. If reels are not stocked, the surgeon may ask the scrub person to wind a standard length onto a rod or other device for this purpose.

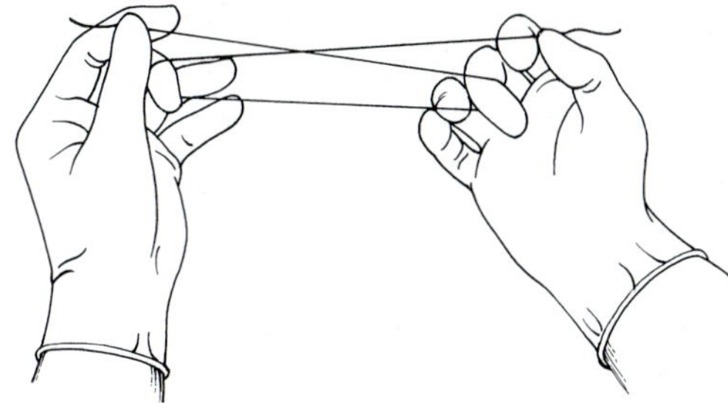

FIGURE 24-7 Scrub person preparing one-third length sutures. One free end of full-length strand is passed from right to left hand. At same time loop is caught around third finger of right hand. Other loop is caught around third finger of left hand while each end is held and suture is adjusted to equal lengths (thirds). Then each loop is cut with scissors.

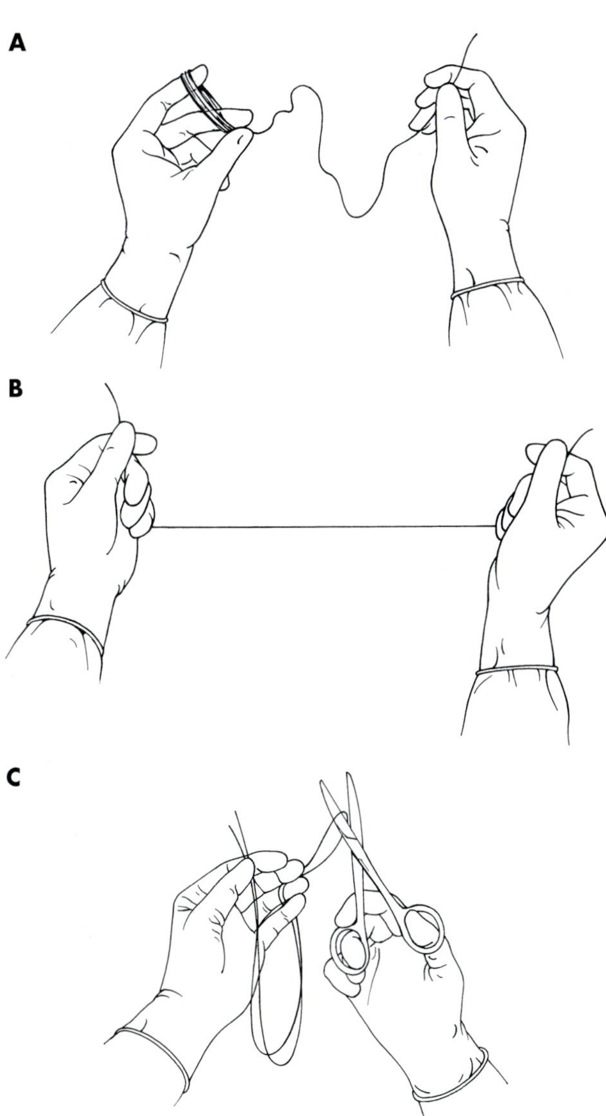

FIGURE 24-6 Sequence of scrub person preparing half-lengths. **A,** Suture loops are separated by fingers of left hand while unwinding. **B,** Full length is gently unwound and straightened before cutting. Scrub person does not pull hard or test strand, but keeps firm grasp on both ends to prevent suture from snapping away and possibly becoming contaminated. **C,** Suture is bent in half, and loop is cut.

Precut Lengths

Most suture materials are supplied in precut lengths ready for use as free ties or for threading. These facilitate handling for the scrub person. They are dispensed individually from some primary packets or may be removed and placed in a fold of the suture book. Packets contain from 3 to 17 strands, depending on the material.

Swaged Needle-Suture

Lengths of sutures are predetermined by the manufacturer; however, the surgeon has a wide variety of choices to meet all suturing needs. The scrub person must remember that a strand can be shortened but not extended. An appropriate length for location of tissue must be handed to the surgeon. A packet may contain one suture strand with single- or double-armed needle(s) or multiple strands with swaged needles. The needle may be armed in a needleholder and withdrawn from the inner dispenser of some packets.

SURGICAL STAPLES

Surgeons can join many tissues with staples. This involves inserting stainless steel or titanium staples through tissues with a stapler, a device specifically designed for this purpose. Some surgical procedures have become simplified or feasible since the advent of surgical stapling techniques. As Hültl recognized in 1908, for stapling to be successful fine wire as the basic material must form a B shape. This shape allows blood to flow through tissues, preventing necrosis secondary to devascularization beyond the staple line. Sufficient pressure must be exerted, however, to provide hemostasis of cut tissues. Length and width of the staples must accommodate tissue being approximated or transected. The number of staples varies with the length of the staple line.

Advantages of Using Staples

Staples can be used safely in many types of tissues and have a wide range of applications.

1. Stapling is a rapid method of ligating, anastomosing, and approximating tissues. The time saved, as compared with suturing techniques, reduces blood loss and total operating and anesthesia time for the patient.
2. Wound healing may be accelerated because of minimal trauma and nonreactive nature of metallic staples.
3. Staples produce an even surface and an airtight, leakproof closure.
4. Staples can be placed through an endoscope.

Stapling Instruments

Each stapler is designed for stapling specific tissues (i.e., skin, fascia, bronchus, gastrointestinal tract, or vessels). The surgeon selects the correct instrument for the desired application. The consequences of an erroneous staple application, however, are much more difficult to correct than those of manually placed sutures. The surgeon must learn when and how to use each instrument. Whether the stapler is reusable or a single-use disposable, the basic technical mechanics of stapling are the same.

Staplers either fire a single staple or simultaneously fire straight or circular rows of staples. A different instrument must be used for each type of firing.

Skin Stapler

To approximate skin edges the stapler fires a single staple with each squeeze of the trigger. Edges of both cuticular and subcuticular layers must be everted, that is, aligned with the edges slightly raised in an outward direction, as close to their original configuration on the horizontal plane as possible. The stapler is positioned over the line of incision so that the staple will be placed evenly on each side. The staple forms a rectangular shape over the incision. As many staples are placed as needed to close the incision. Skin staplers are supplied preloaded with different quantities of staples in varying widths (i.e., crown span). The most appropriate stapler should be chosen for the selected use. For example, an average range of 28 to 35 staples is needed to close most abdominal incisions. More may be needed to close the chest, fewer for an inguinal herniorrhaphy.

Skin staples must be removed, usually 5 to 7 days postoperatively. Extractors are used for this purpose. As it heals, the skin flattens out to form an even surface with excellent cosmetic results if the staples have been properly placed lightly over the skin. Imbedded staples are difficult to remove, and results may be less than desired.

Linear Stapler

Two staggered or side-by-side straight double rows of staples are placed simultaneously in tissue with a linear stapler. This stapler is used throughout the alimentary tract and in thoracic surgery for transection and resection of internal tissues. The tissue is positioned in the straight jaws, of appropriate length, of the stapler. The gap between the jaws must be adequate for the thickness of tissues. A tissue-measuring device may be used for this determination in the gastrointestinal tract in conjunction with a disposable stapler so that the instrument can be adjusted to the appropriate settings for the desired staple height.

When formed, each staple is shaped like a capital letter B. This shape allows staples to hold tissues together without crushing so that tissue perfusion is maintained. The number of staples that will be fired depends on the length of the stapler jaws.

Intraluminal Circular Stapler

With the circular stapler a double row of staggered staples is placed in a circle for intraluminal anastomosis of tubular hollow organs in the gastrointestinal tract. Because the diameter of the lumen of organs in the alimentary tract varies, the surgeon must choose a stapler with an appropriate head size. The number of staples the instrument fires depends on its head size. A circular knife within head of the stapler trims tissue to produce a proper lumen as the stapler is fired. As with the linear stapler, staples form a letter B.

Ligating and Dividing Stapler

A double row of two staples each ligates tissue that is then divided simultaneously between the staple lines with a cutting knife incorporated in the stapler. This stapler is used primarily to ligate and divide omental vessels or other soft tubular structures.

Endoscopic Stapler

Endoscopic staplers are available for ligating and dividing and for linear stapling. The stapling device is passed through an 11- or 12-gauge laparoscopic trocar. It may be reloaded several times with staple cartridges for multiple firings. The stapler is discarded after single patient use.

Reusable Staplers

Reusable, manually operated, heavy mechanical stapling instruments have many moving and detachable parts. They are not always mechanically reliable. They must be precisely aligned to fire accurately. The scrub person is responsible for correctly assembling instruments. The manufacturer's instructions for use and care must be followed to avoid technical failures.

Reusable staplers are supplied with presterilized, disposable cartridges that contain six or more staples. Quantities vary according to the stapler they fit. The number of cartridges needed varies with the procedure and/or design of the instrument. Cartridges are color-coded by the size of staples.

Reusable staplers must be disassembled and cleaned after use. They should be terminally sterilized and then cleaned in an ultrasonic cleaner. They should be steam sterilized *completely disassembled,* according to the manufacturer's recommendations.

Disposable Staplers

Preassembled, sterile disposable staplers eliminate assembling, cleaning, and sterilizing processes. These self-contained, lightweight instruments with integral or reloadable staple cartridges are discarded after single patient use. To avoid unnecessary contamination of a sterile instrument, the package should not be opened until the surgeon determines correct size for intended use of the stapler. The number and size of staples in cartridges vary; length of linear jaws or diameter of circular head varies for internal use. Internal staplers are available with either stainless steel or titanium staples. The surgeon may prefer titanium because it creates less distortion when computed tomography (CT) and magnetic resonance imaging (MRI) are used.

TISSUE ADHESIVES

Conventional suturing and stapling hold tissues in apposition during the healing process. Sutures and staples will not fuse or bond tissues. Ancient Egyptians used resins and gums to hold tissue surfaces together. Research is ongoing for an ideal tissue adhesive that will bond tissue, effect hemostasis, promote regeneration of cells, and serve as a barrier to microbes, fluid, and air. Biologic and synthetic tissue adhesives have extensive potential applications for wound closure and reconstruction.

Biologic Adhesives

Fibrin sealants, most commonly called *fibrin glue,* act as biologic adhesives and hemostatic agents. The components are fibrinogen, cryoprecipitated from human plasma in the presence of clotting factors, and reconstituted thrombin of bovine origin. When applied directly to tissues, thrombin converts fibrinogen to fibrin to produce a clot. Fibrin sealants can be applied to tissues as a liquid, gel, or aerosol spray to control bleeding and approximate tissues technically difficult to approximate by suturing, especially following resections or traumatic injuries of friable or highly vascular tissues such as liver, spleen, and lung. Fibrin glue also may be used for microsurgical anastomoses of blood vessels, nerves, and other structures such as fallopian tubes; for reconstruction of middle ear; to fix ocular implants; to close superficial lacerations and fistula tracts; and to secure some skin grafts. It may be used as a carrier for demineralized bone powder to promote osteoregeneration.

Autologous or Homologous Plasma

Plasma collected from the patient (autologous) or a single donor (homologous) is processed into a cryoprecipitate containing clotting factor XIII to produce fibrinogen. Autologous plasma is obtained preoperatively and prepared either in the blood bank or in the OR. A single donor must be tested for human immunodeficiency virus (HIV) and hepatitis before plasma is processed.

Autologous or homologous fibrinogen is warmed to 98.6° F (37° C) immediately before use. Thrombin is reconstituted to 1000 U/ml. Equal volumes of fibrinogen and thrombin are applied simultaneously.

Pooled-Donor Plasma Fibrin glue commercially prepared from pooled-donor plasma (i.e., blended from multiple donors) has significantly greater bonding strength than autologous or single-donor plasma. The fibrinogen must undergo purification and viral inactivation, however, to prevent transmission of bloodborne pathogens. Used extensively in Europe, this product has not been approved by the FDA for use in the United States.

Synthetic Adhesives

Synthetic gluelike adhesive substances that polymerize in contact with body tissues effect hemostasis and hold tissues together.

Cyanoacrylate

Butyl cyanoacrylate and cyanoacrylate derivatives may be used for skin closure. Degradation of these materials produces toxic by-products that can cause a histotoxic reaction in tissues.

Methyl Methacrylate

Methyl methacrylate is used to augment fixation of pathologic fractures and to stabilize prosthetic devices in bone. It is an acrylic, cementlike substance commonly referred to as *bone cement.* It is a drug supplied in two sterile components that must be mixed together immediately before use. One component is a colorless, highly volatile, flammable, liquid methyl methacrylate monomer in an ampule. This powerful lipid solvent must be handled carefully. The other component is a white powder mixture of polymethyl methacrylate, methyl methacrylate–styrene copolymer, and barium sulfate in a packet. The barium sulfate provides radiopacity to the substance. When the powder and liquid are mixed, an exothermic polymeric reaction forms a soft, pliable, doughlike mass. This reaction liberates heat as high as 230° F (110° C). As the reaction progresses, the substance becomes hard in a few minutes. The mixing and kneading of the entire contents of the liquid ampule and powder packet must be thorough and should continue for at least 4 minutes. The substance must be adequately soft and pliable for application to bone. The completion of polymerization occurs in the patient. After it hardens, it holds a prosthesis firmly in a fixed position.

A hazard to OR personnel has been reported in regard to the use of methyl methacrylate in the operating room. Some personnel have experienced dizzy spells, difficulty in breathing, and/or nausea and vomiting following mixing of methyl methacrylate. The monomer and several of its ingredients are potent allergenic sensitizers when vapor is inhaled. A suitable means of local exhaust should be provided that will collect vapor at the source of mixing at the sterile field and will discharge it into outside air or absorb the monomer on activated charcoal (see Chapter 10, p. 155).

TISSUE REPAIR MATERIALS

Tissue deficiencies may require additional reinforcement or bridging material to obtain adequate wound healing. Sometimes edges of fascia, for example, cannot be brought together without excessive tension. In obese or elderly persons the fascia cannot withstand this tension because of weakness caused by the infiltration of fat. Biologic or synthetic mesh materials are used to fill congenital, traumatic, or acquired defects in fascia or a body wall and to reinforce fascia, as in hernia repair.

Biologic Materials

Cargile Membrane

A thin membrane is obtained from submucosal layer of cecum of the ox. Cargile membrane is rarely used, although it is still commercially available in a 4 × 6 inch (10 × 15 cm) sheet, to cover peritoneum to prevent adhesions, for isolating ligations, as a covering for packing in submucous nasal resections, and as a dural substitute.

Fascia Lata

Strips of fascia lata are obtained from the fibrous connective tissue that covers thigh muscles of beef cattle. In lieu of commercial fascia lata—a *heterogenous graft*—the surgeon may strip a piece of fascia from the patient's thigh—an *autogenous graft*. Fascia lata also is obtained from cadavers and freeze-dried—an *allograft*. Fascia lata contains collagen. It increases the amount of tissue already present and becomes a living part of the tissue it supports. It is used to strengthen weakened fascial layers or to fill in defects in fascia. Since the advent of allografts and synthetic meshes, heterogenous strips are used infrequently.

Synthetic Meshes

Synthetic meshes offer several advantages for reinforcing or bridging fascial or other tissue deficiencies:

1. They are easily cut to desired size for the defect.
2. They are easily sutured underneath the edges of tissue to create a smooth surface.
3. They are pliable to preclude erosion into major structures.
4. They are inert to avoid inflammatory response and to minimize foreign-body tissue reaction.
5. They are porous to allow free drainage of exudate.
6. Fibrous tissue easily grows through openings to incorporate mesh into tissue to maximize tensile strength.

Manufacturer's instructions must be followed for each type of mesh product. Unused mesh should be discarded.

Polyester Fiber Mesh (Mersilene Mesh)

Mesh remains soft and pliable in tissue but has limited elasticity. It is least inert of the synthetic meshes. It is not preferred in the presence of infection or in contaminated wounds because of its multifilament construction. Polyester fibers are knitted by a process that interlocks each fiber juncture to prevent unraveling when cut. However, a minimum of ¼ inch (6.5 mm) of mesh should extend beyond the suture line. Sterile sheets are available in sizes 2½ × 4½ inches (6 × 11 cm) and 12 × 12 inches (30 × 30 cm).

Polyglactin 910 Mesh (Vicryl Mesh)

Mesh is knitted fibers of undyed and uncoated polyglactin 910. Because it is absorbed by hydrolysis, this mesh is intended for use as a buttress to provide temporary support during healing. The mesh acts as a scaffold for ingrowth of connective tissue. It may be used to support a traumatized spleen, kidney, or abdominal wall and to support facial fascia. Absorption is essentially complete between 60 and 90 days. Sterile sheets are available in sizes 10½ × 13½ inches (26.5 × 34 cm) and 5 × 6½ inches (13 × 17 cm).

Polypropylene Mesh (Prolene Mesh, Marlex Mesh)

Knitted mesh of polypropylene has high tensile strength and good elasticity. However, Marlex mesh is stiffer and exhibits greater fiber fatigue than Prolene mesh. Because polypropylene is inert, it may be used in the presence of infection or during healing by second intention. Mesh is used to span and reinforce traumatic abdominal wall defects, incisional ventral hernias, large inguinal hernias, and other fascial deficiencies. It stimulates rapid tissue ingrowth through interstices of mesh. Mesh remains soft and pliable in tissues. It will not unravel when cut. Sterile sheets are available in sizes 2½ × 4½ inches (6 × 11 cm), 6 × 6 inches (15 × 15 cm), and 12 × 12 inches (30 × 30 cm).

Polytetrafluoroethylene (Gore-Tex Soft Tissue Patch)

A sheet of expanded polytetrafluoroethylene (PTFE) may be used to repair hernias and tissue deficiencies that require prosthetic material. This material is flexible, soft, and porous to allow tissue ingrowth. It is not used in the presence of infection. It must be handled only with clean gloves or rubber-shod forceps. Nonsterile patches may be sterilized by steam or ethylene oxide gas according to the manufacturer's instructions.

Stainless Steel Mesh

Available in nonsterile sheets 6 × 12 inches (15 × 30 cm) and 12 × 12 inches (30 × 30 cm), steel is the most inflexible and difficult of the meshes to handle. The sharp edges may puncture gloves. Use wire scissors, not dissecting scissors, to cut it. Steel is opaque to x-ray, which may be a disadvantage for the patient in later life. Also the mesh may fragment and cause patient discomfort.

TISSUE REPLACEMENT MATERIALS

For centuries surgeons have sought materials to replace parts of anatomy. Tissue may be absent or distorted because of congenital deformity, traumatic injury, degenerative disease, or surgical resection. Replacement or substitution of tissue may be possible with biologic dressings or implanted materials or with synthetic prosthetic materials implanted in the body. An overview of types of biologic and synthetic tissue replacement materials is given here. Their uses are referenced in other chapters by surgical specialty or procedures.

Biologic Dressings

A biologic dressing temporarily covers an open surface defect in skin and underlying soft tissues. Although defects are usually the result of trauma such as burns, vascular or pressure necrosis can cause skin ulcers. Open wounds quickly become contaminated. The dressing arrests loss of fluid, reduces or eliminates microbial growth, and minimizes scarring. It promotes production of granulation tissue and epithelialization before healing by second or third intention. A fibrin-elastin biologic bonding adheres the dressing to exposed surfaces. Biologic dressings are dermal replacements. The source determines the type of dressing.

Autograft

Skin is grafted from one part of the patient's body to another part. See the detailed discussion of skin grafts in Chapter 34.

Allograft (Homograft)

Human tissue obtained from one genetically dissimilar person (i.e., unmatched donor) is grafted to another person. This is referred to as an *allograft* or *homograft*. Negative HIV and hepatitis B virus (HBV) status of donor and recipient should be determined and documented before use. Any natural body tissue transferred from one human to another must be infection-free.

Cryopreserved Skin Homogenous skin provides a protective covering that initially acquires, then eventually loses, vascular connection with underlying tissue. A cadaver usually is the source of skin for a dermal allograft. Cryopreservation maintains viability of skin during prolonged storage. Skin is frozen by cooling at a rate of 1° to 5° C (1.8° to 9° F) to −70° C (−94° F), then stored in a liquid nitrogen freezer. Immediately before use, skin is warmed by immersion in sterile water at 42° C (107.6° F), the maximum compatible with cellular viability. Skin should be warmed at a rate of 50° to 70° C (90° to 126° F) per minute. (The patient's own skin can be cryopreserved for prolonged storage for later use as an autograft.) Allografts may be obtained from a skin bank.

NOTE For storage of allografts or autografts up to 14 days, skin may be placed in isotonic saline solution or tissue nutrient medium and refrigerated at 1° to 10° C (33.8° to 50° F).

Amniotic Membrane Prepared from human placenta, amniotic membranes can be used as biologic dressings to promote the healing of burns, skin ulcers, and infected wounds and to cover defects such as spina bifida. The placenta has two loosely connected membranes: amnion is used for partial-thickness wounds, chorion for full-thickness defects. Membranes are harvested by cleaning blood and clots from the placenta immediately after delivery, placing placenta in an iodophor solution, and refrigerating it at 4° C (39° F). Membranes should be stripped from placenta within 36 hours after delivery. Amnion can be used fresh or preserved frozen or dried. It may be obtained from a tissue bank that prepares and stores amniotic membranes.

Heterograft (Xenograft)

Skin obtained from a dissimilar species may be placed on human tissue as a temporary dressing.

Porcine Dermis Porcine (pig) skin is used to cover body surfaces denuded of full-thickness skin until permanent skin grafting can be accomplished. Vascularization does not occur, but the heterograft adheres tightly while reepithelialization proceeds underneath it. It may remain in place for as long as 2 weeks before it dries up and peels off spontaneously. Porcine biologic dressings are available in rolls or strips. They may be prepared fresh for refrigeration, fresh-frozen, irradiated and then frozen, or dried. Some dressings are soaked in an iodophor and should not be placed on a patient allergic to iodine. Dressings must be prepared and used according to the manufacturer's instructions.

Artificial Skin A skin substitute may be prepared from a layer of collagen obtained from the dermis of a calf or pig and coated with autogenous epithelium obtained from the recipient. Another type is synthesized from a bilayered polymeric membrane. The top layer is silicone elastomer. The bottom layer is a porous cross-linked network of collagen and glycosaminoglycan. This artificial skin is biodegradable, but it can be used as a temporary covering that is similar to porcine heterografts.

Biologic Materials

Autogenous tissues may be grafted or transferred from one part of patient's body to another. *Homogenous* tissues or organs may be transplanted from another human. *Heterologous* biomaterials may be used to supplement tissues.

NOTE Standards are set by the American Association of Tissue Banks for screening donors and retrieving, processing, and preserving homogenous tissues, including skin, cartilage, bone, and blood vessels (see Chapter 44, p. 898). Potential donors of allografts must be tested for HIV and HBV. Excluded from donating are persons who are HIV-positive, have a history of hepatitis, have an active infection, or have an immune disorder.

Bone Grafts

A bone graft affords structural support and a pattern for regrowth of bone within a skeletal defect. *Cancellous bone* is porous. Its porosity permits tissue fluid to reach deeper into it than into cortical bone, and thus most of the bone cells live. *Cortical bone* is used for bridging large skeletal defects because it gives greater strength. It may be fixed in the recipient site by means of metallic suture or screws. Bone obtained from the crest of the ilium or a rib is cancellous and cortical bone; cortical bone is obtained from the tibia. The main purpose of a bone graft is to stimulate new bone growth.

Autogenous bone, which is obtained from the patient, usually is taken from the ilium, tibia, or rib cage at the time of the surgical procedure. Calvarial bone from the frontal, parietal, or occipital cranial bones may be harvested for maxillofacial bone grafts. A free bone graft with its vascular pedicle, such as a free fibular graft, may be obtained for revascularization by microvascular anastomosis after removal of dead (avascular) bone. A separate small sterile table may be prepared for the instrumentation required for the donor site. If the recipient area is potentially contaminated, the donor site must not be cross-contaminated from the recipient site.

Homogenous bone, which is obtained from a cadaver, is dead bone. This bone is weaker than autogenous bone, thus requiring a longer time of immobilization. Union occurs from bone regeneration in the recipient with this type of bone graft. It may be desirable, however, to spare patient the added operating time and trauma of removing an autogenous graft.

Composite bone grafts are freeze-dried allografts combined with autogenous particulate cancellous bone and marrow. A crib formed from a cadaver bone (e.g., rib) is packed with the patient's bone particles and marrow. When implanted to reconstruct bony defects, the composite graft induces bone regeneration in the recipient site. The freeze-dried allograft is biodegradable by slow resorption. Eventually it is replaced by mature functional bone.

Decalcified bone and demineralized bone chips or powder, prepared from homogenous bone, also are used to stimulate bone regeneration or to fill defects in bone. This material is sterilized and stored at room temperature. For use, it is soaked in Ringer's lactate solution. The powder then becomes a paste that can be used to fill a depressed area or to caulk an irregularity as in craniofacial reconstruction.

Bone Bank Bone may be preserved and stored in a bone bank until needed. Autogenous bone may be preserved following the surgical procedure by storage in a bone bank for subsequent grafting into the same patient. Bone such as a rib or femoral head may be salvaged from patients (i.e., living donors) who are free of malignancy or infection for a homogenous graft into another person. Bone also may be obtained from cadavers (i.e., nonliving donors).

Bone used for allografts must be clean and sterile. Immediately after removal, bone marrow, fat, and blood are rinsed out with sterile distilled water or normal saline solution. The bone may be put in sterile nested glass jars or double plastic or metal containers. If it is to be used for a homogenous graft, a small piece of bone is put into a sterile Petri dish and sent to the laboratory for culture tests. Bone should never be used until negative results of culture and serology are received. Several methods are used to preserve bone.

1. *Freezing* is the most common method of preserving bone. Bone is quick-frozen in a freezer at −70° C (−94° F) or in liquid nitrogen. If bone will be used within 6 months, it can be stored in a refrigerator freezer at −15° to −20° C (−5° to −4° F). For prolonged storage of more than 6 months, the freezer temperature must be maintained below

−20° C (−4° F) to avoid damage from a buildup of ice crystals. Bone frozen by liquid nitrogen is stored in vapor at about −150° C (−238° F). The container initially is placed on a shelf labeled "not ready for use." It is labeled "sterile" and moved to the freezer compartment labeled "ready for use" when negative results of culture and serology tests are recorded on the identification card. Bone is thawed rapidly immediately before grafting.
2. *Freeze-drying* requires specialized equipment that removes moisture as the freezing process takes place in a condenser with a vacuum cycle.
3. *Ethylene oxide sterilization* ensures safety of bone. It must be aerated for 72 hours before storage at room temperature or in a refrigerator. When protected from air and contamination, sterilized bone can be stored indefinitely, although a 1-year expiration date is recommended if bone is placed in a heat-sealed peel-apart package. In lieu of ethylene oxide sterilization, packaged bone may be shipped in dry ice to a center equipped to sterilize it by irradiation.
4. *Formaldehyde solution*, 0.25% to 1% concentration, may have a bacteriostatic effect around graft site in infected or contaminated wounds, such as in osteomyelitis. During storage, temperature is maintained at 2° to 4° C (35.6° to 39° F) in a refrigerator freezer.

The container must be labeled with donor information (see Chapter 44, p. 898) and not used until laboratory reports are available. The donor must be seronegative for hepatitis B surface antigen and HIV. Bone from a living donor is quarantined for 90 days, awaiting results of a repeat test for HIV.

Heterologous Bone Implant Coraline hydroxyapatite, which is composed of skeletons of sea coral, and collagen may be used to replace facial or cranial bone. This material has hardness, mineral content, and porosity similar to human bone. These implants stimulate bone growth into the porous architecture of the coral.

Organ Transplants

Some whole body organs can be transplanted from one human to another. This is done in an effort to sustain life by compensating for physiologic deficits or inadequate function of vital organs. See Chapter 44 for a complete discussion of transplantation.

Tissue Transplants

Skin and blood vessels are frequently transplanted from one part of the body to another. These are referred to as *autografts* because the patient is both donor and recipient. The transplanted tissue becomes a part of the living tissue in the recipient site. See Chapter 34 for a discussion of grafting techniques and Chapter 40 for a discussion of vascular grafts.

Some tissues can be transplanted from one person to another to restore function, such as the cornea, or to provide support in structures, such as cartilage in nasal reconstruction. These are referred to as *allografts* or *homografts* (see Chapter 44). Some allografts are commercially prepared, such as lyophilized human dura mater and human umbilical cord vein graft.

Human Dura Mater A trimmed and measured piece of dura mater is freeze-dried, sterilized by exposure to ethylene oxide, and stored in a vacuum container. It may be stored at room temperature indefinitely provided the vacuum is maintained. The graft is reconstituted by the addition of normal saline solution to the container for a minimum of 30 minutes. Most of these grafts are used for closure of dural defects, but they may also be used to repair abdominal and thoracic wall and diaphragmatic defects.

Human Umbilical Cord Vein Graft A glutaraldehyde tanning process converts an umbilical vein into an inert, antithrombogenic graft. A polyester mesh covering over the outer surface allows tissue ingrowth and provides added strength. Commercially supplied, a biograft modified human umbilical vein graft is an acceptable graft material for arterial reconstruction when an autogenous saphenous vein is not available. The glutaraldehyde must be thoroughly irrigated from graft with sterile heparinized saline or Ringer's lactate solution before implantation. After rinsing, the graft should remain in sterile heparinized saline solution to keep it moist until implanted. Only noncrushing clamps should be used to avoid damage to the graft during handling.

Heterologous Biomaterials

In addition to porcine skin used as biologic dressings, artificial skin derived from the collagen of a calf or pig, heterologous bone, and other materials derived from animals are commercially prepared for tissue replacement.

Arteriovenous Shunts Enzymatically treated bovine carotid artery heterografts are used for blood access in patients on hemodialysis therapy who have poor blood vessels or in whom it is difficult to create either fistulas or shunts. Femoral arteriovenous bovine shunts can be punctured innumerable times with a low incidence of thrombus formation.

Collagen Collagen is used in its natural form, such as a processed bovine graft and microfibrillar hemostatic powder (see Chapter 23, pp. 471-472), and restructured into membranes or films. It can be injected into middle-to-deep dermis to fill and smooth nasolabial furrows and facial creases. It is implanted to correct soft tissue defects and contours. The duration of effect is 4 to 6 months. Collagen can be altered by a variety of techniques to change its physical properties and duration of action in tissue.

Corium Corium implants are prepared from porcine dermis to replace tissue loss or to support tissues. They can be used as a fascia lata substitute or dural replacement or to repair tympanic membrane, hernia, or bladder sling. Corium will form a collagen matrix to close a defect in soft tissues around teeth. Available in sterile sheets of several sizes, corium implant (Zenoderm) is freeze- or air-dried before sterilization by gamma irradiation. It should not be resterilized.

Synthetic Materials

A *prosthesis* is a permanent or temporary replacement for a missing or malfunctioning structure. Some implants replace vital structures, such as diseased heart valves and blood vessels. Devices such as pacemakers assist the function of vital organs. Other materials are used to repair or replace defects. Prosthetic materials implanted into the body must:

1. Be compatible with physiologic processes
2. Produce no or minimal tissue reaction
3. Be sterile so they will not cause infection or become a culture medium
4. Be noncarcinogenic or other disease causative
5. Have viable and adequate tissue coverage, unless used as a biologic dressing over denuded skin surfaces
6. Have adequate blood supply through or around them
7. Be stable so they will not degenerate or change shape if used for permanent function
8. Contour or conform to normal tissue configuration as desired

Permanently implanted devices can provide support, restore function, and augment or restore body contour. Inorganic substances cannot unite with tissue, however. Their physiologic responses may be predictable. All synthetic materials implanted in contact with blood will activate coagulation and promote the process of thrombosis. The surface of some materials is less thrombogenic (i.e., less likely to form clots) than others. The magnitude of the inflammatory response they stimulate varies in patients. An immune response may cause chronic inflammation from bacterial adhesion. Infection that develops around a prosthesis usually necessitates its removal. Most infections arise from microorganisms inoculated into wound at the time of implantation. Therefore meticulous sterile technique is mandatory. *Prosthetic implants should not be flash-sterilized in steam.* They must be sterilized in a standard cycle for the agent used (see Chapter 13). The cycle should be monitored with a biologic indicator, and a negative spore test result should be confirmed before the implant is used. Many implants are sterilized by the manufacturer.

Carbon Fiber

Pure carbon fibers braided into a strip are used for ligament replacement and articular resurfacing. Inert in tissue, carbon fiber stimulates regrowth of connective tissue and cartilage. The fibers may be braided with polypropylene or coated with a resorbable gelatin or lyophilized dura. The prosthesis should be soaked in normal saline solution before implantation to facilitate handling.

Metal

Stainless steel, a cobalt alloy (with the trade name Vitallium), and titanium are manufactured into prosthetic implants. Used primarily for stabilization of bone, metal implants must be strong enough to withstand the stress of weight bearing or muscular action and must not corrode in body tissues. They are never reused because of the weakening that can occur with use. See Chapter 32 for specific types and uses of metallic orthopaedic implants.

Special care must be taken in handling metal implants to protect the surfaces. A simple scratch on a metal implant can lead to its corrosion in the body. The implant will be bathed continuously by weakly chloride body fluids. If corrosion begins, the implant may fail and have to be removed. It is very important, therefore, that all metal implants be protected from scratches. This can be accomplished by:

1. Wrapping each implant individually, or wrapping sets with each size implant in a separate compartment, for both storage and sterilization. Most prostheses come from the manufacturer in protective coverings or cases. Some of these are suitable for adequate sterilization, with subsequent placement in the sterile field to minimize handling before implantation.
2. Preventing implants from coming in contact with other hard surfaces of metal or glass, either during storage and sterilization or on the instrument table.
3. Not handling or transferring an unprotected implant with any type of forceps.

Implants of one metal should not come in contact with those of another metal because an electrochemical reaction occurs between metals. Two different metals are not implanted in the same patient for this reason. Instruments used for insertion also should be of the same metal as the implant (e.g., a stainless steel screwdriver and screw).

Methyl Methacrylate

A highly refined methyl methacrylate mixture can be molded and shaped to fit a defect in bone. When it hardens, this material looks and feels very much like bone. It is used to repair a skull defect (see Chapter 37, p. 771).

Polyester Fiber

Polyester fibers (Dacron) woven or knitted into seamless cylinders are used to replace major arteries.

Polyethylene

Polyethylene tubing may be inserted into structures, such as fallopian tubes or ureters, to give support during healing or to bridge a defect in tissue continuity. Polyethylene may be combined with silicon to produce a thromboresistant coating for vascular grafts and artificial hearts.

A polyethylene sliding rail, as on a reclosable plastic bag, affixed to polypropylene mesh is used in the manufacture of a surgical zipper. A zipper may be used for temporary abdominal wound closure in the presence of extensive sepsis to allow repeated access to the abdomen.

Implants of porous polyethylene are used for anatomic reconstruction, such as the external ear. The porosity of the implant encourages both soft tissue and vascular ingrowth. Collagen deposited along the framework adds strength. Porous polyethylene is a strong, flexible material that can be molded or shaped to the desired configuration. When dipped into boiling normal saline solution, the material becomes pliable for molding by hand. An implant can also be shaped by cutting with a scalpel blade. Glove powder, lint, and dust particles must not adhere to the implant because they can cause a foreign-body reaction around the implant.

NOTE Sterile normal saline solution can be brought to the boiling point by placing an unopened bottle in a gravity displacement steam sterilizer for 1 minute at 132° C (270° F).

Polytetrafluoroethylene (Teflon, PTFE)

Some prostheses or parts of prosthetic devices are made of the polymer PTFE. It may be woven into a fabric for arterial grafts, extruded into tubing for struts, or molded into a solid configuration for valves or joints. Its lubricity makes it a useful replacement for tissues when motion is desirable.

Silicone

Silicone is one of the most inert of the synthetic polymers used for implantation. It has a durable and nonthrombogenic surface. It is used in many forms: gel, sponge, film, tubing, liquid, and preformed molded anatomic structures. It may be coated with polyurethane or polyester or used as an elastomer to coat polyester. A medical-grade silicone elastomer (Silastic) in one form or another is used in virtually every surgical specialty for tissue reconstruction or replacement. Silicone may migrate from a ruptured or leaking gel- or liquid-filled implant and cause systemic illness.

Complete instructions for cleaning and sterilizing silicone implants before use are supplied by the manufacturer with each type of prosthesis. These instructions must be followed meticulously. Implants are not handled with bare hands, and care must be taken to ensure that they do not pick up lint and dust. Gloves worn during handling must be entirely free of powder. Skin oil, lint, dust, powder, and other surface contaminants can evoke foreign-body reactions around the implant in tissue.

SKIN CLOSURE

In addition to sutures and staples, other materials may be used to hold skin edges in approximation.

Skin Clips

Clips made of noncorroding metal may be used to approximate skin edges. They tend to form more scar tissue than other methods of skin closure, but they may be applied quickly when time is a critical factor and cosmetic result is unimportant. They can be used in the presence of infection or drainage. A specially designed instrument is necessary to apply clips. Skin clips also may be used to secure stockinette or towels to the skin to isolate the incision, particularly on an extremity or cranial incision.

Skin Closure Strips

Adhesive-backed strips of microporous nylon (Proxistrip) or polypropylene (Steri-strip) or rayon acetate are placed at intervals across the line of incision. They may be used to approximate skin edges of superficial lacerations, as the primary closure of skin in conjunction with subcuticular suture, or in conjunction with interrupted skin sutures or staples. Often they are used following early suture or staple removal to support the wound during healing. A skin tackifier, such as tincture of benzoin, may be recommended by the manufacturer for ensuring adhesion to skin.

Sterile strips are available in widths of ⅛, ¼, and ½ inch (3, 6, and 12.7 mm) and lengths from 1½ to 4 inches (3.7 to 10 cm). They are ethylene oxide gas sterilized in peel-apart packets. Skin closure strips:

1. May be used in emergency department on superficial lacerations to eliminate need for sutures that would require local anesthesia for placement and subsequent return of the patient for suture removal.
2. Eliminate foreign-body tissue reaction of suture material in skin.
3. Have enough porosity to permit adequate ventilation of clean or contaminated wounds.

4. Permit removal of sutures within 32 to 48 hours postoperatively. Crosshatch scarring and the possibility of infection are reduced when sutures are removed early. Skin closure strips provide long-term wound reinforcement and support.
5. Permit visibility of the healing wound so surgeon can see how well the wound edges have coapted. Some strips are translucent; others have a color tone or opacity that does not afford this advantage.
6. Minimize skin irritation because they are hyporeactive.
7. Can be applied and removed rapidly.
8. Can be easily cut to meet exact length requirements.

DRUG AND MEDICAL DEVICE LEGISLATION

In 1906 the U.S. government enacted the Pure Food and Drug Act, with the U.S. Department of Agriculture as the enforcing agency to ensure the introduction of safe and sanitary foods to the public. The Food, Drug, and Cosmetic Act of 1938 extended regulation to include the introduction of cosmetics and drugs as well as food, and, to a minimal extent, medical devices. The FDA, within the Department of Agriculture, became the enforcing agency with authority to implement a preclearance mechanism requiring drug manufacturers to provide evidence of safety before a new drug could be sold. Sutures were classified as drugs.

The Kefauver-Harris Drug Amendments of 1962 added strength to the new drug clearance procedures. Drug manufacturers must prove to the FDA the effectiveness as well as the safety of drugs before making them commercially available. These amendments established a mechanism for clinical investigation to evaluate efficacy of drugs. Depending on the nature of a drug, clinical studies often require several years before the FDA approves commercial sale of a product.

The Medical Device Amendments of 1976 gave the FDA regulatory control over medical devices, in addition to the FDA's previous control of drugs. A *medical device* is defined as any instrument, apparatus, or other similar or related article, including any component, part, or accessory, promoted for a medical purpose that does not rely on chemical action to achieve its intended purpose. Under this definition sutures were reclassified as devices. All the wound closure materials discussed in this chapter are classified as devices.

In 1988 the FDA reclassified many devices, including surgical attire, masks, gloves, and drapes, for control under FDA regulations. Medical devices are classified and receive FDA approval before they are marketed. They are classified into one of three classifications.

1. *Class I devices* are subject to general regulatory controls that ensure that they are as safe and effective as similar devices already being sold.
2. *Class II devices* must establish safety and effectiveness performance standards for a new type of product.
3. *Class III devices* are usually life-sustaining or life-supporting implants or external devices. The manufacturer must file for premarket approval before the device is tested clinically to substantiate effectiveness.

A *mandatory* reporting regulation was put into effect in 1984. This regulation requires manufacturers and importers to report to the FDA any death or serious injury to a patient as a result of the malfunction of a medical device. Through the Safe Medical Devices Act of 1990, health care facilities must report directly to the FDA and to the manufacturer the probability that a device caused or contributed to a patient's death, serious injury, or serious illness. Additional requirements for tracking certain permanently implantable devices became effective in 1993. Manufacturers are responsible for tracking devices from the manufacturing facility through the chain of distribution (purchasers) to the end users (patients). Health care facilities that implant and explant (remove) these devices must submit reports to manufacturers promptly after devices are received, implanted, and/or explanted. The manufacturer must be able to provide to the FDA the following specific information regarding:

1. Device
   a. Lot, batch, model, and serial numbers or other identification used by the manufacturer
   b. Date(s) of receipt or acquisition within the chain of distribution
   c. Name(s) of person(s) or supplier from whom the device was received
2. Patient
   a. Date of implantation
   b. Name, address, and telephone number of the recipient patient
   c. Social Security number, if patient's permission is obtained to release his or her Social Security number to the manufacturer
3. Physician(s) who prescribe, implant, and/or explant
4. End-of-life information about the device, as applicable
   a. Date of explantation
   b. Date of patient's death
   c. Date device was returned to distributor or manufacturer
   d. Date device was permanently retired from use or disposed of

Also in 1993 the FDA began the *voluntary* MEDWATCH program to encourage physicians, nurses, pharmacists,

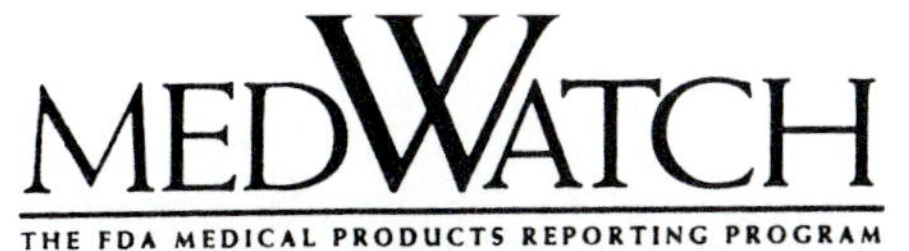

A. Patient information

1. Patient identifier — In confidence
2. Age at time of event: ______ or Date of birth:
3. Sex — ☐ female ☐ male
4. Weight — ______ lbs or ______ kgs

B. Adverse event or product problem

1. ☐ **Adverse event** and/or ☐ **Product problem** (e.g., defects/malfunctions)

2. **Outcomes attributed to adverse event** (check all that apply)
- ☐ death ______ (mo/day/yr)
- ☐ life-threatening
- ☐ hospitalization – initial or prolonged
- ☐ disability
- ☐ congenital anomaly
- ☐ required intervention to prevent permanent impairment/damage
- ☐ other: ______

3. **Date of event** (mo/day/yr)
4. **Date of this report** (mo/day/yr)
5. **Describe event or problem**

6. **Relevant tests/laboratory data,** including dates

7. **Other relevant history, including preexisting medical conditions** (e.g., allergies, race, pregnancy, smoking and alcohol use, hepatic/renal dysfunction, etc.)

C. Suspect medication(s)

1. **Name** (give labeled strength & mfr/labeler, if known)
#1
#2

2. **Dose, frequency & route used**
#1
#2

3. **Therapy dates** (if unknown, give duration) from/to (or best estimate)
#1
#2

4. **Diagnosis for use** (indication)
#1
#2

5. **Event abated after use stopped or dose reduced**
#1 ☐ yes ☐ no ☐ doesn't apply
#2 ☐ yes ☐ no ☐ doesn't apply

6. **Lot #** (if known)
#1
#2

7. **Exp. date** (if known)
#1
#2

8. **Event reappeared after reintroduction**
#1 ☐ yes ☐ no ☐ doesn't apply
#2 ☐ yes ☐ no ☐ doesn't apply

9. **NDC #** (for product problems only)
- -

10. **Concomitant medical products** and therapy dates (exclude treatment of event)

D. Suspect medical device

1. **Brand name**
2. **Type of device**
3. **Manufacturer name & address**
4. **Operator of device**
- ☐ health professional
- ☐ lay user/patient
- ☐ other: ______

5. **Expiration date** (mo/day/yr)

6.
model # ______
catalog # ______
serial # ______
lot # ______
other #

7. **If implanted, give date** (mo/day/yr)
8. **If explanted, give date** (mo/day/yr)

9. **Device available for evaluation?** (Do not send to FDA)
☐ yes ☐ no ☐ returned to manufacturer on ______ (mo/day/yr)

10. **Concomitant medical products** and therapy dates (exclude treatment of event)

E. Reporter (see confidentiality section on back)

1. **Name, address & phone #**
2. **Health professional?** ☐ yes ☐ no
3. **Occupation**
4. **Also reported to**
- ☐ manufacturer
- ☐ user facility
- ☐ distributor

5. **If you do NOT want your identity disclosed to the manufacturer, place an " X " in this box.** ☐

FDA

Mail to: MEDWATCH **5600 Fishers Lane Rockville, MD 20852-9787** *or* **FAX to: 1-800-FDA-0178**

FDA Form 3500 (6/93) **Submission of a report does not constitute an admission that medical personnel or the product caused or contributed to the event.**

FIGURE 24-8 MEDWATCH reporting form.

and other heath care professionals to report adverse events and defects or problems with regulated drugs and devices. The purpose of MEDWATCH is to provide a nationwide standardized system for reporting to the FDA any medical device or drug suspected of causing a patient's death, life-threatening injury or illness, disability, prolonged hospitalization, congenital anomaly, and/or experience that requires intervention to prevent permanent health impairment. The FDA provides a MEDWATCH reporting form (Figure 24-8). Examples of reportable problems include latex sensitivity, malfunction of drug infusion pumps, and failure of an alarm during malfunction of a ventilator.

Surgeons who implant or use medical devices and nurses, surgical technologists, and others who handle them must be adequately instructed in the proper care and handling of all devices to ensure patient safety. Most adverse events occur when devices are misused, are defective, or malfunction. However, an adverse patient reaction can occur when the device functions properly and is used appropriately. The FDA is responsible for investigating a report of an adverse event or product problem and for taking corrective action.

BIBLIOGRAPHY

Anate M: Skin closure of laparotomy wounds: absorbable subcuticular vs. non-absorbable interrupted sutures, *W Afr J Med* 10(2):150-157, 1991.

Bagi P et al: Early local stoma complications in relation to the applied suture material: a comparison between monofilament and multifilament materials, *Dis Colon Rectum* 35(8):739-742, 1992.

Bardaxoglou E et al: Oesophageal perforation: primary suture repair reinforced with absorbable mesh and fibrin glue, *Br J Surg* 81(3):399, 1994.

Clark HC: An improved ligator in operative laparoscopy, *Obstet Gynecol* 83(2):299-301, 1994.

Couig MP, Merkatz RB: MEDWATCH: the new medical products reporting program, *Am J Nurs* 93(8):65-68, 1993.

Curry J: Human fibrin makes effective tissue adhesive, *OR Manager* 10(6):18-19, 1994.

daSilva EG: Suturoscope: a new device that allows endoscopic sutures to be performed with traditional threads, *Surg Endosc* 4(4):220-223, 1990.

Davis MS: Blunt-tipped suture needles, *Infect Control Hosp Epidemiol* 14(1)224-225, 1994.

Device tracking: questions and answers about tracking program; internal tracking system eases employee burden; hospital expands tracking system to comply with law, *OR Manager* 10(4):13-17, 1994.

Edlich RF et al: Scientific basis for selecting surgical needles and needle holders for wound closure, *Clin Plast Surg* 17(3):583-602, 1990.

Edoga JK et al: The endo clip applier—a superior extracorporeal knot pusher in disguise? *Surg Endosc* 7(4):364, 1993.

Elder MJ: Merseline mesh and fascia lata in brow suspension: a comparative study, *Ophthalmic Surg* 24(2):105-108, 1993.

Eppley BL, Sadove AM: Use of bolsters in facial surgery, *J Oral Maxillofac Surg* 48(4):425-426, 1990.

Furst E: The safe medical device act, *J Cardiovasc Nurs* 8(2):79-85, 1994.

Gazayerli MM: The Gazayerli knot-tying instrument or ligator for use in diverse laparoscopic surgical procedures, *Surg Laparoscopy Endoscopy* 1(4):254-258, 1991.

Geis WP, Malago M: Laparoscopic bilateral inguinal herniorrhaphies: use of a single giant preperitoneal mesh patch, *Am Surg* 60(8):558-563, 1994.

Gibson T: Evolution of catgut ligatures: the endeavors of Joseph Lister and William MacEwen, *Br J Surg* 77(7):824-825, 1990.

James JD et al: Technical considerations in manual and instrument tying techniques, *J Emerg Med* 19(4):469-480, 1992.

Kessler DA: Introducing MEDWATCH: a new approach to reporting medication and device adverse effects and product problems, *Gen Hosp Psychiatry* 16(2):96-102, 1994.

Koch FA et al: The safe medical devices act, *AORN J* 55(2):537-548, 1992.

Koninkx PR: An improved needleholder for laparoscopic knot tying, *Fertil Steril* 58(3):640-642, 1992.

Matloub HS et al: Characteristics of prosthetic mesh and autogenous fascia in abdominal wall reconstruction after prolonged implantation, *Ann Plast Surg* 29(6):508-511, 1992.

McLaughlin MJ, McLaughlin BH: Thoracoscopic ablation of blebs using PDS-endoloop in recurrent spontaneous pneumothorax, *Surg Laparoscopy Endoscopy* 1(4):263-264, 1991.

Meddings RN et al: Collagen vicryl—a new dural prosthesis, *Acta Neurol* 117(1-2):53-58, 1992.

Meddings RN et al: Dural prostheses: where do we go from here? *Lancet* 339(8785):127, 1992.

Medical devices: Device tracking: final rules and request for comments, *Federal Register* 58:43442-43455, 1993.

Merriman JA: Legislation: new federal program encourages health professionals to report drug, device problems, *AORN J* 58(3):594-597, 1993.

Nagar H: Stitch granulomas following inguinal herniotomy: a 10-year review, *J Pediatr Surg* 28(11):1505-1507, 1993.

Nathanson LK et al: Safety of vessel ligation in laparoscopic surgery, *Endoscopy* 23(4):206-209, 1991.

O'Connor JJ: Single-operator ligation, *Dis Colon Rectum* 37(7):733, 1994.

Recommended practices: surgical tissue banking, *AORN J* 53(3):768-774, 1991.

Reich H et al: A simple method for ligating with curved and straight needles in operative laparoscopy, *Obstet Gynecol* 79(1):143-147, 1992.

Ritter EF et al: Effects of method of hemostasis on wound-infection rate, *Am Surg* 56(10):648-650, 1990.

Soloman RP, Koch FA: The new implant tracking regulations: defining, implementing, documenting, *AORN J* 58(6):1142-1151, 1993.

Thal R: A technique for arthroscopic mattress suture placement, *Arthroscopy* 9(5):605-607, 1993.

Tian F et al: The disintegration of absorbable suture materials on exposure to human digestive juices: an update, *Am Surg* 60(4):287-291, 1994.

Trott A: *Wounds and lacerations: emergency care and closure,* St Louis, 1991, Mosby.

US Department of Health and Human Services: *Medical device tracking: questions and answers based on the final rule,* USDHSS Pub No FDA 93-4259, Washington, DC, 1993, US Government Printing Office.

Users to report device-related deaths to FDA, *OR Manager* 7(1):1, 13, 1991.

Ward-English L: Suture materials: the surgeon's selection, *Surg Technol* 26(5):16-18, 1994.

Watson S: Surgical cement: friend or foe? *Br J Theatre Nurs* 27(9):4, 1990.

Wound closure manual, Somerville, NJ, 1994, Ethicon.

Zokal F: Made-to-order suture packs, *AORN J* 51(3):817-827, 1990.

SECTION NINE

Postoperative Care of the Patient and Environment

CHAPTER 25

Surgical Wounds

FACTORS INFLUENCING HEALING AND INFECTION

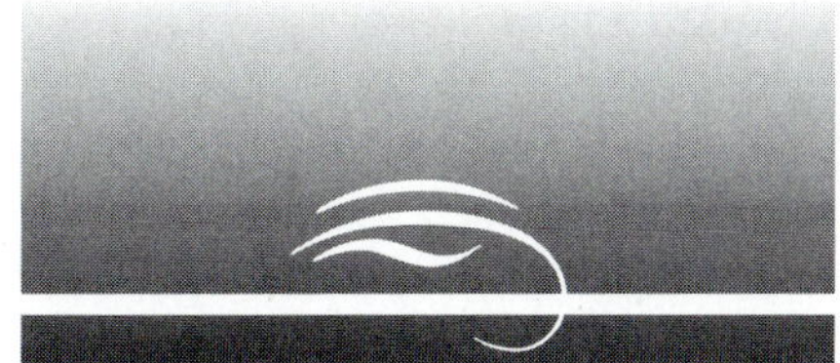

HISTORICAL BACKGROUND

From antiquity, warfare has necessitated some means of controlling hemorrhage and closing wounds. Egyptian papyri dating back to 2100 BC describe how various injuries, including head injuries and fractures, were treated. Early surgeons in India surpassed those of Egypt in their skills in treating fractures and other injuries and in performing plastic surgery. In India military surgeons were responsible for the food and sanitary conditions of the army as well as for treating the wounded.

Early records describe epidemics, purulence, fumigation, and wound management. These early concepts of infection and crude methods to combat it seem strange in light of modern scientific knowledge. Yet the ablest minds of the time worked to develop effective methods to control hemorrhage and infection and to close wounds. They are the forerunners of modern surgery.

After the Middle Ages, surgical techniques improved sporadically. A few surgeons from the twelfth to the nineteenth centuries believed that wounds did not need to suppurate (i.e., discharge pus). Others taught that "laudable pus" was an essential part of the healing process. This almost universally accepted concept persisted in spite of the fact that some pioneering surgeons found that ventilation, sanitation, and heat-treated bed linens reduced the patient infection rate. But acceptance of scientific inquiry was slow, and the inquirer was subject to condemnation and even death.

The concept of contamination by air or fomites did not surface until 1546, when Girolama Francastoro, an Italian physician, held that contagion was caused by the passage of minute bodies, capable of self-multiplication, from the infector to the infected. He was the first to describe typhus fever, a disease prevalent at that time. His theory opened the way to the modern concept of infection and communicable diseases of epidemic proportions.

By the seventeenth century the world had barely begun to discard superstitions. Science was just beginning to emerge. Into such a world, Anton van Leeuwenhoek (1632-1723) was born in Holland. He heard that if one very carefully ground very small lenses out of clear glass, one could see objects much larger than they appeared to the unaided eye. His invention of the microscope was the precursor of many great discoveries. His painstaking work with minutiae was challenged by his contemporaries. By the middle of the century, European rebels stated they would trust only perpetually repeated observations from their own experiments.

Leeuwenhoek's follower was Lazardo Spallanzani (1729-1799), a young Italian who experimented on the multiplication of microbes and their "spontaneous generation." He proved that microbes could live without air. Humanity owes much to these bold, persistent explorers and fighters of death.

Research in wound healing did not occur before the eighteenth century. John Hunter (1728-1793), a Scottish surgeon, recorded observations of healing patterns for the first time. He differentiated primary from secondary healing by calling the first "adhesive inflammation" and the second "suppurative inflammation." He also distinguished between epithelialization and granulation in healing wounds.

Europe was not the only seat of interest in disease, wounds, and infection in the eighteenth century. America was struggling with epidemics as it battled to survive as a new nation. Diseases that are controlled today by inoculations and antibiotics ravaged the Revolutionary Army. Dr. Zabdiel Boylston of Boston introduced inoculation for smallpox in 1721. Some of Washington's troops were inoculated, but many uninoculated soldiers died. Diseases that plagued the losing side frequently tipped the scales of history and were often dreaded more than the enemy.

Dr. Oliver Wendell Holmes (1809-1894), the renowned nineteenth-century physician and poet, wrote in 1843 of the contagious nature of puerperal fever ("childbirth fever"). He expressed the belief that it was carried from patient to patient by nurses and doctors. However, many physicians still believed infection occurred by an act of Providence.

The true pioneer was Ignaz Semmelweis (1818-1865), a Hungarian physician who in Austria established the etiology of puerperal fever, then a major cause of maternal mortality. He required doctors and medical students on his wards to wash their hands in a chlorinated-lime solution before examining patients. In a year's time Semmelweis reduced mortality to one twelfth of its previous level. However, his ideas were not understood, and they created controversy. The great value of his discovery was not recognized by other physicians of his time. Presumably because of this rejection, he was committed to a hospital for the insane and met with an early death.

It was Louis Pasteur (1822-1895), the French chemist and microbiologist, who established the validity of the germ theory of disease. He discovered that fermentation of wine is the result of minute organisms. All previous explanations had been without experimental foundation. He found that heat could halt the organisms' growth. By experimentation in the pure air of the Alps, he destroyed the theory of spontaneous generation of organisms, proving that they came from similar organisms with which ordinary air was impregnated. His discoveries led to his studies of infection and putrefaction in living tissue. He isolated the bacillus of anthrax and developed the Pasteur vaccine for rabies. His greatest contribution was laying the foundation for bacteriology as a science and teaching the role of bacteria in causing disease.

The German physician Robert Koch (1843-1910), also a pioneer in bacteriology, won a Nobel prize for isolating *Mycobacterium tuberculosis.* Every student of bacteriology learns Koch's postulates:

1. A specific organism must be seen in all cases of an infectious disease.
2. This organism must be obtained in pure culture.
3. Organisms from pure cultures must reproduce the disease in experimental animals.
4. The organism must be recoverable from the experimental animals.

These postulates served as guides to the discovery of etiologic agents in many of the most important diseases of humans, animals, and plants.

Before and during the mid-nineteenth century, wounds or injury to an extremity invariably resulted in gangrene. Amputation was routinely performed in an attempt to prevent *septicemia,* a significant invasion of microorganisms into the bloodstream. Infection and pus were to be expected in wounds, whether caused by traumatic injury or surgical procedure.

Joseph Lister (1827-1912), an English surgeon, was the first to recognize the value of Pasteur's germ theory in relation to surgery. He used carbolic acid in the air, in wounds, and on surrounding areas to destroy bacteria. Lister's principle of antiseptic surgery initiated the modern era of surgery.

Reluctantly, surgeons came to accept Lister's principles. One of the best known of these was William Stewart Halsted (1852-1922), an American, who taught the value of antisepsis at Johns Hopkins Hospital in Baltimore. Although Halsted abolished the use of carbolic acid, he made many important contributions that enhanced surgical technique. His principles of tissue handling (see Chapter 24, p. 492) are still followed.

Within reasonable limits, in the absence of hemorrhage and sepsis, wound healing is predictable. However, disregard for the principles of tissue handling and wound management can lead to such complications as hematoma, infection, wound disruption, scarring, stricture, adhesion, and contracture.

DEFINITIONS

Terms relevant to wound healing are found in Box 25-1.

BOX 25-1

Glossary of Terms in Wound Healing

adhesion Band of scar tissue that holds or unites surfaces or structures together that are normally separated.
contracture Formation of extensive scar tissue over a joint.
dead space Space caused by separation of wound edges or by air trapped between layers of tissue.
debridement Removal of damaged tissue and cellular or other debris from a wound to promote healing and to prevent infection.
dehiscence Partial or total splitting open or separation of layers of a wound.
edema Abnormal accumulation of fluid in interstitial spaces of tissues.
evisceration Protrusion of viscera through an abdominal incision.
excision Removal of tissue.
extravasation Passage of blood, serum, or lymph into tissues.
granulation tissue Formation of fibrous collagen to fill the gap between edges of a wound healing by contraction (i.e., second intention).
granuloma Inflammatory lesion.
hematoma Collection of extravasated blood in tissue.
hemostasis Arrest of flow of blood or hemorrhage; the mechanism is by *coagulation,* formation of a blood clot.
incision Intentional cut through intact tissue (syn., *surgical incision*).
ischemia Decrease of blood supply to tissues.
necrosis Death of tissue cells.
scar Deposition of fibrous connective tissue to bridge separated wound edges and to restore continuity of tissues.
seroma Collection of extravasated serum from interstitial tissue or resolving hematoma in tissue.
tensile strength Ability of tissues to resist rupture.
tissue reaction Immune response of body to tissue injury or foreign substances.
wound Injury to tissue, either by intent or accident (syn., *surgical wound, trauma*).
wound disruption Separation of wound edges.
wound healing Body's defense mechanisms to repair tissues. Wounds heal by first, second, or third intention depending on the type of wound. Healing takes place in phases.

TYPES OF WOUNDS

A wound is an injury, either intentional or accidental, that disrupts the continuity of body tissues with or without tissue loss. Wounds may be surgical, traumatic, or chronic.

Surgical Incision and Excision

The surgeon cuts through *intact* tissue for the purpose of exposing or excising tissue. An *incision* is a cut or an opening into tissue. An *excision* is removal of tissue. A sterile sharp scalpel (knife), scissors, or other cutting instrument may be used to separate skin and underlying tissues. Thermal instruments that both cut or vaporize tissue and coagulate surrounding blood vessels are used for incision and excision. Location, length, and depth of an incision must be planned. A safe surgical procedure requires exposure through an adequate incision.

The surgeon spreads the skin taut between thumb and index finger in preparation for making the skin incision. With one stroke of evenly applied pressure on the scalpel, a clean incision is made through skin. A number of factors influence the ease with which a skin incision is made:

1. Sharpness of knife blade
2. Resistance of self-adhering plastic drapes
3. Toughness of skin
4. Thickness of subcutaneous tissue

A clean stroke with a sterile surgical scalpel, followed by attention to all the principles of sterile technique and tissue handling, is the best insurance for primary healing by first intention. However, the direction of the incision may be a factor in wound healing. Wounds heal side-to-side, not end-to-end.

Traumatic Injuries

Following traumatic injury, preservation of life is the first critical concern. No one specific pattern of treatment suits all patients. The patient's general condition is of prime consideration. Injuries are evaluated, and those that pose greatest hazards to life or to return to normal function are cared for first. The primary objective following life support is wound closure with minimal deformity and functional loss. Minor injuries are cared for in the emergency department. Patients with major injuries receive treatment in the emergency department before going to the operating room (OR) as quickly as their conditions warrant.

Traumatic wounds can be considered closed or open, simple or complicated, clean or contaminated. Wound closure is predicated on type, location, severity, and extent of injury.

Closed Wounds

Skin is intact in a closed wound, but underlying tissues are injured. A blister filled with serum or a hematoma of blood and serum may form under the epidermis. Torn ligaments and simple fractures are closed wounds.

Open Wounds

In open wounds the continuity of the skin is broken by abrasion, laceration, or penetration.

Simple Wounds

Continuity of skin is interrupted in simple wounds, but without loss or destruction of tissue and without implantation of a foreign body. These lacerations are usually caused by a sharp-edged object cutting or penetrating at low velocity.

Complicated Wounds

In complicated wounds tissue is lost or destroyed by crush or burn, or a foreign body is implanted by high-velocity penetration. If a penetrating wound was made by an object, such as a knife or bullet, this is not removed until the surgeon explores the wound in the OR. Movement of a foreign object may cause further trauma. The depth of a penetrating wound is irrigated and may be excised. Skin grafting may be required following destruction of dermis.

Clean Wounds

Clean wounds will heal by first intention after closure of all tissue layers and wound edges. The cosmetic care of lacerated areas is important, as is treatment to provide normal function of a part.

Contaminated Wounds

When dirty objects penetrate skin, microorganisms multiply rapidly. Within 6 hours contamination can become infection. Debridement is done to thoroughly wash and irrigate a wound. Devitalized tissue is removed because it acts as a culture medium. For excision of each area of contaminated tissue, clean instruments are used and discarded. Irrigation is continued during tissue excision. After initial debridement to remove foreign bodies, including dirt and dead or devitalized tissue, the wound may be left open to heal by second or third intention. Primary closure is delayed for several days unless the surgeon believes a skin graft or a vascularized flap will remain viable and uninfected. This procedure is attempted only within 4 hours of time of injury.

NOTE Removal of foreign bodies and devitalized tissue is important in preventing tetanus. Tetanus is most likely to occur in deep wounds contaminated by soil or animal feces. The patient must be immunized against the tetanus bacillus. Adsorbed tetanus toxoid (0.5 ml) is given as an initial immunizing dose or as a booster if the patient has been immunized within the previous 5 years. Tetanus immune globulin (human, 250 to 500 units) also should be given to any patient who has a severe wound or who has had the wound more than 24 hours and has not been immunized within the previous 10 years.

Chronic Wounds

Pressure sores and decubitus ulcers may result from compromised circulation over bony prominences for extended periods of time. Venous stasis or inadequate circulation in the legs may cause skin ulcers. Tissue necrosis may occur following radiation therapy. These chronic wounds have tissue loss and usually have heavy bacterial contamination. Topical application of fibronectin, a platelet-derived wound-healing formula, or other preparation of growth factors from patient's own blood may help control infection and promote healing. Growth factors stimulate the growth of tissue, capillaries, and skin. If a wound fails to heal by secondary intention with formation of granulation tissue, debridement and skin grafting may be required.

MECHANISM OF WOUND HEALING

Violation of tissue integrity, either by intent to explore or remove a disease process or to repair traumatic injury, demands understanding the mechanism and factors that influence wound healing. Wound healing is nature's way of restoring continuity and strength to injured or incised tissue.

When tissue is cut, the body's inherent defense mechanisms respond immediately to begin repair. Three types of wound healing are recognized: first intention, second intention, third intention. Each has practical applications in making and closing incisions or traumatic wounds.

First Intention/Primary Union

Healing by first intention is desired following primary union of an incised, aseptic, accurately approximated wound. It shows:

1. No postoperative swelling
2. No serous discharge or local infection
3. No separation of wound edges
4. Minimal scar formation

The rate and pattern of wound healing differ in various tissues. In general, first-intention wound healing consists of three distinct phases:

1. *Lag phase of acute inflammatory response.* Tissue fluids containing plasma, proteins, blood cells, fibrin, and antibodies exude from the tissues into the wound, depositing fibrin, which weakly holds the wound edges together for the first 5 days. Fibrin and serum protein dry out, forming a scab that seals the wound from further fluid loss and microbial invasion. At the same time, fibroblasts, fibrous-tissue germ cells, and epithelial cells migrate from the general circulation. Subsequent adhesion of these cells, a process known as *fibroplasia,* holds the wound edges together. Leukocytes and other white blood cells produce proteolytic enzymes to dissolve and remove damaged tissue debris. Macrophages and neutrophils ingest foreign material, cellular debris, and bacteria.

2. *Healing or proliferative phase of fibroplasia.* After the fifth postoperative day, fibroblasts multiply rapidly, bridging wound edges and restoring the continuity of body structures. *Collagen,* a protein substance that is the chief constituent of connective tissue, is secreted from the fibroblasts and formed into fibers. This results in the rapid gain in tensile strength and pliability of the healing wound. *Tensile strength* is the ability of the tissues to resist rupture. The healing phase begins rapidly, diminishes progressively, and terminates on about the fourteenth day. It may continue for up to 20 days.
3. *Maturation or differentiation phase.* From the fourteenth postoperative day until the wound is fully healed, scar formation occurs by deposition of fibrous connective tissue. The collagen content remains constant, but the fiber pattern re-forms and cross-links to increase the tensile strength. Wound contraction occurs over a period of weeks up to 6 months. As collagen density increases, vascularity decreases, and the scar grows pale.

Second Intention

The mechanism of second-intention healing is wound contraction rather than primary union. Granulation tissue containing fibroblasts forms in the defect and closes it by contraction with secondary growth of epithelium. In this type:

1. Infection, excessive trauma, loss of tissue, or poorly approximated tissue is present.
2. Wound may be left open and allowed to heal from bottom (the inner) toward the outer surface.
3. Healing is delayed.
4. Healing may produce a weak union, which may be conducive to incisional herniation (rupture) later.
5. Risk of secondary infection is proportional to amount of necrotic tissue present in the wound and to compromised immune response in the patient.
6. Scar formation is excessive.
7. Contracture of skin is pronounced.

Grafting may be necessary during the healing process or after healing is complete to fill in a defect, revise a scar, or release a contracture.

Third Intention/Delayed Primary Closure

Suturing is delayed or secondary for the purpose of walling off an area of gross infection or where extensive tissue was removed, as in a debridement or by a traumatic injury. The edges are closed 4 to 6 days postoperatively. In healing by third intention:

1. Two surfaces of granulation tissue are brought together.
2. A deeper and wider scar usually results.

FACTORS INFLUENCING WOUND HEALING

One of the desired outcomes of surgical intervention is for the patient to be free from infection. Clinically, infection is the product of entrance, growth, metabolic activities, and pathophysiologic effects of microorganisms in living tissue. It can be present in the surgical patient preoperatively or can develop as a postoperative complication. Because the factors that influence wound healing correlate with the incidence of infection, they are discussed together.

Physical Condition of Patient

The preexisting physical condition of the patient influences wound healing and the potential for postoperative infection.

General Health

Chronic diseases alter normal physiology. Diseases such as diabetes, uremia, fibrocystic disease, cirrhosis, active alcoholism, and leukemia can delay the wound healing process. Cardiovascular or respiratory insufficiency inhibits tissue perfusion. Oxygenation is essential to wound healing and to inhibit growth of anaerobic microorganisms. Malignant diseases, debilitating injuries, and systemic or localized infections can adversely affect wound healing. Even a brief preoperative illness such as acute appendicitis can influence postoperative healing. Sores, scratches, or unhealed skin wounds indicate the presence of skin sepsis. These and any other remote focus of infection, especially in the respiratory or urinary tracts, may be a contraindication for an elective surgical procedure because they increase the likelihood of wound infection.

Smoking Vasoconstriction caused by smoking decreases blood supply to the wound. Carbon monoxide in smoke binds with hemoglobin and further diminishes oxygenation. Smoking contributes to respiratory complications. This can cause forceful coughing that can raise intraabdominal pressure and create increased strain on an abdominal wound and impair healing.

Age

Loss of skin and muscle tone and elasticity is a natural characteristic of the aging process. The rate of change is variable, however. Thickened connective tissue, decreased subcutaneous fat, diminished capillary blood flow, and reduced vascularity are age-related factors that may delay wound healing. Tension of sutures on aged skin can further inhibit tissue perfusion. Sutures or skin staples should be reinforced with wound closure strips. Newborn infants, especially those who are preterm, and geriatric patients are especially prone to infection.

Nutritional Status

Wound healing is impaired by deficiencies in proteins, carbohydrates, zinc, and vitamins A, B, C, and K. Protein provides essential amino acids for new tissue construction. Carbohydrates are necessary energy sources for cells, preventing excessive metabolism of amino acids to meet caloric requirements. Vitamin B complex is necessary for carbohydrate, protein, and fat metabolism. Vitamin C permits collagen formation. Although Vitamin A and zinc are known to be important in collagen synthesis, their mechanism in wound healing is not well understood. Vitamin K is involved in the synthesis of prothrombin and blood-clotting factors. Copper and iron assist in collagen synthesis. Calcium and magnesium are important in protein synthesis. Manganese serves as an enzyme activator.

Malnutrition, whether primary or secondary to catabolic disease, can be a major factor in wound healing and infection. Impairment of physiologic functions associated with a body weight loss that is greater than 10% and protein energy malnutrition increase the risk of postoperative complications. Liver function, skeletal and respiratory muscle function, overall physical and mental activity, and inflammatory response to wound healing are altered in the malnourished host. Protein and fat deficiency is especially significant in patients with extensive burns or multiple injuries who have greatly increased caloric requirements. Malnutrition caused by anorexia or cachexia has a deleterious effect on wound healing. Hyperalimentation with vitamin, trace element, and mineral supplements preoperatively and postoperatively usually is indicated for malnourished patients (see Chapter 8, p. 111).

Obesity

The bulk and weight of adipose tissue cause difficulty in confining excess fat and securing good wound closure in obese patients. To minimize dead space, the surgeon may place drains and sutures in subcutaneous fat; both may actually potentiate infection. Of all tissues, fat is the most vulnerable to trauma and infection because of its poor vascularity. Many morbidly obese patients, more than 100 lb (45.4 kg) over ideal body weight, have cardiac decompensation and respiratory insufficiency.

Fluid and Electrolyte Balance

The body's system for balancing fluids and electrolytes is extremely complex. As a result of illness, injury, or infection, the patient may not be able to maintain normal fluid and electrolyte balance. Fever associated with infection, for example, can raise fluid requirements as much as 15% for each 1.5° F (1° C) rise in body temperature. Body fluid is *intracellular* (ICF), within cells, and *extracellular* (ECF), outside cells as intravascular plasma and interstitial fluid between cells. The electrolyte content differs (see Chapter 19, p. 380). ECF contains more sodium than ICF; ICF has more potassium than ECF. Changes in this balance can affect kidney function, cellular metabolism, oxygen concentration in the circulation, and hormonal function. Adequate ECF fluid volume is necessary for circulation of blood to tissues.

Hematology

The presence of an abnormal or pathologic condition affecting the blood (see Chapter 23, pp. 482-484) should be carefully evaluated preoperatively. A low hemoglobin level (red cell count) associated with anemia can result in tissue hypoxia, which alters synthesis of collagen and epithelialization. A hematocrit value below 20% lowers oxygen tension in tissues, which disrupts cell regeneration. An elevated leukocyte level (white cell count) indicates the presence of infection in the body.

Immune Responses

The body normally responds at once to repair the inflammatory reaction of the tissues to injury or foreign substances. The cells liberate a tissue extract that starts an immune response for repair of the tissue. This is known as *tissue reaction.* Some foreign materials normally cause more tissue reaction than others. Abnormalities in function of these immune responses, such as an allergic reaction, can contribute to delayed wound healing.

The recipient of a prosthetic implant is susceptible to infection because the immune system concentrates its response around the device, thus increasing the risk of systemic microbial invasion.

Allergic Reaction Hypersensitivity to substances inhaled, ingested, injected, or in contact with skin causes an acute allergic reaction. An antibiotic (e.g., penicillin) cannot be given prophylactically to a patient who is known to be allergic.

Immunosuppressed/Compromised Hosts The patient's immunologic response may be deficient because of a congenital or acquired immunologic disease, drugs, or radiation therapy. Patients of this status, referred to as *immunosuppressed* or *compromised hosts,* are often victims of infection caused by normal but potentially pathogenic flora within their own bodies. They may not present the usual signs and symptoms of infection. Lack of integrity of the immune system, such as leukopenia or defective immunoglobulin synthesis, can be life-threatening.

Drug Therapy

Wound healing occurs basically through collagen synthesis. Agents that interfere with cellular metabolism have a potentially deleterious effect on the healing process. Prolonged high dosage of steroids such as cortisone preoperatively inhibits fibroplasia and collagen formation. Some antineoplastic agents used as chemotherapeutic adjuvants to surgery also may delay systemic wound healing or cause localized tissue necrosis from extravasation at the site of injection. Immunosuppressants are given to transplant patients to prevent organ or tissue rejection. Leukopenia and susceptibility to infection are common sequelae to administration of these drugs.

Radiation Therapy

Healing is delayed if the patient has had radiation in large doses preoperatively. The blood supply in irradiated tissue is decreased. However, little change from the normal healing pattern occurs if radiation has been given in low doses (see Chapter 45) and the surgical procedure is performed within 4 to 6 weeks postradiation.

Intraoperative Considerations

Devitalized tissue caused by laser or electrosurgery is unable to regenerate. Interruption of blood supply and innervation decrease circulation and prevent epithelialization. Excess tension on the suture line that inhibits tissue perfusion prolongs healing time.

Postoperative Complications

Edema, vomiting, or coughing can place stress on the healing wound before fibroplasia takes place. Complications in other parts of the body, far from the surgical site, such as pneumonia, thrombus, or embolus, can inhibit oxygen supply to the wound site. Collagen synthesis is partly a function of the oxygenation of tissues. Therefore oxygen perfusion to tissues contributes to the rate of healing, tensile strength of the wound, and resistance to infection. This is particularly important in arterialized and microvascular tissue grafts and flaps used to cover soft tissue defects (see Chapter 34) and organ transplantation (see Chapter 44). Ischemic tissue is more susceptible to infection than well-vascularized tissue.

Physical Activity

Early ambulation postoperatively is one of the most important factors in recovery for the surgical patient. Ambulation may be started immediately after recovery from anesthesia if the patient's condition does not contraindicate it. Some surgeons exempt only the patient whose blood pressure is not stable, who has a cardiac problem, or whose general condition is poor. If the patient's physical condition does not safely permit ambulation, the surgeon orders otherwise.

Ambulation is started gradually by the patient first turning onto one side. The patient then sits up with feet over side of the bed and then stands on floor for a minute before returning to bed. After repeating this several times, the patient takes a few steps and finally increases the distance walked. Sitting in a chair for prolonged periods is discouraged because this contributes to stasis of blood. The patient must understand the value of early ambulation.

1. It improves circulation, which aids in the healing process and eliminates stasis of blood that may result in thrombus and embolus formation.
2. Patient is better able to cooperate in deep-breathing exercises to raise bronchial secretions; thus pulmonary complications are reduced.
3. Early ambulation decreases gas pains, distention, and tendency toward nausea and vomiting. It helps prevent constipation. Bodily functions return to normal more readily.
4. Increased exercise aids digestion. Thus the patient's oral intake progresses sooner after surgical procedure so less supplementary intravenous fluid is necessary for hydration and nutrition.
5. Early ambulation eliminates the general muscle weakness that follows bed rest.
6. Fewer pain-relieving drugs are necessary.
7. It boosts patients' morale to know they will be out of bed early after the surgical procedure, able to care for themselves, and soon ready to go home. This helps the mental outlook and through it the physical recovery.
8. It shortens hospitalization.

Classification of Surgical Wounds

The surgical site may be clean or contaminated when the surgeon makes the initial incision. A clean site may become contaminated depending on the type of wound, the pathologic findings or circumstances creating the need for the surgical procedure, the anatomic location, or the techniques of the OR team. After wound closure, the circulator should verify the wound classification with the surgeon. This is documented in the patient's intraoperative records. An incident report may need to be completed in the event unusual, extenuating circumstances necessitate a change in the classification of the surgical wound.

Surgical wounds are classified by the degree of microbial contamination. Risk of infection increases in proportion to contamination of the incision and surrounding tissues exposed during the course of the surgical procedure. The wound is classified at the end of the surgical procedure as one of four types (Box 25-2):

1. Clean
2. Clean-contaminated
3. Contaminated
4. Dirty and infected

Surgical Technique

Surgical technique is one of the most important factors influencing wound healing, perhaps more important

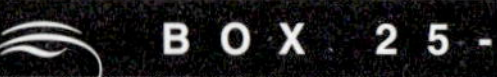

BOX 25-2

Classification of Surgical Wounds

Clean wound (expected infection rate: 1% to 5%)
Elective procedure with wound made under ideal OR conditions
Primary closure, wound not drained
No break in sterile technique during surgical procedure
No inflammation present
Alimentary, respiratory, and genitourinary tracts or oropharyngeal cavity not entered

Clean-contaminated wound (infection rate: 8% to 11%)
Primary closure, wound drained
Minor break in technique occurred
No inflammation or infection present
Alimentary, respiratory, and genitourinary tracts or oropharyngeal cavity entered under controlled conditions without significant spillage or unusual contamination

Contaminated wound (infection rate: 15% to 20%)
Open fresh traumatic wound of less than 4 hours
Major break in technique occurred
Acute nonpurulent inflammation present
Gross spillage/contamination from gastrointestinal tract
Entrance into genitourinary or biliary tracts with infected urine or bile present

Dirty and infected wound (infection rate: 27% to 40%)
Old traumatic wound of more than 4 hours' duration from dirty source or with retained necrotic tissue, foreign body, or fecal contamination
Organisms present in surgical field before procedure
Existing clinical infection: acute bacterial inflammation encountered, with or without purulence; incision to drain abscess
Perforated viscus

than any patient factor. The mnemonic GEM applies to the surgeon:

G *Gentle* tissue handling
E *Expeditious* to minimize surgical time
M *Meticulous* hemostasis and tissue approximation

Dr. John Deaver (1855-1931) of Philadelphia had an apt adage: "If the surgeon cuts well and sews well, the patient gets well." Careful wound management involves the following considerations.

Aseptic Technique

Healthy tissues are able to combat a certain amount of contamination. Microorganisms are normally present in skin and air. Devitalized tissues have little power of resistance. Infection may occur from any one of a variety of causes that results in a breakdown of the wound postoperatively. The surgeon gives meticulous attention to sterile technique throughout the surgical procedure to minimize contamination of the surgical site. The entire OR team carefully carries out aseptic and sterile techniques (see Chapter 12). In addition, many precautions are taken by all OR personnel. Strict adherence to housekeeping techniques, air engineering, sterilization procedures, and all the principles of aseptic technique is necessary. Infection may be caused by a break in the chain of asepsis.

Hemostasis

Complete hemostasis must be achieved to prevent loss of blood, to provide as bloodless a field as possible for accurate dissection, and to prevent hematoma (blood clot) formation. Blood loss is caused by tissue trauma. The extent of dissection and injury can affect healing if delivery of oxygen to the tissues is affected. Healing tissues consume oxygen avidly. Hence any condition that lowers circulatory flow and the delivery of oxygen to the tissues impairs healing. (Hypoxia and hypovolemia are discussed in Chapter 19.) Because they are so critical, the mechanisms and methods of hemostasis are discussed in detail in Chapter 23.

Tissue Handling

All tissues should be handled very gently and as little as possible throughout the surgical procedure. The surgeon makes an incision that is just long enough to afford sufficient operating space. Careful consideration is given to underlying blood vessels and nerves to preserve as many as possible. Retractors are placed to provide exposure without causing undue pressure on tissues and organs or tension on muscles. Trauma to tissue in dissecting, handling with instruments, ligating or suturing may cause edema and necrosis, death of tissue cells, with resultant slow healing. The body must rid itself of necrotic cells before the healing phase of fibroplasia takes place.

Tissue Approximation

Tissue edges are brought together with precision, avoiding strangulation and eliminating dead space, to promote wound healing. Too tight a closure or closure under tension causes *ischemia*, a decrease of blood supply to tissues.

Dead space is caused by separation of wound edges that have not been closely approximated or by air trapped between layers of tissue. Serum or blood may collect in a dead space and prevent healing by keeping cut edges separated. Wound edges not in close contact cannot heal readily. A drain may be inserted to aid in removal of fluid or air from the surgical site postoperatively, or a pressure dressing may be applied over a closed wound to help obliterate dead space. Drains and dressings are discussed on pp. 527-532.

The choice of wound closure materials and the techniques of the surgeon are prime factors in the restoration of tensile strength to the wound during the healing process. Materials used to approximate tissues are discussed in Chapter 24.

Wound Security

Quality of approximated tissue and type of closure material are two factors that determine the strength of the wound. Tensile strength of the tissues themselves varies; some are more friable than others. Drains or catheters may be placed in the wound to evacuate serum or fluid and prevent it from accumulating in the dead space postoperatively. Drainage tubes may cause a weak spot in the incision, and underlying tissue may protrude. Also, drains may provide an inlet for microorganisms as well as an outlet for drainage. When possible, drains are placed through a stab wound in the skin rather than through the surgical incision.

When sutures are used, the suture material provides all the strength of the wound immediately after closure. Closely spaced sutures give a stronger suture line. The strength of a suture should not be greater than the strength of the tissue in which it is placed. To minimize tissue reaction to sutures, the fewest and the smallest sutures consistent with the holding power of the tissues should be used. Inert surgical staples are used to approximate some tissues.

Immediately after closure, tissue along the incision is at about 40% of its original strength. It reaches its greatest strength in 7 to 15 days. The wound is about one-third healed on the sixth postoperative day and two-thirds healed on the eighth day. The condition of the patient, type of surgical procedure, and many other factors may cause variance from the norm. As tensile strength of the wound increases, reliance on other support for wound security gradually lessens.

Wound Management

Providing appropriate conditions for wound healing has been a quest through the ages. In ancient mythology the Greek god Hermes carried a staff entwined with two snakes. This signified the snake's ability to repeatedly shed and regenerate its skin. Although humans do not shed their skin, they can regenerate tissue cells if the wound is protected from accumulations of blood and serum, mechanical injury, impaired circulation, and infection.

DRAINS

The use of devices to drain fluids and pus from the body dates back to the writings of Hippocrates. He wrote of insertion of a hollow tin tube with flushings of wine and tepid oil to treat empyema. This was the first wound drainage system. In the nineteenth century, glass tubes, to be replaced by rubber catheters, were commonly used for gravity drainage. In 1897 Dr. Charles Penrose described a tubular drain made of gutta-percha, the coagulated latex from rubber trees, with a gauze wick inserted through length of the lumen. This latex drain, which still bears his name, is in use today to maintain a vent for the escape of fluid or air or to wall off an area of exudate in the wound. Sump drains, commercially introduced in 1932, offered advantages. Suction drainage has been used since 1947. Closed wound drainage systems, first introduced in 1952, are used to enhance wound healing.

Gravity drainage through various types of tubes vs. capillary drainage through wicking devices historically has been a controversial issue. Even today surgeons do not universally agree on the use of systems currently available. The location and purpose of the drain determine the surgeon's selection from the many types available. Drains may be used prophylactically or therapeutically during the surgical procedure and/or postoperatively.

Intraoperative Drainage

Used prophylactically to evacuate intestinal fluids or urine, intraoperative drainage also helps prevent tissue trauma and restores organs to normal function.

Gastrointestinal Decompression

A plastic or rubber nasogastric tube inserted through a nostril down into the stomach or small intestine removes flatus, fluids, or other contents. The tube has holes in several locations near the tip to permit withdrawal of the contents. Several types of nasogastric tubes are used; most common are the Levin tube into the stomach and the Miller-Abbott tube into the small intestine. A vented tube, such as the Salem sump tube, is preferable for use with nasogastric suction.

To prevent aspiration of stomach contents, the anesthesiologist may insert a nasogastric tube preoperatively to empty the stomach before an emergency surgical procedure. The surgeon may ask anesthesiologist to insert a tube during an intraabdominal procedure for one of the following purposes:

1. Decompression of gastrointestinal tract
2. Relief of distention that obstructs view of surgical site
3. Measurement of blood loss from gastric hemorrhage
4. Evacuation of gastric secretions during intestinal anastomosis

The nasogastric tube may remain in place postoperatively to prevent vomiting and distention caused by decreased peristalsis following anesthesia, manipulation of the viscera during the surgical procedure, or obstruction from edema of tissues at the surgical site. For this purpose the tube is connected to a suction apparatus. The tube also may be used for nasogastric feeding during the healing process after surgical procedure on the upper alimentary canal.

Urinary Drainage

Urethral or ureteral catheters inserted preoperatively provide constant drainage from the bladder or kidneys during the surgical procedure. The purpose may be to keep the bladder decompressed or to prevent extravasation of urine into the tissues around the surgical site during and after genitourinary procedures. Postoperatively the inflated balloon of an indwelling Foley catheter maintains an even pressure on the bladder neck, which may help control bleeding following prostatectomy, for example. An indwelling Foley catheter may be connected to a bladder-irrigation or gravity-drainage system until the bladder resumes normal function postoperatively.

Postoperative Drainage

Drains are used therapeutically in the presence of purulent or necrotic material. Prophylactically they may be inserted to evacuate fluids, including blood, or air from a wound or body cavity postoperatively. Drains are usually placed in a separate small stab wound adjacent to the surgical incision and secured with a nonabsorbable monofilament suture. Drains can stimulate a walling-off process around a surgical site in which subsequent drainage may accumulate. This enhances wound healing by:

1. Eliminating fluid accumulation
2. Obliterating dead spaces
3. Allowing apposition of tissues
4. Preventing formation of hematomas or seromas
5. Preventing tissue devitalization or wound margin necrosis
6. Minimizing a potential source of wound contamination
7. Decreasing postoperative pain
8. Minimizing scarring

The action of drains may be either passive or active.

Passive Drains

Passive drains provide the path of least resistance to the outside. They function by overflow and capillary action through the drain to the absorbent dressing. They are influenced by pressure differentials and may be assisted by gravity.

Penrose Drain A Penrose drain is a thin-walled cylinder of radiopaque latex. The diameter may be ¼ to 2 inches (6 mm to 5 cm), depending on the surgeon's preference. The drain is usually supplied to the sterile field in a 6- to 12-inch (15 to 30 cm) length for the surgeon to cut as desired. Penrose drains are commercially available prepackaged and sterilized. However, if they are prepared for on-site steam sterilization, a gauze wick must be inserted to permit steam penetration of the lumen.

Although Penrose drains are usually used without a wick, the surgeon may prefer the wick of gauze packing left in the lumen to absorb drainage from the wound. This is referred to as a *cigarette drain.* For use without a wick, moisten drain in normal saline solution before handing it to the surgeon. After it is placed into the surgical area and brought out through a stab wound in the skin, the drain is secured with a skin suture, or a sterile safety pin is attached on the outside close to the skin to keep drain from retracting into the wound. The head of the safety pin should be crimped closed with a large forceps to prevent it from opening and piercing the patient.

Constant Gravity Drainage A drain may be inserted for drainage by gravity flow from the gallbladder, bladder, or kidney. Each OR suite has a supply of sterile rubber and/or silicone tubes and catheters. Those used for drains, such as a T-tube, should be radiopaque. Some have inflatable balloons or enlarged bulbous ends (mushroom, malecot, pezzer) to help hold them in place.

A closed or semiclosed system is used to collect drainage. The scrub person keeps end of the tube or catheter sterile until it is connected to sterile end of the constant drainage tubing. Tubing should be connected or clamped as soon as the drain is brought through a stab wound in the skin or a tube or catheter is inserted into an organ. The circulator connects tubing to a drainage bag. Constant drainage bags are marked in gradations from 500 to 2000 ml. The bag must be in a dependent position, lower than site of the drain, to avoid retrograde reflux.

Active Drains

Active drains are attached to an external source of vacuum to create suction in the wound. A constant, gentle, negative-pressure vacuum evacuates tissue fluid, blood, and air through a silicone, polyvinyl chloride, or polyurethane drain. Suction levels vary, depending on the system, to create the negative pressure (less than atmospheric).

Closed Wound Suction Systems These systems are used when it is necessary to apply suction to an uninfected closed wound site in chest wall, as after mastectomy, in upper part of the abdomen, and in areas of joint replacement. They also are placed under large tissue flaps or in subcutaneous spaces in obese patients to eliminate dead space and to hold tissues in apposition.

The sterile plastic drain with tubing connected to a stainless steel trocar is placed in the surgical area. The trocar makes a small stab wound in the skin as it is brought through the underlying tissues. The drain, either round or flat, has several perforations along the length placed in tissues. It also is radiopaque or has radiopaque markings to aid in checking its location on x-ray film, if desired. The tubing is connected to a sterile, self-contained portable container. Several different units are available with containers of different capacities as well as sizes of tubings. Calibrations on side of container measure the drainage, and a line designates when it should be emptied or changed. These units are made entirely or partially of clear plastic so the surgeon can inspect drainage.

The drainage container can be attached immediately after placement of the tubing or after wound closure; then the vacuum is activated. Directions printed on each unit must be followed to activate the vacuum. The amount of suction in these systems varies depending on the method of creating the vacuum. Manually activated spring-loaded devices (Hemovac) and grenade-type or bulb evacuators (ReliaVac, Jackson Pratt) have variable preset suction levels between 30 and 125 mm Hg. A portable battery-powered device (VariDyne) can provide a constant and continuous vacuum at any setting between 10 and 350 mm Hg. With the latter system, the surgeon can determine the suction level on the basis of the material and area to be evacuated. The drainage container does not need to be in a dependent position with closed wound suction systems. An antireflux valve guards against backflow of fluids.

Sump Drains Sump drains may be used for aspiration, irrigation, or introduction of medication. Either flat or round, a sump drain has a double or triple lumen. Usually made of radiopaque silicone, it has large lateral openings to minimize clogging. The drain is brought out through a separate stab wound. Sump drains create equalized negative pressure at the site to be drained, usually in the abdomen. They are connected to a constant drainage system, with or without suction. Irrigation of the surgical site and connection to suction as soon as possible enhance function. Levels of suction between 80 and 120 mm Hg are desirable. The tubing may be attached to a piped-in (wall) or portable vacuum system. The drain must be clamped when not attached to suction or connected to a closed container. It functions as a passive drain if suction is not used and must be in a dependent position.

Chest Drainage Drainage of the pleural cavity ensures complete expansion of lungs postoperatively. Air and fluid *must* be evacuated from pleural space following surgical procedures within the chest cavity. One or more chest tubes are inserted. If the surgeon inserts two, the upper tube evacuates air and the lower drains fluid. After the chest tube is inserted during closure, the end is covered with a sterile gauze until it can be connected to a sterile closed water-seal drainage system. The drainage system must prevent outside air from being drawn into the pleural space during expiration. Water in the collection unit seals off outside air to maintain a negative pressure within the pleural cavity.

Two tubes vent the leakproof top of the collection unit. A short air-outlet tube extends 1 inch (2.5 cm) or more above the stopper to about 3 inches (7.5 cm) below it into the collection unit. The long inlet tube extends from above the stopper, through it, to about 1 inch (2.5 cm) from the bottom of the collection unit. Sterile water is poured into the collection unit to a level 1 to 2 inches (2.5 to 5 cm) above end of the long inlet tube. The circulator marks water level on outside of the collection unit. Clear sterile tubing connects the inlet tube to the tube placed into pleural space. Upon the patient's initial expiration, water rises a short distance up into the inlet tube. With each subsequent inspiration-expiration the water level in the tube fluctuates. If the water level in the tube remains stationary, the chest tube or connecting tubing may be clogged or kinked. *The collection unit must be kept well below chest level to prevent water from entering the chest and to keep the tubing free of kinks.*

Fluid drains by gravity from the chest into the water. The collection unit should be calibrated so that drainage can be measured. Air bubbles through the water and escapes through the outlet tube.

If gravity drainage is not adequate for reexpansion of the lungs, suction may be applied at 15 to 20 cm water pressure to ensure evacuation of air and fluid. This requires the addition of one or two collection units to the system, to act as a pressure regulator, and a suction machine to maintain negative pressure. Disposable chest-drainage units are available commercially, as a single unit or in a series of two or three. Some units have modifications based on the principle described for a closed water-seal system. Follow the manufacturer's direction for use. Be sure the unit is properly connected before the patient leaves the OR.

With some units the chest tube may be clamped during transportation as a safety measure. Check with the surgeon as to whether or not clamping is contraindicated.

Nursing Considerations

Drains, tubes, catheters, drainage tubing, and adapters are used for one patient only; they are never reused for another patient. Aside from aesthetic reasons, the wall absorbs irritating chemicals from the patient's tissues that cause an irritation in the next patient even though it is thoroughly cleaned and sterilized. If not properly handled by the scrub person and circulator, a drain can be a source of wound contamination or irritation. When the surgeon inserts a drain, several considerations should be kept in mind.

1. Drains, tubes, and catheters are kept sterile, ready for the circulator to open if needed. They are available in many styles and sizes. They are usu-

ally patient charge items. Do not open until the surgeon specifies style and size.

2. If patient has a sensitivity to latex, do not use a drain, tube, or catheter made of latex, either entirely or partially.
3. Scrub person keeps end of drain sterile until it is connected to sterile end of drainage tubing. A sterile gauze held with a sterile rubber band may be used.
4. Tubing connections must be physically tight and secured. Do not completely obscure connections by wrapping tape around them.
5. If end of either drain or connecting tubing becomes contaminated inadvertently, wipe the drain off with an alcohol sponge and obtain another sterile drainage tubing.
6. Drain site is dressed separately from the incision site. A nonadherent dressing can be used as the contact layer around drain. Gauze dressings can be slit in a Y shape to fit around the drain.
7. Avoid tension on drain and kinks in drain and tubing. A gentle loop can be made and secured at the time of dressing application.
8. Collection bags or containers connected to passive drains, including chest tubes, must be kept well below level of the body cavity where the drain is inserted and below level of drainage tubing to prevent retrograde flow. Drainage tubing should be positioned so the downward flow is aided by force of gravity.
9. Circulator must check suction level to be certain it is consistent with the surgeon's orders or should activate the suction as appropriate for system being used.
10. X-ray film may be taken to verify placement of the drain or tube.
11. Circulator documents on the intraoperative record the type of drain and its location.

DRESSINGS

Nearly all skin incisions and surgical wounds are covered with a sterile dressing for at least 24 to 48 hours to provide an optimal physiologic environment for wound healing. The dressing serves several functions:

1. To keep incision free of microorganisms, both exogenous and endogenous
2. To protect incision from outside injury, especially in children
3. To absorb the drainage of exudates and secretions from the wound
4. To maintain a moist environment that permits host defense mechanisms to destroy bacteria but prevents destruction of newly formed epithelial cells from dehydration and permits removal without disruption of these cells
5. To give some support to incision and surrounding skin or to immobilize surrounding tissue
6. To provide pressure to reduce edema or to prevent hematoma
7. To conceal the wound aesthetically

A dressing's function is determined by its structure. The overall dressing should be:

1. Large enough to cover and protect the wound site and tissue around it
2. Permeable to gas and vapor, allowing circulation of air to skin
3. Secure to prevent slippage
4. Comfortable for the patient

Types of Dressings

In considering the components to assemble for the dressing, keep in mind the needs of the particular wound. One wound may require a dressing that provides a function different than that needed for another type of wound. The dressing materials should be tailored to location and condition of the wound site.

One-Layer Dressing

A clean incision that is primarily closed with sutures, staples, or skin closure tapes in which no or slight drainage is expected may be covered with an adhering occlusive dressing (such as Bioclusive or Op-Site). These sterile, transparent polyurethane film dressings are available in various sizes. The patient can bathe or shower with these in place. They usually are removed in 24 to 48 hours. Liquid collodion or an aerosol adhesive spray may be used.

Skin Closure Dressing

A transparent plastic film with an adhesive backing (Op-Site) can be placed over the entire length of the incision to hold skin edges in apposition. The film is vented to allow the escape of exudate. An additional wound dressing may be overlaid to further splint and reinforce coaptation of skin edges. These dressings are available in various sizes.

Dry Sterile Dressing

A single or multilayered dressing is applied dry over a clean incision from which no or slight drainage is expected. Dry gauze is not used on a denuded area because it adheres and acts as a foreign body. Granulation tissue will grow into it; bleeding can be reactivated when it is removed. A dry sterile dressing can be applied over a dry wound. It is secured with adhesive tape. A circumferential wrap may be preferred on an extremity, but it must not compromise circulation.

Three-Layer Dressing

When moderate to heavy drainage is expected, a complete dressing consists of at least three layers.

Contact Layer This layer acts as a passageway for the secretion and exudates that emanate from a draining wound. It has a wicking action to help reduce the risk of infection and skin maceration. It must conform to body contours regardless of the site and extent of the wound and must stay in intimate contact with the wound surface for at least 48 hours, yet be nonadherent for painless removal. The contact layer may be:

1. *Nonocclusive.* Nonadherent materials, such as gauze sponges or compressed material on a thin plastic or aluminum film, draw secretions from the wound but remain air permeable. The looser the weave of the material, the more nonocclusive it is.
2. *Semiocclusive.* Hydroactive materials, such as foams, hydrogels, and hydrocolloids, provide a mechanical surface with permeability properties. Some of these agents actually help debride the wound.
3. *Occlusive.* An airtight seal prevents drying of the wound. The dressing is impermeable to air and water but allows passage of exudates. This is usually a fine mesh gauze dressing impregnated with an oil emulsion, such as petrolatum, xeroform, iodophor, antibiotic ointment, or scarlet red. It is nonadherent to skin or wound.

Intermediate Layer This layer absorbs secretions passing through the contact layer. To provide adequate capacity, it should be layered (e.g., with gauze sponges) to the thickness required by the particular wound. It should not be excessively bulky. It must not unnecessarily apply pressure that could compromise circulation.

Outer Layer This layer holds the contact and intermediate layers in proper position. It should be conforming, stretchable to avoid constriction if edema develops, and capable of clinging to itself so it will stay in position without telescoping if mobility is desired. Several materials are used for this purpose.

1. *Adhesive tape* is used most frequently.
2. *Elastic bandage* provides gentle, even pressure to hold bulky dressings in place or to bind a splint onto an extremity. It stretches to conform to body contours, does not constrict, yet gives firm support. The types available include:
   a. Four-ply crinkled-gauze bandage
   b. Cotton-elastic bandage
   c. Cotton-elastic bandage with adhesive on one side, which is especially useful in holding dressings on the chest, because it is firm yet permits chest expansion
3. *Montgomery straps* are used to hold bulky dressings that require frequent changes or wound inspections. These are pairs of adhesive straps in assorted widths with strings attached to one folded end of each strap. The other end of each strap is secured to the skin on each side of the dressing. The strings are tied across the dressing to hold it in place, usually on the abdomen.
4. *Stockinette* is put over the dressing on an extremity before application of a rigid cast used for immobilization. Available in several widths, stockinette is a seamless tubing of stretchable knitted cotton.

Pressure Dressing

Bulky dressings are added to the intermediate layer of a three-layer dressing following many extensive surgical procedures, especially in plastic surgery and surgical procedures on the knee or breast. Pressure dressings are used to:

1. Eliminate dead space and prevent edema or hematoma
2. Distribute pressure evenly
3. Absorb extensive drainage
4. Encourage wound healing and minimize scarring by influencing wound tension
5. Immobilize a body area or support soft tissues when muscles are moved
6. Help provide comfort to the patient postoperatively

Materials used for pressure dressings include:

1. Fluffed gauze
2. Combine pads, which are gauze-covered absorbent cellulose
3. Single-piece bulk dressings, which are available for use on the trunk and extremities and save time in application
4. Cotton rolls, which are used to apply pressure on each side of a knee following a surgical procedure on this joint, for example
5. Foam rubber

Stent Dressing

Stent fixation is a method of applying pressure and stabilizing tissues when it is impossible to dress an area, such as the face or neck. A form-fitting mold may be taped over the nose. Long suture ends can be crisscrossed over a small dressing and tied.

Bolster/Tie-Over Dressing

Dressing materials may be sutured in place to exert an even pressure over autografted wounds to prevent hematoma or seroma formation. Sterile gauze may be rolled into a tubular shape and tied with the ends of the wound closure suture.

Wet-to-Dry Dressing

Dressing materials soaked in sterile normal saline solution are applied to the wound and allowed to dry thoroughly. The dried dressing is then removed, taking adhering tissue layers with it. This process is used to facilitate new tissue growth and is commonly used on burn wounds. This method of debridement is extremely painful, so it is frequently performed in the OR with the patient under general anesthesia.

Wet-to-Wet Dressing

Dressing materials are soaked in sterile normal saline solution or other medicated solution and applied wet. This method provides little mechanical debridement and is less painful for the patient. The dressing material may be changed in the OR or under sterile conditions on the nursing unit.

Application of Dressings

Applying sterile dressings is regarded as part of the surgical procedure. The scrub person and circulator assist the surgeon or first assistant in dressing the wound properly.

1. Circulator opens sterile dressings *after* the final sponge count is completed. Radiopaque sponges are *not* used because they could distort a postoperative x-ray film or cause an incorrect count if the patient's incision must be reopened.
2. Skin surrounding the incision is cleaned of blood with a damp sponge.
3. Surgeon, first assistant, or scrub person should don a clean pair of sterile gloves before applying contact and intermediate layers of dressing or an occlusive film.
4. Incision and wound drainage sites are dressed separately unless the drain comes out through the incision. The scrub person cuts a slit in dressings to go around the drain.
5. Sterile dressings are applied before drapes are removed.
6. Circulator may spray benzoin on the skin around the intermediate layer before adhesive tape is applied to increase its adhesion, if desired by the surgeon.
7. Circulator applies tape or Montgomery straps firmly but not tightly to avoid wrinkling and traction on skin. Traction and wrinkling, rather than sensitivity to the tape, may cause skin irritation.

   NOTE If a patient has a known sensitivity to regular adhesive tape, hypoallergenic tape should be used. It is lightweight, yet strong, sticks well, is porous, and allows skin to breathe.

8. Surgeon or first assistant applies elastic bandages, pressure dressings, stockinette and casts, and stents. The circulator provides the necessary supplies and assists as appropriate. A nursing assistant may help hold the patient's torso or an extremity during application of an elastic bandage or cast.

COMPLICATIONS OF WOUND HEALING

The surgeon gives meticulous attention to sterile technique, hemostasis, tissue handling and approximation, and selection of wound closure materials, including drains and dressings. The entire OR team carries out strict aseptic and sterile techniques to prevent infection and other possible complications of wound healing.

Scar/Surgical Cicatrix

Following the natural process of wound healing, a scar (cicatrix) will remain on the skin surface. To achieve a cosmetically acceptable scar, the surgeon attempts to make the surgical incision along natural creases or within natural skin folds or hairlines. The location and direction of the incision affect scarring. Tension needed for approximation of wound edges during closure and subsequent movement of underlying tissues can affect wound healing and scar formation. Wounds in mobile skin will contract, resulting in a smaller scar.

Hypertrophic scars, which are the result of excessive fibrin formation within the borders of the scar, can develop from too much tension on the wound, poor approximation of wound edges, or infection. Some suture materials may contribute to hypertrophy. Burn wounds are conducive to excessive scarring also. The patient may wish to have an unsightly scar revised at a future time.

Keloids develop when the inflammatory response and fibroblast proliferation are overactive during wound healing. This is an inherited trait, most common among Africans, Asians, and people with dark skin tones or those who freckle. Keloids extend beyond the borders of the scar and can continue to grow and become very large over a prolonged period after the surgical procedure. They may be painful, itchy, and prone to bleeding. They can be excised, leaving a small border of scar tissue. The edges are approximated using skin staples or fine monofilament nonabsorbable suture. If a patient is known to form keloids, an antiinflammatory agent may be injected into tissue before closure. A pressure dressing is useful in prevention of keloid formation.

Nodules and *granulomas* may form in the scar if excess suture material is used. Scar tissue hypertrophies around the suture, in particular the knot. Some patients will extrude suture pieces through their incision line for several months or years postoperatively. This may represent a sensitivity to the suture material.

Adhesions

An adhesion holds or unites two surfaces or structures that normally are separate. Fibrous bands that develop in the peritoneal cavity can hold viscera together, sometimes causing bowel obstruction. The most common cause is previous abdominal or pelvic surgery, but acute appendicitis or peritonitis can cause adhesion formation. Serosal injury caused by abrasion from sponges or gloves, tissue handling, or tissue ischemia may be precipitating factors. Granulomas that form from powder on gloves, lint on sponges, or other foreign material left in the wound also predispose the patient to adhesion formation.

Wound Disruption

Failure of a wound to heal or closure material to secure it during the healing process leads to wound disruption, a separation of wound edges. Disruption usually occurs between the fifth and tenth postoperative day. This is the lag period in healing, the time when the wound is not yet strong. Wound disruption is caused not by a single factor but by a combination of predisposing factors that influence healing.

Although it may occur in any body area, acute wound disruption most frequently follows abdominal laparotomy, surgical incision into the peritoneal cavity. It starts with a small opening in the peritoneum, which allows a wedge of omentum to slip through it. This omentum becomes edematous and extends the opening along the line of incision and upward through other layers of the abdominal wall. Disruption is usually precipitated by distention or a sudden strain, such as vomiting, coughing, or sneezing. Terms used to describe abdominal wound disruption include:

1. *Dehiscence.* Partial or total splitting open or separation of layers of the wound. "Cutting out" of sutures is the most important cause of dehiscence. Strength of tissues and extent of separation determine whether or not the wound must be reclosed.
2. *Evisceration.* Protrusion of viscera through the abdominal incision. Although wound disruption of any degree calls for emergency care, *an evisceration is a catastrophe requiring immediate replacement of viscera and reclosure of the incision.*

Prevention

Factors that may contribute to wound disruption are eliminated to the extent possible preoperatively.

1. Malnutrition and vitamin deficiency are corrected.
2. Obesity is reduced.
3. Anemia is corrected.
4. Surgical procedure is postponed, if possible, if patient has a transient illness, such as cold or influenza.
5. Antibiotics may be given prophylactically. Although antibiotics cannot supplant sterile technique, some can render the surgical field more free of microorganisms than it normally would be, such as in a surgical procedure on the gastrointestinal tract.
6. Patient is taught to breathe deeply and cough without force.

Symptoms

Patients who subsequently experience wound disruption often do not have a smooth course immediately after surgery. They may have undue pain, discomfort, nausea, drainage, slight fever, vomiting, or hiccups. Acute symptoms of wound disruption include:

1. Tachycardia.
2. Vomiting.
3. Abnormal serosanguineous discharge.
4. Change in contour of the wound.
5. Sudden pulling pain during straining. The patient feels something give. Suspect any seepage of serosanguineous fluid after a sudden sharp pain that lasts only momentarily after an effort. Send some of this fluid for culture and sensitivity.

Any of these symptoms should be investigated at once. Examination of the wound may show it gaping somewhat, or viscera may appear at the skin surface.

Treatment at Bedside

1. Place an emergency call for the surgeon. Have a nasogastric tube ready for insertion to relieve distention.
2. Reassure the patient.
3. Apply sterile, moist saline dressings over the wound and a loose binder.
4. Give drugs according to the surgeon's order.
5. Do not give the patient anything by mouth.
6. Prepare the patient for return to the OR. Treatment in the OR consists of secondary wound closure.

Wound Infections

Wound healing can be interrupted by infection at almost any phase. Infection results from introduction of virulent microorganisms into the receptive wound of a susceptible host. Moisture and warmth in the wound create an environment conducive to bacterial growth. Wound infections warrant special attention because many occur in clean wounds as a result of microorganisms introduced at time of the surgical procedure. Secondary contamination is uncommon because fibrin seals the wound within hours after surgical procedure.

INFECTION

The worldwide problem of infection persists to plague patients and physicians alike. Infection is a health hazard of great expense and significance, affecting the final outcome of surgical treatment. The quality of life, both physical and psychologic, can be drastically altered, sometimes permanently, by infection and the associated "d's": *delayed healing, discomfort, distress, dependency,* and *dollars.* Not infrequently, *disability, deformity,* and *disaster* with ultimate *death* are the result of infection.

Clinically, infection is the product of the entrance, growth, metabolic activities, and pathophysiologic effects of microorganisms in living tissue. It can develop in the surgical patient as a preoperative complication following an injury or as a postoperative complication of cross contamination or cross infection.

Process of Infection

Sepsis involves three stages: invasion, localization, and resolution leading to recovery. However, the progress toward recovery may revert to extension of the infection. The characteristics, invasive qualities, and sources of the etiologic microorganism are important in prevention and treatment. Prompt identification of the infecting organism and sensitivity testing are essential so that appropriate antibiotic therapy can be instituted.

Acute bacterial infection is the most common sepsis in surgical patients. A wound infection usually begins between the fourth and eighth postoperative day. Infection usually develops as a diffuse, inflammatory process, known as *cellulitis,* characterized by pain, redness, and swelling. This inflammatory response is the body's initial defense directed toward localization and containment of the infecting organism. Red blood cells, leukocytes, and macrophages infiltrate the cells, with abscess formation (suppuration) often following. An *abscess* is the result of tissue liquefaction with pus formation, supported by bacterial proteolytic enzymes that break down protein and aid in the spread of infection. Fibrolysin, for example, an enzyme produced by hemolytic streptococcus, may dissolve fibrin and delay localization of a streptococcal infection. However, the body attempts to wall off an abscess by means of a membrane that produces surrounding induration (hardened tissue) and heat. Localized pus should be drained promptly.

If localization is inadequate and does not contain the infectious process, spreading and extension occur, causing regional infection. Microorganisms and their metabolic products are carried from the primary invasion site into the lymphatic system, spreading along anatomic planes, causing lymphangitis. Failure of the lymph nodes to hold the infection results in uncontrolled cellulitis. Subsequently, regional and/or systemic infection may develop, characterized by chills, fever, and signs of toxicity. Septic emboli may enter the circulatory system from septic thrombophlebitis of regional veins communicating with local infections. These emboli and pathogenic microorganisms in the blood seed invasive infection and abscess formation in remote tissues.

Sepsis elevates the patient's metabolic rate 30% to 40% above average, imposing additional stress on the vital systems. For example, cardiac output is about 60% above normal resting value. The body's defenses and ability to meet the stress govern whether the infectious process progresses to septic shock (see following discussion) with grave prognosis or whether resolution and recovery are the outcome. Multiple infection sites, the presence of shock, and inappropriate antibiotic therapy result in poor prognosis.

The ultimate resolution of infection depends on immunologic and inflammatory responses capable of overcoming the infectious process. This is associated with drainage and removal of foreign material, including debris of bacteria and cells, lysis (disintegration) of microorganisms, resorption of pus, and sloughing of necrotic tissue. Healing then ensues.

Septic Shock

Septic shock is a state of widely disseminated infection, often borne in the bloodstream (i.e., septicemia). Early septic shock may begin with fever, restlessness, sudden unexplained hypotension, a cloudy sensorium, hypoxia, tachycardia, rapid breathing, and/or oliguria. One or more of these symptoms may be present. Toxic or metabolic by-products increase capillary permeability, permitting loss of circulating fluid into the interstitial fluid. Endotoxins released by bacteria promote vasodilation and hypotension.

Septic shock is most frequently produced by gram-negative bacteria. As shock progresses, the patient develops cold clammy skin, sharply diminished urinary output, respiratory insufficiency, cardiac decompensation, disseminated intravascular coagulation, and metabolic acidosis. The high-risk category comprises patients with severe infection (e.g., peritonitis), trauma, burns, impaired immunologic state, diabetes mellitus, age-extreme patients, or patients who have undergone an extensive invasive procedure.

Treatment consists of control of the infectious process, early administration of antibiotics, fluid-volume replacement, and oxygen. Diuretics, sodium bicarbonate, vasoconstrictors, vasodilators, inotropic agents, or heparin may also be indicated. Corticosteroids may be used, but their use is controversial. A monoclonal antibody may be administered to reduce endotoxins.

CLASSIFICATION OF INFECTIONS

Surgical infections may be classified by source, by clinical factors including pathophysiology, anatomic location, and microbial etiology.

Sources

Incidence and types of infections that occur in surgical patients may be the result of a preexisting localized infectious process, a systemic communicable disease, or an acquired preoperative or postoperative complication.

Community-Acquired Infections

Community-acquired infections are natural disease processes that developed or were incubating before a patient's admission to the hospital or ambulatory care facility.

Communicable Diseases Systemic bacterial, viral, or fungal infections may be transmitted from one person to another. Tuberculosis, hepatitis, human immunodeficiency virus (HIV), and others of major concern are discussed in Chapter 12, pp. 190-194.

Spontaneous Infections Localized infections requiring surgical diagnosis and/or treatment for management, or that occur as adjuvants to medical therapy, include acute appendicitis, cholecystitis, or bowel perforation with peritonitis. Therapy consists of identification of the infection site and causative microorganism, excision or drainage, prevention of further contamination, and augmentation of host resistance.

Nosocomial Infections

Infections that were not present or incubating when the patient was admitted are hospital-associated or acquired (i.e., nosocomial) during the course of health care.

Exogenous An exogenous nosocomial infection is acquired from sources outside the body, such as personnel or environment. These sources are discussed in detail in Chapter 12. Cross contamination occurs when organisms are transferred to the patient from another individual or inanimate object.

Endogenous An endogenous infection develops from sources within the body. Most postoperative wound infections result from seeding by endogenous microorganisms. Disruption of the balance between potentially pathogenic organisms and host defenses permits invasion of microorganisms for which the patient is the primary reservoir. For example, abdominal sepsis may result from enteric flora if the intestine is perforated or transected.

Nosocomial infections may occur as complications of surgical or other procedures performed on uninfected patients. The term also refers to complicating infections in organs unrelated to the surgical procedure, occurring with or as a result of postoperative care. About 35% of all nosocomial infections develop in surgical patients. The majority are related to instrumentation of the urinary and respiratory tracts. Wound infection is the second most common infection. Examples of nosocomial infections are:

1. Urinary tract or respiratory tract infection, infected decubiti
2. Cellulitis or abscess formation related to the surgical procedure, such as intraabdominal abscess following gastrointestinal procedure
3. Thrombophlebitis or peritonitis, regional extensions of postoperative or posttraumatic infections
4. Liver, lung, or visceral abscess following surgical procedure often performed for penetrating injuries or malignant metastases
5. Bacteremia or septicemia, postoperative systemic infection resulting from dissemination of microorganisms into the bloodstream from a distributing focus

Clinical Factors Contributing to Infection

Infection results from the interaction of three elements: organisms, tissues, and host defenses. Stated as an equation, infection equals number of organisms multiplied by virulence and divided by host resistance. Surgery reduces resistance.

Pathogenic Microorganisms

Pathogens must be introduced or already present, then survive and propagate in the wound or other body tissue. Severity of infection depends in part on the size and virulence of inoculum (microbe-containing substance). The infecting organism must reach the host.

Local Factors

Location of surgical site and condition of tissues therein are significant. Necrotic, devitalized avascular tissue or the presence of foreign bodies or accumulated blood enhances infection by providing excellent media for microbial growth. Various body tissues have different powers of resistance. The abdomen, thigh, calf, and buttocks are especially susceptible. The face, scalp, and chest are more resistant. Severe traumatic injuries and debilitating chronic diseases can make all tissues susceptible to infection. Surgical wounds may be:

1. *Uninfected:* heal without discharge
2. *Possibly infected:* inflamed, with no discharge or culture-positive serous fluid
3. *Infected:* suppuration with purulent drainage

Host Defense Mechanisms

The biologic relationships between host defense, trauma of the surgical procedure, and antibiotic therapy are complex. Body responses vary with the type of infecting microorganism, immune response of the patient, severity of infection, and effectiveness of treatment. The general health of the patient influences resistance to microbial invasion.

Adjuvant Factors

Many factors substantially increase the risk of infection. Those associated with the physical condition of the patient are discussed on pp. 523-525 in terms of how they correlate with wound healing. Other factors include:

1. Duration of preoperative hospitalization. Some organisms maintain virulence by passing from patient to patient. The hospital environment is a concentrated reservoir of microorganisms that can colonize in patients, especially those who have received antibiotics. The organisms are rapidly and easily transferred between people and equipment. A noncarrier may become a carrier of an organism that eventually causes an infection of endogenous origin. Studies have shown that the risk of nosocomial infection increases with the length of hospitalization. Same-day admissions and procedures eliminate preoperative hospitalization.
2. Contamination in the surgical wound. Traumatic injuries, such as compound fractures, stab wounds, skin lacerations or abrasions, and burns, quickly colonize with microbial contaminants. Razor cuts and nicks made in the skin during shaving and wet drapes can be sources of contamination around the surgical site.
3. Surgical procedures that involve the genitourinary or gastrointestinal tracts. Some contamination occurs whenever these tracts are opened. The extent of contamination during the surgical procedure is an important factor.
4. Duration of the surgical procedure. The longer the procedure, the greater the chance of contamination and infection. The amount of talking in the OR contributes to airborne inocula.
5. Surgical technique. Injured ischemic tissues, denuded bone, implanted foreign bodies or prosthetic devices have a propensity for microbial invasion. A wound heals faster if tissues are gently handled because fewer cells are destroyed. Necrotic tissue, as from electrosurgery, is microbial media. All invasive techniques are potential contaminants.
6. Intravascular devices. Microorganisms can be introduced into the bloodstream through intravenous infusion and hemodynamic monitoring lines and through intravascular catheters used for diagnostic and therapeutic procedures.
7. Catheters and drains. Closed drainage systems are preferred to minimize microbial migration.
8. Indiscriminate use of antibiotics (see pp. 539-540). Suppression of normal flora of the skin, bowel, and pharynx, which may play a protective role in the defense against pathogenic organisms, may predispose the patient to infection. Antibiotics suppress normal flora.
9. Noncompliance with universal precautions and isolation procedures (see Chapter 12). This may be caused by lack of knowledge of epidemiology on the part of personnel.

In summary, many factors influence the incidence of infection. Exposure of acutely ill patients to the hospital environment, inhabited by virulent antibiotic-resistant organisms, contributes to infection. Many high-risk patients undergo complex and/or prolonged diagnostic and surgical procedures under anesthesia. The accompanying instrumentation and use of medical devices open many portals for microbial entry. Complex therapeutic or supportive procedures, such as invasive monitoring, hyperalimentation, and assisted ventilation, provide microorganisms potential avenues for migration. Continuous urinary catheterization increases the prevalence of urinary tract infection. The concomitant administration of drugs that reduce bodily resistance is a significant factor that favors development of nosocomial infection.

INFECTION CONTROL

Infection control translates knowledge into action. It incorporates the development and maintenance of an attitude of awareness of infection with acceptance of individual and collective responsibility to prevent infection. Although the scope of infection control encompasses the entire hospital, this text focuses on infection control in the surgical patient, primarily control of wound infection that can obviate the benefits of surgical intervention. Infection control concerns keeping number of microorganisms to an irreducible minimum.

The purposes of infection control are to:

1. Minimize infection and eventually to obliterate it
2. Improve wound healing
3. Minimize disability, morbidity, and mortality
4. Reduce the cost of health care

The many aspects of infection control include:

1. Establishment and use of an effective infection control program
2. Recognition of hazards and consistent adherence to established control practices
3. Provision of maximum protection to patients by means of physical barriers to microorganisms and functional measures of control
4. Appropriate use of antibiotic therapy, which includes limiting the use of antibiotics to reduce the development of resistant strains of microorganisms

Infection Control Program

An effective infection control program aims to reduce the incidence of infections and to control sources. Information collected through surveillance serves as a basis for corrective action. This information includes written records and reports of known or potential infections among patients and personnel.

Guidelines and standards for infection control and surveillance are published by the Joint Commission on the Accreditation of Healthcare Organizations in the *Accreditation Manual for Hospitals.* In general, these standards and guidelines include:

1. Establishment of an effective hospitalwide program for surveillance, prevention, and control of infection
2. Establishment of a multidisciplinary committee to oversee the program by reviewing surveillance reports and by approving policies, procedures, and actions to prevent and control infection
3. Assignment of a qualified person(s) to be responsible for management of the infection surveillance, prevention, and control program
4. Provision of written policies and procedures pertinent to infection surveillance, prevention, and control for all patient care departments and supporting services
5. Provision of patient care support services that are adequately prepared to perform all required infection surveillance, prevention, and control functions

Infection Control Coordinator

An infection surveillance, prevention, and control program uses the services of a key person and agent of the infection control committee, the *infection control coordinator.* Because this person is often a registered nurse with special training in epidemiology, microbiology, statistics, and research methodology, he or she may be called an *infection control nurse (ICN)* or *nurse epidemiologist.* The infection control coordinator monitors the environment for infections. The ICN works in close collaboration with the infection control committee. The ICN's duties are:

1. Prompt investigation of outbreaks of disease or infection above expected levels.
2. Prompt identification of origin and cause of outbreaks by epidemiologic study.
3. Acquisition, correlation, analysis, and evaluation of surveillance data and bacterial colony counts. This includes gathering information to compute and classify specific wound infection rates for all invasive procedures. Rates should be entered in the infection control committee record and be available to the department of surgery.
4. Tracking factors that contribute to infection problems.
5. Consultation with directors of critical areas, such as the OR. If an outbreak of postoperative infections occurs, the ICN confers with the OR nurse manager. They review the patients' intraoperative records to determine if the infected patients had the same procedure, same surgical team, or were operated on in the same room. They review antiseptic agents used for skin preparation, antibiotics used for wound irrigation, and other commonalities in patient care. If a patient develops signs and symptoms of infection within the immediate postoperative period, a causative factor in the OR is suspect.
6. Coordination of educational programs for personnel who influence infection control. The ICN is a consultant to all hospital personnel and a liaison officer in dissemination of information on infection control.
7. Assistance in employee health programs in regard to screening, immunizing, and monitoring personal health of personnel.
8. Assistance in development and implementation of improved patient care procedures.
9. Comparison of monthly statistics. There is cause for concern if the monthly reported surgical wound infection rate rises significantly. Reports and data can be helpful in evaluating aseptic practices, if brought to the attention of personnel.
10. Reporting appropriate diseases to public health authorities.
11. Comparison of products for effectiveness. The infection control committee approves disinfectants and antiseptics, for example, based on recommendations of the coordinator.
12. Obtaining information from surgeons about evidence of infection after discharge and conducting retrospective studies for statistical analysis.

In short, the infection control coordinator identifies problems, collects data to find the causes, investigates solutions, and makes recommendations for appropriate hospital policies and procedures to prevent infections. In evaluating infection problems, the ICN attempts to find a common denominator. This often leads to the source of the problem. For example, an outbreak of postoperative respiratory infections would lead to investigation of the cleaning and sterilizing of anesthesia equipment and respirators. Success of the control program depends in part on the information provided by a conscientious staff, including physicians.

Surveillance

The Centers for Disease Control and Prevention (CDC), an agency of the Department of Health and Human Services, is the third largest section of the U. S. Public Health Service. Functioning on both national and international levels, its activities are multifaceted. It carries out a national surveillance of disease incidence and a program, including health education, in prevention of communicable diseases. Through liaison with state and local health departments, the CDC provides assistance and consultation to health care facilities for specific problem solving, analysis of surveillance data, or on-site investigation of a serious outbreak of infections. As part of its commitment to the prevention of nosocomial infections, the CDC furnishes information on how to structure an infection control program.

The CDC sponsors training courses for nurses who wish to work in infection control. Follow-up support is given to trainees in their subsequent work situations, if needed. CDC also is a valuable worldwide resource for information through its many publications. In conjunction with continuous research, CDC establishes guidelines for the prevention of surgical wound infections, control of nosocomial infections, and prevention of transmission of bloodborne pathogens, as well as for handwashing, isolation, and other precautions. Effective action results from applying available information.

Establishment of and conformance to standards are prerequisites for infection control. *Surveillance* involves data collection, analysis, and action or regulatory activities. A statistical database can be correlated with testing to locate a problem or pinpoint changes in infection rates over a period of time. This is accomplished by periodic microbiologic sampling to evaluate procedures and routine testing of essential equipment such as sterilizers. Surveillance that is predicated on an understanding of epidemiology helps to prevent litigation. Measures require:

1. Investigation of every instance in which a patient becomes infected to ascertain if the infection is nosocomial or community-acquired
2. Prompt reporting of infection in any patient to define the incidence and type of infection in the hospital
3. Monitoring of patients, personnel, and environment according to written standards
4. Identification of factors that place a patient at risk
5. Clear definitions of infections, an infection control coordinator, and computerized records that provide statistical comparisons
6. Monitoring of wound infection rate to alert the staff to deviations from normal and to assess the need for changes in procedures because of technologic developments
7. Protection of the patient from reasonable risk for which reasonable control is available

Surveillance data are studied to ascertain trends of infection, high rates associated with specific surgical services, surgeons, or surgical procedures, or clustering in certain areas. A determination must be made as to whether the surgical wound healed without complication (i.e., purulent discharge). On or about the thirtieth postoperative day, the patient should be evaluated. Results obtained by a survey of the surgeons and/or patients are analyzed by the ICN. Computerized surgical data facilitate postoperative statistical analysis to determine accurate infection rates by wound classification. Surveillance provides a basis for improving conditions, procedures, and quality of patient care.

Microbiologic Sampling

Extensive random bacteriologic sampling of personnel and the environment when no problem exists is not recommended by the CDC. Routine culturing of air and equipment has not been found to be beneficial. For results to be purposeful microbiologic sampling is used to:

1. Monitor sterilizers (see Chapter 13, pp. 210-211)
2. Investigate an outbreak of nosocomial infection; type of problem directs type of culture needed for personnel and/or the environment
3. Determine effectiveness of cleaning methods and products
4. Audit an increase in postoperative clean wound infection rate

Infection Rate

Classification of the surgical wound (see Box 25-2, p. 526) provides standardization of records and a resource for comparison of wound infection rates. The information is used to compute the hospital's or ambulatory care facility's infection rate. The overall wound infection rate is the incidence of all types of surgical wounds. This is further differentiated to determine the percentage for clean, clean-contaminated, contaminated, and dirty or infected wounds. Infection rates vary by surgical specialty, type of procedure, length of surgical procedure, individual surgeon, and contributing patient factors. They may reflect the intraoperative care in a facility. Some infections are preventable; others are not. The desired outcome is prevention of infection in clean wounds. Overt tissue destruction can result from infection. The aim should be for a clean wound infection rate of 1% or less.

Reduction in incidence of infection can be attributed to the surveillance of infection, informing surgeons of their infection rates, and implementing infection control measures. The OR staff should be familiar with wound infection statistics. Because most patients are either hospitalized for only a few days postoperatively or not hospitalized at all, evidence of postoperative infection will not be known until after they are discharged from the health care facility. The surgeon is obligated to report an infection that develops in a patient after discharge. Wound sepsis remains one of the prime problems in the surgeon's daily practice.

ANTIMICROBIAL THERAPY

Antimicrobial drugs or agents are a prominent part of the surgeon's armamentarium. *They are adjuvants to, not substitutes for, strict adherence to aseptic and sterile principles and careful surgical technique.*

Antibiotics

Antibiotics act by killing (bactericidal) or inhibiting the growth (bacteriostatic) of bacteria. To be effective, the bacteria must be sensitive to the activity of the antibiotic. Some antibiotics are broad spectrum and attack many aerobic and anaerobic bacteria; others selectively destroy specific species. Antibiotics do not affect viruses and many fungi and yeasts.

The penicillins, cephalosporins, aminoglycosides, and carbapenems are the common categories of antibiotics. The penicillins include natural penicillin G and synthetic or semisynthetic derivatives. Some are rendered inactive by penicillinase, an enzyme secreted by certain bacteria that antagonizes the action of penicillin (e.g., *Staphylococcus aureus*). Several synthetic penicillins are resistant to penicillinase. Cephalosporins also are resistant to penicillinase, but cross-sensitivity may develop between them and the penicillins. They have a broad spectrum of effectiveness and low toxicity. Aminoglycosides are effective against gram-negative organisms (e.g., *pseudomonas, serratia,* and *Escherichia coli*), but they are ototoxic and nephrotoxic in a dose-related manner. Aminoglycosides (acids) precipitate when mixed with heparin and are incompatible with some cephalosporins and penicillins (bases). They should be given at separate times or through separate lines. Adverse effects, such as respiratory arrest, may occur with concurrent use of aminoglycosides and neuromuscular blockers or anesthetic agents. Among the carbapenems, the newest group of antibiotics, imipenem-cilastatin sodium has the broadest aerobic and anaerobic activity of any antibiotic. It is particularly effective against intraabdominal sepsis, with minimal side effects of nausea and vomiting, and susceptible organisms in respiratory and urinary tracts.

The incidence of allergic reactions to penicillin is relatively high. Patients should be questioned about allergies before any drug is administered and closely watched for signs of toxicity as evidenced by skin rash, gastrointestinal disturbance, renal disorder, fever, or blood dyscrasia.

The efficacy of antibiotics is greatly reduced when multiple organisms are involved in an infection. Sufficient risk warrants their use, however. Antibiotics are given:

1. *Therapeutically* to eliminate sensitive viable organisms during a clinical course of infection and in grossly contaminated and traumatic wounds. The choice of antibiotic and the duration of therapy should be determined by clinical factors, that is, pathogen, severity and site of infection, and clinical response. A broad-spectrum drug may be given while awaiting results of cultures and sensitivity tests.
2. *Prophylactically* to prevent the development of infection. Prophylaxis implies that the microorganism is attacked by the antimicrobial agent when it harbors in tissue before colonization takes place. A prophylactic antibiotic is given before surgical intervention, bacterial invasion, or clinically evident infection. These agents are effective as supplements to host defense mechanisms in selected patients. Prophylaxis is recommended for procedures:
   a. Associated with brief exposure to possible infection; evidence indicates that antibiotic can reduce infection (e.g., cystoscopy following cystitis).
   b. Not frequently associated with infection, but occurrence would have disastrous or life-threatening consequences (e.g., clean wounds, insertion of prosthetic implant such as heart valve, vascular graft, or total joint replacement).
   c. Associated with high risk of infection. Organisms are predictable and susceptible to antibiotics (e.g., clean-contaminated wounds such as biliary tract with obstruction, transection of colon).

The probability of infection is determined in the first few hours after bacterial invasion, when capillary permeability and host response are at a peak immediately after bacterial contamination. Therefore timing and duration of drug administration are crucial. To be effective, the prophylactic antibiotic must be present in adequate concentration in tissues at the time of wound creation or contamination. Selection of the appropriate drug and early use are pertinent factors. Antibiotic regimen is governed by site of surgical procedure, potential pathogens to be found, and the patient's history of drug sensitivities. Drugs may be given preoperatively and/or intraoperatively and possibly for a short period postoperatively. The CDC recommends that:

1. Except for cesarean section, parenteral antibiotic prophylaxis should be started within 2 hours before a surgical procedure to produce a therapeutic level during the surgical procedure and should not be continued for more than 48 hours. A 12-hour limit is desirable for most types of wounds. Parenteral use for more than 24 hours increases risk of antibiotic toxicity and development of resistant strains of bacteria or superinfection and does not further reduce the risk of infection.
2. For cesarean section, prophylaxis usually is given intraoperatively after the umbilical cord is clamped.
3. Oral, absorbable prophylactic antibiotics should not be used to supplement or extend parenteral prophylaxis. They should be limited to 24 hours before the surgical procedure when used prophylactically in colorectal operations.
4. Topical antimicrobial products used in the wound should be limited to those agents that will not cause serious local or systemic side effects.

A drastic change in the pattern of life-threatening infections has occurred since the advent of broad-spectrum antibiotics and penicillinase-resistant penicillins. Although gram-positive bacteria (staphylococci, pneumococci, and beta-hemolytic streptococci) continue their pathogenic activity, the resistant gram-negative bacilli, aerobic and anaerobic, deeply concern clinicians. Another grave concern is the increasing incidence of gram-negative infections by bacteria of supposedly low virulence (e.g., *Serratia* organisms), which are capable of causing deep, latent infections. These organisms rapidly colonize in hospitalized patients and are transferred to other individuals by hands or equipment. Many of these organisms develop plasmid-mediated resistance to antibiotics. This means that a bacterium carrying genetic particles (plasmids) that allow it to replicate will not be affected by the antibiotic (i.e., will be resistant to it).

Methicillin-resistant *Staphylococcus aureus* (MRSA) is not plasmid-mediated. However, it is resistant not just to methicillin, a penicillin, but to other categories of antibiotics as well. This resistance has probably developed as a result of overuse of these broad-spectrum agents. Clinically MRSA poses an important nosocomial problem whether by infection of patients or colonization in health care workers. Vancomycin, a highly toxic antimicrobial drug, seems to be effective against MRSA.

Antifungal and Antiviral Drugs

Nosocomial fungal and viral infections also are problematic. Topical antifungal drugs usually control fungus. *Candida albicans* can lead to a fatal opportunistic systemic infection. Candicidin is a specific fungicide for this organism.

Viruses are not usually a risk to a healthy patient undergoing an elective procedure. But patients have died of systemic viremia, sometimes associated with bacteremia or fungemia. Hepatitis and HIV present a unique challenge. Antiretroviral drugs are used to inhibit replication of the HIV.

POSTOPERATIVE WOUND INFECTIONS

A postoperative wound infection may occur in the incision or in deep structures that were entered or exposed. Its nature and severity vary because of local, systemic, technical, or environmental factors. Each factor is important; all are interrelated in clinical infection. Usually a postoperative infection is localized, but severe systemic reaction is possible (see discussion of septic shock, p. 534). The specific pathogen and site of infection determine its gravity. Postoperative wound infections are defined as:

1. *Incisional.* An infection occurs at the site of incision within 30 postoperative days. It involves skin, subcutaneous tissue, or muscle. The incisional area is usually inflamed and sore. Purulent drainage or an organism identified by culture is present. The surgeon usually must open and drain the wound.
2. *Deep wound infection.* An infection occurs at the surgical site within 30 postoperative days if a prosthesis was not implanted or within 1 year around site of an implant. The infection involves tissues or spaces at or beneath the fascia. Pus may be present. The wound may spontaneously dehisce. The surgeon may need to open and drain the wound or remove an implant. Infection involving an implant or gross necrotic tissue is prone to serious sequelae.

Compromised patients and geriatric patients are highly likely to develop endogenous infection. Operations on potentially contaminated areas, such as the gastrointestinal tract, are more apt to result in postoperative infections. The following measures, in addition to those discussed, may help prevent wound infections.

1. Implantation of organisms into surrounding tissue must be avoided if infection is encountered at the surgical site.
2. Potentially contaminated wounds may be irrigated with topical antibiotics intraoperatively.
3. Cultures obtained during surgical procedure should be used for antibiotic-sensitivity testing.
4. Wound closure materials and instruments can be isolated on instrument table so wound is closed

with previously unused instruments to reduce inoculum delivered to incision.

5. Indwelling Foley catheters should be removed as soon as possible to prevent urinary tract infection, which increases in incidence the longer the catheter is in the patient.
6. Special precautions must be taken when prostheses such as heart valves, total joint prostheses, or intraocular lenses are implanted. Infection can have disastrous effects.

Gram-negative bacteria are the primary contaminants in nosocomial infection. They are the predominant flora in the gastrointestinal tract and the primary pathogens in urinary tract, abdominal, and intravenous catheter infections, as well as in pneumonia. These infections carry a high risk of bacteremia and therefore require prompt intervention.

Nonbacterial opportunists such as fungi and viruses are a particular hazard to trauma or burn patients. The likelihood of infection is related to the severity of the injury. Initial gram-positive infection is frequently followed by a virulent gram-negative or fungal infection. Candida is a common fungal colonizer and invader.

Staphylococci species of gram-positive cocci are common pathogens that may occur as normal flora of the skin, hair, and upper respiratory tract. Staphylococcal wound infections acquired in the OR are characterized by pus deep beneath a cleanly healed wound. A red wound accompanied by pus and fever within 7 days after a surgical procedure may indicate such an infection. Infections appearing more than 7 days postoperatively usually were not acquired in the OR.

Streptococci species of gram-positive cocci are found primarily in the upper respiratory tract. Beta-hemolytic streptococci are the pathogenic strain of this group.

Pseudomonas aeruginosa is an aerobic gram-negative bacillus found in water, soil, and intestinal tracts. It has the ability to survive in tap water. It is readily recognized by its bluish-green fluorescent color and characteristic odor.

Difficult to eradicate, these infections, which often progress to septicemia and multiple-abscess formation in the viscera or body areas, can cause death.

Enteric organisms are normally found in the intestinal tract. Gram-negative bacilli are often resistant to long-established antibiotics. Peritoneal contamination can result from visceral manipulation without actually opening or entering the gastrointestinal tract in patients with cancerous lesions. The bowel wall can erode, permitting intestinal organisms to escape into the peritoneal cavity.

Anaerobic organisms thrive in unoxygenated tissues. They outnumber aerobic organisms in the intestinal tract and are less susceptible to antibiotics than are aerobes. Often present in the lower genital tract of females, they cause severe pelvic infection. Anaerobic infections are caused by:

1. *Peptostreptococcus* and *Peptococcus* species.
2. *Bacteroides* and *Fusobacterium* species, the microorganisms most frequently isolated from blood cultures. They are common in the colon.
3. *Clostridium perfringens* and *C. welchii,* which are found in the intestinal tract. These species of highly resistant gas-producing spore formers cause gas gangrene, contributing to high mortality if left untreated.

Investigation of Postoperative Wound Infections

A special form is used to record specific data. Investigation, usually by the infection control coordinator, includes:

1. Analysis of each infection to seek the cause
2. Consultation with all persons who cared for the patient
3. Review of any problem encountered intraoperatively, such as a break in sterile technique
4. Review of possible contributory factors
5. Evaluation of procedures relating to the patient
6. Review of chart, symptoms, and cultures
7. Review of postoperative dressing changes

Prevention of Wound Infection

Prevention of wound infection and successful outcome of surgical intervention are goals of the team administering perioperative care to surgical patients. In summary, preventive measures should focus on:

1. Adherence to aseptic techniques and universal precautions with all patients
2. Control of endogenous infection
3. Use of strict sterile techniques
4. Meticulous surgical technique and wound closure
5. Reduction of exogenous or environmental sources of contamination such as airborne microorganisms
6. Thorough, prompt cleansing and debridement of traumatic wounds
7. Prevention of intraoperative contamination of a wound
8. Appropriate use of prophylactic antibiotics
9. Frequent handwashing
10. Sterile technique for dressing changes
11. Dissemination of wound infection statistics to surgeons and OR staff

Serious sequelae, such as wound disruption or septicemia, may follow wound infection. Therefore they must be assiduously prevented so that wound healing can occur naturally.

Bibliography

Brown KK: Septic shock: how to stop the deadly cascade, *Am J Nurs* 94(9):20-26, 1994.

Brown-Etris M et al: Case studies: considering dressing options, *Ostomy Wound Manag* 40(5):50-52, 1994.

Calligaro KD et al: Comparison of muscle flaps and delayed secondary intention wound grafting for infected lower extremity arterial grafts, *Ann Vasc Surg* 8(1):31-37, 1994.

Claussen DC et al: The timing of prophylactic administration of antibiotics and the risk of surgical wound infection, *N Engl J Med* 326(4):281-286, 1992.

Cuzzell JZ: Choosing a wound dressing: a systematic approach, *AACN Clin Issues Crit Care Nurs* 1(3):566-577, 1990.

Cuzzell JZ, Stotts NA: Wound care: trial and error yields to knowledge, *Am J Nurs* 90(10):53-63, 1990.

Erwin-Toth P, Hocevar BJ: Wound care: selecting the right dressing, *Am J Nurs* 95(2):46-51, 1995.

Fincham JE: Perioperative implications of tobacco use, *AORN J* 56(3):531-538, 1992.

Fowler E et al: Healing with thin-film dressings, *Am J Nurs* 91(3):36-38, 1991.

Gawlikowski J: White cells at war, *Am J Nurs* 92(3):44-51, 1992.

Gerstein AD et al: Wound healing and aging, *Dermatol Clin* 11(4):749-757, 1993.

Giadani MB, Grabski WJ: Cutaneous candidiasis as a cause of delayed surgical wound healing, *J Am Acad Dermatol* 30(6):981-984, 1994.

Gilpin DA et al: Recombinant human growth hormone accelerates wound healing in children with large cutaneous burns, *Ann Surg* 220(1):19-24, 1994.

Goldheim PG: An appraisal of povodine-iodine and wound healing, *Postgrad Med J* 69(3):97-105, 1993.

Groot G, Chappell EW: Electrocautery used to create incisions does not increase wound infection rate, *Am J Surg* 167(6):601-603, 1994.

Kirsner RS, Eaglstein WH: The wound healing process, *Dermatol Clin* 11(4):629-640, 1993.

Koldas T: A simple method for the classic tie-over dressing, *Ann Plast Surg* 28(4):386-387, 1992.

Lazarus GS et al: Definitions and guidelines for assessment of wounds and evaluation of healing, *Arch Dermatol* 130(4):489-493, 1994.

Mertz PM, Ovington LG: Wound healing microbiology, *Dermatol Clin* 11(4):739-747, 1993.

Michie DD, Hugill JV: Influence of occlusive and impregnated gauze dressings on incisional healing: a prospective, randomized, controlled study, *Ann Plast Surg* 32(1):57-64, 1994.

Moy LS: Management of acute wounds, *Dermatol Clin* 11(4):759-766, 1993.

Murray JC: Scars and keloids, *Dermatol Clin* 11(4):697-708, 1993.

Nemath AJ: Lasers and wound healing, *Dermatol Clin* 11(4):783-789, 1993.

O'Hanlon-Nichols T: Clinical savvy: commonly asked questions about wound healing, *Am J Nurs* 95(4):22-24, 1995.

Ondrey FG, Hom DB: Effects of nutrition on wound healing, *Otolaryngol Head Neck Surg* 110(6):557-559, 1994.

Osak MP: Nutrition and wound healing, *Plast Surg Nurs* 13(1):29-36, 1993.

Robinson CJ: Growth factors: therapeutic advances in wound healing, *Ann Med* 25(6):535-538, 1993.

Sawyer RG, Pruett TL: Wound infections, *Surg Clin North Am* 74(3):519-536, 1994.

Shovein J, Young MS: MRSA: Pandora's box for hospitals, *Am J Nurs* 92(1):48-52, 1992.

Silverstein P: Smoking and wound healing, *Am J Med* 93(1A):22S-24S, 1992.

Surratt S et al: Troubleshooting a sump tube, *Am J Nurs* 93(1):42-47, 1993.

Valenta AL: Using the vacuum dressing alternative for difficult wounds, *Am J Nurs* 94(4):44-45, 1994.

Wills RE, Grusendorf PE: Action of antimicrobial agents on the bacterial cell wall, *Surg Technol* 22(1):10-11, 1990.

CHAPTER 26

Postoperative Patient Care

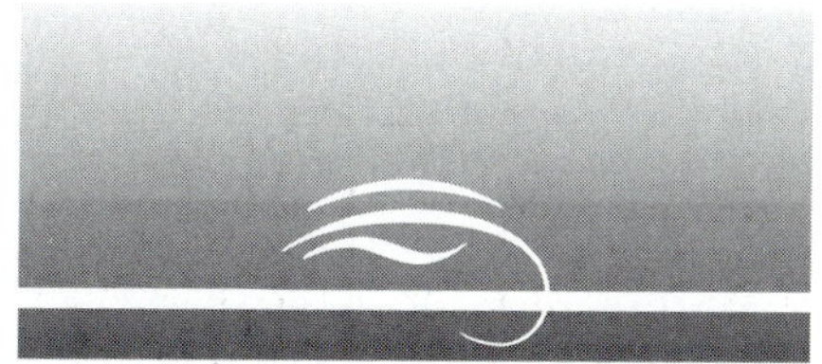

POSTOPERATIVE OBSERVATION OF PATIENT

Surgical procedures are performed in many diverse settings, including surgeons' offices, ambulatory surgery centers, and hospital-based surgical suites and specialty units. The selection of the surgical setting is mainly influenced by complexity of the anticipated procedure, patient's health status, available technology, and financial resources. Postoperatively, regardless of the surgical setting or the procedure performed, the patient should be observed in a controlled postsurgical/postanesthesia environment before transfer to a nursing unit or discharge from the facility. The *postoperative phase* of the surgical patient's perioperative experience begins after the surgical procedure is completed and the patient is admitted to a postoperative recovery area, usually a postanesthesia care unit or an intensive care unit (ICU), or the patient is discharged to his or her home.

The duration and type of postoperative observation and care will vary according to the following:

1. Patient's condition (e.g., alert and oriented vs. unresponsive)
2. Need for physiologic support (e.g., ventilator-dependent compared to awake and extubated)
3. Complexity of the surgical procedure (e.g., open laparotomy compared to laparoscopy)
4. Type of anesthesia administered (e.g., a general inhalation agent compared to local infiltration)
5. Need for pain therapy (e.g., analgesic compared to nerve plexus block)
6. Prescribed period for monitoring parameters to evaluate physiologic status (e.g., stable compared to unstable vital signs)

POSTANESTHESIA CARE

Ideally, an area is designated for the care of postoperative patients. The area may vary in name or location according to its specific function within the health care facility. In some settings where only local anesthetic agents are used, the patient has a brief postoperative observation period in the same room where the procedure was performed. From this room, when the patient is determined to be physiologically stable, he or she is discharged from the facility. Dental, podiatric, and dermatologic offices frequently function in this capacity.

Immediate postoperative patient care is usually given in a designated area of the hospital or an ambulatory care facility. This area may be called the *recovery room (RR)* or *postanesthesia recovery unit (PAR)*. In this text the term *postanesthesia care unit (PACU)* is used to describe this specialized area for patient care during recovery from anesthesia. According to protocol established by the anesthesia and surgical services departments, institutional policies and procedures guide patient care activities in the PACU.

The concept of a PACU has been popular since the early 1940s, when studies on postoperative mortality and morbidity demonstrated that appropriate observation and monitoring could have prevented death in a significant number of postsurgical patients. Causes of death documented within the first 24 hours of anesthetic administration and surgical procedure were obstruction of airway, laryngospasm, hemorrhage, cardiac arrest, and inappropriate administration of medication. Contributing factors included inadequate postoperative patient care, lack of standardized observation parameters, and absence of medical supervision. Postoperative patient care was inconsistent and inefficient. The need for postoperative care performed by appropriately educated registered nurses in a controlled environment was identified.

Postanesthesia Care Unit

Located in close proximity to the operating room (OR), the basic PACU design consists of a large room divided into a series of individual cubicles (spaces) separated by privacy curtains. Each cubicle has a cardiac monitor, pulse oximeter, blood pressure measurement device, suction apparatus, and oxygen administration equipment. Additional supplies include airway management equipment, intravenous fluids and administration sets, dressing reinforcement materials, medications, indwelling Foley catheters and drainage systems, emesis basins, and bedpans. Other equipment, including a cardiac arrest cart with defibrillator, is positioned strategically throughout the room for easy accessibility when needed.

Some facilities include isolation rooms for patients who are highly contagious or highly susceptible to infection. If the PACU does not have a partitioned isolation area, patients may be placed at one end of the room, separated from others by screens or curtains. Isolation procedures should be used in handling bedding and equipment, per institutional policy. All patients have the right to receive the same level of care regardless of extenuating circumstances.

Ideally, cubicle space is allotted per the number of ORs in the OR suite. This allotment may vary between one and one half to two cubicles per OR and is based on the case load, duration of surgical procedures, and room turnover time in the OR. A rapid succession of short procedures could easily fill the PACU and leave no vacancy for additional postoperative patients. This scenario is seen more frequently in facilities where the PACU doubles as a special procedure care unit for ambulatory patients who are receiving nerve blocks for pain therapy. Some institutions allow uncomplicated endoscopies to be performed in the PACU. The rationale behind this practice is that patients having special procedures need to be monitored after a treatment or test for a short period of time by experienced personnel. For some procedures the PACU nurse monitors the patient who is receiving intravenous conscious sedation (see Chapter 18, p. 347) and may assist the physician, thus depleting the available staff for postoperative care.

In larger institutions where prolonged and complex surgical procedures are performed, as for transplantations or multiple trauma, some postoperative patients remain in the PACU for more than 24 hours because of the potential need to return to the OR for an additional surgical procedure. The patient's condition causes the PACU to double as a surgical intensive care unit. Increased patient load and acuity increases the need for adequate staffing, space allocation, education of personnel, and management of resources. Consolidation of facilities and personnel should not jeopardize the delivery of safe postoperative patient care.

Personnel in Postanesthesia Care Unit

Adequate personnel should be available to monitor patients and to provide appropriate care as needed. The education and training of PACU nurses should include knowledge of:

1. Anesthetic agents and their actions (e.g., physiologic depression associated with general anesthesia)
2. Medications and their actions (e.g., narcotics and tranquilizers)
3. Most invasive and minimally invasive surgical procedures (e.g., open laparotomy and laparoscopy)
4. Potential complications related to anesthesia (see Chapter 19, pp. 378-395)

PACU nurses should demonstrate competency in:

1. Physical assessment (e.g., heart and lung sounds)
2. Management of physiologic emergencies (e.g., airway, hemorrhage, cardiac arrest)

Additional competencies should include certification in cardiopulmonary resuscitation (CPR), both basic life support (BLS) and advanced cardiac life support (ACLS).

In 1986 the American Society of Post Anesthesia Nurses (ASPAN) developed specialty certification for PACU nurses. A PACU nurse specializing in the care of patients in hospital-based or extended recovery care facilities may attain certification as a certified postanesthesia care nurse (CPAN) by taking and passing a written examination. Nurses who specialize in postanesthesia care in ambulatory surgery settings can attain certification in ambulatory postanesthesia care (CAPA). The certification is valid for 3 years and can be renewed by passing a written examination or by obtaining continuing education credits.

Other personnel in the PACU may include nursing assistants and licensed practical/vocational nurses (LPN/LVNs). Their duties may vary according to the needs of the department.

Postanesthesia Patient Care

ASPAN, organized in 1980, has established standards of practice for the postoperative care of diverse populations, such as pediatric, adult, and geriatric patients. ASPAN has identified three phases of care, as follows:

1. *Preanesthesia phase.* Focuses on the emotional and physical preparation of patients before a surgical procedure
2. *Postanesthesia phase I.* Focuses on providing immediate postoperative care from an anesthetized state to a condition requiring less acute intervention
3. *Postanesthesia phase II.* Focuses on preparing the patient for self-care or care in an extended-care setting

The goal of postanesthesia care is to assist the patient in returning to a safe physiologic level after an anesthetic has been administered.

Admission to Postanesthesia Care Unit

The circulator should call the PACU nurse before the patient leaves the OR to give the estimated time of arrival in the PACU and to advise of a need to have any special life support equipment on standby for immediate use. As the patient enters the PACU, his or her immediate physiologic and psychologic status is reported to the PACU nurse. Any necessary life support equipment, such as a ventilator, is connected. The PACU nurse connects electrocardiographic electrodes, attaches a pulse oximeter lead, and places a blood pressure cuff on the patient. Many PACUs are supplied with automatic or computerized equipment that provides an immediate display of vital signs and physiologic data. Simultaneously the PACU nurse is assessing the patient and assimilating the data. The flow of activity is fast-paced but directed to the immediate physiologic needs of the patient.

Postoperative Report

The postoperative report provides information from the anesthesiologist (if one was in attendance), the surgeon (or appropriate designee, such as first assistant), and the circulator. Much of the report will be delivered verbally, but postoperative orders and pertinent documentation of the patient's condition and intraoperative care are reinforced in writing. The content of the postoperative report to the PACU nurse should include but is not limited to the following information.

Anesthesiologist's Report

1. Patient's name, gender, age, surgical procedure, and surgeon
2. Type of anesthesia and the patient's reaction(s)
3. Baseline vital signs and summary of vital sign flow during the surgical procedure
4. Allergies and reaction to allergen
5. Any physiologic changes or existing conditions and interventions to counteract them (e.g., diabetes, chronic obstructive pulmonary disease [COPD]), previous myocardial infarction, hypertension)
6. Medications administered preoperatively, intraoperatively, and postoperatively (e.g., preoperative sedation, intraoperative antibiotic, or continuous infusion of medication)
7. Intravenous fluid administration and body fluid output (e.g., blood products, urine, and gastric contents)
8. Specific patient care orders to be performed in the PACU or the immediate postoperative period (e.g., aerosol or mist mask)

Surgeon's Report

1. Postoperative orders pertaining to immediate treatments or therapies to be performed in the PACU or the immediate postoperative period (e.g., passive range of motion device or x-ray film to check placement of central line catheter)
2. Serial diagnostic tests that are to be initiated in the PACU and continued through the immediate postoperative period (e.g., blood counts at specified intervals)
3. Specific interventions pertaining to care of the surgical site (e.g., dressing change or reinforcement)

Circulator's Report

1. Baseline assessment data
2. Positioning and skin preparation
3. Condition of dispersive electrode site
4. Use of specialized surgical equipment, such as laser or endoscope
5. Intraoperative irrigation fluids
6. Administration of medication or dyes in the surgical field
7. Any implants, transplants, or explants
8. Type of dressings and presence of drains and/or stents
9. Any pertinent information not reported by the anesthesiologist or surgeon
10. Location of family member or significant other who may be waiting

The postoperative report will vary according to the type of anesthesia and the surgical procedure, the anesthesiologist's and surgeon's preferences, and institutional policy and procedure. The main emphasis is placed on the needs of the patient in the immediate postoperative period. This continues until the patient is discharged from the PACU.

Patient Care Activities in Postanesthesia Care Unit

Application of physiologic and psychosocial knowledge, principles of asepsis, and technical knowledge and skills are necessary to promote, restore, and maintain the patient's physiologic processes in a safe, comfortable, and effective environment. Particular attention is given to monitoring oxygenation, ventilation, and circulation. PACU care includes maintaining adequate ventilation, preventing shock, and alleviating pain. Postoperative medical orders, coordinated by the anesthesiologist and the surgeon, include monitoring requirements, oxygen and fluid therapies, pain medications, and other special considerations. Patients are evaluated continually by appropriate monitoring methods and frequent observations by registered nurses. Clinical evaluation of each patient's status by listening, watching, and feeling is augmented by electronic monitoring devices.

As in all other patient care areas, universal precautions are carried out for disposal of needles and handling of any item contaminated by blood and body fluids. Handwashing is essential after each patient contact to prevent cross contamination.

Family members are notified when a patient is admitted to the PACU so they will know that the surgical procedure is over. This helps to relieve their anxiety during the hours of waiting. Some facilities allow visitors in the PACU. This is determined by institutional policy.

Documentation in Postanesthesia Care Unit

Observations of respiratory and circulatory functions and level of consciousness are recorded at frequent intervals. Documentation of postoperative physiologic and psychologic status is recorded at the time of any significant event, such as administration of medication, and routinely at 5- to 7-minute intervals for the first hour and at 15- to 30-minute intervals for the second hour and thereafter. Pertinent observations are recorded as appropriate or necessary. Institutional policies and procedures should be followed in documenting PACU care.

Discharge From Postanesthesia Care Unit

Most patients remain in the PACU at least 1 hour or until they have sufficiently recovered from anesthesia so that their vital signs have stabilized and they are capable of reasonable self-care. The patient's condition is scored according to vital signs, activity level, and consciousness. Several standardized formats are available for this purpose. The anesthesiologist assesses the patient as necessary and may determine when the patient is stable enough for discharge from the PACU. The patient is discharged from the PACU and transported to a nursing unit, or an ICU, or is released from the ambulatory care facility.

A physician is responsible for discharge of the patient from the PACU. The anesthesia department and medical staff may approve discharge criteria for the PACU nurse to use to determine readiness for discharge. These criteria should be consistent with the standards of the American Society of Anesthesiologists and the accreditation standards of the Joint Commission on Accreditation of Healthcare Organizations and/or the Accreditation Association for Ambulatory Health Care.

OTHER POSTOPERATIVE CONSIDERATIONS

Unless the surgical procedure was performed in an office or ambulatory care setting (see Chapter 41) or the patient was transferred directly from the OR to the ICU, the patient transfers from the postanesthesia recovery area to progressive stages of self-care before discharge from the hospital. During this postoperative phase of the surgical patient's experience, the perioperative nurse evaluates the effectiveness of preoperative and intraoperative care. Evaluation is the fourth component of the nursing process.

Postoperative Evaluation of Expected Outcomes

Ideally the perioperative nurse who preoperatively assessed the patient and developed and implemented the plan of care intraoperatively will have the opportunity to assess and/or interview the patient postoperatively to evaluate patient care outcomes. An assessment is done in person if possible, or the patient may be interviewed by a follow-up telephone call.

The plan of care should be evaluated in terms of the attainment of expected outcomes. The identification of influencing factors provides a foundation for ongoing improvement of perioperative patient care services. Some considerations for the design of the postoperative evaluation include but are not limited to:

1. Was a preoperative visit made and was it helpful to the patient?
2. Were patient and family adequately prepared for the surgical procedure physically, psychologically, emotionally, and spiritually?
3. What could have been improved?
4. Were all pertinent patient needs, problems, or health status considerations identified in the nursing diagnoses?
5. Did the plan of care address the nursing diagnoses?
6. Did the patient experience any complications?
7. Was preoperative teaching utilized? Was it adequate and helpful?
8. What were the patient's perceptions of the surgical experience?
9. Were the expected outcomes achieved to the patient's satisfaction?
10. To what degree do the patient's observable physiologic and psychosocial responses indicate attainment of expected outcomes?

Evaluation of patient outcomes helps to identify environmental influences and procedural activities that may need to be modified by the OR staff. For example, if the patient developed a reddened pressure area over a bony process, was positioning equipment at fault or was the area unpadded? Reevaluation of products currently being used may be indicated. Injury to skin may be caused by the pooling of prep solutions under the patient, inadequate padding of body prominences, or faulty electrical equipment.

Subjective data received from the patient will help evaluate how much discomfort the patient is experiencing, especially paresthesia, which is a numb, tingling sensation. Neurovascular injuries may be related to positioning on the operating table. The perioperative nurse may suggest comfort measures to help this patient, but an adverse outcome indicates a need to improve positioning procedures for subsequent patients.

The postoperative assessment or follow-up telephone call terminates the direct perioperative nurse-patient relationship. The evaluation of the degree of attainment of expected outcomes completes the perioperative nursing process.

To be successful, a postoperative evaluation program requires the cooperative effort of and input from the PACU, the ICU, perioperative nurses, surgeons, anesthesiologists, nursing unit personnel, and administrative personnel. They should participate in structuring the program at its inception to avoid duplication of action and to promote collegial effort. Many facilities give postoperative patients an evaluation form to complete and return, which provides additional feedback for all members of the health care staff. Postoperative evaluation data may be collected through:

1. Interview and assessment of the patient
2. Conferences with physicians, nurses and other caregivers
3. Review of responses on patient evaluation form

The postoperative evaluation program should be reviewed periodically and revised as necessary. An interdisciplinary conference is an effective medium for the accomplishment of these objectives. An effective perioperative evaluation program and positive patient experiences promote good public relations and demonstrate a caring image of the facility to the public it serves.

DEATH OF PATIENT IN OPERATING ROOM

Although it is an infrequent occurrence, a patient may die while on the operating table. When this happens, the circulator notifies the OR manager immediately. Ideally the surgeon notifies the family when a patient dies in the OR. It may be appropriate to discuss organ donation with the family at this time and to request permission to proceed with organ procurement (see Chapter 44). If circumstances warrant, the surgeon may request permission for an autopsy.

Coroner's Cases

In some states the body of a patient who dies in the OR automatically becomes the property of the coroner. Consent for autopsy is not necessary in this situation. The coroner must give approval for organ procurement and has the right to overrule the wishes of the family.

Individual state law and institutional policy determine the postmortem care of the patient's body. For example, all drainage tubes, implants, and catheters may need to be left in place for removal and examination at autopsy. All medication vials and intravenous solution containers should remain with the body.

In a life-threatening emergency, a patient may be admitted directly to the OR without being undressed or prepared for a surgical procedure. The body of a patient who dies under these circumstances is also considered the property of the coroner, but postmortem care is more complex. Critical medical-legal issues should be taken into consideration if the patient was a suspected victim or perpetrator of violence or was injured in a suspicious manner. All information about the patient's condition, personal effects and attire, and materials discovered during the surgical procedure are considered *forensic evidence*. Forensic evidence is critical for the reconstruction of events involved in a crime or suspected illegal activity. All forensic evidence is preserved according to institutional policy and procedure and is relinquished only to appropriate authorities. Documentation of handling and disposition of evidence is referred to as a *chain of evidence*. This chain is maintained by requiring signatures of all persons who come in contact with forensic evidence. The goal is to attempt to validate that evidence has not been tampered with before reaching the appropriate law enforcement agency.

Intraoperative documentation, another form of evidence, should include a written account of the patient's physical appearance on arrival in the OR, as well as a hand-drawn diagram of any physical markings present before skin preparation, such as penetrating wounds or bruises on the body. Other pertinent data might include unusual odors, such as chemicals, gasoline, or alcohol. Clothing, undergarments, and shoes should be allowed to air-dry before being placed in paper containers for release to the authorities. Items placed in air-tight containers or plastic bags may decay and destroy vital evidence. Bullets, fragments of knives, or other weapon-like implements must be handled according to institutional policy for transport to the appropriate law enforcement agency. Nothing is discarded. A clear documented chain of evidence is frequently difficult to maintain in a crisis, but every attempt is made to document the location from which evidence was taken and its disposition.

Surgical interventions for both the perpetrator and the victim of the same crime are a challenge for the OR team. It may be difficult to deliver objective care to the perpetrator if the victim has died within moments of reaching the OR. Regardless of personal feelings or beliefs, both patients have rights and are entitled to professional care at all times.

After-Death Patient Care

A death may be anticipated, as that of a patient brought to the OR on mechanical life support for organ procurement (see Chapter 44, p. 902). A death may occur as a result of shock following extensive traumatic injuries, exsanguination after rupture of an aortic aneurysm, unsuccessful cardiopulmonary resuscitation following cardiac arrest, or other causes. The circulator's responsibilities after intraoperative death include:

1. Giving after-death care to the body as appropriate or ensuring that forensic protocol is followed before releasing the body to authorities or morgue
   a. Follow institutional policy and procedure.
   b. Be sure identification is correct.
   c. If body is considered part of forensic evidence, it is not washed.
2. Arranging for transportation from OR to the morgue or release to an appropriate authority
   a. Release the body from the OR according to institutional policy and procedure.
   b. Avoid exposing other patients, visitors, and family to removal of the body.
   c. If religious or cultural preference of patient and/or family is known, an appropriate member of the clergy or a spiritual advisor may be consulted concerning postdeath practices.
3. Completing the intraoperative chart and additional documentation as required by institutional policy

Policy may allow the family to view a loved one before the body is transported to the morgue. The room where the viewing takes place should be clean, presentable, and private. The circulator or the circulator's designee should accompany the family and lend support. This person must remain in attendance if the body will be involved in a forensic investigation.

Following a death in the OR, from whatever cause, team members should be given time to express and deal with their feelings about the event. (See discussion of death and dying in Chapter 4, pp. 64-65.)

Bibliography

American Society of Anesthesiologists: *Standards for postanesthesia care*, adopted in 1988, Park Ridge, Ill, The Society.

American Society of Post Anesthesia Nurses: *Standards of nursing practice*, 1994, Richmond, Va, The Society.

Burden N: Telephone follow-up of ambulatory surgery patients is a nursing responsibility, *J Post Anesth Nurs* 7(4):256-261, 1992.

Cushing M: Back to (PACU) basics, *Am J Nurs* 92(7):21-22, 1992.

Dowing K: Certification: accept the challenge, *J Post Anesth Nurs* 6(6):430-433, 1991.

Einhorn GW, Chant P: Postanesthesia care unit dilemmas: prompt assessment and treatment, *J Post Anesth Nurs* 9(1):28-33, 1994.

Feely TW: The design and staffing of a modern post anesthesia care unit, *Curr Rev Post Anesth Nurs* 15(16):131-136, 1993.

Feldman ME: Uncovering clinical knowledge and caring practices, *J Post Anesth Nurs* 8(3):159-162, 1993.

Fetzer-Fowler SJ, Putrycus B: CAPA: your practice, your certification, *J Post Anesth Nurs* 9(4):250-254, 1994.

Hannah BA: Establishing clinical competence in postanesthesia care nursing, *J Post Anesth Nurs* 8(3):187-193, 1993.

Jackson DA: Reflex sympathetic dystrophy: two cases, *J Post Anesth Nurs* 8(5):327-331, 1993.

Litwack KL: *Post anesthesia care nursing*, ed 2, St Louis, 1995, Mosby.

Mamaril M: Standard of care: legal implications in the post anesthesia care unit, *J Post Anesth Nurs* 8(1):13-20, 1993.

Mathias JM: Pain guideline stresses patient involvement, *OR Manager* 8(5):1, 18, 1992.

Muro GA, Easter CR: Clinical forensics for perioperative nurses, *AORN J* 60(4):585-593, 1994.

Odom JL: Airway emergencies in the post anesthesia care unit, *Nurs Clin North Am* 28(3):483-491, 1993.

Rivellini D: Local and regional anesthesia: nursing implications, *Nurs Clin North Am* 28(3):547-572, 1993.

Schramm CA: Forensic medicine: what the perioperative nurse needs to know, *AORN J* 53(3):669-691, 1991.

Simon A: Preparation for recertification, *J Post Anesth Nurs* 7(1):59-61, 1992.

VanRiper S, Luciano A: Basic cardiac arrhythmias: a review for postanesthesia care unit nurses, *J Post Anesth Nurs* 9(1):2-13, 1994.

Vissering TR: Narcotics and implications for the post anesthesia care unit, *Nurs Clin North Am* 28(3):573-580, 1993.

Whitis G: Visiting hospitalized patients, *J Adv Nurs* 19(1):85-88, 1994.

CHAPTER 27

Postoperative Care of the Physical Environment

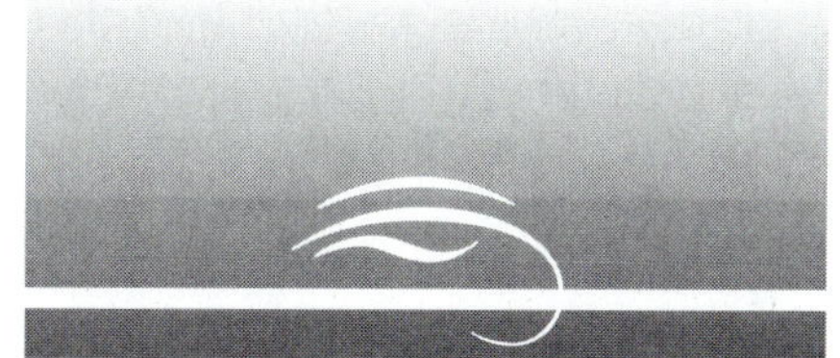

AFTER SURGICAL PROCEDURE IS COMPLETED

Physical facilities influence the flow of supplies and equipment following the surgical procedure. However, basic principles of aseptic technique dictate the procedures to be carried out immediately after a surgical procedure is completed to prepare the operating room (OR) for the next patient. Every patient has the right to the same degree of safety in the environment. In addition, personnel working in the OR suite should be protected. Some patients have known pathogenic microorganisms; others have unknown infectious organisms. Therefore *every patient should be considered a potential contaminant in the environment.* Cleanup procedures should be rigidly followed to *contain and confine contamination,* known or unknown.

The routine cleanup procedure can be accomplished expeditiously by the circulator and scrub person working cooperatively. While the circulator assists with the outer layer of dressing and prepares the patient for transport from the OR, the scrub person begins to dismantle the sterile field before removing gown and gloves. *All* instruments, supplies, and equipment should be decontaminated, disinfected, terminally sterilized, or contained for disposal as appropriate before being handled by other personnel.

ROOM CLEANUP BETWEEN PATIENTS

Room cleanup between patients is directed at the prevention of cross contamination. The cycle of contamination is from patient to environment and from environment to OR personnel and subsequent patients. Exposure to infectious waste is a hazard to all persons who encounter it. After each surgical procedure, the environment should be made safe for the next patient to follow in that room. Institutional policies and procedures for routine room cleanup should be designed to minimize the OR team's exposure to contamination during the cleaning process.

By Scrub Person

Think of the patient as the center, or focal point. The surrounding sterile field and all areas that have come in contact with blood or body fluids are considered contaminated. The primary principles of cleaning procedures are to confine and contain contamination and to physically remove microorganisms as quickly as possible. The sterile field is dismantled by the scrub person. Gown, gloves, mask, protective eyewear, and cap are worn for procedure.

1. Push Mayo stand and instrument table away from operating table as soon as intermediate layer of the

dressing is applied. *Do not contaminate the Mayo stand* until the patient has left the room (refer to NOTE on p. 417, Chapter 20).

2. Assist surgeon and assistant in removing their gowns and gloves. Gowns should be removed before gloves. Grasp both shoulders of gown and pull them downward over arms. Roll outside of gown inward and discard it in a laundry hamper or trash receptacle; reusable woven fabric gown is sent to the laundry, and disposable gowns go into the trash. Using a glove-to-glove technique, grasp cuffs of gloves and pull them inside out over the surgeon's hands. Discard gloves in a trash receptacle.
3. Check drapes for towel clips, instruments, and other items. Be sure that no equipment is discarded with disposable drapes or sent to the laundry with reusable woven fabric drapes. *Roll* drapes off patient to prevent airborne contamination; do not pull them off. Disposable drapes are placed in a plastic bag for disposal. Roll wettest part of reusable woven fabric drapes into center of the bag as far as possible to prevent liquid from soaking through the laundry bag, even though it is waterproof. Soiled drapes, whether disposable or reusable, should be handled as little as possible and with minimum agitation to prevent gross microbial contamination of air by dispersal of lint and debris.
4. Discard soiled sponges, other waste, and disposable items in appropriate impervious trash receptacles.
5. Discard unused sponges and unopened suture packets.
6. Dispose of sharp items safely. Special care should be taken in handling all knife blades, surgical needles, and needles used for injection or aspiration. Remove tip from the electrosurgical handle (pencil). Place these items in an appropriate rigid, puncture-resistant container for either disposal or cleaning to prevent injury and potential risk of contamination. The primary cause of accidental cuts and punctures to personnel, both within and outside of the OR, is disposal of surgical sharps at the end of the surgical procedure. Standardized systems designed specifically for safe handling and disposal of sharps prevent virtually all accidental cuts, punctures, or lacerations.

   Blades and needles are never discarded loose in trash receptacles. These sharp items should be enclosed and secured so they cannot perforate the receptacle. A self-closing adhesive pad designed for this purpose is the safest device to use. Needles can cut through adhesive tape or puncture paper cups, boxes, or suture and blade packets. Sharps in these containers create a hazard. A safe disposal procedure should be implemented and cleaning procedures adhered to.

   a. Remove knife blades from handles. Point the blade toward table away from yourself and other persons in area so if it breaks or slips, it will not fly across the room. Remove blades with a heavy needleholder; *never use fingers.* Never put knife handles in an instrument tray with blades left on them. Other instruments designed for replaceable cutting blades should have blades removed; thereafter they may be handled with other instruments.
   b. Place reusable surgical needles, either on a needle rack or loose, into a perforated box to be terminally sterilized with the instruments. Check the suture book to see that it is not discarded with needles in it.
   c. Place reusable needles used for injection or aspiration in a perforated box with surgical needles. Include those used by the anesthesiologist. Do not attempt to recap them.

   NOTE Whether or not disposable sharps should be terminally sterilized before discarding depends on state regulations or institutional policy. Follow accepted procedure. Steam sterilization in a gravity displacement sterilizer is not possible in a sealed container. The container must allow penetration of steam but also retain its puncture-resistant properties.

7. Remove blood, tissue, bone, and any other gross debris from instruments. *All* instruments, used and unused, must be cleaned, terminally sterilized, or undergo high-level disinfection before they are handled for definitive cleaning and checked for proper functioning before reuse. Instruments should be presoaked and/or prerinsed before processing in a washer-sterilizer or decontaminator. If a mechanical washer is not available, instruments are carefully washed and rinsed by hand and then sterilized or disinfected. Any biologic material remaining on instruments is more difficult to remove after they have been heat-sterilized because it becomes baked on them. The biologic debris inhibits sterilization and disinfection processes. See Chapter 14, pp. 254-257, for a detailed discussion of procedures for dismantling instrument table and for cleaning instruments immediately after the surgical procedure is completed.
8. Load instrument tray with heavy instruments in the bottom. All hinged instruments are opened to expose maximum surface area, including box locks. Instruments designed to be disassembled are taken apart. Carefully space instruments to prevent contact of sharp edges or points with other instruments. Concave surfaces should be turned down.
9. Wash, rinse, and *dry* instruments that cannot be immersed in water or steam sterilized. These instruments are wrapped or placed in closed container

sterilization cases for sterilization in ethylene oxide gas or other agent.

10. Wash, rinse, and *dry* items before immersing them in chemical solution for *high-level disinfection*. Items other than disposables that cannot be sterilized should be disinfected by a process that kills or destroys pathogenic microorganisms, including spores and viruses. Items may include some of the anesthesia equipment (see Chapter 17, pp. 342-343).
11. Put glass syringes, medicine glasses, and other glassware, including those used by the anesthesiologist, into a separate tray. Syringes are separated. Check for disposables and discard them in the trash *without* needles.
12. Place reusable, nondisposable rubber goods and plastic items into tray with instruments if they can be terminally steam sterilized in a washer-sterilizer or decontaminator. They may not be heat stable.
13. Suction detergent-disinfectant solution through lumen of reusable tubing. Thorough cleaning of lumen is difficult to accomplish if biologic debris becomes dry. If reusable tubing is used, it should be wrapped separately for further processing. Disposable suction tubing is recommended and is discarded with other infectious waste.
14. Invert small basins and solution cups over the instruments. Basins and trays too large for the washer-sterilizer or standard instrument sterilizer are washed, dried, and put into plastic bags for transport to the decontamination area. The Mayo tray may be included.
15. Dispose of solutions and suction bottle contents in a flushing hopper connected to a sanitary sewer. Disposable suction units simplify disposal. Wall suction units should be disconnected by the circulator to avoid contamination of the wall outlet. If disposable units are not used, decontaminate contents with disinfectant before hopper disposal. Wash the container. Thoroughly wash plunger and other areas of wall-mounted suction apparatus. Containers are sterilized along with basins and trays.
16. Put instrument trays in washer-sterilizer or decontaminator and/or steam sterilizer, if this equipment is in an adjacent substerile room. The circulator opens doors for the scrub person. If equipment is not in a room that is immediately adjacent, trays should be enclosed in plastic bags to keep instruments moist during transport to the decontamination area in the OR suite or to the central decontamination area on the case cart. The circulator assists with bagging to keep outside clean.
17. Discard all used disposable table drapes in a plastic bag with used disposable patient drapes. Even if they are not obviously soiled, all reusable woven fabric drapes from open packs should be subjected to laundering to replace moisture lost to fabric by sterilization. Therefore, put unused along with used reusable woven fabric drapes in a laundry hamper to be sent to the laundry.
18. Remove gown before removing gloves. The circulator unfastens neck and back closures. Protect arms and scrub clothes from the contaminated outside of gown. Grasp right shoulder of gown with left hand and, in pulling gown off arm, turn sleeve inside out. Turn outside of gown away from body with a flexed elbow. Then grasp other shoulder with other hand and remove gown entirely, pulling it off inside out. Discard gown in a laundry hamper or in a trash receptacle if it is disposable (see Figure 11-22, p. 180).

    To remove gloves, use a glove-to-glove, then skin-to-skin technique to protect clean hands from the contaminated outside of gloves, which bear cells of patient. Gloves are turned inside out as they are removed and are then discarded into trash (see Figure 11-23, p. 180). Wash hands after removing gloves.

By Team

After the patient leaves, the circulator is free to assist with cleanup of the room. Nursing assistants and/or housekeeping personnel may also be available to assist with cleaning. Regardless of which member of the team performs them, specific functions should be carried out to complete room cleanup. The personnel and areas considered contaminated during and after the surgical procedure are:

1. Members of sterile team, until they have discarded their gowns, gloves, caps, masks, and shoe covers (these items remain in the contaminated area; scrub clothes are changed if they are wet or contaminated)
2. All furniture, equipment, and floor within and around perimeter of sterile field; if accidental spillage has occurred in other parts of the room, then these areas are also considered contaminated
3. All anesthesia equipment
4. Stretchers used to transport patients; these should be cleaned after each patient use

Clean, but not sterile, gloves are worn to complete the room cleanup. The scrub person changes gloves after the sterile field is dismantled. Decontamination of environment includes:

1. *Furniture.* Wash horizontal surfaces of all tables and equipment, including anesthesia machine, with a disinfectant solution. Apply disinfectant from a squeeze-bottle dispenser, and wipe with a clean cloth or a disposable wipe that is changed frequently. Spray bottles can cause particles to become aerosolized and should be avoided. All surfaces of mattress, pads, and screw connections of the operating table are included. Mobile furniture can be pushed

through disinfectant solution used for floor care to clean casters.

2. *Overhead operating light.* Overhead light reflectors should be wiped using a clean cloth wet with disinfectant solution. Commercial reflector cleaner also is useful for this purpose. Lights and overhead tracks become contaminated quickly and present a possible hazard from fallout of microorganisms onto sterile surfaces or into wounds during surgical procedures.
3. *Anesthesia equipment.* All reusable anesthesia masks and tubing are *cleaned and sterilized before reusing.* Some of this equipment can be steam sterilized; if not, it may be sterilized by ethylene oxide gas and aerated before reuse. If this method is not available, items should be chemically sterilized according to the sterilant manufacturer's recommendations.
4. *Laundry.* After all cleaning procedures have been completed, cleaning cloths should be discarded or put in a laundry bag if they are not disposable. When all reusable woven fabric items, used and unused, have been placed inside the laundry bag, it is closed securely. To help protect laundry personnel, an alginate bag that dissolves in hot water may be used as the primary laundry bag or as a liner within a cloth bag. Reusable woven fabrics soiled with blood or body fluids are transported in leakproof bags.
5. *Trash.* All trash is collected in plastic or impervious bags, including disposable drapes, kick bucket, and wastebasket liners. Bags should be sturdy to resist bursting or tearing during transport. Trash can be separated into infectious waste, noninfectious trash, and recyclable items. Separate receptacles should be available.

NOTE Double-bagging of laundry and trash is not necessary unless outside of bag has been contaminated. Disposition of potentially infectious waste must comply with local, state, and/or federal regulations for contamination control measures. Appropriately labeled and color-coded leakproof bags for infectious waste and puncture-resistant containers for sharps should be used.

6. *Floors.* Wet-vacuuming with a filter-diffuser exhaust cleaner is the method of choice for floor care in the OR. Machine cleaning is more effective than manual cleaning. If suture material and gross soilage on the floor is great, wet-vacuum equipment may be used dry for the first treatment. The floor is then flooded, half of the room at a time, with a detergent-disinfectant solution. This solution may be dispensed from a pump spray or automatic spraying device attached to a central wet-vacuum equipment system. If portable equipment is used, a spray-type watering can may be used to flood floor, although this method is slower and may wet it unevenly. Hot water may hasten the biocidal action of the disinfectant agent but may also soften tile adhesive. Room-temperature water requires at least a 5-minute contact time for effectiveness.

   Furniture is rolled across the flooded floor area to clean casters. The wet-vacuum pickup is used to pick up solution before furniture is repositioned. Standing platforms are considered part of the floor and may be flooded with solution to be picked up by wet vacuum.

   Exterior of vacuum equipment and tubing is cleaned following each use, with special attention given to cleaning the rubber blade before the next use. If the hose is equipped with a brush attachment, this is washed and sterilized between uses.

   If wet-vacuum equipment is not available, freshly laundered, clean mops can be used. The floor can be flooded with detergent-disinfectant solution. One mop is used to apply solution and one to take up solution. Following *one-time use,* mop heads are removed and placed in a laundry hamper with other contaminated reusable woven fabrics. Mop handles may be stored in the housekeeping storage area until they are needed again. Clean mops and disinfectant solution are used for each cleanup procedure.
7. *Walls.* If walls are splashed with blood or organic debris during the surgical procedure, those areas should be washed. Otherwise, walls are not considered contaminated and need not be washed between surgical procedures.

Cart System Cleanup

All reusable instruments, basins, supplies, and equipment, including suction bottles, are put on or inside case cart. The cart is covered or closed and taken to the central decontamination area outside the OR suite for cleanup. A closed cart, especially if it has been used as the instrument table, is wiped off with a disinfectant solution before it is taken out of the room. A cart with contaminated supplies should be removed from the OR suite via the outer corridor if this is the design of the suite. If dumbwaiters are used, a separate one is provided for the contaminated cart. Clean and contaminated supplies are always kept separated.

The cart is designed to go through an automatic steam cart washer or a manual power wash for terminal cleaning after it is emptied and before it is restocked with clean and sterile supplies.

Room Ready for Next Patient

The cleaning procedures described provide adequate decontamination and terminal sterilization following any surgical procedure. With a well-coordinated team, minimal turnover time between surgical procedures can be accomplished; in an average time of 15 to 20 minutes the room will be ready for the next patient. *Turnover time* includes cleaning up after one procedure and setting up for the next procedure.

DAILY TERMINAL CLEANING

In Operating Room

At completion of day's schedule, each OR, whether or not it was used that day, should be terminally cleaned. Additional and more rigorous cleaning is done in all areas already discussed for cleanup between surgical procedures.

1. *Furniture* is thoroughly scrubbed, with mechanical friction in addition to chemical disinfection. Disinfectants are only adjuncts to good physical cleaning; "elbow grease" is probably the most important ingredient.
2. *Casters and wheels* should be cleaned and kept free of suture ends and debris. Equipment is available that automatically washes stretchers, tables, and platforms and then steam cleans and dries them within a matter of minutes.
3. *Equipment,* such as electrosurgical units, should be cleaned with care so as not to saturate surfaces to the degree that disinfectant solution runs into the mechanism, causing malfunction and requiring repairs.
4. *Ceiling- and wall-mounted fixtures and tracks* are cleaned on all surfaces.
5. *Kick buckets, laundry hamper frames, and other waste receptacles* are cleaned and disinfected; these items are sterilized when feasible.
6. *Floors* are given a thorough wet-vacuum cleaning with wet-vacuum pickup used dry and then wet.
7. *Walls and ceilings* should be checked for soil spots and cleaned as necessary.
8. *Cabinets and doors* should be cleaned, especially around handles or push plates where contamination is common.

Outside Operating Room Itself

1. *Countertops and sinks* in the substerile room should be cleaned. The outer surface of the sterilizer, including the top, should be washed.
2. *Scrub sinks and spray heads* on faucets should undergo thorough cleaning daily. A mild abrasive on sinks removes the oily film residue left by scrub antiseptics. Spray heads, faucet aerators, or sprinklers should be removed and disassembled, if possible, for thorough cleaning and sterilization of parts. Contaminated faucet aerators and sprinklers can transfer organisms directly to hands or items washed under them. *Scrub sinks should not be used for routine cleaning purposes.*
3. *Soap dispensers* should be disassembled, cleaned, and terminally sterilized, if possible, before they are refilled with antiseptic solution. These dispensers can become reservoirs for microorganisms.
4. *Walls around scrub sinks* should receive daily attention. Spray and splash from scrubbing cause buildup of antiseptic soap film around the sink. This film should be removed.
5. *Transportation and storage carts* need to be cleaned with specific attention to wheels and casters.
6. *Cleaning equipment* should be disassembled and cleaned before storage.

WEEKLY OR MONTHLY CLEANING

A weekly or monthly cleaning routine is set up, in addition to the daily cleaning schedule, by the director of environmental/housekeeping services and the OR manager. Any routines for housekeeping are based on physical construction of the department. However, if specific schedules are not established, some areas could be inadvertently missed. Areas to be considered are:

1. *Walls.* Walls should be cleaned when they become visibly soiled. If they are painted or tiled with wide porous grouting, these factors should be considered in planning cleaning routines. Washing walls in the OR and throughout the suite once a week is reasonable, but less frequent time intervals for cleaning may be acceptable if spot disinfection is performed on a daily basis. This requires adequate continuous supervision.
2. *Ceilings.* Ceilings may require regular special cleaning techniques because of mounted tracks and lighting fixtures. The types of fixtures are considered in planning cleaning routines.
3. *Floors.* Floors throughout the OR suite should be machine-scrubbed periodically to remove accumulated deposits and films. Conductive flooring should never be waxed. Rounded corners and edges facilitate cleaning.
4. *Air-conditioning grills.* The exterior of air-conditioning grills should be vacuumed at least weekly. Additional cleaning is necessary when filters are checked and changed.
5. *Storage shelves.* Storage cabinets have been replaced in many OR suites by portable storage carts. Storage areas should be cleaned at least weekly or more often, if necessary, to control accumulation of dust, especially in sterile storage areas.
6. *Sterilizers.* All types of sterilizers should be cleaned regularly as recommended by the manufacturer.
7. *Exchange/vestibular and peripheral support areas.* Walls, ceilings, floors, air-conditioning grills, lockers, cabinets, and furniture should be cleaned on a regular schedule.

CONSIDERATIONS FOR USE OF DISPOSABLE PRODUCTS

Disposable products can be useful in the OR. It is sometimes easier to discard a contaminated item after use than to clean and process it. The use of disposables has become popular, but consideration of the logistics of using them includes determination of the benefits and/or consequences of their use. The production of disposable products often involves the use of natural resources and potential industrial damage to the earth's environment. Disposal of the contaminated item can pose similar problems. Many issues concerning economy including labor costs, storage, delivery, and disposal need to be evaluated on an individual basis. Economy may or may not be shown with the use of disposables.

Pros and Cons of Disposables

A disposable product is *used once* with assurance of safety and effectiveness. It is not salvaged after use; *it is discarded.* The cost of adequately and safely processing supplies is high. This high cost has led to the purchase of many disposable supplies for "one-time" patient use. Some of these are "patient-charge" items, meaning that the cost of these items is added to the patient's bill. Use of patient-charge items requires specific and accurate recordkeeping. It also requires evaluation of the advantages and disadvantages of disposable products to justify the cost to the patient.

Advantages of Disposables

1. When a sterile item is required, proper packaging and sterility must be assured. Sterility is guaranteed by reliable manufacturers as long as the integrity of their packages is maintained. Industry conforms to far more rigid standards of quality control than on-site conditions permit. All sterilized products are tested for sterility before they are distributed to purchasers.
2. Single-use items, such as catheters, are aesthetically more acceptable to patients. More important, disposable products eliminate a potential source of cross contamination.
3. Items such as needles and safety razors ensure more comfort for the patient because they are always new and sharp. Proper function is thus ensured.
4. Standardized service at reduced cost per unit may be provided. Sponges are precounted and sterilized, for example. Packs and trays become standardized and can be customized.
5. Loss and breakage in reprocessing reusable items are eliminated.
6. Labor costs of processing supplies are reduced, particularly in the tedious, meticulous cleaning and packaging of small items, such as needles and syringes.
7. The need for expensive mechanical cleaning equipment is reduced or eliminated.
8. Contaminated used items can be contained for safe disposal. Handling and processing are eliminated.

Disadvantages of Disposables

1. Costly waste occurs if sterile items are contaminated or unnecessarily opened. Extreme care is needed in opening packages to maintain sterility. Handling should not compromise the integrity of wrappings. Even though sterility of products from reliable manufacturers can be assured, their handling and storing may pose a threat to the maintenance of this sterility.
2. Flexibility in complying with requests of individual physicians for special setups is compromised. No allowance is made for deviation from commercially supplied packs or trays, unless customized kits are purchased. Procedures may need to be revised to conform to available items and sets.
3. If a defect is found in one package, it may extend throughout the total lot, requiring replacement of the total supply on hand.
4. Circulator may have to open an increased number of individually packaged items. Some disposable plastic products melt; they cannot be put into instrument sets before steam sterilization.
5. In the event of a disaster or a sudden increase in use, adequate inventory may not be readily available.
6. Expiration date may be required for a potentially unstable product after prolonged storage, such as some disposable trays with medications in them. Unless oldest products are used first, unnecessary costs are incurred if a product is discarded because its time of reliability has expired. All dated products should be routinely checked for expiration.

Other Considerations

Some considerations regarding the use of disposable products that can be argued pro or con include:

1. *Direct labor costs.* Some hospitals have saved money by reducing their labor force through conversion to as many total-disposable systems as possible, such as intravenous therapy, drapes, and special procedure trays. In some geographic areas where efficient labor may be readily available at minimum wage, disposables become more costly than labor. If professional personnel had been used for reprocessing supplies, use of disposable products releases them to give more care to patients and less time to "things."
2. *Storage.* Proper and safe storage facilities should be provided. More storage space or more frequent deliveries may be required to maintain adequate inventories of disposable products.

3. *Disposal.* Disposal may be an ecologic problem. Used items are taken to an incinerator, compactor, or other safe waste-disposal area. Waste should not be allowed to accumulate in the OR suite or in other hospital areas.

Reusing/Reprocessing Disposable Products

Manufacturers use extensive controls and testing procedures to ensure cleanliness, nontoxicity, nonpyrogenicity, biocompatibility, sterility, and function of disposable products. All items must be safe and effective for their intended patient uses. The manufacturer guarantees product stability and sterility for a single use only.

In this era of cost containment, salvage of undamaged disposable items may be attempted. The risks of salvaging items should be evaluated seriously. The health care facility assumes legal responsibility for items it chooses to reuse, reprocess, and resterilize. The manufacturer cannot be held liable for the efficacy of a disposable product or one intended for single use if the user chooses to reprocess it. The burden of liability rests with the processor.

Reuse

Reuse of a *used* disposable single-use item requires cleaning, packaging, and sterilizing, if it will be reused as a sterile item. Some products degrade with use. Many manufacturers have not tested their products for more than one use. To reuse a product, the product should be tested to validate patient safety.

Reprocessing

Repackaging and resterilizing *unused* sterile disposable items may be potentially hazardous. These are items that were opened and not needed, or they are clean but were contaminated in some way (i.e., the original packaging is not intact). Many of these items are very expensive, and salvage seems to be an acceptable alternative. The manufacturer must provide written instructions for resterilization of unused but contaminated items by on-site personnel. Many of these items are heat sensitive. Services that rewrap and resterilize some types of clean unused and undamaged products are available. Such services must guarantee product stability and sterility.

Resterilization

Unopened sterile products may be combined so that only one sterile package or procedural tray needs to be opened rather than many single packages. Or an unsterile part of an item may need to be sterilized for use on the sterile field. The sterilization process must not alter the characteristics of any part of the product. Some products are labeled "do not resterilize." This instruction means that the product will be damaged in the process of resterilization. Manufacturer's recommendations should be followed.

Safety Considerations

Patient safety should be the prime concern in the decision to reuse, reprocess, or resterilize a disposable item. Several questions should be answered.

1. Is the item a noncritical/noninvasive device? Critical items, particularly those that will enter or be in contact with the bloodstream or mucous membranes, present the greatest risks of possible adverse effects. Cleaning of these items should not be attempted.
2. Is the item clean? Many porous materials cannot be thoroughly cleaned after use. If these are not adequately cleaned, microbial growth can predispose patients to infection. Lumens of catheters and tubings are especially difficult to clean. Biologic debris, which interferes with the sterilization process, must be mechanically removed, for example, with a brush that is capable of cleaning the entire length of a lumen.
3. Is the item nontoxic or nonpyrogenic after cleaning and reprocessing? Residues from some cleaning compounds and ethylene oxide (EO) gas are toxic. Water can contain pyrogens. Microorganisms can produce endotoxins. Aeration is required following EO sterilization.
4. Is the item sterile? The sterilization method should be appropriate for materials in the item and in the packaging. The packaging material should allow penetration of the sterilant to all surfaces of the item and should prevent contamination during storage. Sterility should be verified by biologic testing for each type of product that is resterilized.
5. Is the integrity of the product maintained? Physical and/or chemical characteristics may be altered by cleaning agents, the cleaning process, or resterilization. Some materials deteriorate or become brittle, which can affect function.
6. Is the number of times an item has been reprocessed known and controlled? Although this is rare, a manufacturer's written instructions may include the number of times the product may safely be reused or sterilized. The user should ensure that this number is not exceeded. The manufacturer has no control after a product is purchased. If the item is not in its original package, it obviously has been reprocessed. Remember, disposables are intended for single use only.
7. Is the item traceable? Reprocessing of implantable synthetic mesh or graft material should be controlled by lot numbers. The lot number on the product when first obtained from the manufacturer corresponds only with the processes at the point of controlled production. If the product is re-

processed on-site the lot number is no longer valid because the same controls were not in place for subsequent sterilization. Many variables can alter the safety of the product for reuse.

Unless the answer to these questions is a definitive *yes*, the item should not be reused. With or without written instructions from the manufacturer, the health care facility is liable for product stability and sterility of any item it processes and sterilizes.

Custom Packs

A custom pack is a preassembled collection of disposable supplies sterilized as a single unit. The components are specified by the user (i.e., the OR's specifications), for a particular procedure or specialty or a surgeon's preferences. These components are assembled and sterilized by a custom pack supplier or the manufacturer. A pack assembled by a manufacturer will have an assortment of products in a specific category, such as a kit of sutures, ligating clips, and skin staplers or a custom pack of disposable drapes. Many custom packs have approximately a hundred diversified items needed for a specific type of surgical procedure, such as an open heart pack. Care should be taken in handling packs because damage to or contamination of a custom pack may waste many sterile items.

The assembler sterilizes packs with either EO gas or gamma irradiation. All components of the pack must be compatible with the sterilization method. The assembler must adhere to government manufacturing regulations for testing to guarantee product stability and sterility and package integrity.

Using custom packs may be cost-effective for the health care facility. These indirect savings are shared by the materiels management department and the OR.

1. Personnel time (labor costs) for handling supplies is reduced.
   a. Reduces turnover time between procedures by saving time spent gathering and opening supplies. Circulator has more time for direct patient care activities. This may be critical for a trauma patient.
   b. Reduces setup time for scrub person. Items can be prearranged in order of use and with components in proximity, such as suction tubing with tip.
   c. Facilitates transport of supplies into storage or into a case cart system.
2. Storage space requirements are consolidated by storing supplies in bulk rather than individually.
3. Inventory control is facilitated.
   a. Simplifies listing of items in inventory. The supplier may maintain a computerized information system of usage and inventory levels.
   b. Reduces inventory. A minimal backup of supplies can be maintained.
   c. Reduces lost patient charges. Circulator can process one charge for the custom pack rather than itemizing items.
4. Standardization is encouraged by incorporating the basic items routinely used by surgeon(s) into custom packs. This helps to standardize preparations.
5. Infection rate may be decreased. The physical activity of opening supplies can disperse lint and dust into the air. Opening fewer packages decreases this potential environmental hazard.
6. Less environmental waste is generated by packaging material. Fewer disposable wrappers are used.

Many custom pack processors have addressed the problem of changes in surgeon's preferences by offering to supply the packs in small quantities. Changes are incorporated into new stock, thus decreasing the number of pack contents that may not be used. Some manufacturers will replace older or damaged packs for new stock. Evaluation of pack usefulness is ongoing and may change as the types and complexity of surgical procedures change.

RECYCLING

Many surgical supplies are recyclable. Recycling reduces not only the amount of waste in landfills or air pollution but also the amount of virgin resources that are consumed. Paper wrappers and many plastic items that are noninfectious, nonregulated trash can and should be recycled. Recycling in the OR should be an integral part of the overall recycling program of the health care facility. Consideration of recycling potential can be part of the evaluation process in selecting products.

PRODUCT EVALUATION

The user of a product is best qualified to evaluate performance, safety, effectiveness, and efficiency. Before a decision is made to purchase or to standardize a particular item, a clinical evaluation should be conducted to solicit feedback from team members whose work will be affected by the product. This may involve the surgeons or anesthesiologists as well as OR nurses and surgical technologists. Instruction should be provided on the correct use of the item before it is evaluated. To be valid, feedback should be an objective evaluation of function, quality, and use. Does it meet a need? Does it solve a problem? How does it compare with other brands? Several brands of the same product may be evaluated to select the most satisfactory one for the intended purpose and to standardize the inventory.

Many products are used only in the OR; others are also used in other patient care areas. Representatives from all user departments should assist the materiels manager in the selection of products. Most hospitals have a product evaluation committee for this purpose. A representative of the OR staff provides this committee with information regarding quality and effectiveness, on feedback from user staff members.

Once a product has been purchased, the user assumes responsibility for its safety and its proper use for the purpose for which it is intended.

Bibliography

Botsford J, Hixon SK: AORN Special Committee on Environmental Issues reports environmental survey results, *AORN J* 60(4):652-655, 1994.

Breault L, Smith G: Secrets to effective cost management: reduce, recycle, reuse, *Surg Technol* 26(12):18-20, 1994.

Dysart J: Rethinking the earth, *Can Nurse* 86(7):16-17, 1990.

French HM: Blueprint for reducing, reusing, recycling, *AORN J* 60(1):94-98, 1994.

Greaves J: Healthcare and the environment, *Br J Theatre Nurs* 4(3):14-16, 1994.

McVeigh P: The greening of the OR, *AORN J* 56(6):1040-1045, 1992.

O'Neale M: Clinical issues: environmental issues concerning sterile reprocessing, disposal practices, recycling, *AORN J* 55(2):606-609, 1992.

Paech M: Challenging healthcare economics and technology to save the environment, *Int Nurs Rev* 38(4):111-114, 1991.

Pitts CA: Commentary on product evaluation as a research utilization strategy, *Emerg Care* 3(3):14, 1993.

Proposed recommended practices: product evaluation and selection for the perioperative setting, *AORN J* 58(2):357-362, 1993. (Adopted in 1994.)

Raltz S et al: The impact of disposable equipment on room fee reimbursement for endoscopic retrograde cholangio-pancreatography, *Gastroenterol Nurs* 17(1):14-16, 1994.

Recommended practices: environmental responsibility in the practice setting, *AORN J* 58(4):789-795, 1993.

Recommended practices: sanitation in the surgical practice setting, *AORN J* 56(6):1089-1095, 1992.

Richardson M: The standard guide to green nursing: 20 tips to protect the environment, *Nurs Stand* 8(18):50-52, 1994.

Robinson JA: OR time delays: a time management plan that works, *AORN J* 58(2):329-335, 1993.

Weatherly KS et al: Product evaluation process: a systems approach to controlling health care costs, *AORN J* 59(2):489-498, 1994.

SECTION TEN

Surgical Specialties

CHAPTER 28

Diagnostic Procedures

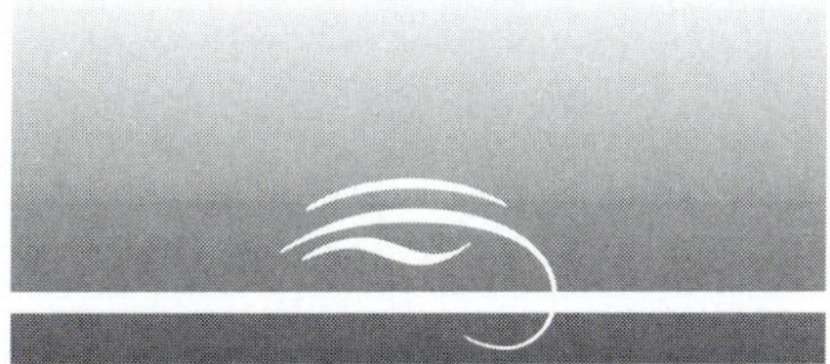

Diagnosis of a pathologic disease, anomaly, or traumatic injury is established before a surgical procedure is undertaken. Many modalities and techniques assist surgeons to assess each individual patient problem, to guide them through the surgical procedure, and to verify results of surgical intervention. The term *diagnosis* refers to the art or the act of determining the nature of a patient's disease. Diagnostic procedures, as discussed in this chapter, include procedures that pertain to establishing a diagnosis or serving as evidence in diagnosis and surgical treatment of pathologic conditions. They will be classified as:

1. *Preoperative*—procedures performed before the patient comes to the operating room (OR) suite or performed in the OR before incision
2. *Intraoperative*—procedures performed in the OR as a part of the surgical procedure
3. *Noninvasive*—techniques using equipment placed on or near the patient's skin but outside body tissues
4. *Invasive*—techniques using equipment placed into a body cavity or vessel and/or substances injected into body structures

Preoperative diagnostic procedures may be noninvasive or invasive; likewise, intraoperative procedures use both techniques. Perioperative nurses and surgical technologists should be familiar with the modalities and equipment necessary to assist with diagnostic procedures. Seven broad categories of modalities are used in diagnosis:

1. *Pathology*—branch of biologic science that deals with the nature of disease through study of its causes, process, and effects (e.g., biopsy, cytology, and histology)
2. *Radiology*—branch of medicine that deals with x-rays, radioactive substances, and ionizing radiations for diagnosis and treatment (e.g., radiographs, scanning, and fluoroscopy)
3. *Magnetic resonance imaging*—use of radio-frequency energy for identifying abnormalities in anatomic structures (e.g., a brain scan)
4. *Positron emission tomography*—form of nuclear imaging used for measuring biochemistry and physiology (e.g., brain and heart scans)
5. *Ultrasonography*—use of sonic energy for studying pulse-echo alterations of anatomic structure (e.g., vascular disease)
6. *Endoscopy*—visual examination of the interior of a body cavity or viscus (e.g., bronchoscopy)
7. *Plethysmography*—measurement of changes in the volume of an extremity or organ caused by blood flow (e.g., oculoplethysmography)
8. *Sensory evoked potentials*—measurement of somatosensory, visual, and/or auditory nerve pathways (e.g., auditory brainstem evoked potential)

PATHOLOGY

Clinical pathology is the use of laboratory methods to establish a clinical diagnosis of the nature of disease. *Sur-*

gical pathology is the study of alterations in body tissues removed by surgical intervention. Methods to obtain tissue and fluid specimens for pathologic examination are always invasive.

Preoperative Pathologic Studies

Preoperatively the surgeon may perform a diagnostic procedure to obtain tissue or fluid samples before scheduling further definitive surgical intervention.

Biopsy

Tissue or fluid removed for diagnosis is referred to as a *biopsy*. The pathologist confirms the diagnosis by histologic and cytologic analysis, the study of cells.

Aspiration Biopsy Fluid is aspirated through a needle placed in a lesion, such as a cyst or abscess, or in a joint or body cavity.

Bone Marrow Biopsy Through a small skin incision or percutaneous puncture, a trocar puncture needle or aspiration needle is placed into bone, usually the sternum or iliac crest, to aspirate bone marrow.

Excision Biopsy Tissue is cut from the body. The surgeon may remove tissue through an incision in mucous membrane. This procedure may be done through an endoscopic instrument. Localization of a lesion in soft tissue (such as the breast) that is to be incised through a skin incision may be guided by xeroradiography or ultrasonography.

Percutaneous Needle Biopsy Tissue is obtained from an internal organ or solid mass by means of a hollow needle inserted through the body wall. Percutaneous puncture into a lesion may be guided by fluoroscopy under image intensification, ultrasound, or computed tomography. Special needles are used; some types are disposable.

1. *Dorsey cannula* resembles a ventricular needle except that it is a bit larger and the end is open. It is used, sometimes through a burr hole, to remove a sample of brain tissue for biopsy.
2. *Franklin-Silverman* biopsy needle is used for obtaining biopsy specimens of thyroid, liver, kidney, prostate, and other organs. It has a 14-gauge thin-wall outer cannula with a beveled obturator. An inner split needle fits into the outer cannula and protrudes beyond the end of it. The distal tips of this split needle are grooved inside. They enter tissue, close on the specimen, and trap it as the needle is withdrawn.
3. *Bernardino-Sones* or a disposable *Chiba* biopsy needle is inserted through chest wall to obtain a biopsy of the lung. This procedure is usually guided by computed tomography to avoid a pneumothorax.

Fine-needle aspiration biopsies are most commonly done to obtain cells from solid lesions in the breast, thyroid, neck, lymph nodes, or soft tissues. Needles may be from 20 to 25 gauge. The needle is manipulated in the mass while suction is placed on the syringe.

Intraoperative Pathologic Studies

Tissue or fluid specimens may be removed immediately before or during the surgical procedure for pathologic examination to determine further therapy.

Cultures

Frank pus is removed from an abscess and may be encountered in other known or suspected areas of infection. Drainage is cultured to enable surgeon to effectively prescribe antibiotics. (See Chapter 20, pp. 421-422, for handling culture specimens during the surgical procedure.)

Frozen Section

Special preparation and examination of tissue can determine whether it is malignant and whether regional nodes are involved. When surgeon removes a piece of tissue and wants an immediate diagnosis, it is placed in a basin or specimen container without any added preservative such as formalin or normal saline solution. Formalin or normal saline solution will alter the freezing process used in the specialized pathologic study. The circulator should alert the pathologist that his or her services will be needed. In some facilities the pathologist comes to the OR suite to do a frozen section, which takes only a few minutes. When the tissue examination is complete, the pathologist will report the results directly to the surgeon in the OR. The patient's consciousness level should be considered during report of pathologic results, especially if the patient is awake. If a malignant lesion is present and the individual situation calls for it, the surgeon proceeds with a radical resection of the affected organ or body area.

Surgical Specimens

All tissue removed during the surgical procedure is sent to the pathology laboratory for verification of diagnosis. (See Chapter 20 for discussion of care of tissue specimens by scrub person, pp. 416-417, and circulator, pp. 421-422.)

Tissue specimens may be stored in a refrigerator in the laboratory or in some other location within the OR suite until they are taken to the pathology department at the end of or at intervals during each day's schedule of surgical procedures. Correct solutions for storage and correct labeling of specimens are critical for accurate diagnosis. Table 28-1 lists types of pathologic specimens.

TABLE 28-1

Pathologic Specimens

TEST	PREPARATION	EXAMPLE
Fluid		
Bacteriology	Anaerobic or aerobic on culture swab in sterile tube	Exudate
Virology	Fresh, in sterile container	Cerebrospinal fluid
Cytology	Fresh or added solution of pathologist's choice in sterile container	Cell washings, urine
Genetic studies	Fresh, in sterile container	Amniotic fluid
Cell count	Fresh, in sterile container	Semen for infertility study
Tissue		
Permanent section	Fresh or added solution of pathologist's choice in sterile container	Diseased organ
Frozen section	Fresh, in sterile container	Margin of malignant lesion
Biopsy	Fresh or solution of pathologist's choice in sterile container	Suspicious lesion
Hormonal assay	Fresh, in sterile container	Breast tissue
Donor tissue	Fresh or added solution of pathologist's choice	Cadaver skin
Calculi	Dry, in sterile container	Gallstone
Ova	Fresh or added solution of surgeon's choice	Human egg for preservation
Muscle	Fresh, extended in special clamp in sterile container	Test for malignant hyperthermia
Nonbiologic specimen		
Foreign body	Fresh, in sterile container	Glass fragments
Projectile from crime scene	Dry, in nonmetalic container	Bullet
Clothing of crime or accident victim	Dry, in porous paper	Underclothes of rape victim
Explanted prosthesis	Dry, in sterile container	Orthopaedic screws or plates

RADIOLOGY

In 1895 Wilhelm Conrad Roentgen discovered x-rays. An *x-ray* is a high-energy electromagnetic wave capable of penetrating various thicknesses of solid substances and affecting photographic plates. X-rays are generated on a vacuum tube when high-velocity electrons from a heated filament strike a metal target (anode), causing it to emit x-rays. The photograph obtained by the use of x-rays may be referred to as an *x-ray film, roentgenogram, radiograph,* or other "-gram" name associated either with the specific technique used to obtain the photograph or with the anatomic structures identified (e.g., mammogram). At first x-rays were used mainly for localization of foreign bodies or visualization of fractures. Today x-rays are also used for diagnostic imaging with fluoroscopy, developed in the 1950s, the scanning techniques of computed tomography introduced in the early 1970s, and digital radiography of the 1980s. Filmless radiologic images may be stored in computerized form if a digital imaging system, developed in the 1990s, is available.

As the science of radiology has advanced, the diagnosis of disease in all surgical specialties has progressed. The treatment to be followed frequently is based on radiologic findings.

Noninvasive Preoperative Studies

The following noninvasive radiologic studies are performed in the radiology department preoperatively. The surgeon may request that the x-ray films or radiographs be sent to the OR for reference during the surgical procedure.

Chest X-Ray Film

Most surgeons consider a chest x-ray film as an extension of the patient's history and physical examination, even though chest disease is not associated with the patient's clinical symptoms. An x-ray study of the chest may be part of the admission procedure for elective surgical patients to rule out unsuspected pulmonary disease that could be communicable or would contraindicate the use of inhalation anesthetics. This procedure may be routine for patients over 40 years of age. It is always a part of the diagnostic work-up in patients with suspected or symptomatic pulmonary abnormalities.

Mammography

A technique for projecting an x-ray image of soft tissue of the breast, mammography is the most effective screening method for early diagnosis of small, nonpalpable breast tumors. Three views of each breast are exposed to conventional x-rays. The procedure may be somewhat painful for the woman because compression is needed for radiologic imaging. Tumors appear on the mammogram as opaque spiculated areas or, occasionally, as areas of punctate calcification.

A needle biopsy device may be used in conjunction with mammography to obtain a tissue specimen from a lesion seen on the mammogram. This technique is called a *mammographic breast biopsy.*

Xeroradiography

For xeroradiography the patient is positioned between an x-ray source and a photosensitive aluminum plate that has an electrically charged selenium surface. The pattern of the charge remaining on plate after exposure to x-ray beam corresponds to densities of tissues and amount of radiation absorbed. A negatively charged blue toner powder is dusted on the plate. A pale blue-on-white image is transferred by photoconduction rapidly and permanently to a sheet of plastic-coated paper. Xeroradiography minimizes radiation exposure, is performed rapidly, and produces detailed images that are easier to interpret than on x-ray film. It is used for diagnosis of disease in anatomic structures such as breast, bone, and larynx and for detection of foreign bodies in soft tissue.

Tomography

In tomography an x-ray beam moves across the body in one direction, usually an arc, to photograph structures in a selected plane of tissue. The roentgenograms show details of structures within this single plane while blurring images above and below the selected plane.

Computed Tomography

In computed tomography special complex and expensive equipment uses an x-ray beam in conjunction with a computer. Because the x-ray beam moves back and forth across the body to project cross-sectional images, the technique is referred to as *computed tomography (CT), computed axial tomography (CAT),* or simply *scanning.* It produces a highly contrasted, detailed study of normal and pathologic anatomy. The x-ray tube and photomultiplier detectors rotate slowly around the patient's head, chest, or body for 180 degrees in a linear fashion along the vertical axis. The computer processes the data and constructs a picture on a cathode-ray tube in shades of gray (on a black-and-white monitor) or in colors that correspond to the density of tissue. Structures are identified by differences in density. This picture is photographed for a permanent record. The computer also prints out on a magnetic disc the numerical density values related to the radiation-absorption coefficients of substances in the area scanned. The radiologist uses this printout to determine whether a substance is fluid, blood, normal tissue, bone, air, or a pathologic lesion. Exact size and location of lesions in the brain, mediastinum, and abdominal organs are identified. CT becomes an invasive procedure when a radiopaque contrast medium is injected intravenously to enhance visualization of the vascular and renal systems to determine the size of an aortic aneurysm or a renal mass. CT presents a hazard to the patient from ionizing radiation and a potential allergic reaction to contrast medium (see pp. 567-568), if used. To ensure proper utilization of this complex equipment, as well as to protect the patient from excessive or unnecessary radiation, the procedure is done under the supervision of a qualified radiologist.

Emission Computed Axial Tomography

In emission computed axial tomography (ECAT) the head of a rectangular field gamma camera rotates 360 degrees around the patient. This capability provides multiplanar images of an organ. A computer program then reconstructs images from these multiple angles and processes them, as in a CT scan. The field of view is enlarged with the ECAT.

Total-Body Scanning

Total-body scanning does not refer to CT but to a scanning procedure following intravenous injection of a radionuclide material (see p. 570). Uptake of the radionuclide within the tissues depends on blood flow. Therefore the imaging procedure may be delayed for several hours after the dose is given, not because it takes long for the material to localize in a tumor or inflammatory lesion where the uptake is high, but rather because differentiation is achieved after washout from normal structures. Scanning may include the whole body or only areas of specific interest. Total-body scanning includes identification of structures in the skeletal and vascular systems for diagnosis of a pathologic process such as metastatic bone tumors or thrombotic vascular disease.

X-Ray Studies for Trauma

In addition to being an aid in determining the extent of traumatic injury, x-ray films and scans may be entered as legal evidence in a court of law to establish injuries sustained by the patient or to justify medical care given. Conventional x-ray films will show:

1. Fractures of bones
2. Presence and location of some kinds of foreign bodies (e.g., bullets)
3. Air or blood in pleural cavity
4. Gas or fluid in abdominal cavity
5. Outline of abdominal and chest organs and any deviation from normal size or location

Invasive Preoperative Studies

Invasive studies require the ingestion or injection of a radiolucent gas, a radiopaque contrast medium, or a radionuclide element before exposure of the patient to radiation. Procedures that require injection of these substances must be performed under aseptic conditions with sterile equipment.

Types of Equipment

Many hospitals have one or more rooms within the OR suite that are equipped for diagnostic as well as intraoperative radiologic procedures. In other hospitals, OR nursing personnel must go to the radiology department to assist with these preoperative diagnostic procedures.

Fixed X-Ray Equipment A fixed overhead x-ray tube with housing may be mounted on a ceiling track for unrestricted movement of the x-ray beam into the desired position over the patient. When not in use, it can be moved against a wall and retracted toward the ceiling. Some units are fixed to specially designed tables, such as the urologic table for cystoscopic examinations (see Chapter 31). The controls, which are in an adjacent room or behind a lead shield, are activated by the radiologist or radiology technician.

Portable X-Ray Machine An x-ray tube mounted on a portable electric- or battery-powered generator of a nonexplosive design may be moved from one room to another in the OR suite. A portable x-ray machine offers the advantages of flexibility in scheduling procedures and availability when and where needed. However, it also has the disadvantage of being a source for cross contamination. All portable equipment should be thoroughly disinfected before being brought into a room and again after use. It should be stored within the OR suite between uses.

Cassette The lightproof holder for x-ray film is referred to as a cassette. The patient is positioned between the x-ray tube and the cassette. Holders for cassettes may be built into or attached to the operating table.

Processing Equipment Conventional x-ray equipment projects a black-and-white image on x-ray film that is developed by a chemical process. Some OR suites have a darkroom where x-ray film is developed after exposure so surgeon can see results of the study without excessive delay. An automatic processor in which film can be developed within 90 seconds to 3 minutes may be available.

Fluoroscope Similar to an x-ray generator, a fluoroscope has an additional screen, composed of fluorescent crystals, which lies in contact with a photocathode. When an x-ray beam passes through this screen, it fluoresces. Fluorescent light sets electrons free from an adjacent photocathode to produce an electron image. Rather than photographing this image of body structures on x-ray film, it is reproduced as an optical image on a luminescent screen. The image can be projected on a television monitor or retained on film or videotape by using a video camera. Known as *fluoroscopy,* examination under a fluoroscope allows visualization of both form and movement of internal body structures. Fluoroscopy is used frequently for both preoperative and intraoperative procedures. It is an invasive technique because a fluorescent substance must be injected or a radiopaque device inserted. Fluoroscopy exposes the patient and personnel to radiation at higher levels than do conventional x-rays when exposure time is prolonged to perform a procedure with visual fluoroscopic control (e.g., cardiac catheterization). Personnel must wear lead aprons during fluoroscopy even though a lead shield is part of the installation. Patients should be protected with gonadal shields.

Image Intensifier The image intensifier amplifies the fluoroscopic optical image projected onto a television screen. The surgeon activates the image intensifier with a foot pedal. Clarity of the image is an aid in diagnosis, particularly of vascular, neurologic, and bone disorders. The surgeon and radiologist can observe the progression of an injected fluorescent substance as it moves through internal structures or the placement of a device into the body. When connected to other closed-circuit television facilities, the image can be transmitted to other rooms for teaching purposes. In addition, the image can be filmed for a permanent record and for teaching. The monitoring screen may be mounted on the ceiling above the operating table to save space in the OR, or it may be portable.

Mobile C-Arm Image Intensifier Designed primarily for orthopaedic procedures, foreign body and calculi localization, and catheter placement, mobile image intensifiers offer the same advantages and disadvantages as do portable x-ray machines. The *C-arm,* so named because of its shape (Figure 28-1), keeps the image intensifier and x-ray tube in alignment; the intensifier is directly under the tube. It can be moved from an

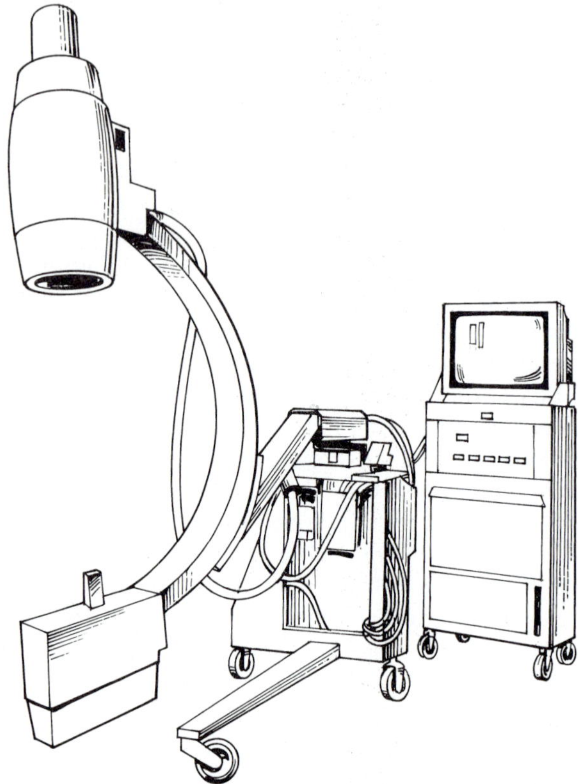

FIGURE 28-1 C-arm keeps image intensifier and x-ray tube in alignment to amplify fluoroscopic optical image.

anterior to a lateral position. Utility of the mobile C-arm image intensifier is enhanced when the system is capable of making electronic radiographs for permanent records. An additional formatting device is required for this function.

Computerized Digital Subtraction Processor Following intravenous injection of a radiopaque contrast medium (see p. 567), the computerized digital subtraction x-ray imaging system visually records perfusion within the cardiovascular system (e.g., extracranial and intracranial vessels). Initially, before contrast medium is injected, fluoroscopic body images are converted to digital data for storage in a memory unit in the processor. Termed the *mask image,* these digitized data are integrated into single or multiple video frames. The video signal is logarithmically amplified and digitized. The mask image is electronically subtracted from subsequent images with the contrast medium. This process removes unwanted background, thus providing optimal visualization of vessels with contrast density that cannot be achieved by other image intensifiers. The resultant images *(digital radiographs)* are displayed on a video screen and can be recorded on film or videotape.

Radiographic Table The tabletop the patient lies on must be made of Bakelite, acrylic, or some other material capable of being penetrated by x-rays (radiolucent). Some operating tables have a tunnel top the length of the table that permits insertion of the x-ray cassette at any area. For fluoroscopy with image intensification, the entire top must be radiolucent because the image intensifier is positioned underneath the table. If the entire operating table is not radiolucent, the foot section can be lowered and a radiolucent extension attached that will accommodate the C-arm.

Procedural and Patient Care Considerations

1. Sterile technique of surgical procedures in general applies also to invasive diagnostic procedures.
2. Each hospital has its own supply list for the procedures routinely performed. It is convenient to keep a stock of routine supplies on a portable cart if procedures are done in the radiology department. In general, the following items should be readily available:
   a. Sterile tray for the specific procedure
   b. Skin prep tray and solutions
   c. Intravenous administration sets and solutions
   d. Local anesthetic agents
   e. Radiopaque contrast material
   f. Sterile gowns, gloves, drapes, and dressings
   g. Extra sterile syringes and needles
   h. Plastic tubing and catheters

   Because an element of risk is associated with some of these procedures, the following items should also be available:
   i. Stimulants
   j. Cardiac resuscitation equipment, including a defibrillator
   k. Oxygen supply and tubing
3. Explanations of procedures should be given to patients to allay fears and to ensure their understanding of the value of the procedure in making a diagnosis. Before the procedure begins, an explanation should be given of the equipment being used and of the necessity to remain quiet while films are being taken.
4. Patients should be carefully observed during all procedures for any change in condition. If a procedure is done under local anesthesia, a registered nurse should monitor the patient's vital signs. A stand-by anesthesiologist may be available to check physiologic status as needed.

Types of Invasive Studies

The most common agents and some of the more commonly performed invasive studies are discussed. Each agent may have many more uses than are described here.

Radiolucent Gases Filtered room air, oxygen, nitrogen, carbon dioxide, or a combination of gases may be injected into body spaces or structures that normally contain *fluid other than blood.* Gases are radiolucent (i.e., transparent to x-rays). Thus gas-filled spaces appear less dense on x-ray film than do surrounding tissues.

The first visualization of the ventricles of the brain was accidental and was reported by W. H. Luckett in 1913. The patient had sustained a skull fracture about 3 weeks previously, and x-ray films showed the ventricles to be filled with air. Luckett explained that the patient, while sneezing, had forced air through fracture lines and lacerated dura, thus filling the ventricles.

Walter E. Dandy, an American neurosurgeon, was the first physician to replace fluid in the ventricles with air and x-ray them. Because most lesions in the brain modify size and shape of ventricles, this procedure aids in localizing a lesion. In 1919 Dandy injected air into the spinal canal to visualize the subarachnoid space. Modifications of his technique are still employed to determine appropriate neurosurgical access to brain lesions.

Ventriculography is the study of the ventricles following injection of gas directly into the lateral ventricles of the brain. It may be used to evaluate a patient with signs of increased intracranial pressure as a result of blockage of cerebrospinal fluid circulation. Ventricular needles or catheters are inserted into one or both lateral ventricles through holes made in the skull. The ventricular needle has a blunt, tapered point that prevents injury to the brain as it is inserted into the ventricle. Openings on the side near the point permit removal of spinal fluid and injection of gas. If the patient is an infant whose suture lines in the skull are not yet closed, needles are inserted through these.

The entire ventriculographic procedure may be done in the OR. Otherwise, the holes are drilled and the ventricular needles or an intraventricular catheter inserted, and the patient is then transferred to the radiology department or diagnostic room within the OR suite. If a lesion is identified, the diagnostic procedure may be followed immediately by a surgical procedure because of the possibility of a further increase in intracranial pressure. If the patient is returned to the unit following the procedure, sterile ventricular needles should accompany the patient. If intracranial pressure becomes too great after gas injection, a needle can be inserted to remove the gas.

Arthrography is the study of a joint following the injection of gas into it. Conventional x-ray films show only the bony structure of a joint. By injection of a gas, injury to cartilage and ligaments may be visualized. A radiopaque, iodinated contrast medium may also be used for a double-contrast study, which is particularly useful in knee arthrograms.

Radiopaque Contrast Media Agents composed of nonmetallic compounds or heavy metallic salts that do not permit passage of radiant energy are *radiopaque.* When exposed to x-ray, the lumina of body structures filled with these agents appear as dense areas. Radiopaque contrast media frequently used for the procedures to be described are listed in Box 28-1. Some of these agents are fluorescent dyes. Most contain iodine. A history of sensitivity to substances that contain iodine, such as shellfish, or other allergies must be obtained before these agents are injected. A test dose of 1 or 2 ml may be given before the dose required for x-ray study. The patient should be observed for allergic reaction throughout the procedure. Signs of reaction may include:

1. Red rash over face and chest
2. Extreme agitation
3. Sudden elevation of body temperature
4. Complaints of muscle, joint, and back pain
5. Respiratory distress

BOX 28-1

Radiopaque Contrast Media

Barium sulfate for gastrointestinal studies
Diatrizoate meglumine, injectable:
- Cardiografin for angiography and aortography
- Hypaque Meglumine, 30%, for urography and CT
- Hypaque Meglumine, 60%, for urography, cerebral and peripheral angiography, aortography, venography, cholangiography, hysterosalpingography, and splenoportography

Diatrizoate sodium, injectable:
- Hypaque Sodium, 25%, for urography and CT
- Hypaque Sodium, 50%, same uses as for Hypaque Meglumine, 60%

Diatrizoic acid, injectable, used as meglumine and sodium salts:
- Hypaque-M, 75%, for angiocardiography, angiography, aortography, and urography
- Renografin for cerebral angiography, peripheral arteriography and venography, cholangiography, splenoportography, arthrography, discography, urography, and CT
- Renovist for aortography, angiocardiography, peripheral arteriography and venography, venocavography, and urography

Ethiodized oil (Ethiodol) for splenoportography and CT
Iodipamide meglumine, injectable:
- Cholografin Meglumine for cholangiography and cholecystography
- Renovue for intravenous excretory urography
- Sinografin for hysterosalpinography

Iohexol (Omnipaque) for myelography
Iophendylate (Pantopaque) for myelography
Ioversol (Optiray) for arteriography and CT
Metrizamide (Amipaque) for myelography and CT
Propyliodone (Dionosil) for bronchography
Sodium iothalamate (Angio-Conray) for arteriography

6. Tachycardia
7. Hypotension
8. Blood-tinged urine
9. Convulsions
10. Loss of consciousness
11. Cardiac arrest

In 1927 Egas Moniz, a Portuguese physician, was the first to perform cerebral angiography. In 1929, in Germany, Werner Forssmann catheterized the right atrium by passing a ureteral catheter into it through a vein in the right arm. He was not successful in his attempt to inject a radiopaque substance through the catheter to visualize the pulmonary vessels. In 1931, Moniz was able to visualize right chambers of the heart and pulmonary vessels using Forssmann's technique. Poor visualization of areas and reactions of patients to the substance discouraged pioneers in this procedure. By 1937 Robb and Steinberg had worked out the technique as it is used today. Now, however, it is enhanced by more sophisticated equipment.

In 1935 the vertebral artery was first exposed and injected, and in 1949 it was first injected percutaneously. Although the latter technique is generally preferred, both methods are used for angiography.

Angiography is a comprehensive term for studies of the circulatory system following injection of a radiopaque substance to permit visualization of a specific blood vessel system. These procedures are useful in the differential diagnosis of arteriovenous malformations, aneurysms, tumors, or vascular accidents due either to traumatic injury or to acquired structural disease.

1. *Aortography* is the study of the aorta and its branches to determine site and size of lesions within the aorta or its major branches such as the renal vascular system. A 7-inch (17.7 cm) × 15-, 16-, or 17-gauge needle may be inserted into the aorta through a translumbar approach with the patient in prone position. The more selective aortographic procedures are performed by positioning a catheter under direct fluoroscopic visualization via the femoral artery into a branch of the aorta.
2. *Arteriography* is the study of the arterial circulation of a specific vascular system. It is identified by reference to the major blood vessel to be injected: right or left carotid or vertebral arteriogram to study cerebral circulation; right brachial artery to study coronary arteries of the myocardium; or right or left femoral arteriogram to study circulation in a lower extremity. Various routes of entrance for a needle or intraarterial catheter exist for injection of these major vessels.
3. *Cardiography* is the study of the chambers in the heart. A catheter is positioned under direct fluoroscopic visualization through one of the great vessels into the heart. Cardiography is done usually in conjunction with other cardiac catheterization procedures. *Cardiac catheterization* includes the recording of pressure measurements within the heart chambers and withdrawing blood samples for analysis (see Chapter 39, pp. 801-802).
4. *Venography* is the study of veins to show inflow, filling, and emptying to determine venous blood flow and valve action.

Techniques and equipment to be used will vary according to specific procedure, but all types of angiography have the following features in common:

1. Access to the vessel to be injected with a radiopaque contrast medium may be made by percutaneous puncture or by a cutdown. An intravenous drip is maintained when the latter approach is used.
   a. Cannulated needles with or without a radiopaque plastic catheter, similar to types used for intravenous infusions, may be used for percutaneous puncture.To prevent backflow of blood, cannulated needles have an obturator that remains in place until the contrast medium is injected. Long catheters have a guidewire to assist threading through the vessel.
   b. Seldinger needle, 18 gauge, has a sharply beveled inner cannula and a blunt outer cannula. The blunt end of the outer cannula prevents trauma to the vessel. After insertion, the inner cannula is replaced with a guidewire and the outer cannula is removed. A 20 cm (approximately 8 inches) vessel dilator is threaded over the guidewire to create a track for a radiopaque catheter. After it is removed, the catheter is positioned and the guidewire is withdrawn. This *Seldinger method* is generally preferred for angiography because blood vessels other than the one punctured can be injected with contrast medium.
   c. Cournand needle has a curved flanged guard that contours to the body. It is particularly useful in carotid arteriography to hold needle in position in the neck during injection.
   d. Robb cannula is blunt, with a large lumen and a stopcock at the hub. It is inserted via a cutdown. It is used with a Robb syringe that has a large opening in the tip for fast injection.
   e. Sheldon needle has an occluded point with an opening at 90 degrees to the lumen. When the vertebral artery is entered, a right-angle injection is made into lumen of the artery.
2. Dosage of radiopaque contrast substances injected into blood vessels is computed for infants and children according to weight. In adults, the dose is measured so that it can be repeated safely for more expo-

sures if necessary. Radiopaque agents dissipate very rapidly in the bloodstream.
3. Radiopaque contrast material should be warmed to body temperature to prevent precipitation and to reduce viscosity.
4. If awake, the patient should be told to expect a warm feeling and possibly a burning sensation when the contrast medium is injected. Procedures may be done under local anesthesia.
5. Plastic tubing, 30 inches (76 cm) long with a syringe on one end and an adapter on the other, is connected to needle or catheter in the vessel to prevent jarring during pressure of injection and to keep hands of the operator out of the x-ray beam.
6. Automatic high-pressure injector may be used instead of injecting contrast medium by hand. This device correlates injection and x-ray exposure. When an automatic injector is used, special high-pressure nylon tubing is used that does not pull apart with pressure. When this tubing is used, a stopcock is placed on the end for closing it off at the syringe connection because nylon tubing cannot be clamped.
7. Automatic seriogram equipment takes rapid multiple exposures while the contrast medium is in sufficient concentration to visualize the vessels. It can be set at ½- to 2-second intervals to take multiple pictures in succession. A roll-film changer, like a movie camera, may also be used. This can be set for multiple exposures per second. These devices are used for angiography with the image intensifier.
8. Digital subtraction angiography converts the x-ray beam into a video screen image (see p. 566). A small amount of contrast medium is injected intravenously. Vessel catheterization is unnecessary and less contrast medium is used. This procedure may be done on an ambulatory basis.

Bronchography is a study of the tracheobronchial tree performed to aid in the diagnosis of bronchiectasis, cancer, tuberculosis, and lung abscess or to detect a foreign body. Location of a lesion can be determined and the surgical procedure planned accordingly. The procedure should be explained in detail to the patient because cooperation is necessary to accomplish the desired result. This radiologic study may be done in conjunction with bronchoscopy (see Chapter 38, pp. 785-786).

Gastrointestinal x-ray studies are performed to identify lesions in the mucosa of the gastrointestinal tract, such as an ulcer or tumor. Inflammatory lesions and partial or complete obstructions caused by a variety of lesions may also be identified. Barium sulfate is either swallowed by the patient or instilled by enema to outline the lumen of segments of the tract to be studied. These studies are done in the radiology department, but surgeons often refer to films during the surgical procedure.

Myelography is a study to identify lesions in the spinal canal. It is helpful to localize a filling defect, a spinal cord tumor, or herniated nucleus pulposus. Most surgeons do not rely entirely on this method of diagnosis; the patient's symptoms and signs are important in making a final diagnosis. Arachnoiditis is a potential complication of intrathecal injection of iophendylate (Pantopaque). Therefore a water-based contrast medium such as metrizamide (Amipaque) may be preferred.

Urography is a comprehensive term for radiologic studies of the urinary tract. Most procedures are performed in the radiology department, but some are done in conjunction with cystoscopic examinations (see Chapter 31, pp. 633 and 644-645).

1. *Cystography* is the study of the bladder following instillation of a contrast medium. It is valuable in detecting ureterovesical reflux, a malfunction of the sphincter valves.
2. *Cystourethrography* is the study of the bladder and urethra to determine whether there is an obstruction or abnormality in contour or position. X-ray films may be taken as contrast medium is injected into the bladder or when the patient voids the material.
3. *Intravenous pyelography* is the study of structures of the urinary tract and kidney function. Contrast medium is introduced intravenously into the circulatory system by rapid injection or slow infusion drip. It is excreted through the kidneys. X-ray films are taken at carefully timed intervals. If the medium is poorly excreted through the kidneys, the last film may be taken as many as 24 hours after injection. Tomograms also may be taken while the contrast material is still in the urinary tract. These procedures are done in the radiology department rather than in the cystoscopy room.
4. *Retrograde pyelography* is the study of shape and position of kidneys and ureters. Contrast medium is injected through catheters placed in each ureter. This procedure is used to visualize renal pelves and calyces.
5. *Ureterography* is the study of one or both ureters to identify position and patency of the lumina. Contrast medium is injected through ureteral catheters (see Chapter 31, pp. 641-642).
6. *Urethrography* is the study of contour and patency of the urethra. Contrast medium may be instilled into the bladder. X-ray films are taken as the patient voids. The medium must flow well but be viscous enough to distend the urethra and provide good detail on the x-ray film. If patient is anesthetized, a very viscous contrast medium is injected into the urethra and films are taken. Because the urethra is quite short, the latter technique is of little value in female patients.

Radionuclides Radioactive elements used in medicine are referred to as *radionuclides.* A *nuclide* is a stable nucleus of a chemical element, such as iodine, plus its orbiting electrons. A nuclide bombarded with radioactive particles becomes unstable and emits radiant energy; it becomes a *radionuclide.* Radionuclides that emit electromagnetic energy are used for diagnostic studies to trace function and structure of most organs of the body. They may be given orally, intravenously, or by infusion. These agents may be used to visualize specific areas rather than radiopaque contrast media in some of the procedures previously described. They are particularly useful in studies of bone marrow, liver, spleen, biliary tract, thyroid, brain, urinary tract, and peripheral vascular system. Because they provide better quantification of arrival times for vascular perfusion above and below lesions, radionuclides may be a more accurate index of the functional significance of a lesion than are other radiopaque contrast media.

Distribution of gamma radioactivity, as from gallium 67 citrate, may be determined by an external scintillation detector. This is referred to as *scintigraphy;* the record produced is a scintigram or scintiscan. A sterile probe may be used intraoperatively to count gamma emissions in cancer cells. A radionuclide, such as iodine 125, and specific antibodies for antigen-producing tumors are injected approximately 3 weeks before the surgical procedure. The computerized display unit emits an auditory signal when the probe detects radioactivity in tissue.

Noninvasive Intraoperative Studies

Noninvasive x-ray films are taken during the surgical procedure most frequently to verify the position of a body structure or a metallic implant or instrument or to identify the presence of a foreign body. The need for x-ray studies can be anticipated, and these studies can be scheduled for:

1. Closed reduction of fractured bones, with or without internal fixation devices
2. Open reduction of hip fractures and fractures of some other bones when internal fixation devices are implanted (see Chapter 32)
3. Stereotactic neuroradiography during neurosurgery to identify landmarks as instruments are introduced into the brain (see Chapter 37, p. 774)

Unanticipated need for x-ray films occurs when a sponge, needle, or instrument is unaccounted for at the time the final count is taken during wound closure. An x-ray film will confirm whether the item is still in the patient. Unless the patient's condition demands immediate wound closure, a film may be taken before closure is completed.

Invasive Intraoperative Studies

The surgeon may wish to inject a radiopaque contrast medium into a blood vessel or other anatomic structure during the surgical procedure to ascertain patency before wound closure or to obtain further guidance for the surgical procedure. Some surgical procedures are performed with the patient positioned on a fluoroscopic table equipped with an image intensifier for radiographic visualization of anatomic structures as the surgical procedure progresses. Examples of procedures that use radiologic control include but are not limited to the following.

Angiography

Intraoperative studies often are essential to assess the results of vascular reconstruction. Angiography is one method of assessment to confirm position and patency of an arterial or venous graft or the quality of a restored vessel lumen. Intraoperative angiography frequently is indicated for these assessments in the peripheral vessels of extremities. After insertion of a bypass graft or endarterectomy, patency of the graft or vessel is checked by pulsations and also by arteriography (see Chapter 40 for further discussion of these surgical procedures).

Angiography is also used at the time of the surgical procedure to identify vascularity or the exact location of some types of lesions in the extremities, brain, and thoracic and abdominal cavities. After injection of radiopaque contrast medium, radiologic studies are made.

Cholangiography

In addition to preoperative diagnostic x-ray studies, some surgeons routinely request radiologic studies in conjunction with cholecystectomy or cholelithotomy (see Chapter 29, p. 586) to identify gallstones in the biliary tract. Other surgeons selectively include cholangiography at time of the surgical procedure in patients in whom they suspect stones might be present or retained in the bile ducts. Conventional x-ray equipment or an image intensifier may be used for these intraoperative studies.

The basic difference between preoperative and intraoperative cholangiography is the site of administration of the radiopaque contrast medium. For preoperative invasive cholangiography, the contrast medium injected intravenously through percutaneous venipuncture is excreted by the liver into the bile ducts. During open surgical procedures the medium is injected directly into bile ducts.

Interventional Radiology

The radiologist may work in collaboration with the surgeon to insert catheters for infusion of pharmacologic and cytotoxic drugs, dilation, or embolization of vessels or organs. Biopsies may be performed percutaneously under radiologic control. Foreign bodies and thrombi may be extracted. Stereotactic radiosurgery using a gamma knife is discussed in Chapter 37, p. 776. Intraoperative radiotherapy is discussed in Chapter 45, pp. 925-926.

Considerations for Patient Safety in Operating Room

All precautions for patient and personnel safety from hazards of radiation exposure should be observed when x-ray films are taken or fluoroscopy is used in the OR. The patient is exposed to the primary beam. Personnel are exposed to scatter radiation in the room. See Chapter 10, pp. 144-148, for a detailed discussion of ionizing radiation hazards. Other factors to be considered for the welfare of the patient are:

1. X-ray film cassette holder, often called a *bucky,* should be properly positioned on the operating table under area to be exposed to the x-ray beam. If table does not have a built-in tunnel or compartment for the cassette, part of the mattress may be removed and the holder, a Bakelite or wooden frame, placed on table in the appropriate section. To check the position of the cassette or C-arm, a scout film or brief fluoroscopic exposure may be taken after the patient is positioned but before the surgical procedure begins. The floor can be marked so that a portable x-ray machine or the C-arm of the image intensifier will be repositioned correctly when films are taken during the surgical procedure. The operating table is positioned under a fixed unit.
2. X-ray tube or C-arm that will extend over the surgical site should be free from dust. It should be damp-dusted with a disinfectant solution before patient arrives and the surgical procedure begins. It may be covered with a sterile drape or sleeve before it is moved over the sterile field.
3. Draping towels may be sutured on rather than secured with towel clips, which might interfere with the view.
4. Sterile technique must be maintained at all times. The scrub person covers the surgical field with a sterile minor sheet to protect it from contamination while the x-ray tube is over it. The circulator removes the sheet after radiographs have been taken.
5. If a lateral x-ray film will be taken, as during fixation of a hip fracture, a lateral cassette holder or C-arm may be positioned before patient is draped and covered with the drape. The circulator raises drape so the radiology technician can place and remove the cassette. Or the holder may be left on the outside of sterile drapes and covered with a sterile Mayo stand cover when technician is ready to swing it into place for the lateral view.
6. Scrub person must enclose cassette with a sterile cover if it will be placed within the sterile field. Disposable covers designed for this purpose are available, or a Mayo stand cover may be used. Be certain gloved hands are well protected in a cuff of the cover while the circulator places the cassette into it.
7. Radiopaque contrast medium used for injection must be sterile. The outsides of ampules or vials must also be sterile if they are placed on the sterile instrument table before contents are withdrawn into a sterile syringe. Warm radiopaque contrast medium to body temperature to overcome viscosity.
8. Remove all instruments and metallic or radiopaque items from the surgical site.
9. Radiologist or radiology technician should be notified well in advance so that he or she is standing by when surgeon is ready. Delays while waiting for radiology personnel prolong the surgical procedure unnecessarily for the patient.

Time, distance, and shielding are the key factors in minimizing radiation exposure. Personnel should stand at least 6 feet away from the x-ray beam and/or wear lead aprons or sternal and gonadal shields. Patients should be protected with gonadal shields if possible.

MAGNETIC RESONANCE IMAGING

Like the CT scan the nuclear magnetic resonance scanner for diagnostic imaging was developed in England and installed there in 1975. Magnetic resonance imaging (MRI), as it is now known, was introduced in hospitals in the United States in 1981. Unlike CT scanning, *MRI does not use radiation.* The patient lies flat inside a large electromagnet. In this static magnetic field, the patient is exposed to bursts of alternating radio-frequency energy waves. The magnetic nuclei of hydrogen atoms in water of body cells are stimulated from their state of equilibrium. As nuclei return to their original state, they emit radio-frequency signals. These signals are converted by a digital computer into two-dimensional color images displayed on a television monitor and recorded on film. Cross-sectional views of the head and all body tissue planes can be obtained. Another computer software system has been developed that produces three-dimensional images.

MRI is based on the magnetic properties of hydrogen in the body rather than on radiodensity of calcium, which is the basis of radiology. MRI looks at both the body's structure and function. It defines soft tissues in relationship to bony and neurovascular structures. It distinguishes between fat, muscle, compact bone and bone marrow, brain and spinal cord, fluid-filled cavities, ligaments and tendons, and blood vessels. The major applications of MRI are detection of tumors, inflammatory diseases, infections, and abscesses and evaluation of functions of cardiovascular and central nervous systems and other organs.

MRI intravenous paramagnetic contrast media, such as gadopenetate, are sometimes used to localize tumors in the central nervous system. These media do not contain iodine, and allergic reactions are rare. All metals can cause artifacts that distort MRI, some more so than others. Titanium ligating clips, for example, create less distortion than do stainless steel clips. Iron-containing pigments used in tattoos and permanent eyeliner alter the image produced. The magnetic field can cause ferromagnetic (iron) components of implants, such as pacemakers and cochlear implants, to malfunction. The magnetic field will also disable metallic devices in the area, such as cardiac monitors and infusion pumps.

POSITRON EMISSION TOMOGRAPHY

Like MRI, positron emission tomography (PET) is a form of nuclear imaging. The rays emitted by an injected radioactive substance are absorbed by detectors inside the donut-shaped scanner. These rays are converted by computer into cross-sectional, three-dimensional images. PET studies provide detailed measurements of an organ's biochemistry and physiologic activity. They are used to study blood flow and metabolic functions, primarily in the brain and heart.

ULTRASONOGRAPHY

Ultrasonography uses vibrating high-frequency sound waves, beyond the hearing capability of human ears, to detect alterations in anatomic structures or hemodynamic properties within the body. The basic component of any diagnostic ultrasound system is its specialized transducer, which is a piezoelectric crystal. The transducer converts electric impulses to ultrasonic waves at a frequency greater than a million cycles per second. These ultrasonic frequencies are transmitted into tissues through a transducer placed on the skin. A water-soluble gel is applied to the skin to maintain airtight contact between skin and transducer because ultrasonic waves do not travel well through air. A portion of the transmitted ultrasonic waves is reflected back as real-time images to a receiving crystal. The transducer, connected to a microprocessing computer, is held on the skin long enough to obtain a graphic recording of the reflected high-frequency sound waves. Uniform imaging of a wide range of body tissues is possible. Ultrasound is not effective in the presence of bone or gases in the gastrointestinal tract. Whether used as a preoperative or intraoperative diagnostic technique, ultrasonography is a rapid, painless, noninvasive procedure that distinguishes between fluid-filled and solid masses.

Preoperative Studies

Alterations in Anatomic Structures

Ultrasonic frequencies are reflected when the beam reaches target anatomic structures of different density and acoustic impedance. The reflected signal is picked up by the transducer/receiver as an echo. The intensity of the returning echo is determined not only by the angle formed between the ultrasound beam and the reflecting surface of the anatomic structure but also by the acoustic properties of that surface. The resulting echo is described in terms of time and intensity. The echo can be displayed on a sonarscope, a cathode-ray oscilloscope, for immediate interpretation of movements and dimensions of structures. The image can be recorded on videotape or printed out to provide a permanent record known as an *echogram* or *sonogram*. Sonograms can be obtained on multiple planes. Ultrasonography is a useful adjunct in the diagnosis of:

1. *Space-occupying lesions in the neonatal brain.* The echoencephalogram will show a shift of the brain caused by tumor.
2. *Lesions in the breast, thyroid, and parathyroid glands and in abdominal or pelvic organs.* Ultrasound can distinguish between a cystic and a solid tumor mass in the kidney, pancreas, liver, ovary, and testis. It is the best imaging method in patients with gallbladder disease.
3. *Emboli, either blood or fat.* Ultrasonography is particularly useful in the early diagnosis of pulmonary embolism. Fat embolus syndrome can develop following long bone fractures.
4. *Fetal maturation.* Fetal head size is an aid in the determination of fetal maturation. This can be measured by ultrasound before an elective cesarean section or to determine the need for C-section if the head is too large for vaginal delivery. Ultrasonography is also used to determine position of fetus and placenta, to identify gender, and to detect fetal abnormalities.
5. *Cardiac defects.* Structural defects, insufficient valvular movement, and blood-flow volumes within the heart chambers and myocardium can be detected. This diagnostic technique is known as *echocardiography*.

Hemodynamic Properties of Peripheral Vascular System

Blood-flow velocity and pressure measurements are possible with ultrasound because moving blood cells produce a sufficient interface with surrounding vessels to independently reflect high-frequency sound waves. The Doppler ultrasonic velocity detector emits a beam of 5 to 10 megahertz (MHz) that is directed through the skin into the bloodstream. A portion of the transmitted ultrasound is reflected from moving particles in the blood. Known as the *Doppler effect,* the reflected sound wave changes in frequency because the source of the sound is in motion. This shift in frequency is proportional to blood-flow velocity. Originally introduced for use in detecting obstruction in arterial blood flow, the Doppler instrument is used extensively to locate and evaluate blood-flow patterns in peripheral arterial and venous diseases or defects.

1. *Arterial disease.* Detection of altered hemodynamics in arterial flow is significant in diagnosis of obstructive or occlusive arterial lesions. For example, the Doppler instrument will indicate regions in the neck where carotid artery blood flow to the brain is obstructed by atherosclerosis. A surgical procedure can be performed to remove or bypass the obstruction to prevent the patient from suffering a cerebrovascular accident (stroke). It also may help the surgeon determine the appropriate level of lower extremity amputation for ischemia caused by peripheral arterial occlusive disease. It is useful in diagnosis of aortoiliac aneurysms.
2. *Venous disease.* Occlusion of superficial or deep veins and the presence of incompetent valves can be located and identified by sounds made by flow of blood through the peripheral venous system. This qualitative information of abnormal venous hemodynamics in patients with varicose veins and thrombotic disease helps the surgeon plan surgical intervention.

Intraoperative Ultrasonography

A sterile ultrasound transducer probe or scan head may be placed on tissue to evaluate vascularity or density. A pathologic condition can be diagnosed or localized. The hand-held transducer must make an acoustic coupling with tissue. Tissues are moistened with sterile normal saline solution, acoustic gel, or peritoneal fluid (if transducer is placed in abdomen). The flexible transducer cable is attached to the ultrasound machine, which has a visible display screen. Permanent recording of images may be made on a videocassette incorporated into the machine. The sound waves may be either continuous or pulsed. A 7.5 MHz focused transducer is usually used. Ultrasonography is less time-consuming and requires less tissue manipulation than other intraoperative diagnostic procedures and does not expose patient to radiation and contrast medium.

Hemodynamics

Ultrasound imaging is used to evaluate adequacy or restoration of blood flow during vascular reconstruction procedures, as of peripheral vessels in lower extremities, hepatic and portal shunts, and carotid arteries. A transesophageal echocardiograph may be obtained during coronary revascularization by placing the transducer in the esophagus. Doppler instruments are frequently used to assess blood flow through reconstructive tissue flaps and grafts and microvascular anastomoses.

Air Embolus

The Doppler instrument can be used to monitor patients during open heart surgery or during procedures on the great vessels in the chest to detect the escape of air into the circulation. Air entering an artery to the brain (cerebral air embolism) may cause brain damage or death. If an air embolism is detected at the time it occurs, therapy can be initiated immediately.

Localization of Lesions

Ultrasound imaging is used for intraoperative localization of subcortical brain lesions, spinal cord lesions, pancreatic and hepatic tumors, pelvic masses, and lesions in other soft tissues to determine whether the lesion is resectable. The exact location of gallbladder and kidney stones can also be identified.

Percutaneous Puncture

The direction and depth of needle punctures to locate lesions in various abdominal organs, such as a pancreatic cyst, can be determined by following the ultrasound beam that is continuously visualized on the sonarscope. The echo from the tip of the needle is easily visible on the scope when the lesion is entered. These procedures are performed to aspirate cytologic specimens for diagnosis.

ENDOSCOPY

Direct visualization within body cavities and structures aids in determination of the appropriate course of therapy for many conditions. Endoscopes are discussed in Chapter 15, pp. 279-285, including their basic design, care, handling, and patient safety considerations. Specific endoscopic procedures are discussed in the following chapters when pertinent to diagnostic and surgical procedures in the appropriate surgical specialties. Box 28-2 lists endoscopic procedures.

Preoperative Endoscopy

Diagnostic endoscopy is frequently performed in conjunction with radiologic studies or to obtain specimens

BOX 28-2

Endoscopic Procedures

angioscopy Heart and major vessels (p. 820)
anoscopy Lower rectum and anal canal (p. 600)
antroscopy Maxillary sinus
arthroscopy A joint, usually the knee (pp. 674-675)
bronchoscopy Tracheobronchial tree (pp. 785-786)
cholangiopancreatoscopy Biliary and pancreatic ducts
choledochoscopy Common bile duct (pp. 586-587)
colonoscopy Colon from ileocecal valve to anus (p. 598)
colposcopy Vagina and cervix (pp. 611-612)
culdoscopy Through vaginal wall into the retrouterine space for visualization of female pelvic tissues, especially the ovaries (pp. 612-613)
cystoscopy Urinary bladder (pp. 641, 644-645)
duodenoscopy Duodenum
esophagoscopy Esophagus (pp. 760-761)
fetoscopy Through abdominal wall and uterus for visualization of fetus in utero (pp. 627-628)
gastroscopy Stomach (p. 529)
hysteroscopy Uterus (p. 613)
jejunoscopy Jejunum
laparoscopy Through abdominal wall for visualization of abdominal organs (pp. 584-585), and female pelvic organs (p. 613)
laryngoscopy Direct visualization of the larynx (pp. 752-753); indirect laryngoscopy is an examination with a laryngeal mirror
mediastinoscopy Mediastinal spaces in the chest cavity (p. 786)
nasopharyngoscopy Nasopharynx
nephroscopy Renal pelvis
ophthalmoscopy Direct and indirect examination of the eye
otoscopy Auditory canal and tympanic membrane
pelviscopy Female pelvic organs (pp. 613-615)
peritoneoscopy Within peritoneal cavity for visualization of abdomonal and pelvic organs
pleuroscopy Pleural cavity
proctoscopy Rectum and anal canal (p. 600)
sigmoidoscopy Sigmoid colon and rectum (p. 598, 600)
sinoscopy Nasal sinuses (p. 738)
thoracoscopy Pleural surfaces (p. 786)
ureteroscopy Ureter (p. 641)
urethroscopy Urethra
vascular endoscopy Arterial or venous lumen
ventriculoscopy Ventricles of the brain

NOTE: From head to foot, nearly every area of the body can be visualized with an endoscope. A description of these procedures is included in the surgical specialty chapters of this text on the page numbers noted above.

for pathologic examination. A radiolucent or radiopaque contrast material may be injected through the endoscope or an accessory before radiologic studies. Fluid and secretions may be withdrawn for culture or chemical analysis. Biopsy specimens are frequently obtained. Direct visualization alone may confirm the presence or absence of a suspected lesion or abnormal condition. This may be enhanced by an ultrasonic transducer at the end of a flexible fiberoptic scope. Endoscopic diagnosis often provides the information necessary to proceed with an open procedure or to cancel an anticipated surgical procedure.

Intraoperative Endoscopy

Vascular endoscopy and visualization of other vessels such as the biliary and hepatic ducts, following either removal or bypass of an obstruction, confirm the patency of the vessel before completion of the surgical procedure. Colonoscopy may be performed intraoperatively to locate soft, nonpalpable tumor masses that will be removed transabdominally. Flexible fiberoptic scopes are used for these procedures. A rigid proctoscope or sigmoidoscope may be inserted transrectally to assess an anastomosis in colon surgery.

Therapeutic procedures are performed through endoscopes without subjecting the patient to an open surgical procedure. Removal of a foreign body, excision of a small tumor or polyp, application of a medication, aspiration of fluid, permanent hemostasis of bleeding, and ligation of a structure are examples of therapeutic procedures. Electrosurgery, cryosurgery, and the laser beam may be used through an endoscope to destroy or remove tissue following confirmation of diagnosis, such as cholecystitis or appendicitis. These therapeutic procedures are often referred to as *minimally invasive surgery.*

PLETHYSMOGRAPHY

In plethysmography pressure-sensitive instruments placed on an organ or around an extremity record variations in volume and pressure of blood passing through tissues. Pen-recorded tracings reflect pulse-wave impulses transmitted from moving currents within arteries and veins. These impulses may be measured, computed by electronic circuits, and displayed as digitalized data. Plethysmography does not identify exact anatomic location, extent, or characteristics of vascular disease. It will quantitatively measure rate of blood flow or degree of vascular obstruction. Four techniques are used.

1. *Oculoplethysmography* is a technique for determining hemodynamically significant carotid artery stenosis or cerebrovascular obstruction. The instrument is placed on each eyeball to

record pulse waves emanating from the cerebrovascular system.

2. *Strain gauge plethysmography* is a technique to evaluate altered venous hemodynamics in deep venous thrombosis and varicose veins. Two pneumatic cuffs are placed on the leg snugly around the thigh and calf or ankle and great toe. A mercury strain gauge attached to plethysmograph is secured around leg or foot between the two cuffs. Cuffs are inflated sequentially for distal arterial occlusion and proximal venous occlusion. Changes in blood-flow volume are measured as the gauge detects changes in circumference of calf or foot caused by sequential inflation and deflation of the pneumatic cuffs.
3. *Venous impedance plethysmography* is a technique to measure venous reflux in lower extremity. Impedance electrodes are attached to the calf under a pneumatic boot. As the boot is inflated, blood is forced proximally out of the veins. Tissues are compressed, causing a concomitant increase in impedance and decrease in calf volume.
4. *Cutaneous pressure photoplethysmography* is a technique to identify peripheral arterial occlusive disease. An infrared light source in a hand-held photoplethysmograph probe is applied to skin with increasing pressure until pulse is occluded. Infrared light is absorbed by blood. Intensity of reflected light changes as volume of blood increases as pressure is released. The probe measures the ability of vascular system to force arterial blood into skin tissue.

SENSORY EVOKED POTENTIAL

Sensory evoked potential (SEP) used to measure neural pathways, involves placement of multiple recording electrodes over peripheral nerves or scalp and ears. The evoked potentials generated in response to stimulation are recorded. Components of the computerized system provide sensory stimulation; acquisition, amplification, and filtering of electrophysiologic signals; signal processing; and display, measurement, and storage of SEP waveforms. These noninvasive measurements may be taken preoperatively to assist in the diagnosis of a pathologic condition, such as acoustic neuroma. The techniques may also be used for intraoperative monitoring (see Chapter 19, p. 378) to assess status of the central nervous system. Multimodality evoked potentials aid in assessment of patients with trauma. Three modalities are used.

1. *Somatosensory evoked potential* is objective evaluation of peripheral and central neural pathways. Pairs of surface or needle skin or scalp electrodes are placed in desired patterns over the appropriate peripheral nerves and areas of the spinal cord and cerebral cortex. These electrodes record somatosensory responses elicited upon application of electrical stimuli, as to the peroneal peripheral nerve at the knee or from over the spinal column or scalp. These impulses along neural pathways are charted to determine if the nerve is functioning properly or if a lesion is impeding impulses to the brain. Testing time can range from 45 minutes to 4 hours, depending on number of peripheral nerves stimulated and sites necessary to assess neural pathways.
2. *Auditory brainstem evoked potential* is a test of the eighth cranial nerve and the auditory pathway to the cerebral cortex. The patient, wearing headphones or earphones, responds to auditory clicks or tones. Multiple electrodes on scalp and ears record responses. This is used to assess the physiologic condition of the brainstem and the patient's hearing threshold.
3. *Visual evoked potential* is a test of responses to visual pattern-reversal stimulation of the optic nerve and its associated pathways to the cerebral cortex. The patient receives stimuli via a television monitor or special eye goggles. Multiple electrodes on scalp and ears record the evoked potentials.

BIBLIOGRAPHY

Bennert KW, Abdul-Karim FW: Fine needle aspiration cytology vs. needle core biopsy for soft tissue tumors, *Acta Cytol* 38(3):381-384, 1994.

Bjare U: Serum-free cell culture, *Pharmacol Ther* 53(3):355-374, 1992.

Bongso A et al: A new lead in embryo quality improvement for assisted reproduction, *Fertil Steril* 56(2):179-191, 1991.

Bright LD, Georgi S: Peripheral vascular disease: is it arterial or venous? *Am J Nurs* 92(9):34-43, 1992.

Burdette-Taylor S, Taylor TG: Wound cultures: what, when, how, *Ostomy Wound Manage* 39(8):26-32, 1993.

Bush WH, Swanson DP: Acute reactions to intravascular contrast media: types, risk factors, recognition, and specific treatment, *Am J Roentgenol* 157(6):1153-1161, 1991.

Davis D, Scarpa N: Transbronchial needle aspiration, *Gastroenterol Nurs* 14(2):80-84, 1991.

Docker CS et al: Intraoperative echocardiography, *AORN J* 55(1):167-176, 1992.

Doillon CJ, Cameron K: New approaches for biocompatibility testing using cell culture, *Internal J Artificial Organs* 13(8):517-520, 1990.

Guthrie BL, Adler JR: Computer-assisted preoperative planning, interactive surgery, and frameless stereotaxy, *Clin Neurosurg* 38(3):112-131, 1992.

Hibner C et al: What is transesophageal echography? *Am J Nurs* 93(4):74-80, 1993.

Hochrein MA, Sohl L: Heart smart: a guide to cardiac tests, *Am J Nurs* 92(12):22-25, 1992.

Husten L: The future for cardiac catheterization labs, *OR Manager* 8(5):23, 1992.

Machi J, Sigel B: Intraoperative ultrasonography, *Radiol Clin North Am* 30(5):1085-1093, 1993.

McConachie NS et al: Computed tomography and magnetic resonance in the diagnosis of intraventricular cerebral masses, *Br J Radiol* 67(795):223-243, 1994.

Plankey ED, Knauf J: What patients need to know about magnetic resonance imaging, *Am J Nurs* 90(1):27-28, 1990.

Plankey ED, Plankey MW: A nuclear approach to cancer detection, *Am J Nurs* 90(6):107-108, 1990.

Raptopoulos V: Abdominal trauma, *Radiol Clin North Am* 32(5):969-987, 1994.

Reading CC: Endorectal sonography, *Crit Rev Diagn Imaging* 33(1):1-28, 1992.

Stevens JK, Miller JI: Transrectal ultrasound, *AORN J* 53(5):1166-1178, 1991.

Thornton KL: Principles of ultrasound, *J Reprod Med* 37(1):27-32, 1992.

Weese DL et al: Contrast media reactions during voiding cystourethrography or retrogradepyelography, *Urology* 41(1):81-84, 1993.

CHAPTER 29

General Surgery

The discipline of general surgery provides the fundamentals for surgical practice, education, and research. The definition of general surgery agreed upon by the American Board of Surgery and the Residency Review Committee for Surgery serves as the basis of graduate education and certification as a specialist in surgery. Inherent in general surgery is:

1. A central core of knowledge of and skills common to all surgical specialties (i.e., anatomy, physiology, metabolism, pathology, immunology, wound healing, shock and resuscitation, neoplasia, and nutrition).
2. Diagnosis and preoperative, intraoperative, and postoperative care of patients with diseases of the alimentary tract; abdomen and its contents; breast; head and neck; endocrine system; and vascular system, excluding intracranial vessels, heart, and vessels intrinsic and immediately adjacent thereto. Also responsibility for comprehensive management of trauma and critically ill patients with underlying surgical conditions.

General surgery provides most of the research in the study of shock, nutrition, fluid and electrolyte balance, wound healing, and infection. The general surgeon in the rural community is experienced in all aspects of trauma and surgical care. In more populous areas, some general surgeons identify areas of special interest, such as breast, biliary tract, gastrointestinal, or colon and rectal surgery. All general surgeons should be competently educated and have the experience to care for traumatic injuries and the most common acute surgical problems of all types.

HISTORICAL BACKGROUND

The earliest time in which surgical procedures were done is not known, but in 5702 BC an Egyptian physician put into writing his knowledge of anatomy. The Greeks were noted for their written records concerning bowel obstruction, hernias, and amputations. Gastric ulcers were recorded as early as the fourth century BC. Hippocrates was recognized as the medical authority for 2000 years.

Revolutionary discoveries by Semmelweis, Pasteur, and Lister marked the beginning of present-day aseptic surgery. The introduction of surgical specialties was the outgrowth of increased knowledge of the etiology of disease and specialized treatment of all parts of the body. *General surgery,* the basis for all specialties, decreased in breadth as specialization increased. The parts of anatomy not specifically delegated to the specialists have remained in the realm of the general surgeon. However, other surgical disciplines depend on general surgeons for clinical collaboration in reconstruction involving the gastrointestinal and vascular systems. The scope of this chapter focuses on procedures commonly categorized as general surgery.

SPECIAL FEATURES OF GENERAL SURGERY

Technologic advances characterize many aspects of surgical practice. The general surgeon of today should be familiar with endoscopic techniques for diagnosis and treatment. Electrosurgery, lasers, and surgical staplers are part of the general surgeon's armamentarium. Patients are best cared for when the surgeon understands the principles of available technologies and has clinical experience in their safe use. The surgeon must be assisted by an equally knowledgeable and skilled team.

1. Malignant lesions account for a large percentage of surgical interventions, especially those of the breast, thyroid, and gastrointestinal tract. The extent of the surgical excision of a lesion may be determined only after thorough exploration during a surgical procedure, sometimes scheduled as an *exploratory laparotomy* or as a *biopsy and frozen section*.
   a. Although the patient has been informed preoperatively of an anticipated procedure, the unknown factor is cause for apprehension. The circulator should convey sincere concern while the patient is awake. A biopsy or endoscopic procedure may be done under local anesthesia, with or without intravenous sedation.
   b. Definitive surgical procedure may be performed on the basis of results of biopsy and frozen section or endoscopic examination while the patient is under anesthesia. The scrub person should be prepared with two draping and instrument setups, depending on the diagnosis established and the surgeon's plan for the surgical procedure. Anticipated equipment and supplies should be available without delay.
2. Types of anesthesia administered are as varied as the types of surgical procedures. Blood pressure, electrocardiogram (ECG), and pulse oximetry should be monitored for all patients.
3. Patients are placed in supine position for most general surgical procedures, but extra padding and accessory positioning aids should be available.
4. Draping for abdominal incisions usually is standardized. Modifications are necessary for other sites.
5. Instrumentation is quite varied and suited to function in a specific anatomic area. For example, gastrointestinal procedures require crushing clamps used to occlude the intestinal lumen before resection and rubber-shod clamps to protect delicate tissues. Included in all procedures are instruments for exposing, dissecting, grasping, holding, clamping, occluding, and suturing. Various lengths of umbilical tape, hernia tape, or thin strips of disposable radiopaque material (vessel loops) may be placed around vessels to retract them. These materials are nontraumatic to blood vessels, nerves, and ureters.
6. Some procedures require minimal access and are adaptable to ambulatory surgery; others are extremely extensive.
7. Electrosurgical unit frequently is used; a laser beam, endoscope, laparoscope, and/or ultrasound transducer may be used.
8. In abdominal and pelvic procedures:
   a. Indwelling Foley or ureteral catheters are often inserted preoperatively.
   b. Nasogastric tube is frequently passed before or during the surgical procedure.
   c. After the abdominal cavity is entered, single free 4×4 sponges should be removed from the field. They are used only folded and secured on a sponge stick. Wet or dry tapes (laparotomy packs) are used in the abdominal cavity. A small dissector (peanut or Kitner) is always clamped in a forceps before it is handed to the surgeon.
   d. Suction should be available and immediately ready to use before the peritoneum is incised, especially in biliary or intestinal procedures or when fluid or blood may be anticipated in the peritoneal cavity.
   e. Before the gastrointestinal or biliary tract is resected, lap packs are used to isolate the area to prevent contamination of peritoneal cavity.
   f. Drain may be exteriorized through a stab wound in the adjacent abdominal wall before closure.
   g. Contaminated items such as those used to anastomose intestinal segments are placed in a discard basin on the sterile field. Only the outside of the basin is touched.
   h. Wound is often irrigated with warm sterile normal saline solution before closure to remove blood and debris.
   i. Retention sutures may be used to give additional strength to wound closure (see Chapter 24, p. 503).
9. Assorted sizes of drains, tubes, drainage bags, and wound suction systems should be available (see Chapter 25, pp. 527-529).
10. Irrigating solutions should be at body temperature when they are used. All radiopaque dyes, anticoagulants, and solutions on the instrument table must be clearly labeled to avoid any error in administration.
11. Blood loss and urinary output are recorded on the intraoperative record.

NECK PROCEDURES

Surgical procedures are conveniently classified by anatomic location. Procedures that involve the head, face, and parts of the neck belong to other specialties.

However, some general surgeons specialize in treatment of tumors in the head and neck region; some specialize in thyroid and parathyroid gland surgery. Cervical and scalene node procedures may be performed by general surgeons. These surgical procedures are discussed in Chapter 36, pp. 758-760.

BREAST PROCEDURES

The *mammary glands* are bilateral organs lying in the superficial fascia of the pectoral area (Figure 29-1). They are attached to the underlying muscles by loose areolar tissue. The breasts extend from the border of the sternum to the anterior axillary line and from approximately the first to the seventh rib.

General surgery on the breast includes diagnostic procedures and those performed for known pathologic disease. Diagnostic techniques include mammography, xeroradiography, ultrasonography, and thermography, as well as the traditional tissue biopsy. A baseline mammogram should be obtained for women between ages 35 to 40 years. Screening mammography may be performed every 1 to 2 years between the ages 40 to 50 and yearly thereafter in high-risk women. Ultrasonography can be used to differentiate between a fluid-filled cyst and a solid tumor. Monthly breast self-examination (BSE) plays an important role in detection of potential breast problems. Premenopausal women are encouraged to examine their breasts 1 week after their menstrual cycle. Menopausal and postmenopausal women should select a monthly date that is easy to remember because their menstrual cycles are not always present or regular. BSE and screening mammography may reveal breast changes that should be investigated by a physician.

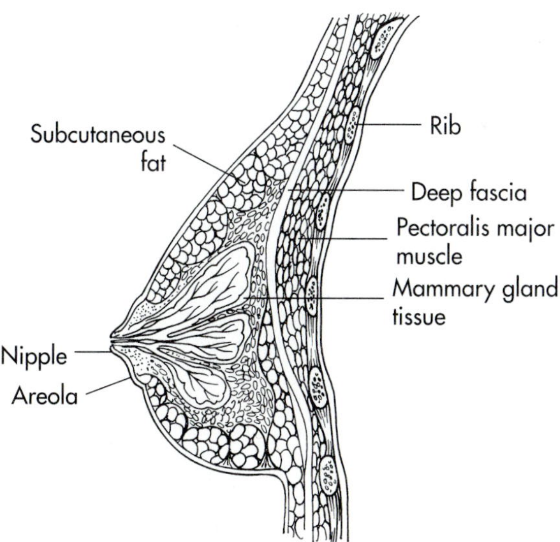

FIGURE 29-1 Sagittal section of normal breast in relation to chest wall and rib cage.

The desired surgical procedure should be determined on an individual basis after careful diagnostic studies and histologic diagnosis. Size, location, and type of diseased tissue or stage of malignancy are important considerations. No single surgical procedure is suitable for all patients.

Incision and Drainage

Surgical opening of an inflamed and suppurative area is most frequently carried out because of infections in the lactating breast. The cavity is usually irrigated and the wound packed and allowed to heal by granulation. The causative organism is often staphylococcus.

Breast Biopsy

To determine the exact nature of a mass in the breast, tissue is removed for pathologic examination. Until proved benign, all breast masses are considered malignant. The size and location of the lesion influence the type of biopsy.

1. *Fine-needle aspiration (FNA).* A 22- or 25-gauge needle attached to a syringe is inserted into the tumor mass. A few cells are aspirated and sent to the pathology laboratory for cytologic studies. This may be done in conjunction with a mammogram (mammographic breast biopsy) or as an office procedure. FNA also may be used to evacuate fluid from benign cysts.
2. *Core biopsy.* A large-bore trocar needle, such as a Tru-cut or Vim-Silverman biopsy needle, is inserted into the mass for this type of incisional biopsy. A core of suspected tissue is withdrawn for histologic examination. Any retrieved fluid is also sent to the pathology laboratory.
3. *Incisional biopsy.* The mass is incised and only a portion is removed for histologic examination.
4. *Excisional biopsy.* The entire mass is removed. The biopsy is carried out because of the presence of a tumor mass detected by palpation, x-ray diagnostic studies, skin changes such as dimpling, and nipple discharge. An excisional biopsy is usually the procedure of choice because it permits examination of the whole mass and avoids entering the lesion with accompanying risk of seeding or implantation of malignant cells.

Preoperatively the surgeon discusses with the patient possible findings and treatment options. The patient may agree to an immediate definitive surgical procedure if results of a biopsy and frozen section warrant it. Two separate prepping, draping, and instruments sets are necessary.

Many women with early operable breast cancer (mass less than 5 cm) opt for limited resection to minimize disfigurement, followed by radiation and chemotherapy. Relationship between tumor and deep tumor-free resection margin remains an important consideration in determination of the most appropriate type of mastectomy (Table 29-1).

Lumpectomy

Lumpectomy, a partial mastectomy, consists of removal of the entire tumor mass along with at least 1 to 2 cm of surrounding nondiseased tissue. This procedure is recommended for peripherally located tumors measuring less than 5 cm.

Breast conservation, the surgical treatment of choice for many women with breast cancer, includes a lumpectomy to excise a primary tumor and axillary node dissection followed by radiation therapy. This approach maintains the appearance and function of the breast. Lumpectomy is contraindicated, however, if breast size precludes postoperative radiation or if negative margins around the tumor cannot be obtained. The surgeon may prefer to perform the lumpectomy first, followed by the axillary dissection. The patient should be reprepped and redraped. A separate set of instruments is used for each procedure to avoid possible tumor cell implantation in the axilla. A transverse incision for axillary dissection, approximately 1 cm below axillary hairline, extends from the pectoralis major muscle anteriorly to the latissimus dorsi muscle posteriorly. Lymphoareolar tissue between these muscles is removed, usually at least 10 lymph nodes.

Segmental Mastectomy

In a segmental mastectomy a wedge or quadrant (quadrantectomy) of breast tissue is removed that includes the tumor mass and the lobe in which it is growing. Some surgeons explore the axilla and take a few lymph nodes for histologic studies.

Simple Mastectomy (Total Mastectomy)

In a simple mastectomy the entire breast is removed but without lymph node dissection. A simple mastectomy may be performed if the malignancy is confined to breast tissue with negative nodes, as a palliative measure for an advanced ulcerated malignant tumor, or to remove extensive benign disease. Skin grafting may be necessary if primary closure of skin flaps would create unacceptable tension. Skin flaps are then loosely approximated, and grafts taken from the thigh are applied to the remaining defect. A latissimus dorsi or rectus abdominus myocutaneous flap may be preferred for reconstruction (see Chapter 34, pp. 711-712).

A subcutaneous mastectomy may be performed for patients with chronic cystic mastitis who have had multiple previous biopsies, patients with multiple fibroadenomas or hyperplastic duct changes, and patients with central tumors that are noninvasive in origin. Removal of all breast tissue is carried out with the overlying skin and nipple remaining intact. A prosthesis may be inserted at the time of the surgical procedure, depending on the surgeon's decision and the patient's wishes (see Chapter 34, pp. 718-719).

Modified Radical Mastectomy

A modified radical mastectomy is usually done for infiltrating ductal and localized small malignant lesions.

TABLE 29-1

Stages of Breast Cancer

STAGE I	STAGE II	STAGE III	STAGE IV
Size			
≤1-2 cm	2-5 cm	≥5 cm	Large and fully integrated with surrounding tissue
Location			
Confined to breast	Breast mass with or without suspicious axillary lymph nodes May or may not extend to pectoral fascia or muscle No distant metastasis	Breast mass with palpable, fixed axillary and/or subclavicular lymph nodes Mass may be adherent to surrounding tissue No distant metastasis	Distant metastasis; extension to skin Lymphedema above or below the clavicle
Surgical options			
Segmental mastectomy	Total mastectomy	Modified or radical mastectomy	Radical or extended radical mastectomy

Breast conservation surgery for stages I and II
Lumpectomy with axillary node dissection and radiation therapy

The term *modified* encompasses various techniques, but all include removal of the entire breast (total mastectomy). In addition, all axillary lymph nodes are resected. The underlying major pectoral muscle is left in place. The minor pectoralis muscle may or may not be removed. Breast reconstruction may be performed immediately or a few days following modified radical mastectomy in patients with small lesions and no metastases (see Chapter 34, pp. 718-719).

Radical Mastectomy

A radical mastectomy is performed to control the spread of malignant disease from large infiltrating cancers. Following a positive finding on tissue biopsy, the entire involved breast is removed along with axillary lymph nodes, pectoral muscles, and all adjacent tissues. During the surgical procedure, skin flaps and extensive exposed tissue are covered with moist packs for protection. The chest wall and axilla are irrigated before closure. Some surgeons prefer to irrigate the mastectomy wound with sterile water instead of sterile normal saline solution to crenate (shrivel or shrink) cancerous cells.

Extended Radical Mastectomy (Urban Procedure)

An extended radical mastectomy is indicated when malignant disease is present in the medial quadrant or subareolar tissue because it tends to spread to the internal mammary lymph nodes. Cancer is a disease that grows deeply as well as laterally. The involved breast is removed en bloc along with underlying pectoral muscles, axillary contents, and upper internal mammary (mediastinal) lymph node chain. This procedure is more difficult than is classic radical mastectomy.

Considerations for Female Breast Procedures

For breast procedure patient is placed in supine position with the involved side close to the edge of the table and arm on the affected side extended on an armboard. The affected side is elevated with a small pillow. The anterior chest is prepped from the chin to the umbilicus and from the axilla on the affected side to the nipple line of the opposite breast. The entire arm on the affected side in included in the prep. General anesthesia is usually preferred for a mastectomy; local infiltrate may obscure a tumor.

Because of the vascularity of breast tissue, laser or electrocoagulation is used for hemostasis. Patients undergoing a mastectomy should be watched for excessive bleeding. The circulator should check with the surgeon about the care of the specimen for the pathologist. The specimen is placed in sterile normal saline solution if estrogen or progesterone receptor studies are to be performed. Formalin is used for permanent sections.

A bulky compression dressing may be applied in the OR. A closed-wound suction system may be inserted, depending on the amount of tissue resected, to remove extravasation of blood and serum and to prevent necrosis of skin flaps.

Patients who have undergone mastectomy are frequently referred to the Reach to Recovery rehabilitative program. In this program, volunteers who have had mastectomies visit patients, share information with them, and give them encouragement.

Reduction of Male Breast

Reduction of the male breast is carried out for *gynecomastia,* a pathologic lesion consisting of bilateral or unilateral enlargement of the male breast. Gynecomastia occurs primarily after the age of 40 years or during puberty and is usually related to alterations in normal hormonal balance. All subareolar fibroglandular tissue is removed, followed by reconstruction of the resultant defect. Some surgeons perform liposuction-assisted procedures to debulk the male breast. Carcinoma can also occur in the male breast.

ABDOMINAL SURGICAL INCISIONS

Surgical opening of the abdominal wall and entering of the peritoneal cavity is called *laparotomy.* Various types of incisions are used, but each follows essentially the same technique. The exact position of the incision is determined before the surgeon begins. The skin and subcutaneous tissue are incised and blood vessels are ligated or electrocoagulated. Fascia covers the muscles anteriorly and posteriorly. The anterior fascia is incised and each muscle layer is separated and/or divided, with bleeding vessels ligated or electrocoagulated. The layers are retracted. The peritoneum is the thin serous membrane that lines the interior of the abdominal cavity *(parietal peritoneum)* and that surrounds the organs *(visceral peritoneum).* It lies beneath the posterior fascia. Both posterior fascia and peritoneum may be cut at the same time, thus exposing the contents of the abdominal cavity (Figure 29-2).

The surgeon chooses the most suitable incision for the procedure to be performed. All incisions incorporate, with varying degrees of success, certain characteristics, including:

1. Ease and speed of entry into the abdominal cavity
2. Maximum exposure
3. Minimum trauma
4. Least postoperative discomfort
5. Maximum postoperative wound strength

Types of Incisions

The two main factors governing incisions are direction and location. Incisions may be vertical, horizontal, or

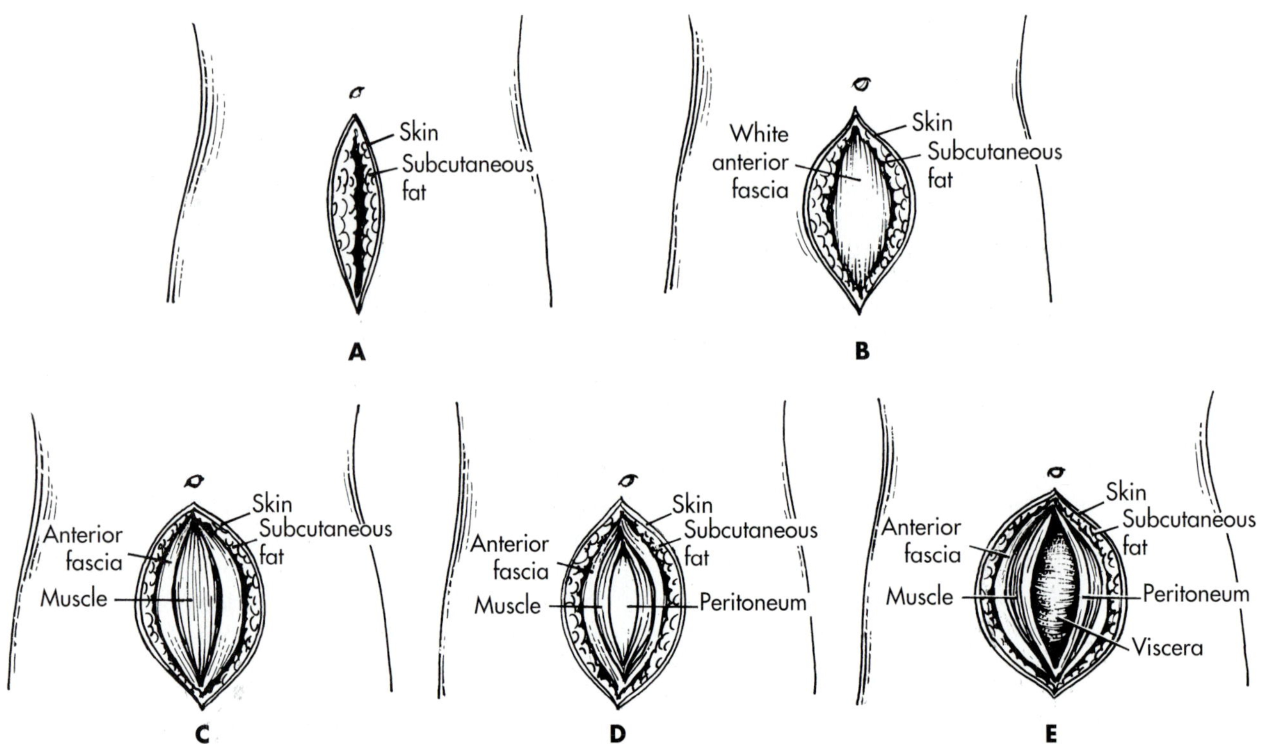

FIGURE 29-2 Dissecting tissue layers of the abdomen. **A,** Subcutaneous fat (yellow). **B,** Anterior fascia (white). **C,** Muscle (red). **D,** Skin through muscle dissected. Thin white peritoneum shown for dissection. **E,** Open peritoneum with viscera beneath.

oblique in various areas of the torso (Figure 29-3). The following incisions are applicable to abdominal or pelvic procedures.

Paramedian Incision

The paramedian incision is a vertical incision about 4 cm (approximately 2 inches) lateral to the midline on either side in the upper or lower abdomen. After skin and subcutaneous tissue are incised, the rectus sheath is split vertically and muscle retracted laterally. This incision allows quick entry into the abdominal cavity with excellent exposure. It limits trauma, avoids nerve injury, is easily extended, and gives a firm closure. Examples of use include access to biliary tract or pancreas in right upper quadrant and to left lower quadrant for resection of sigmoid colon.

Longitudinal Midline Incision

A longitudinal midline incision can be upper abdominal, lower abdominal, or a combination of both going around the umbilicus. Depending on length of the incision, it begins in the epigastrium at level of the xiphoid process and may extend vertically to the suprapubic region. After incision of the peritoneum, the falciform ligament of the liver is divided. *Upper midline incision* offers excellent exposure of the upper abdominal contents and rapid entry, but it is not a strong incision and may disrupt. The *lower midline incision* provides exposure of pelvic organs and rapid entry. It is not as strong as a paramedian incision. Examples of use include an upper midline incision for gastrectomy and a lower midline incision for intestinal resection.

Subcostal, Upper Quadrant Oblique Incision

A right or left oblique incision begins in the epigastrium and extends laterally and obliquely just below the lower costal margin. It continues through the rectus muscle, which is either retracted or transversely divided. Although the incision affords limited exposure except for upper abdominal viscera, cosmetically it provides good results because it follows skin lines and produces limited nerve damage. Although painful, it is a strong incision postoperatively. Examples of use include biliary procedures and splenectomy.

Bilateral incisions joining in the midline may be preferred for stomach and/or pancreas procedures. A bilateral modified subcostal incision, a *Chevron incision,* is made for increased visibility for liver transplantation or resection.

McBurney's Incision

The area just below the umbilicus and 4 cm (about 2 inches) medial from the anterior superior iliac spine

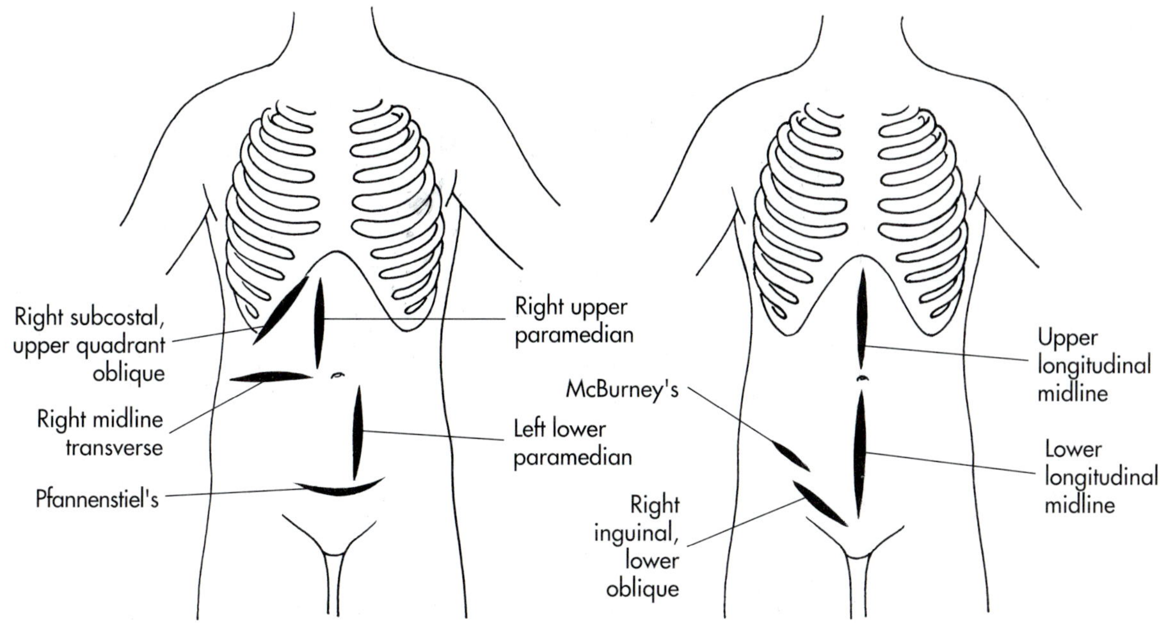

FIGURE 29-3 Abdominal incisions.

marks McBurney's point in the right lower quadrant. A muscle-splitting incision extending through fibers of the external oblique muscle is made. The incision is deepened, and internal oblique and transversalis muscles are split and retracted. The peritoneum is then entered. This is a fast, easy incision, although exposure is limited. Its primary use is for appendectomy.

Thoracoabdominal Incision

With patient in lateral position, either a right or left incision begins at a point midway between the xiphoid and umbilicus and extends across the abdomen to the seventh or eighth costal interspace and along the interspace into the thorax. The rectus, oblique, serratus, and intercostal muscles are divided in the line of incision down to peritoneum and pleura. This converts the pleural and peritoneal cavities into one main cavity, thus allowing excellent exposure for the upper end of the stomach and the lower end of the esophagus (see Figure 38-5, p. 789). Examples of use include esophageal varices and repair of hiatal hernia.

Midabdominal Transverse Incision

The midabdominal transverse incision starts on either the right or left side slightly above or below the umbilicus. It may be carried laterally to the lumbar region between the ribs and crest of the ilium. Intercostal nerves are protected by cutting posterior rectus sheath and peritoneum in the direction of the divided muscle fibers. Advantages are rapid incision, easy extension, provision for retroperitoneal approach, and a secure postoperative wound. Examples of use include choledochojejunostomy and transverse colostomy.

Pfannenstiel's Incision

Pfannenstiel's incision is a curved transverse incision across the lower abdomen within the hairline of the pubis. The rectus fascia is severed transversely and the muscles are separated. The peritoneum is incised vertically in the midline. This lower transverse incision provides good exposure and strong closure for pelvic procedures. Its primary use is for abdominal hysterectomy.

Inguinal Incision, Lower Oblique

An oblique incision of the right or left inguinal region extends from the pubic tubercle to the anterior crest of the ilium, slightly above and parallel to the inguinal crease. Incision of the external oblique fascia gives access to the cremaster muscle, inguinal canal, and cord structures. Its primary use is for inguinal herniorrhaphy.

Wound Closure

Closure is done in reverse order of incision. Each layer is closed with interrupted or continuous sutures (Figure 29-4). Separation of tissues produced by a failure to approximate wound edges closely results in dead space, which delays healing. Absorbable material is usually used if the peritoneum is sutured. Either absorbable or nonabsorbable material is used on muscle and fascia. It may be necessary to place a few absorbable sutures in the subcu-

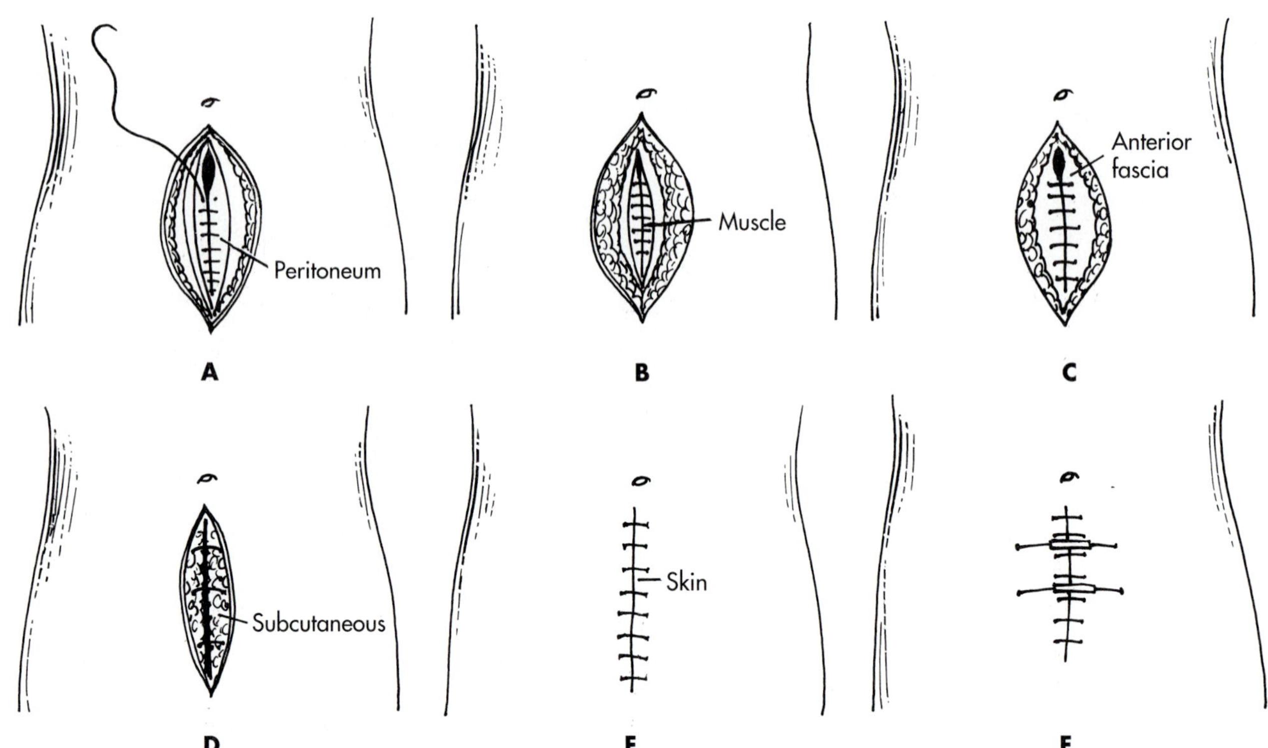

FIGURE 29-4 Suturing incised tissue layers. **A,** Peritoneum (continuous stitch, taper point needle). **B,** Muscle (interrupted stitch). **C,** Anterior fascia (interrupted stitch, cutting needle). **D,** Subcutaneous (not always sutured, taper point needle). **E,** Skin (interrupted stitch, cutting needle). **F,** Retention sutures. Note bumpers to protect skin.

taneous layer. Skin edges are approximated with nonabsorbable suture, skin clips, or staples. Sometimes the suture line is supported by retention or stay sutures.

Many surgeons prefer the Smead-Jones far-and-near technique for abdominal wound closure (Figure 29-5). This is a single layer closure through both layers of fascia, abdominal muscles, and peritoneum with interrupted sutures, either monofilament stainless steel or polypropylene. These sutures resemble the figure 8 when placed. This closure is rapid and strong.

Abdominal wound closure must provide tensile strength to the incision until the wound is healed. It should not inhibit wound healing or promote wound infection. It should be well tolerated by the patient.

Laparoscopy

Rather than incising the abdominal wall to enter the peritoneal cavity, a rigid laparoscope can be used for video-controlled, minimal access, intraabdominal surgical procedures. Lysis of adhesions or inspection of organs may eliminate the need for laparotomy, for example. The gallbladder and appendix can be removed. Needle biopsies, wedge resections, and ablation of some tumors can be performed. Specialized graspers, scissors, sutures, staplers, and ligating clips also can be manipulated through trocars strategically located through the abdominal wall. Laser, electrical, and thermal energy can be directed through secondary ports for cutting and coagulating tissues. Laser may be safer than electrosurgery for procedures close to the bowel where burns are a potential source of injury to internal tissues.

After induction of anesthesia, prepping, and draping, the operating table is tilted about 10 degrees into a slight Trendelenburg's position. A Verres insufflation needle or blunt Hasson trocar is inserted into the peritoneal cavity through a periumbilical incision, about ¼ inch (10 mm), along the lower edge of the umbilicus. The anterior abdominal wall is thinnest at the umbilicus, making this area easiest for penetration of and extraction through a single layer of fascia and peritoneum. The peritoneal cavity is insufflated with carbon dioxide to an intraoperative pressure of 12 to 15 mm Hg. The circulator monitors this pressure during the procedure. It should not fall below 8 mm Hg. After sufficient pneumoperitoneum is established, the patient is placed in a slight reverse Trendelenburg's position. A padded footboard should be in place to prevent the patient from sliding downward on the operating table.

If an insufflation needle is used, it will be replaced by a trocar, usually disposable, inserted straight into

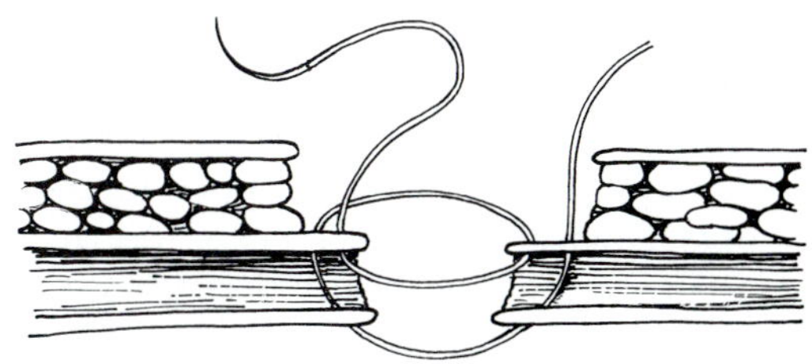

FIGURE 29-5 Smead-Jones figure-of-eight abdominal wound closure technique. (Reproduced by permission of Ethicon, Inc.)

the peritoneal cavity. The trocar sheath matches the size of the rigid laparoscope. A 7 or 10 mm 0-degree telescope is inserted through the trocar for direct visualization within the peritoneal cavity. Secondary 5, 7, or 10 mm trocars are inserted through the abdominal wall under direct vision through the laparoscope. If 10 mm trocars are used, rubber sizing caps can be used to reduce the opening of the sheath for use of smaller endoscopic instruments to prevent the escape of pneumoperitoneum. A sterile camera attached to the laparoscope projects images on video monitors. Usually two monitors, one on each side of operating table, are used. The surgeon views manipulation of instruments inserted through secondary ports. (See also description of procedures for laparoscopy and pelviscopy in Chapter 30, pp. 613-615.)

BILIARY TRACT PROCEDURES

The *gallbladder* is located in the right upper quadrant in a fossa under and immediately adjacent to the right lobe of the liver (see Figure 29-7, p. 592). It is a thin-walled sac with a normal capacity of 50 to 75 ml of bile. Bile secreted by hepatic cells enters intrahepatic bile ducts and progresses to the common bile duct. When it is not needed for digestion, bile is diverted through the cystic duct into the gallbladder, where it is stored. When needed, the gallbladder contracts, emptying bile back into the cystic duct to flow into and through the common duct into the duodenum.

Gallstones, concretions of elements of bile, particularly cholesterol, may be found in the gallbladder or any portions of the extrahepatic biliary duct system. The incidence of stones, referred to as *cholelithiasis,* increases with age and is more prevalent in women than men and in obese persons. Acute or chronic inflammation of the gallbladder, common duct stone *(choledocholithiasis),* carcinoma, or congenital absence of bile ducts *(biliary atresia)* are the most common indications for a surgical procedure. Obstructive jaundice, which is potentially fatal, may be a sign of ductal cholelithiasis or the presence of a neoplasm. Cause of jaundice should be determined and condition relieved to spare patient irreversible progressive liver damage.

The greatest hazards of biliary tract surgery are associated with anatomic relationships of ducts and cystic artery and with pathologic changes in the gallbladder. Complications include hemorrhage and injury to the extrahepatic biliary duct system.

Ultrasonography and computed tomography (CT) scanning are used for diagnosis of gallbladder disease. Oral and intravenous cholecystography may be used for visualization of the gallbladder in the initial evaluation of patients with biliary symptoms. *Endoscopic retrograde cholangiopancreatography* also may be performed, usually by a gastroenterologist, to identify stones, tumor, inflammatory lesions, or an obstruction. With the patient under intravenous sedation and a topical anesthetic to control the gag reflex, a flexible fiberoptic duodenoscope is introduced. Dye is injected to opacify the entire biliary tract and pancreatic duct under fluoroscopy. Some definitive therapy is possible during this procedure, such as retrieval of stones (endoscopic papillotomy), insertion of stents, and sphincterotomy. *Percutaneous transhepatic puncture* is used to biopsy tumors, dilate strictures, or place stents in bile duct and to establish temporary drainage through ducts. Contrast medium can be injected for a cholangiogram.

Cholecystectomy

Removal of the gallbladder, the most common surgical procedure performed on the biliary tract, cures gallbladder disease. Cholecystectomy is done to relieve gastrointestinal distress common in patients with acute or chronic cholecystitis with or without gallstones. It also removes a source of recurrent sepsis. Persistent infection in the biliary tract may cause recurrent stones.

For cholecystectomy, patient is placed in supine position. After induction of general anesthesia, the right upper quadrant may be slightly elevated on a gallbladder rest or pillow, as requested by the surgeon. The table may be tilted slightly into reverse Trendelenburg's position so abdominal viscera will gravitate downward, away from the surgical area.

Open Abdominal Cholecystectomy

The gallbladder usually is exposed through a right subcostal incision, which may be extended over the midline. The incision should be adequate for good exposure of the gallbladder and bile ducts. Following exploration of the abdominal cavity, laparotomy packs are used to wall off surrounding organs. Contents of the gallbladder may be aspirated to prevent bile from spilling into the peritoneal cavity, a potential source for peritonitis, especially if the gallbladder is tightly distended. The cystic duct, cystic artery, hepatic ducts, and common bile duct are accurately identified. After palpation of the ducts for stones, the cystic duct and artery are ligated with hemostatic clips and divided. The gallbladder is freed from the liver and its fossa by blunt dissection and removed. Some surgeons use an Nd:YAG or a Ho:YAG laser for sharp dissection and coagulation. Stones removed as part of the specimen should be sent to the pathology department for analysis and documentation. If bile leakage or hemorrhage was excessive, a sump drain or closed wound suction drain may be placed in the subhepatic space and brought out through a stab wound.

Laparoscopic Cholecystectomy

For laparoscopic cholecystectomy, a rigid fiberoptic laparoscope is inserted into the peritoneal cavity, as described on pp. 584-585. Trocars are inserted through three or four puncture wounds in the right upper quadrant: one or two just right of midline with uppermost trocar slightly below xiphoid and costal margin, and the other midway to the umbilicus; one laterally in anterior axillary line above iliac crest at costal margin; and another in midclavicular line slightly above level of umbilicus 2 cm below rib. Location of puncture sites will vary according to patient size and surgeon preference. A camera attached to the laparoscope allows surgeon to view manipulation of instruments through sheaths of these trocars. Viewing monitors are positioned on each side of head end of the operating table. Fundus of the gallbladder is grasped through lateral port(s) and held by the assistant. After careful dissection, the surgeon ligates and divides the cystic duct and artery with suture loops or clips. Laser, electrocoagulation, or microscissors may be used to transect these structures. The gallbladder is dissected free, most often using an argon, KTP, contact Nd:YAG, or Ho:YAG laser. It usually is aspirated to remove bile and collapse the sac. It may then be removed in one piece or cut into sections and withdrawn through the periumbilical incision.

Common Duct Exploration

Concomitant exploration of the common duct is often but not routinely done during cholecystectomy. Curved stone forceps, small malleable scoops, dilators of various sizes, balloon-tipped catheters, stone baskets, and nylon brushes are useful in clearing hepatic and biliary ducts of stones to prevent their lodging in the duct, with subsequent obstructive jaundice. Palpable stones, jaundice with cholangitis, and dilatation of common bile duct are indications for exploration. A T-tube may be inserted to stent the duct and to provide postoperative drainage. The surgeon may choose other intraoperative techniques to identify unsuspected stones, pathologic conditions, or anatomic variations in the hepatic duct system.

Intraoperative Cholangiograms

X-ray films are taken during either open abdominal or laparoscopic procedures. The radiology department is notified in advance if cholangiography is anticipated. Scout films should be taken when patient is initially positioned on operating table. The table should have a radiographic top or be equipped for x-rays or fluoroscopy. The radiology technician returns to the OR when the surgeon is ready for films. Cholangiograms may be taken after the gallbladder is removed or before the cystic duct and artery are ligated. A radiopaque contrast medium, usually diatrizoate sodium (Hypaque or Renografin), is injected into cystic duct or common bile duct with a 50 ml syringe. Unless fluoroscopy is used, a series of three or four x-ray films are taken. The surgeon injects dye before each exposure through a cholangiocath (a plastic catheter inserted into cystic or common duct), cannula, or direct needle puncture in the common duct. Instruments are removed from field to extent possible to minimize obstruction of structures on the x-ray films. The field is covered with a sterile towel before x-ray tube or C-arm is positioned over patient. Sterile x-ray tube and C-arm covers are commercially available. All other precautions for patient and personnel safety should be observed (see Chapter 10, pp. 144-148, and Chapter 28, p. 571).

Ultrasonography

A sterile ultrasound probe is manipulated along the common bile duct from the liver to the duodenum. The probe transmits high-frequency sound waves as echoes back to the ultrasound unit. These are displayed on a screen as black and white real-time images. The abdominal cavity is irrigated with warm normal saline solution to enhance transmission of ultrasound waves. Density in tissue causes sound waves to echo in altered patterns and directions. Gallstones appear as bright echoes, often with an acoustic shadow. Photographs or a videotape can be obtained to document the findings of ultrasonography. This noninvasive technique takes less time and does not have the radiation hazards of intraoperative cholangiograms.

Choledochoscopy

Intraoperative biliary endoscopy provides image transmission and illumination, thus allowing the surgeon visual guidance in exploring the biliary system. Intrahepatic and extrahepatic bile ducts can be visualized with a flexible fiberoptic choledochoscope introduced into the common duct. To provide distention of biliary tract, normal saline solution must continuously flow through the irrigation channel. Stones are easily seen, usually free-floating under the pressure of the irrigating solution. A flexible stone forceps or basket or a balloon-tipped biliary catheter may be inserted through the instrument channel of either a rigid or a flexible scope to allow manipulation of a stone under direct vision. A biopsy forceps may be inserted to obtain a tissue sample. An Nd:YAG laser fiber may be used through the choledochoscope to crush bilirubin stones in distal common hepatic duct for easy removal.

Cholelithotripsy

Cholelithotripsy is a noninvasive procedure. High-energy shock waves are used to fragment cholesterol gallstones. The procedure is done under intravenous sedation, or general anesthesia. The patient is usually positioned prone, but may be in supine or lateral position, on a lithotripter table or submerged in a water bath. Spark-gap shock waves generated from an electrode pass through a fluid medium into body until they reach the stone. The stone is focused with an ultrasound probe and computer. The shock waves are synchronized with the R waves of the patient's cardiac rhythm monitored by ECG to avoid dysrhythmias. Each shock pulverizes the stone(s) into small fragments, which pass through the bile duct. This passage may be aided by oral administration of deoxycholic acid (ursodiol) taken daily after lithotripsy. This drug dissolves fragments.

Choledochostomy; Choledochotomy

Choledochostomy is drainage of the common bile duct through the abdominal wall. A T-tube is used for drainage. *Choledochotomy* is incision of the common bile duct for exploration and removal of stones. Intraoperative cholangiography may be performed before and after exploration and/or stone removal. The duct is irrigated after removal of calculi. Patency of the duct and of the ampulla of Vater is investigated, often through a choledochoscope. If a neoplasm is found during exploration, resectability is determined. However, many tumors of the liver or pancreas are inoperable.

Cholecystoduodenostomy; Cholecystojejunostomy

Cholecystoduodenostomy or cholecystojejunostomy is done to relieve an obstruction in the distal end of the common duct. These procedures establish continuity, by anastomosis, between the gallbladder and duodenum or the gallbladder and jejunum. Careful evaluation precedes a surgical procedure. These are bypass procedures to avoid further obstructive jaundice, but they do not solve the problem. Common causes of obstruction are calculi, stricture of the duct, or neoplasms of the duct, ampulla of Vater, or pancreas.

Choledochoduodenostomy; Choledochojejunostomy

Side-to-side anastomoses between the duodenum or jejunum and the common duct are carried out for difficult or recurrent biliary or pancreatic obstruction from benign or malignant disease.

LIVER PROCEDURES

The *liver,* the largest gland in the body, is divided into left and right segments or lobes. It is located in upper right abdominal cavity beneath the diaphragm (see Figures 29-6 and 29-7). Part of the stomach and duodenum and the hepatic flexure of the colon lie directly beneath the liver. A tough fibrous sheath, *Glisson's capsule,* completely covers the organ. The tissue within the capsule is very friable and vascular. The hepatic artery, a branch of the celiac axis, maintains the arterial supply. Blood from the stomach, intestine, spleen, and pancreas is carried to the liver by the portal vein and its branches.

The many functions of the liver include forming and secreting bile, which aids digestion, transforming glucose into glycogen, which it stores, and helping to regulate blood volume. The liver is vital for the metabolic functioning of the body. It metabolizes fats, proteins, and carbohydrates and synthesizes cholesterol, excretes biliruben, and secretes hormones. This organ has remarkable regenerative capacity, and up to 80% of it may be resected with little or no alteration in hepatic function. Liver function tests are used to assess the degree of functional impairment and to evaluate liver activity and reserve. Most of these tests involve taking a series of blood samples from the patient for specific studies. Ascites may result from impaired liver function.

Liver Needle Biopsy

A percutaneous needle biopsy may be done to help establish a diagnosis of liver disease. Because the procedure is done under local anesthesia or monitored anesthesia care, the patient should be instructed to take several deep breaths and to hold the breath and remain absolutely still while the needle is inserted. Failure of the patient to cooperate can cause needle penetration of the diaphragm or hepatic injury resulting in hemorrhage, a serious complication. Leakage of bile into the abdominal cavity may produce chemical peritonitis, an additional hazard. After skin preparation and local anesthesia, with the patient supine, a Franklin-Silverman or Tru-cut biopsy needle is introduced into the liver via a transthoracic intercostal or transabdominal subcostal route. The needle is rotated, thus separating a small core of tissue. The needle is withdrawn and the specimen is removed. As soon as the needle is removed, the patient is told to resume normal breathing and is assisted to turn onto the right side to compress the chest wall at the penetration site and thus prevent seepage of bile or blood. Slight bleeding may follow a liver biopsy. Prothrombin time is checked. This method of biopsy is not used if the patient has a blood abnormality.

In selected patients under local anesthesia, a laparoscopic-assisted approach may be used to enhance visualization of the biopsy site. The anterior abdominal wall is elevated with a low volume of carbon dioxide insufflation or a planar lift device without insufflation. The biopsy needle is inserted through the abdominal wall as described. A topical hemostatic gelatin sponge or other topical chemical hemostatic agent is laparoscopically applied to the biopsy site on the liver. The patient remains supine following this procedure.

Drainage of Subphrenic and Subhepatic Abscesses

Abscesses in and about the liver may be caused by a variety of microorganisms or as secondary infections from abdominal organs. They generally are treated by incision and drainage. A catheter may be introduced into the abscess cavity localized on a CT scan. Location of abscess determines the percutaneous approach (i.e., transpleural, subpleural, transperitoneal, or retroperitoneal). Care must taken to avoid contamination of the pleural or peritoneal cavity.

Hepatic Resection

The standard anatomic resections of the liver are right or left lobectomy, right or left trisegmentectomy, and left lateral segmentectomy. Because it is a vital organ, the entire liver cannot be removed without liver transplantation (see Chapter 44, p. 911). Lobectomy or segmental resection is indicated for cysts, benign or malignant tumors, or severe penetrating or blunt trauma. The liver is the most commonly injured abdominal organ. Hepatic parenchymal injuries usually cause intraperitoneal hemorrhage and shock.

Depending on location of lesion to be resected, a right or bilateral subcostal incision or an upper midline incision is made that can be extended as needed for exposure and exploration. Intraoperative ultrasonography is usually used to identify anatomic structures. It is necessary to divide the appropriate ligamentous attachments and to ligate veins and arteries before rotating the liver forward and excising diseased or injured lobes or segments. Lesions that are not accessible for resection may be treated with cryosurgery or a Cavitron ultrasonic aspirator. These techniques may be used in conjunction with resection. An ultrasonic aspirator permits the precise removal of tissue and controls bleeding during resection.

Liver tissue is very friable. Prevention or arrest of hemorrhage is a prime concern. Omental flaps, falciform ligament, or Gerota's fascia flap may be used for coverage and tamponade of bleeding surfaces in conjunction with local hemostatic substances. Microfibrillar collagen or oxidized cellulose is often used to control bleeding. Large, blunt, noncutting needles are used to suture the liver. Drains are usually placed in the wound and brought out through stab wounds. Equipment for blood replacement, portal pressure measurement, and chest drainage should be available.

Portosystemic Shunts

Portal hypertension, bleeding esophageal varices, or massive gastrointestinal hemorrhage may necessitate an emergency surgical procedure for decompression of the portal venous system. Often the patient is alcoholic, with cirrhosis, poor nutrition, and unstable blood volume, or generally is a poor surgical risk. A portosystemic shunt is a vascular anastomosis between portal and systemic venous systems. The surgeon may select one of several techniques for a portacaval or mesocaval shunt. A splenorenal shunt may be performed in conjunction with a splenectomy in patients with portal hypertension and hypersplenism for portal decompression. See Chapter 40, pp. 827-828, for discussion of these shunt procedures.

SPLENIC PROCEDURES

The highly vascular *spleen* is located in the upper left abdominal cavity, is protected by the lower portion of the rib cage, and lies beneath the dome of the diaphragm (Figure 29-6). The capsule of the spleen is covered with peritoneum and is held in place by numerous suspensory ligaments. The splenic artery furnishes the arterial blood supply. The splenic vein drains into the portal system. As the largest lymphatic organ of the body, it has an intimate role in immunologic defenses of the body and acts as a blood reservoir. The functions of the spleen are chiefly concerned with formation of blood elements. Radionuclide scanning and other radiographic studies provide information for diagnosis.

Splenectomy

The most common cause for removal of the spleen is *hypersplenism,* overactivity that causes a reduction in the circulating quantity of red cells, white cells, and platelets or a combination of them. Splenectomies frequently are scheduled at specific times because these patients often require administration of whole blood immediately before a surgical procedure. Often the patients are also receiving steroid treatment, and provisions must be made to maintain therapy during the surgical procedure and postoperatively. Hematologic disorders, tumors, or accessory spleens may also be cause for surgical intervention. In selected patients with benign disease, a laparoscopic approach has been successfully used for splenectomy. Splenic rupture requires an immediate surgical procedure to prevent fatal hemorrhage, and it may necessitate a splenectomy.

A left rectus paramedian, midline, or subcostal incision is used to enter the peritoneal cavity. The spleen is displaced medially by careful manual manipulation. Splenorenal, splenocolic, and gastrosplenic ligaments are ligated and divided. Great care should be exercised

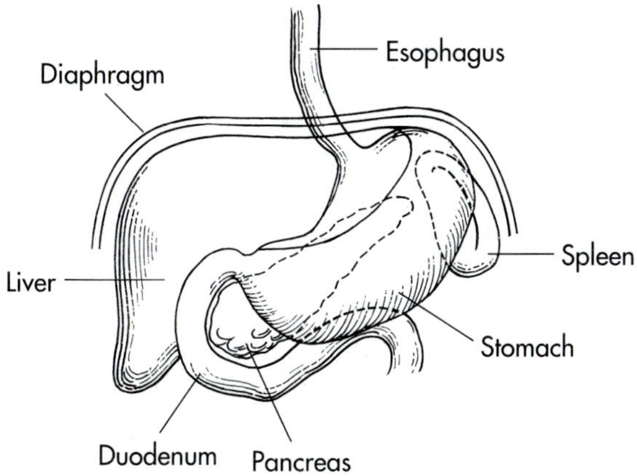

FIGURE 29-6 Organs in upper abdominal cavity.

in ligating the splenic artery and vein because these vessels frequently are friable. Hemorrhage is the principal hazard encountered intraoperatively. After removal of the spleen, careful inspection for bleeding from the splenic pedicle and retroperitoneal space is essential before closure.

Splenorrhaphy

After splenectomy, patients, especially children, are immunologically impaired (i.e., more susceptible to infection), sometimes with catastrophic results. Therefore surgeons attempt to salvage splenic tissue to protect the immune competence following splenic trauma. Splenorrhaphy, splenic repair, can be accomplished in several ways. Once the spleen is mobilized, actively bleeding vessels are ligated and devitalized tissues are debrided. The spleen can then be sutured or stapled along the edge of a partial splenectomy. Microfibrillar collagen or absorbable gelatin sponges can be placed over a small laceration or capsular tear to effect hemostasis. The splenic artery may be ligated. The spleen may be wrapped in omentum or synthetic mesh. Segments can be reimplanted into an omental pouch in the intraperitoneal space to preserve splenic function. A drain, exteriorized through a stab wound, may be inserted in the left subdiaphragmatic space in patients with extensive trauma.

PANCREATIC PROCEDURES

The *pancreas* is both an endocrine and an exocrine gland. Islets of Langerhans comprise the endocrine division and secrete insulin and glucagon, hormones essential to carbohydrate metabolism and storage of calories. Acini and ducts leading from them constitute the exocrine portion that secretes pancreatic juice into the duodenum. Pancreatic juice neutralizes stomach acid. Loss of it results in severe impairment of digestion and absorption of food.

The pancreas lies transversely across the posterior wall of the upper abdomen behind the stomach. The head or right extremity is attached to the duodenum, and the tail or left extremity is in proximity to the spleen (Figure 29-6).

Disorders of the pancreas generally include acute and chronic inflammation, cysts, and tumors. The head of the pancreas is most common site of a malignant tumor. Accuracy in diagnosis of pancreatic problems is difficult, but evaluation by ultrasonography, endoscopic retrograde cholangiopancreatography, and scanning has led to significant improvement in planning surgical treatment. Exploratory laparotomy is the most reliable means of diagnosing and evaluating pancreatic trauma. Pancreatitis is most often associated with pancreatic duct stones, gallstones, or alcoholism. Corrective biliary tract procedures usually alleviate gallstone pancreatitis.

Pancreaticojejunostomy

Pancreaticojejunostomy may be performed for relief of pain associated with chronic alcoholic pancreatitis and pseudocysts of the pancreas. There are several types of procedures for drainage of obstructed ducts or pseudocysts. These procedures involve anastomosing a loop of the jejunum (Roux-en-Y loop) to the pancreatic duct. Hemorrhage and leakage of bile are complications to be avoided.

Pancreaticoduodenectomy (Whipple Procedure)

Pancreaticoduodenectomy, an extensive procedure, is performed on patients with carcinoma of the head of the pancreas or the ampulla of Vater. A gastrointestinal setup is used. The abdominal cavity is exposed through one of several possible anterior incisions, but a long right paramedian incision is usually made. The abdominal and pelvic cavities are explored for distant metastases. Because many vital structures and organs are involved in resecting the diseased portion of the pancreas, careful dissection of vessels is necessary to prevent hemorrhage, which complicates the procedure. Resection includes all but tail of the pancreas, distal stomach, duodenum distal to the pylorus, and distal end of the common bile duct. Several methods of reconstructing the digestive tract are possible, but all include anastomosis of pancreatic duct, common bile duct, stomach, and jejunum. Most surgeons reestablish biliary-intestinal continuity by end-to-side choledochojejunostomy. The stomach and pylorus may be preserved in patients with benign disease or localized, small tumors. After pancreatic and biliary reconstruction, the divided end of the duodenum is anastomosed to the side of the jejunal limb used for the reconstruction. A watertight seal of all anastomoses is essential to prevent peritonitis or pancreatitis. Drains are inserted.

Postoperatively, the most common complications are shock, hemorrhage, renal failure, and pancreatic or biliary fistula. If a fistula should occur, wound suction is continued until the fistula closes. It will generally close spontaneously if adequate nutrition and electrolyte balance are maintained.

Improvements in preoperative and postoperative care and refinement of technical details have increased the survival rate of patients who undergo this potentially hazardous radical surgical procedure.

Pancreatectomy

Subtotal distal pancreatectomy is usually done to resect a benign tumor or for chronic pancreatitis. The distal tail is resected to the head of the pancreas. A splenectomy is usually performed with this procedure because the blood supply to the tail of the pancreas comes from splenic vessels that must be sacrificed.

Total pancreatectomy allows a wide resection of a primary malignant tumor and its multifocal sites in the pancreas. However, the patient will have some endocrine and pancreatic insufficiency.

Pancreatoduodenal Trauma

Combined injuries of pancreas and duodenum from penetrating wounds or blunt trauma are among the most complicated to treat. A midline incision is used to explore the abdomen. Suturing to control bleeding, debriding of devitalized tissue, and draining are initial therapies. Pancreatic fistulas and abscesses are potential complications. Extensive injury of head of the pancreas and duodenum may require pancreaticoduodenal resection with gastrojejunostomy.

ESOPHAGEAL PROCEDURES

The *esophagus* is the musculocutaneous canal between the pharynx in the throat and the stomach in the abdomen. It passes through the thoracic cavity and enters the abdominal cavity through the esophageal hiatus (opening) in the right crus of the diaphragm. It joins the right medial surface of the stomach. Within the abdominal cavity the esophagus lies between the liver anteriorly and the aorta posteriorly and slightly to the left, with the spleen on the left, and between right and left branches of the vagus nerve (Figures 29-6 and 29-7).

Esophageal Hiatal Herniorrhaphy

The abdominal esophagus and a portion of the stomach may slide through the esophageal hiatus into the thoracic cavity when intraabdominal pressure exceeds pressure in the chest. Although the condition, referred to as *hiatal* or *diaphragmatic hernia*, is quite common (see p. 602), a surgical procedure is indicated when resultant esophagitis causes ulceration, bleeding, stenosis, or chest and back symptoms. Reflux esophagitis and sphincter incompetence may also have other causes that necessitate a surgical procedure.

The abdominal approach to correct the problem is through a midline or left subcostal incision. Because visualization of the hiatal area may be difficult, the incision may be extended over the lower rib cage. The patient may be placed in a slight Trendelenburg's position. Organs and vital structures should be protected with moist tapes and gently retracted to expose the hiatus. Long-handled clamps are needed. Following mobilization, the hiatus is narrowed with heavy sutures and the fundus of the stomach is anchored against the diaphragm to prevent recurrent herniation and gastroesophageal reflux. Prevention of reflux is one of the prime objectives of the surgical procedure because it was the cause of the patient's previous esophagitis. Lengthening the intraabdominal esophagus and increasing pressure on the lower esophageal sphincter also help control reflux. Pressure is augmented by wrapping proximal stomach around the gastroesophageal junction, the *Nissen fundoplication* procedure. The fundus of stomach acts as a flap valve to create pressure around the distal esophagus, thus decreasing reflux. As an alternative to fundoplication, some surgeons insert an antireflux collarlike prosthesis around the esophagus just above the gastroesophageal junction.

Laparoscopic Nissen fundoplication, which may be performed in selected patients, has similar advantages to laparoscopic cholecystectomy. The procedure involves mobilizing the esophagogastric junction and repairing the hiatal defect with a continuous suture technique. This is followed by a total fundoplication to fix the anterior margin of the diaphragmatic hiatus proximally and the esophagogastric junction distally. The laparoscopic approach has been successful in treating gastroesophageal reflux as a minimally invasive procedure.

Esophagogastrectomy

Removal of the lower portion of the esophagus and proximal stomach may be indicated to resect malignant tumors, benign strictures, or perforations at or near the esophagogastric junction. A left thoracoabdominal or upper midline incision is made. After the esophagus and stomach are mobilized and divided, an end-to-end esophagogastric anastomosis may be completed with staples and/or sutures. An end-to-side anastomosis with plication of the stomach around the distal part of the esophagus may be preferred. Depending on the extent of esophageal resection, other options for restoring continuity of the alimentary tract may be necessary. See Chapter 36, p. 761, for a discussion of cervical esophageal reconstruction with stomach, jejunum, or colon interposition.

Surgical Procedures for Esophageal Varices

Esophageal varices are tortuous dilated veins in the submucosa of the lower esophagus. They may extend up in the esophagus or down into the stomach. This condition is caused by portal hypertension usually associated with obstruction within a cirrhotic liver. Rupture of esophageal varices can cause massive hemorrhage. The patient may come to the OR with a Sengstaken-Blakemore tube in place to control bleeding by pressure from the inflated balloon in the tube. During the surgical procedure, varices may be sclerosed through an esophagoscope. Sclerosant (see section on sclerotherapy, Chapter 23, pp. 472-473) is injected via needle puncture into each varix. Several injections may be necessary to achieve complete hemostasis. Sclerotherapy is usually attempted before more radical procedures are performed. The lower esophagus may be transected and the distal segment anastomosed with a circular stapler just proximal to the stomach. A portosystemic shunt procedure may be performed for portal decompression (see Chapter 40, pp. 827-828).

GASTROINTESTINAL SURGERY

Advances in surgical management of patients with gastrointestinal problems have lessened the mortality rate, although treatment may be palliative rather than curative.

Interference with the gastrointestinal tract affects its functioning; specific deficiencies may result from gastrointestinal surgery, depending on the site and extent of the surgical procedure. Massive resection of the small intestine can produce long-term nutritional problems, such as weight loss and malabsorption of most nutrients, thus endangering compatibility with life. Metabolic bone disease may follow gastric surgery because of poor absorption of calcium and vitamin D. Patients who have undergone extensive gastrointestinal procedures should have a periodic nutritional evaluation. Biochemical tests monitor nutritional status. These tests include serum proteins, albumin-globulin ratio, and blood urea nitrogen. Body weight is also significant. If caloric intake is inadequate, protein is converted to carbohydrates for energy and protein synthesis then suffers.

Considerations for Gastrointestinal Surgery

Separation of instruments used for resection and anastomosis and for abdominal closure is essential. Two distinct setups may be used, but the single setup, most commonly used, consists of identifying and using only selected instruments and supplies for resection, anastomosis, and abdominal closure and discarding contaminated instruments and equipment from the field after use. Acid secretions from the gastric resection site are very irritating and may cause peritonitis. The intestinal tract harbors many microorganisms. Leakage into the peritoneal cavity can be a source of generalized peritoneal sepsis. Gloves should be changed before closure; gowns also may be changed.

A nasogastric tube is frequently inserted for aspiration of gastric contents or decompression of the intestinal tract. A variety of gastrointestinal tubes should be available for aspiration and irrigation.

Normal saline solution, not sterile water, should be used in abdominal procedures to moisten laparotomy packs. Normal saline is an isotonic solution with the same osmotic pressure as blood serum and interstitial fluid. It will not alter sodium, chloride, or fluid balance because it does not cross cellular membranes. (Hypotonic solutions cause cells to swell; hypertonic solutions cause them to shrink.) Normal saline is used for intraperitoneal irrigation, unless the surgeon prefers to use a solution such as oxychlorosene (Clorpactin XCB). Antibiotics may also be needed for irrigation.

Electrosurgery is used routinely by many surgeons for electrocoagulation of bleeding vessels in the abdominal wall, omentum, and mesentery. Ligating clips or suture ligatures are used for large vessels. Jaws of intestinal forceps should be protected with soft covers, made of rubber or fabric, to reduce tissue trauma. Stapling devices are preferred by most surgeons to mechanically anastomose organs. An intraluminal circular stapler can be used for end-to-end, end-to-side, or side-to-side anastomoses from the esophagus to the rectum (see Figure 29-10, p. 596). A straight linear stapler may be preferred for some gastrointestinal anastomoses and resections. Because the size of the lumen varies in different organs of the gastrointestinal tract, the circulator should not open a sterile disposable stapler until the surgeon determines the appropriate head size or cartridge length for the instrument to be used.

The technical principles that guide the surgeon for all gastrointestinal anastomoses include:

1. Good blood supply
2. No tension
3. Adequate lumen
4. Watertight and leakproof
5. No distal obstruction

A sutured anastomosis produces an inverted suture line with serosa-to-serosa approximation. A stapled anastomosis results in everted mucosa-to-mucosa apposition.

GASTRIC PROCEDURES

The *stomach,* a hollow muscular organ, is situated in the upper left abdomen between the esophagus and duodenum (see Figures 29-6 and 29-7). Anatomically it is divided into the fundus, body, and pyloric antrum. The two borders of the stomach, the *lesser* and *greater curva-*

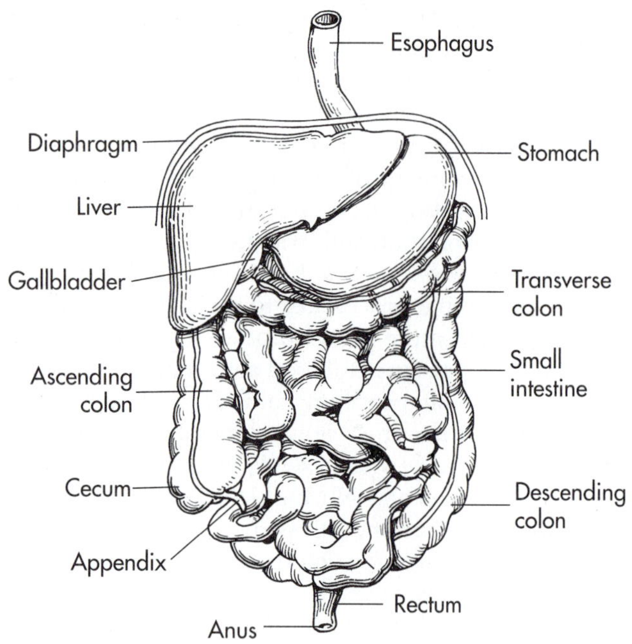

FIGURE 29-7 Abdominal organs within peritoneal cavity.

tures, are important surgically because of their relation to the major vascular and lymphatic systems supplying the stomach. *Omentum,* a double fold of peritoneum attached to the lesser and greater curvatures, loosely covers the stomach and small intestine. The autonomic nervous supply from the vagus nerve controls reflex activities of movement and secretions of the alimentary canal and is significant in rhythmic relaxation of the pyloric sphincter.

Food entering the stomach must be reduced to *chyme,* a semiliquid, to pass through the duodenum and small intestine. Interference of gastric activity or muscular contractions results in gastrointestinal complaints of abdominal pain, nausea, vomiting, hemorrhage, and dyspepsia. Some diseases such as cancer may not produce symptoms until the condition is far advanced. A surgical procedure is indicated when the presence of disease is established following laboratory tests such as gastric analysis, gastroscopy, and/or radiographic studies.

The *dumping syndrome* may be experienced by patients shortly after eating following gastric surgery. This complication occurs because of rapid emptying of food and fluids into the jejunum. It is characterized by nausea, vomiting, weakness, dizziness, pallor, sweating, palpitations, and diarrhea. It may persist for 6 months to a year.

Gastroscopy

Gastroscopy involves passage of a flexible fiberoptic gastroscope. Usually done with the patient sedated, a topical anesthetic is applied in oropharynx to control gag reflex. The operator visually inspects mucosal walls of the stomach. Sometimes tissue specimens are obtained. Bleeding points may be coagulated with laser beam, by electrocoagulation, or with a sclerosing agent.

Gastrostomy

Establishment of a temporary or permanent opening in the stomach may be indicated for gastrointestinal decompression or to provide alimentation for a prolonged period when nutrition cannot be maintained by other means. A gastrostomy tube eliminates incidence of aspiration that may occur around a nasogastric tube. Often the patient is too debilitated to tolerate a major surgical procedure or may have an inoperable esophageal tumor or oropharyngeal trauma. A Foley, Malecot, Pezzer, or mushroom catheter may be inserted percutaneously into the stomach.

Surgical Gastrostomy

With the patient under general anesthesia, the stomach is exposed through a small upper left abdominal or midline incision. The catheter is inserted into the anterior gastric wall and is held in place with purse-string sutures. The catheter is brought out through a separate stab wound in the left upper quadrant. The stomach is sutured to the abdominal wall at the catheter exit site. The surgeon may prefer to place a small-bore catheter into the jejunum rather than the stomach for enteral hyperalimentation following an abdominal procedure on a critically ill patient.

Percutaneous Endoscopic Gastrostomy

While the patient is under intravenous sedation, an endoscopist introduces a fiberoptic gastroscope and insufflates the stomach with air. Light from the scope is directed anteriorly for transillumination through the abdominal wall. The surgeon infiltrates skin with local anesthetic at a selected gastrostomy site, usually about one third of the distance along the left costal margin at the midclavicular line. The catheter is introduced through a small incision and secured with sutures.

Gastric Resections

The stomach may be totally or partially resected for removal of a malignant tumor or for benign chronic ulcer disease. Although surgical resection is the only cure, gastric carcinomas are frequently inoperable because of extended metastases to the liver and surrounding tissues. Palliative procedures may be performed. The appropriate procedure is determined after thorough exploration of the abdominal cavity by the surgeon. Circular staplers are frequently used for anastomosis following resection. Leakage at the site of anastomosis leads to peritonitis. Some surgeons oversew the staple line.

Total Gastrectomy

The entire stomach is excised for malignant lesions through a bilateral subcostal, long transrectus, or thoracoabdominal incision. A total gastrectomy necessitates reconstruction of esophagointestinal continuity by establishing an anastomosis between a loop of jejunum and the esophagus. This anastomosis may be end-to-side with a lateral jejunojejunostomy or end-to-end with a Roux-en-Y jejunojejunostomy. The purpose of the jejunojejunostomy is to prevent reflux of bile and pancreatic fluids into the esophagus. Some surgeons create a jejunal pouch for this purpose.

Subtotal Gastrectomy

Partial resections of the stomach, originally described by Theodor Billroth (1829-1894), are often referred to as *Billroth's procedures.* A benign lesion, usually an ulcer, or a malignant lesion located in the pyloric half requires removal of the lower half to two thirds of the stomach. In a patient with a gastric or duodenal ulcer, the surgical procedure relieves pain, bleeding, vomiting, and weight loss and limits gastric acidity. The peritoneal cavity is entered through a right paramedian or upper midline abdominal incision. A variety of surgical procedures may be used to reestablish gastrointestinal continuity. Anastomosis of the remaining portion of the stomach to the duodenum (gastroduodenostomy, Billroth I, Figure 29-8) or to a loop of the jejunum (gastrojejunostomy, Billroth II, Figure 29-9) is frequently performed. A truncal vagotomy (see discussion to follow) is performed to eliminate the possibility of postoperative peptic ulceration.

Common modifications of the Billroth I procedure are the Schoemaker and the von Haberer–Finney techniques. The Schoemaker procedure involves end-to-end anastomosis of the stomach and duodenum after the lesser curvature of the stomach is sutured to make the anastomosis site the same size as the duodenum. With the von Haberer–Finney method, the lateral wall of the duodenum is brought up to the stomach so that the entire end of the stomach is open for direct anastomosis.

Popular modifications of the Billroth II procedure include the Polya and Hofmeister techniques. These techniques involve variations of end-to-side gastrojejunostomy.

Vagotomy

Chronic gastric, pyloric, and duodenal ulcers that do not respond to medical treatment cause patients severe pain and difficulty in eating and sleeping. Vagotomy may be recommended to interrupt vagal nerve impulses, thus lowering gastric hydrochloric acid production and hastening gastric emptying. *Vagotomy* is division of the vagus nerves. *Proximal gastric vagotomy,* also known as *parietal cell vagotomy,* divides vagal nerves to the proximal stomach but maintains the entire stomach and vagal nerves to the antrum. These nerves inhibit the release of gastrin, a stimulant of gastric secretion.

Truncal vagotomy and *selective vagotomy* require a concomitant drainage procedure because these procedures denervate the stomach. A gastroenterostomy is done with truncal vagotomy, which divides the vagal trunks at the distal esophagus. Antrectomy is performed with selective vagotomy, which transects the gastric branches. Vagotomy with drainage is a compromise procedure restricted to high-risk patients or those with severe duodenal deformity.

Pyloroplasty, enlarging the pyloric opening between the stomach and duodenum, may be done in patients with an obstructing pyloric ulcer or in conjunction with vagotomy to treat bleeding duodenal ulcers. Duodenal dilatation or duodenoplasty may be indicated.

Vagotomy procedures, which are conservative surgical therapies compared with gastrectomy, decrease surgical risk for selected patients with chronic ulcers. It is now known that ulcers caused by the *Helicobacter pylori* organism can be cured with antibiotics.

Gastrojejunostomy (Roux-en-Y Gastroenterostomy)

A procedure may be necessary to reestablish continuity between the stomach and intestinal tract, such as following partial gastrectomy or obstruction of the lower end of stomach caused by an ulcer or a nonresectable tumor. A gastrojejunostomy may be performed to treat alkaline reflux gastritis, postgastrectomy syndromes such as postvagotomy diarrhea, and dumping syndromes. Except in elderly patients, a concomitant vagotomy is necessary to prevent postoperative gastrojejunal ulcer when the acid-forming portion of the stomach is not resected.

A loop of jejunum may be anastomosed to the anterior or posterior wall of the stomach. Both approaches have advantages and disadvantages. In a Roux-en-Y gastrojejunostomy, the jejunum is divided. The distal end is anastomosed to the side of the stomach and the proximal end to the side of the jejunum at a lower level. The result is a Y-shaped double anastomosis that diverts the flow of bile and pancreatic enzymes directly into the jejunum, bypassing the created gastric stoma. An adaptation of a Roux-en-Y anastomosis is also used to drain the biliary tract or other organs, such as the pancreas or esophagus, directly into the jejunum to bypass the stomach and prevent reflux of intestinal contents.

Bariatric Surgery

Interest in the study of morbid obesity, *bariatrics,* has led to the development of subspecialization in general surgery in the field of bariatric surgery. Persons who weigh more than 100 lb (45.4 kg) over their ideal weight, who have no serious disease, and who have failed to lose weight despite years of medical treatment are potential candidates for bariatric surgery.

The physical size of the patient presents special needs with respect to transporting and positioning, selecting instrumentation, and providing psychologic and phys-

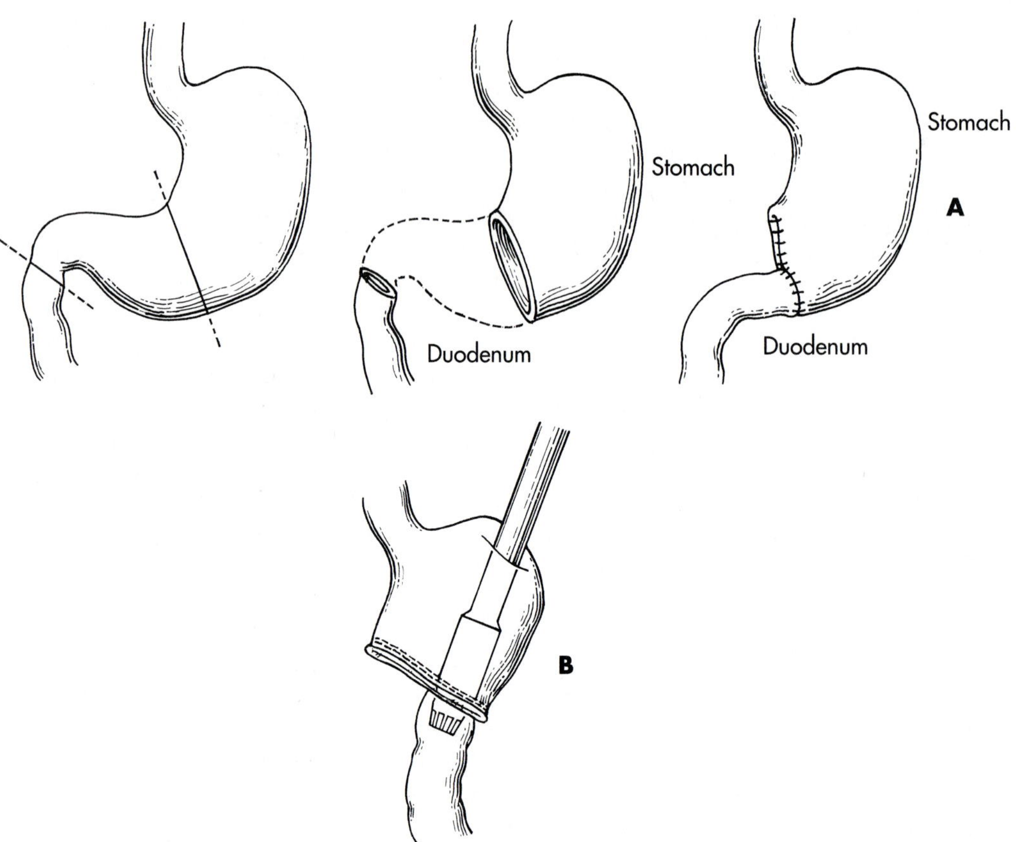

FIGURE 29-8 Billroth I gastroduodenostomy. End-to-end anastomosis of duodenum to stomach may be sutured **(A)** or stapled with an intraluminal circular stapler **(B).**

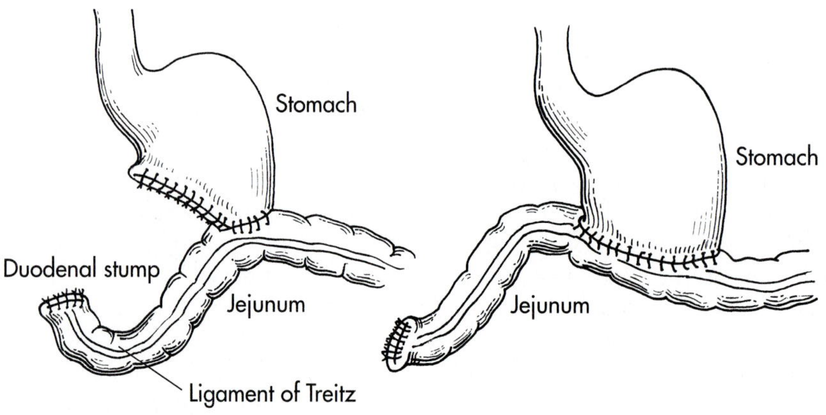

FIGURE 29-9 Billroth II gastrojejunostomy with end-to-side sutured anastomosis of stomach to loop of jejunum.

iologic support. Many morbidly obese patients have medical complications such as hypertension, peripheral vascular disease, cardiac disease, degenerative arthritis, gallbladder disease, or diabetes mellitus. Routine OR procedures usually include the insertion of nasogastric, indwelling Foley urinary, intravenous infusion, and monitoring catheters and application of antiembolic stockings. Respiratory distress is a potential complication during induction of anesthesia; thus intubation while the patient is awake may be the technique of choice. Bariatric procedures for gastric restriction are not without risks. Nutritional deficiencies, anemia, wound infection, and failure of staple lines have occurred postoperatively. The capacity of the stomach is reduced to about 50 ml to restrict food absorption or intake.

Gastric Bypass

In a gastric bypass the size of the stomach is reduced by creating a small pouch in the fundus, the proximal segment. The stomach is transected horizontally with a linear stapler. The proximal jejunum is divided. A Roux-en-Y gastrojejunostomy is constructed between the pouch and the jejunum, bypassing the remainder of stomach, to establish intestinal continuity for the passage of gastric contents. The proximal jejunal segment is anastomosed end-to-side to the distal segment for drainage of gastric, biliary, and pancreatic fluids.

Gastroplasty

In gastroplasty, usually referred to as a *vertical banded gastroplasty,* four linear staple lines are placed vertically on the lesser curvature side of the stomach just left of the gastroesophageal junction. This creates a channel for passage of gastric contents from proximal to distal segments. The stomach is divided between staple lines and oversewn with sutures. The outlet at the end of the staple line is usually reinforced with silicone tubing, a Silastic ring, polypropylene mesh, or a soft rubber drain to prevent dilatation.

INTESTINAL PROCEDURES

Intestines is an inclusive term referring to the continuous muscular tube of the bowel, which extends from the lower end of the stomach to the rectum (see Figure 29-7). Food and products of digestion pass through this section of the alimentary canal during the processes of digestion, absorption, and elimination of waste products. Anatomically, the intestines are divided into the small (upper) and large (lower) intestine, with subdivisions of each.

The small intestine extends from the pylorus to the ileocecal valve. The three sections include the *duodenum* or proximal portion, the *jejunum* or middle section, and the *ileum* or distal portion that joins the large intestine. The *ileocecal valve,* a sphincter muscle, prevents return of material that has been discharged to the large intestine.

The large intestine or *colon* extends from the ileum to the rectum and is generally divided into ascending, transverse, descending, and sigmoid colon. A blind pouch, the *cecum,* is formed where the large intestine joins the small intestine.

The *mesentery,* a peritoneal fold, attaches the small and large intestines to the posterior abdominal wall and contains the blood vessels that nourish the intestines.

Inflammation, intestinal obstruction, and disruption in absorption and motility are disorders that may lead to surgical intervention. Etiologic factors determine the surgical procedure.

Resection of Small Intestine

Tumors, strangulation from adhesions, volvulus, obstruction, and regional ileitis usually are treated by resection of the involved segment. An abdominal incision is made over the suspected or known site of disease. After exposure, clamps are placed above and below the diseased segment of the bowel and mesentery to avoid spillage. The involved area is resected. An end-to-end, end-to-side, or side-to-side anastomosis is done to restore continuity (Figure 29-10). Varia-

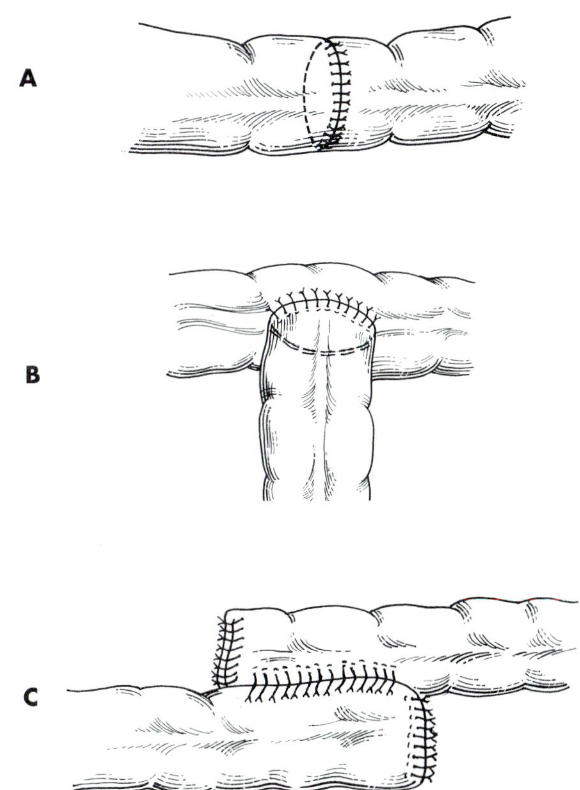

FIGURE 29-10 Intestinal anastomoses. **A,** End-to-end. **B,** End-to-side. **C,** Side-to-side. Shown as sutured anastomoses, they can be done with circular or linear staplers.

tions of this technique are used for other related problems of the small intestine such as extensive perforation. Bowel strangulation and obstruction necessitate an immediate surgical procedure to prevent necrosis, peritonitis, and death.

Hemicolectomy, Transverse Colectomy, Anterior Resection, Total Colectomy

Colitis, diverticulitis, obstruction, and neoplasms are the most frequent reasons for surgical intervention to remove a diseased segment of the colon. Most surgical procedures involve opening the abdomen, walling off the peritoneal cavity, incising and clamping at the points where resection is to be carried out, and finally reestablishing continuity by anastomosis. In selected patients, a laparoscopic approach may be used to mobilize the segment of large or small bowel to be resected. Resected bowel is removed through a small minimal access incision in the abdominal wall. Stomas can also be created with the laparoscopic technique.

The perioperative plan of care includes preoperative administration of intestinal antibiotics, bowel-cleansing methods, and diet restrictions. Intraoperatively, separate instrument technique should be used during the procedure (see considerations on p. 591). Postoperatively, a nasogastric tube inserted before the surgical procedure should remain in place until partial healing of anastomosis occurs and effective peristalsis returns. Fluid and electrolyte balance must be maintained.

Intestinal Stomas

An intestinal *-ostomy* is a surgically created opening, or stoma, from a portion of the bowel to the exterior via the abdominal wall. The procedure may be done to divert intestinal contents so as to permit healing of inflamed bowel, to decompress pressure caused by an obstructive lesion, or to bypass an obstruction such as a benign or malignant tumor. The type and level of the lesion determine whether an ileostomy, cecostomy, or colostomy is indicated. The opening may be permanent or temporary, depending on the cause and course of the disease or obstruction. In patients with a temporary stoma, intestinal continuity is reestablished following healing by closure of the opening in the bowel and anastomosis of the previously resected ends.

Patient acceptance of these procedures is as varied as are an individual's emotional reactions. Each patient requires a rehabilitation plan based on personal needs. These plans should include care of the collection appliance, maintenance of skin integrity, proper diet, odor control, and comfortable, concealing clothing. Patient participation is an integral part of preparation for self-care and enhances self-confidence.

Ileostomy

In an ileostomy, performed for a condition such as chronic ulcerative colitis or following removal of the colon (colectomy), the proximal end of the transected ileum is exteriorized through the abdominal wall. The usual stoma site is located in the midportion of the right rectus sheath approximately 3 cm below the level of the umbilicus. A disk of skin is excised. The anterior and posterior sheaths are incised, and the rectus is divided with a muscle-splitting incision. The proximal end of the ileum is brought out through the peritoneum and muscle to skin. The end is everted and sutured to skin (Figure 29-11). Liquid or semisolid discharge is collected in an ileostomy bag placed over the stoma. Surrounding skin requires special care, such as use of karaya gum, to prevent excoriation and irritation.

Surgical procedures are performed to create a *continent ileostomy.* In the endorectal-ileoanal pull-through procedure, the entire cecum and colon, as well as rectal mucosa (mucosal proctectomy), are resected. The ileum is anastomosed to the anus. Rectal and anal muscles are preserved for anal continence. A pouch is constructed from the terminal ileum proximal to the anal anastomosis to serve as a reservoir for intestinal contents. In the Kock pouch, a nipple valve is created to maintain continency. The patient intubates the valve regularly through an abdominal stoma. In modifications of the classic Kock procedure first described by Nils Kock in Sweden in 1967, either a J-, S-, or W-shaped pouch is created to form an isoperistaltic, ileoanal reservoir at the level of the rectum. A temporary diverting loop or

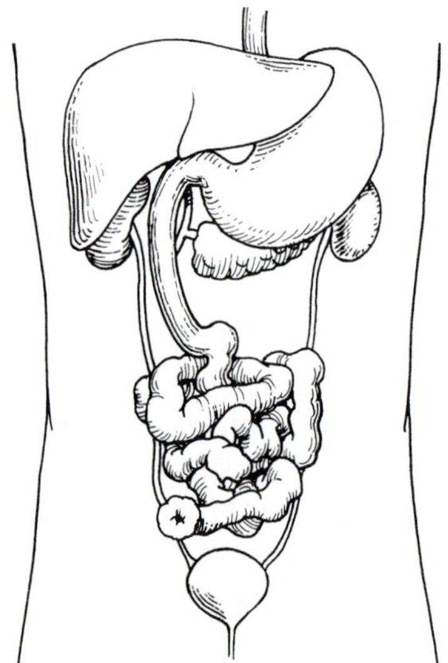

FIGURE 29-11 Ileostomy. Proximal end of transected ileum is brought out through peritoneum and muscle. The end is everted and sutured to skin. Stoma site is in midportion of right rectus sheath below level of umbilicus.

double-barreled ileostomy is brought to the skin for drainage during healing of anastomoses. Subsequently this stoma is closed. Although not without complications, these procedures offer acceptable alternatives to a permanent ileostomy stoma, especially in children and young adults.

Cecostomy

An opening is created in the cecum (cecostomy) and a tube is inserted for decompression of massive distention caused by colonic obstruction. The tube is placed into cecum through the lower right side of the abdomen. Less severe distention may be relieved by suction and irrigation through a colonoscope (see p. 598) and insertion of an intestinal tube through the anus to the cecum. Cecostomy or colonoscopic decompression may precede subsequent colon resection.

Colostomy

An opening anywhere along the length of the colon (colostomy) to the exterior skin surface creates an artificial anus (Figure 29-12). The section of colon to be exteriorized depends on the location of the lesion to be resected or treated. For example, a low anterior bowel resection necessitates a sigmoid colostomy. Either a double-barreled or loop colostomy may be performed. In a *double-barreled colostomy* (Figure 29-12, *B*), the transverse colon is divided and both ends are brought out to the margins of the skin incision. The proximal stoma serves as an outlet for feces, while the distal opening leads to the nonfunctioning bowel. In a *loop colostomy* (Figure 29-12, *C*), a loop of colon is brought out onto the abdominal wall. A plastic rod or ostomy bridge is placed under the loop to hold it out on the exterior abdominal wall. A short length of rubber tubing is connected to each end to stabilize the rod in position. The peritoneum is closed and the wound around the colostomy is sutured. Some surgeons prefer to leave an intestinal clamp in place. This clamp is exteriorized until the stoma is opened, and then it is removed.

Following combined abdominoperineal resection for rectal carcinoma, a permanent colostomy in the sigmoid colon forms an artificial anus. A collection device for fecal material is not needed after a patient's bowel evacuation becomes regulated.

Appendectomy

Appendicitis can occur at any age but is seen most frequently in adolescents and young adults. It may imitate other conditions such as a ruptured ovarian cyst or ureteral calculus. Some appendices are retrocecal, making diagnosis more obscure. Classic symptoms of early appendicitis include right lower quadrant pain, rebound tenderness, nausea, and moderate temperature and white blood count elevation.

Emergency appendectomy is necessary to prevent progression to gangrene and perforation of friable tissue, with subsequent peritonitis. The abdominal approach involves a right lower quadrant muscle-splitting incision over McBurney's point. The blood supply to the appendix is ligated and severed. A crushing clamp is applied to the appendiceal base, which is then

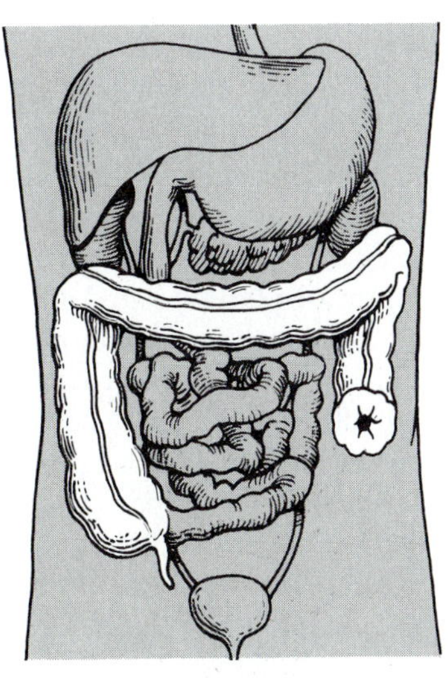

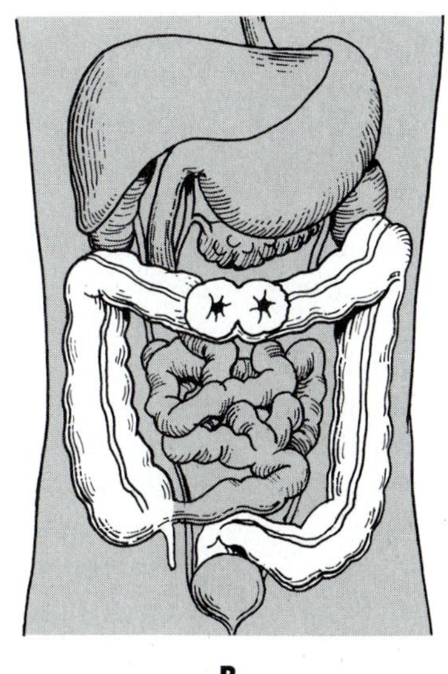

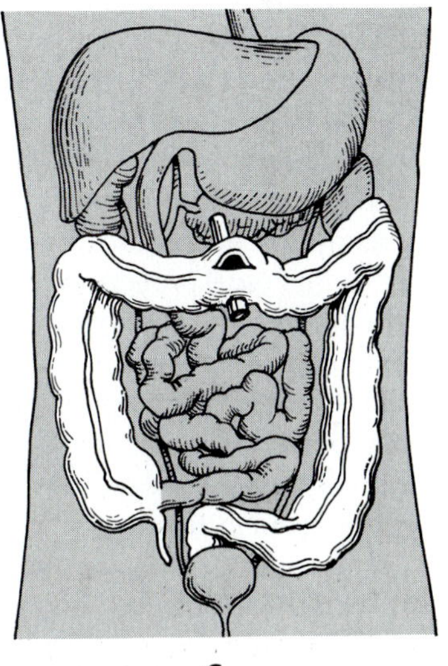

FIGURE 29-12 Colostomy. **A,** Permanent colostomy. Terminal end of descending or sigmoid colon is brought out through peritoneum and muscle and sutured to skin. **B,** Double-barreled colostomy. Both ends of transected colon are brought out to skin. **C,** Loop colostomy. Loop of colon is exteriorized over plastic rod for temporary fecal diversion.

ligated and severed from the cecum. Following amputation, the surgeon may elect to cauterize the stump with phenol and alcohol or wipe it with a sponge soaked with an iodophor (Betadine) to reduce contamination. The stump is then inverted into the cecum as a purse-string suture is tightened around the stump. Because the intestinal tract is laden with bacteria, a culture may be taken in case of future infection.

Drainage is indicated in the presence of an abscess, rupture of the appendix, or any gross contamination of the wound. Usually an appendectomy is an uncomplicated procedure with rapid convalescence unless life-threatening peritonitis results.

Laparoscopic Appendectomy

After insufflation and insertion of a laparoscope through the periumbilical incision (see pp. 584-585), trocars are inserted in the suprapubic area and left lower quadrant. The appendix is elevated and hemostatically freed from the mesoappendix with laser or endoscopic clips or staples. Endoloop ligatures are placed at the base of the appendix. Endoscopic scissors or laser transect it. Grasping forceps are used to place the appendix into an endopouch to prevent extrusion of contents during withdrawal through the periumbilical trocar. The video monitors may be positioned at either side or at the foot end of the operating table.

COLORECTAL PROCEDURES

Colorectal carcinoma is one of the most common abdominal malignancies, with highest incidence in persons over 60 years of age. Incidence of colon cancer is higher in women; rectal cancer is higher in men. Resection of the carcinoma is the surgical procedure of choice, with radiation and chemotherapy as adjuvant therapies or palliation for advanced disease (see Chapter 45). Early diagnosis and prompt treatment of asymptomatic carcinoma improve survival rates.

Diagnostic procedures are routinely performed in patients with bowel or rectal bleeding, chronic diarrhea, or a history of intestinal polyps and/or carcinoma of the colon. Serial guaiac stool tests may detect the presence of occult blood. A barium enema provides a complete radiographic study of the colon. Endoscopic examination is routine. Some therapeutic procedures also may be accomplished with laser or electrocoagulation through endoscopes.

Sigmoidoscopy

Sigmoidoscopy is direct visual inspection of the sigmoid and rectal lumens by means of a flexible fiberoptic or rigid lighted sigmoidoscope. The flexible scope is more comfortable for the patient and gives the surgeon better visualization of the mucosal surface to evaluate the left colon and rectosigmoid. It may be used intraoperatively, as well as for preoperative diagnosis.

The patient is prepared preoperatively with enemas. Placing the patient in the knee-chest or Kraske position allows the sigmoid colon to fall forward into the abdomen. The Sims' or lithotomy position may be used for an extremely obese or extremely ill patient. The surgeon may inflate air to better visualize the mucosal walls. This causes a feeling of desire to defecate, which necessitates reassurance of the patient.

Colonoscopy

Colonoscopy provides visual inspection of the lining of the entire colon. The scope is flexible and consists of two channels, one for suctioning and irrigating and one for operating. Its greatest uses are to examine lumen of the colon and to biopsy tissues in the cancer-prone colon, and especially to search for and excise or ablate polyps. Other indications are for study of inflammatory bowel or diverticular disease, passage of blood in the feces (hemochezia), change in bowel habits, preoperative screen before colostomy closure, confirmation of x-ray findings, and follow-up of patients who had intestinal procedures performed. Argon and Nd:YAG lasers are used through a colonoscope to treat polyps, arteriovenous malformations, and bleeding disorders and to ablate some tumors.

The procedure is contraindicated if the patient is precariously ill or uncooperative. If perforation is likely, relative contraindications may include acute, severe, or radiation inflammatory disease or complete obstruction.

Among the complications are electrical burn during polypectomy, tear or perforation of the colon by tip pressure, tear of the liver or the spleen by air pressure, and tear of diverticuli by introduction of air into them.

Polypectomy

Most surgeons and pathologists agree that adenomatous mucosal polyps in the colon are potentially malignant and should be removed. Polypectomy is usually performed through a fiberoptic colonoscope. Polyps are easily excised at the base. If they are pedunculated, they are cauterized and retrieved for microscopic examination. Electrocoagulation or lasing of the base provides hemostasis. Polyps, which are often familial, may be single or multiple. Some polyps or the involved segment of colon are removed by laparotomy or laparoscopy. The colonoscope may be used intraoperatively to locate polyps. After polypectomy, patients should have annual colonoscopic examinations.

Abdominoperineal Resection

Abdominoperineal resection is an extensive procedure for carcinoma, mainly in the lower third of the rectum. It may extend into the anal canal. Preoperative preparation is meticulous to verify diagnosis, to search for metastasis, and to optimize the condition of the patient.

Before the surgical procedure, a Levin or Miller-Abbott tube is inserted, ureteral catheters are often inserted, and an indwelling Foley catheter is attached to a closed-drainage system.

Two approaches, abdominal and perineal, are required, necessitating preparation and draping of both areas. After resection of the sigmoid, contaminated instruments are removed from the field because the colon is a reservoir of bacteria. Two sets of instruments are necessary. With the patient in Trendelenburg's position, the peritoneal cavity is entered through a lower abdominal incision. Preliminary exploration is done to seek metastases. If the tumor is resectable, the sigmoid colon is mobilized, clamped, and divided. The proximal end of the sigmoid is exteriorized through a stab wound in the left lower quadrant to create a permanent colostomy. The mesentery may be sutured to the abdominal wall to prevent internal hernias. The distal end of the sigmoid is tied to prevent contamination and is placed deep in the presacral space for ultimate removal. The pelvic floor is reperitonealized and the abdomen is closed. Dressings are placed on the abdominal incision and the colostomy.

The second phase of the surgical procedure is closure of the anus with a purse-string suture to prevent contamination and removal of the anus, rectum, rectosigmoid, and surrounding nodes and lymphatics through a perineal incision. Drains are placed and the perineum is closed.

When the abdominal and perineal procedures are done simultaneously, two teams are employed. The patient is initially positioned supine in a modified lithotomy position. This approach reduces operating time and blood loss and provides simultaneous exposure of abdominal and perineal fields.

Patients must be carefully monitored to prevent hypovolemic shock because of the great amount of blood loss from vascular areas and the length of the procedure.

Low Anterior Colon Resection

The sigmoid colon and rectum lie within the bony pelvis, making resection of tumors in the lower sigmoid colon, rectosigmoid, and rectum technically difficult. The objective is to achieve wide local excision with en bloc resection of lymphatics and perirectal mesentery. Intraluminal and linear staplers facilitate colorectal anastomosis in low anterior colon resection. The distal colon is transected after closure with a linear stapler. The intraluminal stapler, with the anvil removed, is introduced through the anus and rectal stump either through or adjacent to the linear staple line. After the anvil is replaced, an intraluminal end-to-end or end-to-side anastomosis with the proximal segment of colon is completed. Total excision of the mesorectum is necessary to prevent recurrence of tumor in the pelvis or at the staple line. A distal tumor clearance of at least 2 cm is necessary. Colorectal continuity is restored and anal sphincter control is maintained with this technique for low anterior colorectal anastomosis without necessity of a permanent colostomy, as with abdominoperineal resection.

ABDOMINAL TRAUMA

Trauma is the major cause of death in persons under 40 years of age. Bleeding from disruption of solid organs or major vessels in the abdomen, including the pelvis, and infection from perforation of a hollow viscus are life-threatening injuries. Blunt and penetrating trauma have different mechanisms of injury. Blunt trauma, caused by direct impact, rapid deceleration, shearing forces, and/or increased intraluminal pressure, can rupture or sever multiple structures, including those that are retroperitoneal. Penetrating injuries involve structures within the path of the weapon; gunshot wounds may also injure adjacent structures by blast effect or cavitation. A stab or gunshot wound of the abdomen can penetrate across the diaphragm into the chest or vice versa. Ultrasonography, angiography, CT, and peritoneal lavage are useful diagnostic tests to assess extent of abdominal injuries and to determine indications for surgical intervention. Injuries to great vessels require an immediate surgical procedure to control bleeding and restore vascular continuity. Major organ injuries mandate laparotomy for repair or reconstruction or to resect severely damaged tissues. Time is a critical factor that significantly influences survival.

Many patients have multiple injuries that affect more than one body system. They require a comprehensive approach to diagnosis and treatment by a multidisciplinary team. The philosophy of trauma management has changed from that of an individual surgeon treating an injured patient in the emergency department and OR to a system that begins at the site of the accident with stabilization by trained personnel and continues with definitive care, including rapid surgical intervention and rehabilitation.

COMPLICATIONS OF ABDOMINAL SURGERY

Patients are particularly prone to pulmonary complications following abdominal surgery. They are also subject to a variety of fluid and electrolyte imbalances because they are generally NPO (nothing by mouth) postoperatively. They may lose sodium, potassium, chloride, and water through nasogastric suction. If great quantities of alkalotic pancreatic secretions are lost through decompression of the small bowel, metabolic acidosis may result. Loss of acidic stomach secretions may lead to metabolic alkalosis.

Peritonitis and wound infection may result after gastrointestinal surgery because of spillage of contaminants from the lumen of the gastrointestinal tract. *Escherichia coli* and *Bacteroides fragilis* are the most common organisms. *Clostridium perfringens*, the chief cause of gas gangrene, can also be found in the intestinal tract. Wound infection can cause wound disruption (see Chapter 25, p. 533), and/or formation of scar tissue. The latter is enhanced by peritonitis or postoperative radiation therapy. Increased intraabdominal pressure even years postoperatively may induce an incisional hernia through an old scar that has weakened (see p. 602).

Adhesions are the most common cause of postoperative intestinal obstruction. They are caused by an outpouring of fibrin from traumatized tissues that causes intestinal surfaces to stick together, thus limiting mobility. Foreign bodies in the peritoneal cavity can produce granulomas that stimulate fibrin. Glove powder, lint from sponges, and some powerful antibiotics can produce granulomas. Some patients must return to the OR for lysis of adhesions. Adhesions may present a contraindication for future laparoscopic surgery.

ANORECTAL PROCEDURES

Hemorrhoids, abscesses, fissures, and fistulas are frequently indications for surgical intervention. The anal region is well supplied with nerves, and these procedures often cause much discomfort. Patients are also sensitive and embarrassed because of the surgical site. Following rectal surgery, patients may have initial difficulty voiding and usually experience considerable pain, requiring medication and sitz baths.

Anoscopy, Proctoscopy, Sigmoidoscopy

Endoscopic diagnostic procedures such as anoscopy, proctoscopy, and sigmoidoscopy are used to visually examine the mucosa of the anus, rectum, and sigmoid. Sigmoidoscopy is routinely done before rectal surgery. Fiberoptic equipment has aided in early detection and treatment of tumors, polyps, and ulcerations.

Hemorrhoidectomy

Hemorrhoidectomy is surgical removal of varicosities of veins or prolapsed mucosa of the anus and rectum that do not respond to conservative treatment. Hemorrhoids are classified as *internal*, occurring above the internal sphincter and covered with columnar mucosa, or *external*, appearing outside the external sphincter and covered with skin. Often both types are present in the patient. External hemorrhoids cause pruritus and pain. The internal type frequently bleed and may become thrombosed and edematous. Rectal bleeding cannot be assumed to be from hemorrhoids but requires thorough investigation to rule out gastrointestinal disease.

The usual procedure consists of dilating the sphincter, ligating the hemorrhoidal pedicle with suture ligatures, and excising each hemorrhoidal mass. A laser, electrosurgical, or cryosurgical unit may be employed. Kraske position usually is used, with patient's buttocks retracted by hemorrhoid straps fastened to edges of the operating table. Some surgeons prefer to position female patients in lithotomy to avoid contamination of the vagina with bloody anal fluid. Petrolatum gauze packing may be inserted in the anal canal, or a compression dressing and perineal binder are applied at completion of the surgical procedure.

As an alternative to a surgical procedure, McGivney rubber-band ligation of internal hemorrhoids as an office procedure is popular. After infiltration of local anesthetic, the hemorrhoid is visualized with an anoscope and grasped with the ligating instruments. Two bands are placed around the base of each hemorrhoid. Sloughing of the avascularized hemorrhoid occurs in 7 to 10 days.

Incision and Drainage of Anal Abscess

Localized infection in tissues around the anus results in abscess formation. Early incision and drainage are essential to prevent infection from spreading.

Fistulotomy, Fistulectomy

An anal fistula often develops after incision and drainage or spontaneous drainage of an anorectal abscess. A fistulous tract may be opened (fistulotomy) to allow drainage and healing by granulation, or the tract may be excised (fistulectomy). Injection of a dye or use of a probe and grooved director aids in identifying the tract. Fistulas can be excised with a laser beam.

Fissurectomy

When a benign ulcerative lesion occurs in the lining of the anal canal, the anus is dilated and infected tissue is excised. Some fissures can be vaporized with a laser. Fecal incontinence caused by damage to the anal sphincter is a potential complication that the surgeon tries to avoid.

Treatment of Rectal Tumors

Surgeons prefer to resect a small rectal cancer instead of performing a radical surgical procedure. Many cancers within 20 cm of the anal verge are amenable to local treatment with endoscopic, laser, or cryosurgical technique. Electrosurgical cutting and coagulating can also be combined to remove superficial anorectal and pararectal lesions. For electrosection, the lesion should be small, mobile, and polypoid, with no palpable lymph nodes. The procedure may be done for palliation to relieve bleeding, painful sphincter spasms (tenesmus), or severe constipation (obstipation). Sometimes interstitial radiation therapy is used for small anorectal squamous cell carcinoma. Protocol may include external radiation, but bleeding lesions do not respond well to radiation.

Tumors in the upper half of the rectum may be excised through an operating rectoscope. This long, tubular instrument improves the surgeon's visual image by incorporating a binocular stereoscope. The procedure is called *transanal endoscopic microsurgery* (TEM). Carbon dioxide is insufflated to hold the walls of the rectum open. Tissue graspers, a high-frequency knife, suction, needleholders, and other instruments can be inserted through ports in the airtight eyepiece on the rectoscope. TEM may be used to remove benign lesions and some malignant tumors.

EXCISION OF PILONIDAL CYST AND SINUS

A painful draining cyst with fistulous tract(s) may occur in soft tissues of the sacrococcygeal region. When it becomes infected, drainage is necessary to relieve pain, swelling, and suppuration. The cyst and sinus tracts must be *excised* or *marsupialized* to prevent recurrence. Marsupialization is suturing of cyst walls to the edges of the wound, following evacuation, to permit the packed cavity to close by granulation. A Z-plasty may be preferred for primary closure to produce a strong transverse scar, or the wound may be closed with a rotational pedicle flap (see Chapter 34, p. 711). Surgical judgment determines whether primary closure or healing by granulation is chosen. A compression dressing is applied.

HERNIA PROCEDURES

A *hernia* is the protrusion of an organ or part of an organ through a defect in supporting structures that normally contain it. A hernia may be congenital, acquired, or traumatic. Most occur in the inguinal or femoral region; however, umbilical, ventral, and hiatal hernias also occur.

A hernia is usually composed of a sac (covering), hernial contents, and an aperture (opening), but in some locations a sac is absent.

When hernial contents can be returned to the normal cavity by manipulation, the hernia is called *reducible*. If the hernial contents cannot be reduced, it is called *irreducible* or *incarcerated*. Bowel present in an incarcerated hernia not only may lack adequate blood supply but may also become obstructed. This is referred to as a *strangulated* hernia. An immediate surgical procedure is necessary to prevent necrosis of the strangulated bowel.

Inguinal Herniorrhaphy (Hernioplasty)

An inguinal hernia is often repaired under local anesthesia. An oblique inguinal incision on the affected side is extended through external oblique aponeurosis. The hernia sac is emptied of its contents, ligated, and excised. The floor of the inguinal canal is reconstructed. Sometimes prosthetic mesh is needed to reinforce a large or recurrent defect. Repair depends on whether the inguinal hernia is indirect or direct.

Indirect

In an indirect hernia the peritoneal sac containing intestine protrudes through the internal inguinal ring and passes down the inguinal canal. It may descend all the way into the scrotum. Indirect inguinal hernia, more common in male patients, originates from a congenital defect in the fascial floor of the inguinal canal.

Direct

A direct hernia protrudes through a weakness in the abdominal wall in the region between the rectus abdominis muscle, inguinal ligament, and inferior epigastric artery. This hernia is the most difficult type to repair and appears more frequently in men. An acquired weakness of the lower abdominal wall, a direct inguinal hernia often results from straining, such as heavy lifting, chronic coughing, or straining to urinate or defecate. Prompt surgical repair prevents possible discomfort and threat of later complications.

NOTE In both indirect and direct inguinal herniorrhaphy in male patients, the spermatic cord and blood supply to the testis must be protected from injury. If herniorrhaphies are performed bilaterally, severance of the cords will cause sterility. Infarction of a testis can occur if the blood supply is compromised.

Laparoscopic Repair

Either an indirect or direct reducible inguinal hernia may be repaired through a laparoscopic procedure. This is particularly advantageous for repairing bilateral or recurrent hernias. A transabdominal preperitoneal or intraperitoneal approach may be used, or an extraperitoneal procedure can be done. Polypropylene mesh is inserted to reinforce the wall of the inguinal canal. This is stapled in place.

Femoral Herniorrhaphy

Femoral herniorrhaphy involves repairing the defect in the transversalis fascia below the inguinal ligament, as well as removing the peritoneal sac protruding through the femoral ring. The transversalis fascia is normally attached to Cooper's ligament, which prevents the peritoneum from reaching the femoral ring. To repair this defect it is necessary to reconstruct the posterior wall and close the femoral ring. These hernias appear more frequently in women.

Umbilical Herniorrhaphy

Repair of an umbilical hernia consists of closing the peritoneal opening and uniting the fasciae above and below the defect to reconstruct the abdominal wall surrounding the umbilicus. This type of hernia, seen most frequently in children, represents a congenital defect of protrusion of the peritoneum through the umbilical ring. It also may be acquired by women following childbirth.

Ventral (Incisional) Herniorrhaphy

Impaired healing of a previous surgical incision, usually a vertical abdominal one, may cause an incisional hernia. Often the result of weakening of abdominal fasciae, projections of peritoneum carrying segments of bowel protrude through fascial perforations. It is necessary to reunite the tissue layers to close the defect. After excising the old scar, the peritoneal sac is opened, the hernia is reduced, and the layers are firmly closed. If existing tissue is not sufficient for repair, synthetic mesh may be used to reinforce the repair. Incisional hernias are sometimes the aftermath of postoperative hematoma, infection, or undue strain.

Ventral hernias have a high recurrence rate when mesh is placed on the outside of a large repair. Through an intraabdominal laparoscopic approach, omentum can be placed over the mesh or peritoneum can be put back over the mesh.

Hiatal (Diaphragmatic) Herniorrhaphy

A hiatal hernia results when a portion of the stomach protrudes through the hiatus of the diaphragm. The *hiatus* is the opening for the esophagus through the *diaphragm,* which is the chief muscle of respiration. A weakening in the hiatus permits violation of the muscular partition between the abdomen and chest. Symptoms largely are caused by inflammation and ulceration of the adjacent esophagus, resulting from reflux of gastric juices from the herniated stomach. Symptoms include pain, blood loss, and difficulty in swallowing (dysphagia). Diagnosis is made by radiologic and endoscopic studies.

Surgical treatment is appropriate when medical therapy fails to alleviate the problem. Surgical approach may be via the abdomen or chest, or thoracoabdominal. Each approach offers certain advantages. The abdominal approach is generally preferred (see p. 590). However, the better view of the hiatal region afforded by opening the chest may favor this approach (see Chapter 38, p. 792).

AMPUTATION OF EXTREMITIES

Amputation is the total or partial removal of any extremity. Necessity for amputation is associated most frequently with massive trauma, presence of malignant tumor, extensive infection, and vascular insufficiency. (See Chapter 44 for discussion of replantation of traumatically severed extremities.) Orthopaedic or vascular surgeons may perform these procedures.

In preparing the patient for a lower extremity amputation, expose both legs for comparison before skin preparation in addition to checking the chart. *Be absolutely certain the correct leg is prepared.*

Many lower extremity amputations are done under spinal anesthesia. Ensure that the specimen is never, at any time, within the patient's sight. Follow policy in regard to patient's permission for disposal of an extremity.

Two types of amputation generally are performed, *open (guillotine)* and *closed.*

The guillotine procedure, rarely performed, is regarded as an emergency procedure. Tissues are cut circularly with the bone transected higher to allow soft tissues to cover the bone end. Blood vessels and nerve endings are ligated, but the wound is left open. The surgical procedure frequently is followed by prolonged drainage and healing, muscle and skin retraction, and excessive granulation tissue. A second procedure is often required for final repair. Patients who are severely ill or toxic or who experience severe trauma, such as an extremity caught under an immovable object, are candidates for this procedure.

The conventional flap or closed type of amputation is more desirable. Fashioning curved skin and fascial flaps before amputation of the bone allows for deep and superficial fasciae to be approximated over the bone end before loose skin closure. Drainage by catheter or suction apparatus may or may not be required. The wound usually heals in about 2 weeks.

Amputations of Lower Extremity

Amputations of the lower extremity are classified as above the knee (AK), below the knee (BK), toe, transphalangeal, transmetatarsal, and Syme's amputation. The level of amputation is determined by the patient's general health, vascular status, and rehabilitative potential.

Above-Knee Amputation

Amputation at the lower third of the thigh is selected when gangrene or arterial insufficiency extends above the level of the malleoli. Mid-thigh amputation involves circular incision over the distal femur, creating large anterior and posterior skin flaps, transecting fasciae and muscles. Vessels and nerves such as the femoral and sciatic, respectively, are ligated and severed. Sharp bone edges of the stump are smoothed by filing. The wound is well irrigated with sterile normal saline solution before closure of tissue layers. Hemostasis is important to prevent massive hemorrhage or painful hematoma. Depending on the surgeon's preference, drains may be used. A noncompressive dressing is applied. A longer time is required for rehabilitation than after BK amputation because AK amputation is a more extensive procedure. A prosthesis is generally fitted 4 to 6 weeks after amputation.

Below-Knee Amputation

Amputation at the middle third of the leg provides for more functional prosthesis fitting and reduction of phantom limb pain. It also permits a more natural gait. An *immediate postoperative prosthesis* (IPOP) can be applied in the OR. The IPOP dressing requires a stump sock, felt and lamb's wool for padding, twill Y straps that are attached to a fitted corset, and a rigid plaster dressing. This dressing not only protects the stump but aids in controlling the weight placed on it. The prosthesis is metal and provides a pull on the stump. The pylon (foot) may be attached before the patient returns to the unit. However, if the patient is obese or debilitated, weight bearing may be delayed for several days.

Toe, Transphalangeal, and Transmetatarsal Amputations

Toe and partial foot amputations are generally performed for gangrene and osteomyelitis.

Syme's Amputation

Syme's amputation is usually performed for trauma and involves the distal part of the foot. The amputation is above the ankle joint. The skin of the heel is used for the flap.

Hip Disarticulation and Hemipelvectomy

Hip disarticulation and hemipelvectomy involve total removal of the right or left pelvis, including the innominate hipbone, along the ipsilateral lower extremity. Division of bone may be carried through the sacroiliac joint, or a portion of iliac bone and crest may be preserved. An internal hemipelvectomy includes removal of innominate bone with adjacent muscles. The large defect created may be covered by a myocutaneous flap of quadriceps femoris muscle and overlying skin and subcutaneous tissue. The neck of the femur rests against soft tissues. These radical procedures are indicated for malignant bone or soft tissue tumors and extensive traumatic injuries. Specialized prosthetic devices are available to permit ambulation.

Amputations of Upper Extremity

Amputations of Hand

Hand amputations usually result from trauma and include part or all of the distal phalanges of the digits. Attention is directed to keeping the hand as a working unit when one or more fingers are removed. Every effort should be made to save the thumb because the smallest stump is better than a prosthesis. (See section on digital transfer in Chapter 34, p. 713.)

Forearm and Forequarter Amputation

Wrist, elbow, and humerus disarticulations are radical procedures performed for malignant tumors or extensive trauma.

Rehabilitation

Postoperative considerations for any amputation include control of bleeding and phantom limb sensations, stump care, immediate fitting and functional terminal prosthesis, exercises to prevent flexion contractures, and ambulation or use of a hand or arm.

The loss of an extremity involves major adjustment psychologically and physically. The rehabilitative process, so important, is often affected by the emotional reactions of the amputee. Patients with an early postoperative prosthesis have a more positive outlook about their loss. Being able to walk the first postoperative day or soon thereafter (which will depend on the surgeon's orders for the weight-bearing program in the case of a leg amputee) boosts morale. This in turn aids in ambulation.

Phantom limb pain is particularly distressing to many patients. Nerves have been severed, but the patient has the sensation that the amputated part is still present. This sensation is often associated with painful paresthesia (i.e., tingling, prickling, tickling, or burning). The pain is real. It usually responds to aspirin, acetaminophen (Tylenol), or a similar agent, but narcotics may be necessary to control pain.

The combined efforts of the patient, family, and interdisciplinary professional personnel are needed for successful rehabilitation.

Bibliography

Alston RC: Ileal pouch-anal anastomosis procedure, *Surg Technol* 23(5):9-13, 1991.

Beachley M, Farrarr J: Abdominal trauma: putting the pieces together, *Am J Nurs* 93(11):27-34, 1993.

Braasch JW, Gasbarro KA: Fibrous bile duct obstructions, *AORN J* 52(4):818-826, 1990.

Brumm JA, Crim BJ: Biliary lithotripsy: a smashing solution, *Today's OR Nurse* 12(4):4-8, 1990.

Bunt TJ: Physiologic amputation, *AORN J* 54(6):1220-1224, 1991.

Butler RW: Managing the complications of cirrhosis, *Am J Nurs* 94(3):46-49, 1994.

Campbell AD, Ferrara BE: Toupet partial fundoplication, *AORN J* 57(3):671-679, 1993.

Chin AK et al: Gasless laparoscopy using a planar lifting technique, *J Am Coll Surg* 178(4):401-403, 1994.

Cooperman AM: *Laparoscopic cholecystectomy: difficult cases and creative solutions*, St Louis, 1992, Quality Medical Publishing.

Darzi A et al: Laparoscopic assisted surgery of the colon, *Endosc Surg Allied Technol* 1(1):13-15, 1993.

Deters GE: Managing complications after abdominal surgery, *RN* 50(3):27-32, 1987.

Front ME et al: Common bile duct strictures, *AORN J* 52(1):57-67, 1990.

Geis WP, Malago M: Laparoscopic bilateral inguinal herniorrhaphies: use of a single giant preperitoneal mesh patch, *Am Surg* 60(8):558-563, 1994.

Goldman J, Kirshenbaum G: Laparoscopic laser cholecystectomy, *Surg Technol* 23(1):16-19, 1991.

Gonzalez-Cortes SB, Procuniar CE: Laparoscopic inguinal herniorrhaphy, *AORN J* 60(3):419-430, 1994.

Hansen VA et al: Splenic salvage vs splenectomy, *AORN J* 53(6):1519-1528, 1991.

Hashizume M et al: Laparoscopic splenectomy, *Am J Surg* 167(6):611-614, 1994.

Heidrick R: Low anterior resection of rectal carcinoma, *Surg Technol* 23(3):10-13, 1991.

Hilmer DM: Technical considerations of bariatric surgery in the superobese, *Surg Technol* 26(7):8-12, 1994.

Jackson DC et al: Endoscopic laser cholecystectomy, *AORN J* 51(6):1546-1552, 1990.

Jamieson GG et al: Laparoscopic Nissen fundoplication, *Ann Surg* 220(2):137-145, 1994.

Johnson JR: Caring for the woman who's had a mastectomy, *Am J Nurs* 94(5):25-31, 1994.

Jones WG et al: Pancreatic injuries: diagnosis, treatment, *AORN J* 53(4):917-933, 1991.

Junge T: Endoscopic inguinal herniorrhaphy, *Surg Technol* 25(5):10-13, 1993.

Jurf JB et al: Cholecystectomy made easier, *Am J Nurs* 90(12):38-39, 1990.

Khoo RE et al: Laparoscopic loop ileostomy for temporary fecal diversion, *Dis Colon Rectum* 36(10):966-968, 1993.

Knobf MT: Early-stage breast cancer: the options, *Am J Nurs* 90(11):28-30, 1990.

Kuzmak LI et al: Surgery for morbid obesity, *AORN J* 51(5):1307-1324, 1990.

LeBlanc KA, LeBlanc ZZ: Gastrointestinal end-to-end anastomosis, *AORN J* 51(4):986-993, 1990.

Lichtenstein IL et al: Hernia repair with polypropylene mesh, *AORN J* 52(3):559-565, 1990.

Long TD, Sandler J: Outpatient hernia repair, *AORN J* 52(4):801-816, 1990.

Lyerly HK, Mault JR: Laparoscopic ileostomy and colostomy, *Ann Surg* 219(3):317-322, 1994.

Mason DS et al: Roux en Y gastric bypass: surgical treatment of morbid obesity, *AORN J* 58(6):1113-1135, 1993.

Mathias JM, Patterson P: Applications for laparoscopic surgery growing, *OR Manager* 8(10):1, 9-12, 1992.

Matthews K: Endoscopic cholecystectomy: a new approach, *Today's OR Nurse* 12(8):17-20, 1990.

McGinnis C, Matson SW: How to manage patients with a roux-en-Y jejunostomy, *Am J Nurs* 94(2):43-45, 1994.

McKernan JB, Laws HL: *Laparoscopy and the general surgeon*, Somerville, NJ, 1990, Ethicon.

Morris PB et al: Outpatient carbon dioxide laser mastectomy, *AORN J* 55(4):984-992, 1992.

Morrison CW et al: Cholecystectomy: a surgical perspective, *Surg Technol* 23(1):11-14, 1991.

Nyhus LM et al: Inguinal hernia repair, *AORN J* 52(2):292-304, 1990.

Payne JH et al: Laparoscopic or open inguinal herniorrhaphy? A randomized trial, *Arch Surg* 129(9):973-979, 1994.

Phillips E et al: Laparoendoscopy and partial resection of the small bowel, *Surg Endosc* 8(6):686-688, 1994.

Rogalla CJ: Pancreatic duct calculi, *AORN J* 53(6):1506-1517, 1991.

Sam KL et al: Radical gastrectomy: the role of the RN first assistant, *AORN J* 58(4):749-763, 1993.

Scannell D: Liver resection, *Surg Technol* 26(12):8-11, 25, 1994.

Shoaf BA, Apelgren KN: Intraoperative endoscopy of the small bowel, *AORN J* 51(3):776-782, 1990.

Smith A: When the pancreas self-destructs, *Am J Nurs* 91(9):38-48, 1991.

Smith EB: Pancreatoduodenectomy: a complicated solution, *Today's OR Nurse* 12(9):6-11, 1990.

Spiro CM et al: Diverticular disease, *AORN J* 59(3):625-634, 1994.

Stein P, Zera RT: Breast cancer, *AORN J* 53(4):938-964, 1991.

Stengel JM, Dirado R: Laparoscopic Nissen fundoplication to treat gastroesophageal reflux, *AORN J* 61(3):483-489, 1995.

Steuer K: Hepatic resection, *AORN J* 52(2):230-250, 1990.

Stillman A: Laparoscopic cholecystectomy: an electrosurgical approach to biliary disease, *AORN J* 57(2):429-436, 1993.

Thompson S: Ultrasonography: intraoperative diagnoses of choledocholithiasis, *AORN J* 51(4):983-985, 1990.

Tsoi EK et al: Laparoscopy without pneumoperitoneum: a preliminary report, *Surg Endosc* 8(5):382-383, 1994.

Weinstein SM: Phantom pain, *Oncology* 8(3):65-70, 1994.

Willis DA et al: Gallstones: alternatives to surgery, *RN* 53(4):44-50, 1990.

Wyman A et al: Surgery for gastric cancer, *Dig Dis* 12(2):117-126, 1994.

Zuro LM et al: Laparoscopic colotomy, polypectomy, *AORN J* 56(6):1068-1073, 1992.

Zuro LM et al: Transanal endoscopic microsurgery, *AORN J* 56(3):466-475, 1992.

CHAPTER 30

Gynecologic and Obstetric Surgery

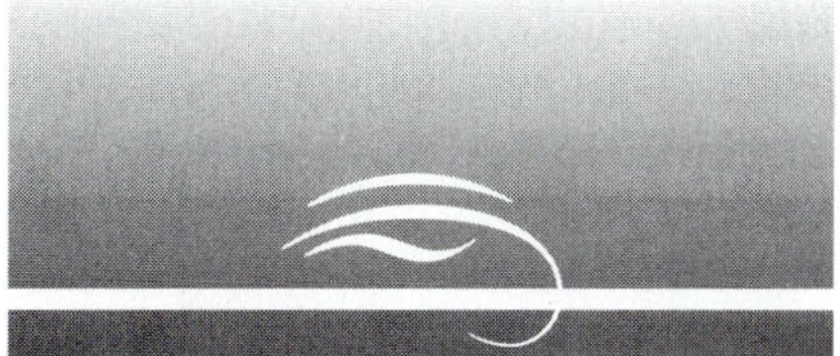

From its inception in 1930, the American Board of Obstetrics and Gynecology has emphasized the inseparability of the two phases of this specialty because of their anatomic and physiologic relationships. *Gynecology,* commonly referred to as "gyn" (GYN), is the science of diseases of the female reproductive organs. Gynecologic surgery includes certain problems of the female genitourinary tract. *Obstetrics* (OB) concerns the care of women during pregnancy, labor, and puerperium (period from delivery to time the uterus regains normal size, usually about 6 weeks). Although all surgeons certified by the Board are competent in both disciplines, some limit their practice to either obstetrics or gynecology. Specialty certification boards have also been established in gynecologic oncology, endocrinology and infertility, and perinatal medicine. This text limits discussion to the most common surgical procedures performed by gynecologists and/or obstetricians in the operating room (OR).

HISTORICAL BACKGROUND

Obstetric care, left to the mother herself or to a midwife, was neglected until the Renaissance. In prehistoric cultures, the woman squatted on a bed of leaves, delivered, chewed off or cut the umbilical cord, bathed the infant in a stream, wrapped it in hide, and resumed her womanly duties. Up through the Dark Ages, based on the Biblical decree, "In sorrow shalt thou bring forth children," it was believed that pregnant women should suffer. Some were attended by midwives. The first book on obstetric care was written by the German physician Eucharius Rösslin in 1513. But it was the treatise of François Mauriceau published in Paris in 1668 that became the basis of obstetrics. He is known as the founder of modern obstetrics and gynecology.

Ancient interest in diseases of women is recorded in the Egyptian *Ebers Papyrus* of the sixteenth century BC. Hippocrates described problems of menstruation and puerperal infection and advocated intrauterine douches. During the Greco-Roman period, Soranus of Ephesus, who practiced in Rome between 98 and 138 AD, described uterine disease and treatments. For centuries his writings were regarded as authoritative.

The practice of gynecology was limited, bound by tradition, and even regressed during medieval times. New interest developed in the Renaissance. In 1566, Caspar Wolf of Switzerland issued an encyclopedia of gynecology entitled *Gynecia.* In 1663 the Dutch surgeon Hendri von Roonhuyze published the first book on surgical gynecology having modern connotations. He described extrauterine pregnancy, uterine rupture, and vesicovaginal fistula.

In the eighteenth century, progress was made, particularly in England. Practitioners advocated the treatment of ovarian cysts. But surgical gynecology did not become an independent specialty until the early nineteenth century.

In 1809 Ephraim McDowell of Kentucky successfully removed an ovarian cyst by an abdominal approach without benefit of modern anesthesia and aseptic techniques. A limited variety of gynecologic procedures such as oophorectomy and salpingectomy were developed by succeeding pioneers. The first successful vaginal hysterectomy was performed in 1818.

The practice of dilating the cervix for a variety of purposes was known since the days of Hippocrates. Many instruments were used. In 1879 Alfred Hegar developed the metal cervical dilators that bear his name and are still commonly used.

Early male gynecologists fought public prejudice against exposure of female organs, even for examination. Clergy, midwives, and physicians attempted to deter their practice. Opposition to the progress of surgery in general eventually was overcome. Use of the speculum was a notable advance for gynecologists.

Obstetricians and gynecologists were influential in introducing the concept of periodic health examination on a large scale. Obstetricians aim to protect the pregnant woman and unborn fetus from unnecessary complications. The intent of gynecologists is to discover and treat pelvic disease, especially carcinoma, in the early stages.

ANATOMY AND PHYSIOLOGY

The genitourinary system comprises the organs, glands, secretions, and other elements of reproduction. Components of the female reproductive system are both external and internal organs.

External Genitalia

Vulva is a collective term for the female external genitalia. This sensitive, delicate area is highly vascular, with an extensive lymph supply and rich cutaneous sensory innervation. It includes the following.

Labia Majora

The labia majora are two large folds, or lips, containing sebaceous and sweat glands embedded in fatty tissue covered by skin. They join together anteriorly in a fatty pad, the *mons veneris,* which overlies the pubic bone. In the adult female this area is covered with hair. Sebaceous secretions of the labia lubricate the proximal area. The labia majora atrophy and hair follicles decrease in number after menopause, making the labia minora more prominent.

Labia Minora

The labia minora or small lips, lying within the labia majora, are flat folds of connective tissue containing sebaceous glands. Anteriorly these labia split into two parts. One part passes over the clitoris to form the protective prepuce or foreskin. The other passes under the clitoris to shape a *frenulum,* a fold of mucous membrane. Posteriorly they join across the midline to form the *fourchette,* a fold of skin just inside the posterior vulvar commissure.

Clitoris

The clitoris, an erectile organ, is the female homologue of the penis. The mucous membrane covering the glans contains many nerve endings. The urethra opens just below the clitoris.

Vestibule

The vestibule is the space, or shallow elliptical depression below the clitoris, enclosed by the labia minora. The fourchette bounds it posteriorly. Urethra, vagina, and bilateral ducts from Bartholin's glands open into the vestibule.

Bartholin's Glands

Small bilateral Bartholin's glands lie deep in the posterior third of the labia majora, within the bulbocavernosus muscle. The mucus secretion is a coital lubricant.

Hymen

The hymen is a thin vascularized connective tissue membrane that surrounds and may partially or completely occlude the vaginal orifice. It varies individually in thickness and elasticity. The central aperture permits passage of menstrual flow and vaginal secretions.

Perineum

The perineum is a diamond-shaped wedge of fibromuscular tissue between the vagina and the anus. It is divided by a transverse septum into an anterior urogenital triangle and a posterior anal triangle. It consists of the perineal body and perineal musculature. With fibers of six muscles converging at its central point, the perineum forms the base of the pelvic floor and helps support the posterior vaginal wall. These muscles are the bulbocavernosus (vaginal sphincter), the two superficial transverse perineal, the two levator ani, and the external anal sphincter. The levators ani are the largest muscles and, in contrast to the other superficial muscles, are deep. The most important muscles in the pelvis, the levators ani (pelvic diaphragm), form a hammock-type suspension from the anterior to the posterior pelvic wall, beneath the pelvic viscera. These muscles retain the organs within the pelvis by offering resistance to repeated increases in intraabdominal pressure, such as coughing, respiring, bearing down in labor, and straining at stool.

Internal Genital Organs

The internal organs (Figure 30-1) lie within the pelvic cavity, protected by the bony pelvis. Bones and ligaments form the pelvic outlet. The dilated cervix of the uterus and the vagina constitute the birth canal.

Vagina

The vagina is a thin-walled, fibromuscular tube extending from the vestibule obliquely backward and upward to the uterus, where the cervix projects into the top of the anterior wall. Constituting a copulatory and parturient canal, the vagina is capable of great distention. The bladder lies anteriorly to it, the rectum posteriorly. It is lined with mucous membrane and contains glands that produce a cleansing acid secretion.

The anterior vaginal wall is shorter than is the posterior. The upper third of the posterior wall is covered by peritoneum reflected onto the rectum. Normally the anterior and posterior walls relax and are in contact. However, the lateral walls remain rigid because of the pull of the muscles and therefore are in close contact with pelvic tissues.

A rich venous plexus in the muscular walls makes the organ highly vascular. Uterine and vaginal arteries supplying the area are branches of the internal iliac artery. Branches of the vaginal artery extend to the external genitalia and the adjacent bladder and rectum. Lymphatic drainage is extensive. The upper two thirds of the vagina drains into the external and internal iliac nodes, the lower third into the superficial inguinal nodes.

The *vault*, dome or upper part of the vagina, is divided into four *fornices*, or arches (Figure 30-2). During digital pelvic examination, the gynecologist can palpate pelvic contents through the thin walls of the vault. The anterior fornix, in front of the cervix, is adjacent to base of the bladder and distal ends of the ureters.

The *pouch of Douglas* (retrouterine cul-de-sac) directly behind the larger posterior fornix lies behind the cervix. This pouch separates the back of uterus from the rectum: anteriorly by the uterine peritoneal covering, which continues down to cap the posterior vaginal fornix; and posteriorly by the anterior wall of the rectum. Lateral uterosacral ligaments embrace the lower third of the rectum. The floor of the pouch, about 7 cm above the anus, is formed by reflection of the peritoneum from the rectum to the upper vagina and uterus. The posterior fornix is the route of entry for a number of diagnostic or surgical procedures because the pouch of Douglas, the lowest part of the peritoneal cavity, is separated from the vagina only by the thin vaginal wall and peritoneum of the fornix.

The lateral fornices lie on either side of the cervix, in contact with anterior and posterior sheets of the broad ligaments surrounding the uterus. Proximal structures are the uterine artery, ureters, fallopian tubes, ovaries, and sigmoid colon.

Uterus

The organ of gestation, the uterus, receives and holds the fertilized ovum during development of the fetus and expels it during childbirth. Resembling an inverted pear

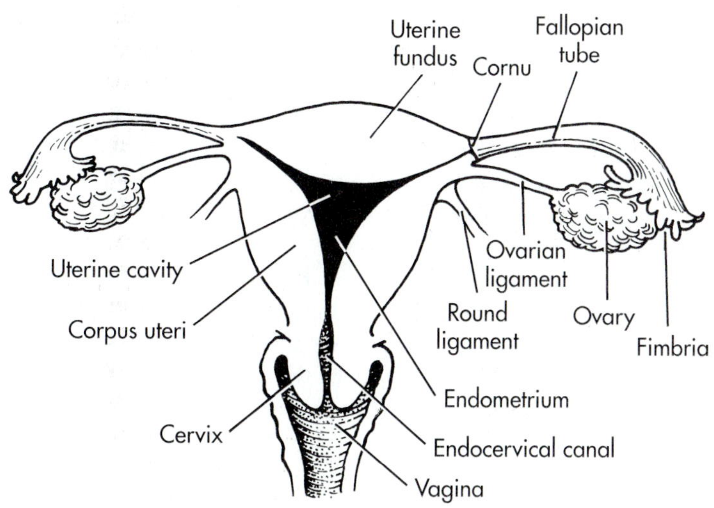

FIGURE 30-1 Female reproductive system.

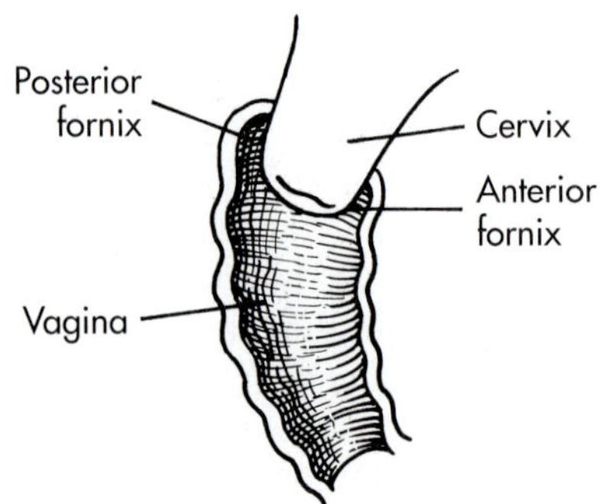

FIGURE 30-2 Cervix in vaginal vault.

in shape, this hollow muscular organ is situated in the bony pelvis. It lies between the bladder anteriorly and the sigmoid colon posteriorly. It is divided by a slight constriction into a wider upper part, the body or *corpus uteri,* and a narrower lower part, the *cervix uteri* or ectocervix that protrudes into the vagina (Figure 30-2). The corpus meets the cervix at the *internal os.* Peritoneum covers the corpus externally; the endometrium lines it internally. This mucous membrane is uniquely adapted to receive and sustain the fertilized ovum. The *fundus,* or domelike portion of the uterus, lies above the uterine cavity.

The *uterine cavity,* flattened from front to back, is roughly triangular in shape in the nonpregnant female. The upper lateral angles extend out toward openings of the fallopian tubes, which enter through the uterine walls at the *cornua.* The apex of the triangle is directed downward to the cervix. The cavity within the cervix, the *endocervical canal,* narrows to a slit at the end where the cervix communicates with the vagina via the *external os.* The *endocervix* is the glandular mucous membrane of the cervix. The corpus and cervix are considered individually in relation to disease and therapy because they differ in structure and function.

As the incubator and nurturer of the developing embryo, the uterus is capable of expansion. Much of the bulk of the corpus consists of involuntary muscle, the *myometrium,* composed of three layers. The inner layer prevents reflux of menstrual flow into the tubes and peritoneal cavity, which could result in endometriosis. It also contributes to the competency of the internal os sphincter to prevent premature expulsion of the fetus. The middle layer encloses large blood vessels. These muscle fibers act as living ligatures for hemostasis after delivery. The outer layer has expulsive action, ejecting menstrual flow and clots, aborted embryo, or the fetus at term.

Usually the uterus lies forward at a right angle to the vagina and rests on the bladder. Although the cervix is anchored laterally by ligaments, the fundus may pivot about the cardinal ligaments widely in an anterior-posterior plane. Mobility rather than position is the criterion for normality.

Fallopian Tubes (Salpinges)

The fallopian tubes, small, hollow musculomembranous tubes, sometimes called *oviducts* or *uterine tubes,* run bilaterally like arms from each side of the upper part of uterus to the ovaries. Near each ovary, the open end of each tube expands into the *infundibulum,* which divides into *fimbriae,* fingerlike projections that sweep up the *ovum* (the female reproductive cell) as it is expelled from the ovary. Ciliated cells move the ovum toward the uterus. The lumen of the tube becomes very narrow where it penetrates the uterine wall to reach the uterine cavity. Contractions in the muscular walls change shape and position of the tubes. At ovulation they move the fimbriated ends into close apposition with ovarian surfaces.

Ovaries

The ovaries are oval-shaped and lie in a shallow peritoneal fossa on the lateral pelvic walls from which they are suspended by the infundibulopelvic ligaments. They are attached to the posterior layer of the broad ligament by the *mesovarium,* a peritoneal fold, and to the uterus by the *ovarian ligament,* a fibromuscular cord.

The ovaries, counterpart of the male testes, give rise to ova. Each ovary consists of a center of cells and vessels surrounded by the *cortex,* the main portion that contains the stroma or fibrous framework in which the ovarian follicles are embedded. Of the approximately 200,000 primordial follicles present at birth, less than 400 are likely to produce a mature ovum *(graafian follicle)* during the reproductive years. A serous covering derived from peritoneum surrounds the ovaries.

In addition to producing ova, the ovaries, which atrophy after menopause, produce female sex hormones.

The ureters course along the peritoneum and lie close to the ovarian blood supply.

Muscles and Ligaments

Muscles and ligaments support the uterus and fallopian tubes in the normal position in the center of the pelvic cavity.

Broad Ligaments Bilateral broad ligaments are composed of a broad double sheet of peritoneum extending from each lateral surface of the uterus outward to the pelvic wall. Between these two layers of peritoneum, the fallopian tubes are enclosed in the free upper borders (mesosalpinges) with the tubal ostia opening directly into the peritoneal cavity.

Round Ligaments The round ligaments are fibromuscular bands that extend from the anterior surface of the lateral borders of the fundus to the labia majora.

They run beneath the peritoneum and anterior sheet of the broad ligament down, outward, and forward through the inguinal canal to the labia.

Cardinal Ligaments The lower portion of the broad ligaments, the cardinal ligaments are attached to the lateral vaginal fornices and supravaginal portion of the cervix. They act as a supportive pivot.

Uterosacral Ligaments The uterosacral ligaments are peritoneal folds containing connective tissue and involuntary muscle. They arise on each side from the posterior wall of the uterus at the level of the internal os, pass backward around the rectum, and insert on the sacrum at level of the second sacral vertebra. They pull on the cervix to keep the uterus anteverted and, through the cervix, the vagina in position as well.

Physiology

The function of the female reproductive organs is to conceive, nurture, and produce offspring. The development and function of these organs are influenced by the hormonal secretions of the ovaries and adrenal, thyroid, and pituitary glands. The organs also affect sex characteristics.

The physiologic cycle prepares the womb for the fertilized ovum. Hormone production stimulates the endometrium and breasts, resulting in thickening and increased blood supply.

Each month during the years from puberty to menopause, one of the ovaries produces on its surface a follicle from within. When the matured graafian follicle ruptures, it discharges the enclosed ovum, which enters the fallopian tube at the fimbriated end. The process of maturation and discharge of the egg is called *ovulation*, a fertile period that lasts several days. Changes in cervical mucus and vaginal epithelium also accompany ovulation. Union of the ovum with a viable mature male germ cell *(spermatozoon)*, which has ascended to the fallopian tube from the vagina, results in *fertilization*. The fertilized ovum normally proceeds to the cornu of the uterus, where it enters to implant in the endometrium within 14 days of fertilization. The ensuing pregnancy will last approximately 266 days or 9 calendar months if carried to full term.

The ovarian hormone estrogen together with progesterone cause a sequence of changes in the endometrial lining of the uterus to prepare for implantation of the fertilized ovum. Estrogen also produces the development of secondary sexual characteristics. Progesterone is responsible for maintaining pregnancy until hormones from the placenta assume this role.

Menstruation, the end result of lack of fertilization, is the periodic discharge of blood, mucus, disintegrated ovum, and uterine mucosa formed during the cycle. The duration of the menstrual period varies but averages 3 to 5 days. The amount of blood lost varies greatly. The menstrual cycle, time between onset of each period, is approximately 28 days. Regularity of menstruation can be disturbed by disease conditions and emotions in addition to onset of pregnancy. This physiologic cycle continually recurs throughout the reproductive life of the woman. Assessment of the female patient should include documentation of the date of the last menstrual period (LMP). The possibility of pregnancy should be taken into consideration if the female patient is within childbearing age. A surgical procedure and/or the administration of anesthetic agents could be hazardous to a developing embryo (see Chapter 8, pp. 116-122 for discussion of the pregnant surgical patient).

GYNECOLOGY

The emotional preparation of gynecologic patients presents a special challenge to the OR team. Anticipation of physical exposure, potential loss of sexual function, infertility problems, or termination of pregnancy can create severe anxiety. Some surgical procedures terminate reproductive capability and produce menopause. Patients must be able to express concerns, ask questions, and receive reassurance and support.

Examination Under Anesthesia

Bimanual examination of the pelvis with the patient in lithotomy position and relaxed from anesthesia usually precedes vaginal and abdominal gynecologic surgical procedures. This allows the surgeon to thoroughly assess the size, outline, consistency, position, and mobility of the uterus, fallopian tubes, and ovaries. The examination also helps the surgeon determine the stage of malignancy and whether a lesion is resectable, especially in women experiencing pain or nervous tension or those who are obese. The vaginal vault is prepped and the examination is performed before abdominal preparation for laparotomy.

Special Features of Gynecologic Surgery

Diagnostic and surgical procedures may be carried out through a vaginal or abdominal approach, or the two approaches may be combined. Each requires a different position and different preparation, drapes, and setup. Surgical techniques for abdominal procedures discussed in Chapter 29 apply to gynecologic surgery. However, diagnostic and surgical procedures are often combined and done in one surgical procedure. In both vaginal and abdominopelvic procedures:

1. Spinal, epidural, or more commonly, general anesthesia is used. An epidural catheter may be inserted preoperatively for postoperative pain control.
2. Patient is catheterized in the OR unless she has an indwelling catheter. Usually a Foley catheter is in-

serted after the administration of anesthesia to prevent the bladder from becoming distended during the surgical procedure and to record urinary output. The circulator should check the collection bag regularly and report evidence of blood. This could indicate injury to the bladder or ureters. Insertion of a cannula directly into the bladder (suprapubic cystostomy) provides an alternative indwelling drainage system in selected patients.
3. Electrosurgical unit is frequently employed, with either monopolar or bipolar electrodes.
4. Argon, carbon dioxide, and Nd:YAG lasers are used, usually in conjunction with a colposcope (pp. 611-612) or laparoscope (p. 613) and the operating microscope. See Chapter 15, pp. 274-278 for discussion of laser safety.
5. Closed-wound suction drainage, or another type of drain, may be used to prevent hematoma or serum accumulation in the pelvis and/or the wound.
6. Prophylactic anticoagulation with heparin, antiembolic stockings, and early ambulation are especially important in pelvic surgery because of the anatomic relationship of deep major vessels to the surgical field. In addition, lithotomy position slows circulation. Postoperative thrombosis is a serious complication.

Vaginal Approach

1. Patient is in lithotomy position.
2. Instrumentation must be of sufficient length for use within the vaginal canal and uterine cavity (e.g., long curved dressing forceps for insertion of vaginal packing). In addition to cutting, holding, clamping and suturing instruments, vaginal setups include *dilatation and curettage (D&C) instruments* (Table 30-1).
3. Laser or cryosurgical unit may be used to remove hypertrophied tissue or certain benign neoplasms.
4. Suction system, including a Poole suction tip with guard, tubing, and collection canister, is part of the setup.
5. Sponges should be secured on sponge forceps in deep areas. Long narrow sponges with radiopaque markers on the end are used for packing off abdominal viscera in vaginal procedures. All counts are very important in these procedures.
6. Vaginal packing is inserted following certain procedures. Antibiotic or hormone cream may be applied to the packing during insertion. The packing should be recorded on the patient's chart and removed at the surgeon's order.
7. At completion of the surgical procedure, a perineal pad is placed against the perineum between the patient's legs.

TABLE 30-1

Instruments for Dilatation and Curettage

PURPOSE	INSTRUMENTS
To expose	Vaginal speculum Posterior retractor Weighted posterior retractor Narrow lateral Heaney retractors
To grasp and hold	Single- and double-toothed tenaculi
To measure uterine cavity	Uterine sound (graduated probe)
To dilate cervix	Graduated dilators Goodell dilator
To scrape tissue	Sharp and blunt, large and small uterine curettes
To obtain specimen	Endometrial biopsy suction curette
To carry sponges	Sponge forceps
To remove polyps and biopsy tissue	Polyp and biopsy forceps
To insert packing	Uterine dressing forceps

Abdominal Approach

1. Supine or Trendelenburg's position is used for abdominopelvic procedures. Preparation and drapes are the same as for abdominal laparotomy.
2. When a large abdominal mass is present or the pelvic organs are pushed from their normal relationships, ureteral catheters may be inserted before the surgical procedure to facilitate identification of the ureters in proximity to or within the area of dissection. Inadvertent severing of the ureters during the procedure greatly increases postoperative morbidity and mortality if the injury is not immediately detected and corrected.
3. Instrumentation includes basic laparotomy setup with the addition of long instruments for deep manipulations within the pelvis.

Combined Vaginal-Abdominal Approach

If vaginal and abdominal surgery is indicated, a combined procedure is planned. For example, the patient may be scheduled for a total abdominal hysterectomy with anterior vaginal colporrhaphy. In such instances the vaginal procedure is performed first. Then the patient is removed from lithotomy position, repositioned in supine position, and the abdominal prep and surgical procedure are carried out.

1. Because of the possibility of infection, separate sterile setups are used for vaginal and abdominal procedures performed concurrently.

2. Vaginal preparation precedes exploratory pelvic laparotomy in readiness for the unexpected or for a D&C scheduled to precede an abdominal procedure. A separate sterile prep table is used for the external genitalia and vagina. Another sterile setup is used for the abdominal prep.

DIAGNOSTIC TECHNIQUES

The gynecologist employs both noninvasive and invasive diagnostic techniques. Some are performed as office or ambulatory procedures, especially those using the vaginal approach.

A pelvic examination includes inspection and palpation of external genitalia; bimanual abdominovaginal and abdominorectal palpation of the uterus, fallopian tubes, and ovaries; and speculum examination of the vagina and cervix. This inspection is augmented by a cytologic study of smears of cervical and endocervical tissue obtained by scrapings. The *Papanicolaou (Pap) smear* has significantly increased diagnosis of cervical cancer and premalignant lesions. Characteristic cellular changes in cervical epithelial cells are identified. Cytologic aspiration from within the endocervical canal may reveal unsuspected carcinoma of the endometrium, tubes, or ovaries and occult cervical cancer.

Schiller's test involves staining the vaginal vault and cervical squamous epithelium with Lugol's solution. Glycogen in normal epithelium takes up the iodine. Abnormal tissues, with little or no glycogen, do not stain brown and thereby pinpoint sites for biopsy. Abnormal cytologic findings are an indication for further evaluation by histologic tissue study.

NOTE Uterine cancer consists of two entities: cervical cancer and endometrial cancer. These differ by age groups, types, and consequences. *Cancer of the cervix* appears most often in association with coitus at an early age, multiple partners, nonbarrier contraceptives, poor sexual hygiene, a chronically infected cervix, or a history of sexually transmitted diseases. These include infection with herpes simplex virus, human papilloma virus, cytomegalovirus, *Chlamydia trachomatis,* and *Trichomonas vaginalis.* A higher frequency of abnormal Pap smear findings are associated with these infections and with herpesvirus and papilloma virus, which produce condylomata, identified as possible causes of carcinoma. Cancer of the endometrium, more common than cervical cancer, occurs primarily in postmenopausal women. It is often associated with obesity, low parity, late menopause, hypertension, and diabetes mellitus.

Biopsy of Cervix

Uterine cancer may not present symptoms in the early stage and may progress to invasion before discovery. Intermenstrual *(spotting)* or postmenopausal bleeding may be the first visible sign. The condition may be suspected by results of cytologic examination or visual inspection, but diagnosis must be made by biopsy.

Excisional Biopsy

In excisional biopsy, an attempt is made to excise the entire cervical lesion or section of a vulvar lesion.

Incisional Biopsy

Incisional biopsy involves use of a scalpel, punch biopsy, or other instrument to obtain tissue for diagnosis but not to remove the lesion. If a malignancy is diagnosed, additional evaluation and further treatment must be carried out by surgery and/or radiation therapy.

Cone Biopsy (Conization of Cervix)

Patients diagnosed by Pap smear as having severe cervical dysplasia or intraepithelial carcinoma of the cervix require conization to remove the lesion and rule out invasive carcinoma. The biopsy, obtained with a laser, scalpel, or cervitome *(cold knife conization),* includes the squamocolumnar junctions of the ectocervix (transformation zone) and is tapered to include the endocervical canal to the level of the internal os. Most of the lesions categorized as cervical intraepithelial neoplasia (CIN), dysplasia, and carcinoma in situ are found in this area. Conization of the cervix provides the most comprehensive specimen to diagnose a premalignant or malignant lesion. Multiple blocks and sections are examined by the pathologist to determine the extent of invasive disease.

Complications include hemorrhage, infection, cervical stenosis, incompetent cervix, and infertility. The cutting beam of the carbon dioxide laser to obtain a cone biopsy minimizes these risks. Hemostasis must be secured with sutures as needed.

Fractional Curettage

Tissue is obtained for histologic examination by scraping the uterine cavity. Fractional curettage differentiates specimens between the endocervix and the endometrium. The cervix may be biopsied, if indicated by Schiller's test, in association with curettage. A small curette is introduced into endocervical canal, which is scraped from internal to external os. The specimen is placed on a Telfa pad, and both are put into a container. This scraping precedes cervical dilatation to avoid dislodging tissue from above. After dilatation (see D&C, p. 617), a curette is inserted into the uterine cavity for curettage of the endometrium. The endometrial specimen is placed in a separate container from those obtained by endocervical curettage.

Colposcopy

Illumination and binocular magnification afforded by the *colpomicroscope* permit identification of abnormal epithelium to target for biopsy. The colposcope has a cool intense white light that can be fitted with a green filter to improve visualization of the vascular pattern. With the colposcope positioned in front of the vulva, without touching patient, the colposcopist can focus light through a speculum on the ectocervix, the lower part of the cervical canal, and the vaginal wall. The cervix is wiped with 3% acetic acid to eradicate mucus and to facilitate viewing the surface and vasculature. Biopsies are always taken for histologic confirmation of diagnosis. Endocervical curettage may also be performed. A camera can be attached to a colposcope to photograph lesions.

Vaginal condylomas and adenoses, preinvasive lesions of the cervix, cervical dysplasia, CIN, and other vaginal and cervical lesions can be treated by laser with the colpomicroscope. Visualization is excellent, unobstructed by instruments. Condylomata appear as white raised areas when exposed to acetic acid. The laser permits selective destruction of large areas of vaginal epithelium without vaginal and cervical stenosis. It cuts, coagulates, seals, and sterilizes simultaneously. This results in less blood loss, shorter period of vaginal discharge after treatment of the cervix, and lower incidence of infection than in other surgical treatment modalities. Electrosurgery or cryosurgery are other options to ablate lesions.

Culdocentesis and Colpotomy

Culdocentesis

In culdocentesis blood, fluid, or pus in the cul-de-sac is aspirated by needle via the posterior vaginal fornix for suspected intraperitoneal bleeding, ectopic pregnancy, or tuboovarian abscess.

Posterior Colpotomy (Culdotomy)

In posterior colpotomy a transverse incision is made through the posterior vaginal fornix into the posterior cul-de-sac to facilitate diagnosis by intraperitoneal palpation, inspection of the pelvic organs, or determination of free fluid, blood, or pus in the pouch of Douglas. Pus from a pelvic abscess or blood, possibly a sign of ectopic pregnancy or ruptured ovarian cyst, is evacuated. Tubes and ovaries are inspected. If they are normal, the incision is closed. A drain may be inserted.

Some surgical procedures, such as aspiration of an ovarian cyst or sterilization by tubal ligation, can be performed through the incision, although exposure and visualization are limited. A tube or ovary is sometimes removed through the vagina.

Tubal Perfusion

To test tubal patency, methylene blue or indigo carmine dye in a solution of normal saline is introduced into the uterine cavity via a 50 ml syringe or intravenous tubing attached to a cervical cannula. The surgeon views the ends of the fallopian tubes through a laparoscope. Dye seen coming from one or both tubes indicates patency.

Uterotubal Insufflation (Rubin's Test)

Uterotubal insufflation may be used to test patency of the fallopian tubes. It usually is done as an office procedure to study infertility. The test may be therapeutic in relieving minor obstructions. Contraindications include genital tract infection, possible pregnancy, and uterine bleeding.

A cannula with an airtight seal is inserted into the cervicouterine canal and connected to an insufflation apparatus. Carbon dioxide is introduced slowly under controlled flow. A relationship exists between tubal patency and pressure required to force gas through tubes into the peritoneal cavity. Resistance to flow (i.e., back pressure) is measured on a mercury manometer. A Rubin's test precedes, never follows, a curettage to prevent gas embolism. Irritation before total absorption of carbon dioxide from the peritoneal cavity causes referred pain in the shoulders.

Hysterosalpingography

Radiologic study of the uterus and tubes may afford further evaluation of infertility following repeated negative Rubin's test. Patient is placed in lithotomy position. The vagina is prepped. The cervix is grasped with a single-tooth tenaculum. A cannula is inserted into the cervical canal, and 10 ml of a water-soluble radiopaque contrast media is instilled with a syringe through the cannula. This contrast medium ascends into the corpus uteri and tubes to yield information about structure and function. Serial x-ray films may be taken to assess postprocedural tubal spillage. In some patients, tubal spasms prevent immediate passage of the contrast media through the tubes. Iodine-based contrast media is contraindicated in a patient with iodine allergy.

PELVIC ENDOSCOPY

Pelvic endoscopy is an established part of the gynecologist's diagnostic and therapeutic armamentarium. It permits detailed intraperitoneal inspection of the pelvic organs without laparotomy. These procedures are not without danger, however. Inadvertent perforation of hollow viscus and infection are major hazards. Operator expertise, careful patient selection, adequate anesthesia, and safe equipment are essential. *Pelvic endoscopy is a sterile procedure.*

Two approaches are employed for direct visualization of pelvic organs and adjacent structures: vaginal and abdominal.

Culdoscopy

A culdoscope is introduced into the peritoneal cavity via the posterior vaginal fornix and pouch of Douglas. Some gynecologists prefer culdoscopy to investigate ovaries or posterior surfaces in the lower pelvis. Local or caudal anesthesia is used. Patient is placed in knee-chest or lithotomy position. With posterior lip of the cervix held by a tenaculum and retracted anteriorly, the uterus is elevated while counterpressure is applied to the posterior vaginal wall by the speculum. This maneuver stretches the posterior vaginal fornix while a trocar and cannula or sheath penetrate the thin wall and enter the pelvis between the uterosacral ligaments. When the trocar is removed with the cannula in place, air enters the cul-de-sac because of the negative intraabdominal pressure produced by the knee-chest position. Air displaces the bowel, and the scope may be inserted through the cannula.

At completion of the procedure the culdoscope is removed. Before the cannula is removed, the operating table is straightened and the patient flattened while as much air as possible is evacuated by hand pressure on the abdomen. Some surgeons place a suture in the puncture site.

Hysteroscopy

A rigid fiberoptic hysteroscope, introduced vaginally, provides direct inspection of the interior of the uterus to diagnose or treat intrauterine disease. Adequate dilatation of the uterine cavity is a prerequisite for viewing endometrial surfaces. High viscosity fluid, such as 5% glucose in water or dextran, is instilled to provide distention. Visibility is further enhanced with a video camera and monitor screen.

The hysteroscope is used most commonly for *endometrial laser ablation* to stop or decrease uterine bleeding. With the Nd:YAG laser for deep photocoagulation, the endometrium is destroyed, producing scarring of the uterine lining. The tip of the laser fiber can be held away from tissue (blanching technique) or in contact with endometrium (dragging technique). A specialized electrosurgical rollerball electrode is an alternative method to using a laser. The entire endometrial lining is treated from fundus to about 4 cm above the external cervical os. This can provide relief from menorrhagia (i.e., excessively heavy menses).

The hysteroscope also may be used to identify and remove polyps and submucous fibroids, lost intrauterine devices (IUDs), or intrauterine adhesions.

NOTE Air or gas is *never* used for uterine insufflation or laser fiber cooling during hysteroscopy because of the risk of air or gas embolism. Also, 32% dextran 70 in dextrose (Hyskon) is not used as an irrigant for endometrial laser ablation because of systemic effects of fluid absorption through open capillaries.

Laparoscopy

A 7 mm fiberoptic laparoscope with a 0-degree angle lens inserted into the peritoneal cavity permits direct observation of pelvic and abdominal organs and peritoneal surfaces. This technique may be used to diagnose ectopic pregnancy; inspect the ovaries for evidence of follicular activity; visualize pelvic masses; and determine the cause of pain, internal bleeding, infertility, endocrinopathies, or amenorrhea. It often eliminates the need for laparotomy because many pelvic diseases such as endometriosis, adhesions, and ovarian cysts may be identified and treated through the laparoscope and its accessory instrumentation. Surgical procedures such as tubal sterilization by electrocoagulation with or without division or partial resection, placement of a metal clip or silicone ring on the tube, or biopsy can be performed. Laparoscopy may also be used to recover ova for in vitro fertilization (see pp. 628-629).The argon laser will pass through the working channel of the sheath to ablate endometrial implants. The carbon dioxide laser may be used to vaporize tissue in conjunction with the operating microscope attached to the laparoscope. Special instrumentation may be needed for microsurgical procedures.

Pelviscopy

Pelviscopy, as developed in the 1970s by Kurt Semm in Germany, differs from laparoscopy in two respects: a 10 or 12 mm rigid pelviscope with a 30-degree angle lens replaces the standard 7 mm laparoscope with a 0-degree angle, and instrumentation is capable of intraabdominal hemostasis and suturing. The 30-degree angled telescope gives a stereoscopic perspective for a better view of size, depth, and mobility of organs. The larger lumen allows a wider field of vision. The gynecologist-endoscopist can perform myomectomy, salpingectomy, oophorectomy, hysterectomy, and other procedures such as tuboplasty and incidental appendectomy without the need for a large abdominal incision.

Procedure

The increasing popularity of minimally invasive surgery has led to the expansion of laparoscopy to pelviscopy. The technique for using both types of scopes is essentially the same. The surgeon and assistant manipulate instruments through trocar sheaths. A video camera and monitor are used for optimal visualization. Frequently, procedures are recorded as part of the permanent record. Most equipment is capable of taking still photographs also. Both sterile and nonsterile equipment is needed.

Sterile endoscopic equipment includes:

1. D&C instrument tray, including uterine manipulator/cannula (Hulka tenaculum, Cohen/Jarcho cannula, or Hasson/Humi inflatable cannula).
2. 20 ml Luer-Lok syringe.
3. Endoscope.
4. Verres needle, 80 mm or 120 mm for insufflation through abdominal puncture; 150 mm for insufflation through cul-de-sac in obese patient.

5. Appropriate sized trocars and insulated sheaths with sealing caps to prevent gas leakage.
6. Insufflation tubing with in-line filter.
7. Aspiration cannula, biopsy forceps, and graduated probe. Most are insulated and compatible with monopolar electrosurgical unit.
8. Bipolar grasping forceps (Kleppinger forceps).
9. Suction/irrigation tubing.
10. Endoscopic needleholders, sutures, clip appliers, and staplers. These may be needed for more complex procedures.
11. Electrosurgical probe or endocoagulator, and/or laser fiber.

Nonsterile endoscopic equipment includes:

1. Insufflator with full tank of carbon dioxide (CO_2) and a compatible disposable hydrophobic filter.
2. Fiberoptic light source.
3. Video camera and monitor(s).
4. Laser and/or electrosurgical unit. Only solid-state electrical generator should be used with the endoscope. High peaks of voltages from spark-gap generators may cause excessive tissue destruction.

Usually general anesthesia is administered. The patient is placed in modified lithotomy position with stirrups adjusted so legs are at 45-degree angles to axis of the operating table. The abdomen is prepped, followed by perineal and vaginal prep. An indwelling Foley catheter is inserted. The patient is draped for a combined abdominovaginal procedure. The sterile drapes must provide two exposures (i.e., an abdominal opening and a perineal opening) and cover the legs.

A tenaculum may be placed on the cervix. A cannula is inserted for instillation of methylene blue or indigo carmine to determine tubal patency and for manipulation of the uterus during the procedure to provide greater visibility. A D&C may be performed as part of the conclusion of the procedure after the injection of dye.

Insertion of the scope is preceded by pneumoperitoneum to produce abdominal distention. The infraumbilical midline area is most commonly used if no scars, with possible adherent viscera beneath, are present. This area is preferred because it has no abdominal wall vessels that might be injured. The firm attachment of the fascia to the peritoneum facilitates entry. However, great care must be taken to avoid injury to the great vessels or intraabdominal organs.

To produce pneumoperitoneum, a Verres needle may be introduced percutaneously into the peritoneal cavity. This spring-loaded needle has an outer sharp hollow cannula with an inner blunt retractable stylet with a two-way stopcock at the base for control of gas flow. Some surgeons prefer to incise the infraumbilical margin through the fascial and peritoneal layers and insert a blunt Hasson trocar and sleeve for insufflation. This method decreases the risk of perforated viscus. Insufflation tubing is attached to convey carbon dioxide from the insufflation apparatus to the patient. Carbon dioxide is used as the insufflation medium because it is nontoxic, highly soluble in blood, and rapidly absorbed from the peritoneal cavity. The gas is introduced into the cavity under a controlled high flow of 12 to 14 mm Hg pressure until the volume insufflated ranges between 2.5 and 4.5 L. The flow rate and volume are monitored by the circulator and surgeon. Overdistention must be avoided to prevent respiratory impairment and subcutaneous emphysema. After the desired pneumoperitoneum is established, the insufflator is switched to a maintenance flow of 3 to 4 L at 14 mm Hg pressure. Electronic sensors in the device maintain the pneumoperitoneum at a constant level during periods of irrigation and suction.

The patient is placed in 15-degree Trendelenburg's position to shift the abdominal organs cephalad. A small periumbilical skin incision is made in the anterior abdominal wall. Through it, a trocar and sheath are introduced into the peritoneal cavity via puncture. The sharp tip of the trocar must be carefully guided to avoid inadvertent perforations. Some trocars and sheaths have spring-loaded end guards that cover the sharp tip and protect underlying structures after penetration of abdominal tissue layers. The trocar is removed and the scope of the same caliber is inserted through the sheath, which remains in the cavity. Before use, warming tip of scope in warm towels or normal saline solution can prevent fogging of distal lens of the endoscope by intraperitoneal temperature and moisture. (Sterile antifog solution is commercially available.) The fiberoptic cable is connected to endoscope and the light source. Because of the potential fire hazard to drapes, the light source is not activated until attached to the scope. The gas tubing is connected to the inflow valve. The video camera is draped and connected to the endoscope.

Although an operating scope permits insertion of accessory instruments, these may be introduced through one or two additional 5 or 7 mm insulated trocar(s) and sheath(s) inserted through small incision(s) in the lower and/or lateral abdomen. These trocars may be inserted into the peritoneal cavity under direct vision through the endoscope, which offers good transillumination for the puncture when the room lights are dimmed, or visualization on the video monitor. The suction/irrigation tubing is attached to a side port on an accessory sheath.

Intraabdominal ligation is achieved with loops of chromic or plain surgical gut (Endoloop ligatures). After the applicator is passed through the scope, the loop is placed around the tissue and pulled taut. An endoscopic swaged needle-suture is passed in a needleholder for suturing. Intracorporeal (inside body) and extracorporeal (outside body) knotting techniques are used to secure sutures (see Chapter 24, p. 502). Endoscopic ligating clips and staples also are used for ligation and tissue approximation. Hemostasis also may be accomplished with a laser fiber, an electrosurgical probe, or an endocoagulator (see discussion of argon beam coagulator, Chapter 23, p. 479). The endocoagulator uses directed heat at a temperature around 212° F (100° C) for coagulation of protein by thermal conduction rather than high-frequency current.

At completion of the surgical procedure, the carbon dioxide and light sources are turned off, accessory instruments and sheaths are removed, and the patient is returned to supine position. Hemostasis is surveyed before the scope is removed from the primary puncture site. The valve of its sheath closes to prevent escape of intraperitoneal gas into the room air. The pneumoperitoneum contains aerosolized blood and body fluids and should be evacuated through the suction tubing into the suction canister. Electrosurgical plume also should be suctioned from the peritoneal cavity because it binds with hemoglobin and causes the arterial oxygenation to decrease. The patient can become hypoxic. The skin incisions are sutured and small dressings or adhesive bandages (Band-Aids) are applied.

The patient requires close monitoring by the anesthesiologist because increased intraabdominal pressure may lead to cardiovascular disturbances from vagal reflex. This reflex is caused by stretching of the peritoneum, retention of carbon dioxide, or compression of the inferior vena cava.

Postoperative shoulder pain may follow the use of pneumoperitoneum. This is referred pain caused by pressure on the diaphragm, which is somewhat displaced by carbon dioxide during the procedure. Slight elevation of the head after recovery from anesthesia relieves this pain. Although numerous complications have been reported, the most common are perforation of the intestine or major blood vessel, hemorrhage from a biopsy site, gas embolism from intravascular injection, and burns of the abdominal wall and bowel. Some injuries, such as viscus puncture or thermal damage, may not be immediately apparent. Symptoms may not be present until 48 to 72 hours postoperatively when tissue necrosis or sloughing occurs.

VAGINAL PROCEDURES

The vaginal wall, cervix, and uterus may be approached with the patient in lithotomy position. Tumors, benign or malignant, may be confined to any one of these structures or may involve adjacent tissues. Herniation or fistula formation may require repair of the vaginal wall and adjacent structures. Excision or repair may require a combined vaginal-abdominal procedure.

Vaginal Wall

Excision of Adenosis Lesion

A biopsy taken from an epithelial tumor should be studied histologically to rule out adenocarcinoma. Vaginal adenosis and gross cervical abnormalities, as well as clear cell adenocarcinoma of the vagina, have occurred in female offspring of women who received diethylstilbestrol (DES) or similar synthetic estrogen during the first trimester of pregnancy to avoid spontaneous abortion. Adenosis may be treated with laser (see section on colposcopy, pp. 611-612).

Vaginectomy

Vaginectomy (partial or complete) is performed for carcinoma in situ or carcinoma of the vagina. Vaginoplasty is necessary for reconstruction. External radiation and radium application (see Chapter 45), with possible eventual pelvic exenteration (p. 620), are the treatment for advanced invasive malignancy. The proximity of the bladder and rectum makes therapy difficult.

Radical vaginal or abdominal hysterectomy and vaginectomy with extraperitoneal lymphadenectomy sometimes are combined for carcinoma of the upper and middle thirds of the vagina if the bladder or rectum is not involved.

Vaginoplasty

A vagina may be constructed in patients with congenital absence of an entire vagina or, more commonly, those with stenosis after radiation therapy or after surgical removal of the vagina. Care must be taken to avoid damage to the urethra, bladder, and rectum. The vaginal space is created by blunt and sharp dissection. If a large part of the surface of the space is denuded, a skin or amnion graft is shaped around a vaginal mold. The mold is placed in such a way that the graft will take. With the use of dilators to prevent stenosis and estrogen cream to assist in epithelization of the cavity, an adequate functional vagina can be created in many patients. A pseudovagina is created for transsexual surgery (see Chapter 31, p. 651).

Procedures for Repair of Pelvic Outlet

Injury to muscles and fascial layers of the perineum and/or genital tract, usually during childbirth, may result in extensive vaginal relaxation. Manifestation of perineal hernias may be delayed until later years, when generalized loss of elastic tissue develops. Downward pressure is exerted on other structures, such as the bladder. Moderate to severe degrees of herniation of viscera require surgical intervention to restore pelvic floor integrity and sphincter competency. Vaginal plastic procedures for genital prolapse consist of narrowing and reconstructing the damaged pelvic floor. Vaginal repairs are referred to as *vaginal plastic procedures*.

Anterior Colporrhaphy (Kelly's Procedure) Anterior colporrhaphy is performed for prolapse of the anterior vaginal wall to repair *urethrocystocele,* a herniation of the bladder into the vaginal canal. The wall is incised and a strip of redundant vaginal mucosa is excised, the extent of which depends on the severity of the prolapse. The bladder is dissected free from the vaginal septum and returned to normal position by suturing the pubocervical ligaments beneath it. Approximation of the pubococcygeus muscles provides further suburethral support. The vaginal wall is closed with sutures. By improving support to the bladder neck region, restoring the posterior urethrovesical angle, and narrowing the urethral opening, stress incontinence (urine leakage with coughing, sneezing, or laughter) is relieved. The surgical procedure also prevents voiding difficulty and recurrent cystitis that accompanies retention of urine caused by a cystocele bulging below the bladder neck.

Posterior Colpoperineorrhaphy Repair of the posterior vaginal wall for *rectocele,* a herniation of the rectum into the vagina, consists of a triangular excision of redundant vaginal mucosa and separation of the vagina from the rectum. Support is reestablished by suturing together rectovaginal fascia, as well as the levator ani, as high as possible. Perineal muscles are reconstructed to restore continuity of support. A lacerated perineum may also be sutured. The surgical procedure relieves fecal incontinence and/or constipation.

Repair of Enterocele An abnormally deep hernial sac may contain a segment of intestine, referred to as an *enterocele,* or cul-de-sac hernia. Repair consists of opening the sac, reducing its contents, excising the sac, closing the aperture or weakness that allowed the sac to descend into the rectovaginal septum, and strengthening the normal anatomic coverings. Approximation of the uterosacral ligaments and levator ani in the midline removes the cul-de-sac defect.

Repair of Prolapsed Uterus or Procidentia Various surgical procedures correct and restore support. Correction of prolapse anteverts the uterus and shortens an elongated cervix and cardinal ligaments. In the Manchester colpoperineorrhaphy, for example, the cervix is amputated and the cardinal ligaments united in front of it. The anterior vaginal wall is plicated and the posterior pelvic floor is reconstructed. Often cystocele and rectocele are present and are simultaneously repaired. In complete prolapse both the cervix and uterine body protrude through the vaginal aperture and the vaginal canal is inverted. Bleeding ulceration of exposed tissues may ensue. Vaginal hysterectomy (pp. 617-618) is done for severe prolapse or prolapse accompanied by stress incontinence when childbearing is no longer desired. A vaginal pessary to support a retrodisplaced or prolapsing uterus may be inserted in a woman who presents a poor surgical risk.

Repair of Vaginal Eversion Outward protrusion of the vagina can occur following obstetric or surgical trauma or from inherent weakness in vaginal muscle tone, particularly in postmenopausal years. The fascia of the vagina is attached to the sacrospinous ligament, located within coccygeus muscle. The resultant scarring and fibrosis fixates the vagina in a normal anatomic position.

Colpocleisis (Le Fort Procedure) Colpocleisis, obliteration of the vagina by denuding and approximating the anterior and posterior walls, is generally reserved for elderly patients or those who present a poor surgical risk.

Procedures for Repair of Genital Fistulas

A fistula is an abnormal communication between a part of the genital canal and either the urinary or intestinal tract. Various dye tests, cystoscopy, and pyelography help pinpoint a urinary tract fistula. Injury during parturition, surgical trauma (especially radical procedures for cancer), penetrating extension of cervical carcinoma, and radiation necrosis are common etiologic factors.

Repair of Vesicovaginal Fistula A vesicovaginal fistula, which develops between the bladder and vagina, is the most common type of genital fistula. A small opening permits seepage of urine, although the patient may void normally. Total incontinence may result from a large fistulous aperture and cause irritation of the vagina, vulva, and thighs. Through a vaginal approach, the anterior vaginal wall is dissected free. The fistula to the bladder is closed, and the bladder to vagina attachment is reestablished. The repair should be made with at least three layers of tissue. The bladder should be decompressed by an indwelling Foley catheter for at least 14 days. Antibiotics may be administered judiciously to prevent infection in the healing site.

If the vesicovaginal fistula is high in the vagina, a better result will be obtained by entering the bladder via suprapubic incision for direct repair rather than using a vaginal approach. Care must be taken not to occlude ureteral orifices. This is accomplished by insertion of ureteral catheters, which can be removed following the procedure. Attention is given to excision of any infected tissue, closure with multiple layers, and bladder decompression by catheter.

Repair of Ureterovaginal Fistula A ureterovaginal fistula is between the ureter and vagina; its repair depends on location. If the fistula is near the junction of the ureter and the bladder, the ureter can be divided above the defect and reimplanted in the bladder. If the fistula is not proximal to the bladder, it can be excised and the severed ureteral ends anastomosed. Occasionally a nephrectomy on the involved side is necessary.

Repair of Urethrovaginal Fistula A urethrovaginal fistula is between the urethra and vagina; repair consists of layered closure. If the neck of the bladder is involved, the area must be reconstructed. This may include transplantation of the bulbocavernosus muscle.

Repair of Rectovaginal Fistula A fistula between the rectum and vagina may follow episiotomy or obstetric perineal lacerations, vaginal or rectal surgery, radiation therapy, trauma, or infection. Fecal incontinence and fecal material in the vagina are characteristic, although the anal sphincter is intact. Preoperative bowel preparation, including prophylactic antibiotic therapy, is important because of the contaminated surgical area. A temporary colostomy may be advisable before the surgical procedure to divert the fecal stream from the repair site. With a vaginal approach, a plastic repair of the perineum is done. Scar tissue and the fistulous tract are excised, and the edges of the perineal muscles and fascia are approximated.

Cervix

Surgical treatment of an abnormal cervix should be preceded by tests to rule out early malignant change.

Cauterization

The cervix may be cauterized by laser or electrocautery to treat chronic inflammation and/or leukorrhea (i.e., vaginal discharge).

Trachelorrhaphy

Lacerations of the cervix may result from childbirth. Repair (i.e., trachelorrhaphy) involves reconstruction of the cervical canal as necessary. A vaginal plastic setup is used.

Conization

Cervical dysplasia can occur in females 15 years and older; the peak incidence is between ages 25 and 35. Employed therapeutically for chronic inflammation and for premalignant lesions in women of childbearing age, conization may be performed by scalpel, electrosurgery, or laser. Laser conization is used to treat severe dysplasia and carcinoma in situ. Loop electrosurgical excision procedures (LEEP) use a stainless steel or tungsten loop electrode to excise a central core of tissue from the transformation zone of the endocervical canal. Large loop excision of the transformation zone (LLETZ) is performed with minimal bleeding and few complications. These procedures may be performed in the OR or office setting with local anesthesia. Future childbearing is unaffected. Although the specimen is comparable in size to a cold knife conization, the specimen has superficial dessication and may be inferior in quality.

Amputation

The cervix may be amputated to remove an intraepithelial cancer. However, because this procedure leaves the corpus uteri, which may become cancerous, most surgeons prefer total hysterectomy to cervical amputation.

Uterus

Dilatation and Curettage (D&C)

The most frequently performed gynecologic procedure, dilatation of the cervix and curettage of the uterus (D&C), is done for diagnostic and/or therapeutic purposes. The main purpose of a D&C is to establish the cause of abnormal uterine bleeding so that the gynecologist can plan definitive treatment. The procedure is mandatory in women with postmenopausal bleeding or symptoms suggestive of endometrial cancer, even when cytologic smear findings are negative. It may be performed in infertility studies or to confirm preoperative diagnosis before amputation of the cervix or hysterectomy. D&C is performed therapeutically to relieve dysmenorrhea by cervical dilation only, to remove polyps or benign endometrial pathologic conditions, to remove residual tissue and arrest bleeding following incomplete abortion, or to perform voluntary or therapeutic abortion before the thirteenth week of pregnancy. A regional paracervical block or general anesthesia is required.

With the anterior lip of the cervix held in a tenaculum and the posterior vaginal wall retracted, a small curette is introduced into the endocervical canal, which is scraped from the internal to the external os. A uterine sound is then introduced into the uterus to determine the length and direction of the intrauterine cavity. It is important that the surgeon know the shape and position of the uterus to avoid perforation and injury to it and to other pelvic organs, the primary complications. Successively larger dilators are then passed through the cervix and internal os to permit insertion of a curette into the uterine cavity for curettage of the endometrium. Submucous fibroids are usually discernible as the curette passes over them. Exploration of the fundus with a polyp forceps usually extracts any polyps present in the endometrium.

Vaginal Hysterectomy (Standard)

Vaginal hysterectomy is performed for severe uterine prolapse or prolapse accompanied by stress incontinence and for patients with pelvic relaxation or history of myomata, irregular uterine bleeding, or a treated premalignant lesion.

The uterus is removed through the vagina, with incision of the vaginal wall and the pelvic cavity. Urinary incontinence, enterocele, and/or rectocele may be simultaneously repaired by anterior and posterior colporrhaphies and with reconstruction of the pelvic floor. Advantages of the procedure include restoration of normal anatomic relationship and preservation of vaginal function. The ovaries are not usually removed. Contraindications are immobility of pelvic organs, large uterus, a pathologic condition such as ovarian mass, or pelvic cancer.

The vaginal wall is incised anteriorly and the bladder is separated from the cervix. The incision is continued around the cervix. The peritoneal cavity is entered through the posterior cul-de-sac and the anterior uterovesical pouch. Ligaments supporting the uterus and uterine vessels are ligated and cut. The fundus is delivered, the upper pedicles sutured, the uterus removed, and the peritoneum closed. Suturing the cardinal and uterosacral ligaments together and to the vaginal vault supports the vault and prevents prolapse of the vagina. Potential complications include injury to the ureters, bowel, or bladder, and massive hemorrhage from the uterine vessels. An unopened laparotomy setup should be available.

Radical Vaginal Hysterectomy (Schauta's Procedure)

A surgical approach to early carcinoma of the cervix, radical vaginal hysterectomy does not permit pelvic lymph node dissection but is useful in selected patients (e.g., obese patients). It includes vaginal removal of the uterus, upper third of vagina, parametria, fallopian tubes, and ovaries. Damage to the ureters or bladder is a potential complication.

Laparoscopic-Assisted Vaginal Hysterectomy

In laparoscopic-assisted vaginal hysterectomy (LAVH), an abdominal endoscopic approach is used to dissect the uterus from its supporting ligaments and vasculature. Endoscopic clips, linear staplers, sutures, electrosurgery, or a laser may be used to enhance hemostasis. Once the intraperitoneal attachments of the uterus are ligated and divided, a vaginal approach is used to separate the bladder from the anterior aspect of the uterus as in a standard vaginal hysterectomy. Direct visualization of the bladder flap dissection through the endoscope from above enables the surgeon to avoid damage to adjacent structures. The uterine vascular pedicles are ligated vaginally. In the *Heaney technique*, the uterus is inverted and removed fundus first through a posterior colpotomy. The uterosacral ligaments are sutured to the posterior aspect of the vaginal cuff, and the colpotomy is closed. This method is used in moderate prolapse of the uterus. In the *Döderlein technique*, a nonprolapsed uterus is inverted and removed fundus first through an anterior colpotomy. This technique provides greater visibility of the uterine vessels and a more effective vaginal suspension. LAVH is the procedure of choice when a minimally invasive procedure is desired, when salpingo-oophorectomy may be necessary, and when the uterus is only moderately enlarged.

ABDOMINAL PROCEDURES

The open abdominal approach may be used for a fixed or enlarged uterus, exploration, inflammatory disease, and most malignant lesions of the uterus, fallopian tubes, and ovaries. This approach permits inspection of pelvic and abdominal organs, as well as lymph glands for biopsy or treatment. Open laparotomy or minimally invasive endoscopic procedures are performed as appropriate to achieve desired outcomes.

The contents of the vagina may enter the peritoneal cavity if the vaginal vault is transected. Therefore the vagina should be prepped before an abdominal procedure and always before a uterine procedure. An indwelling Foley catheter usually is inserted to decompress the bladder. A D&C may be performed while the patient is in lithotomy position. Because the patient may be placed in Trendelenburg's position so that abdominal organs will gravitate away from the pelvis, her knees must be over lower table break when she is repositioned. Watch patient's hands to avoid trapping them in the joints while table sections are being manipulated.

Abdominal Cavity

Pelvic Exploration

Exploratory pelvic laparotomy or endoscopy performed for diagnosis may be followed immediately by a therapeutic procedure. Significant pelvic pain, uterine bleeding, or a pelvic mass are frequent indications for differential diagnosis from abdominal disease. A pelvic exploratory laparotomy is always done to diagnose and accurately assess the stage of ovarian cancer. A vertical midline incision from the symphysis to midway between the umbilicus and the xiphoid allows exploration of the peritoneal cavity for evidence of metastases.

The appendix may be removed incidentally unless the patient's condition precludes this. The patient should be informed preoperatively that this procedure may be performed at the discretion of the surgeon. The rationale is that the procedure will preclude appendicitis, necessitating another surgical procedure for the patient in the future.

Uterus

Endometrial cancer is essentially a disease of perimenopausal or postmenopausal years. It is characterized by intermittent spotting between menstrual periods or after menopause or steady bleeding from the uterine lining. Postmenopausal bleeding is considered to be caused by cancer until proved otherwise. Patients with confirmed malignant lesions may be treated by preoperative radiation to decrease the tumor mass and slow the progression of disease.

Medical, psychosocial, and sexual ramifications must be considered when contemplating removal of the uterus, a hysterectomy. Medically the procedure may be lifesaving in patients with malignant lesion or severe hemorrhage. The gynecologist has an obligation to consider the individual patient's attitudes when more than one mode of therapy is available as an alternative to hysterectomy. Signaling as it does the end of the patient's reproductive potential, hysterectomy may cause psychologic stress and a sense of incompleteness, even though sexual responsiveness is not dependent on the uterus. Patients whose families are complete, however, may welcome reproductive sterilization.

Abdominal Hysterectomy

The uterus is removed through an abdominal incision and opening of the peritoneal cavity. The most frequent indication for abdominal hysterectomy is leiomyofibroma, commonly known as *benign fibroids* or *myomas.* Fibroids are composed of muscle and fibrous connective tissue. They may be single or multiple and most often are present in the wall of the uterus. Some may be attached by a pedicle or protrude into and distort the uterine cavity. Fibroids, which are usually slow growing, are treated conservatively if they are small and present no problems. The tumor ceases to grow at menopause. If symptoms such as menometrorrhagia, bladder or bowel pressure, pelvic discomfort, or rapid tumor growth develop, surgical treatment is essential. Differential diagnosis includes dysfunctional bleeding caused by disturbed endocrine function, tubal or ovarian masses, and pelvic cancer. In addition to these indications, hysterectomy is performed for uterine prolapse, extensive endometriosis, and cervical or uterine cancer. Various types of hysterectomy are performed.

Total Abdominal Hysterectomy (Panhysterectomy) The entire uterus, including the cervix, is resected. Normal ovaries are preserved for hormone production whenever possible in women under 45 years of age. Studies have shown that after hysterectomy, women have a 20% increased risk for ovarian cysts within 5 years of the surgical procedure. Bilateral oophorectomy followed by hormone replacement therapy has eliminated the need for subsequent surgery for ovarian pathologic conditions.

The abdominal peritoneal cavity is entered through a vertical midline or transverse Pfannenstiel's incision. Vertical incision facilitates exploration. The patient is placed in deep Trendelenburg's position. Incision through the uterine peritoneum is carried out laterally. The abdominal organs are retracted and protected with laparotomy packs moistened with warm normal saline solution. The fallopian tubes and round and broad ligaments are clamped, cut, and ligated. The ovaries, when not removed, are suspended to avoid adherence to the vaginal vault. With the uterus forward, posterior sheets of the broad ligaments are incised, the ureters are identified, and the uterine vessels and uterosacral ligaments are clamped, divided, and sutured. All uterine-supporting ligaments must be divided and ligated. The bladder is mobilized from the cervix and vagina, the vaginal vault is incised, and the cervix is dissected from the vagina. After the uterus is removed, the connective tissue ligaments are anchored to the vagina. The vaginal mucosa and muscular wall are approximated by absorbable sutures or staples, and the bladder, vault, and rectum (i.e., pelvic floor) are reperitonealized (i.e., covered with peritoneum). Abdominal layers are closed as for laparotomy.

NOTE

1. When the surgeon is closing the vaginal vault following removal of the uterus, the needle, suture, needleholder, or stapler and all instruments used on the cervix and vagina are considered contaminated. The scrub person holds the specimen basin to receive them and does not touch them. Separate instruments are used for abdominal closure.
2. Complications of hysterectomy include injury to the ureters, with possible fistula formation or renal failure, injury to the bladder or bowel with fistula formation, or massive hemorrhage from damage to major vessels.

Laparoscopic-Assisted Abdominal Hysterectomy The uterus can be mobilized through a minimally invasive abdominal endoscopic procedure (see pelviscopy procedure, pp. 613-615). All of the uterine vascular pedicles are ligated and divided abdominally rather than vaginally as in LAVH (p. 618). The uterus is taken out below, however, through a culdotomy, an incision into the rectouterine portion of the peritoneal cavity between the rectum and the posterior surface of the uterus. The vaginal cuff is repaired laparoscopically from above. Laparoscopic-assisted abdominal hysterectomy affords less morbidity, blood loss, pain and discomfort, and faster recovery than an open abdominal hysterectomy.

Wide Cuff Hysterectomy Wide cuff hysterectomy is removal of the total uterus and a generous cuff of the vagina. Surgeons employ this procedure for cervical carcinoma in situ or early stromal invasion (microinvasion) if invasion is less than 5 mm and no tumor cells appear within lymphatic or vascular channels. Preservation of ovaries depends mainly on the patient's age.

Radical Hysterectomy With Pelvic Lymph Node Dissection (Radical Wertheim's Procedure) The radical Wertheim procedure may be performed for early stages of invasive cervical cancer and sometimes for endometrial cancer. It involves wide en bloc removal of paracervical, parametrial, and uterosacral tissues (uterus, tubes, ovaries, ligaments), and at least the upper third of the vaginal canal. Bilateral pelvic lymph nodes and channels surrounding the external iliac artery and vein, the hypogastric artery and vein, and the obturator fossae are also dissected and removed.

Some surgeons perform a *modified Wertheim's procedure* for microinvasive carcinoma. This is somewhat less extensive than is the radical procedure and may omit lymphadenectomy.

Because radical hysterectomy involves excision of paracervical and paravaginal tissue, bladder innervation is disrupted. This results in bladder dysfunction postoperatively, sometimes for as long as 6 months. Bladder complications are related to the extent of dissection.

Hysterosalpingo-oophorectomy Fallopian tubes and ovaries are removed along with the uterus. This procedure may be done for endometrial, tubal, or ovarian cancer; excessive vaginal bleeding; or large fibroids. In postmenopausal women when total hysterectomy is indicated, bilateral salpingo-oophorectomy is often performed to avoid future ovarian pathologic conditions.

Myomectomy

In myomectomy, single or multiple fibroid tumors are removed from the uterine wall in premenopausal women who may still desire pregnancy. The procedure is especially adaptable to pedunculated tumors, which may become necrotic from interference with the blood supply. Removal of large submucous fibroids may require opening the uterus.

Pelvic Exenteration

An ultraradical procedure for invasive persistent carcinoma, exenteration is not performed for palliation but only when a possibility of cure exists. The extent of the disease determines the amount of exenteration. In *anterior exenteration,* the reproductive organs and the distal part of the ureters, bladder, and vagina are removed. This modification is performed for cancer of the cervix, vagina, or vulva with extension to the bladder. The ureters are diverted to an ileal conduit while the bowel remains intact. *Posterior exenteration* removes the reproductive organs, sigmoid colon, and rectum. It is done for cervical carcinoma involving the rectum or advanced rectal carcinoma involving the uterus and posterior vaginal wall. The urinary system remains intact; fecal diversion is by colostomy. *Total or complete exenteration,* rarely performed, involves en bloc dissection of the bladder, reproductive organs, perineum, rectum, and pelvic lymph nodes. Two setups are needed: abdominal and perineal. These mutilative procedures change structure, function, body image, and sex life and should be preceded by intensive physical and psychologic preoperative preparation.

Numerous complications may occur involving any major system. Anesthesia and procedural times are long. Blood replacement and extensive monitoring are essential. Multiple stoma and gross pelvic defect with much dead space predispose the woman to infection; therefore wound drainage is used. Vascularized omental and myocutaneous flaps are used to fill pelvic defects (see Chapter 34).

Fallopian Tubes

The fallopian tubes are also referred to as the *uterine tubes, oviducts,* and *salpinges.*

Tubal Ligation

Tubal ligation should be considered a permanent method of reproductive sterilization because reversal cannot be guaranteed. Thorough preoperative counseling of the patient and her husband or partner should preface this procedure. A number of surgical techniques are used for tubal ligation. They are essentially similar in removal of a portion of the middle part of the fallopian tube on each side for pathologic confirmation and ligation of both the distal and proximal ends to prevent the cut ends from growing together. Frequently performed by laparoscopy, tubal ligation by open abdominal approach may be done alone, in conjunction with other indicated abdominal surgery, or in patients in whom laparoscopic technique is contraindicated. Ligation may be performed through a small transverse incision in the pubic hairline area. This is referred to as *minilaparotomy.* Tubal ligations are often performed immediately following cesarean delivery and closure of the uterine wall (see pp. 626-627). No additional instruments are required other than those used for the C-section.

The *Pomeroy technique* of ligation is the most reliable, provides a surgical specimen of each tube, and causes minimal tubal destruction. Tube is tied with suture material and a section is removed. The tube eventually pulls apart, destroying passage between ovary and uterus.

Sterilization may also be performed following vaginal delivery on the first to third postpartum day through an infraumbilical incision. In the cauterization technique, the bipolar electrosurgical electrode transects and seals the ends of the fallopian tube or excises a section of tube and seals the ends. Application of a stretchable Silastic band (Fallope-ring) or a ligating (Hulka) clip may also produce occlusion. In some patients, however, Pomeroy and other occlusion techniques may be reversible by a subsequent reparative procedure. An estimated 1% of sterilized women will seek reversals because of sterilization at an early age, remarriage, or death of a child.

Tuboplasty

Removal of an obstruction may restore tubal patency to reverse infertility caused by diseased, damaged, or occluded tubes. Microsurgical techniques with fine suture materials and lasers have vastly improved results of tubal reconstructive procedures. Success depends on the extent of abnormal tissue or tubal destruction and/or the site of obstruction. Location of previous ligation and normality of tissues at severed ends of tubes will influence reversibility of a tubal ligation. Although tubal patency may be restored, abnormal function may persist in tubes damaged by pelvic inflammatory disease (PID). The chance of successful uterine pregnancy may remain limited. The risk of a tubal pregnancy can increase following tuboplasty. Preoperative assessment may include a hysterosalpingogram to determine the length and patency of tubal segments and/or laparoscopy with tubal dye perfusion or ultrasound imaging with installation of sterile normal saline solution to demonstrate patency. Contraindications for tuboplasty include active infection or disease and a tube that is less than 3 cm long.

Tuboplasties are microsurgical procedures performed through an abdominal incision. They include the following options.

Salpingolysis Adhesions caused by an inflammatory process, such as a ruptured appendix or ovarian cyst, may surround the fallopian tubes. The tubes may function normally following lysis of adhesions.

Salpingostomy Tubal mucosa and/or fimbria may become occluded secondary to PID or other infectious process. A salpingostomy creates an opening in a distally obstructed tube. A carbon dioxide laser beam may be used through the microscope to open fimbriated ends and to divide adhesions in blocked tubes. An incision in a tube also may be performed to evacuate an early small tubal pregnancy.

Tubal Anastomosis A proximal obstruction in the tube is resected. The remaining patent segment is then reimplanted into the uterus and anastomosed at the cornu. Salpingitis usually occludes the tube near the cornu, which may need to be shaved to reach healthy tissue. A previous sterilization procedure usually occludes the mid-isthmus. This anastomosis will be midtubal in the ampulla.

Salpingectomy, Salpingo-oophorectomy

Removal of a fallopian tube, *salpingectomy*, is often performed in association with partial or total removal of the corresponding ovary, *salpingo-oophorectomy*. Procedures may be unilateral or bilateral. Indications are extensive damage from PID or endometriosis, cysts, primary adenocarcinoma of the tube and ectopic pregnancy (pp. 624-625). Total abdominal hysterectomy and bilateral salpingo-oophorectomy may be performed for bilateral disease. Removal of a large tuboovarian abscess is essential to prevent rupture and dissemination of pus in the abdominal cavity.

Ovaries

Ovarian pain usually is referred to the lower abdomen just above either groin, making differential diagnosis from abdominal disease pertinent. Pelvic endoscopy, ultrasonography, and computed tomography (CT) scan assist diagnosis. An ovarian mass requires exploration for evaluation. The mass may be a cyst or a tumor. Ovarian tumors may be benign or malignant, cystic or solid. Epithelial ovarian cancer begins as a cystic intraovarian growth. It usually is asymptomatic until malignant cells have spread into the peritoneal cavity. Disease is usually confined to the peritoneal cavity and retroperitoneal lymph nodes, but advanced ovarian carcinoma can obstruct the urinary and intestinal tracts. Ovarian cancer is the leading cause of gynecologic cancer deaths in the United States.

Benign cysts, more common than tumors, may arise from the graafian follicle, corpus luteum, or epithelium (dermoid). As they grow in size, ovarian cysts can cause menstrual disturbances, pain, and abnormal uterine bleeding. They may leak contents into the peritoneal cavity causing irritation, or they may rupture causing massive bleeding that necessitates immediate laparotomy.

Cysts or solid tumors, even if asymptomatic, should be removed as a precaution because they may degenerate into a malignant lesion, increase in size, or lead to twisting of the pedicle. The type of procedure depends on the type of cyst or tumor, the age of patient, and the importance of childbearing potential.

Incision or Biopsy

The surgeon incises an ovary to obtain tissue for frozen section. If a cyst or tumor is found in one ovary, the gynecologist transects the other ovary to rule out a neoplasm. Biopsies also may be taken from paraaortic and pelvic lymph nodes.

Removal of Ovarian Cyst

A procedure to remove an ovarian cyst may be scheduled as an oophorocystectomy, cystoophorectomy, or ovarian cystectomy. Many benign ovarian cysts and tumors are treated by local excision with preservation of the ovary. A large cyst may be aspirated before removal. Immediately after removal, the surgeon incises the cyst for examination to determine its character because gross appearance as well as frozen section are important. If there is reasonable assurance that the lesion is benign, removal of only the cyst or resection of a diseased portion (e.g., endometrioma) is justified, with preservation of normal tissue.

Oophorectomy

The most frequent indications for removal of an ovary, oophorectomy, are benign ovarian tumors. Many gynecologists believe that cystadenomas and all solid benign ovarian tumors should be treated by unilateral salpingo-oophorectomy because of the difficulty of clean dissection and the questionable assurance of their benign nature. In postmenopausal women, both ovaries, tubes, and uterus are removed to avoid future cancer.

If there is a strong probability or proof of malignancy in any ovarian cyst or mass, total hysterectomy and bilateral salpingo-oophorectomy are usually performed, regardless of age. Partial or complete omentectomy may be included because the rich blood supply of omentum contributes to rapid metastases. The extent of the surgical procedure is determined by the lesion. In malignant tumors a differentiation is made between primary and metastatic ovarian cancer, which influences treatment. As much tumor is removed as possible, a procedure referred to as *debulking*, for management of advanced ovarian cancer. An ultrasonic aspirator may be used for debulking. The procedure may require resecting parts of small and large intestines and urinary tract. Following debulking, most patients receive chemotherapy. This often is followed by a "second-look laparotomy" to reassess the peritoneal cavity for further palliative or therapeutic therapy.

Muscles and Ligaments

Urinary Stress Incontinence Procedures

Urinary stress incontinence is the sudden, involuntary, and intermittent release of urine as a result of muscular changes around the proximal urethra, bladder neck, and bladder base. Differential diagnosis from fistulas, bladder neuropathies, and primary lesions is established by urethroscopy, cystometrogram, and urodynamics (see Chapter 31). Surgical correction attempts to restore support. Three basic approaches are used. *Anterior colporrhaphy* with plication (i.e., reducing the size of the bladder neck) often is satisfactory (p. 616). In a *urethral sling* procedure, a musculofascial sling is placed beneath the bladder neck and urethra; usually this is a combined vaginal and abdominal procedure. *Urethral suspension* procedures reposition the urethra and bladder neck retropubically by suspending the urethra in a plane with the symphysis pubis through a transverse abdominal incision. Sometimes a combined abdominoperineal approach is necessary for urethral suspension. Variations of these procedures have been devised, including an endoscopic suspension of the bladder neck. See Chapter 31, pp. 645-646, for discussion of other procedures for urinary incontinence.

Marshall-Marchetti Krantz Vesicourethral Suspension After mobilization through an extraperitoneal abdominal approach into the prevesicle space, the urethra and bladder neck are suspended to the posterior border of the symphysis pubis. Sutures are placed through the anterior vaginal wall on each side of the urethra and brought through the periosteum on the posterior surface of the symphysis pubis. Sutures also may be placed adjacent to the bladder neck and through the rectus muscle fascia to suspend the bladder neck. This procedure may be performed in conjunction with other pelvic surgery. It is 85% effective in the treatment of stress incontinence in women. A suprapubic catheter may be used for bladder drainage for 48 to 72 hours postoperatively. Urinary retention is a common complication for up to 7 days.

Abdominal Complications

Injuries to ureters, which can lead to loss of renal function if unrecognized, can occur during the surgical procedure because of their relationship to pelvic structures. The surgeon must identify and isolate the ureter(s) on the affected side(s) to prevent accidental crushing or kinking.

Adhesions following pelvic surgery can cause infertility, intestinal obstruction, and/or chronic abdominal pain. The surgeon may place a biodegradable fabric (Interceed Absorbable Adhesion Barrier) over tissues and pelvic organs before closing the peritoneal cavity. This satinlike, knitted fabric acts as a physical barrier to prevent adhesion formation during the healing process. Within 8 hours the fabric becomes a gelatinous protective coating. This is completely absorbed within 28 days.

VULVAR PROCEDURES

Benign growths, although rare, consist mainly of fatty and fibrous tumors. These are excised if large. Suspicious lesions should be removed for pathologic examination. Cancerous lesions may be multicentric, with the majority found on the labia majora and a lesser percentage on the labia minora, vestibule, clitoris, and posterior commissure. Vaginal smears should be taken to determine the presence of metastatic growth to the vaginal wall. Treatment depends on size of primary lesion, involvement of nodes, and extent of metastasis. Mutilative procedures require emotional adjustment to permanent change.

Vulvectomy

Wide local excision of a single, well-localized area with no premalignant changes elsewhere may be done. Punch biopsies may be obtained. Leukoplakia and preinvasive lesions of the vulva may be treated with a laser or ultrasonic aspirator.

Simple Vulvectomy Without Node Dissection

The labia majora and minora, part of the mons veneris, and the hymenal ring, including the clitoris, may be removed for premalignant lesions and early microinvasive cancer of limited penetration. The clitoris and perianal region are spared if the lesion is small. Incision must be wide to avoid local recurrence.

Total Vulvectomy

Basal cell carcinoma usually does not metastasize but is often locally extensive and prone to recur. Treatment consists of wide total vulvectomy, also without node dissection.

Radical Vulvectomy With Bilateral Inguinal-Femoral Lymphadenectomy

Radical vulvectomy is performed for invasive vulvar cancers or melanoma and is usually done in one stage. Resection lines may vary depending on location and size of the lesion. Because the procedure involves abdominal and perineal dissection, both areas, including thighs to knees, are prepped. Structures generally removed include all from the anterior surface of the pubis to perianal region posteriorly, with wide lateral excision beyond the vulva, to fascial depth. More specifically, large areas of abdominal and groin skin, labia majora and minora, the mons, clitoris, Bartholin's and periurethral glands, and bilateral inguinal lymph nodes are removed en bloc. Inguinal skin flaps are retained for closure. Deep pelvic node dissection is carried out if frozen sections determine that these nodes are cancerous. If the vagina, urethra, and/or anus are involved, they are also removed. Anal involvement may require a colostomy.

Lymphadenectomy is carried out with the patient in supine position. Two teams may perform bilateral dissection. The patient is then placed in the lithotomy position for vulvectomy. Reconstruction of the pelvic floor and vaginal walls may be necessary. The legs are abducted for easier approximation of subcutaneous tissue during primary closure with sutures or staples. Closed wound suction drainage is used postoperatively to avoid fluid collection beneath skin flaps. A pressure dressing is applied.

Bartholin's Glands

Obstruction of the secretory duct of Bartholin's gland may be caused by inflammation. A cyst may be prone to secondary infection or abscess formation.

Marsupialization of Bartholin's Cyst

A cyst enlarges as mucous secretions accumulate. Marsupialization establishes drainage from within the vagina by creation of a new enlarged ductal opening. The cyst is incised linearly in the region of the normal opening and evacuated. The edges of the vaginal mucosa and cyst wall are sutured together to produce epithelialization so that the cyst cannot recur. An abscess may be drained.

Sex Reassignment

Sex transformation (gender transformation) is an established phenomenon in modern society. The patient shows an anxious desire to change from one physical status to another. A sex change, however, requires a stable personality, psychiatric counseling for feasibility, and careful preparation and support. The patient also changes legal identity and social status. Although most transformations are from male to female (see Chapter 31, p. 651), female to male cross gender is also possible in satisfactory candidates; however, the management of this change is more complex. A treatment schedule of hormonal substitution (i.e., androgens [male hormone] in the female patient) is begun well in advance of the procedure.

In a one-stage, female-to-male procedure, bilateral subcutaneous mastectomy, total abdominal hysterectomy, and bilateral salpingo-oophorectomy are performed. Three additional stages are necessary to complete the transformation. These are:

1. Urethral reconstruction, to the tip of enlarged clitoris
2. Transfer of the labia for penile lengthening and scrotal construction
3. Prosthetic testicular implantation

An understanding, nonjudgmental, unembarrassed attitude on the part of health care personnel can help the patient adjust psychologically, as well as recover physically, after the radical change. Consideration should be given to the patient's family and significant others because they, too, must adjust. The patient in the role of his or her birth sex may have married and produced children. In addition to confusion about parental roles, the patient may experience rejection or revulsion from offspring. Referral for family and individual counseling should be included in the plan of care.

Obstetrics

Diagnostic techniques such as ultrasonography, specialization in fertility problems, and techniques of fetal monitoring and management have brought significant changes in the field of reproductive biology. Consequently, OR nursing personnel become involved in the care of obstetric patients both in elective and emergency procedures. The pregnant woman experiencing trauma or an acute surgical disease, such as appendicitis, presents challenges to the OR team. The well-being of the fetus depends on maternal physiologic factors. Anesthesia and positioning are especially critical concerns. (See Chapter 8, pp. 116-122, for discussion of the pregnant surgical patient.)

Threatened Pregnancy

Cerclage

A tape is placed around an incompetent internal cervical os in an attempt to retain a pregnancy. The procedure is employed following diagnosis of an incompetent cervix from a history of rapid, painless, second- or early third–trimester spontaneous abortions in apparently normal pregnancies. Preferably elective in patients with typical history, cerclage is performed between 12 and 14 weeks of pregnancy. Occasionally it may be an emergency procedure when the cervix is dilating and membranes are bulging, as long as membranes have not ruptured or premature labor has not begun.

Shirodkar Procedure A small incision is made in the anterior vaginal mucosa at the level of the bladder reflection and at the posterior cervico–cul-de-sac junction. A tunnel under the cervical mucosa is then made to join the anterior and posterior incisions. A polyester (Mersilene) tape is drawn around the internal os and tied. The knot is secured posteriorly to prevent erosion into the bladder. Mucosal incisions are closed. At term the patient usually undergoes a cesarean section.

McDonald Procedure The polyester tape is placed around the cervix with a circumferential running stitch without mucosal dissection. The tape can be removed at term for vaginal delivery.

Aborted Pregnancy

Termination of pregnancy may be spontaneous or induced. (See section on ethical issues associated with abortion in Chapter 4, p. 62.) Implantation of a fertilized ovum can be intrauterine or extrauterine. The procedure will depend on the location and gestational age of the fetus. Ultrasonography examination may be used to determine the stage of intrauterine pregnancy.

Some patients are psychologically repulsed by the word *abortion*. They may associate the word with elective termination regardless of natural causes or therapeutic need. Religious or personal beliefs may influence decision making about a pregnancy that cannot continue to full term. In some circumstances the patient may accept and understand the word *miscarriage* and feel freer to select appropriate treatment options without fear of reprisal or rejection. Consideration for the support of psychologic coping mechanisms of the patient in crisis is more important than using absolute words such as abortion.

Suction Curettage

Intrauterine contents can be aspirated for deliberate termination or for incomplete spontaneous abortion within the first 20 weeks of pregnancy.

Uterine Evacuation A small flexible plastic tip or cannula is inserted into the uterus of a woman who is less than 8 weeks pregnant. Suction created by drawing back on a large syringe attached to the cannula is sufficient to evacuate contents of the uterus. Disposable equipment for suction curettage not requiring dilatation or anesthesia is commercially available.

Dilatation and Evacuation (D&E) Between 8 and 16 weeks, the cervix must be dilated. Cervical dilatation is adjusted to the stage of pregnancy and the necessary cannula. A laminaria tent (i.e., a cone-shaped plug) may be inserted preoperatively to gradually dilate the cervix, usually for 4 to 24 hours. The laminaria, removed before the procedure, is gentler than instrument dilatation, which can cause cervical tearing. A vacuum aspirator-cannula is connected by tubing to an electric vacuum pump. With gentle suction the specimen is collected in the vacuum bottle and removed for examination.

Following an incomplete abortion, it is vital to remove all retained products of conception to prevent infection, especially from anaerobic bacteria, which may progress to septic shock (see Chapter 25, p. 534). A D&C setup is used. The removed tissue is sent for culture and pathologic examination.

Ectopic Pregnancy

A fertilized ovum may become implanted outside the uterus. Referred to as an *ectopic pregnancy*, rarely does this fetus develop to term. Although it may reach the ovary, abdominal cavity, or cervix uteri, the ovum usually implants in a fallopian tube. Symptoms of tubal pregnancy are abdominal pain and menstrual irregularity. Diagnosis is made by ultrasonography, laparoscopy, or by detection of blood in the cul-de-sac by aspiration (see discussion of culdocentesis, p. 612). Hemorrhage results from extensive trauma to the tube and mesosalpinx. The patient often goes into severe shock. An immediate surgical procedure and blood replacement are mandatory. *Ruptured ectopic pregnancy is a true obstetric/gynecologic emergency.* The affected tube and fetus are removed, the pelvic cavity is aspirated, and bleeding is stopped. Removal of the associated ovary depends on the extent of damage from the rupture.

If an ectopic pregnancy is diagnosed by laparoscopy before rupture, conservative surgery may be able to restore fertility. Tubal pregnancy can be removed through a linear salpingostomy or by segmental resection, followed by tuboplasty. Laparoscopic or pelviscopic techniques may be used. Some ectopic pregnancies can be managed through a vaginal colpotomy incision or abdominal minilaparotomy.

Cesarean Section

Commonly referred to as *C-section,* a cesarean section is a method of delivery by abdominal and uterine incisions. Cesarean delivery may take place in the obstetric labor and delivery suite or in the OR suite. Pregnancy and labor produce many physiologic alterations. Both the mother and the newborn have specific needs requiring comprehensive care. To promote a positive experience the OR team must be cognizant of these physiologic and psychologic needs and of the reasons for abdominal delivery. C-section is a significant family event. Partners or support persons may be permitted in the OR, and mothers are usually awake.

The frequency of cesarean section is attributed mainly to diagnosis and management of uterine dystocia (ineffective labor), failure to progress, and fetal monitoring for detection of fetal distress. C-section is performed when safe vaginal delivery is questionable or immediate delivery is crucial because of threatened well-being of the mother or fetus. Indications may include hemorrhage, placenta previa, abruptio placentae, toxemia, fetal malpresentation, cephalopelvic disproportion (CPD), chorioamnionitis, genital herpes in the mother within 6 weeks of delivery, fetal distress, or prolapsed cord.

Cesarean delivery may be scheduled or an emergency. Severe unexplained complications during late pregnancy or labor that adversely affect the mother or fetus (e.g., massive third-trimester bleeding or severe fetal distress) create an emergency. For these patients, preparations must be rapid. The patient easily senses a loss of control, especially if she participated in a childbirth education program for vaginal delivery. She needs special support. Most mothers fear more for the survival of the fetus than for themselves.

Admission procedures vary. Some hospitals admit an elective patient the morning of surgery. The patient is prepared by maternity personnel and taken to the OR or to an OR in the delivery suite. An emergency patient may go directly to the OR from the labor area. The trend is to perform C-sections in the obstetric suite. In any situation the pediatrician and neonatal personnel from the nursery are notified before the procedure to resuscitate and care for the infant in the OR. Sterile pediatric equipment and supplies must be available instantly. Notification is a responsibility of the circulator and/or obstetrician. The circulator must also communicate with the postpartum obstetric unit where the patient will go.

Oxygen consumption increases about 20% during pregnancy and as much as 100% above normal during labor in response to the increased metabolic demand. Hypoxia and hypercapnia develop rapidly. Fetal oxygenation varies in direct relation to that of the mother in normal and abnormal situations. In treating fetal distress, continuous 100% oxygen is administered to the mother until delivery or relief of the distress. Hypoventilation and hyperventilation are potentially harmful because they induce hypoxemia and hypercapnia in both the mother and the fetus. Maternal hypotension and hypovolemia diminish uterine blood flow and fetal perfusion. Hypoxia and acidosis threaten fetal well-being. The mother is safeguarded by appropriate anesthetic technique and selection of drugs. The fetus is protected by adequate uteroplacental perfusion and fetal monitoring by trained personnel. The patient should not be left alone in the holding area or OR. The fetal heart rate and uterine contractions are monitored continually. *The procedure involves the care of two patients.*

Setup

Routine laparotomy skin prep, drape, and setup are used for C-section. Instruments are essentially those for a major gynecologic laparotomy with the addition of delivery forceps, cord clamp, and aspirant bulb for the infant. A Foley catheter provides intraoperative bladder drainage.

Position

Uterine displacement to the left during transport and until after delivery is necessary to shift the uterus away from pelvic vessels. Positional effect on cardiac output is of major importance in avoiding maternal hypotension and maintaining fetal well-being. In the supine position the enlarged uterus compresses the inferior vena cava and aorta, resulting in diminished venous return to the heart, stroke volume, and cardiac output. The patient is positioned supine with the right side slightly elevated by a wedge to tilt the uterus to the left. The OR table may be tilted 30 degrees to the left. Slight Trendelenburg's position assists venous return.

Anesthesia

Anesthesia is selected on an individual basis. Regional anesthesia is advantageous in diabetic patients because of reduced metabolic expenditure, low incidence of vomiting, and earlier return to oral intake. It is also advantageous for the patient with asthma or sickle cell anemia. General anesthesia is advised when the mother or fetus is in jeopardy and delivery is crucial, as in the presence of hemorrhage or severe fetal distress. The choice also depends on the reason for the surgical procedure, degree of urgency, and the patient's condition and wish. A cesarean section can be done with local anesthesia in an extreme emergency when an anesthesiologist is not immediately available. The anesthesiologist chooses the method safest for mother and fetus. Gastric motility and emptying is inhibited by fear, pain, labor, and narcotic administration. Patients requiring emergency surgery may have eaten recently. *A pregnant patient should always be regarded as having a full stomach.*

Spinal or epidural anesthesia allows the mother to see her newborn in the OR. It also reduces neonatal depression and risk of maternal aspiration. Hypotension is treated with intravenous infusion and/or ephedrine given IV. Ephedrine, mephentermine (Wyamine), and metaraminol (Aramine) do not cause undesired uterine vasoconstriction. Other vasopressors can cause fetal hypoxia. Placentally transmitted drugs depressant to the fetus are avoided. A single injection of morphine may be given through the epidural catheter at conclusion of the surgical procedure. With injection into the pain path, the drug significantly reduces postoperative pain for 24 to 36 hours with minimal side effects.

General anesthesia provides more rapid induction, less hypotension, greater cardiovascular stability, and better control of the airway and ventilation. Preoxygenation precedes induction. Rapid-sequence induction and intubation are used. Cricoid pressure during intubation occludes the esophagus to prevent regurgitation. Induction to delivery (I-D) and uterine incision to delivery (UI-D) intervals must be minimized. I-D time is directly related to fetal hypoxia. UI-D intervals greater than 3 minutes may lead to lower pH of blood and depression of the infant from altered uteroplacental perfusion. All efforts are made to deliver the newborn as rapidly as possible consistent with safety to minimize anesthesia and surgical time and to protect the fetus. With general anesthesia, all preparations, such as patient skin prep, draping, gowning, and gloving, are done before induction of anesthesia.

Incision and Delivery

A low transverse Pfannenstiel's or low midline vertical incision is made in the skin and underlying tissue layers. The length varies with size of the fetus. Dissection is expeditious. The uterine incision is made by one of the following methods:

1. *Low transverse (Kerr incision).* The bladder is dissected off the uterus and retracted gently downward. The lower uterine segment is entered through a low horizontal curvilinear incision. This approach causes less intraoperative blood loss and decreased chance of rupture with subsequent pregnancy.
2. *Low vertical midline (Krönig incision).* An 8 cm vertical incision is made in the lower uterine segment after the bladder is separated and retracted away. This incision is used when the fetus is small, preterm, and in the breech position. It is used also when cesarean hysterectomy may be performed following delivery.
3. *Classic uterine incision.* The uterus is incised vertically above the attachment of the bladder. The bladder is not dissected off the lower uterine segment. This approach is rarely used but may be necessary for a fetus in transverse presentation or for multiple fetuses. It may be indicated for a low anterior placenta, varicosities of the lower uterine segment, or cervical cancer. A major disadvantage is the high incidence of rupture with subsequent pregnancy.

As the uterus is incised, suction must be ready for amniotic fluid. Retractors are removed and the fetal head or the presenting part is gently delivered as pressure is applied to the fundus (Figure 30-3). Immediately on emergence of the head, the nares and mouth are aspirated with a bulb syringe to clear them of amniotic fluid. Newborns delivered by C-section have respiratory secretions. Delivery is completed and the umbilical cord is double-clamped and cut. The newborn is transferred via a sterile sheet to the neonatal resuscitation team. The circulator or neonatal team member who receives the newborn should wear gown and gloves until all blood and amniotic fluid are wiped off the baby. Risk of exposure to blood and amniotic fluid warrants the same adherence to universal precautions as any other contacts with blood and body fluids.

After delivery of the shoulders, IV oxytocin is administered to the mother to promote uterine contraction, minimize blood loss, and facilitate expulsion of the placenta and membranes. The placenta is delivered, visually inspected, and placed in a specimen basin. The

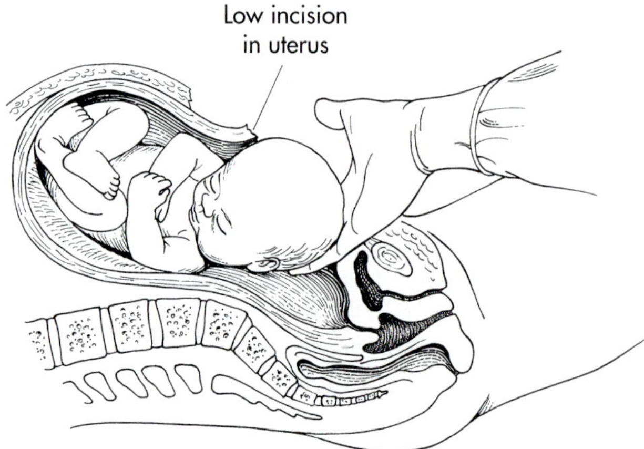

FIGURE 30-3 Cesarean delivery after incising uterus and fetal membranes. As head is lifted through low uterine incision, pressure usually is applied to fundus of uterus through abdominal wall to help expel fetus.

uterine fundus is palpated for firmness and massaged as necessary to prevent hemorrhage from relaxation. The patient is returned to a horizontal supine position. The uterine incision is closed with staples or absorbable sutures, and hemostasis is ensured. After inspection of the pelvic organs and possible tubal ligation, the peritoneum and abdominal incision are closed.

Intraoperative assessment is the same as for any major surgical patient. However, sponges, tapes, and needles are counted before closure of the uterus and again before closure of the peritoneum and skin.

Postpartum surveillance of the patient is essential. Lochia is observed. Abnormal bleeding, such as rapid saturation of the perineal pad, is reported and recorded. Nurses' notes should include the mother's contact with the infant, emotional reaction to the surgical procedure, and persons in attendance, in addition to physical assessment data.

Neonate

Immediate postdelivery care is given in the OR by the neonatal team. The baby is taken to the nursery after careful examination by a pediatrician. The neonate traditionally has been evaluated by the Apgar score, acid-base status, and neurobehavioral examination. The Apgar score is an excellent screening tool for vital functions immediately (at 1- and 5- minute intervals) after birth, but subtle effect of drugs may be overlooked. The Neurologic and Adaptive Capacity Score does not use noxious stimuli but emphasizes neonatal tone. Drugs that will produce significant neurobehavioral changes in the newborn must be avoided during labor and delivery.

In the newborn, the apical or umbilical pulse is the most accurate. Oxygenation is extremely important. Too little oxygen, hypoxia, can lead to intracranial hemorrhage, brain damage, or necrotizing enterocolitis. Too much oxygen, hyperoxia, administered at a rate in excess of 40% concentration, can cause bronchopulmonary dysplasia or retrolental fibroplasia.

Father or Support Person in Operating Room

Paternal or support-person participation in the birthing process is well-established for vaginal delivery to provide support to the mother, a family-centered birth, and immediate bonding with the infant. However, the presence of the father or support person in the OR during cesarean delivery is not universal. Hospitals adopting this policy report favorable experiences. The presence of the father or support person during the surgical procedure must be approved by the obstetrician. This person is informed of the conditions permitting and excluding his or her presence. Those who have attended a structured childbirth education course have more understanding of pregnancy and birth. In compliance with hospital policy, donning of OR attire and supervised washing of hands with an antiseptic agent before entrance to the OR are mandatory. The father or support person sits by mother's head. He or she may accompany the baby to newborn examining area after delivery. If the condition of the newborn and mother permits, they may rejoin the mother in the OR for bonding.

Prenatal Testing

Potentially useful for management of some congenital developmental disorders or genetic defects, prenatal diagnostic studies are performed during pregnancy in selected patients. Fetal anomalies are found in 2% of all women tested. Disorders in the fetus may be cause for induced abortion, elective cesarean delivery, or intrauterine fetal surgery.

Ultrasonography

Ultrasound is the standard tool for fetal imaging in utero. Ultrasonography, a noninvasive technique, permits accurate location of placenta and reliable diagnosis of structural defects (e.g., hydrocephalus or spina bifida).

Blood and Chorionic Villus Sampling

Ultrasound is also used for catheter or cannula guidance to obtain percutaneous umbilical blood samples or transcervical chorionic villus samples. Through direct fetal blood samples, anemia and some metabolic and chromosomal abnormalities can be diagnosed and treated in utero. Intravascular blood transfusions can be given to correct fetal anemia. Chorionic villi are a source of fetal genetic information. When obtained between the eighth and twelfth weeks of gestation, chorionic villi can aid in accurately diagnosing some enzymatic defects and in detecting the gender of the fetus.

Amniocentesis

Amniotic fluid is aspirated from the amniotic sac under ultrasound direction at 16 to 20 weeks of gestation for chromosomal analysis. This highly accurate test is indicated for known or suspected risk of chromosome abnormality because of advanced maternal age, known parental translocation carrier, or history of previous pregnancy with chromosomal defect in the fetus or infant. Maternal serum alpha-fetoprotein measurement can predict neural tube disorders (e.g., myelomenigocele) in the fetus.

Fetoscopy

Fetoscopy permits direct visualization of the fetus. A fiberoptic needle scope (fetoscope) is inserted into the amniotic cavity to view fetal parts, to obtain a biopsy of skin, or to sample fetal blood. The fetoscope is 1.7 mm in diameter with a visual field of 70 degrees. To ensure an adequate volume of amniotic fluid, fetoscopy is done after 16 weeks of pregnancy. Because of the intent to view specific structures, the position of the fetus must first be determined and the procedure performed under sonographic-assisted visualization. Placental localization is important, especially in the area of umbilical cord insertion. Hemoglobinopathies and coagulation problems (e.g., hemophilia) may be rapidly diagnosed by aspiration of fetal blood from the placenta or umbilical cord. Congenital skin disorders and albinism may be detected by biopsy. Direct viewing of the fetus may reveal characteristic abnormalities of various congenital syndromes. The procedure is not without complications and should be performed only by trained physicians when genetic information is critical.

Intrauterine Fetal Surgery

Improvement and expansion in prenatal diagnosis have led to rapidly developing antenatal surgical intervention, *intrauterine fetal surgery*. The aim is to provide optimal prenatal development, a crucial factor in determination of ultimate health. For example, diagnostic screening by sonogram during gestation reveals abnormalities heretofore diagnosed after delivery. Some medical disorders can be treated in utero. Other conditions fall within the province of the surgeon. Prerequisites for fetal therapy include accurate diagnosis, known pathophysiology, workable treatment, and technical capability. Radiologists, perinatologists, pediatric surgeons, anesthesiologists, perioperative nurses, and surgical technologists comprise fetal surgery teams. (See section in Chapter 42, p. 868.)

Most correctable malformations may be detected in utero but are best remedied by a surgical procedure after delivery at term. The full-term infant is a better surgical risk than is the fetus. Other anomalies, such as giant omphalocele or conjoined twins, can cause dystocia or require cesarean delivery. Surgical treatment in utero is reserved for fetuses in whom impaired organ development could be normal if treated (e.g., obstructive hydrocephalus, diaphragmatic hernia, or hydronephrosis caused by urinary tract obstruction). As these complex procedures are attempted, perioperative nurses and surgical technologists participate in coordination of efforts intraoperatively.

ASSISTED REPRODUCTION

Infertility, the inability to conceive a child after a year or more of repeated attempts, can be emotionally devastating. Both partners undergo extensive testing to determine possible organic or functional causes. These may include structural defect in either partner, past or present infections, genetic and/or immunologic abnormalities, or endocrine imbalance or deficit. In the female, a hostile cervix, antibodies to sperm, endometriosis, or exposure to DES in utero may prevent conception. Tubal occlusion is the most frequent cause of infertility. A male partner may have an inadequate number, quality, or mobility of sperm or an absence of live spermatozoa in semen. When conventional infertility therapy has failed to produce a pregnancy, other options are available to assist in achieving pregnancy and birth of a mature live infant.

In Vitro Fertilization

In vitro fertilization (IVF) refers to removal of the ovum from the prospective mother, fertilization and incubation in the laboratory, and subsequent embryo transfer to the uterus. In vitro means "in glass." Fertilization literally takes place in a culture dish or test tube. The first birth from in vitro fertilization and embryo transfer occurred in England in 1978.

Patient Selection

IVF is accepted therapy for women with severely damaged or nonfunctioning fallopian tubes, for men with scarce or absent sperm, or for infertility of unknown cause. Contraindications include uterine myoma, only one cornu, or a septate uterus. The female must have a normal uterine cavity, an accessible ovary, and evidence of ovulation. These factors are evaluated by pelvic ultrasonography and serum estrogen levels. A laparoscopy, endometrial biopsy, and hysterosalpingogram may be part of preoperative testing. Semen analysis is done to check sperm count of the male partner.

Induction of Ovulation

IVF is coordinated with timing of the ovulatory cycle. The medical protocol is prescribed for the individual couple. From day 2 or 3 of the menstrual cycle through day 6 or 7, the woman takes fertility drugs to stimulate growth and maturation of ovarian follicles. These drugs are a combination of clomiphene citrate, a synthetic hormone, and human luteinizing and follicle-stimulating hormones. Follicular growth is monitored daily, beginning about the eighth day, by ultrasonography and serum estrogen levels. The fluid-filled follicles on the surface of the ovaries contain ova (oocytes). When the largest follicle reaches a diameter of 15 to 20 mm, the woman is given human chorionic gonadotropin (HCG) intramuscularly to stimulate final maturation and induce release of the follicle. Ova harvested from the graafian follicle must be mature or they will not divide normally and fertilize properly. Maturation of several ova improves chances of retrieving at least one.

Ovum Retrieval

The patient is scheduled for retrieval of mature ovum or ova about 35 hours after HCG injection before spontaneous ovulation occurs. Ovum retrieval may be accomplished through transvaginal, transvesicle, or transabdominal approach, with ultrasound used as a guide. The procedure is done with the patient under general anesthesia or intravenous sedation to relieve pain and decrease anxiety. *Ultrasonographic transvaginal ovum retrieval* is usually the procedure of choice, but the approach depends on accessibility to the ovary. With the patient in lithotomy position, the ultrasound probe with an aspiration needle guide attached is advanced through the cervix, uterus, and fallopian tube to the ovary. The needle guide is directed toward the follicle, as seen on a monitoring screen. The follicle is punctured with a 14-inch × 17-gauge needle. Follicular fluid is aspirated into a 5 ml syringe.

Extensive scarring in tubes may make ovaries inaccessible via the transvaginal approach. For a transvesicle approach, the ultrasound probe is inserted through urethra and posterior bladder wall to the ovary. With the patient in supine position, a probe can be inserted percutaneously through the abdominal wall to reach the ovary in the pelvic cavity.

If the ultrasonographic approach is unsuccessful or not preferred, ova can be retrieved by *laparoscopy.* The surgeon visualizes the ovaries. The follicle is punctured with an 8-inch × 14-gauge needle and aspirated directly into a test tube through a catheter attached to the needle. All instruments used for retrieval must be kept at a normal physiologic temperature of 98.6° F (37° C), including syringes or tubes and flushing solution. After completion of aspiration, the syringe or test tube is handed to circulator. To avoid contamination, fluid should not be exposed to the environment, including light. Dimmed room light also enhances the surgeon's view on the monitor. The circulator labels the specimen and sends it immediately to the laboratory for confirmation of ovum retrieval while instrumentation is still in place. If the report is negative, the search for another ovum continues until the laboratory gives a positive response of retrieval. The procedure may be repeated on the contralateral ovary. Many surgeons prefer to retrieve at least three ova for fertilization.

Fertilization

The aspirated ovum is placed in a culture dish containing a nutrient mixture similar to tubal secretions at midcycle, which prepares it for fertilization. Fresh semen obtained an hour or so before the woman undergoes ovum retrieval, or previously collected frozen sperm from a partner or donor, is added. The culture dish is incubated for 40 to 48 hours for fertilization to take place. Cell division is detected by microscopic examination. When the embryo reaches the four-to-eight cell stage of development, it is ready for transfer to the uterus. Multiple oocytes can be fertilized and embryos stored frozen for later implantation if desired.

Embryo Transfer

About 48 hours after retrieval, the woman returns for embryo transfer. She is placed in knee-chest position. Anesthesia is unnecessary. A catheter prepared in the laboratory, containing the embryo in culture medium, is inserted into the uterus. The patient remains in the knee-chest position for at least an hour to allow the embryo to gravitate to the upper uterine fundus. Immediately following embryo transfer, an injection of progesterone is given. Necessary for implantation, injections are given daily for the next 12 to 15 days. The embryo must implant itself into the uterus to become a fetus and to grow and develop. The woman's own ovarian function sustains early gestation, as confirmed by ultrasonography.

Failure to implant may result from escape of the embryo from the uterus with removal of the catheter, excess uterine contractility, inadequate luteal phase affecting the endometrium, mechanical disturbance of the endometrium, or encapsulation of the embryo in blood or mucus.

Gamete Intrafallopian Transfer

The procedure for gamete intrafallopian transfer (GIFT) is similar to IVF but is always done laparoscopically. The woman must have at least one patent, functional fallopian tube. Ovulation is induced as described for IVF. Laparoscopy is scheduled 34 or 35 hours after injection of HCG. Fresh semen is obtained from the partner at least an hour before this procedure. The embryologist prepares the culture medium with live sperm.

Ovum retrieval via laparoscope is accomplished as described for IVF. The follicular fluid is sent immediately to the laboratory where an embryologist selects two or three ova. These and the sperm, along with the culture medium, are loaded into a catheter and sent back to the OR. The surgeon passes the catheter through the laparoscope and injects fluid into the ampulla of the fallopian tube. One or both tubes may receive an injection.

Other procedures, such as laser vaporization of endometriosis or lysis of adhesions, may be performed while the surgeon waits for the catheter. Additional ova may be inseminated and cryopreserved for IVF if GIFT is unsuccessful. Many implants may precede conception; it may never be successful.

Artificial Insemination

In vivo fertilization by artificial insemination of sperm may provide a reproductive option for a fertile woman. Homologous insemination deposits the partner's sperm into the upper vagina, cervical canal, or uterine cavity. Whole ejaculate is used when the man is unable to deposit sperm into the partner's vagina because of psychologic or physiologic factors. Washed sperm are used for intrauterine injection. Semen or sperm may be frozen and stored in a sperm bank for future use if reproductive capacity is threatened as by illness.

Donor insemination involves the same techniques, but sperm are obtained from a donor other than an infertile partner. Donors are screened for sexually transmitted diseases, including infection with human immunodeficiency virus (HIV) and hepatitis B virus (HBV). Genetic screening also may be required. Donor sperm may be sought when the partner has a genetically transmitted disease or defect. The couple may have concerns about donor selection.

Artificial insemination must be coordinated with the recipient's ovulation for conception to occur. Assisted reproduction, as well as infertility surgery, fulfills hopes for many couples worldwide.

Bibliography

Adair CD et al: Bilateral tubal ectopic pregnancies after bilateral partial salpingectomy, *J Reprod Med* 39(2):131-133, 1994.

Apgar BS et al: Diagnostic hysteroscopy, *Am Fam Phys* 46(5 suppl): 19S-24S, 1992.

Apgar BS et al: Loop electrosurgical excision procedure for CIN, *Am Fam Phys* 46(2):505-509, 1992.

Berek JS, Hacker NF: *Practical gynecologic oncology*, ed 2, Philadelphia, 1994, Williams & Wilkins.

Berger PH, Saul HM: Radical hysterectomy, *AORN J* 52(6):1212-1222, 1990.

Bloomfield PI et al: Pregnancy outcome after large loop excision of the cervical transformation zone, *Am J Obstet Gynecol* 169(3):620-625, 1993.

Deardorf MA: Practical innovations: increasing multipuncture laparoscopic instrument longevity, *AORN J* 54(2):357-360, 1991.

DeChurney AH, Pernoll ML: *Current obstetric and gynecologic diagnosis and treatment*, ed 8, Norwalk, Conn, 1994, Appleton & Lange.

Dressner N et al: Refusing to terminate a life-threatening pregnancy, *Gen Hosp Psych* 12(5):335-340, 1990.

Emergency Care Research Institute: Exercise caution during intrauterine laser surgery, *Today's OR Nurse* 12(7):35, 1990.

Emergency Care Research Institute: The entry of abdominal fluids into laparoscopic insufflators, *Hazard: Health Devices* 21:180-181, 1992.

Hollands P: In vitro fertilization, *Br J Theatre Nurs* 27(2):9-10, 1990.

Jackson KD: Endometrial ablation with rollerball electrode, *AORN J* 54(2):265-282, 1991.

Kazmierczak S: Caesarean birth: a breath of life, *Surg Technol* 22(3):20-23, 1990.

Kolker A, Burke BM: Grieving the wanted child: ramifications for abortion after prenatal diagnosis of abnormality, *Health Care Women Int* 14(6):513-526, 1993.

Levine AH: Fetal surgery: in utero repair of congenital diaphragmatic hernia, *AORN J* 54(1):16-32, 1991.

Martin DY: An alternative to hysterectomy, endometrial laser ablation, *Br J Theatre Nurs* 27(5):10-11, 1990.

Mayeaux EJ Jr, Harper MB: Loop electrosurgical procedure, *J Fam Prac* 36(2):214-219, 1993.

McBride WZ: Spontaneous abortion, *Am Fam Phys* 43(1):175-182, 1991.

McCormick KA et al: Urinary incontinence in adults, *Am J Nurs* 92(10):75-93, 1992.

Millard S: Emotional responses to infertility: understanding patient's needs, *AORN J* 54(2):301-305, 1991.

Murdoch JB et al: The outcome of pregnancy after CO_2 laser conization of the cervix, *Br J Obstet Gynecol* 101(3):277, 1994.

Orcutt S: Total abdominal hysterectomy, *Surg Technol* 25(10):8-12, 1993.

Rabar FG: Gamete intrafallopian transfer: another approach for the treatment of infertility, *AORN J* 53(6):1466-1475, 1991.

Raz S: *Atlas of transvaginal surgery*, Philadelphia, 1992, Saunders.

Reed TP, Saade G: Microcolposcopy: how and when to do it, *J Reprod Med* 38(9):725-728, 1993.

Reinhardt M: Ectopic pregnancy rupture, *Am J Nurs* 94(7):41, 1994.

Rosenfeld JA: Emotional responses to therapeutic abortion, *Am Fam Phys* 45(1):137-140, 1992.

Schneider D et al: Safety of midtrimester pregnancy termination by laminaria and evacuation in patients with previous cesarean section, *Am J Obstet Gynecol* 171(2):554-557, 1994.

Shapiro P: Pelviscopy for ectopic pregnancy: a safer and quicker alternative, *Today's OR Nurse* 12(6):6-10, 1990.

Smith CD: Clinical issues: . . . filters for laparoscopic insufflators, *AORN J* 56(1):126-128, 1992.

Soderstrom RM: *Operative laparoscopy: the masters' techniques*, New York, 1993, Raven Press.

Turner RJ et al: Analysis of tissue margins of cone biopsy specimens obtained with cold knife, CO_2 and Nd:YAG lasers and a radiofrequency surgical unit, *J Reprod Med* 37(7):607-610, 1992.

Ulmer BC: Cervical intraepithelial neoplasia: etiology, diagnosis, treatment, *AORN J* 59(4):851-860, 1994.

Vasilev SA, Liming PR: Ectopic pregnancy, *AORN J* 54(5):1030-1039, 1991.

Wheeler SR: Psychosocial needs of women during miscarriage or ectopic pregnancy, *AORN J* 60(2):221-231, 1994.

White J: The laparoscope, *Br J Theatre Nurs* 27(2):13, 1990.

White MC et al: Patient care after termination of pregnancy for neural tube defects, *Prenat Diag* 10(8):497-505, 1990.

CHAPTER 31

Urologic Surgery

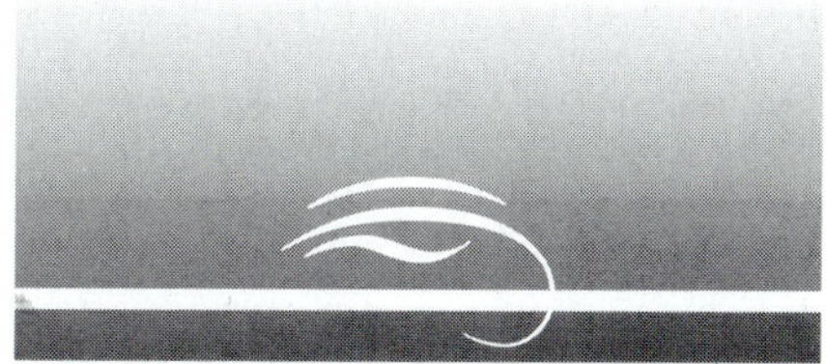

Urology is defined as that branch of medicine and surgery concerned with the study, diagnosis, and treatment of abnormalities and diseases of the urogenital tract of the male and the urinary tract of the female. The practice of urology involves, aside from routine diagnostic and surgical work, special knowledge and skills in the treatment of pediatric urologic problems, infections of the urinary tract, infertility and sterility, male sexual problems, renal dialysis and renal transplantation, renal hypertension, endocrine problems as they relate to the adrenal, testes and prostate, and cancer immunology and therapy. Because of shared responsibility in patient care with pediatricians, internists, nephrologists, endocrinologists, surgeons, and chemotherapists, close association with specialists in these disciplines is essential.*

HISTORICAL BACKGROUND

Writings from about 3000 BC tell of urinary diseases. The earliest known specimen of a bladder stone was found in the grave of an Egyptian dating back to 4000 BC. Around 2000 BC people in India are known to have suffered from bladder stones. Removal of a stone from the bladder through an incision is one of the earliest known surgical procedures. It was often performed by itinerant lithotomists, who flourished from the time of Hippocrates to the early eighteenth century. Hippocrates wrote that stone removal should be left to those trained for such work. For centuries this surgical procedure was not considered a part of medicine.

Although enlarged prostate glands were noted in the time of Hippocrates, attempts to remove part of them perineally or to tunnel through them with a sharp instrument were extremely dangerous.

Urethral sounds and bronze catheters were found in the ruins of Pompeii, buried since 79 AD. Metal catheters were used until the advent of rubber ones in the late nineteenth century.

The first urologists were mainly venereologists and "instrumenteurs" of the urethra. Urology advanced as a science with the invention of the microscope in the seventeenth century. Attempts to visualize the interior of the bladder were not made until the early nineteenth century. But the source of light and the instruments were inadequate. In 1876, Nitze, an Austrian, developed an instrument that is the basis of our modern cystoscope and urologic endoscopy.

Urologists have contributed to the evolution of medicine in general. Swick's development of intravenous pyelography is the foundation of modern angiography. Huggins opened a new vista to oncology when he identified that prostatic cancer was not fully autonomous. The use of antibacterial drugs by urologists freed all physicians from time-consuming treatment of venereal disease. Urology has been and continues to be a supporting specialty within medicine and surgery and is interdependent with other specialties.

*American Board of Urology.

ANATOMY OF URINARY TRACT

The urinary system provides the vital life-sustaining functions of extracting waste products from the bloodstream and excreting them from the body. Organs of this system include bilateral kidneys and ureters, the bladder, and the urethra (Figure 31-1). An obstruction to blood flow in the renal arteries or in any part of the urinary system can cause renal damage, ultimately resulting in uremia (biochemical imbalance) or renal failure, if undiagnosed and untreated. Vascular hypertension, tumors, infection, trauma, and other systemic or neurogenic disorders are of major concern to the urologist.

Kidneys

The *kidneys* are large bean-shaped glandular organs located bilaterally in the retroperitoneal space of the thoracolumbar region behind the abdominal cavity. Each kidney is enclosed in a thin fibrous capsule. The *renal parenchyma,* the substance of the kidney within the capsule, is composed of an external cortex and internal medulla. The *medulla* consists of conical segments called *renal pyramids.* Each pyramid and its surrounding cortex form a lobe. Within these pyramids are the essential components of renal function: the nephrons.

Each *nephron* consists of a glomerulus, glomerular capsule, and tubules. A *glomerulus* is an aggregation of capillaries formed by an afferent branch of the renal artery. These capillaries unite to form an efferent vessel. This capillary network is enclosed in a *glomerular capsule* (capsule of Bowman), which is the dilated beginning of the *renal tubule.* From the capsule, the tubule becomes tortuous and forms the proximal convoluted tubule. The distal portion forms the descending and ascending limbs of the *medullary loop* (loop of Henle). Nitrogenous wastes, salts, toxins, and water filtered from the capillary network form urine that flows through the medullary loop into the collecting tubule. The collecting tubules converge at the papilla (apex) of each renal pyramid. Urine flows continuously from each papilla into a *calyx.* Each kidney has between four and thirteen minor calyces leading into two or three, rarely four, major calyces that form the renal pelvis. The *renal pelvis* forms the dilated proximal end of the ureter.

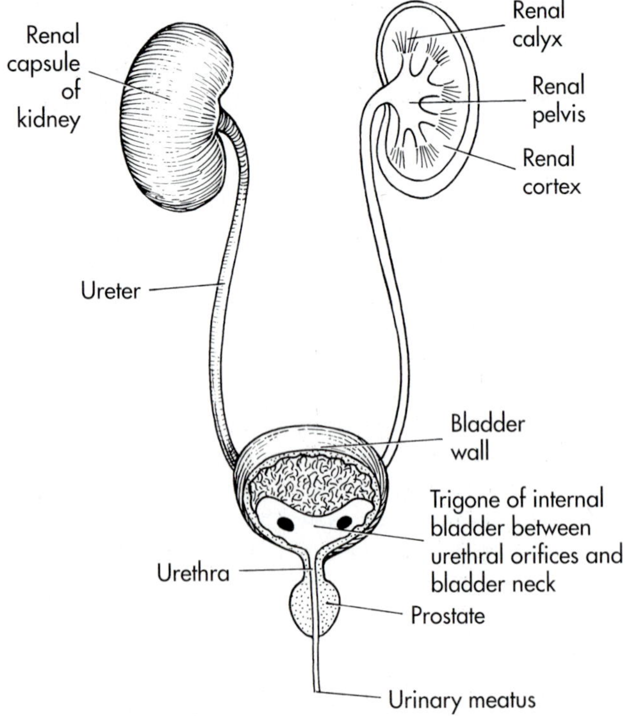

FIGURE 31-1 Male urinary tract.

Ureters

The *ureters* are connecting tubes, 4 to 5 mm in diameter and about 12 inches (27 to 30 cm) long, between the kidneys and bladder. They lie bilaterally beneath the parietal peritoneum and descend along the posterior abdominal wall to the pelvic brim. From there, they pass along the lateral wall of the pelvis and curve downward, forward, and inward along the pelvic floor to the bladder. The wall of each ureter is composed of mucous membrane, longitudinal and circular muscles, and an outer layer of fibrous and elastic tissue. Slow, rhythmic, peristaltic contractions carry urine from the kidneys to the bladder.

Bladder

The *bladder* is a hollow muscular reservoir lined with mucous membrane located in the anterior pelvic cavity behind the symphysis pubis. The ureters enter the bladder wall obliquely on each side. The triangular area between ureteral and urethral orifices is called the *trigone.* Valves formed by folds of mucous membrane in the bladder wall prevent backflow of urine into the ureters. Urine collects in the bladder until nerve stimulus causes micturition (urination) through the urethra. This stimulus opens the muscle fibers that form an internal sphincter at the *bladder neck,* the vesicourethral junction.

Urethra

The *urethra* in the male is about 8 inches (20 cm) long and consists of three portions: prostatic, membranous, and cavernous. The *prostatic urethra* passes from the bladder orifice to the pelvic floor through the prostate gland. The *membranous urethra* passes through the pelvic floor to the penis. The *bulbous* and *anterior urethra* pass through the penis to the external urethral orifice. The membranous and anterior urethra also serve as a passageway for secretions from the male reproductive system.

The female urethra is about 1½ inches (3.5 cm) long. It is firmly embedded posterior to the clitoris and anterior to the vaginal opening. Females are predisposed to urinary tract infections because the urethra is anatomically located near the vagina and the anus, both of which have resident flora that can cause infection if introduced into the urethra. Mechanical injury during coitus also may be a contributing factor.

UROLOGIC ENDOSCOPY

Cystoscopic diagnostic and some conservative urologic procedures approached through the urethra are performed in an especially designed and equipped area, often referred to as the *cysto room* or *suite*. This may be within the OR suite or in the urology clinic. X-ray control booths and developing units are adjacent to or within the area. Because x-ray procedures are frequently performed, walls and doors of the room should be lead-lined.

All safety regulations apply in the cysto room, just as they do elsewhere in the OR suite, to protect the welfare of the patients and personnel. All lighted instruments and electrical equipment should be checked for proper function before and after each use. Personnel who must remain in the room with the patient while x-ray films are taken should wear lead aprons. Patients should be protected with gonadal shields whenever feasible.

Proper OR attire is worn by all personnel entering the room. Most urologists don a water-repellent apron before scrubbing, unless sterile water-repellent gowns are provided. The urologist wears sterile gown and gloves. Procedures performed in the cysto room must maintain a sterile field. Adherence to principles of aseptic technique should be practiced to prevent nosocomial urinary tract infection.

Urologic Table

A urologic table differs from the standard operating table in that it provides an x-ray unit, a drainage system, and knee supports. Urologic radiographic studies use conventional x-rays, fluoroscopy and image intensification, and tomography. The imaging system is an integral part of the urologic table. Some tables have a built-in automatic film handling system; others have a film cassette holder; some adapt to a C-arm (see Chapter 28). The drainage system may have a drainage pan with tubing to drain port or single-use drainage bags. Under-knee/calf supports provide patient comfort in lithotomy position. Tables are equipped with hydraulic or electric controls to adjust height and tilt. Some have tray attachments for the light source and electrosurgical unit, as well as hooks for irrigating solution containers.

Patient Preparation

1. Patient may be encouraged to drink fluids before coming to the cysto room, unless the procedure will be done under general or regional anesthesia. Fluids ensure rapid collection of a urine specimen from the kidneys.
2. Frequently, procedures are done without anesthesia, with topical agents, or with local infiltration anesthesia. The patient should be reassured that the procedure usually can be performed with only mild discomfort. Respect the patient's modesty, and try to avoid embarrassing him or her.
3. Patient is assisted into lithotomy position with knees resting in padded knee supports. Pads avoid undue pressure in popliteal spaces. Some cystoscopic procedures are performed with the patient in supine position.
4. Drainage pan is pulled out of the lower break of the urologic table after the patient's legs are positioned on knee supports and foot of the table is lowered.
5. Pubic region, external genitalia, and perineum are mechanically cleansed with an antiseptic agent according to routine skin preparation procedure (see Chapter 22). Warm the solution according to the manufacturer's recommendations before applying it to an unanesthetized patient. Temperature of the solution should not exceed 110° F (57° C) or burns could result.
6. Topical anesthetic agents are instilled into urethra at end of the prep procedure. A viscous liquid or jelly preparation of lidocaine hydrochloride, 1% or 2%, may be used. This medium remains in the urethra rather than flowing into the bladder.
   a. *For female.* The female urethra is most sensitive at the meatus. Thus a small sterile cotton applicator dipped into the anesthetic agent and placed with cotton tip in the meatus is sufficient. It is removed when the urologist is ready to introduce an instrument.
   b. *For male.* A disposable cylinder with an acorn tip is used for intraurethral insertion. The agent is injected into the urethra and the penis is compressed with a penile clamp for a few minutes to retain the drug.
7. Sterile stainless steel filter screen is placed over the drainage pan. The patient is draped as for other perineal procedures in lithotomy position. The urologist may want to have access to the rectum. A disposable O'Connor sheet may be used. This has a synthetic rubber rectal sheath that protects the finger during rectal palpation. The perineal sheet has two fenestrations: one exposes genitalia; the other fits over the screen on the drainage pan. A gauze filter is incorporated into this latter fenestration in a disposable cystoscopy drape.

The urologist may prefer to wear a sterile disposable plastic apron over his or her gown. Attached to the table, this provides a sterile field from the urologic table to the urologist's shoulders. A receptor kit that attaches to the apron eliminates the need for the drainage pan. Tissue specimens are collected as irrigating fluid passes through a collecting basket.

Urologic Endoscopes

Urologic endoscopic instruments and catheters are available in sizes to suit infants, children, and adults. The size of these instruments and catheters is measured on the *French scale:* the diameter in millimeters multiplied by 3. Ureteral catheters are available in sizes 3 to 14 French, as described on pp. 641-642. The smallest is 1 mm in diameter times 3, or 3 French.

Specific endoscopic equipment is required for each procedure. All rigid urologic endoscopes have the same basic components.

Sheath

The hollow sheath may be concave, convex, or straight in configuration at the distal end inserted into the urethra. The other end has a stopcock attachment for irrigation. Sizes range from 11 French for infants to 30 French for adults. Within the sheath, space is provided to accommodate instruments for work in the bladder or urethra. Other instruments and catheters can be inserted through the sheath into the ureters and/or kidneys for diagnostic or therapeutic procedures.

Obturator

The stainless steel obturator, inserted into the sheath, occludes the opening and facilitates introduction into the urethra without trauma to the mucosal lining.

Telescope

Telescopes are complex precision optical systems. Each telescope contains multiple, finely ground optical lenses that relay the image from the distal end inside the bladder or urethra to the ocular (eyepiece) of the urologist. Additional rod-shaped elements (i.e., field lenses) are between each pair of relay lenses. Properly spaced throughout the length of the telescope, the lenses give an undistorted clear vision at the desired angle with some magnification. All telescopes are stainless steel with a Bakelite ocular. Some have operating or working elements incorporated into them.

Telescopes are costly, delicate instruments that must be handled gently at all times. The optical systems provide several angles of vision:

1. Direct forward or 0-degree vision is useful for viewing the urethra and for use with the optical urethrotome.
2. Right-angle or 30-degree vision is most suitable for viewing the entire bladder and for ureteral catheterization.
3. Lateral, which deviates 70 degrees but includes right angle in line of vision, is used for wide-angle viewing within the bladder.
4. Foroblique, which is a forward vision with an oblique view somewhat in front of right angle, is used to examine the urethra and for transurethral surgical procedures.
5. Retrospective, which provides an approximate 55-degree angle of retrograde vision, is used to inspect the bladder neck.

Light

The light source may be either a fiberoptic bundle or an incandescent bulb (see Chapter 15, p. 280). This may be an integral part of the sheath or the telescope. A cord connects the instrument to a fiberoptic projection lamp, rheostat, or battery. Fiberoptics have replaced most incandescent lamps.

Types of Urologic Endoscopes

Many different urologic endoscopes and accessories are in use, including nephroscopes introduced into the kidney and cystoscopes introduced through the urethra into the bladder. Verify with the urologist the type and size of the available endoscopes preferred for the examination and/or treatment before placing instrumentation on the sterile instrument table. The endoscopes and accessories most commonly used in the cysto room are described.

Brown-Buerger Cystoscope The stainless steel sheaths range in size from 14 to 26 French. Size 21 French is used most frequently in adults with a right-angle examination telescope for routine inspection of the bladder. Size 24 or 26 French is used to accommodate larger instruments and catheters that cannot be used through size 21. The sheath contains the light carrier.

A Brown-Buerger cystoscope set usually consists of two sheaths, one concave and one convex, each with its own obturator, and two or three right-angle telescopes. Along with the basic examination telescope, the set may have a combination operating and double catheterizing telescope (i.e., a convertible telescope), or the operating and double catheterizing functions may be in separate telescopes. The convertible operating and catheterizing telescopes have a small deflectable lever on the distal end to aid in directing ureteral catheters or flexible stone baskets into the ureters (see pp. 641 and 642). All corresponding parts of each set must be the same French size.

McCarthy Panendoscope The stainless steel sheaths range in size from 14 to 30 French. These are used most frequently with the foroblique telescope for viewing the urethra. Other telescopes are available for bladder visualization. The telescopes are interchangeable with all sizes of sheaths. A bridge assembly is required to fit the telescope properly to the sheath. The light is supplied through the telescope.

Wappler Cystourethroscope The Wappler cystourethroscope combines the functions of the Brown-Buerger cystoscope and the McCarthy panendoscope. The stainless steel sheaths range in size from 17 to 24 French. The foroblique and lateral telescopes, which also supply the light, are interchangeable with all sheaths. A visual obturator may be used to permit visualization and irrigation during introduction of the sheath into the urethra.

Resectoscope The resectoscope uses electric current to excise tissue from the bladder, urethra, or prostate. Components of this instrument include the sheath, obturator, telescope, working element, and cutting electrode. The sheath, usually 24 to 28 French, must be made of Bakelite or fiberglass to prevent a short circuit of the electric current. If the short beak post sheath is used with a wide-angle telescope, a Timberlake obturator must be used to introduce the sheath into the urethra.

The working element of the resectoscope, inserted through the sheath, has a channel for the telescope and cutting electrode. The types of working elements differ by the method in which the cutting electrode moves.

1. The *Iglesias* resectoscope uses a thumb control on a leaf spring-lock mechanism. The working element can be adapted for simultaneous irrigation and suction to control hydraulic pressure in the bladder.
2. The *Nesbit* resectoscope uses a thumb control on a spring.
3. The *Baumrucker* resectoscope uses finger control on a sliding mechanism.
4. The *Stern-McCarthy* resectoscope uses a rack and pinion to move the loop forward and back. This requires two hands.

The cutting electrode is the most critical component of a resectoscope. Because it must both cut and coagulate tissue, the electrode must be stabilized in the working element so that it retracts properly into the sheath after each cut. The electrode has a cutting loop from which electric current is passed through tissue, an insulated fork, an insulated stem, and a contact that is inserted into the working element. Several loop sizes are available; the stem is usually color-coded by size. Loop size corresponds to French size of the sheath. The electrode is malleable; therefore it must be checked before use to be certain insulation is intact and the loop is not broken. Electric current is applied only when the loop is engaged in tissue and inactivated after a cut is completed. The sheath can be charred if electric current is maintained after the cutting loop has been retracted into it. Disposable loop electrodes are commercially available.

Conductive lubricants should never be used on the sheath. They may provide a pathway for electric current. Cleanliness of the sheath and all other components is essential to proper function.

Endoscopic Accessories

Ureteral catheters (pp. 641-642), bougies, filiforms and followers, stone baskets (p. 641), and sounds are part of the urologist-endoscopist's armamentarium. Other accessories are used to remove tissue or calculi (stones).

Electrodes

In addition to the cutting loops used with the resectoscope primarily for transurethral resections (TUR), other types of electrodes with tips of various shapes are used in the bladder. These are inserted through the operating telescope of the Brown-Buerger cystoscope or Wappler cystourethroscope. They are used mainly for fulguration of bladder tumors, coagulation of bladder vessels to control bleeding following biopsy, and ureteral meatotomy. More electric current is needed when working in solution, as in the bladder, than in air. The power control settings on the electrosurgical unit should be as low as possible, however. All precautions and safeguards for the use and care of electrosurgical equipment apply to urologic procedures (see Chapter 15, pp. 269-270). A spark-gap generator should be used for transurethral resection and fulguration, which require high-voltage arcing described as spray coagulation (see Chapter 23, p. 478).

Lasers

Argon and Nd:YAG lasers can be adapted for use with urologic endoscopes. These are particularly useful for ablation of hemangiomas and vascular tumors in the bladder and kidneys. The argon-pumped tunable dye laser is used for photodynamic therapy on solid bladder tumors. A pulsed dye laser will fragment calculus in a ureter.

Irrigating Equipment

Continuous irrigation of the bladder is necessary during cystoscopy to:

1. Distend bladder walls so the urologist can visualize them
2. Wash out blood, bits of resected tissue, or stone fragments to permit continuous visibility and collection of specimens

A sterile disposable closed irrigating system is used because it prevents airborne contamination of the solution. Two to four or more liters of sterile irrigating solution may be needed for a single examination. Disposable tandem sets may be used to connect several containers together. Tandem sets allow for a continuous flow and for replacement of containers without interruption of flow. Sterile disposable irrigating tubing is connected to the irrigating solution container before it is hung on a hook on the urologic table, in the ceiling, or on a stand placed beside the table. The solution container should be at a level 2½ feet (0.75 m) above the table: a lower level decreases flow; a higher level increases hydraulic pressure with consequent fluid absorption by patient's tissues. Tubing should be filled with solution before it is attached to the sheath of the cystoscope or resectoscope. The plastic tubing from the container to the instrument is for individual patient use only.

Sterile isosmotic irrigating solutions that are nonhemolytic and nonelectrolytic are generally preferred by most urologists. However, sterile distilled water may be used for observation procedures and during resection or fulguration of bladder tumors. If a sufficient amount enters the circulation through open blood vessels, water may hemolyze red blood cells. As much as 3 to 6 L of solution may be absorbed during a transurethral prostatectomy. Minerals in water or saline act as a conductor and disperse the current when the electrosurgical unit is used. Saline must *never* be used.

Isosmotic solutions of 1.5% glycine, an amino acid, or sorbitol, an inert sugar, premixed in distilled water are commercially available in 1.5 and 3 L containers. A glycine solution, Urogate or Uromatic, is more commonly used for transurethral resection.

During the procedure, the flow of solution into the endoscope is controlled by the stopcock on the sheath where the tubing attaches. Rubber tips or nipples are used to seal other openings on the instrument to prevent escape of solution during a procedure. The openings through which catheters or instruments are to be inserted are closed with tips containing a hole. The accessory can be inserted through this hole with the seal maintained.

When the urologist wishes, the irrigating solution flows away from the instrument into the drainage pan through the filter screen. Solution drains from the pan, through the tubing, and into a collecting bucket that is emptied after each patient use. Some cysto rooms have floor drains. These may be a source of environmental contamination unless cleaned thoroughly. If large quantities of solution are used, observe the level of drainage into the bucket to avoid overflow onto the floor or around the foot pedal of the electrosurgical unit.

Evacuators

Evacuators may be attached to the endoscope to irrigate the bladder and to aspirate stone fragments, blood clots, or resected tissue. The two most commonly used types are the Ellik and Toomey. Stone or tissue fragments collected in the evacuator are retrieved and sent to the pathology laboratory.

1. *Ellik Evacuator.* The Ellik is a double bowl-shaped glass evacuator containing a trap for fragments so that they cannot be washed back into the sheath of the endoscope during irrigation with pressure on the rubber-bulb attachment.
2. *Toomey Evacuator.* The Toomey is a syringe-type evacuator with a wide opening into the barrel. It may be used with any endoscope sheath. A metal adapter permits its use with a catheter.

Care and Preventive Maintenance

1. Adequate sterilization is mandatory; therefore all endoscopes and reusable accessories must be free of debris and residue.
   a. Disassemble all parts and open all outlets.
   b. Clean all parts in a warm nonresidue liquid-detergent solution. Clean the interior of sheaths and openings with a soft brush.
   c. Rinse in clean water, and dry thoroughly.
   d. Wipe lenses gently with a soft, dry cloth.
2. When cleaning inside of a sheath or telescope, take care not to break the glass window over the light. These windows should be inspected each time the endoscopes are used because the urethra may be lacerated by a broken window.
3. Place endoscopes on a towel, to act as padding, in a sink, on countertops, and in trays to protect them from hard surfaces during handling and storage.
4. Check function of all moving parts, clarity of vision through telescopes, and patency of channels through instruments and catheters.
5. Keep sets of sounds, bougies, and filiforms and followers together so urologist will have a complete range of sizes readily accessible.
6. After cleaning, wrap items for sterilization. Flexible instruments should be protected by a rigid container.
7. Clean, dry stone baskets may be sealed in a peel-open package and sterilized in ethylene oxide gas. Retractable stone baskets are sterilized in the open position.
8. Principles and methods of sterilization discussed in Chapter 13 apply to urologic instrumentation. Steam-sterilizable items should be steam sterilized. However, with the exception of nylon and rubber catheters, bougies and nonflexible stainless steel instruments that do not have lenses, urologic endoscopes, and accessories are sterilized in ethylene oxide gas or activated glutaraldehyde or peracetic acid solution. All items should be sterilized after cleaning and then placed in sterile storage. Aeration following ethylene oxide sterilization is essential for Bakelite parts of endoscopes and for woven and synthetic materials.
9. If sterilization between patient uses is not feasible, high-level disinfection may be the method of choice for processing urologic endoscopic instruments.

SURGICAL PROCEDURES IN URINARY TRACT

Many patients seen by urologists are in the preadolescent and older age groups. Congenital and common pediatric problems are discussed in Chapter 42. This discussion focuses on adult problems. Most of these occur in men over 50 years of age with prostatic disease.

The genitourinary tract is often referred to as the *GU tract*. An open surgical procedure is performed only after conservative treatment fails or examination of the GU tract confirms a condition that does not yield to this treatment. Fortunately, most urologic conditions can be diagnosed and treated conservatively through a urologic endoscope and its accessories. The urologist performs open surgical procedures to repair, revise, reconstruct, or remove organs when a congenital or acquired condition does not respond to conservative therapy. Obstructive and neuromuscular disorders are common problems in the urinary tract. Renal calculus disease and tumors in the urinary tract are most commonly diagnosed in middle age. These conditions may cause obstruction and subsequent infection in the kidneys, ureter, or bladder.

Kidney

Ren is the Latin word for kidney; hence the adjective *renal* and combining forms of *ren-* and *reno-* pertaining to the kidney.

Definitive renal surgical procedures are justified for management of renal neoplasms, large cystic lesions that compromise renal function and/or produce obstruction, inflammatory diseases that necessitate drainage, or renal vascular disease. Chronic degenerative disease or severe traumatic injury can produce irreparable damage to renal cells. Computed tomography and magnetic resonance imaging identify the site, size, and extent of tumor involvement. Ultrasonography and intravenous urograms differentiate solid from cystic disease. Radionuclide scan may indicate renal function. Arteriograms and venograms indicate the extent of renal vascular disease.

The kidney is usually approached posteriorly with patient in a lateral position (see Figure 21-9, p. 446). The kidney rest is raised, and the table is flexed until flank muscles become tense. After patient is secured in position, the table is tilted in Trendelenburg's position until the flank is horizontal to floor. A flank incision is made parallel to and just below or over the eleventh or twelfth rib. The twelfth rib may be removed. The retroperitoneum is opened to expose kidney.

The kidney can be approached anteriorly through a transverse, subcostal, or midline incision. A thoracoabdominal incision may be preferred in obese patient or to reach lesion in the upper pole. These incisions, with patient in supine position, are frequently used for exposure of the aorta and vena cava for renovascular procedures. An anterior approach may be advantageous when prompt control of blood supply is important in renal trauma.

Nephrectomy

Removal of a lobe or the entire kidney is indicated when tumor, disease, or traumatic injury has resulted in the absence of renal function.

The entire kidney can be removed through a laparoscope. The organ is dissected, fragmented, and aspirated. Vascular pedicles are stapled. This alternative technique is used primarily for benign renal disease.

Partial Nephrectomy or Heminephrectomy

Partial excision may be sufficient when a lobe has been destroyed by localized disease or injury but the remainder of the kidney is functional. The vascular supply to the segment to be removed must be identified, ligated, and divided. The parenchyma of the lobe is resected from the capsule by blunt dissection. The renal pelvis and remaining capsule are closed.

Radical Nephrectomy The renal vessels are dissected free, ligated, and divided. Prerenal fat and fascia are dissected to deliver the kidney. The ureter is divided and ligated close to the bladder. The renal pedicle is ligated and divided, and the kidney is removed. Massive hemorrhage from renal artery and veins is a potential complication, as is injury to adjacent structures (i.e., inferior vena cava, aorta, duodenum on the right side or spleen on the left side).

Nephrectomy is performed in the OR on a living donor (unilateral) or on a cadaver donor (bilateral) to procure kidney for transplantation. Meticulous dissection is necessary to free the kidney, its blood vessels, and the ureter with minimal trauma. The ureter is dissected free and transected while the renal blood supply remains intact to ensure adequate urinary output. This surgical procedure may last longer than the usual nephrectomy.

Bilateral Nephrectomy Removal of both kidneys may be indicated before transplantation for a patient maintained on chronic dialysis (see pp. 638-639) who has severe hypertension. Following kidney transplantation, if rejection is uncontrollable, the patient may require transplant nephrectomy and return to chronic hemodialysis. This is less likely following transplantation from a live donor than from a cadaver. Kidney transplantation is discussed in Chapter 44, pp. 908-909.

Nephrostomy or Pyelostomy

Incision through the renal parenchyma or into the renal pelvis may be necessary to establish temporary or permanent drainage when an obstruction prevents the flow of urine from the kidney. A tube placed in the kidney exits through the skin. A cutaneous nephrostomy tube may be used to drain a kidney postoperatively during healing following renal reconstruction or revascularization. Silastic tubes placed internally through a cystoscope eliminate the need for an open surgical procedure for temporary urinary diversion. More frequently this is done percutaneously (see percutaneous nephrostolithotomy, p. 639) under fluoroscopic or ultrasound guidance by a radiologist and/or urologist. A plastic disk is applied to skin to secure the catheter. Tubing is connected to a leg bag to avoid tension on the catheter.

Pyeloplasty

Revision or reconstruction of the renal pelvis is performed to relieve an anatomic obstruction in the flow of urine by creating a larger outlet from the renal pelvis into the ureter. This may be done to repair or excise damaged tissue so that kidney function will be restored without a partial or total nephrectomy.

Either a rigid or a flexible fiberoptic nephroscope may be used to visually inspect the renal collecting system. A laser fiber may be used to treat some tumors.

Renal Revascularization

Stenotic lesions of renal arteries are surgically correctable causes of hypertension. Renovascular reconstructive procedures (renal angioplasty) are designed to improve blood flow through the stenotic area to the kidney or to bypass the stenotic area. Revascularization procedures may have a dual purpose: to correct hypertension and to preserve renal function. The patient is in supine position for these procedures because the renal arteries are approached through an abdominal incision.

In Situ Vascular Reconstructive Techniques Renal artery obstruction most often occurs from atherosclerotic stenosis at the origin of the artery or fibromuscular dysplasia (abnormal development) confined to the main renal artery. The obstruction is most often resected and replaced by an aortorenal-saphenous vein bypass graft. A reversed segment of proximal saphenous vein, gently distended and irrigated, is anastomosed first to the aorta and then to the renal artery. Prosthetic woven Dacron grafts may be used rather than an autogenous vein graft for renal artery bypass combined with distal aortic replacement. (See Chapter 40, pp. 821-822 for discussion of vascular prostheses.) Segmental resection of diseased arterial segments with primary end-to-end anastomosis may be performed. However, thromboendarterectomy is more frequently performed than is the latter procedure. All these procedures may be performed bilaterally or as staged bilateral renal artery reconstructions. Percutaneous transluminal angioplasty may be preferred to these open procedures (see Chapter 40, pp. 822-823).

Ex Vivo Extracorporeal Kidney Surgery When stenotic disease or another obstructive lesion extends into branches of the renal artery, in situ reconstruction may be difficult, hazardous, or impossible. In these patients, temporary nephrectomy with microvascular repair followed by autotransplantation of the kidney may be performed. This is referred to as *workbench surgery.* The kidney is completely mobilized from the retroperitoneal space. If one kidney is to be reconstructed, the ureter can remain intact and reconstruction is performed on a sterile bench (Mayo tray) placed over the patient's lower abdomen. For bilateral reconstruction, one kidney is detached from its ureter to permit complete removal from the abdomen. A second team works on the contralateral kidney while the other kidney is reconstructed at an adjacent dissecting bench (table).

Extracorporeal perfusion is necessary for renal preservation during reconstruction. This may be accomplished either with perfusion of cold Ringer's lactate or other hyperosmolar solution by gravity flow or with a continuous hypothermic perfusion through a Belzer pump machine. Or simple cold storage in saline slush may be used for renal preservation.

A kidney may be autotransplanted into the patient's groin or pelvis for revascularization of the kidney, removal of renal tumors or calculi, or repair of ureteral injuries.

Traumatic Injury

If a kidney is ruptured or injured by blunt trauma, a bullet, or a stab wound, fatal or near-fatal hemorrhage may be associated with the accident. This requires an immediate surgical procedure. The surgeon makes every effort to save kidney tissue and the ureter. A Foley catheter is inserted to keep an output record and to check for the presence of hematuria preoperatively and postoperatively. Gross hematuria preoperatively usually indicates injury to the bladder or urethra. Kidney damage is diagnosed by the presence of blood seen microscopically.

Renal Dialysis

End-stage renal disease and acute renal failure are potentially fatal conditions unless they can be controlled or reversed. Uremia and hypertension develop if renal failure is prolonged. *Renal dialysis* is the procedure of removing waste products and excess intravascular fluid from the body of a patient in acute or chronic renal failure by diffusion through a semipermeable membrane. This may be accomplished either by *hemodialysis* or by *peritoneal dialysis.* The treatment modality alleviates the acute manifestations of uremia and controls many of the chronic long-term complications of end-stage renal disease. Grossly undernourished and anemic patients with severe electrolyte imbalances must be adequately stabilized by dialysis before kidney transplantation. Some patients will be on dialysis for the remainder of their lives. Therefore patients undergoing chronic dialysis must have a means of access established for long-term maintenance.

Hemodialysis

Waste products are removed from the blood through the semipermeable membrane of a *dialyzer* (artificial kidney machine). An arteriovenous (AV) shunt or fistula is created subcutaneously in either an arm or a leg to provide access to the patient's circulation. The Quinton-Scribner double-lumen shunt, developed in 1960, consists of two tips attached to tubing. One tip is placed in the artery and the other in a nearby vein. Tubing from each tip is exteriorized through a subcutaneous tunnel to the skin and connected. Still used for acute access, variations and modifications of this basic external shunt are used to create an AV conduit; some have self-sealing devices to minimize potential problems of clotting and infection.

An anastomosis, usually between the radial artery and the cephalic vein in the forearm, creates an arterialized peripheral vein that permits dialyzer connections to be made by venipuncture. Needles are placed in the venous limb of the AV fistula for blood outflow and return. The Brescia-Cimino radiocephalic AV fistula, first described in 1966, is easiest to construct and has the least complications. If creation of an AV fistula by direct anastomosis is not feasible, a biologic or synthetic graft may be interposed between the artery and the vein. Preserved human umbilical vein, saphenous or other autologous vein, bovine carotid artery heterograft, and polytetrafluoroethylene (PTFE) grafts are used.

Peritoneal Dialysis

A Tenckhoff silicone catheter is placed into the peritoneal cavity for acute, intermittent, or continuous peritoneal dialysis. A paramedian incision is usually used to place a section of the catheter in subcutaneous tissue. The catheter has one or two cuffs to anchor it in subcutaneous tissue and to block bacterial invasion along the catheter into the peritoneal cavity. Dialysate is instilled over a period of time into the peritoneal cavity to draw solutes from body fluids into dialyzing solution. The patient may perform this routine at home, usually during the evening hours several times per week. This process selectively removes electrolytes, metabolites, toxins, and water normally excreted by the kidneys. Dialysate, warmed to body temperature, is instilled, allowed to remain for a specified number of hours and then withdrawn by a cycling machine or by gravity drainage. A Y-set disconnect system attached to catheter allows separation of inflow and outflow. Peritonitis is always a potential complication. Infection is frequently treated by adding antibiotics to the dialysate. Heparin is added to prevent fibrin clots in the catheter.

A patient being treated with peritoneal dialysis may come to the OR for an unrelated surgical procedure. Respiratory excursion may be impaired by pressure of retained dialysate under the diaphragm. Slight reverse Trendelenburg's position may alleviate respiratory discomfort. Additional suction containers should be available if the abdomen must be evacuated while the patient is in the OR. Fluid removed from the peritoneal cavity is measured, and the appearance and volume are recorded on the intraoperative record.

Patients with chronic renal failure can tolerate extensive surgical procedures with minimal complications. Their management in the OR must include strict attention to maintenance of a patent dialytic access shunt, fistula, or catheter; careful monitoring of fluid and electrolyte balance; and avoidance of postoperative infections. Following kidney transplantation, the patient may require postoperative dialysis; thus access must remain patent during and after the surgical procedure.

Urolithiasis (Urinary Calculus)

A renal calculus, a kidney stone, is a solid deposit or deposits (calculi) of minerals and salts that accumulate in the renal collecting system. Calculi may form as a result of a metabolic disorder. More commonly, they are concentrations of excess substances such as calcium oxalate, calcium phosphate, or uric acid in the blood that are filtered through the kidneys or crystals of salts that form around fragments of organic matter as from chronic infection. Renal colic is perhaps the most intense pain experienced by human beings. It is caused by a calculus or fragments of calculi partially or completely obstructing the calyces or renal pelvis. Renal calculi frequently dislodge and move from the renal pelvis into the ureter. A nidus, such as infection or an exposed suture postoperatively, can be the focal point for formation of a calculus in the ureter. If calculi are small enough, they will pass into bladder and be voided. Those that remain lodged, causing obstruction to outflow from any part of the urinary tract, must be removed. Preservation of renal function is the primary objective of surgical procedures for urolithiasis. *Lithotomy* is removal of a calculus. *Lithotripsy* is fragmentation of a stone followed by removal. *Chemolysis* is dissolution with a chemical substance.

Percutaneous Nephrostolithotomy or Nephrolithotripsy

A guidewire inside a transluminal angioplasty needle is introduced, under fluoroscopy, through the flank into the renal pelvis. The access point is carefully closed. This may be done in the radiology department under local anesthesia. In the OR, dilators are placed over the guidewire to enlarge a nephrostomy tract for introduction of a nephrostomy tube or nephroscope. The patient is placed in a modified prone position to slightly elevate the surgical side.

Renal calculi may be removed with stone forceps or baskets, or they may be fragmented with a lithotriptor. Lithotripsy is necessary for large calculi such as a staghorn calculus, which branches from the renal pelvis into the calyces and may extend into the ureter. Size, density, composition, and location will influence the urologist's choice of lithotripsy.

Ultrasonic Lithotripsy Ultrasonic waves will shatter calculus into fragments. Either a rigid or flexible fiberoptic nephroscope is inserted percutaneously. This procedure is usually done with the patient under spinal or general anesthesia. A hollow metal ultrasonic probe, which emits high-frequency sound waves, is inserted through the nephroscope. The probe is visually placed in contact with calculus that is localized in the renal pelvis as identified on x-ray film or by fluoroscopy. As ultrasonic energy is absorbed, the calculus fragments. The shattered particles are aspirated by suction through the probe. A nephrostomy tube may be placed in the renal pelvis for temporary drainage postoperatively. The nephrostomy tube is usually removed after 2 weeks.

Electrohydraulic Lithotripsy An electrohydraulic lithotriptor creates an electric discharge in fluid. This discharge is transformed into a hydraulic shock wave. A calculus disintegrates when the probe is directed at it. Larger fragments may be removed with Randall stone forceps; smaller ones are flushed out with irrigation. A tube is left in the nephrostomy tract for continued irrigation for several days after lithotripsy. This procedure may be performed with local anesthesia with intravenous sedatives and analgesics.

Nephrolithotomy or Pyelolithotomy

A large staghorn renal calculus that does not dislodge from the calyces or renal pelvis may have to be removed through an open incision. A nephroscope may be used during the surgical procedure for direct visual examination of the nephrons to locate and remove residual calculi. Ultrasound may also be used to identify retained fragments. Localized hypothermia provides the surgeon with a bloodless surgical field and extends the period of time in which the renal artery may safely be clamped without loss of renal function during the search for and extraction of calculi.

Percutaneous Chemolysis

Hemiacidrin may be instilled through a small nephrostomy tube to alkalinize cysteine and uric acid calculi and to dissolve debris remaining following other lithotomy procedures.

Extracorporeal Shock-Wave Lithotripsy

Immediately before a noninvasive extracorporeal shock-wave lithotripsy (ESWL) procedure, many patients are scheduled for cystoscopy. A ureteral stent may be inserted to facilitate passage of stone fragments (see p. 642). The ureteral stone may be manipulated back up into the renal pelvis. An x-ray film may be taken to check the location of the calculus.

Waterbath Lithotripsy After receiving continuous epidural or general anesthesia, the patient is positioned in a gantry (a hoist) and hydraulically lifted into a tub filled with degassed, demineralized water. The calculus must be visualized by fluoroscopy to focus shock waves. Rapid, high-voltage sparks, discharged within an ellipsoid reflector at the bottom of the tub, generate shock waves. These waves are focused and transmitted through water to enter the body. The impact of the waves against the calculus liberates high-energy mechanical stresses that cause fragmentation. Over a period of 45 to 60 minutes, up to 1500 shock waves are produced. After each series of 150 to 200 waves, focus on calculus is rechecked by fluoroscopy. Each shock wave is synchronized with the patient's respirations and resting phase of the heartbeat. The electrocardiogram (ECG) monitors R waves to avoid disrupting cardiac rhythm. A loud report sounds in the room each time a spark is fired. Both the patient and personnel must wear protective earplugs.

Tubless Lithotripsy Under local anesthesia or transcutaneous electric nerve stimulation (TENS), the patient is positioned on the table over a shock-wave generator. Spark-induced shock waves may be transmitted through a water cushion that contains an electrode and curved reflector. Patient's back is in contact with the cushion. This shock-wave energy is generated electromagnetically and focused with an acoustic lens. Fragmentation of calculus is verified with intermittent fluoroscopic images or x-ray films.

Shock waves also may be produced by piezoelectric transducers activated by an electronic generator. These transducers are mounted on a bowl-shaped spherical dish. A soft fluid membrane over this dish maintains contact with patient's skin. Ultrasound images, produced from an ultrasound localization system, are used to position stone at focal point of the shock waves.

ESWL equipment may be located in the OR suite adjacent to or in the cysto room, in a separate unit, or housed in a mobile van. Because this equipment is very expensive, patients are referred to regional centers. A mobile van may serve several hospitals within the region. OR nurses may be assigned to assist with ESWL.

Percutaneous Ureterolithotomy

A calculus lodged in the renal pelvis or upper tract of the ureter can be extracted or fragmented through a ureteropyeloscope, as described for percutaneous nephrolithotomy and lithotripsy.

Transurethral Ureteroscopic Lithotripsy or Lithotomy

A urologic endoscope can be introduced transurethrally for direct visualization and lithotripsy or for extraction of a calculus obstructing a ureter. Ultrasonic and electrohydraulic lithotripsy can be performed, as described, through a ureteroscope.

Laser Lithotripsy A pulsed dye laser beam is directed through a flexible fiberoptic ureteroscope to a calculus in the lower tract. The fine tip of the laser fiber probe must extend beyond the end of the scope to come in contact with the calculus. The energy generated through the intermittent laser pulses fragments calculus by mechanical action. This procedure may be done with the patient under epidural or general anesthesia.

Ureteral Stone Extraction A flexible-shaft, basket-type stone dislodger *(stone basket)* is inserted into the ureter through a cystoscope in the bladder for extraction of ureteral calculus. Several types of stone baskets are available, including the Dormia, Johnson, Levant, Pfister-Schwartz, and Lomac. These have a fine wire or nylon basket that can be expanded through the shaft to ensnare a calculus located in lower third of the ureter.

Stone baskets must be cleaned promptly after use in a nonresidue liquid-detergent solution to remove debris. Removable parts must be disassembled. Debris should be brushed *away* from the junction of basket and shaft with a small soft brush. During cleaning, inspection of the basket wires is critical. If they are cracked or broken at the end closest to the shaft, the basket may be passed into the ureter, but it cannot be withdrawn without trauma.

Ureterolithotomy

If a calculus fails to pass spontaneously through the ureter or cannot be removed with a stone basket, an open surgical procedure may be necessary. The patient is positioned for a lateral flank incision below the twelfth rib if the calculus is high in the ureter near the kidney. An abdominal incision is used to reach one in the lower segment near the bladder. When exposed, the ureter will be dilated proximal to the calculus and collapsed distal to it. The surgeon makes a small incision directly over the calculus and extracts it from the ureter with a stone forceps.

Cystolithotomy and Litholapaxy

Calculi usually can be removed from the bladder through the urethra. Crushing a urinary calculus in the bladder is referred to as *litholapaxy* or *lithotrity.* A lithotrite, introduced into the bladder through the urethra, is used to pulverize and remove calculi. This may be an instrument with hinged jaws, an ultrasound lithotriptor, or an electrohydraulic lithotrite. The electrohydraulic lithotrite generates energy shock waves at the tip of a flexible probe inserted through a cystoscope. With either instrument a telescope enables the urologist to work under vision. The stone fragments are irrigated from the bladder.

If a litholapaxy is unsuccessful or contraindicated, the removal of a calculus by incision into the bladder may be necessary. This surgical procedure is a *cystolithotomy.*

NOTE Following removal from any location in the GU tract, urinary calculi should be placed in a dry container and sent to the pathology laboratory for chemical analysis.

Ureter

The ureters are the vital anatomic structures for the flow of urine produced in the kidneys to the bladder. An obstruction to urinary flow must be corrected or diverted. The ureters may be approached either through an endoscope or through open incision.

Ureteral Endoscopy

Both rigid and flexible, short and long, fiberoptic *ureteroscopes* allow direct visualization of ureteral tumors, calculi, and strictures. These scopes are introduced percutaneously or cystoscopically. Tumors can be biopsied. Strictures can be corrected by balloon dilatation. Ureteral calculi can be extracted with stone baskets or forceps or fragmented using ultrasound or laser.

Percutaneous endoscopic techniques can be used in conjunction with cystoscopy. *Complete cystoscopy* implies that the procedure extends beyond the bladder into the ureters. This procedure may be performed for:

1. Drainage of the renal pelvis for differential diagnosis or renal function
2. Insertion of ureteral catheters to provide constant drainage for one or both kidneys or to outline ureters for a difficult pelvic surgical procedure
3. Insertion of a ureteral stent for internal drainage of an obstructed ureter
4. Transluminal dilatation of a ureteral stricture
5. Manipulation and removal of calculus
6. Ureteral meatotomy to enlarge the opening of one or both ureteral orifices into the bladder

Endoscopic instruments introduced into the urinary bladder were discussed on pp. 634-636. Only accessories used for diagnostic or therapeutic procedures within the ureters are mentioned here.

Ureteral Catheters Made of flexible woven nylon or other plastic material, ureteral catheters range in caliber from size 3 to 14 French and are about 30 inches (76 cm) long. Sterile, prepackaged disposable catheters are available. Most are radiopaque so that they can be visualized on x-ray film.

The urologist visualizes the ureteral orifice through the cystoscope. The catheter is inserted through the scope and introduced into the ureter. The catheter has graduated markings in centimeters so urologist can judge the distance the catheter has been inserted. The urologist will request size and style of catheter tip best suited for the intended purpose. The most common tips are shown in Figure 31-2.

1. *Whistle tips,* which are used for drainage, as ureteral markers, or for injection of radiopaque contrast medium for retrograde pyelography (see Chapter 28, p. 569). Largest sizes are used to dilate ureters to facilitate passage of a calculus.
2. *Olive tips,* which may be used for the same purposes as whistle tips.
3. *Round tips,* which may be preferred for drainage.
4. *Flexible filiform tips,* which may be used to bypass an obstruction for drainage.
5. *Blassuchi curved tips,* which may be used to bypass a ureteral stricture more easily than straight tips.
6. *Braasch bulb with whistle tips,* which are preferred to dilate the ureter or to inject contrast medium for a ureterogram (see Chapter 28, p. 569).

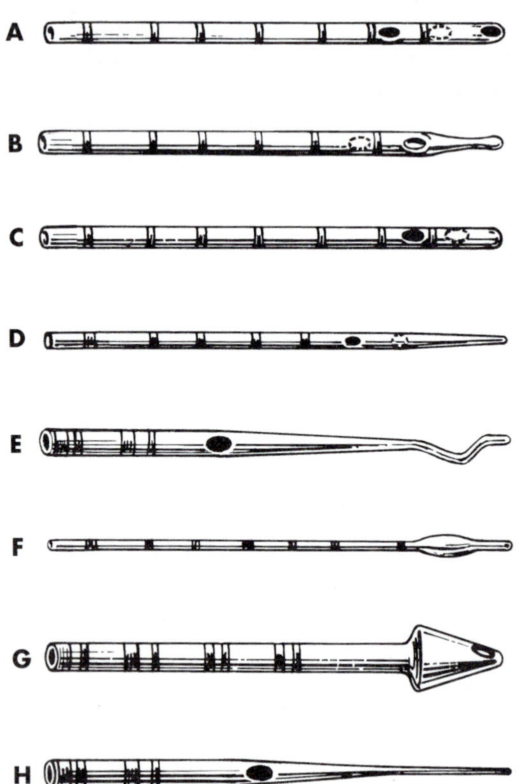

FIGURE 31-2 Ureteral catheter tips. **A,** Whistle. **B,** Olive. **C,** Round. **D,** Flexible filiform. **E,** Blassuchi curved. **F,** Braasch bulb. **G,** Acorn/cone. **H,** Garceau tapered.

7. *Acorn* or *cone tips,* which may be preferred for a ureterogram.
8. *Garceau tapered tips,* which are used to dilate ureters.

If left indwelling to provide drainage, ureteral catheters must be attached to a sterile closed urinary drainage system. Because they are smaller in diameter than standard urinary drainage catheters, an adapter must be used. This may be a small rubber tip or nipple placed on one end of a straight connector or both ends of a Y connector. The catheters are put through the hole in the tip(s). The other end of the connector is attached to a constant drainage system with a piece of sterile tubing.

A separate drainage system for each catheter may be desired by the urologist. Each drainage container must be labeled to identify right and left ureteral catheters.

Ureteral Stent An indwelling stent is inserted for long-term drainage in a wide variety of benign and malignant diseases causing ureteral obstruction. A stent also may be indicated for temporary drainage. Several types of stents are used. They are made of durable and biocompatible silicone, polyurethane, or other copolymer. The stent may have a collar, a double-J configuration, pigtail, or coil to minimize migration up into the renal pelvis or down into the bladder. The stent is passed through the cystoscope and over a guidewire into the ureter. It remains fixed for internal urinary drainage. Some types of stents are used to identify ureters and provide external drainage intraoperatively, as described for ureteral catheters.

Urinary Diversion Procedures

The ureters may be permanently or temporarily transplanted to maintain excretion of urine from the body but to divert flow away from the bladder. Bilateral transplantation for permanent urinary diversion is performed when neoplasm, chronic infection, congenital anomaly, trauma, or other cause impairs bladder function. The procedure follows completion of a total cystectomy (removal of bladder), a radical cystoprostatectomy in a male patient, or radical hysterectomy with salpingo-oophorectomy and cystectomy in a female patient, with or without pelvic lymphadenectomy. The ureters may be implanted into the intestinal wall, but more commonly they are transplanted to an isolated loop or segment of intestine that becomes a conduit for urinary flow. Ideally, a urinary reservoir collects and stores urine and expels it under voluntary control (i.e., functions as the lower urinary tract). The upper urinary tract should be protected from reflux of urine, which can lead to kidney infection. Normal renal function and electrolyte balance must be preserved. These objectives are not easily attained. Various procedures are used for urinary diversion.

Continent Reservoir An intestinal pouch is created with bilateral antirefluxing ureteroenteric anastomoses. This high-capacity (up to 800 ml), low-pressure pouch provides an intraabdominal reservoir (neobladder) for storage of urine. A one-way outflow valve provides continence (i.e., ability to control function). A cutaneous stoma also may be created (Figure 31-3) to empty the reservoir. The procedure is performed through a low midline incision. Several techniques are used to create the reservoir from a segment of ileum. Anastomoses may be stapled or sutured to reestablish intestinal continuity.

Although it is a lengthy surgical procedure, the resultant quality of life for the patient makes a continent reservoir, to prevent involuntary urinary leakage, the procedure of choice unless contraindicated by the patient's tolerance or pathologic condition.

KOCK POUCH A U-shaped pouch is created from a segment (70 to 80 cm [28 to 32 in]) of ileum. Nipple valves are created on two sides by intussusception (i.e., a portion of ileum is ensheathed in another portion). The afferent inflow valve prevents reflux. The ureters are anastomosed end-to-side distally near this inflow valve. The efferent outflow valve provides continence. Absorbable staples and/or mesh are used to help stabilize the valves. The reservoir will gradually increase in capacity to as much as 750 to 800 ml of urine. The patient does not wear a collection device but needs to use a catheter every 4 to 6 hours to empty the reservoir through the exteriorized cutaneous stoma.

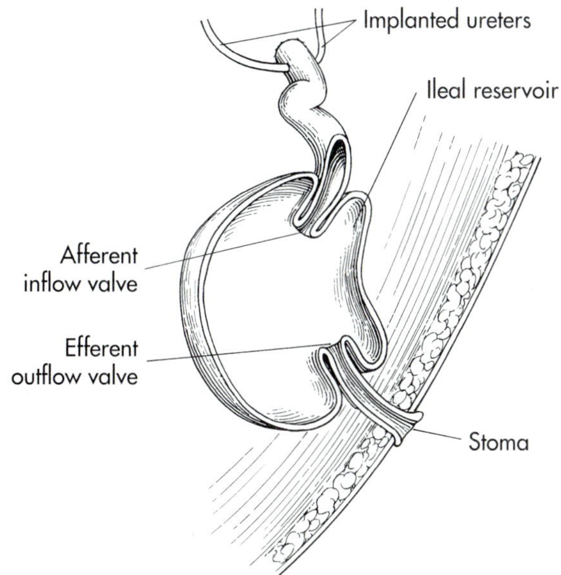

FIGURE 31-3 Ileal reservoir created from segment of ileum with ureters implanted distal to inflow valve. Exteriorized stoma allows self-catheterization through continent outflow valve. A continent reservoir includes implanted ureters, afferent inflow valve, ileal reservoir, efferent outflow valve, and stoma.

INDIANA POUCH A pouch is constructed by mobilizing a segment (15 to 20 cm [6 to 8 in]) of terminal ileum, cecum, and ascending colon. The ureters are anastomosed to the colonic segment, inferiorly on each side of the pouch, to prevent reflux. The terminal ileum is exteriorized to form a continent stoma for self-catheterization.

CAMEY POUCH An ileocystoplasty can be performed on male patient if a U-shaped segment (about 40 cm [16 in]) of ileum reaches the urethra at the pelvic floor without tension. The ureters are anastomosed through small enterostomies to distal ends of mobilized and divided ileum. A urethroileal anastomosis in the midsection of the ileal reservoir allows the patient to void through the urethra. Spontaneous contraction around the outflow valve at the site of anastomosis maintains continence. Micturition occurs by relaxation of perineal muscles and a Valsalva maneuver (i.e., a forced expiratory effort).

MAINZ POUCH A reservoir is formed by mobilizing a segment (10 to 15 cm [4 to 6 in]) of cecum and ascending colon and detubularizing (opening out flat) two small segments of equal length of terminal ileum. The walls of the pouch are formed by anastomoses of ascending colon and cecum with the ileal segments. The ureters are implanted into the ascending colon in an antirefluxive manner. This pouch can be anastomosed to the urinary bladder remnant after partial cystectomy to increase capacity. Continent diversion can be achieved by inverting the appendix into the cecum and exteriorizing the intussuscepted appendiceal mucosa to form a continent stoma for self-catheterization. In the absence of a healthy appendix, an additional segment (8 to 12 cm [3 to 5 in]) of ileum can be used to create a continent stoma.

Ileal Conduit Popularized by Bricker in the 1950s, both ureters are anastomosed to an isolated segment of the terminal ileum near its proximal end. The distal end is everted and sutured to a predetermined stomal site on the skin, usually on the right side of the abdomen below the waist. A urinary collection appliance is secured over the stoma before the patient leaves the OR. An ileal conduit with an incontinent external stoma (Figure 31-4) creates the psychologic stress of an altered body image for the patient, but it may be the procedure of choice for the patient who will receive systemic chemotherapy following radical cystectomy (see p. 645). As a secondary procedure after chemotherapy, an incontinent ileal conduit may be converted to a continent ileal reservoir.

Ureterosigmoidostomy Ureters may be anastomosed to a nonrefluxing segment of sigmoid colon. Urine diverted into the colon may cause physiologic complications, making this alternative for permanent urinary diversion the least desirable therapeutically. The patient retains an intact body image, however.

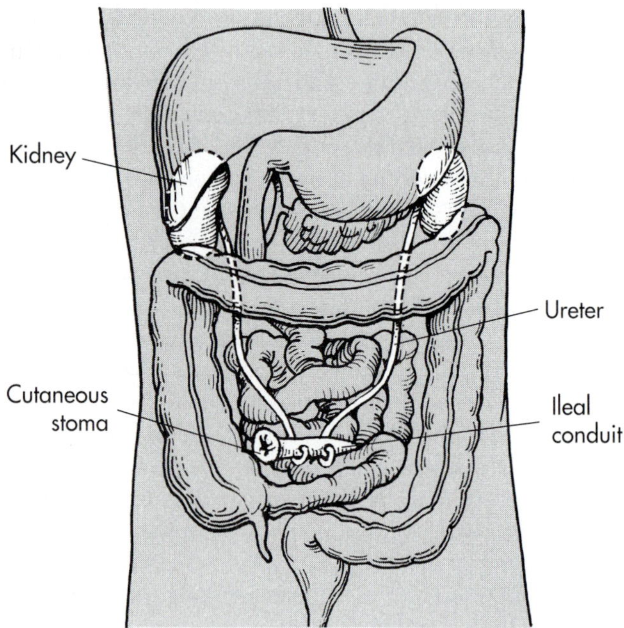

FIGURE 31-4 Ileal conduit created from isolated segment of ileum with ureters anastomosed to segment between closed end and external stoma. Urinary collection device must be placed over incontinent stoma. Incontinent urinary diversion carries urine from kidneys through implanted ureters and ileal conduit to stoma.

Cutaneous Ureterostomy The end of the ureter closest to the bladder is brought through the abdominal wall to the skin. Ureterostomy can be performed unilaterally or bilaterally with a single cutaneous stoma or a double-loop stoma. The patient must be fitted postoperatively with an appliance for collection of urine directly from the ureter to the exterior of the body. This procedure may be performed as a temporary emergency measure following trauma to the bladder, such as a ruptured bladder.

Ureteroneocystostomy

Implantation of the ureters into the bladder wall can be performed to relocate the ureters into a different site for correction of ureterovesical reflux, to reestablish urinary flow following temporary diversion or ureteral injury, or to establish urinary flow from kidney transplant following bilateral nephrectomy and ureterectomy.

Ureteroureterostomy

Anastomosis of two segments of one ureter is usually performed to reestablish ureteral continuity following traumatic injury. A ureteral catheter may be inserted as a stent and the ureter sutured over it. This procedure, or *transureteroureterostomy anastomosis,* may be indicated to bypass a ureteral stricture or to eliminate ureteral reflux that also may be the result of trauma to a ureter. Injury to a ureter can occur as a complication of pelvic or abdominal surgical procedures, as well as from external penetrating wounds. Ideally a transureteral anastomosis can be made 2 to 4 cm above the pelvic brim because ureters are close at this point and the recipient ureter has a straight course into the bladder.

Vesicopsoas Hitch Procedure

Loss of a large segment of middle or distal ureter can result from trauma or ureteral resection for tumor or stricture. A vesicopsoas hitch may be the procedure of choice when the length of the remaining ureter is insufficient for ureteroneocystostomy or ureteroureterostomy. Through an extraperitoneal approach into the retroperitoneal space, the bladder is mobilized. It is attached (i.e., hitched) to the psoas muscle to reposition the bladder cephalad. The segment of proximal ureter is brought through and sutured to the bladder wall. The kidney also may be mobilized and attached to the psoas muscle if too much tension will be placed on ureterovesical anastomosis.

Bladder

The bladder may be opened through a suprapubic incision when a neoplasm, calculus, obstruction of the bladder neck, or traumatic injury is not amenable to treatment through the cystoscope. Diagnosis is usually established through *urodynamics,* the study of bladder function, and direct visualization via cystoscope.

Cystometrogram

A cystometrogram measures voiding pressure within the bladder to determine muscle tone and to check nerve supply. A calibrated recording tidal irrigator cystometer is used. When 350 ml of solution is put into the bladder, the patient should feel a desire to void. Carbon dioxide gas is used with some electronic transducers or radio pressure gauges. Normal maximum capacity is 450 to 550 ml. Normal pressure is 40 to 50 ml of water. If the problem is neurogenic, cystometric findings are not higher than normal. If the problem is a hypertonic bladder, they are higher than normal.

Cystoscopy

Cystoscopy is a visual examination of the interior walls and contents of the bladder. The term is used broadly because various concurrent procedures may be carried out by using specially designed instruments through the cystoscope.

Plain cystoscopy is a routine examination of the bladder. Complete cystoscopy and litholapaxy have been described. In conjunction with plain cystoscopy, the following procedures may also be performed within the bladder.

1. Biopsy of a tumor with a flexible-shaft biopsy forceps to obtain specimens
2. Cystogram for diagnostic x-ray studies (see Chapter 28, p. 569) after injection of contrast medium into the bladder
3. Fulguration of a tumor by use of an electrode (see p. 635) to destroy tissue
4. Resection of or incision into a bladder neck obstruction with electrosurgical equipment (see section on resectoscope on p. 635)
5. Coagulation of hemangioma with argon laser, vaporization of a superficial tumor of the bladder wall with Nd:YAG laser, or photodynamic therapy to a solid tumor with argon-pumped tunable dye laser (see Chapter 45, p. 921)
6. Removal of a foreign body with flexible-shaft foreign-body forceps
7. Insertion of interstitial radionuclide seeds (see Chapter 45, pp. 923-924)

Suprapubic Cystostomy

In suprapubic cystostomy urinary drainage from the bladder is established via a catheter inserted through a suprapubic incision or trocar puncture into the bladder. If the bladder or urethra is injured by trauma associated with bony and soft tissue injuries of the pelvis, the bladder may be drained with a catheter placed above the pubic arch. This method of drainage is also preferred following some ureteral, bladder, prostatic, and urethral surgical procedures to decrease tension on sutures, to ensure a patent route for urinary drainage, and to minimize urinary retention. A suprapubic catheter also can be used when the surgeon wants the patient to void some urine voluntarily via the urethra if maintenance of urethral function and tone is desired, as following bladder or vaginal repairs. Suprapubic catheters are connected to a sterile closed constant drainage system before the patient leaves the OR. The most commonly used catheters for cystostomy drainage are:

1. Foley, 30 ml balloon, French sizes 20, 22, or 24.
2. Foley, 5 ml balloon, French size 24, three-way irrigating catheter. The third lumen can be used for continuous irrigation.
3. Bonanno suprapubic catheter.

Cutaneous Vesicostomy

In cutaneous vesicostomy urinary drainage is established directly from the bladder into a collecting device affixed on the abdomen rather than through a suprapubic catheter. The bladder is opened through a transverse suprapubic incision and a flap is raised at the dome. A skin flap is raised in the midline of the abdomen below the umbilicus. The bladder flap is sutured to the defect created in the skin and then covered with the skin flap. A transparent adhering skin dressing and collection device form a seal around the resultant bladder stoma. Cutaneous vesicostomy may preserve renal function and/or improve upper urinary tract structure in patients with neurogenic or atonic bladder, urinary incontinence, or bladder outlet obstruction.

Cystotomy, Cystoplasty

An incision into the urinary bladder through a suprapubic incision (cystotomy) may be performed to repair (cystoplasty) a bladder laceration or rupture as a result of trauma or a bladder wall defect. Various techniques are used to restore capacity and function of the bladder. Free fascial grafts, seromuscular grafts, myouterine flaps, and segments of stomach, ileum, or sigmoid colon are used to close defects. The defect may be covered with peritoneum, omentum, lyophilized human dura, gelatin sponge, or a biodegradable or synthetic material to stimulate regeneration of tissue. The bladder is also incised to perform a Y-V plasty to relieve a stricture or contracture of the bladder neck by broadening the outlet of the bladder into the urethra.

Cystectomy

The bladder is removed (cystectomy) for invasive malignant disease. Radical total cystectomy with en bloc pelvic lymph node dissection is usually performed. The neurovascular bundle, required for erection, may be preserved in a male patient, or a penile prosthesis may be implanted at a subsequent surgical procedure (see p. 651). Salvage or partial cystectomy with intraoperative radiation therapy (see Chapter 45, pp. 925-926) may be an alternative to total cystectomy. If a urinary diversion procedure (previously described) has not been performed before removal of the bladder, transplantation of the ureters into the skin or into the intestinal tract for urinary drainage is required at the time of cystectomy. A gastrocystoplasty may be the procedure of choice following partial cystectomy, especially in a patient with impaired renal function.

Urinary Incontinence

Involuntary, uncontrollable voiding may accompany congenital or acquired physiologic conditions, such as loss of bladder control following spinal cord injury or neurogenic disease. Urinary incontinence may develop in male because of loss of sphincter control following prostatectomy (see pp. 649-650) and in female following obstetric injury, radiation therapy, or severe pelvic fractures. Surgical intervention is often necessary for *stress incontinence* (i.e., the intermittent leakage of urine as a result of sudden increase in intraabdominal pressure, as during coughing or sneezing), on weakened urethral sphincter muscles at the bladder neck. Various surgical procedures are performed as determined by urodynamics. Gynecologists perform some bladder suspension procedures (see section on Marshall-Marchetti Krantz suprapubic vesicourethral suspension, Chapter 30, p. 622); urologists perform other procedures. Laparoscopic approaches have been developed for bladder neck suspension with use of synthetic mesh and titanium staples. Surgical procedures that suspend, support, or reposition the bladder can correct urinary incontinence or improve urinary continence.

Stamey Procedure

In the Stamey procedure sutures are placed on both sides of urethrovesical junction from anterior rectus fascia into the vagina. The patient is positioned in a modified lithotomy position so legs extend laterally to flatten the lower abdomen. Short suprapubic incisions, right and left of midline, are extended to anterior rectus fascia. Vagina is incised transversely and dissected from urethra to expose trigone of the bladder. The urethrovesical junction is located by palpation of balloon of Foley catheter inserted into the bladder. A Stamey straight or angled needle is passed through the rectus fascia, along internal vesicle neck, and out through vaginal incision. A cystoscope is inserted to ascertain correct needle placement without injury to the bladder. A heavy nylon suture threaded onto the needle is drawn from vagina to suprapubic incision. The needle is inserted again. Vaginal end of suture is passed through a 1-cm length of polyester tubular graft before it is threaded onto needle. When suture is drawn to the abdominal wall, it establishes a suspending loop on one side of the bladder neck. The suture is tied over the anterior rectus fascia with enough tension to elevate bladder neck by traction on adjacent vaginal fascia. The procedure is repeated on contralateral side. The cystoscopic equipment should be set up on a separate sterile table because contamination of the eyepiece is unavoidable.

Pereyra Procedure

In the Pereyra procedure the bladder neck is elevated with sutures suspended from the anterior rectus fascia. The primary difference between this procedure and the Stamey procedure is that a Pereyra ligature carrier needle is passed blindly down through retropubic space and out into the vagina. Both procedures relocate the proximal urethra and bladder neck into the zone of intraabdominal pressure without necessity for open pelvic surgery. The Pereyra procedure is used for uncomplicated recurrent urinary stress incontinence and is 80% effective for long-term resolution of urinary leakage.

Artificial Urinary Sphincter

A prosthesis may be implanted to apply pressure to the urethra to maintain continence between periods of voiding. The pressure-regulating mechanism has a balloon, cuff, and pump constructed of silicone rubber. A balloon with desired predetermined pressure is positioned intraabdominally beside the bladder. The cuff encircles either the bladder neck or bulbous urethra, depending on the preferred surgical approach. The pump is placed in the subcutaneous tissue of the scrotum (in male) or labium (in female). A control assembly lies subcutaneously adjacent to external inguinal ring. Tubing connects the components. A radiopaque isotonic solution is used to fill the prosthesis. When a patient squeezes the pump, solution is transferred from cuff into balloon, thus releasing pressure on the urethra to permit urine to flow.

Teflon Injection

Teflon paste (Polytef) may be injected into tissues surrounding the urethra proximal to the external sphincter. The injection swells the tissue, narrowing the urethra sufficiently for sphincteric control. This is done in selected patients with moderate to severe urinary incontinence, such as in a male following transurethral resection or in a female in whom a suspension procedure has been unsuccessful. The injection is made transurethrally with a flexible syringe through a fiberoptic cystourethroscope. A suprapubic catheter is used for 3 to 5 days postoperatively to allow some voluntary passage of urine from the urethra. Postoperative complications include urinary retention, urethral fistulas, and Teflon granulomas. Studies have shown this method to be 88% effective in providing major improvement in urinary control. Collagen may be injected rather than Teflon paste.

Bladder Flap Urethroplasty

When urodynamics show a resistance to urinary flow in a female with neurogenic bladder, a bladder flap urethroplasty procedure is advisable. A lesion of the nervous system causes dysfunction of the bladder.

Urethra

The urethra functions as the outlet for urine to pass from the bladder. Obstruction or dysfunction of the urethra may cause urinary retention or incontinence. Enlargement of the prostate may cause obstruction. Gonorrhea, other disease processes, or traumatic injury may cause a stricture. Problems associated with congenital displacement of the urethra are discussed in Chapter 42, p. 859.

Perineal Urethrostomy

When indwelling or intermittent urethral catheterization is contraindicated in a male patient with an obstructed or traumatized urethra, urinary drainage may be established through a perineal incision. An indwelling catheter is inserted into the bladder through an incision into the membranous urethra.

Urethral Dilatation

Periodic dilatation may be necessary for weeks to years following infection or trauma that has caused a urethral stricture. Either balloon dilators, woven filiforms and followers, bougies, or metal sounds are used. If the latter are preferred, curved metal sounds are used to dilate a male urethra; straight sounds are used on female. A short urethral stent may be inserted.

Urethrotomy

An Otis urethrotome may be used to cut into a urethral stricture. After the instrument is passed into the urethra, the blade is released to cut the stricture. If a specimen of the urethra is taken for biopsy, a rigid biopsy forceps is used through a cystourethroscope. This scope also is used with a laser to open a urethral stricture.

Urethroplasty

Reestablishment of continuity without stricture is the ultimate objective following traumatic urethral injury, usually associated with pelvic fracture in male. Scrotal-inlay urethroplasty or another method of urethral reconstruction is usually delayed until the extent of injury can be fully evaluated by urethrograms. A suprapubic cystostomy catheter, inserted as an emergency measure, can maintain urinary drainage for several weeks to months. Insertion of a urethral catheter into a ruptured urethra in the immediate posttraumatic period can produce periurethral infection, stricture, and other irreparable damage.

ENDOCRINE GLANDS

Two pairs of glands in the endocrine system are of primary interest to the urologist: the adrenal glands in both sexes and the testes in the male.

Adrenal Glands

The adrenal glands secrete substances that help regulate fluid and electrolyte balance, influence metabolism and sexual organs, and assist the body in coping with stress. These glands are located in the retroperitoneal spaces immediately above the superior pole of each kidney. Total or partial excision of one or both adrenal glands is usually performed by the urologist. However, in some hospitals, this surgical procedure has become the province of endocrinologic surgical specialists.

Adrenalectomy may be indicated for the removal of a benign, malignant, or metastatic tumor within the adrenal medulla or to eliminate adrenal hormonal secretions. The adrenal glands are a rich source of estrogens. Bilateral adrenalectomy may be performed as supplemental treatment of advanced prostatic or breast cancer to reduce the hormonal environment within the body. Estrogens may stimulate recurrence or metastasis from prostatic or breast cancer.

For a unilateral adrenalectomy, the adrenal gland is usually approached posteriorly through a lateral incision into the retroperitoneal space. Usually the twelfth rib is resected on right side because the adrenal gland lies above the kidney, behind the liver. The surgeon may also prefer a posterior approach for a bilateral adrenalectomy with the patient placed in a modified prone position for bilateral incisions. Other surgeons prefer an anterior thoracoabdominal or transabdominal incision into the retroperitoneal space with the patient in supine position. The circulator must verify with the surgeon the preferred position before the patient is positioned, prepped, and draped. The thoracoabdominal incision may be preferred to extend the incision across the costal margin into the eighth or ninth intercostal space for exposure and exploration of the extraadrenal paraganglion system, depending on the preoperative diagnosis.

Testes

The *testes* are the pair of male reproductive glands suspended in the scrotum that after sexual maturity are the source of spermatozoa. They also secrete hormones that influence growth and development, sexual activity, and secondary sex characteristics. When both testes are excised, the castrated patient becomes sterile and deficient in male hormones.

Bilateral orchiectomy may be performed as adjunctive therapy in patients with prostatic cancer to alter the hormonal environment. Control of the disease following this relatively simple procedure is attempted before the urologist considers adrenalectomy. Psychologic preparation is important to help the patient accept sterilization and other body changes, such as breast enlargement, which may occur as a result of alteration in the hormonal system.

Bilateral oblique incisions in the inguinal canals extend into the upper anterior surface of the scrotum over the testes. Following ligation of the spermatic cords at the external or internal inguinal rings, the testes are removed from the scrotum. Silicone rubber prostheses may be implanted in the scrotal sac to improve cosmetic appearance for psychologic rehabilitation of the patient.

MALE REPRODUCTIVE ORGANS

The primary functions of male reproductive organs are procreation, sexual gratification, and hormone secretion. Organs are both internal and external (Figure 31-5).

Testes

The testes are both hormonal glands and male reproductive organs. Disorders in or around one (or both) testis that inhibit sexual activity, reproductive capability, or cause discomfort in the scrotum may necessitate a surgical procedure.

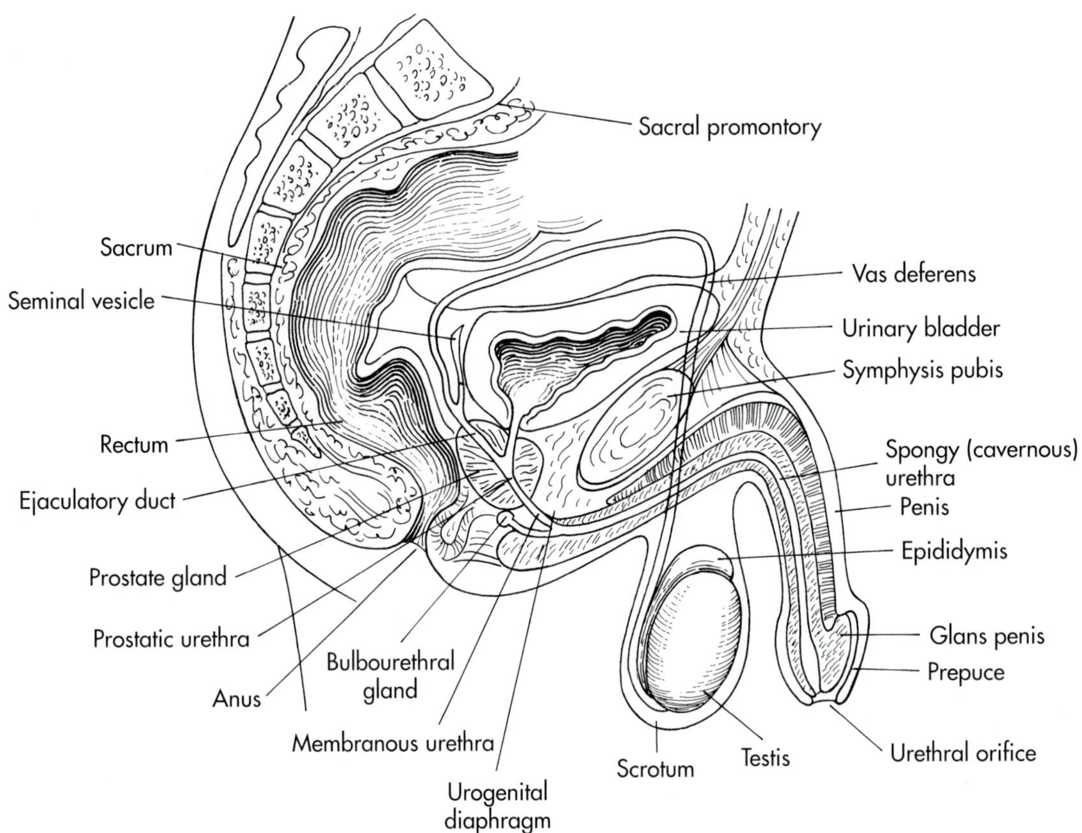

FIGURE 31-5 Male reproductive organs in sagittal section.

Unilateral Orchiectomy

Removal of one testis does not sterilize the patient. This procedure (unilaterally as described for bilateral orchiectomy) may be indicated following traumatic injury or infection, but it is more commonly performed to remove a tumor. Primary testicular tumors may be right- or left-sided; germ cell tumors may develop bilaterally. Accurate histologic findings and clinical evaluations of the type of tumor and stage of disease are mandatory for determination of appropriate therapy. Computed tomography and lymphangiography or lymphoscintigraphy are valuable diagnostic tools. Unilateral radical orchiectomy, via an inguinal incision, may be followed by radiation or chemotherapy and retroperitoneal lymph node dissection. The spermatic cord and vas deferens are ligated and divided separately at the internal ring so that these structures can be identified if further dissection is needed for metastatic disease.

Retroperitoneal Lymphadenectomy A transabdominal midline incision is made for exposure of lymph nodes and sympathetic nerve fibers in the paraaortic plane, usually along anterolateral aspect of the aorta in the retroperitoneal space. Unilateral lymphadenectomy usually is done on ipsilateral (same) side as the tumor unless regional metastases have spread via lymphatic invasion; then a bilateral dissection is indicated. If possible, neurovascular bundles from the hypogastric plexus going to corporeal tissues of penis are preserved. These nerve fibers are identified and placed in vessel loops before lymphadenectomy is carried out, thus allowing preservation of ejaculatory function.

Scrotal-Testicular Trauma

An injury may require exploration of the scrotum to ligate bleeding vessels or to insert a Penrose drain. Infection is likely to develop following a penetrating wound; thus extraperitoneal spaces in the scrotum must be drained thoroughly.

Hydrocelectomy

A *hydrocele* is an accumulation of fluid in sac of the tunica vaginalis of the testis. Through an anterior incision into the scrotum, the hydrocele sac is dissected away from the testis and removed from the scrotum.

Varicocele Ligation

Dilation of spermatic veins of the pampiniform plexus of the spermatic cord can cause a soft, elastic, often uncomfortable swelling in the scrotum. This condition, known as *varicocele,* occurs more frequently on the left side. It can cause loss in testicular mass and a decrease of sperm density associated with male infertility. Ligation of the spermatic vein can improve sperm count if the testis has not atrophied.

The spermatic vein is ligated above the inguinal canal lateral to the inferior epigastric vessels or in the retroperitoneal space lateral to the iliac artery. In the latter approach, a transverse abdominal incision starts at the anterior superior iliac spine and extends toward the lateral aspect of the rectus abdominis muscle. The hemiscrotum must be manually emptied of all blood before the vein is ligated or the varicocele may persist postoperatively.

Laparoscopic approaches have been developed for spermatic vein ligation. The internal inguinal ring is located laparoscopically and the spermatic cord and blood vessels are identified. The spermatic vein is dissected free and ligated with two endoscopic clips. The vein is cut between the clips with endoscopic scissors. Most patients are able to return to work within 2 days of the procedure.

Vas Deferens

The *vasa deferentia* are the small fibromuscular excretory ducts that carry sperm upward through the spermatic cords from the epididymides lying along the upper portion of each testis to the seminal vesicles, the pouchlike glands in front of the urinary bladder near the prostate gland. Interruption of or obstruction to a vas deferens inhibits normal spermatogenesis.

Vasectomy

Elective bilateral vasectomy is an established method of male sterilization. This is usually performed as an ambulatory surgical procedure. A segment of each vas deferens is removed. Cut ends are either ligated with suture or clips or fulgurated by coagulating epithelium of lumen, depending on preference of the urologist. Techniques vary, but all patients should be informed that spontaneous regeneration of a severed vas deferens does occur in a small percentage of patients.

Vasovasostomy

Recannulization of the vas deferens for restoration of fertility requires a nonobstructed anastomosis. The tough 2 mm outer diameter with an inner diameter of 1 mm or less at the distal end plus dilatation of the proximal end makes precise anastomosis under the operating microscope preferable to nonmicrosurgical techniques in which it is difficult to see the lumen of the vas deferens on the distal side. One-layer anastomosis and splinting techniques for vasectomy reversal often result in a stricture caused by scarring within lumen of the vas deferens that inhibits passage of sperm. After a scrotal incision exposes vas deferens above and below the site of previous ligation, the two ends are cut to excise scar tissue and to open lumen. Under magnification of the operating microscope, interrupted sutures are placed in mucosal lining of the lumen to create a fluid-tight anastomosis. Muscularis is approximated separately. A carbon dioxide milliwatt laser may be used to weld tissue to overcome scarring and stricture that may be associated with suturing. Sperm counts return to normal soon after the surgical procedure.

Prostate Gland

A musculoglandular organ encased in a fibrous capsule, the *prostate gland* surrounds the posterior urethra at the bladder neck. It is divided into five lobes. Normal function of this gland provides secretions to the seminal fluid for sperm mobility during ejaculation.

Although this gland normally weighs 20 g, it will enlarge to some degree in most men by the time they reach 50 years of age. Enlargement of the prostate gland can obstruct the urethra. Difficulty in voiding most often brings men with prostatic disease to a urologist. The entire gland or one or more lobes can be resected from its capsule transurethrally. Prostatectomy can also be performed through a suprapubic or retropubic abdominal approach or a perineal incision. A radical prostatectomy, performed through a retropubic abdominal or perineal incision, includes extirpation of the prostate, periprostatic tissue, seminal vesicles, and vas ampullae en bloc. The approach and procedure depend on the urologist's preference for removing the type of pathologic condition. Transrectal aspiration, core biopsies, or ultrasonography help establish diagnosis. Prostatic carcinoma may be treated by surgical removal, interstitial and external beam radiation, chemotherapy, and/or hormonal therapy. Management depends on stage of the disease and age and condition of the patient. Carcinoma of the prostate is the second most common cause of cancer-related deaths in American men. Benign prostatic hypertrophy/hyperplasia (BPH) is a common indication for prostatectomy in men over 50 years of age.

Transurethral Prostatectomy

Transurethral resection (TUR), also referred to as transurethral resection of prostate (TURP), is removal of all or part of the glandular tissue within the prostatic capsule by electroresection. A *resectoscope* (see p. 635) is introduced into the prostatic urethra. Using alternating currents through the cutting loop electrode, the urologist resects tissue and coagulates bleeding vessels. The bladder must remain filled during resection. Nonconducting, isosmotic glycine irrigating solution is used; 10 to 12 L may be needed (see irrigating equipment, pp.

635-636). Resected tissue is collected in an Ellik or other evacuator. After the surgical procedure, tissue fragments must be sent to pathology department for analysis and weighing. The urologist may insert a three-way 30 or 50 ml Foley catheter. The inflated balloon compresses vessels around the bladder neck to help control bleeding. The third lumen provides a means for continuous irrigation postoperatively to prevent formation of clots in the bladder.

Benign nodular hyperplasia of glands under 50 g in size is the usual indication for TUR. This approach has potential complications of impotence and urinary incontinence. The technique is one of the most difficult for a urologist to master. Although electroresection is used most commonly, transurethral incision of small prostate glands (less than 25 g), balloon dilatation of prostate, and cryosurgery are other invasive techniques for treating BPH. TUR may be done for diagnosis or treatment of localized cancer.

Suprapubic Prostatectomy

The suprapubic approach for prostatectomy is limited almost exclusively to removal of a large benign hypertrophied gland over 50 g. Through a midline vertical incision above the symphysis pubis, the superior bladder wall is opened to expose the prostatic urethra. The prostatic lobes are enucleated with a finger inserted through an incision into the mucosa of the urethra. This procedure may be termed *transvesicocapsular prostatectomy* because the prostatic capsule is approached through the bladder. Hemostatic agents are usually packed into the extremely vascular prostatic fossa to help control bleeding. Pressure from the Foley catheter balloon inserted after closure of the urethra also helps obtain hemostasis. A cystostomy tube is inserted to facilitate urinary drainage from the bladder during the healing process.

Retropubic Prostatectomy

In retropubic approach the prostate gland is exposed below the bladder neck through a vertical or transverse abdominal incision above the symphysis pubis. The gland is removed through an incision in the prostatic capsule; this is a *transcapsular prostatectomy*. The periprostatic tissue, seminal vesicles, and vas ampullae also may be excised.

Radical Retropubic Prostatectomy A limited pelvic lymph node dissection is performed for carcinoma with no evidence of spread beyond the prostatic capsule. This radical procedure may be carried out as initial curative therapy or following transurethral prostatectomy. After dissection of lymph nodes, one of two approaches may be used to totally remove the prostate.

1. *Campbell technique.* An incision is made at the bladder neck and the urethra is transected. The prostate and periprostatic tissue are widely dissected anterograde from the bladder. The bladder neck is reconstructed for the vesicourethral anastomosis. The patient will be impotent because the nerves responsible for erection are transected. A penile prosthesis may be implanted (see p. 651).
2. *Walsh technique.* The prostate is resected retrograde beginning at the urethra, working back to the bladder neck. Dissection is carried out close to the prostatic capsule to preserve the neurovascular bundle and thus maintain potency. The vesicourethral anastomosis is completed.

Perineal Prostatectomy

The perineum affords the most direct open surgical approach to the prostate through a relatively avascular field. With the patient in an extreme lithotomy position, the perineum is incised above the anal sphincter. The rectum may be dissected from the posterior surface of the prostate, or dissection may be carried out between the external anal sphincter and the rectum. The perineal approach may be used to enucleate the prostate gland from its capsule or for radical cystoprostatectomy. This latter procedure includes removal of the entire prostate gland, its capsule, seminal vesicles, and a portion of the bladder. The classic radical perineal prostatectomy with pelvic lymph node dissection may be the surgical procedure of choice to reduce morbidity of prostatic carcinoma.

Transperineal Prostatic Cryoablation

Transperineal prostatic cryoablation is performed in the cysto room with the patient under general or spinal anesthesia. The entire prostate and periprostatic tissues are frozen. With patient in lithotomy position, an ultrasound probe is placed in the rectum for guidance in positioning five cryoprobes. Each cryoprobe is placed transperineally through a hollow sheath inserted in a small (18-gauge) needle puncture site. Liquid nitrogen is delivered to each probe from the cryosurgical device/console. Care must be taken to avoid freezing the rectum. Warm water is run through a urethral catheter to keep the urethra warm to prevent sloughing, a potential complication of transurethral cryosurgery. The prostate gland, including tumor cells, is destroyed. Transperineal cryoablation offers an alternative to radical prostatectomy in selected patients with cancer of the prostate.

Pelvic Lymphadenectomy

For pelvic lymphadenectomy, either a low abdominal incision into the extraperitoneal space or a laparoscopic approach may be used. Lymph nodes are dissected bilaterally from the iliac vessels, the obturator spaces, and the hypogastric vessels. These nodes may be examined by frozen section to detect early and subtle metastases from prostatic carcinoma. If several nodes are positive for cancer, the patient is unlikely to benefit from radical prostatectomy. If nodes are negative, the urologist may proceed with a radical retropubic prostatectomy. Pelvic lymphadenectomy also may be done as a staged procedure before radical perineal prostatectomy. If feasible, at least one neurovascular bundle is preserved.

Penis

The *penis* is the male organ of copulation. Because it contains the urethra, a deviation or malformation in structure may affect normal urinary flow from the bladder. Surgical procedures to repair congenital anomalies of the penis and circumcision are discussed in Chapter 42, pp. 859-860 because these procedures usually are performed during infancy and childhood.

Impotence

The cause of erectile impotence can be classified as *organic* or *psychogenic*. Patients must be thoroughly evaluated by a urologist and properly selected for surgical therapy. Most procedures for impotence are performed with the patient under regional anesthesia. Consideration for the patient's privacy should be included in the plan of care.

Dorsal Vein Ligation Failed erection can be caused by inadequate filling or inadequate storage of blood in the erectile tissue of the corpus cavernosa of the penis. Some patients are able to achieve erection but unable to maintain it for more than a few minutes because of a cavernosal leak. The diagnosis is made by dynamic infusion cavernosometry and cavernosography. In selected patients with this condition, the urologist may elect to ligate the dorsal vein and several collateral vessels of the penis to delay the venous return from the erectile tissue to sustain erection.

Penile Prosthesis Implantation of a *penile prosthesis* can enable some impotent men to achieve a satisfactory return of sexual activity. Penile prosthetic implants are of three types: semirigid silicone, semiflexible silicone-braided silver, and an inflatable hydraulic device.

1. The Small-Carrion semirigid prosthesis consists of two foam-filled silicone rods inserted into the corpus cavernosum on each side of the penis, usually through a vertical incision in the perineum underneath the scrotum. The suitable-size prosthesis is selected from lengths available. The prosthesis maintains a permanent semierection.
2. The Finney Flexirod is similar to the Small-Carrion prosthesis except that it is hinged at the penoscrotal junction when implanted. This allows the penis to hang in a dependent position when an erection is not desired.
3. The Jonas prosthesis is constructed of malleable braided silver and silicone. It is semiflexible.
4. The Scott-Bradley inflatable hydraulic device is inserted through a midline incision extending from the base of the penis to a point midway between the symphysis pubis and the umbilicus. Silicone cylinders are implanted into each corpus cavernosum. Tubing connected to these cylinders at the base of the penis is brought into the left inguinal canal, the prevesical space, and the right inguinal canal, where it is connected to tubing from the pump-release mechanism placed in the scrotum. A reservoir, filled with a radiopaque solution, is sutured into the abdominal fascia of the prevesical space. Tubing from this reservoir is also connected to the pump-release mechanism. To achieve erection of the penis, the patient squeezes the pump in the scrotum.

Penectomy

The penis is partially or completely resected because of neoplasm or trauma. Partial penectomy may allow the patient enough length for upright voiding. In some patients cosmetic reconstruction may be possible. Invasive disease may necessitate complete penectomy, including removal of scrotum and testes. Reconstruction following complete penectomy includes urethral diversion to the perineum. The plan of care should include consideration for psychologic counseling.

Transsexual Surgery

Transsexual surgery may be the only acceptable alternative for a patient who is psychologically possessed with the desire to physically and emotionally become a member of the opposite sex. This type of surgery presents extreme challenges to the urologist and gynecologist. Surgical techniques have been developed to eliminate the obvious external genitalia of a male by dissection of penile structures, shortening of the urethra, and removal of the testes. The penile and scrotal skin are preserved for construction of a pseudofemale vaginal orifice. This procedure is done as the final stage following change of secondary sexual characteristics by hormonal and/or surgical therapy to produce breast enlargement, suppression of beard and body hair, redistribution of adipose tissue, voice change, and removal of pronounced thyroid cartilage (Adam's apple). This final stage of transsexual surgery, from male to female, creates a vagina by inverting the hollow penis into the hypogastrium between the new urethral orifice and the rectum. Because the nerve endings from the penis are intact, the newly constructed vagina is capable of experiencing orgasm postoperatively. The prostate and seminal vesicles are retained so that orgasm with emission is possible. The scrotal skin forms the labia.

POSTOPERATIVE COMPLICATIONS

Oliguria, the diminished capacity to form urine, is frequently seen postoperatively. Water and sodium are conserved by antidiuretic hormone, aldosterone, epinephrine, and norepinephrine secreted during stress. This decreases urinary output. Dehydration, shock, cardiac failure, renal failure, or third-space loss such as edema or ascites may contribute to oliguria. Because prolonged oliguria may result in renal failure, urinary output of less than 30 ml an hour should be reported to the surgeon. Treatment depends on the cause.

The patient should be watched for infection following all urinary tract procedures because of the introduction of instruments and catheter. Cloudy urine, dysuria, frequency, urgency, and pain or burning on urination are symptoms of urinary tract infections. Damage to bladder sphincters from instrumentation or urethral infection may lead to incontinence. Sharp abdominal pain following cystoscopy or manipulation of a ureter to remove calculi may suggest peritonitis from bladder or ureteral perforation. Susceptibility to infection accompanies urinary diversion.

BIBLIOGRAPHY

Arai Y et al: Long-term followup of the Kock and Indiana pouch procedures, *J Urol* 150(1):51-55, 1993.

Burger R et al: The appendix as a continence mechanism, *Eur Urol* 22(3):255-262,1992.

Cass AS: Nephrectomy: a review of surgical approaches, *Today's OR Nurse* 12(6):16-21, 1990.

Cavas M, Makay S: The Indiana pouch: a continent urinary diversion system, *AORN J* 54(3):494-509, 1991.

Cleeve J: A common problem: a study of a patient undergoing transurethral resection of bladder tumour, *Br J Theatre Nurs* 28(1):3-8, 1991.

Cohen JK, Miller RJ: Thermal protection of urethra during cryosurgery of prostate, *Cryobiology* 31(3):313-316, 1994.

Cubler-Goodman A: Endoscopic lithotripsy for urinary calculi: treatment alternatives, *AORN J* 58(5):954-960, 1993.

Cubler-Goodman A et al: Flexible ureteroscopy: patient care, indications, *AORN J* 54(6):1211-1219, 1991.

Cumes DM: Transurethral prostate resection, *AORN J* 58(2):302-311, 1993.

Cumming J, Pryor JP: Treatment of organic impotence, *Br J Urol* 67(6):640-643, 1991.

Das S: Penile amputation for the management of primary carcinoma of the penis, *Urol Clin North Am* 19(2):277-282, 1992.

Denson CE: Ureteral stents, *AORN J* 51(5):1293-1306, 1990.

Dos Reis JM et al: Penile prosthesis surgery with the patient under local regional anesthesia, *J Urol* 150(4):1179-1181, 1993.

Eldh J: Construction of a neovagina with preservation of the glans penis as a clitoris in male transsexuals, *Plast Reconstr Surg* 91(5):895-900, 1993.

Emmert GK et al: Primary neoplasms of the penile shaft, *South Med J* 87(8):848-850, 1994.

Fisch M et al: Seven years experience with the Mainz pouch procedure, *Arch Espan Urol* 45(2):175-185, 1992.

Fisch M et al: Sigma-rectum pouch: Mainz pouch II, *Urol Clin North Am* 20(3):561-569, 1993.

Fisch M et al: The Mainz pouch II, *Eur Urol* 25(1):7-25, 1994.

Fisch M et al: The Mainz pouch II: Sigma-rectum pouch, *J Urol* 149(2):258-263, 1993.

Freedman AL et al: Long-term results of penile vein ligation for impotence from venous leakage, *J Urol* 149(5):1301-1303, 1993.

Holschneider CH et al: The modified Pereyra procedure in recurrent stress incontinence: a 15-year review, *Obstet Gynecol* 83(4):573-578, 1994.

Jordan GH et al: Penile prosthesis implantation in total phalloplasty, *J Urol* 152(2):410-414, 1994.

Karram MM et al: Artificial urinary sphincter for recurrent/severe stress incontinence in women, *J Reprod Med* 38(10):791-794, 1993.

Kenney L: Extracorporeal shock wave lithotripsy, *AORN J* 56(2):251-263, 1992.

Kerfoot WW et al: Investigation of vascular changes following penile vein ligation, *J Urol* 152(3):884-887, 1994.

Klein EA: Partial and total penectomy for cancer, *Urol Clin North Am* 18(1):161-169, 1991.

LaFollette SS: Kidney cancer, *AORN J* 56(1):31-48, 1992.

Lasater SJ: Cancer of the penis, *AORN J* 56(1):19-30, 1992.

Lasater SJ: Testicular cancer: a perioperative challenge, *AORN J* 51(2):513-526, 1990.

Lotenfoe R et al: Periurethral polytetrafluoroethylene paste injection in incontinent female subjects: surgical indications and improved surgical technique, *J Urol* 149(2):279-282, 1993.

Lowe A, Gabriel LS: Laser lithotripsy: patient care, staff education, *AORN J* 58(5): 961-969, 1993.

Martin JP: Transrectal ultrasound: a new screening tool for prostate cancer, *Am J Nurs* 91(2):69, 1991.

Mathias JM: New technology: cryoablation for prostate cancer, *OR Manager* 11(2):8-9, 1995.

McLoughlin J et al: Surgical treatment of venous leakage, *Eur Urol* 23(3):352-356, 1993.

Moore S et al: How to irrigate a nephrostomy tube, *Am J Nurs* 93(7):63-67, 1993.

Moore S et al: Nerve-sparing prostatectomy, *Am J Nurs* 92(4):59-64, 1992.

Moore S et al: Treating bladder cancer: new methods, new management, *Am J Nurs* 93(5):32-39, 1993.

Newton M et al: Prostate cancer: staging through laparoscopic lymphadenectomy, *AORN J* 59(4):823-836, 1994.

Onik GM et al: Transrectal ultrasound-guided percutaneous radical cryosurgical ablation of the prostate, *Cancer* 72(4):1291-1299, 1993.

Opjordsmoen S et al: Sexuality in patients treated for penile cancer: patients' experience and doctors' judgement, *Br J Urol* 73(5):554-560, 1994.

Ou CS et al: Laparoscopic bladder neck suspension using hernia mesh and surgical staples, *J Laparoendoscop Surg* 3(6):563-566, 1993.

Politano VA: Transurethral Polytef injection for post-prostatectomy urinary incontinence, *Br J Urol* 69(1):26-28, 1992.

Rauscher JA, MacLeod SR: Laparoscopic spermatic vein ligation: a new technique to treat varicoceles, *AORN J* 57(3):664-670, 1993.

Rauscher JA, Parra PO: Vesico-psoas hitch procedure: a method of repairing ureteral injuries, *AORN J* 52(6):1177-1186, 1990.

Rauscher JA et al: Camey procedure: a continent urinary diversion technique, *AORN J* 54(1):34-44, 1991.

Rauscher JA et al: Kock pouch: an internal ileal reservoir for continent urinary diversion, *AORN J* 56(4):666-678, 1992.

Ronk LL, Kavitz JM: Perioperative nursing implications of radical perineal prostatectomy, *AORN J* 60(3):438-446, 1994.

Roobottom CA et al: Endosonographic monitoring of transurethral cryoprostatectomy, *Clin Radiol* 48(4):241-243, 1993.

Salter MJ: Aspects of sexuality for patients with stomas and continent pouches, *J Enterostom Nurs* 19(4):126-130, 1992.

Saver CL: Transurethral balloon dilatation of the prostate: an option for patients with benign prostatic hypertrophy, *AORN J* 56(6):1049-1060, 1992.

Schivai RC et al: Erectile function and penile blood pressure in diabetes mellitus, *J Sex Marital Therapy,* 20(2):119-124, 1994.

Shandera KC, Thompson IM: Urologic prostheses, *Emerg Med Clin North Am* 12(3):729-748, 1994.

Stein P: Perioperative considerations of vascular access for dialysis, *AORN J* 60(6):947-958, 1994.

Tan LB et al: Traumatic rupture of the corpus cavernosa, *Br J Urol* 68(6):626-628, 1991.

Teimann D et al: Artificial urinary sphincters: treatment for post-prostatectomy incontinence, *AORN J* 57(6):1366-1379, 1993.

Toto KH: Acute renal failure: a question of location, *Am J Nurs* 92(11):44-53, 1992.

Vancaillie TG, Schuessler W: Laparoscopic bladder neck suspension, *J Laparoendoscop Surg* 1(3):169-173, 1991.

Walker GT, Texter JH: Success and patient satisfaction following the Stamey procedure for stress urinary incontinence, *J Urol* 147(6):1521-1523, 1992.

Wespes E et al: Objective criteria in the long-term evaluation of penile venous surgery, *J Urol* 152(3):888-890, 1994.

Willis D: Taming the overgrown prostate, *Am J Nurs* 92(2):34-40, 1992.

Witt MA et al: The post-vasectomy length of the testicular vasal remnant: a predictor of the surgical outcome in microscopic vasectomy reversal, *J Urol* 151(4):892-894, 1994.

Young MJ et al: Penile carcinoma: a twenty-five year experience, *Urology* 38(6):529-532, 1991.

CHAPTER 32

Orthopaedic Surgery

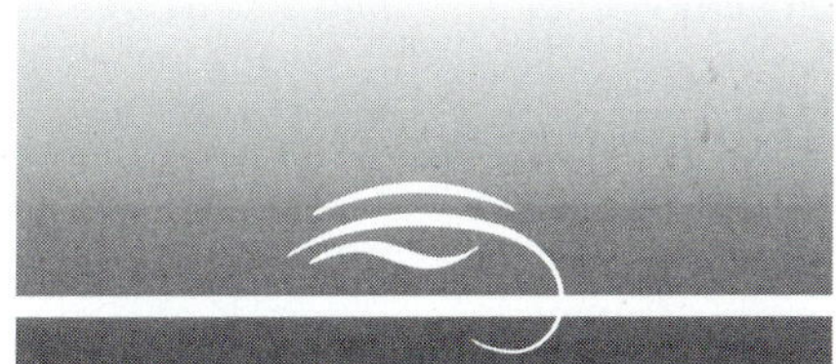

The word *orthopaedics* is derived from two Greek words: *orthos* (ορδος, straight) and *pais* (παιδι, child). As the name implies, orthopaedics began with the treatment of crippled children by means of rest, braces, and exercise. Even today conservative, noninvasive medical and physical methods nearly always are used if possible to restore form and function. However, patient care must be individualized. As a branch of medicine and a contemporary surgical specialty, orthopaedics is: "concerned with the diagnosis, care, and treatment of musculoskeletal disorders—that is injury to or disease of the body's system of bones, joints, ligaments, muscles, and tendons."*

Degenerative diseases and disabilities affecting the musculoskeletal system cause loss of function and impair activity of many individuals, especially the aged. Congenital deformities are frequent. Consequently, orthopaedists treat a disproportionate number of geriatric and pediatric patients in comparison with their ratio in the general population.

Orthopaedics depends on many disciplines to help evaluate and treat patients. Diagnostic imaging, bioengineering, electrobiology, genetics, microbiology, oncology, and transplantation are but a few of these.

HISTORICAL BACKGROUND

Records tell of the treatment of fractures in Egypt 4500 years ago. Mummies have been found with splints still in place. Some of these were made from the bark of trees; others were strips of linen impregnated with a gluelike substance. Egyptian mummies and murals show evidence of crippling diseases. One drawing, over 800 years old, shows a man using a crutch.

Hippocrates described scoliosis, congenital dislocation of the hip, and clubfoot. His writings included the accumulated knowledge of past centuries; thus many of the treatment methods he advocated date back beyond his time. Almost all the principles of treating fractures currently followed are included in his book *On Fractures.* Hippocrates discussed the use of traction, countertraction, bandages, splints, and treatment of compound fractures. He used mixtures of gelatinous substances and clay to coat bandages. He recognized the necessity of immobilizing a joint above and below a fracture. He described the proper position of fixing joints for the best possible future function. He wrote that exercise strengthens but inactivity wastes a part. He advocated mobilization of fractures as much as possible to prevent atrophy. For centuries much of the wisdom in the books of Hippocrates was ignored or forgotten, then rediscovered.

Galen described muscles and their function as a motor system directed by the brain through nerves. He named the spinal deformities still known as lordosis, scoliosis, and kyphosis.

In the sixteenth century, Ambroise Paré described appliances to support or correct orthopaedic conditions. He wrote a book on dislocations. His description of fractures of the spine was the beginning of modern spinal surgery.

*American Academy of Orthopaedic Surgeons.

Modern orthopaedic surgery began to evolve in the eighteenth century. The earliest known institute for treatment of skeletal deformities was founded in Switzerland in 1780. The development of orthopaedic surgery has been enhanced by governmental and societial expenditures for the care of the crippled and disabled and by the growth of hospitals and rehabilitation centers.

Of the orthopaedic surgeons in the late nineteenth century, no one contributed more to the development of the specialty than Charles Fayette Taylor (1827-1899). His investigations in *kinesiatrics* (movement therapy) and surgical mechanics contributed to the undertaking of exercise and rest in the treatment of musculoskeletal disorders. Fundamental concepts of these and other early teachers have not changed; their methods of treatment have changed as new knowledge has been gained and materials have been improved. Knowledge of skeletal tissue led orthopaedists to attempt surgical procedures on tendons and joints. An increased knowledge of bone regeneration, the concept of aseptic technique, the discovery of x-ray technology, the introduction of sulfonamides and antibiotics, and the development of instrumentation and appliances all have contributed to the advancement of orthopaedic surgery.

The multidisciplinary approaches of physics and biology created a surge of interest in neuromusculoskeletal science and technology for orthopaedic surgery. Attempts were made in the 1950s to replace the components of the hip joint. In 1959 John Charnley suggested in England that methyl methacrylate, used in dentistry, might be used to hold prosthetic components in place. The field of biomechanics really began to develop, however, when Charnley introduced the low-friction torque prosthesis for total hip replacement in 1962. Since then the principles of biomechanics have revolutionized orthopaedic surgery.

MUSCULOSKELETAL SYSTEM

Structures that make up the musculoskeletal system provide bony shape, support, and stability, protect vital organs, and enable parts and the body as a whole to move. The musculoskeletal system includes bones, cartilage, joints, ligaments, muscles, and tendons. The orthopaedic surgeon is concerned primarily with these structures in the upper and lower extremities, including the shoulder and hip joints, and the vertebral column.

Bones

The human skeleton (Figure 32-1) has 206 separate *bones,* including 32 in each upper extremity and 31 in each lower extremity. The cortex (outer layer) of bone is compact, dense, hard, and strong but slightly elastic connective tissue. This cortical osseous (from Latin *os,* meaning bone) tissue surrounds porous, spongy cancellous tissue. Bones are classified according to shape as long, short, flat, and irregular. The humerus in the upper arm, radius and ulna in the forearm, femur in the thigh, and tibia and fibula in the lower leg are long bones. The bones in the hand and foot are short bones. The scapula and patella are examples of flat bones. The vertebrae are irregular bones.

Periosteum, a strong fibrous membrane, covers bone, except at joints. The blood supply penetrates through periosteum and osseous tissue into cancellous tissue. Red bone marrow, found in porosities of cancellous bone, is vital to the production, maintenance, and disposal of blood cells. The center of the shaft of a long bone, the *medullary canal,* contains yellow fat bone marrow.

Cartilage

Cartilage, a smooth, relatively hard, compressible connective tissue, cushions most articular (joint) surfaces at the ends of bones. It does not have a direct blood supply. Rather articular cartilage derives its nutrition from synovial (lubricating) fluid.

Joints

Bones give stability, but the body must bend and flex for locomotion. The ends of bones come together at *joints.* The articular cartilage and construction of the joint prevent bones from scraping against each other. Tough, fibrous connective tissue forms the outside capsule of the joint. The synovial fluid contains macrophages and white blood cells that keep the joint free of debris and bacteria that could interfere with mobility. Joints are classified by variations in structure that permit movement (Figure 32-2). Hip and shoulder are ball-and-socket joints; knee, ankle, elbow, and phalangeal joints of fingers are hinged; the wrist is a condyloid joint; and the thumb is a saddle joint. The proximal and distal bone ends are held securely in place by the joint capsule attached to both bone shafts and by ligaments.

Ligaments

Ligaments are bands of flexible, tough fibrous tissue that join the articular surfaces of bones and cartilage. They become strong when the parallel configuration of their collagen fiber is oriented against the forces applied to them, for example, as the cruciate ligaments that stabilize the knee joint.

Muscles

The human body has hundreds of *muscles.* The fibers of muscles contract, causing movement of parts and organs of the body. Muscles are classified as smooth (involuntary) or striated (voluntary). Skeletal muscles are striated (see Figure 32-1). They have a rich vascular supply because muscles require oxygen to perform functions of locomotion. They contract when an eletrochemical impulse from the brain crosses the myoneural

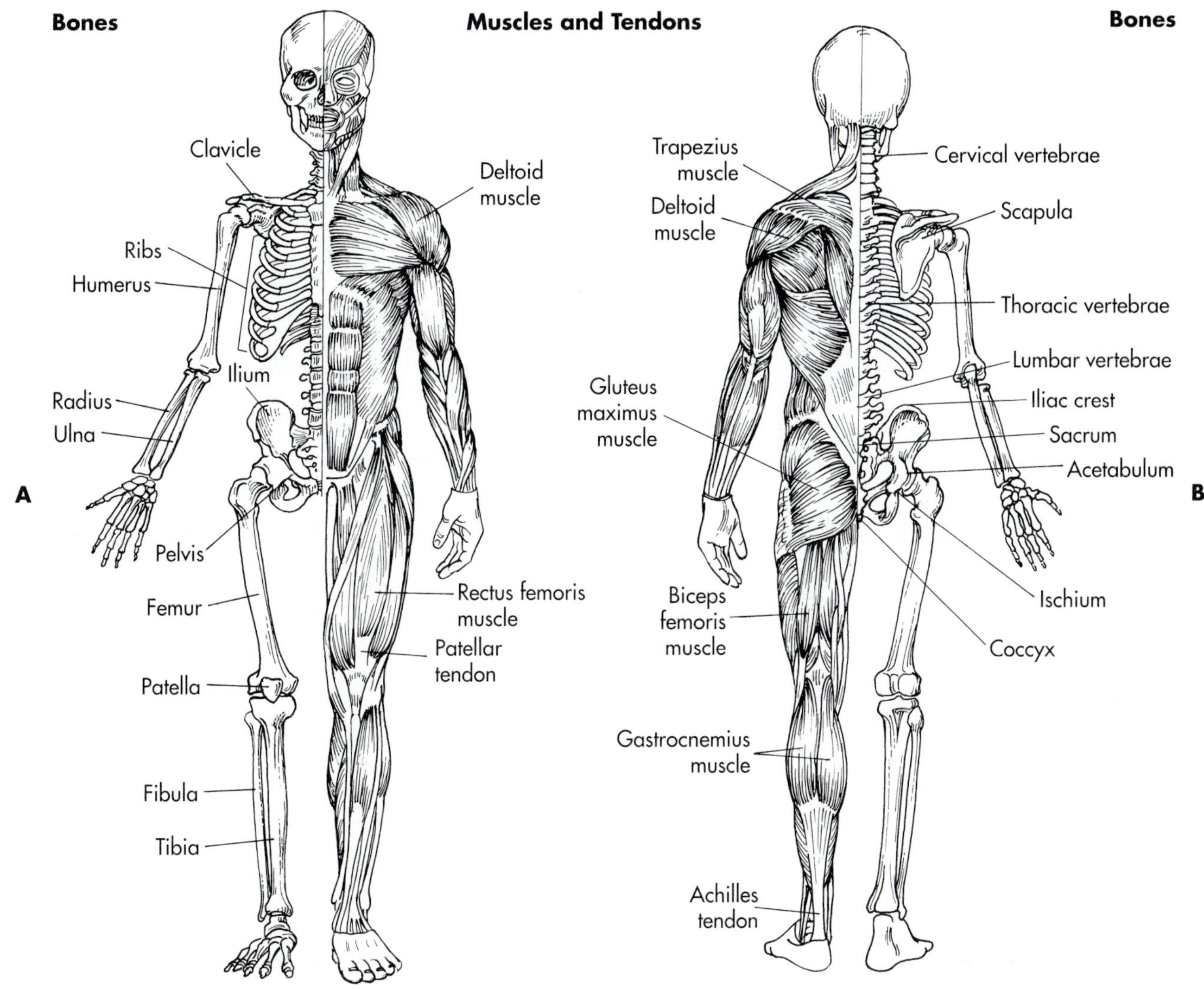

FIGURE 32-1 Musculoskeletal system. **A,** Anterior view. **B,** Posterior view.

junction, causing fibers to shorten. Groups of muscles work together (i.e., contract simultaneously to bring about body movement).

Tendons

Tendons are bands of extremely strong, flexible fibrous tissue that attach muscles to bones (see Figure 32-1). They are encased in the synovial membrane sheath of movable joints.

SPECIAL FEATURES OF ORTHOPAEDIC SURGERY

The orthopaedic surgeon, also referred to as an *orthopaedist* or *orthopod,* attempts to restore function of the musculoskeletal system lost as a result of injury or disease. Surgical procedures may be performed to repair traumatic injuries, such as fractures, dislocations, torn ligaments, or severed tendons. Other procedures reconstruct joints, eradicate a benign or malignant disease process, or correct postural disabilities. Procedures to correct congenital deformities are discussed in Chapter 42, pp. 860-861.

In addition to conventional x-rays, computed tomography (CT), magnetic resonance imaging (MRI), and bone densitometers allow evaluation of conditions amenable to surgical correction. Arthroscopy (see pp. 674-675) enhances diagnosis and treatment of joint disorders, especially those caused by sports injuries. Highly sophisticated implants and instrumentation make many orthopaedic procedures possible. However, a large percentage of the surgical procedures involve contaminated traumatic wounds or tissues highly susceptible to infection.

Osteomyelitis, infection in bone, typically occurs after bone is injured in an accident or is involved in a sur-

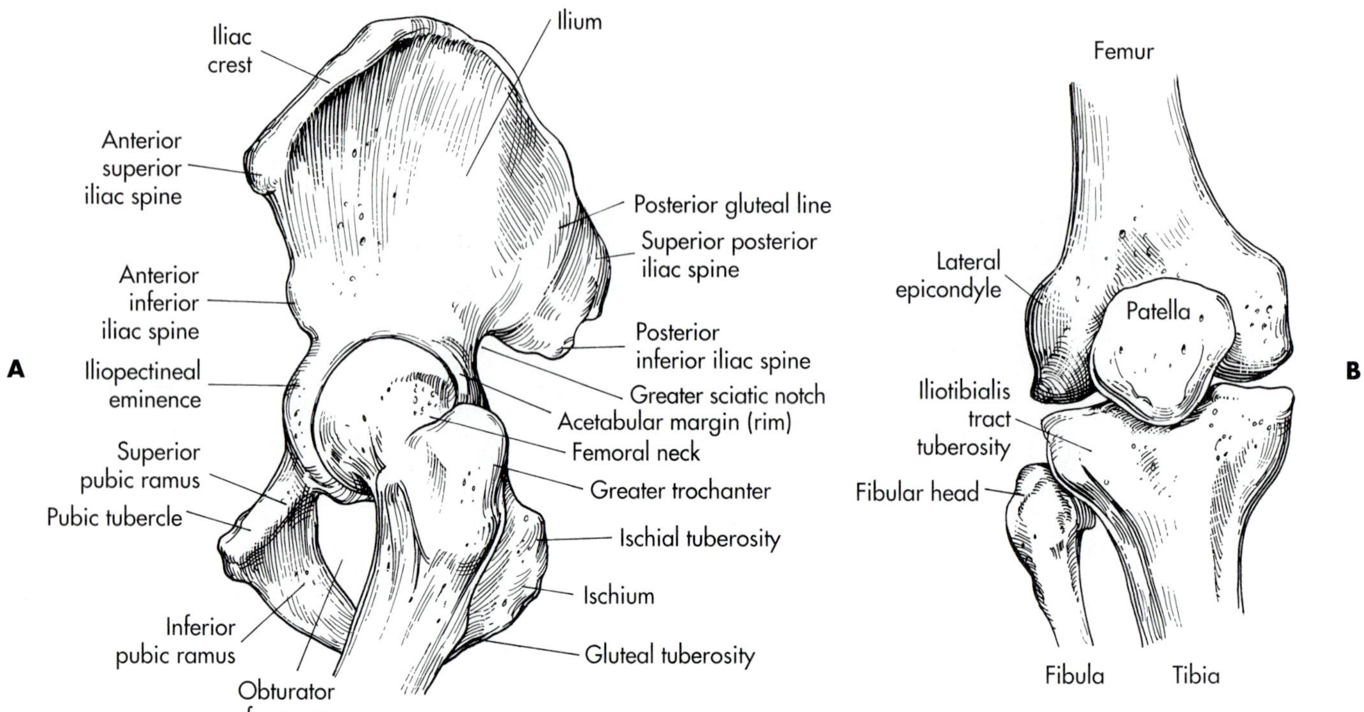

FIGURE 32-2 Joints. **A,** Ball-and-socket hip joint. **B,** Hinged knee joint.

gical repair. Microorganisms may harbor in a hematoma or in soft tissues and spread directly to bone. Acute osteomyelitis may cause nonunion of fractures. Chronic infection may remain for life; it may cause loss of an extremity. Posttraumatic, postoperative, and nosocomial wound infections are leading causes for amputation. Chronic osteomyelitis is often associated with peripheral vascular disease. Meticulous attention to sterile technique is critical in all orthopaedic procedures to prevent or at least minimize the devastating effects of infection. Sterility of implants and fixation devices is absolutely essential.

Precautions also must ensure protection for the orthopaedic surgeon and team, especially when caring for a trauma victim. Manipulation of sharp bony fragments and instrumentation can be hazardous. Transmission of hepatitis, human immunodeficiency virus (HIV), and other bloodborne pathogens are of particular concern to orthopaedists. In addition to universal precautions recommended by the Centers for Disease Control and Prevention (CDC) (see Chapter 12, pp. 198-199), the American Academy of Orthopaedic Surgeons recommends:

1. Wearing of protective attire
   a. Knee-high, waterproof shoe covers or boots. Blood and body fluids frequently get on the floor and lower legs. Shoe covers should be removed and changed if they become contaminated.
   b. Water-impervious gowns or waterproof apron under gown. Copious irrigation frequently is used.
   c. Double gloves at all times and/or additional protection for fingers. Cloth gloves or glove liners may be worn between latex gloves in cases of trauma and major reconstructive procedures when sharp instruments and mechanical devices are used.
   d. Full face shield when splatter is anticipated. Powered bone instruments can produce a fine mist. A space suit–type helmet (see p. 663 and Chapter 12, p. 197) should be considered when powered bone instruments are used.
2. Avoiding inadvertent penetration of skin of personnel during the surgical procedure
   a. Use instrument ties and other nontouch suturing and sharp instrument techniques whenever possible.
   b. Pass sharp instruments on tray or magnetic mat, not hand-to-hand.
   c. Announce when instruments are being passed.
   d. Cover exposed internal wires and pins that extend through the skin with appropriate tubing, cork stoppers, or plastic caps.
3. Clean gowning and gloving (i.e., the scrub person should change contaminated gloves before gowning and gloving another team member during the surgical procedure).

Instrumentation

Each orthopaedic procedure must have the correct instrumentation for *that* particular bone, joint, tendon, or other structures the orthopaedist will encounter. An instrument used on a hip procedure is not appropriate for a hand. Orthopaedic instruments are heavy, often large and bulky, resembling carpentry tools, but also delicate. Each instrument has a specific purpose and requires special care and handling. Orthopaedic instruments can be divided into categories by functional design.

Exposing Instruments

To expose a bone or joint, special retractors and elevators are used (Figure 32-3). Retractors are contoured to fit around the bone or joint without cutting or tearing muscles. Periosteal elevators are semisharp instruments used to strip periosteum from bone without destroying its ability to regenerate new bone.

Grasping Instruments

Grasping instruments are required to hold, manipulate, or retract bone. Bone-holding forceps should be selected appropriately for size of the bone in the surgical field. Bone hooks are used for retraction and leverage (Figure 32-4). Heavy clamps are needed to hold smaller bones or to grasp a joint capsule, such as a meniscus clamp for fibrocartilage in the knee.

Cutting Instruments

Cutting instruments are used to remove soft tissue around bone; to cut into, cut apart, or cut out portions of bone; and to smooth jagged edges of bone. The orthopaedist's armamentarium includes osteotomes, gouges, chisels, curettes, rongeurs, reamers, bone-cutting forceps, meniscitomes, rasps, files, drills, and saws (Figure 32-5). These have sharp edges. Take extra care not to nick or damage cutting edges; always protect them on

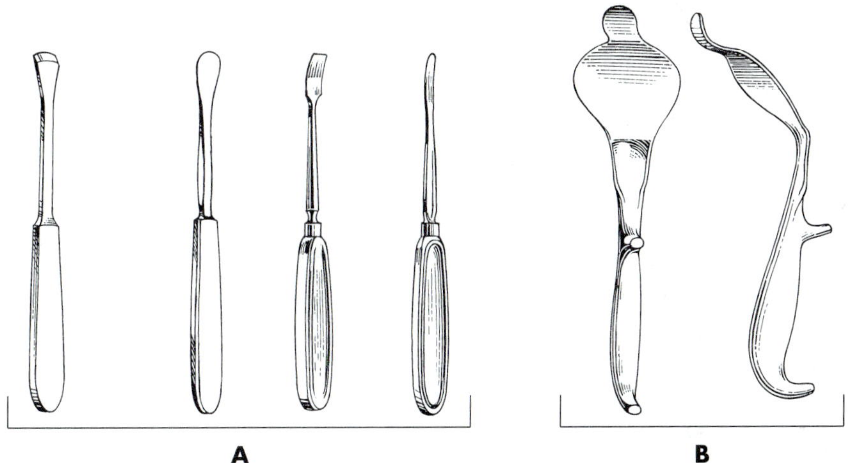

FIGURE 32-3 Exposing instruments. **A,** Periosteal elevators. **B,** Bennett retractor.

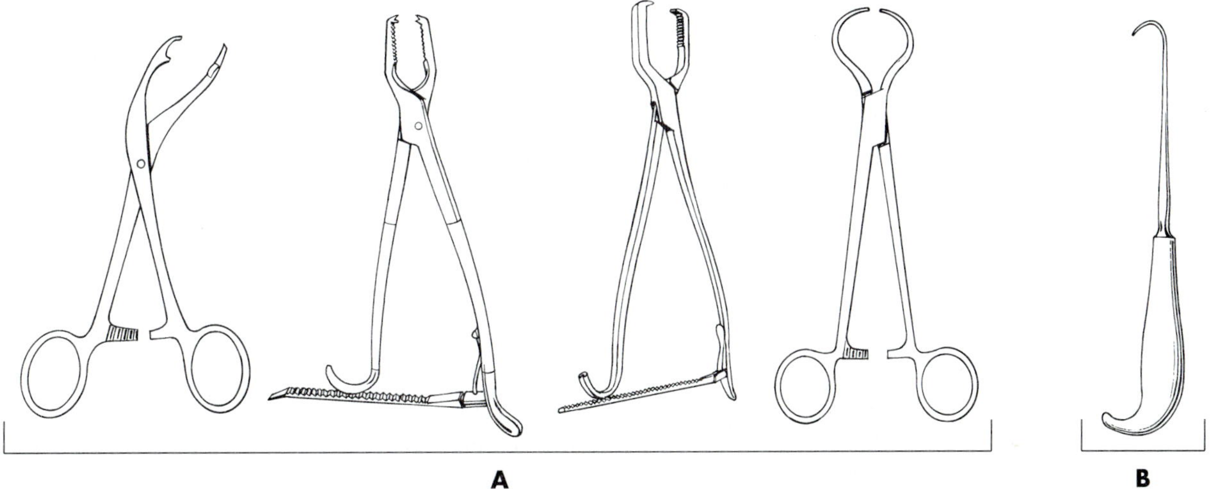

FIGURE 32-4 Grasping instruments. **A,** Bone-holding forceps. **B,** Bone hook.

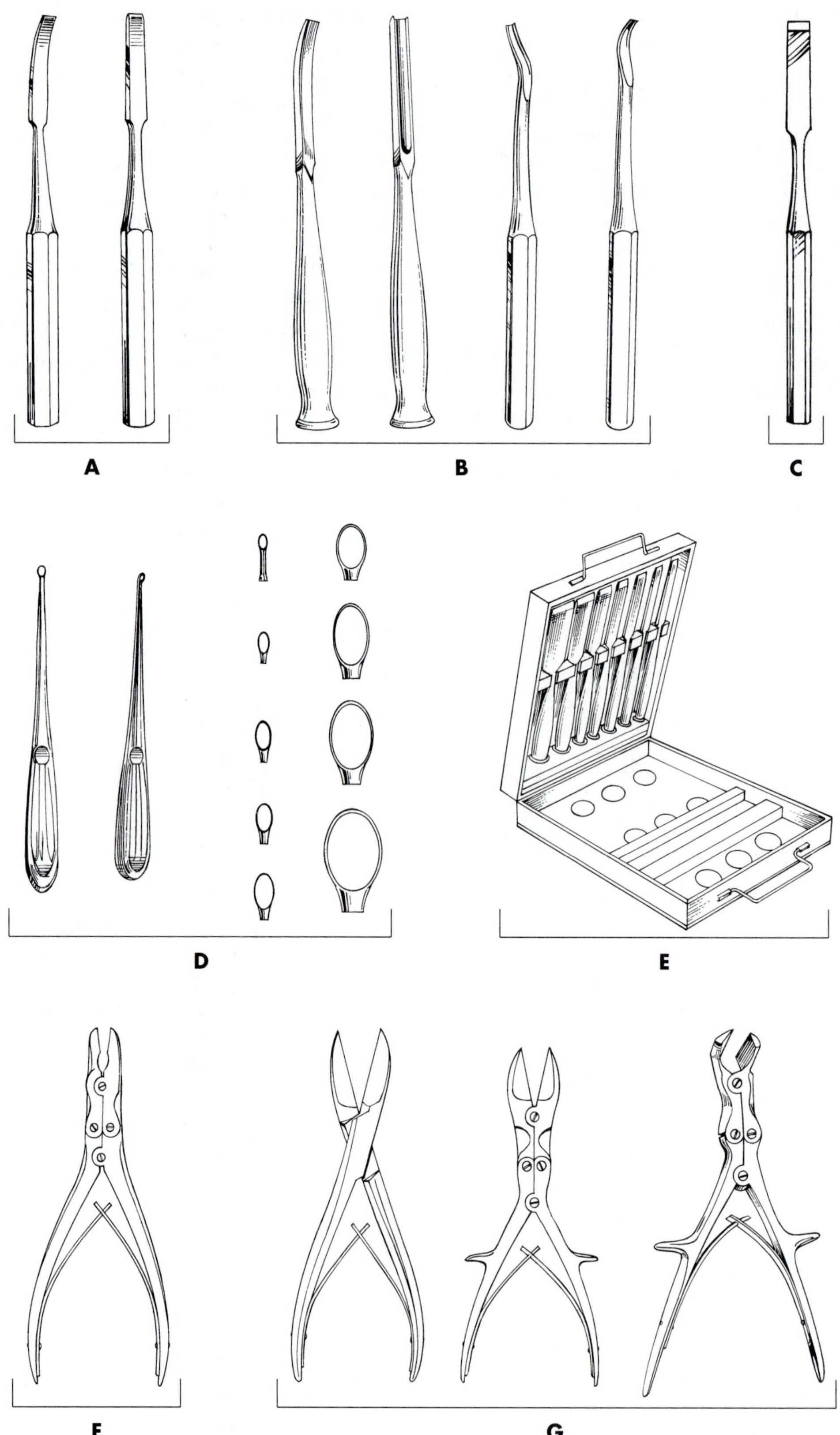

FIGURE 32-5 Cutting instruments. **A,** Osteotome, curved or straight tapered blade. **B,** Gouge, curved, straight, or angled tip. **C,** Chisel, straight blade. **D,** Curette, with assortment of sizes of cutting loops. **E,** Sterilizing case for set of osteotomes, gouges, chisels, or curettes. **F,** Rongeur. **G,** Bone cutter, straight or angled blade.

the instrument table and during cleaning, sterilizing, and storing. Fitted sterilizable racks (Figure 32-5, *E*), trays, foam towels, or canvas cases are used to keep sets together by sizes (e.g., osteotomes, gouges, chisels, and curettes), as well as to protect cutting edges.

NOTE Cutting instruments must be sharp. Osteotomes, chisels, gouges, and meniscitomes can be sharpened by operating room (OR) personnel with hand-held hones or a honing machine designed for this purpose. Most manufacturers provide a service for sharpening and repairing instruments. Curettes, rongeurs, and reamers should be returned for sharpening. Small drill bits and saw blades usually are discarded when dulled.

Power-Driven Cutting Instruments Instruments powered by electricity or compressed air or nitrogen offer precision in drilling, cutting, shaping, and beveling bone. The instrument may have rotary, reciprocating, or oscillating action. Rotary movement is used to drill holes or to insert screws, wires, or pins. Reciprocating movement, a cutting action from front to back, and oscillating cutting action from side to side are used to cut or remove bone. Some instruments have a combination of movements and can be changed from one to another with hand controls. In some the change may be made by adjusting the chuck forward or backward and locking it into desired position. Powered instruments increase speed and decrease fatigue of manually driven drills, saws, and reamers. They also reduce blood loss from bone by packing tiny particles into cut surfaces. They are not used without some inherent dangers, however. See Chapter 14, pp. 261-263, for complete discussion of powered instruments.

Implant-Related Instruments

Drivers, clamps, and retractors are used for inserting, securing, or removing fixation and prosthetic implants. Each type of implant requires its own instrumentation. Instruments used for insertion or extraction of metallic implants must be of the same metal as the implant to prevent galvanic reaction.

Items Used Frequently

The items to be discussed are handled frequently, although they are not used in every orthopaedic procedure.

Bone Grafts

When necessary to provide structural support, a piece of bone from one part of the skeletal system may be obtained from the patient to reinforce another part of the skeletal system. Autogenous cancellous and cortical bone is obtained from the crest of ilium and cortical bone from tibia. Free vascularized fibular grafts may be preferred to replace avascular (dead) bone or large segments of long bones following trauma or tumor resection. Autogenous bone may not have adequate shape or strength or may not be available in sufficient quantity, or the orthopaedist may deem it undesirable to subject patient to a secondary incision or added operating time. Homogenous bone (an allograft), a heterologous bone implant of coraline hydroxyapatite, or a bone graft substitute of tricalcium may be used. (See discussion of bone grafts in Chapter 24, pp. 510-511.) Donors, both living and cadaver, should be tested for HIV antibody before a bone allograft is transplanted. Living donors should be retested 90 days after procurement if possible. Persons who are HIV-positive, have any immune disorder or active infection, and have a history of hepatitis are excluded as donors. The probability of transmission of HIV in frozen or freeze-dried bone is remote. Secondary sterilization by ethylene oxide or ionizing radiation may increase the margin of safety but will reduce the biologic effectiveness of the graft.

Soft Tissue Allografts

Cartilage, ligaments, and tendons obtained from cadavers may be frozen or freeze-dried for use to augment soft tissue repairs.

Fixation Devices

External and internal fixation devices are used to stabilize or immobilize bone, usually following skeletal injury. External devices provide temporary support during healing (see pp. 666-667). Many types of screws, plates, and nails are used for temporary or permanent internal fixation of fractures or bone segments following a reconstructive procedure (see pp. 667-669). Devices also are used to stabilize the vertebral column (see p. 679).

Prosthetic Implants

Prosthetic implants are used to permanently replace bone, joints, or tendons. They are made of nonmagnetic and electrolytically inert metals such as stainless steel, cobalt, and titanium alloys or of polymers such as silicone and polyethylene. Some modular implants are made of several materials. Others have a polymeric or porous coating for tissue ingrowth over a portion of the implant (see total joint replacement, p. 671). Methyl methacrylate, bone cement, may be used to reinforce fixation or to increase strength of implant (see pp. 671-672 and Chapter 24, pp. 507-508). An orthopaedic implant must withstand stresses within the internal environment. Fatigue strength, corrosion resistance, biocompatibility, and biomechanics are critical factors in selecting an implant.

Because of the high cost of implants and fixation devices, the inventory is kept as low as possible, yet large enough to ensure availability when needed. These expensive implants are usually patient-charge items; they cannot be reused even if temporarily implanted. After measurements are taken, an implant of the correct size, shape, and design is selected from the sets available. Only the one to be used is handled, without the others being touched.

An infection around a fixation or prosthetic implant may require its removal, often resulting in permanent deformity or disability. Sterility at the time of implantation is imperative. Some implants are supplied sterile by the manufacturer. Others must be packaged and sterilized. Manufacturers may provide instructions for the recommended method of sterilization. Aeration time may be recommended following ethylene oxide sterilization. Reprocessing is appropriate only if an implant has not been implanted or contaminated by blood or body fluids. *Implants should not be flash sterilized;* that is, do not steam sterilize at a high temperature for a short time (see Chapter 13, p. 214). Only standard cycles should be used. Some implants cannot withstand the heat of steam sterilization; ethylene oxide must be used. Follow the manufacturer's recommendations. Each sterilization cycle containing an implant(s) should be biologically tested and the implant(s) not used until a negative test result is known.

Implants made of or coated with polymers should be wrapped in an appropriate plastic or combination paper and plastic wrapper to prevent contamination with lint or other debris. Do not remove a metal implant from a package with an instrument. The surface could be scratched. An implant with a scratched or dented surface cannot be used because an electrolytic reaction will occur in the body. Powder-free gloves should be worn by team members who handle prosthetic implants. (See the discussion of synthetic materials in Chapter 24, pp. 512-513.)

Specifics about the device or prosthesis implanted must be recorded in the patient's intraoperative record. This includes the type, size, and other identifying information such as manufacturer's lot number.

Lasers

Although not used as commonly as in other surgical specialties, lasers are used in some orthopaedic procedures. They are useful in confined areas, as through an arthroscope, to minimize bleeding. Lasers are described in detail in Chapter 15, pp. 270-279.

Carbon Dioxide Laser Methyl methacrylate can be vaporized with a carbon dioxide (CO_2) laser to remove a cemented joint implant during a revision arthroplasty. The CO_2 laser cannot be used in a fluid environment. A joint must be insufflated with gas; the distention medium is carbon dioxide. The vaporization of cellular water destroys soft tissue. The CO_2 laser is useful in arthroscopic surgery for sculpturing articular cartilage and for synovectomy. The joint must be irrigated to remove charred tissue.

Holmium:YAG Laser Used primarily in the knee, ankle, shoulder, and elbow, the Ho:YAG laser is approved for all joints except the spine. The 2.1 μm wavelength with low penetration depth combined with pulsed high energy is delivered through a fine fiberoptic fiber. The Ho:YAG laser acts on water in cell without charring or damaging tissue extensively. It can ablate dense cartilage, bone, and soft tissue. It is used through an arthroscope to cut, shape, smooth, and sculpt cartilage and tissues in joints.

Neodymium:YAG Laser The Nd:YAG laser is used primarily in arthroscopy of the knee and shoulder joints on articular cartilage. It vaporizes protein and bonds collagen. It can be used for percutaneous disk procedures. Delivered fiberoptically, the Nd:YAG laser may have a reusable sapphire tip or a disposable, single-use ceramic contact tip. The Nd:YAG beam may be passed through a potassium-titanyl-phosphate (KTP) crystal, which has good cutting properties, to vaporize protein.

Bone Wax

Used for hemostasis in bone (see Chapter 23, p. 477), bone wax is placed on the instrument table and opened as requested. Check the orthopaedist's preference card before opening the packet.

Nerve Stimulator

A nerve stimulator is used occasionally to verify neural tissue during a partial nerve resection to control spastic muscles. When the popliteal nerve, for example, is given a slight shock with the nerve stimulator, the foot jerks. Both direct electric current and disposable battery-operated stimulators are available.

Sutures

Ligaments, tendons, periosteum, and joint capsules are fibrous tissues. They are primarily tough, stringy collagen and contain few cells and blood vessels. As a result, they heal more slowly than do vascular tissues. Nonabsorbable materials are generally used to suture ligaments, tendons, and muscles involved in movement of the bony skeleton. Absorbable suture is generally preferred to suture periosteum. Check the surgeon's preference card before opening suture packets.

Casts and Braces

A cast or brace is a means of obtaining external fixation of a fracture or a part following tendon repair, arthrodesis, or other type of surgical procedure. It is the means of putting a part at rest or attempting to correct an injury or abnormality. Cast application in the OR is discussed in detail later in this chapter (see pp. 679-682).

Cast Room Casts are applied in the cast room, sometimes referred to as the *plaster room.* Many closed, noninvasive procedures are performed here, particularly those requiring general or regional anesthesia, when a cast room is located within the OR suite. This frees the OR for open, invasive surgical procedures. It also keeps plaster dust from the individual ORs, an important aspect of aseptic environmental control. Following an open surgical procedure, the patient can be wheeled on the operating table into the cast room for application of a cast, if the patient is not endangered.

Ultraclean Air System

Special care must be used to carry out strict asepsis. Infection is the most serious, dreaded, and costly complication of orthopaedic surgery. Therefore many orthopaedists prefer to operate within an ultraclean air system, especially for total joint replacement procedures. Laminar airflow, as described in Chapter 12, pp. 196-197, is used more frequently by orthopaedic surgeons than by other surgical specialists.

A surgical isolation bubble system or patient isolation drape may be used to isolate the sterile field from personnel and equipment (see discussion of plastic isolator in Chapter 22, p. 467). Surgical helmets are available that isolate airborne contaminants from each team member. Hoses exhaust air. This system can be used independently or in conjunction with a laminar airflow system.

Isolation suits are fully contained gowns with acrylic plastic face shields and a battery-powered air filtration system. Because the suits retain heat, the OR may be kept at 70° F (21° C) for the comfort of team members. The patient should be placed on a hyperthermia mattress to prevent hypothermia.

Orthopaedic Table

An orthopaedic table, often referred to as the *fracture table*, is used for many surgical procedures requiring traction, image intensification or conventional x-ray control, and/or cast application. The many available attachments make possible any desired position and traction on any part of the body. The table can be raised, tilted laterally, or put into Trendelenburg's or reverse Trendelenburg's position. Attachments are designed not only for stabilizing the patient in the desired position but also for exerting traction to help reduce a fracture, and for providing a means of evaluating diagnosis or therapy by radiologic control. Bakelite or other material that does not interfere with radiographic studies is used for attachments that might otherwise obscure the findings.

Essential standard component attachments on all models of orthopaedic tables include three-section patient body supports, lateral body brace, sacral rest, and traction apparatus. Optional accessories are available to accommodate the types of procedures performed and the model of the table. When the orthopaedic table will be used:

1. Consult the surgeon's preference card, procedure book, and manufacturer's manual for attachments needed for each desired position.
2. Check the patient's height and weight.
3. Assemble the necessary attachments. Pad all parts of the table and attachments to prevent pressure on joints, sacrum, and perineum.
4. Attach the standard components and accessories to the table frame so that all is in readiness for positioning the patient when the orthopaedist arrives. The patient may be anesthetized before positioning is completed.

X-Ray Control

Conventional x-ray equipment and image intensifiers frequently are used during orthopaedic procedures. Considerations for patient safety and personnel protection described in Chapter 10 apply to the use of radiologic control for invasive or noninvasive orthopaedic procedures performed in the OR suite. Special positioning and draping techniques may be necessary, especially when a C-arm image intensifier is used.

Often both anteroposterior (AP) and lateral views are necessary to assess the alignment of a bone or to determine the position of a fixation device or prosthetic implant. X-ray films or recorded fluoroscopic images document the work of the orthopaedist.

Special Considerations

1. Although unit beds and wheeled equipment should not enter the OR suite, in the interest of the patient's comfort and safety this rule is relaxed for some orthopaedic patients, such as patients in traction apparatus. Beds, frames, and stretchers can be decontaminated in the vestibular/exchange area.
2. A cast should be removed preoperatively in the cast room. If the OR suite does not have a cast room, a cast may be bivalved in the patient's room and then removed in the OR. Cover sterile tables with a large sterile sheet while the cast is being completely removed to prevent airborne contamination from plaster dust.
3. Positioning on the orthopaedic table for some surgical procedures requires an extra amount of activity. When possible, position these patients in the cast room before transporting them into the OR, thereby avoiding dispersal of lint and microorganisms into the air that could settle on sterile tables.
4. Positioning of the patient intraoperatively and postoperatively should be directed by the surgeon. *Immobilization* and good body alignment contribute to patient comfort. Pillows or other supports should not cause pain, impair function of unaffected muscles and joints, or compromise circulation.
5. Transcutaneous electric nerve stimulator (TENS) may be used for postoperative analgesia. The electrode pads are affixed to the skin along sides of the incision when dressing is applied. Before application, skin should be cleansed with water. (Saline is a conduc-

tor, so it cannot be used for cleansing.) The wires are connected to the stimulator in the postanesthesia care unit (PACU) or after recovery from anesthesia. The patient can be taught preoperatively how to use the TENS for relief of pain postoperatively.

6. Electrostimulation promotes cellular responses in bone and ligaments. Mechanically stressed bone generates electric potentials related to patterns of bone regeneration. If stimulated, healing may accelerate. Both internal direct-current stimulators and external pulsating electromagnetic field or electrical capacitor devices are used to stimulate bone and neural regeneration, revascularization, epiphyseal growth, and ligamental maturation.

EXTREMITIES

Although instrumentation varies by procedure and the size of structures involved, basic techniques apply to handling both upper and lower extremities.

General Considerations

1. A sterile irrigating pan is placed under an extremity to catch solution if an open wound is to be cleansed, irrigated, and debrided, as for compound fracture (see Chapter 22, pp. 453-454).
2. A pneumatic tourniquet is usually used for a surgical procedure on or below the elbow or knee to provide a blood-free field. The tourniquet cuff is applied before the extremity is prepped. However, *it is not inflated until draping is completed.* Always check the pressure setting with the surgeon before inflating a tourniquet. Ischemia time is a critical factor in patient safety. Notify the orthopaedist of the time lapse after the first hour and every 15 minutes thereafter throughout tourniquet inflation. (See discussion of tourniquets in Chapter 23, pp. 474-476.) Document tourniquet time.

   An Esmarch's bandage may be applied before the pneumatic tourniquet is inflated to force blood from the extremity.
3. An extremity is always held up for skin preparation. See that the area under it is dry before draping (see Chapter 22). Prevent prep solution from running under the tourniquet cuff.
4. A self-adhering incise drape may be used as the first drape applied. It may be impossible to drape adequately with self-adhering plastic drapes or fenestrated sheets. If the extremity must be manipulated during the surgical procedure, the entire circumference must be draped. A limb or split sheet may be used.
5. Stockinette may be used over a self-adhering plastic drape or to cover skin. This is cut with dressing scissors over the line of the incision. The cut edges may be secured over skin edges with skin clips if a plastic drape is not used. A medicine cup is a handy receptacle for these clips after removal. The scrub person holds this at the field to receive clips as the orthopaedist removes them. They must be counted.

   A self-adhering incise drape eliminates the need for either stockinette and metallic skin clips or towels and towel clips that might interfere with the interpretation of x-ray films or image intensification.
6. A fluid-control drape collects blood and irrigating fluids in a pouch to prevent strike-through of and runoff from drapes. Fluids can be drained or suctioned for disposal. Blood may be suctioned for autotransfusion if blood loss is more than 400 ml, as in some hip procedures.
7. After a surgical procedure on a knee joint, a pressure dressing is usually applied to prevent serum accumulation. This may be a Robert Jones dressing, which includes a soft cotton batting roll, sheet wadding, and cotton elastic bandage. A cotton roll, or other bulky material, may be placed on each side of the knee and held in place with sheet wadding. A four-ply, crinkled-gauze bandage or cotton elastic bandage over this provides even, gentle pressure. Depending on the surgical procedure, a plaster splint or other type of knee immobilizer may be preferred.
8. After a surgical procedure on a shoulder, the arm may be bound against the side of the chest for immobilization. An absorbent pad or a large piece of cotton or sheet wadding is placed under the arm to keep skin surfaces from touching because they may macerate. The arm is held in a shoulder immobilizer that supports the humerus and wrist, or it may be bound firmly to the side of the chest with a cotton elastic bandage.
9. An extremity is elevated on a pillow placed lengthwise. This facilitates venous return, decreases swelling, and minimizes pressure on nerves. The hand should be elevated above level of the heart; the toes must be higher than the nose.

Types of Procedures

Preoperative assessment of an acute or a chronic disability affecting the musculoskeletal system of an extremity includes evaluation of the extent of bony or soft tissue involvement with or without concomitant neurovascular compromise. Assessment for signs and symptoms of neurovascular impairment in an extremity includes the 6 *p*'s: *p*allor, *p*ulses, *p*ain, *p*arasthesia, *p*uffiness, and *p*aralysis.

Because they are the essence of adult orthopaedic surgery and are caused either by trauma or by a degenerative disease process, procedures on the following major anatomic classifications of structures will be discussed:

1. Fracture of bones
2. Reconstruction of joints
3. Repair of tendons and ligaments

FRACTURES

Intact bones are essential to the stability and mobility of upper and lower extremities. A comminuted (splintered) or fractured (broken) bone can cause malfunction and pain. Fractures vary by cause, location, and type of fracture line and extent of injury.

1. *Traumatic.* The impact, forced twisting, or bending of an accidental injury can break one or more bones in the body. Traumatic fractures can occur when bone has become fatigued from overwork or has inadequate muscle support during exertion; a *stress fracture* may result as in the tibia or fibula of an athlete. Traumatic fractures are either closed or open.
   a. *Closed fracture.* Sometimes referred to as a *simple fracture,* broken fragments do not protrude through adjacent tissue to puncture the skin (Figure 32-6, *A*).
   b. *Open fracture.* Also referred to as a *compound fracture,* either the proximal or distal end of bone, or both, protrudes from the fracture site through adjacent tissues and skin (Figure 32-6, *B*). Because of the risk of infection developing in the exposed bone, an open fracture is a surgical emergency.
2. *Pathologic.* Demineralization of bone as from osteoporosis or the aging process and primary or metastatic malignant bone disease can spontaneously fracture a bone without undue stress. Although technically simple fractures, pathologic fractures may require more than simple fixation of bone fragments. Bone allografts or heterografts may be needed. Methyl methacrylate bone cement may be used to increase the strength of a fixation implant or as an adjunct to fill a bone defect as following removal of a tumor around a pathologic fracture. A compound made from collagen protein mixed with ceramic material may serve to stimulate creation of cartilage and osteoblasts, bone-forming cells.

A fracture heals in stages by a slow process of *osteogenesis,* the formation of bone. Healing begins with a hematoma, the blood clot that serves as a fibrin network for subsequent cellular invasion. Cells proliferate from the fracture site into fibrin to form a *callus,* a deposit of fibrous connective tissue and cartilage. Formation of a callus is dependent on the periosteum and an adequate blood supply in surrounding tissues. Periosteum, which heals fairly rapidly, contributes to the vascular network of the callus. *Osteoblasts* form a matrix of collagen that enters the callus. Known as the *osteoid,* this matrix calcifies to bridge the fracture site and thus unite the bone. Throughout life, osteoblasts build new osteocytes, bone cells, while osteoclasts tear down or remodel bone structures. This process allows osteoblasts to rebuild new bone. The process slows with age, especially in menopausal women whose calcium level is decreased. Therefore healing time depends partially on age of patient, but it also depends on extent of injury to surrounding tissues, blood supply to bone, amount of displacement and bone loss, and method of realignment.

Mechanical means are used to reduce a fracture and immobilize the parts, maintaining the fragments in proper alignment. Fractures must be handled gently with support above and below the site to prevent further trauma. A physician assumes responsibility for sup-

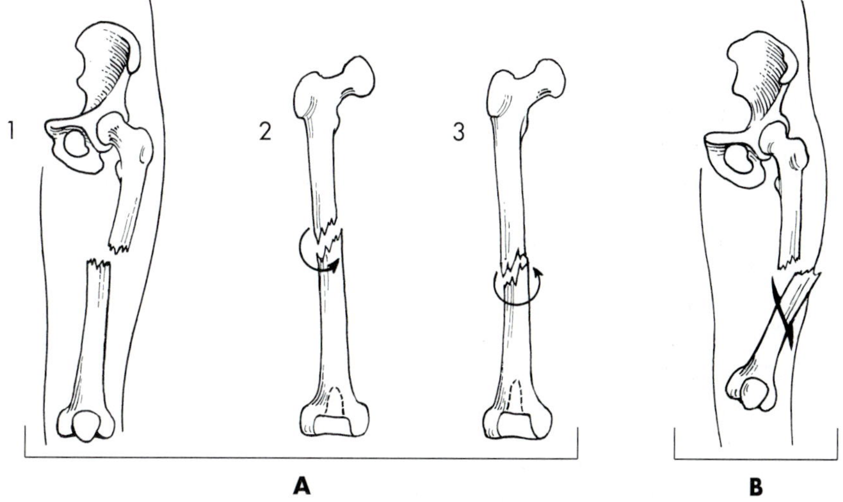

FIGURE 32-6 Fractures of a long bone. **A,** Simple closed fractures: *1,* transverse break runs across bone; *2,* oblique break runs in slanting direction across bone; *3,* spiral break coils around bone. **B,** Compound open fracture protrudes through skin.

porting the fracture site during transfer of patient to or from a stretcher, bed, or table. Other personnel must be instructed regarding the special care needed to move a patient. The orthopaedist removes or directs removal of temporary splints, traction, or pneumatic counterpressure device (see Chapter 23, pp. 473-474). Adequate personnel must be available so that the patient can be lifted gently. All lifters should be on the affected side because this helps support the fracture during transfer.

In treating a fracture, the orthopaedist seeks to accomplish a solid union of bone in perfect alignment, to return joints and muscles to normal position, to prevent or repair vascular trauma, and to rehabilitate the patient as early as possible. Treatment of fractures usually includes three distinct phases: reduction, immobilization, and rehabilitation. The methods of treating fractures include:

1. Closed reduction with immobilization
2. Skeletal traction
3. External fixation
4. Internal fixation
5. Electrostimulation (see p. 664)

Closed Reduction

A fracture may be manipulated (set) to replace the bone in its proper alignment without opening the skin. This technique is referred to as a *closed reduction*. Many fractures of the lower leg or arm can be treated by closed reduction. When both leg bones are fractured, fibula fractures are generally disregarded and attention is directed to the tibia.

Often performed in the emergency department, the patient may come to the cast room in the OR suite for closed reduction under anesthesia and application of a device for immobilization. A plaster, fiberglass, or other lightweight synthetic cast (see pp. 679-682), cast-brace, or molded plastic fracture-brace may be used to hold the reduced fracture site in alignment during union.

Skeletal Traction

Traction is the pulling force exerted to maintain proper alignment or position. In skeletal traction, the force is applied directly on the bone following insertion of pins, wires, or tongs placed through or into the bone. A small sterile setup is required. Traction is applied by means of pulleys and weights. Weights provide a constant force; pulleys help establish and maintain constant direction until the fractured bone reunites.

Forearm or Lower Leg

A Kirschner wire, either plain or threaded, or a Steinmann pin is drilled through the bone (preferably cortical) distal to the fracture site. For forearm fractures the wire or pin must be strong enough to prevent side-to-side, angular, and rotary motion while the fracture is healing. A traction bow is attached to the protruding ends of the wire or pin. The pulleys are fastened to this bow. The ends of the wire or pin are covered with corks or plastic tips to protect the patient and personnel from the sharp ends.

Finger

A fine Kirschner wire may be drilled through the distal phalanx. The ends may be attached to a banjo splint. Or a cast may be applied to the forearm with a loop of heavy wire incorporated in it that fans out beyond the fingers. The Kirschner wire is fastened to this loop by a rubber band.

External Fixation

External fixation devices are used for the treatment of selected types of skeletal injuries, especially to the pelvis and extremities, with marked soft tissue loss and instability. Skeletal pins and connecting bars permit rigid fixation, but with access to devitalized skin and soft tissue for wound management, especially for open injuries of tibia. Fixation devices used for unstable pelvic fractures allow early ambulation. Controlled fracture motion is not detrimental and may provoke an external callus response at the fracture site.

Femur and Tibia

External fixation applies tension and compression forces to bone. Tension stimulates bone growth. Compression helps control infection and promotes union in fractures without bone loss. External fixators can also be used for correcting bone deformities and for lengthening the femur and tibia following osteotomy for limb-length discrepancy (see Chapter 42, p. 860). Several types of devices, used on lower extremities, allow the patient to ambulate.

Stabilization Bar Two or more pins or screws, parallel to each other, are inserted into the cortex of each fragmented section of bone. These may be connected to a metal bar, such as the dynamic axial fixator, that runs parallel to the bone on one side of the leg, or the pins may protrude through the leg and be clamped onto bars on both sides, such as a Hoffman external fixation system.

Ilizarov Technique Particularly useful for salvaging infected and nonunion fractures, the Ilizarov external fixator frame consists of a series of stainless steel rings connected by rods, nuts, and bolts. It can be assembled in various configurations and lengths. Wires are inserted percutaneously through the bone and connected under tension on both sides of the rings. Usually two wires are attached to each ring, at the proximal and distal levels, to stabilize bone fragments. The placement of wires is checked under C-arm fluoroscopy. Threaded rods are placed parallel to each other and in line with the longitudinal axis of the bone to connect and stabilize rings. The system has more than 120 interchangeable components, including wrenches, pliers, and wire cutters. Wire insertion is a sterile procedure. The frame is assembled on the sterile field. It weighs about 8 lb (3.6 kg) when assembled.

Internal Fixation

Internal fixation is necessary for fractures that are not amenable to closed reduction and stabilization with cast or brace immobilization, skeletal traction, or external fixation methods. The fracture must be reduced to align fragments. *Open reduction* exposes the fracture site for realignment under direct visualization; closed reduction sometimes precedes the insertion of an internal fixation device. If vascular structures have been traumatized, internal fixation followed by vascular repair may be necessary to restore arterial tissue perfusion and adequate venous drainage. The procedure may be performed under regional block anesthesia, especially in patients in poor physical condition such as an aged person or a patient who has suffered multiple trauma. Intravenous (IV) sedation may be given to dull the patient's awareness of the sound of drills and mallets.

Excellent results can be obtained with internal fixation of a fracture soon after it occurs. This method provides firm immobilization and close approximation of the fragments so that the gap between the ends is not too great for the callus to bridge. It reduces to a minimum space between fragments and movement at the fracture site. Healing seems to take place faster. The patient starts nonweight-bearing exercises and progresses to ambulation early, which reduces joint stiffness and muscle atrophy and prevents a long period of rehabilitation.

Screws, Plates, and Nails

Many types of rigid fixation implants are available. The orthopaedist chooses the type best suited to serve its purpose. The implant may remain permanently, or it may be removed after the fracture has healed, especially in a young person. For example, a plate can cause a stress fracture from the shielding forces exerted over time along its rigid edges on the less rigid underlying bone. If osteomyelitis develops, an implant must be removed.

Screws, plates, nails, rods, and pins are made of stainless steel 316L, titanium or cobalt alloys. These metals are nonmagnetic and electrolytically inert. Only one kind of metal is used in a patient. The instrumentation used to implant it must be of the same metal. Semirigid carbon-fiber–reinforced plastic plates are also used in some situations. Biodegradable screws and rods provide stability during osteogenesis. An implant may be affixed to cortex of the bone or inserted into the bone through the fracture site. The type and size of implant(s) must be documented in the patient's record.

Screws Screws alone may be used for fixation of an oblique or spiral fracture of a long bone. Screws must be long enough to penetrate both cortices. Hard cortical bone gives the best fixation and two cortices generally hold better than one. Screws are available in various lengths and diameters. Not all screws have the same type head, for example, single slot, cross slot, concave cross slot, hexagon, and Phillips head (Figure 32-7). The correct screwdriver must be used with each type screw.

Compression Plate and Screws Many fractures requiring open reduction are rigidly fixed through the compression method. Compression plates are heavy and strong. They are held in place by specially designed cortical lag screws. The threads of these screws are deeper than are those on other types of screws and are farther apart, which allows a larger amount of bone between the threads. This construction gives maximum holding power and rigid fixation. A compression instrument may be used. It is connected to the end of the plate and then fastened to the bone with a short screw. When the nut on the compression instrument is tightened, the bone fragments are brought tightly together. The remaining screws are put into the plate and the fracture is fixed. Screws alone are used only in selected situations. A cast may or may not be applied.

Following open reduction of an acetabular fracture, a compression plate may be bent to conform to the con-

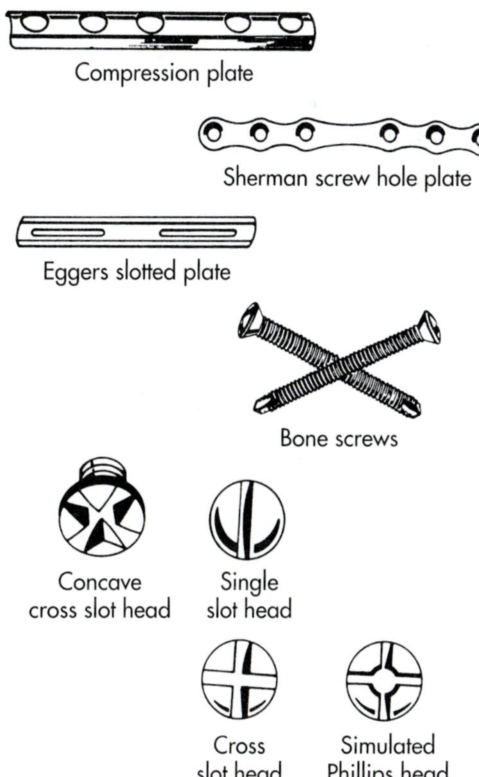

FIGURE 32-7 Fixation plates and screws. (Reproduced by permission of Ethicon, Inc.)

tour of the acetabulum and secured with long cortical and cancellous lag screws.

Eggers Plate and Screws The plate is slotted, which permits the muscle tone of the extremity to keep the ends of the fragments pressed closely together. The pressure stimulates osteogenesis.

Sherman Plate and Screws The appropriate sized plate is fitted to the contour of the bone, by bending slightly if necessary, before applying the screws. With a drill guide, holes for the screws are drilled with an electric or air-powered drill in the center of the screw hole and perpendicularly to the plate. The drill bit should be slightly smaller than the screws. The screws should pass through both cortices of the bone.

Nails An intertrochanteric or subtrochanteric fracture of the neck of the femur may be treated by inserting a nail, compression screw, or multiple pins through the neck into the head of the femur. Many different types of nails are used. They are usually inserted over or alongside a guidewire. The nail may form a continuous angulated unit with a plate that fits on the outer lateral cortex of the femur, or the plate may be attached and the nail, screws, or pins inserted separately. Screws secure the plate to the shaft of the femur before or after the nail is inserted, depending on the design of the implant. Some of the more commonly used implants are:

1. Smith-Petersen cannulated nail with a McLaughlin adjustable plate
2. Jewett cannulated nail and plate unit (a Jewett overlay plate may be used with this implant)
3. Neufeld nail and plate unit
4. Deyerle plate and multiple pins
5. Lag screw with compression tube and plate (Figure 32-8)

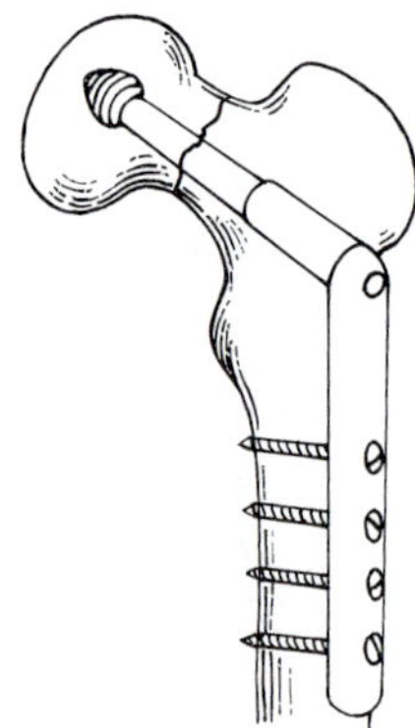

FIGURE 32-8 Compression hip screw for fixation of fracture of femoral neck.

6. Massie sliding nail and tube assembly
7. Ken sliding nail
8. I-Beam (Sarmenito) nail

The patient is usually positioned on the orthopaedic table. The orthopaedist and assistants assume responsibility for moving and positioning the patient. Figure 32-9 shows the position for nailing the left hip. If portable x-ray machines are used, one is on the unaffected side for an AP view, and one is at foot of table for a lateral view. Film for AP view is placed on cassette holder from the unaffected side. The procedure may be performed with fluoroscopic image intensification with C-arm rather than conventional x-ray machines. All sterile tables are positioned on the affected side. The orthopaedist may sit to operate.

Intramedullary Nailing

An intramedullary nail, rod, or pin is driven into the medullary canal through the site of the fracture. This brings the ends together for union, splints fracture, and eases pain. It permits early return of function so that the patient can be ambulatory. Intramedullary implants also provide a method of holding fragments in alignment in comminuted fractures. Rigid implants are usually used for pathologic fractures or impending fracture of diseased bone. Flexible intramedullary rods may be preferred for some traumatic fractures, particularly femoral fractures. The length, size, and shape of the nail or pin depend on the bone to be splinted. The most commonly used appliances include:

1. Kuntscher nail, for femur
2. Hansen-Street pin, for femur
3. Zickel intramedullary rod and hip nail, for femur—a particularly strong implant for stabilization of pathologic fractures
4. Knowles pin, for femur
5. Sampson rod, straight or curved, for femur
6. Enders nail, for femur, tibia, or humerus
7. Schneider nail, for femur, tibia, fibula, ulna, or radius
8. Lottes nail, for tibia
9. Rush pin, for all long bones
10. Steinmann pins, for clavicle, humerus, or ulna

The patient with a femoral or tibial fracture is positioned on the orthopaedic table. This permits traction as needed to maintain reduction. Figure 32-10 shows the position of the patient for intramedullary nailing of the left tibia. The C-arm image intensifier is used for fluoroscopic control. The fracture may be reduced with visual exposure of the fracture site or by closed reduction. In some situations the medullary canal must be reshaped or enlarged before an implant is inserted. The implant may be removed after union at the fracture site

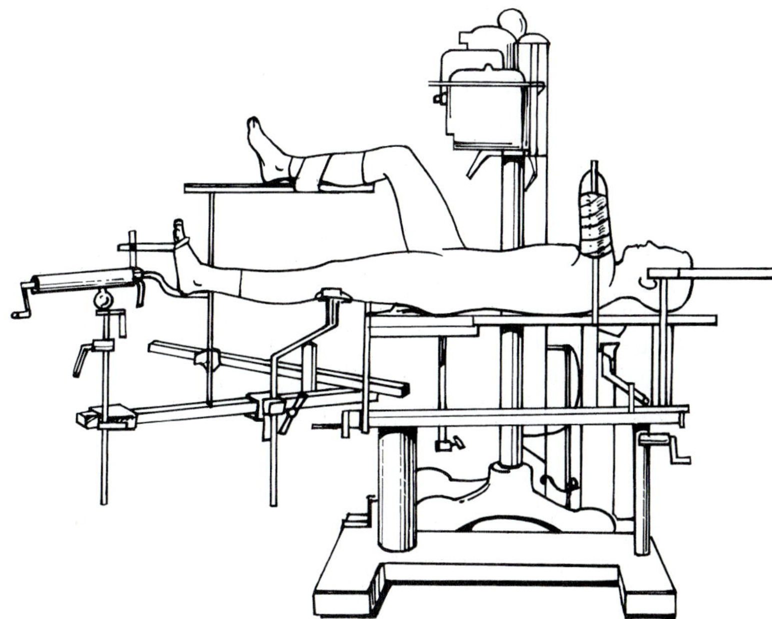

FIGURE 32-9 Position on orthopaedic table for nailing left hip. Note arm on affected side suspended from screen to remove it from surgical field. Note traction on affected leg and support under knee. Elevated right leg permits x-ray tube to be adjusted under it for lateral view.

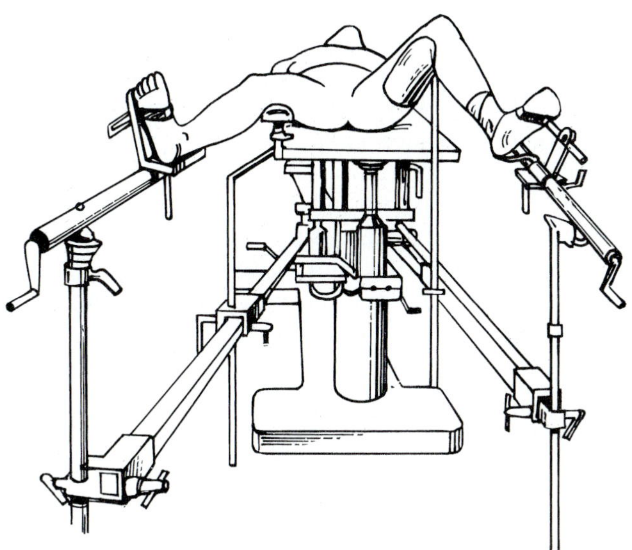

FIGURE 32-10 Position on orthopaedic table for intramedullary nailing of left tibia. Note left foot anchored to footholder and knee resting on elevated curved knee rest. Right foot is anchored and knee rest adjusted for support of leg.

has taken place, especially if it causes pain. If nonunion occurs, the implant may need to be removed.

Interlocking Nail Fixation After closed reduction of the fracture, an intramedullary rod or nail is inserted the length of the shaft of a long bone without exposing the fracture site. This technique is *closed intramedullary nailing* and may be used for transverse or short oblique fractures of the midshaft of the femur or tibia. An incision is made to expose the femoral trochanter or tibial tuberosity. To stabilize more oblique, comminuted fractures and those beyond the midshaft region, transfixion screws are also used with locking nails. These screws pass through the cortices of the bone and holes in the intramedullary nail. This method of *closed interlocking nail fixation* may be static or dynamic, depending on the location and configuration of the fracture. In the static method, screws are inserted in both the proximal and distal fragments; in the dynamic method they are proximal or distal. Several types of interlocking nail systems are available, such as the Grosse-Kempf, Brooker-Wills, and Russell-Taylor systems. All systems prevent gliding and rotation of fragments, as well as shortening of the limb from bone loss.

JOINT RECONSTRUCTION

Joint function depends on the quality of its structures. Articular cartilage covers the two ends of bone where they meet to form the joint. Bones are held securely in place at their articulation by ligaments and the joint capsule attached to both bone shafts. The synovial membrane lining the joint capsule secretes synovial fluid to lubricate the joint. When injured or altered by arthritis or other degenerative disease, normal joint motion is impaired and/or painful.

Dislocations

Dislocation of one or more bones at a joint may occur with or without an associated fracture. Tendons, ligaments, and muscles are deranged. The articular surface of the bone is displaced from the joint capsule. The force of displacement damages the capsule and tears ligaments and surrounding tissues. Blood vessel and nerve damage can occur, impeding circulation and causing changes in sensation and muscle strength. Closed reduction, with or without skeletal traction, may be necessary at the time of an acute injury. If closed reduction fails to *stabilize* the joint and prevent recurrence, open reduction and internal fixation may be necessary. Surgical procedures to stabilize chronic recurrent dislocations are most frequently performed on the shoulder.

Arthrodesis

Fusion of a joint may be achieved by removing the articular surfaces and securing bony union or by inserting a fixation implant that inhibits motion. Arthrodesis may be performed following resection of a recurrent benign, potentially malignant, or malignant lesion that involves the ends of the bones and joint. After resection of the diseased portion of the bones, the joint may be stabilized with a *bone graft* or an *intramedullary fixation implant*. This procedure is performed most frequently for lesions in the distal femur and proximal tibia around or including the knee joint. Arthrodesis may also be performed to relieve osteoarthritic pain or to stabilize a joint that does not respond to other methods of treatment following injury, such as instability of the thumb. Because arthrodesis limits motion, other joint reconstructive procedures are usually attempted first.

Triple arthrodesis of the ankle is performed to correct deformity or muscle imbalance of the foot. The subtalar, calcaneocuboid, and talonavicular tarsal joints are fused. Staples are sometimes used to hold bones together.

Arthroplasty

Arthroplasty, reconstruction of a joint, may be necessary to restore or improve range of motion and stability or to relieve pain. This may be done by resurfacing, reshaping, or replacing the articular surfaces of the bones.

Cup Arthroplasty of Hip

The hip joint is disarticulated by removing the head of the femur from the acetabulum. The femoral head is smoothed with a bone rasp to a spherical shape. The acetabulum is reamed to the configuration of a perfect hemisphere. A metallic cup is implanted into the acetabulum to provide a smooth surface for joint movement. Reamers must be correlated to the size of the cup to ensure proper articulation. Then the femoral head is placed back in the socket.

Femoral and Humeral Head Replacement

A metal prosthetic implant can replace the femoral or humeral head and neck (Figure 32-11). These prostheses have a shaft that is driven into the medullary canal of the bone. The head of the bone is removed. The neck is shaped or removed as necessary for accurate placement of the prosthesis. A reamer may be used to enlarge the canal for insertion of the prosthesis. These prostheses are used:

1. To mobilize the joint in arthritic patients
2. To replace a comminuted fractured head when soft tissue attachments are destroyed
3. To replace the head if avascular necrosis or nonunion occurs following reduction of fractures

A free vascularized fibular graft may be preferred to decompress the femoral head, provide structural stability, and vascularize bone in an area of avascular necrosis. This procedure preserves the femoral head rather than replacing it with a prosthesis after removal of dead bone. The peroneal artery and vein are preserved with the graft. Under the operating microscope, these vessels are anastomosed to branches of the femoral circumflex vessels. Restoration of vascularization prevents progression of necrosis and stimulates osteogenesis, new bone formation.

Femoral Head Surface Replacement

As an alternative to femoral head replacement, a concentric metal shell is cemented over the femoral head. A high-density polyethylene shell is cemented into the acetabulum. Surface replacement is reserved for young adults with good femoral and acetabular bone stock to relieve severe hip pain and disability. Patients with sclerotic, well-vascularized subchondral bone of hypertrophic osteoarthritis, for example, may be candidates for this procedure. Resurfacing induces healing and reduces stress on the hip joint.

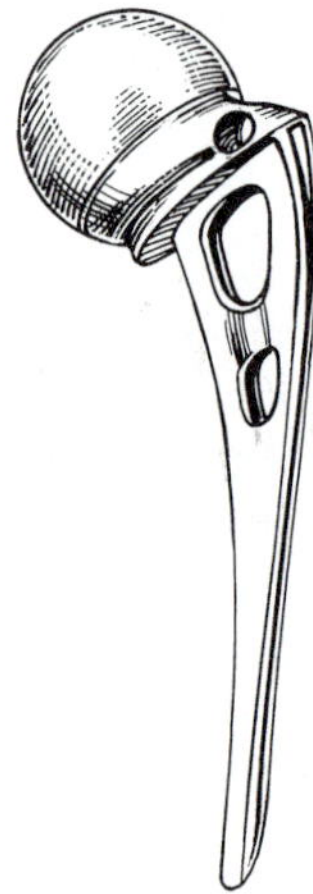

FIGURE 32-11 Prosthesis to replace femoral head and neck. Shaft is driven into medullary canal of femur.

Total Joint Replacement

Any joint in the extremities can be replaced with a prosthetic implant. The orthopaedist's goal in total joint arthroplasty is to alleviate pain and to create functional mobility and stability. The prosthesis must maintain normal anatomic relationships and biologic fixation to bone. Correct alignment and fit of component parts are crucial aspects of their function. Although prosthetic implants for some joints have not been as well developed as are those for others, total joint replacement is an accepted therapeutic modality, especially for the hip, knee, and elbow joints. Usually performed to improve mobility and relieve pain of severe arthritic joints, total joint replacement may be indicated when other therapeutic measures have failed to correct a congenital defect, traumatic injury, or degenerative disease. A functional design for a prosthesis must consider a combination of load bearing, strain-stress, and kinetics in association with the pathologic condition. Positioning of the prosthesis influences the distribution of stress and rate of wear.

The bones on both sides of the joints are replaced or resurfaced. Both component parts must be solidly anchored to avoid movement of the prosthesis and wear on surrounding tissue. All movement must be between the smooth articulating surfaces of the prosthesis. Various alloys, ceramics, and high-density polyethylene or silicone are used; component parts of many prostheses are made of more than one material. Metal to plastic joints are self-lubricating. Natural synovial fluids help lubricate other types. The rate of wear on parts must be low so the prosthesis will remain functional over a period of many years (the exact number is undetermined). The major complication of total joint arthroplasty is loosening of the prosthetic components over time, particularly in weight-bearing joints of obese patients and active persons. Configuration, surface features, and the method of fixation of component parts influence mechanical stability of an "artificial" joint. The orthopaedic surgeon must consider:

1. *Biomechanics.* Ideally, a prosthesis provides full range of motion. The support provided by cartilage, ligaments, and articular capsule surrounding the prosthesis influences its stability. Two types of prostheses are used.
   a. *Constrained* prosthesis provides a stable joint but restricts motion to a single plane or limits motion in all planes.
   b. *Nonconstrained* prosthesis allows gliding and shifting motions resembling normal range of motion, but it is inherently unstable.
2. *Biophysical components.* A total joint prosthesis has at least two components, one for each side of the articulation. To determine the size and shape of components to fit patient, measurements of bones that form the joint may be obtained preoperatively by developing templates (i.e., patterns on grids) from the patient's x-ray films. If templates have not been obtained, x-ray films and measurements must be taken at the surgical field. The surgeon also takes trial measurements at the site to verify the correct selection of the implant.
   a. *Solid components* have a predetermined configuration. The orthopaedist must select the most appropriate size from those available. Bone may need to be reshaped to accommodate prosthesis.
   b. *Modular systems* have interchangeable components so that the orthopaedist can customize the prosthesis at the operating table. For example, the width, depth, or length can be adjusted to patient's anatomy. A quick-setting Silastic mold may be formed for precise matching in three dimensions. The mold is sent to a laboratory where the prosthesis is customized with use of a laser scanner and a computer-guided milling machine.
3. *Fixation.* The bone into which the component part is implanted and the surface of the prosthesis will determine method of fixation.
   a. *Press-fit fixation* relies on direct bone-to-prosthesis contact. This can be achieved by a variety of methods, including reshaping bone to size and/or configuration of implant, and/or securing threads, pegs, or screws on the prosthesis into bone.
   b. *Biofixation* refers to a surface on the implant that allows tissue ingrowth for stability. Ingrowth is defined as the development of bony tissue in an empty hole. A portion of the implant has a porous or rough surface. Bone grows into pores or interstices. Many types of coatings are used, such as tricalcium phosphate or coraline hydroxyapatite sprayed on the surface. Others have a porous material such as polysulfone bonded to the metal. Surfaces that are porous enough for bone ingrowth without greatly expanding the surface area or weakening the implant are most desirable. These *cementless prostheses* require a precise fit in bones. They are particularly suited for young, active patients. The joint usually is immobilized for a period of time until ingrowth begins.
   c. *Methyl methacrylate fixation* uses a self-curing thermoplastic acrylic cement to provide long-term fixation. Three different preparations of polymethyl methacrylate, commonly referred to as *bone cement*, are available. The powder and liquid components are mixed at the instrument table immediately before insertion into the intramedullary canal of a long bone or socket of a

joint (see pp. 673-674). Bone cement is injected in a state of low viscosity under pressure to fill the interstices of bone. When the implant is placed, the cement fills the space around it for a secure fit. This is the method of choice for most patients over 65 years of age because it allows early ambulation. Cement can crack or break and cause loosening of the prosthesis over time.

d. *Hybrid fixation* refers to a combination of fixation methods. Some components are cemented; some are press fitted or held by screws or other noncemented technique.

e. *Bone grafts* may be needed to replace bone loss around joint. Either autologous or fresh frozen homologous bone may be used.

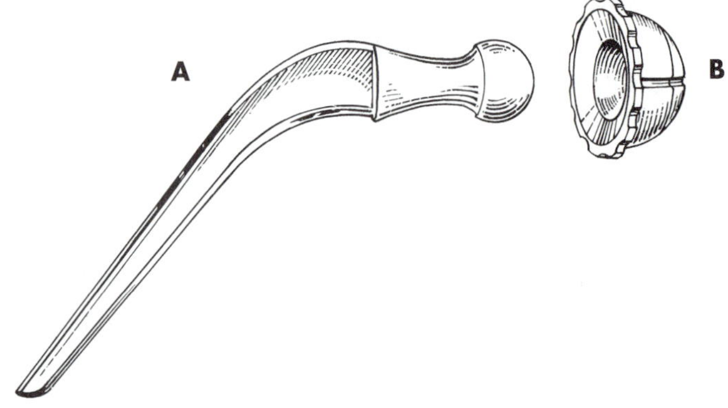

FIGURE 32-12 Components of total hip replacement prosthesis. **A,** Metallic stem with femoral head. **B,** Acetabular cup.

Total Hip Replacement Total hip prostheses have greatly reduced the number of arthroplasty procedures previously described, especially in patients older than 50 years of age with degenerative hip disease. Several types and sizes of prostheses are available. Each has its own advantages and disadvantages. The orthopaedist must select the appropriate one for each patient's particular condition.

With the patient supine on the radiographic operating table, an incision about 10 inches (25 cm) long is made along the lateral aspect of the thigh to remove the greater trochanter. Removal of the greater trochanter facilitates exposure to prepare sites for the insertion of the prosthesis. However, its removal can cause abductor muscle weakness, instability, and other complications. Therefore some orthopaedists prefer an anterior approach to the hip joint with the patient in supine position; others prefer a posterior approach with the patient in lateral decubitus position. With all approaches the femur is dislocated from the acetabulum. The femoral head is removed at the neck and replaced with a prosthesis. This may be a metal, usually titanium, head on a metallic stem that is seated into the medullary canal of the femur. Before the femoral prosthesis is inserted, the acetabulum is reamed to the configuration of the cup-shaped acetabular component (Figure 32-12). This may be high-density polyethylene or metal with a smooth, rough, or porous outer surface. The inner surface is smooth to articulate with the smooth finish on the head of the femoral prosthesis. The acetabular component is fixed in the socket. Then the femoral prosthesis is positioned. This sequence is reversed if a Silastic mold is made for a customized femoral component.

A computer-assisted surgical robot may be used to help the orthopaedist plan the surgical procedure, select the most appropriate type and size of hip prosthesis, and to prepare the surface of the bone. A drill in the end of the robotic arm precisely drills the cavity in the femur to hold the implant stem.

Total Knee Replacement Insertion of a total knee prosthesis may be indicated to provide for mechanical deficiencies in the function of the knee. The patient, usually older than 60 years of age, may have significant chronic pain and joint destruction as a result of arthritis, an inflammatory condition, or an autoimmune disorder. One or both knees may be affected. Bilateral total knee replacement can be performed safely in a patient who has the ability to actively participate in postoperative rehabilitation. Selection of the appropriate prosthesis from among the types available depends on the deformity of the femorotibial articulation, patellofemoral articulation, and the structure of the cruciate and collateral ligaments. The prosthesis consists of a multiradius femoral component, a modular tibial component, and a patellar component. The tibial and patellar components of high-density polyethylene articulate with the polished metallic surface of the femoral component.

With the patient supine on the operating table, the knee is maintained in a flexed position. Numerous commercial devices are available for this purpose. The pneumatic tourniquet cuff is placed on the thigh before prepping and draping. A vertical midline incision is made over the front of the knee. After the distal femur and the proximal tibia are cut, a trial prosthesis is inserted. The knee is taken through a range of motion to assess alignment, ligament balance, and patellar positioning before the components are fixed in place. To achieve stability, permanent bone ingrowth into a porous-coated or rough surface implant is desirable. Prostheses of this construction may not require bone cement for fixation. Hybrid fixation is used for others.

Total Ankle Replacement Rheumatoid arthritis and posttraumatic osteoarthritis are the most common causes of ankle degeneration. Ankle joint replacement may be indicated as an alternative to arthrodesis in selected patients, usually older than 60 years of age, to relieve pain and secondarily to increase motion and provide stability in the tibiotalar joint. With the patient in supine position, an anterior incision may be made from base of the second metatarsal to crest of the tibia. A posterior approach, with patient in prone position, may be preferred for wider exposure of anatomic structures. Procedures vary depending on the type of prosthesis to be implanted. The nonconstrained type allows normal dorsiflexion, plantar flexion, and rotation of foot but is inherently unstable; the constrained type restricts motion to a single plane but is inherently more stable. The tibial components of both types are high-density polyethylene, and the talar components are metal. They are cemented in place.

Total Metatarsophalangeal Joint Replacement Hallux rigidus and hallux abductus valgus deformities can lead to pain and altered gait. By joint replacement the deformity can be realigned with stability and motion. Several types of implants are available. The Silastic hinge toe, a double-stemmed silicone prosthesis with a hinge, is popular to restore motion of the great toe and lesser metatarsophalangeal joints.

Total Shoulder Replacement Shoulder replacement may be indicated for severe destruction by disease or posttraumatic degeneration of humeral articular surface with resultant loss of motion, instability, and pain. The prosthesis replaces the humeral head and resurfaces the glenoid cavity, the articular surface of the scapula. Preferred if ligamentous or capsular support is sufficient, a nonconstrained prosthesis has a plastic component for the glenoid socket and a metal humeral head. Only the articular surfaces are replaced with these gliding metal-to-plastic components. A stable fixed-fulcrum constrained prosthesis with interlocking components may be required to prevent dislocation. The patient is placed in semi-Fowler's position for these surgical procedures.

Total Elbow Replacement Prosthetic replacement may be indicated to correct intraarticular problems within the elbow joint, especially one with severe surface damage. Surface replacement with a nonarticulating constrained prosthesis provides internal stability. A hinged or articulated nonconstrained capitellocondylar prosthesis improves the functional range of motion in the humeroulnar articulation. Both the metallic humerus and ulnar components are cemented in place following shaping of the bones. High-density polyethylene bushings facilitate articulation of the hinge assembly connecting the humoral and ulnar components.

Total Wrist Replacement Silicone rubber implants are used to replace the radiocarpal joint in the wrist, primarily to improve function. A resection arthroplasty is done, usually from an anterior approach. The proximal row of carpal bones (i.e., scaphoid and lunate) and the trapezium are resected. Stems of the flexible, hinged implant are inserted into the intramedullary canals of radius proximally and capitate carpal bone distally. A silicone cap is placed over distal end of the ulna. Flexion and extension of the wrist are possible through free sliding of stems within the medullary canals. Some other types of prostheses have fixed stems.

Trapeziometacarpal Joint Replacement A metal ball-to-plastic socket prosthesis restores function of the thumb. This prosthesis is cemented in place.

Metacarpophalangeal Joint Replacement Known as *implant replacement arthroplasty* for small joints in the hands, the head of affected metacarpal or proximal phalanx is removed. The silicone rubber implant bridges the excised joint. One stem fits into the medullary canal of proximal metacarpal and the other into distal phalanx. The hinged body of the implant keeps the bones separated and mobile.

Nursing Considerations in Joint Arthroplasty

Patients of all ages have debilitating and painful arthritis; many are over 65 years of age. Attention must be paid to support all joints during moving and positioning these patients. Other unique aspects of joint replacement should be kept in mind.

1. Prosthesis must be handled carefully.
   a. Use only instruments specifically designed for implantation of prosthesis.
   b. Avoid dents and scratches.
   c. Avoid glove powder and lint. Silicone implants should not be placed on fabrics; place the implant in a metal basin or transfer it directly to the surgeon.
   d. Open sterile packages just before use, after the orthopaedist determines the size and style.
2. Bone cement, if needed, must be mixed by the scrub person immediately before use.
   a. Follow manufacturer's instructions for handling this material. The scrub person should know by feel and appearance when the cement is of the correct consistency. A practice session is helpful before mixing for the first time during an actual surgical procedure.
   b. Avoid excessive exposure to vapors. In addition to irritation to eyes, soft contact lenses may be damaged if worn. A scavenging system should be used. A fume evacuator, if used, may need to be recharged before and after use (see Chapter 10, p. 155).

c. Avoid getting lipid solvent on gloves. It can diffuse through the latex to cause allergic dermatitis.
d. Cement is poured into a syringe for injection into the intramedullary canal, as for hip or shoulder joints. Cement may be shaped manually for hinged joints.
e. Room temperature can affect the time necessary for cement to set.

3. Silastic mold, if used to customize the prosthesis, must be prepared at the sterile field. Scrub person mixes catalyst and silicone quickly and thoroughly and then pours the mixture into injector tube immediately before it is inserted into bone. The customized prosthesis must be steam sterilized when it arrives from the laboratory. A standard sterilization cycle, not flash sterilization, is used.
4. Air-powered drills, saw, and reamers must be properly connected with adequate pressure. Check the pressure in tanks of compressed air or nitrogen before the surgical procedure begins. It must be more than 500 lb.
5. Suction tubing must be kept open and collection containers changed as necessary to maintain suction for irrigation during the surgical procedure.
6. Blood loss should be appropriately monitored. It can be extensive during total hip arthroplasty. Blood may be salvaged from the sterile field and processed, as through a cell saver, for autotransfusion (see Chapter 23, p. 486).
7. Closed-wound suction drainage usually is used, especially following hip, knee, and shoulder arthroplasty.
8. Exhaust system for personnel must be functioning properly if the surgical procedure is performed within an ultraclean air system (see p. 663).
9. Traffic through the OR should be restricted to minimize air turbulence if laminar airflow is not installed. Infection is a major potential hazard of all bone and joint surgery. It can be both disabling and expensive.
10. Type of prosthesis used must be documented, including manufacturer's identifying information. The label of a sterile implant can be affixed to the patient's record.

Arthroscopy

Arthroscopy, the visualization of the interior of a joint through an arthroscope, allows diagnosis and conservative treatment of some cartilaginous, ligamentous, synovial, and bony surface defects. Most frequently used for definitive treatment of meniscal, articular cartilage, and ligamentous defects in the knee, an arthroscope may be used in the shoulder, elbow, wrist, hip, and ankle. Fiberoptic arthroscopes have diameters ranging from 1.7 to 6 mm to accommodate the size of the joint. Angles of the viewing lenses also vary from 30 to 90 degrees.

Sterile irrigating solution, either Ringer's lactate or normal saline solution, at room temperature is necessary to distend the joint, although some arthroscopists prefer air or carbon dioxide. The solution is injected initially via needle and syringe. Then through a small stab wound, a cannula is inserted into the medial aspect of the knee, for example, for inflow of irrigation. Outflow tubing is connected to the metal sheath of the arthroscope. It can be attached to suction or placed in a drainage bucket and allowed to drain by gravity.

The sheath (sleeve) over a sharp trocar is inserted through a stab wound in the skin at the selected site of entry for the arthroscope. When the trocar penetrates the capsule, the capsule and synovium form a tight seal around the sheath. The sharp trocar is replaced with a blunt obturator to advance the sheath into the joint. The obturator is removed and the arthroscope inserted through the sheath. The inflow and outflow irrigating tubes are connected to the stopcocks on the sheath.

An operating arthroscope may have a channel for passage of long, thin, manually operated instruments such as probes, hooks, scissors, knives, punches, and grasping forceps. Or these instruments may be manipulated through separate puncture sites (portals) into the joint under visualization through the scope. Power-driven shavers are also used to smooth rough articular cartilage or bony surfaces. A pulsed energy Nd:YAG, Ho:YAG, or CO_2 laser may be adapted to some arthroscopes for use in a confined area and to minimize bleeding. A video camera attached to the eyepiece allows projection of the view to a closed-circuit television monitor so that the surgeon can manipulate instruments more comfortably than by squinting through the eyepiece. Some cameras attach to the side of a beam splitter on the scope. Daylight film should be used with fiberoptic lighting.

Nursing Considerations for Arthroscopy

1. All metal components are steam sterilized. Some optical systems and fiberoptic cords can be steam sterilized; others require gas sterilization. Foam-lined sterilizing cases are recommended to protect the optics. If a solution of activated glutaraldehyde or peracetic acid is used, the arthroscope must be rinsed in sterile distilled water before use. Follow manufacturer's recommendations for sterilization of the arthroscope and its component attachments.
2. Scrub person checks all sterile equipment and instruments while setting up.
   a. Check arthroscope for clean lenses and unbroken optics.
   b. Check patency of inflow and outflow irrigation stopcocks and ports.

c. All component parts must be the correct size; optics, trocar, and obturator must fit securely into the sheath. Surgical instruments must pass through the channel. Fiberoptic cord must fit the arthroscope and projection lamp.
d. Inspect the edges of cutting instruments, such as blades, burrs, knives, and scissors, under magnification. Blades must be sharp, set properly, and glide smoothly.
e. Assemble power equipment. Rings must fit tightly. Forward and reverse rotating actions must function smoothly. Blades must be locked properly. The power source should be checked.

3. Circulator checks all nonsterile equipment (i.e., fiberoptic projection lamp, video equipment, laser).
4. Video camera and cable must be enclosed in a sterile cover unless the camera has been sterilized. Scrub person and circulator coordinate draping.
5. Extremity must be firmly supported in a leg or arm holder that allows flexion of the joint. A tourniquet is applied for arthroscopy of the knee, ankle, elbow, or wrist.
6. Patient is prepped and draped as for any *sterile* procedure on the extremity (see Chapter 22), with extra precautions to provide a waterproof barrier against contamination by irrigating solutions.
7. Circulator hangs containers of irrigating solution on an IV pole at least 3 feet (1 m) above the joint to ensure adequate hydrostatic pressure to keep the joint distended and to maintain the flow of the irrigating solution. Two to four 3000 ml containers may be needed. Extra containers should be available in the room. The solution is maintained at room temperature to avoid hyperemia from warm solution, which may appear as inflammation of synovium, or blanching, which produces an avascular appearance from cold solution.
8. Equipment must be appropriately attached after the patient is draped.
   a. Scrub person secures drainage tubes, fiberoptic cord, suction, air-power cables, etc., to drapes in a location that will not impede movement of the extremity.
   b. Circulator attaches tubings to irrigating and suction systems, cords to power sources, etc.

Arthrotomy

Arthrotomy (i.e., incision into a joint) may be necessary to remove bone or cartilage fragments or to repair a defect in the synovium or joint capsule. *Synovectomy* may be the procedure of choice for relief of pain and control of inflammation in a rheumatoid arthritic joint. If a joint is ankylosed (fused), fibrosed, or deranged, open arthrotomy rather than arthroscopy may be necessary. Occasionally during arthroscopy, an injury or disease process that cannot be adequately treated requires arthrotomy while the patient is anesthetized, or it may be performed at a later time. In the knee, for example, potential neurovascular complications may preclude arthroscopic repair.

Bunionectomy

Hallux valgus, a lateral deviation in position of great toe, increases prominence of the adjoining metatarsal head. Pressure at base of the first metatarsophalangeal joint causes inflammation that creates formation of an *exostosis* or *bunion* beneath the bursa and joint capsule. A bunionectomy is done to remove a painful exostosis and to functionally or cosmetically correct the deformity. A capsulotomy must be performed to enter the first metatarsophalangeal joint. The procedure may be done under local infiltration anesthesia and IV sedation. A pneumatic tourniquet around the ankle provides hemostasis, unless contraindicated in a patient with a circulatory problem in the foot. One of several procedures may be selected.

1. *Keller arthroplasty.* The proximal third of the proximal phalanx of the great toe is resected. A silicone implant may be placed in the intramedullary canal to stabilize the metatarsophalangeal joint.
2. *Metatarsal osteotomy.* The metatarsal alignment is corrected by moving the metatarsal head laterally.
3. *McBride operation.* The abductor tendon is fixed to the lateral portion of the metatarsal neck, and the sesamoid bone is excised.
4. *Silver bunionectomy.* The medial aspect of the exostosis is removed from the first metatarsal head.

NOTE Bunionectomies are only one of many procedures performed by podiatrists, as well as orthopaedists in the treatment of foot-related disorders, including degenerative diseases and injuries of the foot and ankle.

Neurolysis

Neuropathy caused by entrapment of a nerve produces tingling, numbness, and a burning sensation with radiating pain and compromise of function. Known as a *tunnel syndrome,* this most frequently occurs in the wrist from entrapment of the median nerve (i.e., *carpal tunnel syndrome*). It may originate from compression of the radial nerve in the lower arm (i.e., *radial tunnel syndrome*) or from the posterior tibial nerve in the foot (i.e., *tarsal tunnel syndrome*). The cause of formation of scar tissue or adhesions around the nerve may be unknown, or it may be related to trauma or inflammatory disease. *Neurolysis,* freeing of the nerve from the surrounding structures, relieves pain and restores sensation and function. For example, in the wrist, the transverse carpal ligament overriding the median nerve is incised. A segment may be excised, and a synovectomy may be performed to relieve the symptoms of carpal tunnel syndrome. Release of the median nerve also may be accomplished endoscopically.

REPAIR OF TENDONS AND LIGAMENTS

Tendons and ligaments may be severed, torn, or ruptured. These injuries are frequently seen in athletes. Total or partial avulsion of the major ligaments and tendons torn from their attachments in or around an extremity joint requires repair to stabilize the joint.

Tendons can be lengthened, shortened, or transferred. When a surgical procedure is indicated, tendon repair is a meticulous but tedious procedure. *Tenorrhaphy,* close apposition of the cut ends of tendons, particularly extensor tendons, is imperative to successfully restore function. Tendons heal slowly. Stainless steel suture is widely used in tendon repair because of its durability and lack of elasticity. A tendon may be wrapped in a silicone membrane to prevent adhesions after repair. Artificial tendons are made of a polyester center covered with silicone rubber. A double-velour polyester prosthesis is used for ligament repair of a shoulder separation.

Hand Surgery

Hand reconstruction has become a subspecialty of both orthopaedics and plastic surgery. (See Chapter 34, p. 713, and Chapter 44, pp. 912-913, for discussion of transfer and replantation of severed digits.) Tendon surgery is within the realm of orthopaedic surgeons; however, many plastic surgeons also perform tendon repair and transfer for hand reconstruction. Restoration of function is the goal of the hand surgeon. The orthopaedist often manages surgical correction of fractures and rotational deformities of the fingers. *Tenosynovectomy,* excision of the tendon sheath, may be performed to release arthritic contractures.

Sports Medicine

Sports medicine deals with the anatomic, biochemical, physiologic, and psychologic effects of motion, strength, and coordination on physical activity. Public awareness of and orthopaedists' concern about athletic injuries have led to the development of sports medicine centers that emphasize physical conditioning, injury prevention, and rehabilitation of athletes. Sports medicine is a rapidly growing area of orthopaedics, primarily as a result of interest in exercise among the general population. The intensity of a sports activity places physical demands on the musculoskeletal system that can result in injury. Most injuries involve ligaments, tendons, and muscles rather than broken bones. Most injuries, such as a strained muscle or tendon, do not require surgical intervention. Magnetic resonance imaging is a reliable method of assessing intraarticular injuries, either acute or chronic. The knee, shoulder, and ankle are most prone to athletic injuries of ligaments and dislocations of joints. Arthroscopy is useful in the diagnosis and treatment of some injuries. Others require open surgical reconstruction to regain joint stability. For example, a complete ligament tear usually requires surgical repair. Some procedures combine arthroscopy and arthrotomy. Postoperative rehabilitation aims to restore range of motion, to minimize muscle atrophy, and to reestablish muscle endurance and joint position. The patient should commit to a long-term conditioning program to prevent reinjury.

Knee Injuries

The knee is the most vulnerable joint to both contact and noncontact sports injuries. Hyperextension, for example, can result from a noncontact activity. Contact sports can result in a combination of injuries to the cruciate and collateral ligaments, meniscus, and posterior capsule.

Anterior Cruciate Ligament Knee stability is influenced by the dynamics of the anterior and posterior cruciate ligaments. Injuries to these ligaments are the most common and most serious types of knee injuries. The anterior cruciate ligament (ACL) can be partially or completely torn, ruptured, or avulsed. The extent of the injury determines the method of reconstruction. Arthroscopically, the ACL may be transferred into the posterior aspect of the lateral femoral condyle and secured with sutures, staples, or screws.

After an autograft is harvested through an open incision, the knee may be reconstructed through the arthroscope. One technique places a bone-patellar tendon-bone autograft and fixes it with cancellous or interference bone screws into tibial and femoral tunnels. In another method a composite of autogenous musculus semitendinosus with a polypropylene ligament augmentation device sutured to it extends from the tibial attachment across the joint and is stapled to the distal femur. In the open Insall procedure, a bone-block graft with an iliotibial band of fascia lata is secured to the tibial tubercle.

Artificial ligamentous substitutes may be preferred for ACL reconstruction. These materials also are used to stabilize torn or ruptured ligaments in the ankle. Expanded polytetrafluoroethylene can be secured with screws. Homograft ligaments also are used. Woven bovine collagen, a bovine and carbon fiber material, or a partially absorbable matrix of polylactic acid polymer and filamentous carbon may be used as a scaffold for new collagenous tissue ingrowth for disrupted ligaments. Concomitant partial menisectomy or meniscal repair may be performed with ACL reconstruction.

Meniscus Partial meniscectomy or repair of a meniscal tear may be done by open arthrotomy or closed arthroscopy. Neurovascular injury is a potential complication of these procedures. Patients selected for arthroscopy usually have a single vertical longitudinal tear that can be debrided. Localized synovium can be abraded. Sutures must be placed to reduce displacement and stabilize the meniscus.

Ankle Injuries

Rupture of the Achilles tendon can occur spontaneously during a physical activity, such as basketball or racquet sports, usually from indirect trauma. A gap is palpable at the back of the ankle. Severed ends of the tendon may be brought together through an open or percutaneous repair with heavy (size No. 2) nonabsorbable suture.

Ankle arthroscopy may be the procedure of choice to place internal fixation devices or to remove osteophytes, bony outgrowths in the joint after healing of ankle fracture.

Shoulder Injuries

Many anterior glenoid labrum and minor rotator cuff tears, the most common acute injuries, can be repaired arthroscopically. Some recurrent dislocations also can be stabilized with sutures, staples, or screws. For a major rotator cuff tear, an open Bankart repair usually is necessary to suture the labrum and reattach the glenohumeral ligament. An open Putti-Platt correction for recurrent dislocation will limit external rotation of the shoulder.

VERTEBRAL COLUMN

The bony structure of the vertebral column extends from the foramen magnum at the base of the skull to the coccyx. The 33 vertebrae, which provide support for the body, vary in size and are classified according to location: 7 cervical vertebrae are in the neck; 12 thoracic vertebrae articulate with the ribs; 5 lumbar vertebrae are posterior to the retroperitoneal cavity; 5 sacral vertebrae are fused to form the sacrum; and 4 fused coccygeal vertebrae form the coccyx. An intervertebral disk is held between each cervical, thoracic, and lumbar vertebral body by the annulus fibrosus and posterior longitudinal ligament. The disk itself, a fibrocartilaginous substance known as *nucleus pulposus,* acts as a shock absorber or cushion between the vertebrae. Each vertebra has an anterior body with a thick pedicle on each side that connects the vertebral body to transverse winged-shaped processes. Laminae, thin layers of bone, connect these to the posterior spinous process to form the vertebral arch that surrounds foramen (opening) of the spinal canal. The spinal cord passes through this canal in the cervical and thoracic vertebrae to the level of the second or third lumbar vertebrae. Pairs of spinal nerve roots branch out from the spinal cord to each side of these bodies from under each lamina. (See anatomic landmarks in vertebral column in Figure 32-13 and Figure 18-1, p. 349.)

To determine the mechanism of an injury or deformity or the location of a lesion, the vertebral column can be anatomically divided into three equal columns.

1. The *posterior column* includes the laminae, facet joints, spinous processes, and posterior ligamentous complex.
2. The *middle column* includes the posterior walls of vertebral bodies, anterior longitudinal ligaments, and anterior annuli fibrosus.
3. The *anterior column* includes the anterior vertebral bodies, anterior longitudinal ligaments, and anterior annuli fibrosus.

Because of the proximity of the vertebral column to the spinal cord, both orthopaedists and neurosurgeons perform surgical procedures in this area. Orthopaedic procedures on the back are usually performed to excise vertebral lesions, to relieve pressure on the spinal cord, to stabilize the vertebral column, or to correct gross deformities. Primary neoplasms such as a giant cell bone tumor, bone cyst, hemangioma or osteoid osteoma, and metastatic tumors can occur in vertebrae. Osteomyelitis, spondylolisthesis (a condition in which one lumbar vertebra slips onto another), and degenerative diseases such as arthritis and osteoporosis may cause severe low back pain unresponsive to nonsurgical treatment. Fracture, with or without dislocation of one vertebra or more, may be reduced by traction, internal fixation, or excision of bony fragments. Scoliosis, a progressive curvature of the spine, may be stabilized.

For diagnosis of spinal conditions, CT detects abnormal bone. CT and MRI evaluate spinal injuries. MRI and myelography (see Chapter 28, p. 569) outline soft tissue abnormalities, such as disk degeneration, protrusion, or rupture. Because it is noninvasive and seems as effective, MRI is replacing myelography.

Surgical procedures to relieve low back pain or to stabilize the spinal column are most commonly performed by orthopaedic surgeons. The use of intraoperative spinal cord monitoring with cortical and spinal somatosensory and motor evoked potentials (see Chapter 19, p. 378) increases the safety of these procedures. Dermatomal mapping and "wake-up" tests also are reliable techniques for monitoring spinal cord function. In the latter test the patient must be *awake* enough to respond to the surgeon's command to move the foot.

Diskectomy

Intervertebral disk injuries usually occur between the lumbar vertebrae, often caused by lifting heavy objects or by the stress of twisting the spine. The nucleus pulposus can herniate or rupture through a tear in the annulus fibrosus

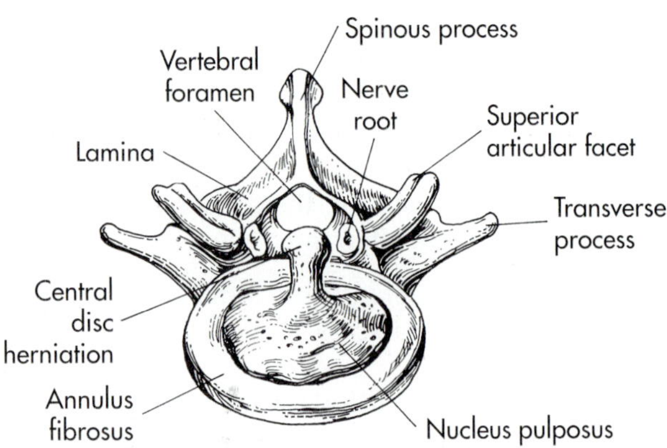

FIGURE 32-13 Vertebra. Superior view with herniation of nucleus pulposus.

and posterior ligament (Figure 32-13). This protrusion, referred to as a *herniated disk* or *ruptured* or *slipped disk*, compresses the spinal nerve roots or spinal cord within the spinal canal against the vertebra. This causes pain from the lumbar or sacral region to the lower back. Pain may radiate down the sciatic nerve pathway to the leg. During the surgical procedure, the herniated nucleus pulposus or ruptured portion of the annulus fibrosus is excised.

Lumbar Laminectomy

A laminectomy is usually carried out through a vertical midline skin incision with patient in prone or lateral position. For prone position, the patient may be positioned on a Hastings or Andrews frame or on a spinal table. The extent of the incision depends on the number of laminae to be removed. The fascia and muscles are retracted to expose spinous processes and laminae. These are cut off with a rongeur to expose the intervertebral disk. The herniated part of the disk and any loose fragments are removed from the intervertebral space.

Microdiskectomy

A unilateral, one-level diskectomy is performed under the operating microscope. Microdiskectomy permits exposure of the herniated nucleus pulposus without extensive manipulation of paraspinal muscles or removal of a large section of lamina. The skin incision is shorter than required for a standard laminectomy.

Ligamentum Flavotomy

The ligamentum flavum is the yellowish elastic tissue that connects laminae of adjoining vertebrae. It is incised and retracted laterally. The disk is removed. Then the ligamentum flavum is sutured back in place. Some orthopaedists prefer this simple, limited diskectomy rather than laminectomy for selected patients.

Percutaneous Lumbar Diskectomy

Percutaneous lumbar diskectomy is an endoscopic procedure to remove a focal bulge-type herniated disk, usually at the level of L4-5. It is done under local anesthesia, usually with IV sedation, because the patient must be alert enough to assess radicular pain in the leg. The patient may be either in a prone or in a lateral decubitus position. A trocar is inserted through skin and soft tissue into the disk capsule. Under fluoroscopic control, a cutting probe (Nucleotome) is inserted through the outer cannula. The herniated nucleus pulposus is excised and aspirated to relieve pressure on the spinal nerve root.

Spinal Stabilization

Immobilization of vertebrae in segments of the vertebral column may be necessary to treat chronic, degenerative diseases of the spine. Progressive instability, especially in the upper cervical spine, may lead to compression of the spinal cord with resultant neurologic deficit. After decompression of the spinal cord or excision of a bone tumor or following trauma, the vertebral column may need stabilization to protect the spinal cord or to relieve pain. Surgical alignment is indicated for scoliosis or other curvature when it progresses to cosmetic deformity, when pain becomes a handicap, or when cardiopulmonary functions are decreased. (See Chapter 42, p. 861, for discussion of scoliosis in children.)

Spinal Fusion

Spinal fusion may be indicated following spinal injury or excision of bone to stabilize the vertebral column. Either a posterior or an anterior approach may be used to place the bone grafts. A combined anterior and posterior spinal fusion may be required for severe deformities. The anterior fusion is performed first. Unless the lesion or bone fragment to be removed is on the right side of the vertebral column, an anterior thoracolumbar approach is through an incision with the patient in a right lateral position (left side up). A retroperitoneal incision is made for an anterior lumbar approach. These approaches are safer on the left side because the surgeon works near the aorta, which is more resistant to inadvertent injury than is the vena cava on the right.

Bone grafts are placed in the intervertebral spaces or along the spinous processes to bridge over or to stabilize the defect. The rib removed for an anterior thoracolumbar approach is used for grafting. Homogenous cancellous bone from the bone bank may be needed to provide a larger quantity of bone than can be obtained from the rib or an autogenous graft from the crest of the patient's ilium. Cancellous bone rather than cortical bone is usually preferred for spinal fusion. Bone grafts may be used with or without internal fixation devices. The goals of spinal fusion are to achieve stability, rigidity, and correction of deformity. The combined use of internal fixation devices with bone grafts may facilitate postoperative care and early ambulation.

Internal Fixation

Complex procedures are performed for sublaminar wiring, transpedicle screw fixation, and internal vertebral stabilization or fusion. Many spinal implant systems are available. All have a common goal of immobilizing spinal segments; each offers significant biomechanical advantages, but all have potential complications. The surgeon chooses the most appropriate device for the location, approach, and type of deformity and instability. For example, the posterior body and ligamentous structures in cervical spine may be disrupted by a flexion-compression type of injury. Interspinous wiring and bone grafting provide posterior neck fusion for stability. In the thoracolumbar spine, transpedicular screw and plating systems can be used in conjunction with spinal fusion in treatment of fractures, spondylolisthesis, and idiopathic scoliosis. Cotrel-Dubousset rods, hooks, and screws, Harrington or Moe rods and hooks, Luque rods and sublaminar wires, or Wisconsin spinous process wires may be used to provide decompression of spinal nerve roots and vertebral alignment following posterior thoracolumbar spinal fusion. Kaneda, Zielke, Dwyer, or Dunn devices are used when an anterior approach is preferred. Each device has its own set of instrumentation; these are not interchangeable.

CAST APPLICATION

A *cast* is a rigid form of dressing used to encase a part of the body. It supports and immobilizes the part in optimum position until healing takes place. A cast usually includes the joints above and below the affected area. It may suffice as a conservative mode of treatment, as for fractures. It can be fitted to any body contour or position and can be worn for months. Requisites of a cast are that:

1. It must fulfill its intended function of maintaining position of the desired parts.
2. It must not be too tight and must have no pressure areas. *Postapplication pain is an important symptom and must be promptly investigated.* Circulation may be impaired.
3. It must not be too loose. It must be as light as possible, yet strong enough to withstand usage.
4. It must be comfortable, with no binding or chafing.

Padding Under Cast

Padding is usually placed under the cast and serves several functions.

1. It absorbs inevitable ooze from the wound following an open surgical procedure. Sterile padding is put on over the dressing before applying the cast.
2. It protects the wound and the patient's skin.
3. It protects bony prominences.

Materials used for padding include:

1. *Stockinette.* A seamless tubing of knitted cotton 1 to 12 inches (2.5 to 30.4 cm) wide, stockinette stretches to fit any contour snugly.
2. *Sheet wadding.* A glazed cotton bandage 2 to 8 inches (5 to 20 cm) wide is available as a sheeting. It is used over stockinette or in place of it.
3. *Soft roll.* A soft roll of thin cotton batting has some stretch for smooth contour.
4. *Felt.* Sheeting made of wool or blends of wool, cotton, or rayon available in thicknesses ranging from $\frac{1}{8}$ to $\frac{1}{2}$ inch (3 to 13 mm), felt is cut into desired sizes to fit bony prominences. Felt pads are applied over sheet wadding. The plaster adheres to pads and prevents them from slipping.
5. *Foam rubber.* Available as a sheeting $\frac{1}{4}$ to 1 inch (6.4 to 25 mm) in thickness, foam rubber may be used in place of felt.
6. *Webril.* Webril is a soft, lint-free cotton bandage. The surface is smooth but not glazed, so that each layer clings to the preceding one and the padding lies smoothly in place.

Plaster Casts

Plaster is gypsum or anhydrous calcium sulfate. It is finely ground to break up the crystals and is then heated to drive out the water. When water is added again, recrystallization takes place and the plaster sets. It was first used as a method of splinting fractures in the nineteenth century.

Plaster bandages and splints are made of crinoline or other fabric, with the plaster powder entrapped in the meshes. These are available in rolls or strips 2 to 8 inches (5 to 20 cm) wide. Plaster splints are either supplied precut or made from rolls as the need arises. Usually six or eight thicknesses of the desired length are used. To provide added strength, splints are applied over areas that may weaken from extra strain. Plaster bandages and splints are available with three types of plaster.

1. *Slow setting* requires up to 18 minutes to set. It is used in large casts requiring more time to apply and mold. It permits blending of the layers.
2. *Medium setting* requires up to 8 minutes to set. This type is used in average-size casts.
3. *Fast setting* requires 4 to 5 minutes to set. It is advantageous for small casts on children who are difficult to keep in position. Many orthopaedists prefer fast-setting type in all kinds of casts; it is the most universally used type of plaster.

Application of Plaster

1. Spread a disposable plastic or nonwoven fabric sheet on the floor around the table to catch drips.

2. Protect the table. If the orthopaedic table is used, spread a sheet over table parts after the patient is suspended.
3. Protect patient's hair with a cap.
4. Use a disposable plaster pail or a plastic liner bag in a plaster bucket.
5. Fill bucket with water at room temperature. Water warmer than 70° to 75° F (21° to 24° C) will speed setting time and may cause excessive loss of plaster from the fabric. More important, plaster will get even hotter than its normal exothermic reaction if dipped in hot water.
6. Don nonsterile disposable gloves to protect hands from irritation by lime content.
7. Remove outer wrapping. Start soaking plaster only when the surgeon is ready to apply it. Keep just ahead in soaking it. Have the next roll ready when needed, but do not prepare several rolls ahead. They may harden and, if used, can produce an ineffective laminated cast. Avoid waste.
8. Hold the bandage under water in a vertical position to allow air bubbles to escape from the rolled end. When air bubbles stop rising, it is soaked through. Compress ends between fingers and palm of each hand to remove excess water. This procedure prevents telescoping during use.
9. Open the end about 1 inch (2.5 cm), and hand to the surgeon.
10. Fanfold a strip once toward the center, before soaking, leaving the ends free to grasp. When soaking, grasp an end in each hand, press hands together and submerge strip in water for a few seconds; remove it and pull strip taut by the ends. It may seem drippy, but the layers blend together well when quite wet.
11. Ask the surgeon if another roll will be needed before soaking it when the cast appears near completion.
12. Handle the cast with flat open hands, never fingers, and support the patient in such a way that he or she cannot attempt to bend an incorporated joint. Wet plaster has only one third to one half its ultimate strength when dry. The person who supports an extremity while a cast is being applied takes care not to make finger-pressure areas in plaster that will damage tissue under it.
13. Elevate an extremity on a pillow until the cast hardens. If it is laid on a hard surface, flat pressure areas may be pressed onto it.
14. Clean up as much as possible while the cast is being applied. Wipe plaster off equipment as well as off the patient before it dries. It is easy to remove when still damp; after it dries it must be scraped off. A cast dryer, if used, hastens drying.
15. Avoid splashing plaster on furniture, walls, and floor.
16. Clean equipment and table thoroughly. If sink has a plaster trap, all plaster drip can be washed down the sink and contents of the bucket poured into the sink. If there is no plaster trap, leave bucket until plaster in the bottom hardens; then empty water and throw the plaster pail or plastic liner bag into the trash. Clean a reusable bucket as soon as finished with it.

Casts Commonly Used

Cylinder A circular cast, made by wrapping the plaster bandages around an extremity, is used after closed or open reductions of fractures, after some surgical procedures for immobilization, or for the purpose of resting a part of an extremity.

Walking Cast A rubber walking heel or polyurethane sole is applied to the sole of a cylinder cast for ambulation. Use of a lower extremity helps to maintain strength and muscle tone and to prevent atrophy.

Hanging Cast A cylinder is applied to the arm with the elbow flexed. It extends from the shoulder over the hand, leaving the thumb and fingers free. A wire loop is incorporated at the wrist. A strap through this loop and around the neck suspends the arm. The weight of the cast provides needed traction on the humerus.

Shoulder Spica Applied to trunk, arm, and hand, leaving fingers and thumb free, a spica cast is used after some surgical procedures on the shoulder or humerus or for a fracture of the humerus. The orthopaedic table may be used for its application, or the patient may sit on a stool with the surgeon supporting the arm in the desired position.

Hip Spica A hip spica cast is applied to the trunk and one or both legs following some hip procedures and fractures of the femur. The orthopaedic table is used. The sacrum rests on a sacral rest. The perineal post provides countertraction. Attachments may be used to support the legs of an adult.

Minerva Jacket A Minerva jacket is applied from the hips to the head. If the head is to be completely immobilized, it is included in the jacket. The plaster is molded to fit around the face and lower jaw. A part of the plaster at the back of the head is cut out. It is used for fractures of cervical or upper thoracic vertebrae. The orthopaedic table is necessary.

Body Jacket A body jacket extends from the axillae to the hips to immobilize vertebrae. Application of this cast usually requires the orthopaedic or Risser table with the necessary attachments, although sometimes the patient may stand on the floor. Traction may be applied by an overhead sling. If an open surgical procedure is to be performed with the patient in a body cast, a cast cutter must be at hand in case of respiratory difficulty. However, a body cast is usually bivalved before a patient is given an anesthetic.

NOTE An opening is always made over the abdomen of a Minerva or body jacket to allow space for lung expansion and decompression of abdominal distention that normally occurs with ingestion of food. A folded towel may be placed over the abdomen before the stockinette is pulled over the body. This is removed when the opening is made in the cast to allow more space between the body and cast.

Plaster Shell A body jacket is cut along each side, into anterior and posterior parts. The parts may be fastened together by heavy straps with buckles, or the patient may rest in one while the other is removed temporarily.

Wedge Cast A wedge-shaped portion is cut from the cast. The edges are brought together and held with plaster reinforcement. This cast is used to overcome angulation in a fracture.

Plaster Splint Six or more thicknesses of plaster of the desired width and length may be applied to the posterior part of an extremity and secured with gauze or cotton elastic bandage. Excess water is pressed from the plaster splint after it is immersed in water. A splint may be used for immobilization of a fracture of the ulna or fibula.

Hairpin or Sugar-Tong Splint A splint twice as long as the lower arm and hand is used for a fracture of the ulna or radius. After the plaster is soaked, it may be covered with stockinette. Starting with one end on the back of the hand, the splint is placed around the flexed elbow. The palm of the hand and fingers rest on the other end of it. It is secured with a bandage.

Abduction Hip Splint An abduction hip splint keeps hips in constant abduction. If desired for postoperative management, it is applied immediately after a hip procedure.

Plaster Rope Plaster rope may support the arm in a shoulder spica or join legs in a bilateral hip spica. It is made by twisting a wet roll of plaster bandage into a rope as it is unwound, fanfolding to the desired length and drawing it through cupped hand to blend the strands. A wooden splint may be incorporated into the rope for reinforcement.

Molds Molds are made as plaster patterns for removable metal or leather braces for the body, neck, or extremities.

Trimming, Removing, and Changing Casts

Rough edges of plaster are trimmed off and the edges of a cast are covered with stockinette or adhesive tape to protect the patient's skin. Instruments specifically designed for cutting through plaster must be used for trimming or removing casts. These include:

1. *Plaster knives,* which have short slightly curved blades.
2. *Plaster scissors,* which are heavy bandage scissors.
3. *Electric cast cutter,* which is an oscillating saw. It cuts the cast but not the stockinette or other padding under it because the padding moves with the oscillations. The patient's skin also moves somewhat and is not injured if touched lightly, although care should always be taken not to touch the skin. One model has a vacuum attached to pick up the plaster dust created by the saw. A carbide steel blade is recommended for cutting fiberglass cast (see discussion on next page). A regular blade dulls quickly and can result in an inadvertent burn to patient.
4. *Cast spreader,* which is a long-handled instrument that has thin serrated jaws that can be inserted in the cutting line to pry open the cast.
5. *Cast bender,* which is a heavy forceps-type instrument used to bend a small portion of the edge of a cast away from an area, such as a portion of a jacket away from the mouth and chin, to give freer movement.

Sharp plaster knives or scissors are usually used to trim casts. For large casts the electric cast cutter may be used, for example, to cut an opening over the abdomen of a body jacket. In a hip spica, adequate space is provided for use of the bedpan without soiling. If it is necessary to cut a "window" (i.e., a small opening in a cast to remove sutures or to inspect an area), it is put back in place and secured with a few turns of plaster bandage. An opening in a cast encourages swelling of the tissues under it, known as *window edema.*

When the edema in a wound under a cast recedes, the cast does not furnish as much immobilization as may be desired. The cast is usually changed at this stage. A cast may be changed periodically during long-term immobilization because muscles atrophy with disuse. The cast becomes loose as muscle size decreases.

Skin sutures are removed at time of a cast change if cast was applied following surgical procedure. A sterile suture removal tray should be ready for use when requested. Sterile sheet wadding may be needed to cover the wound after sutures are removed and before another cast is applied.

If the patient has been in a cast for some time, the skin is apt to be oily, somewhat soiled, and rough. If the surgeon wishes the skin cleansed before applying another cast, only superficial dirt can be removed. Scrubbing off oily scales may cause irritation. Usually skin is not washed but rubbed with cold cream or powdered with talc before applying sheet wadding and a new cast.

Provide a large plastic-lined trash container in which to put the wrappings, trimmings and removed cast during cast application and removal. (This can be sealed and taken directly for disposal with minimal environmental contamination.)

Wash knives, scissors, cutter, spreader, and bender promptly after use. Before putting instruments away, apply oil to all instrument joints to prevent rust and corrosion.

Fiberglass Casts

A woven fiberglass tape impregnated with a water-activated polyurethane resin can be used for casting or bracing. Polypropylene stockinette is applied over the patient's skin. Polypropylene web wrap may be used for extra padding over bony prominences and pressure points. The person applying the cast must wear gloves or coat hands with a silicone hand cream to facilitate smoothing and blending the layers of the fiberglass tape and to prevent resin pickup on the hands. The resin is activated by warm water. The tape is applied in the same manner as plaster.

The cast is lighter, thinner, yet stronger and more porous for better ventilation than is a plaster cast. The outside may get wet without deterioration. X-rays penetrate synthetic materials better than they do plaster to evaluate the healing process. A combination of plaster and synthetic resin on a gauze backing produces a thinner, more waterproof cast that weighs less and is as strong as a plaster cast. Because of these advantages, casting tapes are preferred by many orthopaedic surgeons for extremity casts.

ORTHOPAEDIC CART

For closed reduction of fractures, traction, and postoperative applications, many orthopaedic appliances must be available and at hand when needed. An orthopaedic cart can provide the necessary items for these situations. The items may vary somewhat at different hospitals, but many will be universally used. The cart can be taken wherever needed in the OR suite. One shelf should be kept for sterile items:

1. Suture removal trays
2. Webril and soft roll
3. Assorted gauze dressings and bandages
4. Skin antiseptic agents

Another shelf should contain nonsterile items:

1. Pulleys and attachments for beds
2. Ropes, weights, and carriers
3. Felt padding and foam rubber
4. Arm and shoulder immobilizers
5. Pelvic slings and rods
6. Assorted sizes of gauze and muslin bandages, stockinette, sheet wadding, soft rolls, etc.
7. Stapler
8. Safety pins
9. Cold cream and talcum powder
10. Disposable plaster pail or bucket with plastic liner bag
11. Plastic bag for trash
12. Assorted sizes of plaster rolls and splints
13. Cast cutters, knives, scissors, spreaders, and bender

Splints, overhead traction bars, shock blocks, footdrop stops, and other bulky items are obtained from the cast room as needed.

COMPLICATIONS FOLLOWING ORTHOPAEDIC SURGERY

Thromboembolism is the most common postoperative complication of orthopaedic surgery, particularly if the patient must be immobilized for an extended period. Fat embolism is possible following fracture of a long bone. Pneumonia can be fatal for elderly persons. Urinary tract infection and skin breakdown also are potential problems, particularly in the elderly patients. As previously emphasized, wound infection can be devastating.

BIBLIOGRAPHY

AAOS Task Force on AIDS and Orthopaedic Surgery: *Recommendations for the prevention of human immunodeficiency virus (HIV) transmission in the practice of orthopaedic surgery,* Park Ridge, Ill, 1989, American Academy of Orthopaedic Surgeons.

Alexander W: Hips while-u-wait: designing total hips during surgery, *Today's OR Nurse* 12(7):14-17, 1990.

Allen GJ: Arthroscopic Bankart repair of the shoulder, *Surg Technol* 23(2):6-11, 1991.

Allen GJ: Bone grafting in fracture management, *Surg Technol* 26(8):8-12, 1994.

Allen GJ: Meniscal repair in the knee, *Surg Technol* 25(7):8-12, 1993.

Alston R: Bilateral patellar tendon rupture, *Surg Technol* 26(11):8-11, 1994.

Anderson BA: Endoscopic carpal tunnel release, *AORN J* 57(2):413-428, 1993.

Bach BR et al: Surgical arthroscopy for anterior cruciate ligament reconstruction, *Today's OR Nurse* 12(2):4-9, 1990.

Banitt L: Total elbow arthroplasty procedure, *Surg Technol* 24(4):8-11, 1992.

Barrett JB, Bryant BH: Fractures, *AORN J* 52(4):755-771, 1990.

Binski D et al: The Ilizarov external fixation system: the new perioperative challenge, *Today's OR Nurse* 12(8):6-11, 1990.

Boyd GS: Free fibular graft to the hip for avascular necrosis, *Surg Technol* 25(3):8-12, 1993.

Bradley JP et al: Achilles tendon ruptures, *AORN J* 55(4):994-1008, 1992.

Brazytis KE, Hergenroeder PT: Arthroscopic ankle surgery, *AORN J* 55(2):492-502, 1992.

Campbell TD: Anterior cruciate ligament reconstruction: using patellar tendon grafts, *AORN J* 51(4):944-966, 1990.

Caruthers BL: Hemilaminectomy with lumbar diskectomy, *Surg Technol* 23(6):8-11, 1991.

Clevenger SW: Miller/Galante total knee systems, *Surg Technol* 24(2):26-29, 1992.

DeSisto S: Endoscopic automated percutaneous lumbar diskectomy, *Surg Technol* 27(1):8-12, 1995.

Driscoll AH: When your patient wears an Ilizarov device, *Am J Nurs* 93(6):63-65, 1993.

Duckworth MA, Marquez RA: Carbon dioxide laser arthroscopy, *AORN J* 54(4):716-729, 1991.

Dykes PC: Minding the five Ps of neurovascular assessment, *Am J Nurs* 93(6):38-39, 1993.

Everett CL et al: Arthroscopic dissecans, *AORN J* 55(5):1194-1209, 1992.

Gaehle KE et al: Adult lumbar scoliosis, *AORN J* 54(3):546-560, 1991.

Gaehle KE et al: Thoracolumbar burst fractures, *AORN J* 55(3):721-731, 1992.

Gregory B: *Perioperative nursing series: orthopaedic surgery,* St Louis, 1994, Mosby.

Klinger DL: Acetabular fractures, *AORN J* 61(1):157-178, 1995.

Lenke LG et al: Lumbar disk herniation, *AORN J* 59(6):1230-1248, 1994.

Lester VS et al: Total knee arthroplasty, *AORN J* 58(4):731-746, 1993.

Mathias JM: Robot helps perform hip surgery, *OR Manager* 9(1):10-11, 1993.

Neighbors JH: Spinal stabilization: an anterior approach, *Surg Technol* 24(6):8-12, 1992.

Nussman DS, Poole RC: Rescue and recovery in traumatic hip dislocation, *Am J Nurs* 91(11):34-38, 1991.

Pellins TA: How to manage hip fractures, *Am J Nurs* 94(4):46-50, 1994.

Preksto D: The Kaneda device: a new stabilization system, *AORN J* 55(3):734-746, 1992.

Ross BR et al: Anterior cruciate ligament: history, anatomy, and reconstruction, *Surg Technol* 24(2):14-29, 1992.

Roth M: Metacarpophalangeal joint implant arthroplasty, *AORN J* 60(6):929-942, 1994.

Sherk HH: *Lasers in orthopaedics,* Philadelphia, 1990, JB Lippincott.

Snyder SJ, Kapp K: Arthroscopic evaluation and treatment of rotator cuff pathology, *AORN J* 56(2):225-241, 1992.

Valentine WA et al: Ilizarov external fixation, *AORN J* 51(6):1530-1545, 1990.

Wallace DJ: Elder care: managing arthritis in elderly, *AORN J* 51(4):1074-1080, 1990.

CHAPTER 33

Ophthalmic Surgery

HISTORICAL BACKGROUND

Disorders of the eye have plagued human beings since time immemorial. None has been as well-documented as the *cataract*, an opacification of the crystalline lens of the eye. The word *cataract*, originally derived from the Greek word *kataraxtos* (καταρραχτος), was translated in Arabic to mean "mist of a waterfall." Throughout history cataract has been called by various names, such as "pearl of the eye."

Awareness of cataract probably extends back at least 3000 years. The finding of Bronze Age (2000-1000 BC) instruments such as those used for an ancient couching treatment helps substantiate this belief. Couching consisted of striking a blow to the front of the eye with a sharp instrument to spontaneously dislocate the opacified lens and push it back into the vitreous cavity. Light then entered the pupil. Couching was used by the Hindus, Greeks, Romans, and Arabs.

A treatise written centuries before Christ by the reknowned Hindu surgeon, Shusruta, taught that a disorder of eye fluids caused an opacity of the lens. Hippocrates wrote that pupils of the eyes sometimes became distorted, taking on the color of the sea.

In the early Christian era, Celsus differentiated between incipient (beginning) and mature cataracts. Galen thought the white opacity to be partly in the lens and partly in the aqueous humor in the form of a membrane floating between the lens and the iris. That belief was held, and couching was practiced sporadically until the mid-eighteenth century when J. Daviel, a French surgeon, performed the first deliberate lens removal. Extracapsular cataract extraction was the accepted technique during the first half of the twentieth century until an intracapsular technique became popular in the mid-1940s.

The first corneal transplant in which a scarred cornea was replaced with a clear cornea was performed around 1817. It failed because heterologous tissue was used instead of homologous tissue. The first reported successful full-thickness graft of full corneal depth to remain clear was transplanted in 1905. Although attempted in the interval, corneal transplantation did not become an established technique until after World War II. Since then, the technique has been refined to produce a high rate of favorable outcomes.

Fruitless attempts were made in the early eighteenth century to implant lenses. The modern era of implantation of plastic intraocular lens evolved from an incidental observation. Surgeons in England noted a lack of reactivity to fragments of plastic from shattered plane canopies that penetrated the eyes of fighter pilots in World War II. Posterior chamber lenses placed in the 1950s produced disappointing long-term results mainly because of dislocation. These lenses subsequently had to be removed because of inadequate fixation. The first series of anterior chamber lenses placed in front of the iris sometimes produced delayed corneal damage. The iris-supported lenses were designed to avoid this complication, but they are seldom used because of mechanical problems such as dislocation and corneal irritation. However, modifications of the design of anterior chamber lens have reduced complications. Since the 1960s the posterior chamber lens has attained greatest popularity.

The development of fluorescein angiography, visualization of the entire retinal vascular tree by injection of a fluorescing dye, has expanded the knowledge of retinal and choroidal physiology and disease, resulting in improved therapy.

The advent of ophthalmic lasers that provide ablation of pathologic conditions with light energy was a great step forward. Laser therapy obviates the need for some surgical procedures for many patients. Initially used primarily for vascular diseases such as diabetic retinopathy, laser use has expanded to include corneal reshaping and treatment of glaucoma and secondary membrane. Ophthalmologists pioneered the use of medical lasers and operating microscopes.

The main causes of blindness are retinal disorders, glaucoma, and cataract. A substitute system for vision in the eye, one of the most intricate organs in the body, does not exist, but modern ophthalmic techniques can cure or greatly improve many types of impaired vision. Ocular disorders may be the initial manifestations of systemic disease. Early detection and referral on the part of an alert ophthalmologist can be life-preserving as well as sight-preserving.

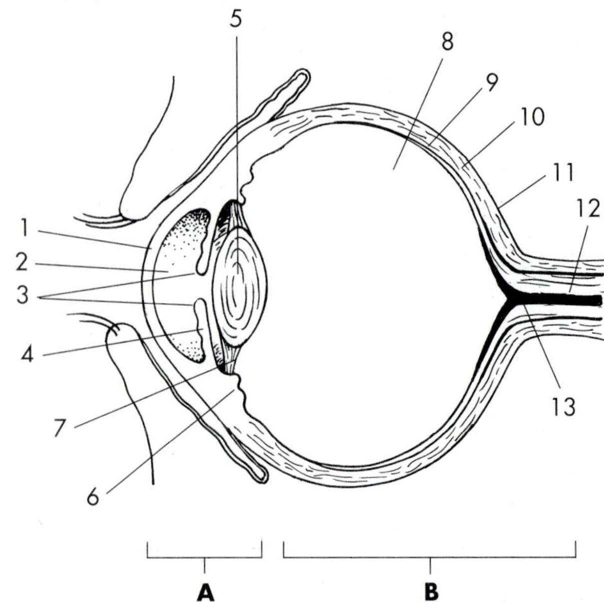

FIGURE 33-1 Anatomy of the eye. **A,** Anterior segment: *1,* cornea; *2,* anterior chamber; *3,* pupil; *4,* iris; *5,* lens; *6,* ciliary body; *7,* zonule. **B,** Posterior segment: *8,* vitreous body; *9,* retina; *10,* choroid; *11,* sclera; *12,* optic nerve; *13,* central retinal artery.

EYE

A thorough understanding of the anatomic structure and physiology of the eye is fundamental to comprehension of the surgical procedures (Figure 33-1).

Anatomy

The *globe,* or *eyeball,* is situated within the bony orbit surrounded by a padding of fatty tissue. Its position is maintained by extraocular muscles and fascial attachments. The *sclera,* the white outer tissue layer of the globe, is contiguous with the transparent avascular *cornea* anteriorly. The *conjunctiva* is the mucous membrane that lines the inner side of the eyelids and the exposed portion of the sclera except for the cornea.

The *anterior segment* of the eye includes the cornea, the anterior chamber filled with aqueous fluid (humor), the circular pigmented iris, and the lens. The lens consists of clear, transparent gelatinous protein encased in a capsule. It is supported by a series of suspensory ligaments called *zonules.* The portion of the eye lying beyond the lens, the *posterior segment,* contains the vitreous fluid, which must be clear for vision, the retina, and the choroid linings, which are the vascular nourishing layers.

Physiology

The function of vision requires:

1. Visual apparatus
2. Source of light
3. Intact neurovascular communication with the brain
4. Interpretation by the brain of what is seen

The eye resembles a camera with a compound lens system. Light rays emanating from an object in the field of vision are transmitted to the eye, where they traverse the optical system to get to the retina. The retina corresponds to the film of the camera. The area of highest sensitivity for details is called the *macula,* which is located approximately in the center of the retina at the posterior pole.

The *optical system* is comprised of the transparent cornea, or window of the eye; the aqueous fluid behind the cornea; the pupil, or opening in the colored iris; and the lens. The naturally flexible lens focuses light rays by bending them to form an image on the retina, the innermost layer of the eye that contains the visual-nerve endings. These sensory cells translate patterns of light into nervous impulses, which are transmitted to the brain via the optic nerve. The cells are connected to nerve fibers, which converge toward the brain to become the optic nerve. The occipital portion of the brain interprets the light-ray images registered on the retina. The intensity of light is automatically determined by the size of the pupil, which is controlled by the iris muscles. The iris action functions like the shutter of a camera.

OCULAR SURGICAL PROCEDURES

Surgical treatment of the eye can be divided for convenience into two main classifications:

1. *Extraocular,* conditions affecting the exterior surface of the eye or the orbit
2. *Intraocular,* conditions pertaining to the interior contents of the eye

Extraocular Procedures

Eyelid

Excision of Neoplasm of Lid Tissue may be excised with a knife, by electrodesiccation (high-frequency electric current), or by cryosurgery. An extremely common but benign tumor of the lid is the *chalazion,* a cystic alteration of one of the oil-secreting meibomian glands in the lid. The resulting accumulation of oil forms a hard tumor of the lid, requiring excision. This is usually an office or ambulatory surgical procedure.

Following removal of a malignant lesion of the lid, repair employs plastic procedures such as Z-plasty and sliding flaps from adjacent areas and full- or partial-thickness flaps from the opposing lid to close the defect (see Chapter 34).

Correction of Ptosis Ptosis, drooping of the upper lid, may be acquired in adults, although it is more commonly congenital (see Chapter 42, p. 862). An incision on the front or back surface of the lid exposes the levator muscle. This muscle is dissected free of its adjacent attachments, and a variable amount is excised in proportion to the degree of ptosis. Fasanella-Servet is a popular surgical procedure for correcting a minor degree of ptosis.

Repair of Acquired Malformation of Lid Conditions such as senile ectropion or entropion most commonly affect the lower lid. *Ectropion* is a condition in which either lid is *everted* (turned out) so as to expose the conjunctival surface. *Entropion* is the opposite condition in which the lid margin is *inverted* (turned in). Frequently the lashes then abrade the cornea. Various procedures may be employed to correct both conditions.

Blepharoplasty Common results of aging are stretching of the eyelid skin and bulging of orbital fat from between the muscle fibers of the lids. Both cause cosmetic disfigurement or "baggy lids," and in extreme cases may obstruct vision. Redundant fold(s) of skin and herniated pockets of fat are removed. Defects in the muscle layer are repaired (see Chapter 34, p. 715).

Lacrimal Apparatus

Lacrimal Duct Dilatation Lacrimal duct dilatation is performed for excessive tearing. A series of probes, graduated in size, are introduced one by one into the duct system to permit freer drainage of tears.

Dacryocystectomy Extirpation or removal of the lacrimal sac is performed for chronic dacryocystitis. It does not reestablish the tear-drainage system.

Dacryocystorhinostomy Construction of a new opening into the nasal cavity from the lacrimal sac is done to correct congenital malformation of or trauma to the nasolacrimal duct. A new tear-drainage system is constructed.

Extraocular Muscle Procedures

Procedures on oculomotor muscles, those that control eye movement, are performed to correct misalignment that interferes with the ability of the two eyes to remain in simultaneous focus on a viewed object. The surgical procedures correct muscle imbalance by strengthening a weak muscle or by weakening an overactive one. Although commonly performed on children (see Chapter 42, p. 862), muscle procedures may be required in adult patients for:

1. Untreated childhood strabismus (squint)
2. Unsatisfactory result from a childhood surgical procedure
3. Trauma to the brainstem or to the orbit with resultant muscle injury or paralysis
4. Systemic disease, such as thyroid exophthalmos, and muscle paralysis
5. Cerebrovascular accident (CVA) with resultant muscle paralysis

Orbital Procedures

Decompression Decompression is the treatment for severe exophthalmos, protrusion of the eyeball(s), that does not respond to medical treatment.

Orbital Tumors Exploration may be approached through a lateral wall or roof of the orbit, depending on the location of the tumor. The procedure may involve a multidisciplinary team of surgeons (see Chapter 36, p. 745).

Procedures for Removal of Eye

Following removal of an eyeball, the patient is fitted with an artificial eye to restore cosmetic appearance. A spherical implant, such as silicone, plastic, tantalum, or hydroxyapatite, may be used to line the orbit and provide support for a prosthetic eye. The eye muscles are sutured to the implant, thereby providing natural movement, allowing growth of surrounding tissue, and preventing the lower lid from sagging. The type of prosthesis that can be used depends on the procedure for removal of the eyeball.

Enucleation Enucleation is the complete removal of the eyeball and severing of its muscular attachments. Muscle stumps are preserved. The space between them forms a pocket for the spherical plastic artificial eye prosthesis. Overlying fascia and conjunctiva are closed to hold the prosthesis in the socket. Contraction of eye muscles causes the prosthesis to move in the socket, simulating normal eye movements.

Evisceration Evisceration removes the contents of the eyeball only, leaving the outer sclera and muscles intact for attachment to a prosthesis. This procedure reduces the danger of transmission of intraocular infection to the orbit and brain. Predisposing factors include destruction of the eyeball by injury or disease and absolute glaucoma (hard blind eye).

Exenteration Exenteration is the removal of the entire eye and orbital contents, including tendon, fatty, and fibrous tissues. It is done for a malignant tumor of the lids or the eyeball that has extended into the orbit. Extensive plastic reconstruction is necessary before fitting an artificial eye.

Intraocular Procedures

Many ophthalmic surgeons subspecialize in *anterior segment surgery* on the cornea, iris, and lens or in *posterior segment surgery* on the vitreous body, retina, and sclera. Both types of surgery require specialized instrumentation. The operating microscope is used for intraocular procedures by most surgeons.

Corneal Procedures

Although it consists of resilient tissue, the continually exposed cornea is especially susceptible to injury and infection.

Cauterization Cauterization with chemicals or heat is sometimes used for corneal ulceration that does not respond to antibiotics. This is sometimes performed for herpes simplex virus infections of the corneal epithelium. It may be used in conjunction with topical antiviral agents.

Pterygium Pterygium is a benign growth of conjunctival tissue over the corneal surface. Although usually slow growing, pterygia can become fairly aggressive, especially in southern climates. A significant decrease in visual acuity secondary to induced astigmatism and corneal scarring can result from the abnormal growth. A popular surgical technique devised for its eradication is the *bare sclera method*. This involves excision of the entire pterygium, leaving an area of bare sclera. Beta radiation may be used as an adjunct to surgical treatment.

Corneal Transplantation (Keratoplasty) The damaged cornea may be removed and replaced with healthy cornea from a human donor (Figure 33-2). This procedure is indicated when scars or opacities on the cornea reduce or destroy vision by preventing transmission of a clear image. The cornea must be clear to permit light to enter and focus on the retina. Corneal opacity may result from degenerative changes, scars from chemical burns, perforated corneal ulcers, trauma, or edema following a cataract surgical procedure. In addition, ocular surgery such as phacoemulsification, vitrectomy, and intraocular lens implantation potentially can damage corneal endothelium. Keratoplasty is the most successful transplantation procedure, with considerably less rejection phenomenon than other tissues, except bone, because the cornea is avascular. The greatest advance in technique to reduce the rate of rejection and restriction of activity during convalescence has been the use of the operating microscope and microsutures. Continuous 10-0 or 11-0 nylon sutures are left in situ with minimal tissue reaction. Two types of grafts are used:

1. Full-thickness, the common type, in which the entire thickness of the cornea is replaced, usually 6.5 to 8 mm in diameter (penetrating keratoplasty)
2. Partial-thickness or lamellar, less popular, in which only the top layer of the cornea, not its entire depth, is replaced (lamellar keratoplasty)

An opaque cornea is an optically nonfunctioning one. The goal is to provide recipients with the highest quality corneal tissue. Fresh, healthy cornea cut from the promptly enucleated eye of a relatively young donor within 4 to 6 hours of death is considered the best for transplantation. It should be inserted in the recipient eye, which has a healthy retina and optic nerve, as soon as possible to preserve viability and to prevent opacity. However, the acceptable times for collection of tissue after death and transplantation may vary among eye banks.

Donor tissue criteria include the following:

1. Consent for enucleation must conform with state laws. Responsibility for obtaining legal consent may rest with the person who will perform enucleation. A certified eye bank technician may enucleate eyes.
2. Medical information about the potential donor is evaluated. Some conditions that preclude use of donor tissue are unknown cause of death, previous intraocular surgery, Reye's syndrome, lymphosarcoma, rabies, and transmissible diseases

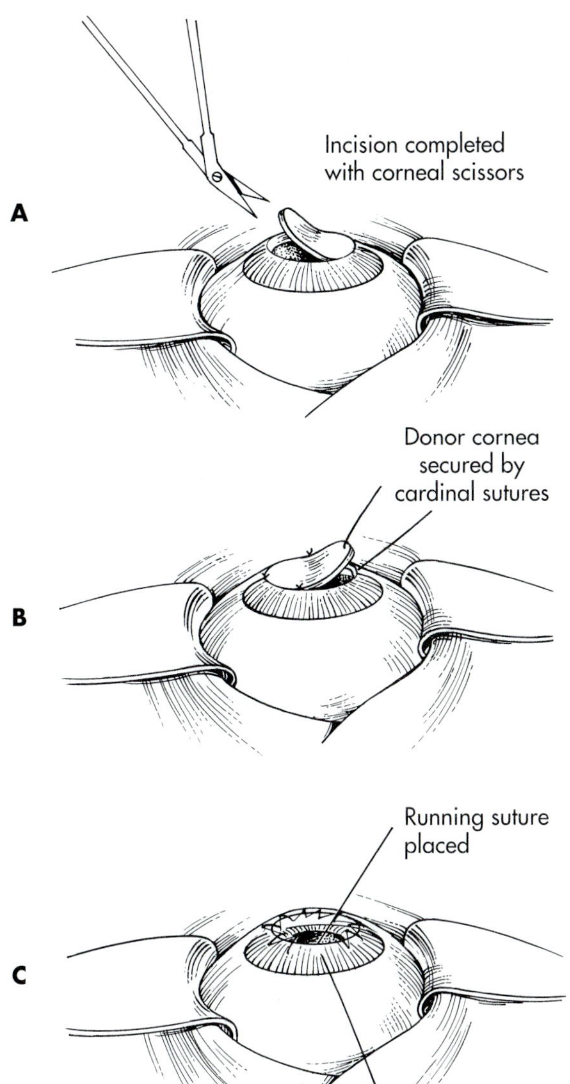

FIGURE 33-2 Corneal transplantation (keratoplasty). **A,** Damaged cornea is excised with corneal scissors. **B,** Donor cornea is secured by cardinal sutures. **C,** Continuous suture remains in situ.

such as hepatitis, human immunodeficiency virus (HIV), and Creutzfeldt-Jakob disease. Donor information must be documented on the donor screening form that accompanies the tissue. A copy should be filed at the eye bank.

3. Endothelium, the very sensitive inner single layer of corneal cells, must be kept intact for eventual transparency of the graft. Either the whole donor globe is removed, or the cornea with scleral rim is excised for transplantation. Sterile technique, removal of as much conjunctiva as possible from the donor globe, avoidance of damage or contamination of the removed eyes, and the use of appropriate transport containers and preservation methods are important factors to optimize the success of the transplant.
4. Eyes are cooled as soon as possible to prevent deleterious effects. Placement of ice bags over the eyes promptly after death slows the metabolism of corneal cells. Generally, the sooner enucleated eyes are refrigerated or corneas removed from the globe, the better the quality of the donor tissue will be. An interval exceeding 5 hours from enucleation to storage is considered unsatisfactory by many corneal surgeons. Enucleated eyes are placed in a controlled environment at the eye bank.
5. Cornea is carefully evaluated for epithelial defects, clarity, presence of any foreign body, or evidence of jaundice or infection. Endothelial cells can be counted, which is a determining factor in estimating prognosis. The higher the count and the more regular the cellular pattern, the better the tissue. Age is not a deterrent if tissue is acceptable for transplantation, but donors younger than age 80 are preferred. The evaluation form must be completed and must accompany tissue. The transplant surgeon also may receive specular microscopic photographs of the endothelium.

Donor tissue preservation methods include the following:

1. Preservative medium. Favored by many eye banks, McCarey-Kaufman (M-K) medium allows storage for 72 to 96 hours. Antibiotics may be added to the medium, but this does not ensure sterility. In the OR the surgeon should inspect container before using the cornea. The cornea should not be used and the eye bank should be notified if medium is turbid or contaminated, such as by a crack in the container. If cornea is used, the remaining corneoscleral rim should be placed in culture medium and sent to the laboratory for culture. However, incidence of positive culture is low. Other preservative medium, such as Dexsol or Optisol that may provide better cellular viability, may be preferred.
2. Refrigerated whole eyes. Rarely used, whole globes can be stored for 24 to 36 hours in a moist chamber at 39° F (4° C).
3. Tissue culture medium. This method has not become widespread because of problems with sterility, which requires strict observation by a laboratory technician and microbiologist. The donor epithelium must not be injured during the process.
4. Cryopreservation. Both cryopreserved corneal and scleral tissue can be used for transplantation or for patching purposes. Use generally is limited to emergency procedures when fresh tissue is not available. Usually this tissue is used less than 6

months after cryopreservation. Precise freezing and defrosting methods are of crucial importance in prevention of injury to the endothelium. When the solution is thawed, the team should work rapidly because of extreme time limitation because corneal metabolism resumes with defrosting. Tissue should be placed immediately within its natural anatomic environment to enhance the potential for successful grafting.

Regardless of the storage method, tissue preferably is used as soon as practical after donation. In the operating room (OR), adequate preparation, teamwork, and standardized transplantation procedure are imperative. The recipient eye is trephined to receive the donor cornea. A separate sterile donor table is set for the surgeon to use in preparing the donor tissue to the exact measurement needed for the recipient eye. Also a tissue recipient information form is completed following a surgical procedure. This form indicates how the tissue was utilized. It is mailed to the eye bank where it is kept on file. If the tissue is contaminated, the donor number and source can easily be traced. Forms include recipient medical information; previous keratoplasties; date, type, and details of the current surgical procedure; and estimate of success.

Available corneal tissue is in limited supply, which places restraints on transplantation. Numerous eye banks in the United States constitute the Eye Bank Association of America, which is tangentially associated with the International Eye Bank. These groups are central clearinghouses for distribution of accessible tissue. They follow a stringent code of ethics in their functions to inform the public of the need for eye donations, procure donated eyes, assist in optimum use of donor corneas locally, or arrange for transportation to an area of greater need. Tissue procurement is facilitated by:

1. Distribution of donor forms from eye banks and organ donation organizations such as Life Bank.
2. Organ donation consent affixed to driver licenses. Family consent is still required before procurement.
3. Education of medical and health care personnel to alert them to ask families of deceased patients for donations. Some state laws require donation request.

Phototherapeutic Keratectomy (PTK) Scar tissue is removed from the cornea with an excimer laser. This restores vision that has been blocked by scars caused by infection, injury, or an inherited condition. This procedure may obviate the need for a corneal transplant.

Refractive Keratoplasty (Corneal Reshaping) Refractive keratoplasty includes a group of surgical procedures that are designed to alter the shape and refractive power (i.e., focusing power) of the cornea to minimize the optical problems of myopia, aphakia, keratoconus, hyperopia, and astigmatism.

1. *Radial keratotomy* reduces myopia (nearsightedness) by making multiple small radial incisions in the cornea to approximately 90% of its depth. These incisions allow stretching and flattening of the anterior corneal surface to reduce corneal curvature and bring light to a focus closer to, or on, the retina. This flattening corrects the refractive error.

   The procedure is performed on patients who have occupational requirements for a visual acuity level without use of glasses or contact lenses, such as certain airline, police, and firefighter positions. The procedure also may be performed for cosmetic reasons. Potential complications include perforations of the cornea; permanent corneal scarring; glaring or variable vision; injury to the lens, causing cataract; and infection. Long-term results, although somewhat unpredictable, are improved with microsurgical techniques. The procedure should be limited to patients with healthy eyes. Only low amounts of nearsightedness can be corrected with this procedure.
2. *Keratomileusis* and *keratophakia* procedures modify corneal refractivity by inserting a lathed button of corneal tissue into the cornea, using a computerized technique. If the patient is the donor *(keratomileusis),* the anterior lamellae of the cornea are removed, reshaped by cryolathing, and then sutured in place. For *keratophakia,* the tissue is obtained from another donor and may be preserved. The lenticule is cryolathed during the surgical procedure, inserted intralamellarly into the recipient cornea, and sutured in place.

   These surgical procedures require a highly specialized experienced team and costly equipment, the cryolathe for shaping the corneal button, and the computer. Research is ongoing to develop other materials that may be used in place of human tissue as a donor lenticule in keratophakia. Very high water content plastic similar to continuous-wear contact lens material has been utilized.
3. *Epikeratophakia* is performed to correct extreme refractive errors such as aphakia (absence of lens inducing extreme hyperopia), myopia, or keratoconus (cone-shaped cornea causing extreme astigmatism). The recipient corneal epithelium is removed, and a previously cryolathed and preserved donor button of corneal tissue is sutured onto the corneal surface of the recipient.
4. *Corneal sculpting (photorefractive keratectomy)* is performed to reshape the corneal surface or to remove scars or other surface irregularities. The ex-

cimer laser is used to reshape the front corneal contour to correct nearsightedness, farsightedness, and astigmatism. The laser beam removes minute amounts of corneal tissue with each pulse wave without burning through or heating the tissue.

5. *Hyperopic thermokeratoplasty* uses a heated needle or the Ho:YAG laser to permanently change the shape of the cornea to correct farsightedness. Use of the heated needle is declining because the Ho:YAG laser can be calibrated to a more precise depth so that it does not penetrate through the full thickness of the cornea. The thermal effect shortens collagen fibers in the periphery of the cornea, thus changing the way light is refracted as it enters the eye. The central portion of the cornea steepens, causing a temporary overcorrection that stabilizes 4 to 6 months postoperatively.

Iris Procedures

Excision of Prolapse Prolapse may follow eye laceration or a surgical procedure on the anterior segment. Fresh prolapses may be reduced mechanically during the surgical procedure or pharmacologically with drugs. Older prolapses should be excised to avoid intraocular infection.

Procedures for Glaucoma Glaucoma is a disease characterized by an abnormally increased intraocular fluid pressure; it often involves the iris. If uncontrolled, glaucoma progresses to atrophy of the optic nerve, hardening of the eyeball, and blindness. The incidence of glaucoma in persons over 40 years of age increases with each decade. There is a familial predisposition to the disease.

Intraocular pressure (IOP) is estimated in one of three ways:

1. *Schiötz' tonometer* records the depth of indentation of the cornea by a plunger of known weight. The degree of indentation is calibrated on the tonometer to correspond to the IOP. The normal numerical value is 10 to 22 mm Hg. This tonometer can be sterilized for use in the OR for preoperative pressure measurement.
2. *Applanation tonometer* attached to the biomicroscope (slit lamp) records the force required to flatten a specified area of cornea. Normal value is 10 to 21 mm Hg. This is considered to be the most accurate method.
3. *Air puff device* measures the force of a reflected amount of air blown against the cornea.

Persons suspected of having glaucoma undergo additional testing. Tonography continuously measures the rate of aqueous outflow with an electric tonometer. Visual fields detect diminished peripheral vision. Gonioscopy determines structure of the angle.

Two basic types of glaucoma are classified anatomically by the size of the angle between the iris and the cornea: *narrow-angle* or *angle-closure glaucoma* and *wide-angle* or *open-angle glaucoma.* If the angle is narrow, the iris may mechanically obstruct outflow of aqueous. This will cause the pressure within the eye to rise and precipitate an attack of acute glaucoma, an emergency situation that is very painful. Surgical intervention, usually a laser iridotomy, affords relief. It is always necessary to widen the angle for this condition and reduce pressure to avoid damage to the optic nerve. Surgical iridectomy occasionally is necessary.

Wide-angle or open-angle glaucoma, the most common, is a chronic type, often of insidious onset, which may cause permanent visual loss before it is detected. The obstruction is not mechanical but a physiologic lack of ability to filter aqueous. Surgical procedures for this type of disease are performed only if medical and laser therapy are unsuccessful. Laser therapy to trabecular meshwork (trabeculoplasty) offers an alternative to conventional surgical procedures for some glaucoma patients (see optical lasers, pp. 701-702). One of the following surgical procedures may be preferred.

1. *Iridectomy,* excising a sector of iris, or *iridotomy,* cutting a small opening in the iris, is done to deflate the mechanical obstruction, thus increasing drainage by permitting the normal outflow of aqueous from the posterior to the anterior chamber. Another use of iridectomy is to create a new optical pupillary opening to improve visual acuity in patients with corneal or lens opacity caused by injury or cataract not associated with glaucoma.
2. *Filtering-type procedures,* of which there are many variations such as *trephining* and *trabeculectomy,* create an artificial fistula between the angle of the anterior chamber and the subconjunctival space to bypass the usual blocked outflow channels. Iridectomy is usually performed as part of the procedure to eliminate blockage of the fistula by the underlying iris. The Nd:YAG laser may be used to reopen filtering sites that have scarred closed following previous surgery for glaucoma. The Ho:YAG laser may be used to create an opening in the sclera, a *sclerostomy,* to promote filtration.
3. *Cyclodialysis, cyclodiathermy,* and *cyclocryotherapy* are performed to diminish aqueous secretion by the ciliary body. Cyclodialysis involves severing the blood supply of the ciliary body. Cyclodiathermy and cyclocryothermy use the application of heat or cold, respectively, for the same purpose.

Secondary glaucoma is often a complication of inflammation such as iritis, which usually responds best to medical treatment. On the other hand, neoplasm, vascular obstruction, trauma or hemorrhage, and other causes of obstruction to aqueous drainage may require surgical intervention. Treatment is directed to the primary cause.

Congenital glaucoma, from an inherent defect in the trabecular meshwork or a systemic disorder, manifests soon after birth. (See discussion of goniotomy in Chapter 42, p. 862.)

Cataract Procedures

A cataract is an opacification of the crystalline lens or its capsule, or both. The more or less opaque lens does not transmit clear images to the retina. Symptoms are related to the location and configuration of the opacity. The cause may be known metabolic or systemic disease, toxic material, radiation, trauma, or genetic factors, or the etiologic factors may be unknown. With advancing age, persons are more prone to develop degenerative cataracts. Although cataracts often develop in both eyes, each cataract tends to mature at a different rate and only one is removed at a time. Most ophthalmologists perform cataract surgery as ambulatory surgical procedures.

Cataracts may be classified as:

1. Congenital (see Chapter 42, p. 862)
2. Senile or primary
3. Secondary, resulting from local or systemic disease or eye injury

Surgical removal, followed by appropriate optical rehabilitation, is the only treatment. The surgical procedure is determined by the patient's age and type of cataract. The procedure is performed according to visual requirements, general health, and the potential for rehabilitation. Cataract extraction is the most frequently performed of all surgical procedures in adults. The advent of microsurgery revolutionized the procedure.

Extracapsular Extraction The lens is delivered through a small incision made in the region of the *limbus,* the junction of the cornea and sclera. The anterior capsule is incised with a cystotome (a miniature hook-shaped knife) or with a bent 25-gauge needle. The nucleus is delivered by manual expression, or it may be aspirated by phacoemulsification (see later discussion). The remaining cortex is extracted by irrigation-aspiration, sparing the posterior capsule, which is left in place. Automated mechanical irrigation-aspiration devices usually are used. Some surgeons prefer a manual technique using a two-way cannula and syringe. The wound is closed with a few sutures.

Extracapsular extraction with preservation of the posterior capsule revolutionized the practice of artificial lens implantation (see pp. 694-695). The implant can be placed at the time of cataract extraction. It resides in the posterior chamber behind the iris, resting on the posterior capsule. Thus the implant is positioned in almost the identical location of the lens it replaces.

The physiologic advantage of extracapsular cataract extraction, with or without phacoemulsification and/or lens implant, is protection of the vitreous and retina by the clear posterior lens capsule, which then serves as an anatomic barrier between the posterior and anterior segments of the eye. Occasionally the posterior capsule will remain opaque. Nd:YAG laser capsulotomy or discission/needling is performed at a later date to provide an optically clear opening.

The following innovations have enhanced the advantages of extracapsular extraction:

1. Operating microscope with coaxial illumination to clearly view posterior capsule during aspiration.
2. Phacoemulsifier to remove nucleus through a tiny (3 to 3.5 mm) incision. The smaller wound facilitates healing and causes less distortion of corneal curvatures.
3. Automated irrigation-aspiration system with electronic sensor to remove all cortex remnants. This minimizes local foreign protein reaction.
4. Nd:YAG laser to atomize posterior capsule opacity. The laser achieves a better result than discission/needling, which requires a second surgical intervention. The laser can be used immediately postoperatively or the procedure can be delayed. The laser can be used under a drop of local anesthetic without an incision and blood loss.
5. Intraocular lens designed to achieve insertion into the posterior chamber through a small incision.

Intracapsular Extraction The entire lens, intact within its capsule, is delivered through a moderately sized incision made in the region of the limbus. Before delivery, an iridectomy or multiple iridotomies are performed, chiefly to prevent iris prolapse and to preserve communication between the anterior and posterior chambers. The lens is grasped by mechanical forceps, suction device, or cryoextractor, depending on surgeon's preference.

A miniaturized, sterile disposable cryoextractor facilitates removal of fragile or dislocated cataracts. The cryoprobe freezes onto the surface of the cataract, thus obtaining secure adherence. The freezing technique greatly reduces the inadvertent rupture of capsule during extraction. The scrub person should have a balanced salt solution (BSS) irrigator available for use in case it is necessary to unfreeze unintentional attachment of the cryoextractor to the iris or cornea. The wound is closed watertight with multiple sutures, commonly 10-0 nylon.

With intracapsular lens extraction, no remnant remains in the visual axis that might proliferate or opacify to obstruct vision. The success rate for regaining vision is high, but the procedure's popularity has waned. Fluorescein angiography has identified a number of patients who developed cystoid macular edema postoperatively, resulting in marked loss of visual acuity. Intracapsular extraction may also be followed by retinal detachment, which is discussed later in this chapter.

Linear Extraction Linear extraction is performed in young adults. A small incision is made through the limbus. The anterior capsule is incised and the major portion of it excised with a cystotome. The soft cataractous material is irrigated from the anterior chamber.

Phacoemulsification Although the aspiration technique is commonly used in young persons, it was not successful in adults with senile cataracts until the late 1960s. At that time a sophisticated machine, the *phacoemulsifier,* was developed to break up (fragment) and remove firm, insoluble lens nuclei. This machine, with components for ultrasonic vibration and irrigation-aspiration, permits extracapsular extraction through a very small incision in the limbus. All functions are controlled by foot pedal.

The handpiece of the phacoemulsifier consists of a disposable hollow titanium alloy needle surrounded by a silicone sleeve. The needle is inserted into the anterior chamber following removal of the anterior capsule with a cystotome. The activated needle breaks up the lens with ultrasonic vibrations. While the lens is thus emulsified, a constant flow of BSS irrigating solution through the sleeve prevents heat buildup. The irrigation-aspiration flow is automatically regulated to maintain anterior chamber depth. The aspirator removes the fragments. After the cortex (material surrounding lens nucleus) is removed by irrigation-aspiration, the posterior capsule may be polished with an instrument to remove any residual cortex. The posterior capsule is left intact unless an opacity remains, in which case it may be incised during the initial surgical procedure or at a future time. The limbal incision is closed with one stitch.

Appropriate checks should be made before use of the handpiece and for integrity of the vacuum and irrigating systems. The linear motion of the ultrasonic vibrations is created by electrical impulses. Two types of phacoemulsifiers are in use. In the magnetostrictive machine, the electrical impulses create a magnetic field. The handpiece should be disassembled for cleaning and sterilizing in ethylene oxide gas or high level disinfection and then reassembled on sterile field before use. In the newer piezoelectric machine, electrical impulses stimulate crystals to produce mechanical energy. This generates heat. A cooling pump circulates coolant, either fluid or air, through the power cord. The handpiece is steam sterilizable as a single unit. The scrub person and circulator work closely with the surgeon to monitor the various functions of the machine in use to avoid error. They should also observe the transparent tubes for flow of aspirate. Aspirated fluid is contaminated and is discarded postoperatively in the same manner as all blood or body fluid.

Phacoemulsification has certain *advantages:*

1. It dramatically shortens convalescence. The patient usually returns to full activity in 1 or 2 days.
2. It employs a small incision and minimal suture, which promotes healing.
3. It retains the posterior capsule of the lens to preserve a more physiologically normal condition. The occurrence of post–lens extraction edema and retinal detachment is thereby diminished.
4. The posterior capsule supports an implanted intraocular lens. Postoperative astigmatism is minimized.

The procedure also has *disadvantages:*

1. It is not suitable for all patients. Contraindications are corneal disease, dislocated lens, shallow anterior chamber, difficult-to-dilate pupils, and completely hard, stonelike cataracts.
2. It requires special techniques, which if not thoroughly mastered, may precipitate surgical complications, such as temporary or permanent corneal damage (opacification), prolapse of lens into the vitreous, and vitreous loss.
3. It may injure the cells because of the necessary substantial amount of anterior chamber irrigation. Corneal cells are very sensitive to manipulation and can respond by loss of function.
4. It requires meticulous technical monitoring of the machine. Usual precautions for use of electrical equipment are also observed.

Rehabilitation Following Cataract Extraction Rehabilitation consists of substitution for the missing part, the lens, so that the optical system can function to focus incoming light on the retina. Patients with no optical substitute see only blurred objects of large size with no detail. Rehabilitation may be accomplished by spectacles (glasses), contact lens, or intraocular lens implantation.

Spectacle correction of *aphakia,* the absence of the lens, provides focusing of light. However, because the *spectacle lens* is approximately 2 cm in front of the original lens, it magnifies images so that they are approximately 35% larger than those the patient saw before development and extraction of the cataract. This magnification requires considerable readjustment to judge distances. Also, peripheral areas are distorted. Spectacle type of replacement is intolerable in patients who have good vision in the unaffected eye, because attempts to fuse the dissimilar images of the two eyes cause double vision.

A *contact lens* rests on the cornea only 2 to 3 mm from the original lens. Consequently it causes only 7% magnification and provides a full, undistorted field of vision. A contact lens is often used to replace the optical deficiency caused by cataract extraction. It is difficult for some elderly persons to handle and care for contact lenses because of lack of manual dexterity, arthritic hand and finger joints, or visual defects in the opposite eye. For these patients, an *implanted intraocular lens* offers a feasible and popular alternative.

Implantation of Intraocular Lens

An intraocular lens (IOL) is implanted in almost the identical position of the original lens and therefore does not change size of the retinal image. Spatial displacement as seen by the aphakic eye and narrowing and distortion of the visual field are eliminated, thereby producing early visual rehabilitation. With spatial displacement, orientation in space is changed. Objects are not where they appear to be. An IOL is intended to remain in situ permanently. The implant is usually inserted through the same incision used to remove the defective, natural lens. This is called *primary insertion.* Some surgeons prefer to implant the lens at a later time; this is referred to as *secondary insertion.* The type of IOL used is contingent on the type of cataract extraction the surgeon chooses. Anterior chamber lenses are inserted in conjunction with intracapsular cataract extraction. Posterior chamber lenses require extracapsular extraction. IOL implantation is a microsurgical procedure.

Prescription of the implanted lens (refractive power) involves complex preoperative calculations based on the patient's corneal curvature as determined by keratometer readings, anterior chamber depth, and eyeball axial length. Ultrasonography is helpful in making these determinations preoperatively. The information obtained is fed into a computer that automatically calculates refractive power of the IOL to be selected.

Numerous IOLs of different shapes and sizes are available. The optical portion of a hard lens is made of an inert plastic, polymethyl methacrylate with or without an ultraviolet blocker, polished to a microscopic smoothness. Flexible lenses are made of silicone elastomer. The fixation portion has springlike supports or loops, called *haptics,* made of plastic, usually polypropylene. Some lenses are secured with polypropylene sutures. Lenses differ in design and method of fixation. They can be classified according to placement or method of fixation.

Anterior Chamber (Angle Fixation) The lens consists of a band of plastic long enough to traverse the anterior chamber from one angle to the other. The optical portion is centrally located in the anterior chamber, in front of the pupil. The pupil remains mobile because iris adhesions are not required for fixation. Although anterior chamber lenses are sometimes inserted primarily, they are popular lenses for secondary insertion.

Posterior Chamber (Capsular or Ciliary Body Fixation) Posterior chamber lenses are placed behind the iris and pupil where the patient's own lens had been. Placement of the IOL in the most normal physiologic position results in stabilization of the iris; less irritation of the uveal tract; reduced tendency to iritis, secondary glaucoma, and cystoid macular edema; and stabilization of the optics. Posterior lenses permit safe dilatation of the pupil if necessary to examine or treat posterior structures of the eye, such as the retina.

With capsular fixation, the lower loop of the haptic is inserted into a pocket of capsule created during extraction of the cataract. The lens does not touch the iris. The pupil is free to move.

With ciliary fixation, the haptics are placed between the iris and posterior capsule. They rest on the corona (inner rim) of the ciliary body.

Pros and Cons of IOL Implantation The final decision to implant an artificial lens rests with the surgeon, who should exercise good judgment to avoid serious complication.

Indications for implantation are:

1. Elderly patients with disabling bilateral cataracts and others who cannot adapt to contact lens
2. Patients with occupations having specific visual requirements (e.g., airplane pilots) or difficult working environment (e.g., ranchers in a dusty area)
3. Children with traumatic cataract, thus preventing amblyopia

Contraindications are:

1. Impossibility for follow-up to observe patient for late complications
2. Ocular conditions such as poorly controlled glaucoma or previous retinal detachment
3. Diabetic proliferative retinopathy
4. Poor result in previous implant
5. Patient anxiety in regard to the procedure
6. Young patients with congenital cataracts
7. Endothelial corneal dystrophy
8. Cataracts associated with recurrent iritis

Advantages are:

1. Superior spatial orientation and binocular vision
2. Permanent device unless complications develop
3. Additional option for postcataract refractive correction
4. Unrestricted pupillary dilatation if necessary

Complications are:

1. Corneal damage or latent edema.
2. Prolonged inflammation such as iritis or vitritis.
3. Cystoid macular edema.
4. Secondary cataract (i.e., opacification of the anterior vitreous) from recurrent iritis.

5. Corneal opacity although this is rare with posterior implants.
6. Dislocation or malposition of the lens, which can damage cornea, but fortunately rarely occurs. For repair, type of approach depends on amount of dislocation. With the anterior approach, an anterior vitrectomy is performed to remove vitreous in front of the lens, followed by removal or repositioning of lens. With the posterior approach, the vitrector is used to remove lens through the pars plana (see p. 697).

Retinal Procedures

Following accidental or surgical trauma, or in some degenerative diseases, defects can occur in continuity of the retina. *Retinopathy* is a noninflammatory degenerative disease of the retina. Retinal changes can occur in the diabetic patient (i.e., *diabetic retinopathy*). Diabetes can affect every part of the eye, causing lens changes (cataract), palsied extraocular muscles, glaucoma, or corneal problems. A person who has been a diabetic for more than 15 years has a significant likelihood of having some form of retinopathy, which generally occurs bilaterally. Severity may differ from one eye to the other. The dense network of capillary vessels in the retina makes the eyes vulnerable to microvascular disease. *Retinopathy* is classified as:

1. *Background or nonproliferative.* Bulges or microaneurysms form in retinal capillary walls, eventually permitting leakage and deposition of exudates. Intraretinal hemorrhages occur and are reabsorbed. Disease is confined to the retinal surface. Progressive changes in capillary membranes lead to blockage of capillaries, resulting in retinal ischemia. Deterioration then progresses to the proliferative stage.
2. *Proliferative.* In an effort to relieve retinal anoxia, new blood vessels emerge from the retina and form in the surrounding tissues (i.e., *neovascularization*). These fragile vessels may rupture spontaneously, producing hemorrhage into the retina and/or vitreous humor. The eventual result may be partial or complete blindness. Panretinal photocoagulation (PRP) is one method of eliminating abnormal vascularization. PRP consists of the application of hundreds of laser burns to the peripheral retinal tissue to partially destroy it. The retinal metabolic need for oxygen is thereby reduced. After neovascularization has occurred, laser therapy is less effective in delaying or stopping the destructive process. Therefore early diagnosis and treatment are crucial. In an effort to prevent new vessel formation, lasers are used to cauterize minute hypoxic areas of tissue before damage occurs.

Laser (see optical lasers, pp. 701-702) is used for diabetic retinopathy and other retinopathies such as central serous retinopathy with swelling of the macula, angiomas and hemangiomas, aneurysms, and small tumors and for cauterizing bleeding vessels. Laser light is absorbed selectively by three pigments in the retina: macular xanthophyll, hemoglobin in retinal and subretinal blood vessels, and melanin in retinal pigment epithelium. Laser therapy is not effective in correcting severe retinal damage or detachment.

Repair of Detached Retina The retina can become separated from its surrounding nourishing layer, the choroid. Detachment (i.e., separation) may occur in any region of the retina. *Primary retinal detachment* is characterized by a hole in the retina. *Secondary detachment* is characterized by fluid and/or tissue behind the retina, not necessarily accompanied by a hole. Seepage of vitreous fluid into the potential space between retina and choroid causes the retina to become detached. Serious visual disturbance results. Secondary detachment may result from displacement of the retina by blood, fluid, or tumor. Enucleation is usually indicated for tumor.

Reattachment is effected only by surgical intervention. The retinal defect is sealed off. Often the subretinal fluid is drained. The specific procedure to achieve retinal reattachment is determined by the type and location of the detachment.

1. *Diathermy.* Traditional procedure involves *diathermy coagulation* to an area of the sclera overlying the region of the retinal defect. The resultant localized inflammation acts to seal off the break. Coagulation is delivered by a specialized shortwave diathermy unit.
2. *Cryosurgery.* Some surgeons prefer *cryosurgery* because of the type of adhesion obtained. Therapeutic applications of cryosurgery are basically similar to diathermy. Tissue reactions superficially resemble each other. Cryosurgery is frequently used for anterior tears.
3. *Scleral buckling.* Internal elevation of the sclera may be increased by the *scleral buckling procedure.* This technique involves implantation of a wedge of silicone episclerally or intrasclerally. An encircling band of silicone may be used to keep constant external pressure on the buckle.
4. *Intraocular gas tamponade.* Injection into the vitreous cavity of room air or absorbable inert gas can be used to create an intraocular tamponade. Room air absorbs after 5 days. Inert gases such as short-acting sulfahexafluoride (SF_6), intermediate-acting perfluoroethane (C_2F_6), or long-acting perfluorooctane ($C_3 F_8$) are sometimes used to approximate the retina to the choroid (i.e., flatten the retina against the choroid). With *pneumoretinopexy,* the patient remains in a seated position for a su-

perior tear or prone for a tear near the macula. The position is maintained for several weeks postoperatively so that the gas bubble successfully rises to close the retinal hole. The length of time and position is determined by the ophthalmologist according to each individual patient's need. Pneumoretinopexy is less invasive than scleral buckling for securing a retinal detachment.

5. *Intraocular fluid tamponade.* Silicone oil has been approved by the Food and Drug Administration (FDA) for use as a vitreous substitute to secure a retinal detachment that cannot be corrected through conventional surgical intervention. Silicone oil is used for long-term intraocular tamponade. It is removed by the ophthalmologist several months postoperatively.
6. *Laser therapy.* Laser therapy can be used to secure the retina, except in severe detachment. A laser is frequently used to secure small posterior tears. (See discussion of laser therapy that follows.)

Glaucoma and infection are potential postoperative complications. Glaucoma may be caused by congestion of the uvea by the buckle, increased IOP, or movement of injected gas from the desired site causing blockage of outflow channels of aqueous humor. Infection is evident by swelling, purulent drainage, and loss of optical clarity.

Laser Therapy The laser delivery system employs the binocular microscope of the slit lamp, thus providing stereopsis and greater magnification (see Chapter 15, pp. 286-288 and 290). The nature of the laser beam permits extremely rapid delivery of radiant energy that produces a sharply defined burn. The small lesion it produces can be placed close to macula. Exposure can be as brief as one hundredth of a second and the treated area as small as 50 μm (less than 2/1000 inch) in diameter. Because of this short exposure time, immobilization of eye is unnecessary unless treated area is close to the macula. The macula is the central region of the retina with the clearest visual acuity. Accidental injury may result in loss of central vision. Pupillary dilatation is essential to avoid macular burn.

The *argon laser* is effective in treating retinal holes or tears and diabetic retinopathy. The *krypton laser* can be used to treat lesions closer to the macula and to treat retinal bleeding. The krypton spectrum is poorly absorbed by the red pigment of hemoglobin. Therefore it may be used effectively to treat retinal bleeding in the presence of blood in vitreous humor. Under these circumstances the argon blue laser would be ineffective because of absorption by even a small amount of blood. Similarly, the krypton laser can be used to treat lesions much closer to the center of the macula, the zone of the most distinct vision of the retina, because of its poor absorption of yellow pigment of the retina.

Photocoagulation A retinal hole not surrounded by any detachment may be prophylactically sealed by xenon or laser photocoagulation. These therapeutic modalities, usually performed in an ophthalmic treatment area rather than in the OR, were the outgrowth of traumatic retinal burns caused by watching eclipse of the sun.

The *xenon arc photocoagulator* uses an intense source of multiwavelength light furnished by a xenon tube. This is optically focused and concentrated into a delivering device that is basically an indirect ophthalmoscope. The latter can also be used to view the area to be treated as well as to aim the light beam. The light may be directed to any of the pigmented (light-absorbing) layers of the eye, such as the iris or retina. These darker layers readily absorb the xenon tube's white light. The optical system of the eye is used in the process of focusing the light beam on the desired area. The amount of power and exposure time are completely controlled by the operating ophthalmologist. Vitreous shrinkage possibly leading to an inoperable detachment can be a complication. The pupil of the eye under therapy is dilated to give maximum visibility to the surgeon. The eye is immobilized by local anesthesia to prevent undesired movement, which could result in burn to an area other than the one desired. Also, pain from intensity of the heat is prevented.

Vitrectomy

Vitrectomy is the deliberate removal of a portion of vitreous humor, also called *vitreous body,* that fills the space between the lens and the retina. Therapeutically it is performed for vitreal opacities, vitreal hemorrhage, and certain types of retinal damage or detachment. In addition to other causes, endophthalmitis (i.e., inflammation of internal tissues of eyeball) and the presence of an intraocular foreign body may result in vitreal opacity. Generally candidates for vitrectomy have substantially impaired vision and complicated conditions preoperatively.

Whereas aqueous fluid is a clear liquid, vitreous is normally a transparent, gelatinous, viscid material containing fibrils. The vitreous helps give shape to the eyeball, in addition to serving a refractive function. It permits light rays to pass through it to the retina after the rays have traversed the lens. Diagnostically, removal of a small amount of vitreous provides a sample for microbiologic study in suspected endophthalmitis. The procedure also provides tissue for biopsy to establish the diagnosis of intraocular tumors.

Alterations in vitreous can have serious consequences. Loss of vitreous during surgical procedures is a dreaded complication, particularly of cataract extraction. Subsequent to retinal hemorrhage, common in diabetic patients, bands of scar tissue may opacify the vitreous as well as adhere to the retina near the original bleeding vessel. Traction on the retina by these bands or further cicatrization (scarring) can lead to retinal tears or detachment. Persistent hemorrhage, lasting over a year, is permanent. It will not absorb spontaneously.

For years the vitreous was considered an inaccessible, inoperable area. Research and the advent of microsurgery changed this belief. Loss of vitreous from the posterior segment during the surgical procedure is rendered relatively innocuous if the anterior segment is cleared of vitreous. Thus no residual strands are present to cause traction effects or to block visual function. Also, the eye tolerates subtotal vitreal excision in the posterior segment if the vitreous body is proportionately replaced with BSS.

Vitrectomy is a microsurgical procedure that lasts 2 to 3 hours and requires a skilled retinal surgeon. It is performed with a vitreotome (vitrector) such as the Ocutome or Microvit. These devices, which incorporate a micromotor, terminate in a needlelike tube that contains a cutting mechanism for severing abnormal adhesions and cutting obstructive tissue into small pieces. In addition, the vitreotome has auxiliary connections for aspiration of vitreous, debris, or blood in the posterior segment and for replacement with BSS via a separate infusion catheter to maintain adequate IOP. A fiberoptic light source or pic is inserted into vitreous to illuminate the posterior portion of the globe. Various vitrectomy systems are available, but all have cutting, suction, infusion, and illumination systems.

The scrub person and circulator should assemble and check equipment before the surgical procedure begins. The vitreotome handpiece is attached to sterile tubing, which is connected to a power console. While one person activates various switches, the other tests suction vacuum and cutting function. Test suction at maximum pressure. Place tip in sterile saline and activate until fluid reaches the collection bottle. *Then lower pressure* to the surgeon's preference. To assess cutting, activate switch and check tip visibly and audibly for movement. The infusion catheter is primed with solution of surgeon's choice to remove air bubbles that could disturb the view in the posterior segment. Consult the manufacturer's manual.

Local anesthetic is administered unless the patient's condition necessitates a general anesthetic. Two approaches to the vitreous body are:

1. Through the posterior segment, via the pars plana (i.e., the anterior attachment of the retina). Because the pars plana has no visual function, entry is relatively nontraumatic, with least chance for retinal detachment. The anterior segment remains intact; IOP is maintained. This approach is used to incise opacified vitreous, old hemorrhage, or bands of scar tissue, thereby giving a clear view of the retina and restoring visual function.
2. Through the anterior segment, via incision at the limbus (i.e., junction of the cornea and sclera). A large corneal section is folded back and the vitreous is exposed through the pupillary opening. This approach is used for removal of vitreous inadvertently displaced into the anterior chamber during cataract removal to avoid postoperative complications. The vitreous volume is replaced with BSS. Anterior vitrectomy also is used to correct retinal traction in retinopathy (retrolental fibroplasia) in premature infants.

The procedure is intricate, requiring special equipment. The surgeon may request bipolar cautery with a Charles clip attachment for actively bleeding intraocular vessels. A handheld contact lens placed onto the cornea enhances view of the posterior chamber. This may be held by the assistant. Some lenses have a handle through which continuous infusion can be run to keep the cornea moist. The lens must be precisely positioned. Success of the procedure may depend on the surgeon's view. Occasionally, lensectomy is performed during vitrectomy to facilitate view of the posterior segment.

After removal of vitreous, before wound closure, and with the retina in clear view, the latter is inspected for defects such as holes or vascular abnormalities. If these are found, treatment is applied by means of endocryotherapy, a freezing application delivered by intraocular probe, or endophotocoagulation, photocoagulation delivered by an intraocular device. These maneuvers may be accompanied by injection of air or inert gas to push the retina into physiologic position.

Postoperatively these patients may experience considerable pain, requiring medication, ice packs, and steroid eye drops for treatment of inflammation. After vitrectomy, patients have aphakia if the lens was removed for visualization of the posterior segment and will eventually need optical correction such as that needed after cataract extraction. Vitrectomy can significantly improve vision.

Complications of vitrectomy include iatrogenic retinal damage, vitreous hemorrhage, or cataract formation from damage to the lens. A secondary surgical procedure may be required to repair the retina (e.g., a scleral buckling procedure or intraocular tamponade). No present treatment for retinopathy is without danger. To save vision, some tissue is destroyed or sacrificed.

EYE INJURIES

Various forms and degrees of trauma may occur as a result of injury. *All types of injury require immediate appraisal by an ophthalmologist.* Delay of even minor injuries may result in temporary or permanent loss of vision. Complications include hemorrhage, infection, iritis or tears of the iris, retinal tears or detachment, macular edema, and secondary cataract. Treatment may be immediate, or secondary, if delay is necessary because of life-threatening injuries. Improved surgical management, such as vitrectomy and microsurgery, have reduced the loss of severely injured eyes. The optical result is especially crucial in patients with bilateral eye injuries. Patients with eye injuries should be kept supine if possible until seen by the ophthalmologist.

Evaluation of the injury may necessitate sedating or anesthetizing the patient to prevent further damage at examination. Pressure to the eye must be avoided because bone fragments may be displaced or globe contents emptied.

Injuries may be simple, involving only the external layers, or compound, including inner structures. They may be nonpenetrating, usually caused by a blunt object, or penetrating, caused by a sharp object. The more structures involved, the more difficult it is to salvage an eye.

Treatment, determined by type or combination of injuries, aims to:

1. Promote healing and prevent anatomic distortion by reparative techniques
2. Preserve maximum vision and/or restore it
3. Control pain, by medication
4. Prevent infection and inflammation by antibiotic and steroid administration

Nonpenetrating Injuries

Burns

Burns may be caused by ultraviolet radiation, such as sunlamps or sunlight, or by electric flash. These burns are basically self-limited but rarely surgical. *A chemical burn constitutes an emergency.* Initial treatment consists of flooding the cornea with water. Alkali burns may be further neutralized by prompt irrigation of epithelium-denuded cornea with ethylenediaminetetraacetic acid (EDTA). This is especially important if discrete particles of alkali are superficially imbedded within tissue. EDTA deactivates an enzyme, collagenase, and neutralizes soluble alkali such as sodium hydroxide (lye). Severe burns may be treated with specific amino acids, EDTA, or acetylcysteine (Mucomyst) to inhibit continuing destruction of the cornea by collagenase, but they often progress to corneal opacity and blindness.

Contusions of Globe

Contusions may or may not require surgical treatment. If hemorrhage is present, treatment consists of bed rest and antiglaucoma therapy to keep IOP controlled. It is not unusual for a secondary hemorrhage to occur on the third or fourth day after injury. If the IOP remains high, blood staining of the cornea and damage to the optic nerve may result. It is then sometimes necessary to perform a *paracentesis,* an incision into the anterior chamber to drain the blood. If an organized clot is found, judicious irrigation may supplement incision.

Penetrating Injuries

Lacerations of the globe may occur with or without a retained foreign body and with or without prolapse of ocular contents. In injuries to the globe, an ophthalmic surgeon should repair tissues adjacent to the eye, in addition to the eye wound.

With this type of injury there is the possibility of an eventual *sympathetic ophthalmia,* inflammation of the uninjured eye. Antitetanus therapy should be included in the treatment of these injuries.

Vitrectomy and lensectomy have rendered salvageable some massive injuries that formerly were inoperable. Such injuries include extensive lacerations with cataract formation, vitreous hemorrhage, and retinal damage.

Without Foreign Body

Eyelid Laceration Lacerations are repaired according to anatomic principles. Plastic repair involves approximation of the anatomic layers. Penetrating wounds such as animal bites are debrided. If the laceration includes the lacrimal canaliculus (duct for passage of tears), special probes are used to identify the proximal portions for rejoining. Lacerations of the lacrimal canaliculus may be repaired by suturing over either of two types of stents. The Quickert-Dryden tubing consists of a length of flexible silicone with a malleable metal lacrimal probe swaged onto each end. One end of probe is inserted through the upper lid canaliculus; the other end is inserted into the lower lid canaliculus. Both exit via the tear sac and nasolacrimal canal into the nose. The lacerated canaliculus is then sutured over the tubing, which is removed after healing takes place. Some surgeons prefer the rigid Veirs stainless steel rod. This is inserted into the lacerated canaliculus. A suture swaged to one end permits withdrawal of the rod after healing.

Conjunctival Laceration Conjunctival laceration is usually debrided and, unless large, permitted to heal without suturing. If it is large, with loss of conjunctival tissue, sutures or rotating flaps of conjunctiva may be necessary for repair.

Corneal and Scleral Lacerations A small corneal laceration may be covered with a protective soft contact lens to seal it and hold the edges together. A larger wound requires accurate appositional sutures best placed under the operating microscope. The microscope is especially useful for irregular, complicated, or multiple tears.

Some irregular corneal lacerations not easily closed by direct suturing may be closed and the leak stopped by application of cyanoacrylate glue. Usually a soft contact lens is placed as a bandage over the freshly glued cornea. A conjunctival flap can be placed to achieve a similar seal, but it is used less frequently. A large laceration may require a penetrating keratoplasty as an emergency procedure to ensure the integrity of the eye.

Adequate exploration, particularly of a scleral wound, is necessary to determine the extent of injury as well as to ensure uncovering of the entire wound for repair. In instances of vitreous fluid presentation or loss, it is preferable to remove the fluid from the wound and the anterior chamber with the vitreotome before proceeding with repair. This is done to prevent undesirable vitreous adhesions from developing postoperatively.

Prolapse of Iris Prolapse of the iris or other uveal tissue is usually excised, except in very early clean wounds where repositioning it may be attempted.

Posterior Rupture of Globe Rupture usually involves herniation of retinal and uveal tissue into the orbit. Although such injuries are self-healing, the eye is irreparably damaged. This injury usually results in enucleation. *Avulsion* (tearing) of the optic nerve produces permanent blindness even though the rest of the globe may be intact.

With Foreign Body

Extraocular injuries are usually not extensive. An intraocular foreign object is removed very gently under sterile conditions to avoid secondary infection and further trauma. A corneal foreign body is removed with a sharp probe (spud), and the surrounding rust ring is taken off with a rotating burr. The type, size, and position of other intraocular foreign bodies should be determined accurately before removal. Localization is accomplished by:

1. Direct vision with ophthalmoscope
2. Computed axial tomography (CAT)—the most accurate method
3. Berman locator, a small but extremely sensitive version of a mine detector, which may indicate exact location of a ferrous metallic foreign body
4. X-ray study, using a contact lens containing radiopaque landmarks (Sweet's localizer)

Fragments of ferrous metals can often be retrieved by using the attraction of a strong electromagnet. In some cases these foreign bodies can be withdrawn along the path of entry. Nonmagnetic foreign objects present a more serious problem. Frequently they may be secured only by passing a delicate forceps into the globe. Such instrumentation is combined with partial vitrectomy, thus obtaining satisfactory results.

In summary, traumatic injuries may introduce infection or produce severe inflammatory reaction in greater degree than do elective surgical procedures. Proper early treatment is indicated to save vision. Early reintervention, before scar formation, may be necessary in some patients.

CONSIDERATIONS IN OPHTHALMIC SURGERY

The ophthalmic patient faces impairment or loss of vision if the outcome of surgical intervention is unfavorable. Special features of ophthalmic surgery aim to prevent such a loss. Surgical procedures on the eye are extremely delicate, requiring precision instrumentation, a steady hand, and quiet surroundings.

Operating Microscope

Most ophthalmic surgeons use the operating microscope for intraocular procedures. The microscope, all accessory equipment, and microinstruments should be set up and checked before the surgical procedure. The outcome of the procedure depends on the condition of the instruments. The tips of these expensive, fragile microinstruments should be protected and handled as carefully as fine jewelry before, during, and after use. (See Chapter 14 and Chapter 15, pp. 291-293.)

When the operating microscope is used, the operating table should be mechanically secure and the patient's head stabilized. Inadvertent movement is not tolerated because of the minute surgical field. The headrest should be narrow so it does not obstruct the surgeon's approach to the surgical site from sides of the vertical column of the microscope. The patient is instructed about the importance of remaining still during the surgical procedure. The patient could easily move out of the field of vision under the microscope or precipitate a complication.

The assistant observes the surgical procedure through an assistant's ocular. If the assistant observes a potentially unsatisfactory situation that the surgeon cannot observe from his or her position, the assistant should bring this to the surgeon's attention. Some scrub persons are trained to first assist.

Ophthalmic Drugs

Many drugs are critical to the preparation of the eye for the surgical procedure. The patient is prepared as ordered. These orders often contain common abbreviations that identify the eye(s) to receive drops: OD, right eye; OS, left eye; and OU, both eyes. A registered nurse instills medications, as well as anesthetic drops, as ordered, before skin preparation. *To instill eye drops:*

1. Wash hands.
2. Identify correct medication, eye, and patient.
3. Explain the procedure to patient.
4. Tilt patient's head back. Tell the patient to look up. While gently pulling down on the lower lid, instill medication on inner aspect of the lower lid, in the middle third. Release the lid while the patient slowly closes the eye to retain the drop. Let the patient close the eye between repeated drops. Gen-

tly blot excess fluid to prevent drainage into the tear duct, nose, and stomach. Some medications, such as atropine, may have a systemic effect. In small infants or young children, systemic absorption is avoided by applying finger pressure over the lacrimal sac region (inner canthus) of both eyes simultaneously for a minute. In a struggling child, have the patient tilt the head back and close both eyes. Instill the medication at the inner canthus. The drop will roll into the eye as child reopens it.
5. Only the specified number of drops are administered.
6. Read the label on the vial each time before instillation.
7. Each patient should receive a fresh, single-use, disposable vial that is discarded after use.

Mydriatic or Miotic Drugs

Medications may be given to alter the size of the pupil.

1. *Mydriatic drops:* 2.5% or 10% phenylephrine hydrochloride (Neo-Synephrine) to dilate the pupil.
2. *Mydriatic-cycloplegic drops:* 1% cyclopentolate hydrochloride (Cyclogyl), 1% atropine, and 0.25% scopolamine hydrobromide (Isopto-Hyoscine) to dilate the pupil and paralyze the ciliary body, diminish reaction to trauma, and prevent anterior synechiae (e.g., iris adhering to the lens). These drugs are longer-acting than phenylephrine.
3. *Miotic drops:* 2% pilocarpine hydrochloride to constrict the pupil.

Local Anesthesia

Except for children and selected patients, local anesthesia is used. Most surgical procedures are scheduled as *monitored anesthesia care (MAC)* or *attended local.* An anesthesiologist is present to monitor the patient and to administer oxygen and/or supplement the local anesthetic if necessary. Intravenous (IV) midazolam (Versed) and/or fentanyl (Sublimaze) or propofol (Diprivan) is often given to relax the patient. Tolerance to procedures is increased because of sedative effects of these agents. If general anesthesia is used, usual general anesthesia routines are followed. Local anesthesia consists of:

1. *Topical instillation* of anesthetic drops. Drug used may be 0.5% proparacaine hydrochloride (Ophthaine), 0.5% tetracaine hydrochloride (Pontocaine), or 2% lidocaine hydrochloride (Xylocaine).
2. *Local infiltration* of the lids and tissue around the eyes (Van Lint method) or O'Brien block of the facial nerve, the seventh cranial nerve, for lid akinesia or paralysis of extraocular muscles. A 25-gauge × 1½ inches (3.8 cm) needle for the Van Lint method or ½ inch (12.7 mm) for the O'Brien block with a 2 ml syringe are commonly used.
3. *Retrobulbar block.* A popular solution consists of a mixture of equal parts of 2% or 4% lidocaine hydrochloride and 0.75% bupivacaine hydrochloride with hyaluronidase (Wydase), 3.75 units/ml for penetration. One drop of epinephrine hydrochloride 1:1000 may be added to 10 ml of the solution to prolong the anesthetic effect for cataract extraction. A 25-gauge × 1½ inches (3.8 cm) needle with a sharp rounded point (e.g., Atkinson needle) and a 5 ml syringe usually are used. The needle is inserted by the surgeon behind the eyeball into the muscular cone, the common origin of the extraocular muscles, to obtain anesthesia of the globe and paralysis of the muscles. The patient is asked to look up and away from the injection site and is told that a slight burning sensation may accompany injection. Up to 5 ml of solution may be slowly and carefully injected.

   Retrobulbar block may be followed by intermittent massage of eye to soften it, to lower IOP, and to facilitate surgical manipulation during cataract extraction, especially when intraocular lens insertion is contemplated. Massage is continued until the IOP is lowered to a satisfactory level (e.g., 10 to 12 scale reading on sterile Schiötz' tonometer [see p. 691]).

   Some surgeons apply the Honan balloon pressure device to soften the eyeball after a retrobulbar block. A small inflatable balloon is placed directly over the closed eyelid and is secured with a strap around the head. The balloon is inflated to 30 to 40 mm Hg for 5 to 10 minutes to lower intravitreal pressure. An absolutely quiet eye is mandatory, especially at high magnifications of the microscope. When general anesthesia is used, some surgeons administer a retrobulbar block for immobility and to lower IOP.
4. *Peribulbar anesthesia.* An alternative to retrobulbar injection, injections are made in the soft tissue adjacent to each side of the globe rather than behind it. A greater amount of the same anesthetic solution is used. Adequate anesthesia is obtained without risk of retrobulbar hemorrhage.

Ophthalmic Solutions

Emphasis is placed on the need for extreme and constant care with *ophthalmic solutions.* Nearly all are colorless and may be in similar receptacles. *Solutions are immediately and individually labeled* by the scrub person. *Identity must not be confused* because an error could result in total, irrevocable blindness for the patient. If identification is missing, discard the solution. *Solutions for intraocular use must be separated from all others.* Ideally they should be filtered with micropore filters. *Sterile solutions commonly used* include the following:

1. On a separate table, before the patient is prepped and draped:
   a. Local anesthetic. Hyaluronidase (Wydase) 5 to 7 units/ml of anesthetic solution is sometimes added to expedite spread of the anesthetic through the tissue and to create more profound anesthesia.
   b. Epinephrine hydrochloride 1:1000 (1-2 ml) with an eye dropper, for hemostasis. After a drop is added to the topical local anesthetic, this container is removed from the table so that the medication is *never* inadvertently injected.
   c. Small 30 ml sterile bottles of BSS to which an irrigating cannula may be attached are commercially available for irrigating the anterior chamber and for keeping the cornea moist.
2. On the instrument table:
   a. Acetylcholine chloride (Miochol) to irrigate the anterior chamber after insertion of a posterior chamber IOL to rapidly constrict the pupil. It may also be used during cataract surgery.
   b. Steroids for topical application or subconjunctival injection of methylprednisolone acetate suspension (Depo-Medrol 80 mg/ml or Depo-Kenalog), dexamethasone (Decadron), or betamethasone (Celestone) at conclusion of surgical procedure to diminish inflammatory response and to prevent corneal graft rejection.
   c. Antibiotic for topical application or subconjunctival injection (e.g., gentamicin sulfate solution or cefazolin [Ancef, Kefzol]) following intraocular procedures to prevent infection.
   d. Mannitol 15%, 2 g/kg body weight IV, as an osmotic agent to draw fluid from the eye to lower IOP.
   e. Sodium hyaluronate (Healon), a viscous jelly, sometimes used in anterior segment surgery to occupy space and prevent damage when opening anterior capsule and to prevent adhesion formation.
   f. Alpha-chymotrypsin (Alpha Chymar), an enzyme solution, to soften the zonules holding the lens, before intracapsular cataract extraction to facilitate extraction of lens.
3. Epinephrine 2 ml of 1:10,000 added to 500 ml BSS, used as irrigation to maintain pupil dilatation intraoperatively (e.g., in vitrectomy and extracapsular cataract extraction). Dosage may vary among surgeons. Preservative-free solution is commercially available. The container of solution is hung on an IV pole for use with the irrigation/aspiration machine.

The surgeon should check with the anesthesiologist before using medications intraoperatively. Epinephrine or other sympathomimetics may have side effects when used with some anesthetic agents. Also, medications that may induce vomiting are avoided. Any straining or gross movement may cause intraocular hemorrhage, a sudden rise in IOP resulting in loss of vitreous, or expulsion of ocular contents through the wound. All can cause blindness.

Optical Lasers

Use of an optical laser is often a safe alternative to conventional surgery for ablation of a pathologic condition. The color and wavelength of each laser determine which part of the eye it can best treat. Specific wavelengths destroy disease in tissues whose pigments are capable of discriminating absorption of that wavelength. Conversely, the selected wavelength should be only minimally absorbed by vital adjacent tissues to be preserved. The ophthalmologist controls the power, intensity, and direction of the laser beam. The beam precisely cauterizes tissue and blood vessels, preventing bleeding. Each laser has selective uses.

1. *Blue-green argon:* for retinal detachment, tear or hole, diabetic retinopathy, and macular neovascular lesions; laser trabeculoplasty, to lower IOP and facilitate aqueous outflow in selected patients with open-angle glaucoma; iridotomy, in place of iridectomy by incision, to create a small opening in the iris that allows aqueous to enter the anterior chamber (angle-closure glaucoma). Laser use may reduce the threat of endophthalmitis, a serious postoperative complication. Adherence of the iris to laser treatment sites (synechiae) is a complication of laser trabeculoplasty. A portable laser is available for intraoperative use. It permits surgeons to work inside the eye rather than through it while the patient is under general anesthesia.
2. *Red-yellow krypton:* for blood vessel aberrations of the choroid, common to senile macular disease in which abnormal vessels damage adjacent nerve tissue; for lesions in the perimacular region, the laser beam passes through cloudy vitreous hemorrhage; for retinal vascular diseases, such as proliferative diabetic retinopathy and retinal detachment.
3. *Invisible pulsed neodymium (Nd:YAG):* for preoperative anterior capsulotomy before extracapsular cataract extraction; posterior capsulotomy (discission) after extracapsular cataract extraction to make an opening in an opaque capsule and thus permit light to reach the retina; lysis or severing of strands of vitreous and/or fibrous bands in the posterior segment that cause cystoid macular edema. Cloudy areas of tissue interfering with vision are painlessly pushed aside,

resulting in immediate improvement in sight. Rather than producing the effect by absorption, energy is released almost entirely at the point of focus. Problems in both anterior and posterior parts of the eye are treatable (e.g., with optical iridectomy and photocoagulation of retinal disorders). The Nd:YAG laser does not require the target tissue to be pigmented for effectiveness as do the visible light lasers.

4. *Visible excimer:* for shaping the cornea, as in lamellar keratectomy, to correct refractive disorders.
5. *Invisible holmium:YAG (Ho:YAG):* for sclerostomy to create opening in sclera that promotes filtration for glaucoma. It can also be used for corneal sculpting.

Advantages of laser therapy are:

1. Minimal possibility of infection. Treatment is noninvasive and sterile, an advantage to diabetic and susceptible patients.
2. Minimal pain, requiring only topical anesthetic unless many retinal areas are treated with high-energy laser.
3. Performed as an ambulatory procedure.
4. Appropriate amount of energy is concentrated in very small area.
5. Highly flexible light, which seems to do little damage to the clear media it traverses.
6. Selective absorption. Ideally, only desired tissue is affected.
7. Useful in poor-risk surgical patient or one who had previous unsuccessful surgical procedure.

Other Considerations in Ophthalmic Surgical Patients

Impaired vision may produce prolonged severe stress and alter the patient's self-image. Most patients are elderly. Reassure them, exercise patience, give directions clearly, anticipate needs, and check comfort level.

1. Urinary urgency can be a problem in elderly patients or those receiving diuretic medication. Although the patient should void before coming to the OR, offer a bedpan before transfer to the operating table. Severe urinary urgency can cause increased IOP during the procedure. *Strain and gross movement are dangerous and to be avoided.*
2. Surgeon and circulator verify the intended surgical site with the patient as well as with office records. To avoid error, after confirmation some surgeons also place an indelible mark on the side of the patient's neck that corresponds to the affected eye. A small, removable sticker can be used for the same purpose.
3. Patient is positioned supine on the operating table so that head and body are aligned. The top of the head is in line with the edge of the table for accessibility. The head is stabilized in a ring-shaped pillow (donut). Patient's gown is untied at the neck to prevent pressure. The head should not be turned greatly in either direction. Any obstruction to venous circulation can cause undue increased IOP, which can produce loss of vitreous humor when the eye is opened. The table is tilted so patient's head is elevated by 5 to 10 degrees to assist venous return from the head. For long procedures, an egg-crate or gel pad mattress may be placed on the table.
4. Skin preparation and draping procedures are performed as per routine (see Chapter 22). Sterile plastic drapes are often placed over woven textile drapes to contain lint, especially before lens implantation. A patient with a drape over the face is often apprehensive and afraid of suffocating. The drape can be placed over a Mayo stand or clipped to an IV pole to create a tentlike space above the patient's nose and mouth; this helps eliminate the feeling of claustrophobia. Oxygen is delivered via nasal prongs or insufflated to the facial area beneath the drape at 6 to 8 L/min.
5. Provide a quiet, stimulant-free environment for the awake patient receiving local anesthesia.
6. Some surgeons use a sterile, opaque pupillary shield to protect the patient's retina from phototoxic damage caused by prolonged exposure to the illumination of the microscope. The patient has no defensive blink reflex to protect the retina from light exposure. Some scopes have a sensor near the surgeon's eyepiece that dims the light source when he or she is not directly looking into the scope. When the surgeon is positioned at the eyepiece, the light resumes the desired intensity.
7. Prepare for emergencies by anticipating problems. Fast action can make the difference between a seeing or nonseeing eye postoperatively. Potential complications are:
   a. Systemic reaction to medication or local anesthetic drugs and cardiac arrest
   b. Loss of vitreous, which requires removal of vitreous from the anterior chamber with a vitreotome to prevent prolapse of wound, severe inflammation, or updrawn pupil
   c. Expulsive hemorrhage; expulsion of ocular contents, which requires a sharp knife, such as a Beaver blade or Wheeler knife, for fast cutdown into the pars plana area and an 18-gauge needle or cannula attached to a syringe to aspirate blood and reduce pressure in an effort to save the eye and vision
   d. Instrument failure (hand aspiration devices should be available for immediate use)

8. Wide variety of fine-sized absorbable and nonabsorbable sutures are used. The scrub person follows the manufacturer's recommendations for handling these delicate materials and needles with appropriate needleholders. Special techniques are used in microsurgery.
9. Sponges are of precut compressed cellulose on sticks.
10. No foreign material should be introduced into the surgical wound. In intraocular procedures, no portion of any instrument or item intended to enter the eye should be touched by a gloved hand. Intraocular lenses are soaked and rinsed in BSS and sometimes lubricated with sodium hyaluronate (Healon) before insertion to remove any debris or impurity.
11. Inflammation should be kept as minimal as possible because even slight inflammation may result in total functional loss. Steroids are often administered locally, subconjunctivally, and sometimes systemically. The eye may respond violently to the slightest amount of trauma.
12. Antibiotic drops are often instilled topically for 24 hours preoperatively and postoperatively.
13. At conclusion of surgical procedure, a sterile eye pad is applied. A protective shield is secured over it to guard against mechanical injury.
14. Patient should not be permitted to participate in move from the operating table following intraocular procedures, which will prevent a sudden rise in IOP and/or dislocation of the IOL.
15. Arm restraints are essential for infants and young children. Restraints are applied to adults only under extreme circumstances, such as disorientation. Use of siderails is standard procedure for all patients having ophthalmic surgery.

The tendency is toward ambulatory surgery or short hospitalization. A most important aspect of postoperative care is to inform the patient not to get out of bed alone. A fall or injury to the eye can nullify an otherwise successful surgical procedure. The patient must not do anything to increase IOP (e.g., bend over at the waist or lift heavy objects). Deep breathing postoperatively is encouraged, but coughing is avoided because it could increase IOP and rupture the suture line. The patient should report any pain, swelling, redness, or discharge postoperatively. The outcome of ophthalmic procedures includes a cosmetic as well as a functional aspect.

Bibliography

Ai E, Gardner TW: Current patterns of intraocular gas use in North America, *Arch Ophthalmol* 111(3):331-332, 1993.

Bochow TW et al: Pneumatic retinopexy perfluoroethane (C_2F_6) in the treatment of rhegmatogenous retinal detachment, *Arch Ophthalmol* 110(12):1723-1724, 1992.

Boker T et al: Results and prognostic factors in pneumatic retinopexy, *Ger J Ophthalmol* 3(2):73-78, 1994.

Caramella F: Silicone oil as a vitreous substitute in vitreoretinal surgery, *J Ophthalmic Nurs Technol* 13(5):241-242, 1994.

Cataract guideline downplays surgery, tests, *OR Manager* 9(5):21, 1993.

Charpentier DY et al: Radial thermokeratoplasty is inadequate for overcorrection following radial keratotomy, *J Refract Corneal Surg* 10(1):34-35, 1994.

Clinical guidelines: cataract surgery and its alternatives, *Am J Nurs* 93(7):59-61, 1993.

Dausch D et al: Excimer laser photorefractive keratectomy for hyperopia, *J Refract Corneal Surg* 9(1):20-28, 1993.

Durrie DS et al: Holmium:YAG laser thermokeratoplasty for hyperopia, *Refract Corneal Surg* 10(suppl 2):S277-S280, 1994.

Effert R et al: Retinal hemodynamics after pars plana vitrectomy with silicone oil tamponade, *Ger J Ophthalmol* 3(2):65-67, 1994.

Geggel HS: Problems following radial keratotomy, *Ophthalmic Surg* 24(4):286, 1993.

Haight MG: No greater gift, *J Ophthalmic Nurs Technol* 10(1):28-29, 1991.

Irvine AR, Lahey JM: Pneumatic retinopexy for giant retinal tears, *Ophthalmology* 101(3):524-528, 1994.

Koch PS: Managing the torn posterior capsule and vitreous loss, *Int Ophthalmol Clin* 34(2):113-130, 1994.

Kowalski CK: Cataracts at any age, *Home Healthcare Nurse* 12(2):43-46, 1994.

Kuhn PL: Phacoemulsification, *Surg Technol* 22(5):7-12, 1990.

Langseth FG: Levator aponeurosis surgery: surgical correction for blepharoptosis, *AORN J* 54(4):731-741, 1991.

Maguen E et al: Results of excimer laser photorefractive keratectomy for the correction of myopia, *Ophthalmology* 101(9):1548-1556, 1994.

Martinelli AM: Glaucoma, *AORN J* 54(4):743-757, 1991.

Price MJ: Glaucoma screening, *J Ophthalmic Nurs Technol* 9(5):203-205, 1990.

Sandler RL: Clinical snapshot: glaucoma, *Am J Nurs* 95(3):34-35, 1995.

Saroya JS et al: Vitrectomy for intraocular foreign body removal, *Indiana J Ophthalmol* 40(2):38-40, 1992.

Schein OD et al: Variation in cataract surgery practice and clinical outcomes, *Ophthalmology* 101(6):1142-1152, 1994.

Schepens CL: Management of retinal detachment, *Ophthalmic Surg* 25(7):427-431, 1994.

Sommer A et al: Developing specialtywide standards of practice: the experience of ophthalmology, *QRB* 16(2):65-70, 1990.

Szerenyi K et al: Keratitis as a complication of bilateral, simultaneous radial keratotomy, *Am J Ophthalmol* 117(4):426-467, 1994.

Tornambe PE: Pneumatic retinopexy: current status and future directions, *Int Ophthalmol Clin* 32(2):61-80, 1992.

Updegraff SA et al: Pupillary block during cataract surgery, *Am J Ophthalmol* 117(3):328-332, 1994.

Wiedemann P et al: Reconstruction of the anterior and posterior segment of the eye after massive injury, *Ger J Ophthalmol* 3(2):84-89, 1994.

CHAPTER 34

Plastic and Reconstructive Surgery

Tissue transplantation and repositioning, as well as tissue removal or replacement, are the art of the plastic surgeon. Skin, mucous membranes, fat, cartilage, tendons, nerves, blood vessels, and bone can be transferred either locally or from remote parts of the body. However, the results depend not only on the skill of the plastic surgeon but also on the age, health status, skin texture, bone structure, extent of the defect, and healing capacity of the patient. Approximately 50% of all plastic surgery may be done as ambulatory procedures, many under local anesthesia with sedation. The surgeon performs the simplest and safest procedure that will meet the patient's expected outcome.

Plastic surgery is defined as:

> Surgery dealing with restoration of wounded, disfigured, or unsightly parts of the body. It includes cosmetic surgery or cosmetic corrections not necessarily related to the physical health or safety of the patient. The word "plastic" in its classic sense means "giving form or fashion to matter." As used in plastic surgery, the word bears no relationship to the current concept of plastic materials and products.*

Autografts, allografts, or prosthetic implants may be used to improve or restore contour defects or functional malformations caused by congenital, developmental, disease, or traumatic disfigurements.

Elective surgical procedures desired by an individual in an attempt to improve appearance for psychologic well-being are classified as aesthetic or cosmetic surgery. Thus the plastic surgeon's hand extends to alteration of cosmetically unacceptable body contours, as well as to repair and reconstruction of tissue injuries. Plastic surgeons have a philosophy about how tissues can be handled and a technique for handling them that heals the patient's body and mind, limited only by the surgeon's ingenuity. They attempt to restore both function and appearance.

General plastic surgeons practice their art on virtually any part of the body. Some plastic surgeons limit their practice to specific areas, such as the head and neck, hand, or breast. Some specialize in reconstructive surgery to restore function; others specialize in aesthetic procedures to alter cosmetic appearance. Many specialists in a specific part or organ of the body also perform plastic surgery. Otolaryngologists operate on the ears and nose. Ophthalmologists may repair eyelids. Orthopaedists correct deformities of hands and feet. Gynecologists repair the vaginal vault. Dermatologists remove skin lesions. The surgeon specifically trained in the art of plastic surgery frequently is a member of a multidisciplinary team, as described in Chapter 36, to assist with the repair of defects and/or restoration of function.

*The American Society of Plastic and Reconstructive Surgeons, Inc.

HISTORICAL BACKGROUND

Plastic surgery was probably the first form of surgery. Egyptian papyrus scrolls tell of skin grafts and pedicle flaps to replace deficiencies as early as 3500 years ago. Egyptian mummies have been found with artificial ears and noses. In India more than 2000 years ago, the Hindus became skilled in transferring tissue to form noses for those who had lost them as a punishment. Ancient records verify other attempts to improve appearance.

During the fourteenth and sixteenth centuries, restorative procedures for the nose, lips, and ears were described by Italian surgeons. However, further development of the art of reconstruction did not occur in Europe until the nineteenth century. The German surgeon, Edward Zeis, first used the term *plastic surgery* in his book published in 1863. Other German and French surgeons before and after Zeis described free grafts, tissue transfers, and methods to repair soft tissue defects.

In the twilight of the nineteenth and the dawn of the twentieth centuries, descriptions of "featural surgery" were brazenly advertised by "cosmetic surgeons," often with unwarranted claims of success. Charles Conrad Miller (1880-1950) has been called both "the father of modern cosmetic surgery" and "an unabashed quack." Practicing in Chicago, Miller began around 1904 to improvise surgical procedures to alter facial features. He did them in his office with the patient receiving local anesthetic.

Vilray Papin Blair became a prominent plastic surgeon when he published in 1906 the results of closed ramisection of the mandible for micrognathia and prognathism. Within a short time, physicians from all over the United States and Europe sent patients to Blair for jaw reconstruction and other facial surgery.

Sir Arbuthnot Lane, a contemporary of Miller and Blair, was doing cleft lip, cleft palate, and some mandibular surgery in England. When Blair arrived in England in 1918 as chief consultant in maxillofacial surgery for the American armed forces, he visited the center Lane had established for treating soldiers with facial injuries. The work being done there by Harold Gillies impressed Blair. The high quality of work at this and other centers during World War I on facial injuries, burns, and reconstruction of other injured parts of the body did much to establish plastic surgery as a surgical specialty.

During World War II the development of military plastic surgery centers led to rapid progress in the rehabilitation of casualties with maxillofacial and hand injuries. Plastic surgeons worked closely with other specialists in treating many types of war injuries. They found that by replacing lost skin with grafts, fractures under these areas healed better and more quickly and parts returned to normal function sooner.

Today's plastic surgery is largely the refinement of techniques developed during World Wars I and II to restore men disfigured by the ravages of war. These techniques are not only imaginative but precise. They are imaginative because plastic surgeons reshape and replant living tissue and augment tissue with prosthetic implants.

Plastic surgery has been called the "surgery of millimeters" because of the critical margin between good and poor cosmetic results. Each millimeter lack or excess of tissue can have an extreme psychologic impact on the patient. If the patient thinks his or her appearance has improved, personality and self-image improve and others respond more positively to him or her.

Plastic surgery has been extended by increased knowledge of the principles and techniques of microvascular and microneural anastomoses for replantation and transplantation of tissue.

PSYCHOLOGIC SUPPORT FOR PLASTIC SURGERY PATIENTS

Physical appearance affects self-image and self-esteem. Children can develop inferiority complexes and introverted personalities because of congenital malformations in body structure or deformities caused by trauma. The defect may not affect physiologic function but may predispose the person to psychologic crippling if not corrected to the individual's satisfaction.

Adults who are dissatisfied with their body image may believe that a change in personal appearance will solve their social, marital, sexual, or business problems. The plastic surgeon must assess the patient's psychologic status, motivations, and expectations before scheduling a surgical procedure. Realistic goals must be set. The patient should be emotionally stable and aware of the potential outcomes. Psychologic assessment and preparation are advisable preoperatively and are essential before surgical procedures that will result in disfigurement.

Many extensive reconstructions for severe deformities are done in stages, often over a period of months. These patients require prolonged psychologic support and encouragement.

Plastic and reconstructive surgery, either therapeutic or cosmetic, evokes emotional responses from the patient, family or significant other, and the health care team. Anticipation of the final outcome, which can be seen by the patient and others, often creates temporary psychosocial reactions such as depression and isolation. Positive reassurance of progress in improvement of physical appearance and during emotional crises is essential throughout the perioperative period. Perhaps the surgeon-nurse-patient-family relationship is closer when a person undergoes alteration of physical appearance than with other types of surgery. The patient may be physically healthy but may suffer alterations in self-esteem related to perception of a defect in appearance. Care must be given in a manner that protects the self-esteem of the patient and respects the dignity of the family. This requires communication, understanding, and empathy. Preoperative teaching and discharge planning prepare the patient and his or her family for postoperative rehabilitation.

SPECIAL FEATURES OF PLASTIC AND RECONSTRUCTIVE SURGERY

Scars are inevitable whenever skin is incised or excised, either intentionally by the surgeon's scalpel or accidentally by trauma. The plastic surgeon attempts to minimize scar formation by meticulous realignment and approximation of underlying tissues and wound edges. The plastic surgeon makes the incision along natural skin lines whenever possible. Many plastic procedures involve only the subcuticular tissues and skin (see anatomic layers in Figure 34-1, p. 709). Reconstructive procedures, however, may include manipulation of underlying cartilage, bone, muscles, tendons, nerves, and blood vessels.

Most plastic surgeons ask their patients not to take aspirin or smoke for at least 2 weeks before an elective surgical procedure. Aspirin has an anticoagulant action that can affect bleeding. Smoking causes vasoconstriction that can affect wound healing. Photographs are usually taken preoperatively and postoperatively so patient can compare the difference in body appearance.

General Considerations

1. Pressure points must be protected during prolonged procedures. Microvascular plastic and reconstructive surgical procedures may take 12 to 18 hours to complete. The patient should be positioned on an egg-crate mattress or gel pad. Bony prominences should be well-padded to prevent tissue necrosis.
2. Sterile dye, such as methylene blue, gentian violet, Bonney's blue, or brilliant green, is often used to outline areas for incision. This can be done with a sterile marking pen after the skin is prepped.
3. Exposure of both sides for comparison is usually required for surgical procedures on the face, ears, and neck.
4. Draping often exposes much skin surface, which is unavoidable. A fenestrated sheet frequently cannot be used. The opening does not give adequate exposure, especially for skin grafting procedures. Use towels, self-adhering plastic sheeting, and minor and medium sheets under and around the areas, according to needs, to drape as much of the patient as possible. Drapes can be secured with towel clips, skin staples, or sutures.
5. Local anesthesia is used for many surgical procedures on adults. Epinephrine may be added to help localize the agent, prolong the anesthetic action, and provide hemostasis. Short 26- or 30-gauge needles are used for injection.
6. Nos. 15 and 11 scalpel blades are routinely used to cut small structures. A hemostatic scalpel may be used to incise skin and cut through soft tissues, especially in vascular areas.
7. Instruments must be small for handling delicate tissues. Iris scissors, mosquito hemostats, fine-tipped tissue forceps, and other small-scale cutting, holding, clamping, and exposing instruments are part of the routine plastic surgery setup. Microinstruments are needed for microsurgical techniques (see Chapter 15, pp. 291-293).
8. Nerve stimulator may be used to help identify nerves, especially in craniofacial, neck, and hand reconstruction procedures.
9. Bone, cartilage, or skin grafts may be needed. Homografts may be obtained from the tissue bank rather than the patient's own tissues.
10. Silicone or other prosthetic implants may be used in plastic surgery to reconstruct soft tissue and cartilage defects. They cannot be used unless there is adequate soft tissue coverage. They cannot be used in an infected area. (See Chapter 24, p. 513, for discussion of handling silicone implants.)
11. Suture sizes range from 2-0 through 7-0, depending on location and tissue, with sizes 8-0 through 11-0 sutures for microsurgery. The material used varies according to the personal preference of the surgeon. Synthetic nonabsorbable and absorbable polymers are used more commonly than natural materials because they engender less tissue reaction.
12. Swaged needles of small wire diameter with sharp cutting edges minimize trauma to superficial tissues. An appropriately fine-tipped needleholder must be used with these delicate, curved needles.
13. Skin staples may be used to close skin or to secure skin grafts.
14. Skin closure strips may be used as skin dressing with sutures or to supplement closure with skin staples.
15. Closed-wound suction drainage is frequently used to hold flaps against underlying tissue.
16. Fine-mesh gauze may be used for the contact dressing. This may be impregnated with petrolatum or an oil emulsion, with or without medication, to cover denuded areas. Several types of sterile nonadherent dressings are commercially available. Dry gauze is not used on a denuded area because it adheres and acts as a foreign body; granulations grow through it.

17. Pressure dressings may be used following extensive surgical procedures to splint soft tissues and prevent contractures. The mild pressure keeps fluid formation in tissues or under a skin graft to a minimum. Commercial dressings for various body areas are preferred by some plastic surgeons. (See Chapter 25, p. 531, for types of pressure dressings.)
18. Stent fixation is a method of obtaining pressure when it is impossible to bandage an area snugly, as the face or neck. A form-fitting mold may be taped over the nose. Long suture ends can be tied crisscrossed over a dressing to immobilize it and exert gentle pressure.

Categories of Plastic Surgery

Four main categories of problems are treated by plastic surgeons.

1. Congenital anomalies, especially in structure of the face and hands. The most commonly corrected anomalies are discussed in Chapter 42.
2. Cosmetic appearance, especially of the face and breasts.
3. Benign and malignant neoplasms, especially those leaving large soft tissue defects. Resection of extensive tumors other than those involving the skin or head and neck are not usually within the province of the plastic surgeon initially, but the patient may be referred for reconstructive surgery and rehabilitation. Frequently reconstructive procedures are done in conjunction with another specialty surgeon at the time of tumor resection.
4. Traumatically acquired disfigurements, especially facial lacerations, hand injuries, and burns. The objective of the plastic surgeon is to restore function, as well as body image.

Tissue may be approximated, supplemented, excised, transferred, or transplanted. Many procedures are done in stages before complete reconstruction and restoration of function are achieved. Tissue flaps and grafts, prosthetic implants, and external prosthetic appliances may be required for functional and cosmetic restoration as a result of ablative surgery or trauma.

GRAFTING TECHNIQUES

Denuded areas of the body are resurfaced by transplanting or transferring segments of skin and other tissues from an uninjured area to the injured area. The plastic surgeon prefers to transfer tissues of compatible color, texture, thickness, and hair-bearing characteristics. Soft tissue autografts are used whenever possible. They are classified by the source of their vascular supply, essential for viability, as:

1. *Free graft.* Tissue is detached from the donor site and transplanted into the recipient site. It derives its vascular supply from the capillary ingrowth from the recipient site.
2. *Pedicle flap.* Tissue remains attached at one or both ends of the donor site during transfer to the recipient site. The vascular supply is maintained from the vessels preserved in the pedicle of the donor site.
3. *Free flap.* Tissue, including its vascular bundle, is detached from the donor site and transferred to the recipient site. Microvascular anastomoses between arteries and veins in the flap or autograft and recipient site establish the vascularity necessary for viability.

Deformities caused by loss of soft tissue substance such as trauma of accidental injury, tumor resection, or radiation therapy may require a graft to fill in deficiencies and restore contours or to cover tendons and bones. Free grafts, pedicle flaps, and free flaps may be taken from various areas of the body to reconstruct soft tissue defects.

Free Skin Grafts

The epidermis, including the basal layer of the dermis that generates new skin, is transplanted from a donor site to a recipient site in which it becomes a part of living tissue in that area. Adherence to healthy underlying tissue and adequate vascularity are necessary for graft survival. A fibrin layer forms to bind the graft to the recipient site and to provide nourishment until vascularization is established in the graft. The depth of the graft (Figure 34-1) will vary according to its purpose.

1. *Split-thickness graft.* The epidermis and half of the dermis to a depth of 0.010 to 0.035 inch (0.3 to 1 mm) are removed. The donor site heals uneventfully unless it becomes infected. Split-thickness grafts are widely used to cover large denuded areas on the back, trunk, and legs.
2. *Full-thickness graft.* The epidermis, dermis, and occasionally subcutaneous fat at a depth greater than 0.035 inch (1 mm) are removed or elevated. Full-thickness grafts inhibit wound contraction better than split-thickness grafts and generally are preferred on the face, neck, hands, elbows, axillae, knees, and feet.

The desired thickness of a free skin graft is predetermined by the plastic surgeon before the skin is incised. The appropriate cutting instrument is selected to obtain the graft.

Dermatomes

A dermatome is a cutting instrument designed to excise split-thickness skin grafts. The thickness of the graft can be calibrated by adjusting the depth gauge. The width of the graft is determined by the width of the cutting blade. Blades are detachable and most are disposable, which always ensures a sharp new blade for every patient. The length of the graft may be limited by the type of dermatome used.

Oscillating-Blade Type Dermatomes may be electric or air-powered with compressed nitrogen or air. The length of the graft is limited only by the donor site. The surgeon checks the adjustable depth gauge before cutting the graft (Figure 34-2, *A*). The oscillating-blade dermatome is not usually used on the abdominal wall where underlying support is not firm. The oscillating blade, free of vibrations, takes an accurate graft from other donor sites.

NOTE Extreme care should be used in handling these precision dermatomes. If electric, the circulator should remove the foot pedal as soon as the graft is taken. If air-powered, the scrub person and surgeon should place a thumb under the lever on the handle while preparing the instrument for use. These dermatomes *cannot be immersed in water* or put in a washer-sterilizer or ultrasonic cleaner. Follow manufacturer's instructions for use, care, and sterilization.

Drum Type Padgett and Reese dermatomes consist of one half of a metal drum, which is one half of a circle (Figure 34-2, *B*). A metal handle through the center of the drum has an arm on each end. These arms hold the bar that carries the blade. The bar swings around the drum to cut the graft. The size of the graft is limited by the width and length of the drum. An adhesive must be placed on both the skin surface and the drum to keep the skin in contact with the drum. The knife blade is moved from side to side as slight tension is exerted on the skin by rotating the drum. The drum-type dermatome is used on flat, open areas because it is bulky. Its use is limited by body contour and amount of skin on the donor site.

Dermatome tape must be used with the Reese dermatome. Packaged sterile, the tape has an adhesive coating on each side covered with a paper backing. Remove the backing on one side, and apply to the drum with care to line up the edges of the tape and the drum. After the backing paper is removed from the other side

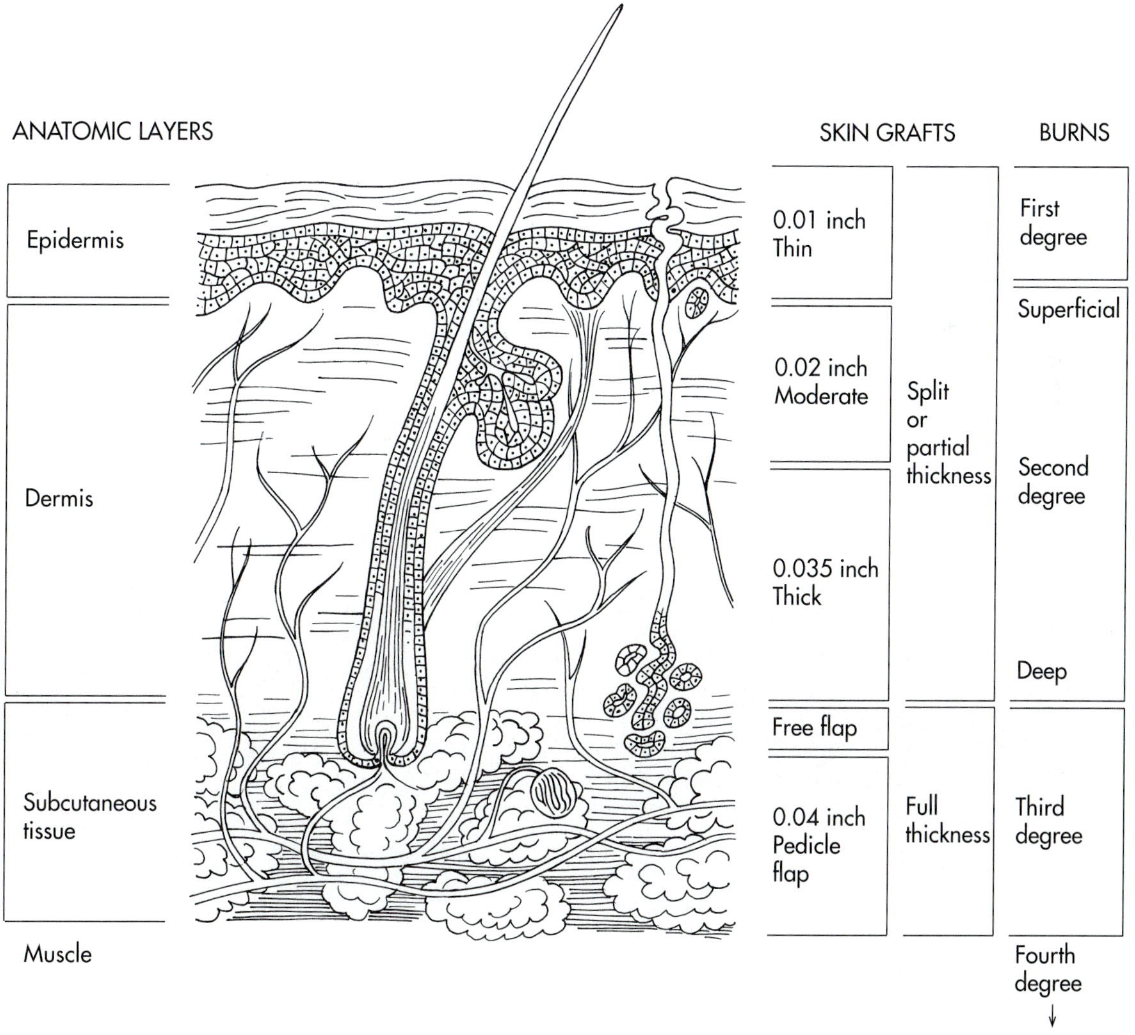

FIGURE 34-1 Cross section of skin and subcutaneous tissue, relative thickness of skin grafts, and categorization of burn injury.

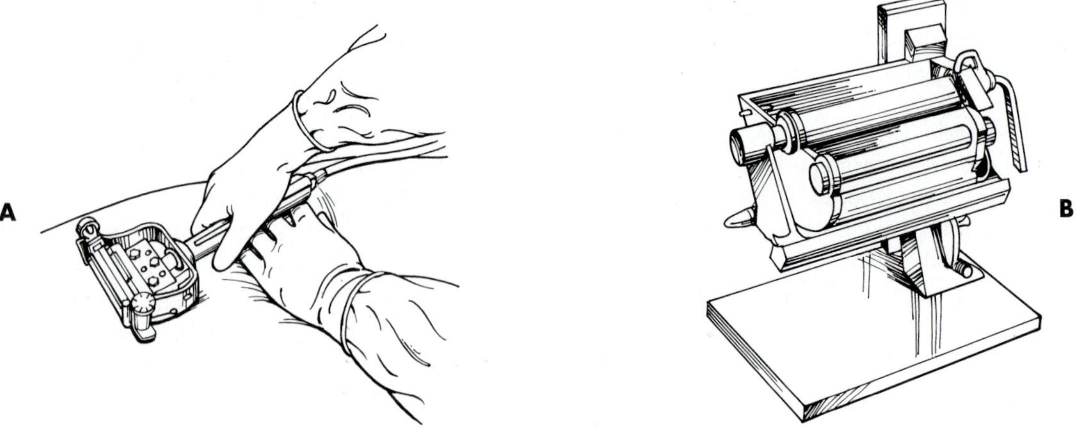

FIGURE 34-2 Dermatomes. **A,** Powered oscillating-blade type dermatome with depth gauges on each side of blade. **B,** Drum-type dermatome to manually cut skin graft.

of the tape, the drum is placed on the skin, which adheres to it.

NOTE When handling a drum-type dermatome, *always* grasp the blade carrier to prevent its swinging around the drum and seriously injuring your hands. Leave the dermatome in the rack when not in use or until the blade is removed.

Kinds of Free Skin Grafts

Split-Thickness Thiersch Graft Removed with a free-hand skin-graft knife or dermatome, Thiersch grafts are used to cover superficial defects. The surgeon may use sutures or skin staples along the edges of the graft to hold it to underlying subcutaneous tissue. This prevents movement and helps obliterate dead space in the recipient site. The skin of the donor site regenerates rapidly, and the same area can be used again in 2 or 3 weeks if necessary, or sooner if a thin graft is taken from an infection-free donor site.

SPLIT-THICKNESS MESH GRAFT A mesh graft makes it possible to obtain a greater area of coverage from a split-thickness skin graft. After removal with a dermatome, the graft is placed on a plastic derma-carrier, cut side down. This is a rigid base to keep the graft spread out flat while it is put through a mesh dermatome. This instrument cuts small parallel slits in the graft. When expanded, the slits become diamond-shaped openings (Figure 34-3). This permits expansion of the graft to cover an area three times as large as the original graft obtained from the donor site. The mesh graft can be placed over the recipient site with slight tension. The increased edge exposures are conducive to rapid epithelialization. The mesh allows serum to escape through the openings. If a mesh dermatome is not available or is not feasible to use, slits can be made with a knife blade in the donor graft to accomplish the same purposes.

Full-Thickness Wolfe Graft A Wolfe graft is cut exactly to the size and shape of the recipient site with a skin-graft knife. It is sutured into place under normal skin tension. Full-thickness grafts are used on face, neck, or hands to fill in superficial denuded areas and over joints to prevent contractures. This graft does not become viable readily on granulated surfaces, and the amount that can be transferred is much more limited than in a Thiersch graft.

NOTE To ensure viability, the donor graft must be held in apposition to healthy tissue in the underlying recipient site. The surgeon tacks the edges of the graft with sutures or staples. The middle portion may be "quilted" (i.e., affixed)

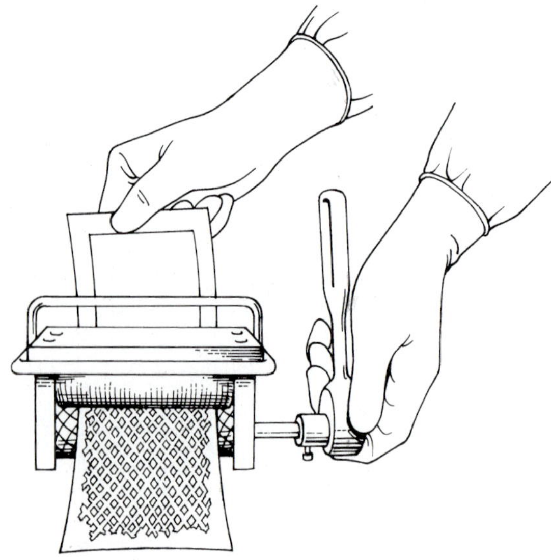

FIGURE 34-3 Split-thickness skin graft being passed through mesh dermatome. Mesh graft expands to obtain greater coverage of recipient graft area.

with sutures or staples. The graft is covered with a pressure dressing.

Free Composite Grafts

A composite graft usually includes skin, subcutaneous tissue and cartilage, bone, or other tissues. Viability of the graft depends on ingrowth of the vascular system from the recipient site.

Free Omental Grafts

A free graft of omentum can be used to provide contour in a soft tissue defect in the face or neck, to resurface an area such as the scalp, to provide vascular support for bone and skin grafts around prosthetic materials, and to control wound infection as in the chest wall. Omentum will localize inflammation and wall off infection. It will not resorb when grafted. Omentum resected from the peritoneal cavity can be transplanted to an avascular area if sufficient blood vessels are available for microvascular anastomoses to the gastroepiploic artery and vein in the graft. Split-thickness skin grafts cover the omental graft.

Pedicle Flaps

Creation of a pedicle flap may be the procedure of choice to reconstruct deformities of soft tissue loss that will create, or have created, an obvious aesthetic or functional disability for the patient. The *pedicle,* which is the attachment of elevated tissue to the donor site, must contain a vascular bundle to maintain blood supply to tissue. Pedicle flaps are constructed from several types of tissues and sources of the vascular bundles. Flap survival seems to depend on a reduction in vascular resistance or an increase in arterial perfusion pressure, or both. Several techniques are used to monitor circulation in the flap intraoperatively and postoperatively (see pp. 713-714).

Arterialized Skin Flap

A full-thickness skin graft contains a vascular bundle within subcutaneous tissue and skin. Arterialized flaps may be:

1. Those with axial vasculature from axial vessels that supply a fairly definite area of skin and subcutaneous tissue. A direct cutaneous artery flows through the length of the flap.
2. Those with random or local vasculature from subdermal plexus. Random flaps do not have a specific blood vessel within the flap. These are usually small flaps created around the head or neck.
3. Those with both axial and random vasculature. A deltopectoral flap, for example, has axial vessels from the sternal region and random vessels in the deltoid area.

Depending on proximity of the recipient site to the donor site, the pedicle flap will be one of the following types.

Rotational Flap One end of flap is rotated and sutured to the recipient site to cover a denuded area. The flap tissue is obtained from an area near the recipient site. Arterialized skin pedicle flaps with axial vasculature are rotated in a one-stage procedure. Random rotational pedicle flaps can be used in the face because vascularity is sufficient in the head and neck.

Cross-Finger Flap Tissue at donor site is undermined and rotated to cover a small defect in an adjacent digit.

Tissue Expansion Flap

The epidermal surface area can be increased by implanting a tissue-expanding device subcutaneously close to the defect. Available in many sizes and shapes, the device has a soft, pliable silicone pouch connected by tubing to a self-sealing inflation reservoir. After insertion under a designated area for the skin flap, the pouch is filled with saline by injecting small amounts into the reservoir. Rapid expansion may be achieved immediately in the head or neck area or gradually over a period of weeks to months in other areas. Natural physiologic skin expansion occurs. The dermis stretches and thins while the epidermis duplicates itself without changing thickness. Tissue will increase to about one and one-half times the width of the device. The vascular network that develops produces more viable tissue than that of other pedicle flaps. The tissue has similar color, texture, and thickness as the recipient site. The expanded tissue is advanced or transferred to cover a defect, helping to minimize scarring and donor site deformity. Tissue expansion flaps are used for scalp and facial defects, breast reconstruction, and other soft tissue defects. They can be used for closure of large donor site defects.

Myocutaneous (Musculocutaneous) Flap

Pedicle myocutaneous flaps allow safe and rapid transfer of tissue over long distances to cover large defects and vital structures. They are used, for example, to close soft tissue defects in the lower extremities, to cover pressure sores on paraplegics, and to reconstruct contour following head and neck resection and mastectomy.

A myocutaneous flap incorporates the muscle with its overlying fascia, subcutaneous tissue, and skin. It receives a vigorous blood supply from the vascular pedicle that supplies the underlying muscle (Figure 34-4). It may include a neurovascular bundle with nerve fibers to innervate the muscle in the flap. Usually done as a one-stage procedure, myocutaneous flaps can be created from the following and other muscles:

1. Trapezius
2. Sternocleidomastoid
3. Platysma
4. Latissimus dorsi
5. Pectoralis major

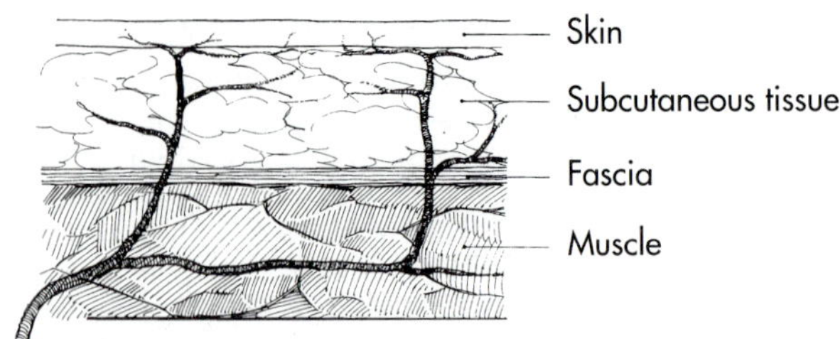

FIGURE 34-4 Myocutaneous flap. (From Ruberg RL, Smith DJ Jr: *Plastic surgery: a core curriculum,* St Louis, 1994, Mosby.)

6. Rectus abdominis
7. Gracilis
8. Gluteus maximus
9. Tensor fascia lata
10. Biceps or quadriceps femoris

Myocutaneous flaps revolutionized reconstructive surgery and stimulated the imagination of plastic surgeons.

Fasciocutaneous Flap

Mobilized fascia, subcutaneous tissue, and skin are transferred as pedicle flaps similarly to the way myocutaneous flaps are transferred. The donor site may need to be covered with a split-thickness graft.

Muscle Flap

A divided section of a muscle with its proximal blood supply intact can be rotated over a soft tissue defect, such as an ulcer on the leg or buttock. A muscle flap may be covered with a split-thickness skin graft.

Neurosensory Flap

Sensory nerves may remain intact in a flap with other tissues or be restored by microneural anastomosis or by nerve grafting. Preservation of nerves in a vascularized flap becomes important when sensation is critical to function, as in the hand, foot, and buttocks.

Omental Flap

Omentum is mobilized from the peritoneal cavity, without compromise of the vascular pedicle, to cover an infected mediastinal wound or a defect in the chest wall, such as following resection for irradiation necrosis or neoplasm. Vascularity of donor omentum revascularizes the reconstructed chest wall recipient site. Split-thickness skin grafts, which may be mesh grafts, cover the omental flap. If additional rigidity is needed to restore the chest wall, polypropylene mesh may be sutured inside the rib cage to supplement strength of the omental flap.

Microsurgical Free Flap Transfer

Composite free flaps or grafts of tissue are resected and transplanted from one area of the body to another to cover a denuded area, to restore function, or to restore body contour. Microsurgical techniques allow one-stage transfer of tissues. The main artery and vein supplying donor tissues must be anastomosed to vessels in the recipient site under the operating microscope. Often two teams work simultaneously at donor and recipient sites. These are lengthy, tedious procedures often taking 8 to 12 hours to complete.

Fasciocutaneous Graft

Free grafts of fascia with overlying skin, with or without underlying muscle, may be transferred. For example, temporalis fascia may be transplanted into another area in the face.

Free Muscle Graft

Free island grafts of functional muscle can be resected and transplanted to replace motor function in another area. Although a small percentage of the graft survives, significant regeneration of muscle occurs. Free muscle, transferred by microvascular techniques and covered with a split-thickness skin graft, promotes healing of infected wounds.

Vascularized Muscle Pedicle Free Flap

In a multistaged procedure, a myocutaneous flap is raised at the donor site and allowed to develop a new isolated vascular system before free transfer to a recipient site. The vascular system in the muscle underlying the skin flap branches out to supply the skin. At the final stage, the newly vascularized muscle pedicle is dissected free from the donor site. The donor site may need to be covered with a split-thickness graft. Under the operating microscope, arteries and veins in the flap are anastomosed to vessels at the recipient site. Two teams may complete the final stage: one to prepare and close the recipient site and the other to free the flap and close the donor site. The advantage of this type of flap is that the surgeon can select donor skin that will best provide color, texture, bulk, and contour at the recipient site, such as on the face.

Neurovascular Free Flap

Fascicles of nerves must be anastomosed to restore sensation, as well as microvascular anastomoses of arteries and veins to maintain viability of the donor tissue. A neurovascular free flap, also known as a *sensate flap,* may be taken from the scapular region. Many surgeons use the scapular flap because it is easy to dissect, has a long vascular pedicle, and creates a minimal donor site deformity. Other donor sites include the medial and lateral thigh and the lateral aspect of the upper arm.

Digital Replantation or Transfer

Microneurovascular techniques are used for replantation of traumatically amputated digits (see Chapter 44, pp. 912-913). Less common is the toe-to-thumb transfer, called the *free wraparound neurovascular flap,* performed when an amputated thumb cannot be salvaged. Skin from the dorsum of the foot, great toe including tendons and bone, and second toe web space are transferred as a sensate flap to the hand. After bone fixation and tendon anastomoses, arterial and venous circulation is established under the microscope. Digital nerves are anastomosed to reinnervate sensation and function. Other toes can be similarly transferred for finger reconstruction.

Free Autogenous Bone Graft

Vascularized autografts of bone are superior in strength and are less prone to deossification and structural weakness than conventional bone grafts. Anastomosis of the vascular bundle with a free rib, for example, may increase the chance of survival of the donor bone graft in a poorly vascularized recipient site.

Composite Myoosteocutaneous Free Flap

A composite flap of skin, muscle, and bone provides soft tissue bulk, internal structural support, and external coverage in one-stage reconstruction of compound defects following head and neck resection. The skin and iliac crest on a vascular pedicle from the deep circumflex artery may be preferred. The scapula and tissue from the upper arm provide an alternative donor site. Or the skin, soft tissue, and latissimus dorsi muscle along with a portion of an underlying rib may be dissected free, preserving the thoracodorsal vessels for anastomosis at the recipient site. Other donor sites include the radial forearm and the fibula with dorsalis pedis muscle.

Free Revascularized Intestinal Autograft

A segment of small intestine, usually jejunum, can be mobilized and transferred into the neck to reconstruct the cervical esophagus (see Chapter 36, p. 761). The mucous membrane of a jejunal graft remains moist, soft, and pliable. This may be useful in reconstruction of an oral mucosal defect.

General Considerations for All Tissue Autografts

1. Hyperthermia blanket or a water mattress is placed on the operating table to keep the patient warm. Room temperature should be increased to 75° to 80° F (24° to 27° C).
2. Skin may be prepped with a colorless antiseptic agent so plastic surgeon can see true skin color and assess vascularity of the donor graft.
3. Donor and recipient sites are prepped and draped separately, but concurrently. Care is taken that cross contamination does not occur from one site to the other.
4. Recipient site is covered with a sterile drape until the surgeon is ready to apply a free graft or pedicle flap if preparation of donor site will be the first procedure. If the recipient site must be prepared to receive the donor graft or flap, the donor site is covered.
5. Separate sterile instrument table is prepared for the donor site. This includes appropriate instruments for obtaining the graft or flap and dressings for the donor site. Two surgical teams may work simultaneously.

NOTE *Always* put a dermatome on a separate, small sterile table, never on the recipient instrument table. Handle dermatomes carefully so the depth gauge is not disturbed.

6. Grafts must be kept moist by covering them with a sponge wet with normal saline. A free flap should be kept in iced saline slush until the recipient site is prepared.
7. Operating microscope and appropriate microinstruments must be in readiness for microvascular and microneural anastomoses. For these long procedures, the patient should be positioned on an eggcrate mattress or gel pad.
8. Tissue viability must be ensured. A sterile device may be needed during the surgical procedure to identify major blood vessels underlying a graft. Assessment of patency of vessels and perfusion of the flap is possible through several types of monitoring.
   a. Doppler probes. A laser Doppler probe is placed on the recipient site preoperatively to obtain baseline measurements for comparison with postoperative measurements. The microcomputer machine has a digital readout. Ultrasonic Doppler probes also may be buried in tissues for monitoring.
   b. Photoplethysmographic disk. A disk applied to the flap surface measures reflected light from pulsatile blood flow changes in tissue. A change in blood volume in tissue produces a corresponding change in amount of light reflected. These changes are amplified and displayed on an oscilloscope.
   c. Fluorometer. A fluorescing dye is injected intravenously, and fluorescence is measured with a fluorometer for perfusion of flap. Fluorescein and an ultraviolet Wood's lamp are used occasionally to check patency and perfusion. The room must be darkened to see fluorescence. A photomultiplier may be used to amplify skin fluorescent emission.

d. Thermocouple probe. Patency of microvascular anastomosis can be assessed by temperature in surrounding tissues.
9. Hemostasis is obtained during the surgical procedure by warm saline packs, pressure, or thrombin.
10. Dressings over grafts vary by surgeon preference. Stent fixation to obtain pressure on the grafted area may be preferred. Some plastic surgeons omit pressure dressings and use an exposure technique on grafts so they can watch graft and incise a hematoma if necessary. The graft is kept covered with sterile, moist saline gauze dressings to keep the skin moist until revascularization occurs. Synthetic adhesive dressings that are moisture and vapor permeable are impermeable to liquid and bacteria. Healing under these occlusive dressings may be more rapid and less painful than at donor sites covered with fine mesh gauze. A cast frequently is applied to immobilize extremities during migration or transfer of pedicle flaps.

HEAD AND NECK RECONSTRUCTION

Some plastic surgeons specialize in head and neck oncology or reconstruction, or both. Others limit their practice to aesthetic, cosmetic surgery.

Soft Tissue Reconstruction

Defects in soft tissues of the face or scalp, usually as result of trauma, may be reconstructed by advancement of tissue expanded from an adjacent area. This technique ensures consistent skin color, texture, and hair-bearing characteristics. Other types of grafts or flaps may be necessary or preferred.

Craniofacial Surgical Procedures

The plastic surgeon usually heads the multidisciplinary team that performs the complex craniofacial procedures discussed in Chapter 36, pp. 745-747. Many of the concepts developed for these procedures are applied in less complicated surgical procedures. A variety of extracranial osteotomies, with or without bone grafts, reshape the bony framework. These maneuvers, plus reconstruction of soft tissues, contour facial deformities. The desired aesthetic and functional results can be obtained only by painstakingly careful dissection and repositioning with the utmost patience and cooperation of all operating room (OR) team members.

Maxillofacial and Oral Surgical Procedures

Plastic surgeons reconstruct *soft tissue* defects around and in the mouth that are caused by trauma or surgical resection. Those maxillofacial procedures involving bony structures that may also be performed by plastic surgeons are discussed in Chapter 36, pp. 747-749. Congenital deformities are discussed in Chapter 42, p. 864.

Transfacial Nerve Grafting

Restoration of the quality of facial expressions in a patient with severe facial nerve paralysis can be accomplished by transfacial nerve grafting. Segments of nerve grafts are brought through tunnels across the lips from the normal side of the face to the paralyzed side. These are anastomosed to the distal facial nerve on the normal side and then to the proximal branches of the injured nerve on the paralyzed side. The overpull of the mouth and lower face toward the normal side is balanced when the nerve graft is anastomosed between fascicles of the intact facial nerve innervating the facial muscles to the same fascicles on the denervated side. If the facial muscle has been paralyzed for a prolonged period, serratus muscle from the chest wall may be transplanted and innervated by the facial nerve.

Repair of Lacerations of Lip or Mouth

Wound edges of the lip(s) and/or mucosa in the mouth are carefully sutured to repair lacerations.

Excision of Leukoplakia

Chronic irritation can result in an abnormal whitening of the mucous membrane of the lip and tongue (leukoplakia), a lesion primarily seen in heavy smokers. Dissection or carbon dioxide (CO_2) laser is used to resect a precancerous lesion.

Excision of Tumor of Lip

Excision of a lip tumor may be minor, with V-wedge excision, or extensive, depending on the stage of malignancy. Extensive lesions require a flap procedure for reconstruction.

Lip Reconstruction

Lips can be adequately reconstructed by a variety of techniques to restore sensation and motor function following trauma or surgical resection. Lip cancer is the most common type of cancer in the upper respiratory and digestive tracts. Surgical procedures to reconstruct lips may be classified as:

1. Those amenable to repair by primary closure of the remaining lip segments.
2. Those that can be closed with a full-thickness cross-lip flap from the opposite lip.
3. Those that require arterialized or myocutaneous flaps from adjacent cheek or nasolabial tissue.
4. Those that necessitate distant flaps. Arterialized and innervated myocutaneous flaps from the forehead or deltopectoral region may be used. These require staged procedures. Free microvascular composite grafts are done in one stage.

The ideal repair yields a lip that is not tight and that has a good vermilion border, an adequate sulcus, good sensation, and good muscle tone.

Aesthetic Procedures

Procedures are not always performed for cosmetic appearances alone. They may restore function as well as correct a facial deformity or defect.

Blepharoplasty

Redundant skin and/or protruding orbital fat is excised to correct deformities of the upper or lower eyelids of one or both eyes. *Blepharochalasis,* loss of elasticity of the skin of the eyelids, can occur at any age and usually is of unknown cause. *Dermatochalasis* primarily involves hypertrophy of the skin of the upper lids. Resection of the excessive redundant skin removes the mechanical visual obstruction caused by these two conditions. *Protrusion of intraorbital fat* into the lids is the most common eyelid deformity. It is often familial, sometimes seen in patients as young as in their twenties. This fat is removed from the compartments in the upper and/or lower lids to correct the deformity. This may be associated with dermatochalasis. A free graft of cartilage and mucosa from the nasal septum may be necessary to reconstruct lower eyelid defects following excision for tumor. *Hypertrophy of the orbicularis muscle* appears as a horizontal bulge below the lower lid margin. A skin-muscle flap resection may be performed. A surgical procedure for lifting the eyebrows will secondarily correct a hooding deformity of the upper lids caused by ptosis of the eyebrows.

These procedures are usually performed with local anesthesia. An upper lid incision is made in a natural skin fold; an incision in the lower lid is just under the eyelash line (Figure 34-5). The patient should wear dentures to the OR because facial contour is distorted without them. The surgeon could remove too much or too little redundant skin.

Because of proximity to eyes, protrusion of periorbital fat may impair vision. Oculoplastic procedures may be performed by an ophthalmologist as mentioned in Chapter 33, p. 687. Through a conjunctival incision, subconjunctival fat may be removed with a CO_2 laser. An eyelid procedure also may be necessary to protect the eye in a patient with facial nerve paralysis caused by trauma or tumor resection. A gold weight, between 0.05 to 1.2 g, or a spring can be inserted in the upper eyelid under local anesthesia. This protects the eye by allowing the eyelid to blink.

Otoplasty

Deformities of one or both external ears of an adult are usually the result of burns or traumatic avulsion. A segment of external ear that is partially or completely amputated often can be reattached to the remaining segment and buried beneath a flap of postauricular skin. The area over a completely severed auricular cartilage, which cannot be sutured back in place, is covered with a split-thickness skin graft initially. Later reconstruction may include insertion of cartilage taken from a patient's rib cage, a cartilage homograft (allograft), or a porous polyethylene or silicone prosthetic implant. The porous implant allows vascular and soft tissue ingrowth that reduces the risk of infection and extrusion, potential complications with a silicone implant. The graft or implant is buried beneath a segment of turned-down temporoparietal fascia. Then the area is covered with a split-thickness skin graft from the scalp or a full-thickness graft from the opposite postauricular area.

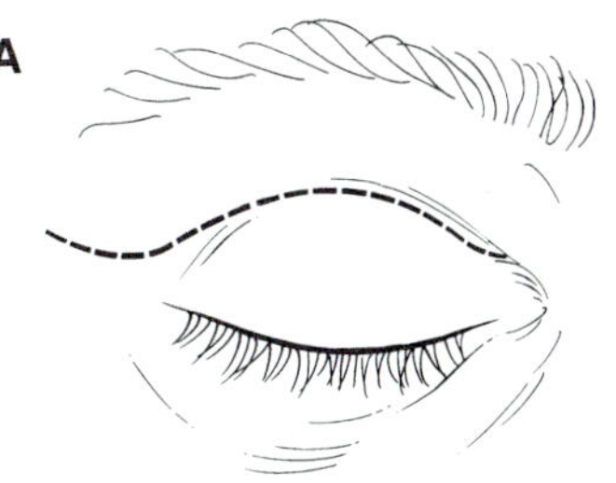

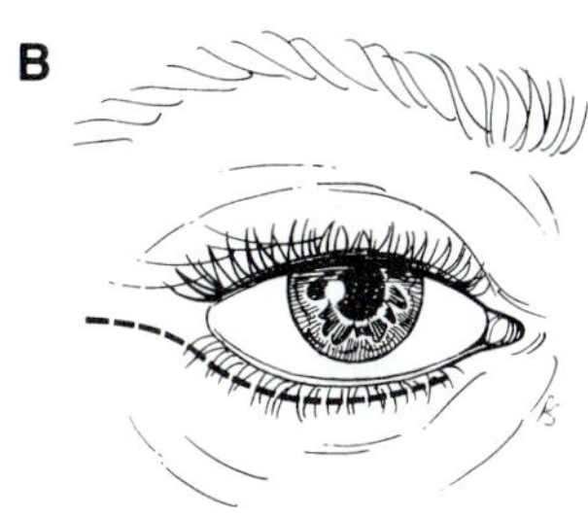

FIGURE 34-5 Incisions for blepharoplasty. **A,** Upper eyelid. **B,** Lower eyelid. (From Ruberg RL, Smith DJ Jr: *Plastic surgery: a core curriculum,* St Louis, 1994, Mosby.)

Rhinoplasty

Reshaping of the nose, although usually performed for cosmetic alteration desired by the patient, may be necessary to correct defects caused by trauma or surgical resection of neoplasms. Subtle changes with limited nasal reduction or augmentation of the nasal tip with the patient's own nasal cartilage can result in an aesthetically attractive and physiologically normal nose in most patients. Through an intranasal incision, the nose can be shortened or narrowed by rearranging, reshaping, and/or removing bone and cartilage. This may be done to relieve breathing problems. Nasal packing and a nasal splint support the structures postoperatively.

A free composite graft or pedicle flap may be necessary to close a large tissue defect. Bone or cartilage grafts may be needed for skeletal support. Prosthetic reconstruction for partial or total loss of the nose may be the procedure of choice.

Mentoplasty

Shape and size of the chin can be altered for aesthetics and/or functional bite disorders. (See discussion of orthognathic surgery in Chapter 36, p. 749.) The mandible can be repositioned forward or backward to change alignment in relation to the maxilla. Sections are removed to reduce size, or osteotomies are made to reshape the chin. *Micrognathia*, an abnormally small jaw, is augmented with bone or cartilage grafts or a silicone implant or by advancing the mandible. Lip incompetence, the inability to bring lips together without tension, may be corrected during the same surgical procedure.

Rhytidoplasty

Commonly referred to as a *face lift*, rhytidoplasty involves extensive dissection from above the ear, both in front of and behind the pinna, downward along the jaw line and upper neck (Figure 34-6, *A*). The skin is freed from underlying fascia. Wrinkles and folds caused by the normal aging process smooth out as the skin is lifted up and sutured in place. Dissection beneath the platysma muscle, referred to as the submuscular aponeurotic system (SMAS) procedure, minimizes the amount of skin undermined. The platysma is sutured back to the mastoid (Figure 34-6, *B* and *C*). Redundant skin is trimmed away. Frequently other procedures, such as blepharoplasty or rhinoplasty, accompany this surgical procedure. Meticulous hemostasis is essential to prevent hematoma formation, the foremost complication of rhytidoplasty. Hypotensive anesthesia may be used to help reduce this incidence. Closed-wound suction drainage is frequently used with or without a pressure dressing applied after the surgical procedure.

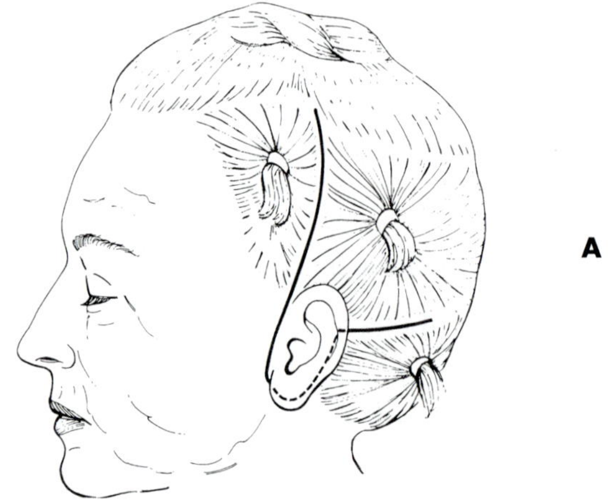

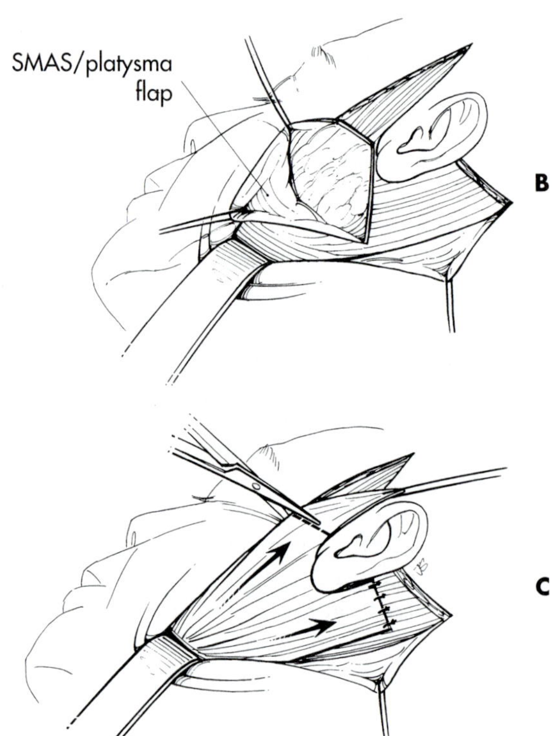

FIGURE 34-6 Rhytidoplasty (face lift). **A,** Incision from above ear and in front of and behind pinna. **B,** Dissection beneath and elevation of platysma flap (SMAS procedure). **C,** Platysma muscle is sutured back to mastoid. (From Ruberg RL, Smith DJ Jr: *Plastic surgery: a core curriculum,* St Louis, 1994, Mosby.)

Soft Tissue Augmentation

Fat transplantation may be done by microlipoextraction and injection of the patient's own tissue. Fat cells are withdrawn from the lower abdomen, hips, or thighs into a syringe through a hypodermic needle. The fat then is injected into areas around the lips or eyes to smooth wrinkles or into hollow spaces in the cheeks or other facial defects. This procedure may be done in conjunction with a rhytidoplasty. The correction may not be permanent because some of the fat cells will die.

A purified form of bovine dermal collagen can be injected for the same purposes. A series of injections of small amounts of the collagen are deposited to fill small soft tissue defects or to smooth out wrinkles.

Hair Replacement

Hair follicles can be transplanted from well-endowed areas of the scalp to bald or balding areas. Hundreds of micrografts (4.0 mm) and minigrafts (4.5 mm) are randomly scattered over the entire bald area to change the hairline. A new hairline can be initially established with rotational flaps from other parts of the scalp. This may necessitate tissue expansion. If hair loss is not complete, hair follicle grafts complement and thicken the existing hair. Several transplantation sessions may be necessary to achieve the final result the patient is seeking.

NOTE Because of vascularity in the head, patients are advised not to take aspirin or aspirin-containing medications for at least 2 weeks before surgical procedures on the face or head. The anticoagulant effect of aspirin can promote excessive bleeding. Hypotensive anesthesia may be used during the surgical procedure to help control bleeding.

Neck Dissection

Dissections for tumors originating in head or neck regions are discussed in Chapters 35 and 36. Following primary resection by a laryngologist, head and neck oncologist, or oral surgeon, the plastic surgeon may be called on to reconstruct the resultant defect. Or the plastic surgeon may be the primary surgeon who resects a tumor or lesion approached through the oral cavity or neck, followed by an immediate reconstruction.

RECONSTRUCTION OF OTHER BODY AREAS

Adipose Tissue

Lipectomy is an excision of excessive fat and redundant skin from the upper arms, abdomen, buttocks, thighs, or other body areas.

Liposuction

Localized areas of fat deposits are removed by suction-assisted lipectomy, known as *liposuction,* to alter body contours. Some surgeons prefer to inject target tissue with 0.25% lidocaine with 1:400,000 epinephrine to reduce blood loss during the surgical procedure. A blunt, hollow, curved or straight metal cannula (Mercedes cannula) measuring 1.5 to 6.0 mm with multiple openings in the distal shaft connected to negative pressure suction is inserted through a small skin incision. The cannula moves back and forth along the axial plane, parallel to skin surface, to bluntly dissect and aspirate cores of fat in a honeycomb pattern. This pattern allows for uniform tissue contouring. A laser beam may be used through the cannula to vaporize fat rather than suction it out. The laser diminishes bleeding by coagulating vessels. The patient's hematocrit level decreases by 1% for each 150 cc of fat removed by conventional liposuction.

Liposuction may be used in conjunction with abdominoplasty. It is also used to remove fat from the neck and chin, upper arms, breasts, flanks, buttocks, thighs, knees, and ankles. It can be used to defat transfer flaps and to treat some forms of lymphedema and lipomas. The amount of fat removed must not exceed the ability of the overlying skin to contract and is limited to 1500 cc. Large fluid volume shifts follow lipectomy. The incisions are sutured, and compression garments are worn for 10 days to 2 weeks postoperatively to control edema.

Abdominoplasty

Abdominoplasty includes excising excess, lax abdominal wall skin and adipose tissue and tightening abdominal wall musculature. This is usually a cosmetic procedure referred to as a *tummy tuck.* Physical discomfort or the inability to perform personal hygiene because of a large panniculus that hangs like an apron over the lower abdomen and genital region may be a functional indication for the procedure. Its purpose is not to make an obese person thin. The most suitable patient has ideal weight and good health. Causes of the abdominal wall laxity include pregnancy, marked weight loss, and the aging process.

Preoperatively, the primary incision line is marked along a natural skin fold using a marking pen with the patient in a standing position. After the administration of anesthesia, the head and foot of the operating table are elevated 15 to 20 degrees to anteflex the patient's torso and decrease abdominal tension. The surgeon chooses either a low transverse incision from one anterior superior iliac spine to the other or a combination transverse/secondary vertical incision (Figure 34-7). The typical area of dissection extends subcutaneously to the costal margins and xiphoid process superiorly and mid-to-lateral axillary lines laterally. The umbilicus is preserved and repositioned in the abdominal wall after the rectus muscle is tightened (plicated) and excess skin, subcutaneous tissue, and fat are resected. When wound closure is completed, the abdominal wall should be flat and smooth. Closed suction drainage, bulky pressure dressing, and an abdominal binder are used to prevent hematoma formation and eliminate dead space.

Postoperatively, the patient remains on complete bed rest with the head and foot of the bed flexed for 24 hours and then may ambulate progressively.

Breast

Breasts can be enlarged, reduced, or reconstructed. Unilateral augmentation or reduction is sometimes performed to correct asymmetry of breasts.

Augmentation Mammoplasty

A bilateral mammoplasty usually is performed for aesthetics on a woman who desires larger breasts. Inflatable implants are inserted under either breast tissue or underlying pectoralis muscles and then filled with sterile saline solution through self-sealing valves.

The breast implant can be inserted through a periareolar, transaxillary, inframammary, or supraumbilical endoscopic approach. The *periareolar* incision, made around the outside border of the lower half of the areola, is the most difficult for insertion of the implant, but it leaves the most inconspicuous scar. The *transaxillary* incision in the axilla does not scar the breast. The *inframammary* incision, the most common, is made transversely along the submammary fold. The implant is in-

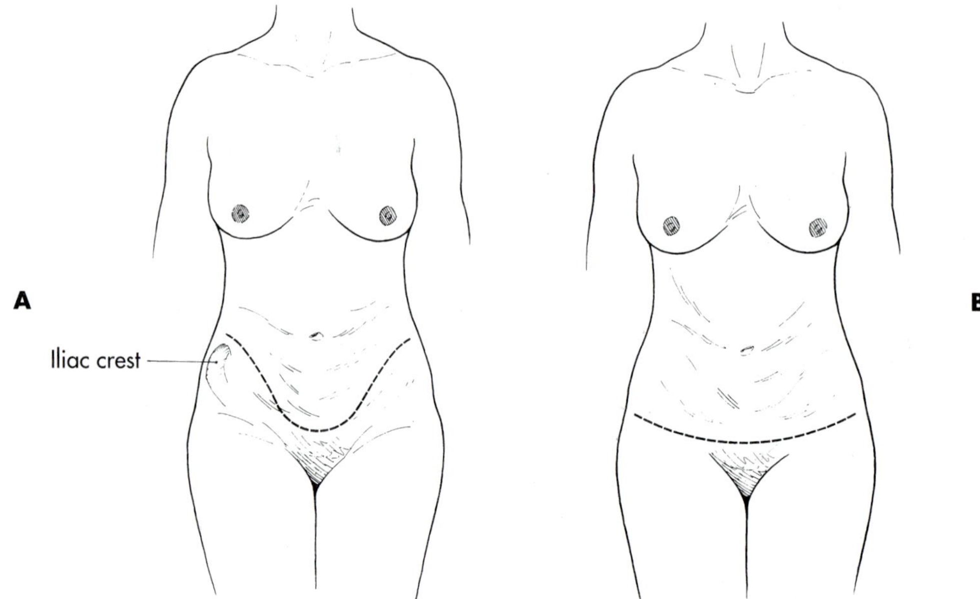

FIGURE 34-7 Abdominoplasty incisions. **A,** Medial to iliac crest for patient who desires high "French cut" swimsuit. **B,** In natural abdominal skin crease fold below iliac crest. (From Ruberg RL, Smith DJ Jr: *Plastic surgery: a core curriculum,* St Louis, 1994, Mosby.)

serted into a pocket formed between the mammary gland and pectoralis muscle or under the muscle.

An implant can also be inserted through a *supraumbilical endoscopic approach.* This technique eliminates an incision into the breast. A single incision is made in the superior border of the inner aspect of the umbilicus. An endoscope is inserted between the fascia and subcutaneous tissue up to the breast. The endoscope permits visual placement of a deflated expander between the breast tissue and the pectoralis muscle. The expander is filled with sterile saline solution, through a fill tube, to create a pocket for the implant. After insertion through the endoscope into the pocket, the deflated implant is inflated with sterile saline solution and the fill tube is removed.

Most implants are supplied sterile by the manufacturer. Manufacturers' instructions for sterilization of nonsterile implants must be followed. Sterile packages should not be opened by the circulator until the surgeon selects the appropriate-sized implants. Silastic sizers are frequently used to make this determination. The implant identification card should be put in the patient's chart and each implant's catalog and lot number recorded.

The woman with breast implants may be excluded from routine screening mammography programs (see Chapter 28, p. 564). Additional radiologic images must be taken to visualize all of the breast tissue. Ultrasonography frequently is performed at the same time to confirm the integrity of the implant. Studies have shown that the risk of rupturing the implant is not increased by compression during mammography if performed according to the American College of Radiology standards.

Capsular contraction, hematoma, infection, and skin necrosis are potential complications following prosthetic implantation for breast augmentation performed either unilaterally or bilaterally. Because of reported incidences of rupture and leakage, with the development of autoimmune disease, implants containing silicone gel are not used for aesthetic/cosmetic breast augmentation unless women are enrolled in a controlled clinical study.

Removing a ruptured or leaking silicone implant frequently is complicated by intracapsular adhesions. Control of bleeding points is critical to prevent silicone emboli in open blood vessels. This necessitates meticulous capsular dissection and hemostasis during removal of the implant shell, as well as irrigation with copious amounts of sterile saline solution to remove viscous silicone from the wound.

Reconstructive Mammoplasty

Breast reconstruction following mastectomy psychologically helps the patient cope with an altered body image. The type and timing of reconstruction are influenced by the patient's psychologic response to mastectomy, the type of mastectomy, and the patient's diagnosis and prognosis. Technical maneuvers of the general surgeon at the time of mastectomy will influence the possibility of an aesthetically acceptable result following breast reconstruction by the plastic surgeon.

To reconstruct breast contour, an implant may be inserted beneath the muscle layers at the time of subcutaneous mastectomy. Following modified radical or radical mastectomy, the wound should be well-healed, the scar mature, and the skin well-vascularized before implantation. A prosthesis can be implanted only when reliable skin is available to cover it. Skin flaps should be cut as thickly as consistent with a curative mastectomy. If sufficient skin flaps are not available, the plastic surgeon may transfer a pedicle skin flap from the abdomen or back to the chest wall.

Immediate breast reconstruction, or a delay of only a few days, after a modified radical mastectomy can be psychologically advantageous in women who have small lesions and no metastases. A latissimus dorsi myocutaneous flap may be used with an inflatable implant. A vertical or transverse rectus abdominis myocutaneous (TRAM) island flap with the vascular bundle from the superior epigastric vessels can be used without an implant. These flaps can also be used weeks to months after mastectomy for reconstruction. Aesthetically the end result is a semblance of a breast in weight and consistency. An areola and nipple complex may be constructed in a second-stage surgical procedure. A form of tattooing may be used to create natural color and shading resembling the nipple-areola complex.

The techniques described may be contraindicated in markedly obese patients and in some patients because a sufficient amount of autogenous tissue is not present for breast reconstruction. Another option is to place a tissue expander under the pectoralis muscle. When desired expansion is achieved, usually slightly larger than the other breast, the expander can be replaced with a permanent prosthesis. One type of expander/mammary prosthesis has a detachable reservoir and tubing to convert the expander into a permanent prosthesis. If this technique is not an option and the patient does not have adequate tissue in the lower abdomen or back, a microvascular free-flap transfer may be the procedure of choice. The vascular pedicle from a transverse abdominis rectus, superior gluteal, or inferior gluteal myocutaneous free flap may be anastomosed to the axillary or thoracodorsal vessels.

Reduction Mammoplasty

Hyperplasia of the breasts is reduced by resection of skin and glandular tissue. Reduction mammoplasty is usually sought by women for comfort, as well as aesthetic improvement of body image. The nipple-areola complexes are mobilized and transferred intact with the underlying breast tissue, maintaining the blood and nerve supply. The excess skin and glandular tissue may be excised with a scalpel, dermatome blade, or laser. Because breast tissue is very vascular, attention to hemostasis is important. The CO_2 laser offers the advantage of coagulating small blood vessels and sealing lymphatics as tissue is incised. A hemostatic scalpel can be used for the same purposes.

Hand

The plastic surgeon is dedicated to salvaging injured tissues whenever possible. Surgeons who subspecialize in hand reconstruction frequently use the operating microscope. Microsurgical revascularization and primary nerve repair salvage many traumatized hands that have lost their blood supply and sensation. Neurovascular island flaps also reinnervate and revascularize digits. Other traumatic hand injuries can be repaired by resurfacing with free skin grafts or pedicle flaps. Lacerated tendons are sutured or grafted. Hand reconstruction is also performed to correct joint deformities of degenerative diseases or for secondary release of contractures. Silicone rubber prosthetic implants may be used to replace metacarpophalangeal joints. (See Chapter 32, p. 664, for general considerations pertaining to surgical procedures on an extremity.)

Scars

Scar formation, the body's mechanism for healing wounds, is inevitable whenever skin is incised or injured. The plastic surgeon attempts to make a scar a fine line and as level and smooth as possible at the time of primary wound closure or as a secondary scar revision.

Scar Revision

The plastic surgeon can excise an aesthetically displeasing scar, realign wound edges, and resuture or close them with anticipation of a better cosmetic result. The direction of a scar can be changed to be less conspicuous in the natural skin lines. Scars are frequently revised following extensive reconstructive procedures or following a laceration with or without soft tissue trauma, particularly a facial scar. Z-plasty, W-plasty, M-plasty, Lazy-S, Y-V–plasty, and other techniques are used to improve the appearance of a hypertrophied or prominent scar.

Keloid formation, an abnormal deposition of collagen in healing skin wounds, presents a particularly difficult problem for the plastic surgeon and a psychologic problem for the patient. Keloids may require excision and grafting. The administration of a lathryrogenic agent and colchicine to inhibit cross-linking of newly synthesized collagen following grafting may prevent development of recurrent keloid formation. The argon laser also is used in treatment of keloid scars to reduce blood supply to the scar and to alter balance of collagen synthesis and lysis.

Dermabrasion

Dirt and cinders can become embedded in the dermis from a brush-burn injury. The plastic surgeon may use a wire brush or sandpaper to scrub out dirt and irrigate it from the area with warm saline solution. Sandpapering is also done to improve acne scars. This procedure is not always satisfactory if many pitted scars are too deep to reach or there are changes in the pigment of scars. Some plastic surgeons prefer to use chemical preparations, such as phenol, trichloroacetic acid, or alpha-hydroxy acid, to produce dermal peeling for a skin-smoothing effect in selected patients with facial scars or fine wrinkles. The patient is advised to avoid direct sun exposure for at least 6 months. Patients with fair complexions and thin skin have more favorable results than those with dark, oily complexions because the chemicals used decrease melanin in the skin and cause discoloration.

A high-speed dermabrader with rotating tips covered with diamond dust can be used on moderately damaged or tattooed skin. The rotating speed is controlled by regulation of pressure from the compressed nitrogen-gas power source. Older dermabraders have narrow bands of waterproof, steam sterilizable sandpaper mounted on an electric, air-powered, or battery-operated drill.

Facial resurfacing also can be accomplished with the CO_2 laser. The depth of beam penetration is controlled by the focus of the beam. Full-face laser resurfacing promotes continuity of skin color and texture rather than spot removal of facial scars.

Skin Cancer

Because overexposure to sunlight is the primary cause of skin cancer, most skin cancers occur on areas of the face, neck, and ears. Basal cell carcinoma, squamous cell carcinoma, and malignant melanoma are the three types of skin cancer. Certain types of nevi are skin lesions that may be precancerous and, therefore, should be removed. Skin lesions may be removed by a plastic surgeon or dermatologist by:

1. Excision and closure with sutures, grafts, or flaps
2. Punch biopsy with closure by secondary intention
3. Cold knife excision for frozen section
4. Electrosurgical curettage and electrodesiccation
5. Cryosurgery
6. Laser surgery
7. Radiation therapy

Mohs micrographic surgery is a technique used to excise advanced, recurrent, or poorly defined basal cell or squamous cell carcinomas of the skin with minimal excision of normal tissue. The bulk of the clinically evident tumor is excised initially. Then the lesion is resected by serial tangential excision (i.e., underlying tissue layers are removed with 1 to 3 mm borders). Each layer is numbered and charted for size and location. A map of the corresponding margins of each layer is drawn. The tissue is frozen, cut into sections, and examined microscopically. The patient may be allowed to leave the operating room and wait in a waiting room for the results. The surgeon removes additional layers of tissue or extends dissection until microscopic examination determines all cancer cells have been removed. Then the wound is closed. Small wounds may be left open to heal by secondary intention. Others may be sutured or covered with rotational myocutaneous flap from an adjacent area. Large denuded areas may require a split- or full-thickness skin graft. If a cartilage graft is needed, cartilage may be transferred from the auricle (pinna) of the ear to the transplant site.

Mohs surgery is not used for excision of malignant melanomas. Primary melanomas are treated according to their anatomic site and level of cutaneous penetration. A wide margin of normal tissue is excised around the melanoma. Skin grafts often are required. Regional lymph node dissection may be indicated to control metastatic disease.

BURNS

Skin and underlying tissues can be destroyed by thermal, chemical, or electrical injury. Burns are open wounds. As in other injuries, initial treatment is aimed at saving the patient's life. Then the treatment is directed toward preserving or restoring to normal, or as near normal as possible, the patient's bodily functions and appearance as rapidly as possible. Depending on the depth, extent, and location of the burn, reconstruction may extend over long periods of time, from months to years. The patient must be helped to accept the disfigurement; thus rehabilitation from a psychologic standpoint is important. Psychotherapy as well as surgery and physiotherapy may be necessary to promote as early a return to normalcy and usefulness as possible.

Classification of Burn

Severity of injury is determined by location and the cause of the burn. The Abbreviated Burn Severity Index (ABSI) is a five-variable scale used to evaluate burn injury severity and probability of survival. The five variables are sex, age, presence of inhalation injury, presence of full-thickness burn, and percentage of total body surface burned. An ABSI score of 2 to 18 is calculated by summation of coded values for each variable. Burns are classified by depth and extent as soon after injury as possible. The depth of a burn is classified by the degree of tissue involvement (see Figure 34-1, p. 709).

First-Degree Superficial Burn

Only the outer layer of the epidermis is involved in a first-degree burn. Superficial erythema, redness of the skin, and tissue destruction occur, but healing takes place rapidly.

Second-Degree Partial-Thickness Burn

All epidermis and varying depths of the dermis are destroyed in a second-degree burn. This is usually characterized by blister formation, pain, and a moist, mottled red or pink appearance. Hair follicles and sebaceous glands may be destroyed. Reepithelialization can occur provided the deepest layer of the epithelium is viable. However, superimposed infection can interfere with healing. Thickened scars form following healing of deep second-degree burns.

Third-Degree Full-Thickness Burn

The skin with all its epithelial structures and subcutaneous tissue is destroyed in a third-degree burn. This is characterized by a dry, pearly-white, or charred-appearing surface void of sensation. The destroyed skin forms a parchmentlike *eschar* over the burned area. If removed or left to slough off, eschar leaves a denuded surface that can extend to the fascia. Third-degree burns require skin grafts for healing to occur unless the area is small enough for closure by reepithelialization.

Fourth-Degree Burn

Sometimes referred to as *char burns,* fourth-degree burns may damage bones, tendons, muscles, blood vessels, and peripheral nerves. An electrical burn, for example, causes damage much deeper than is apparent on the skin surface. Often necrotic muscle and bone must be excised.

Estimation of Burn Damage

Two methods are used to estimate the total percentage of body surface burned and the percentage of each degree of burn.

Lund-Browder Chart

The percentage sizes of the head and lower extremities differ in infancy, childhood, and adulthood. According to the guidelines of the Lund-Browder chart (Figure 34-8), the percentage of burn is estimated on the basis of age in addition to anatomic location of the burn.

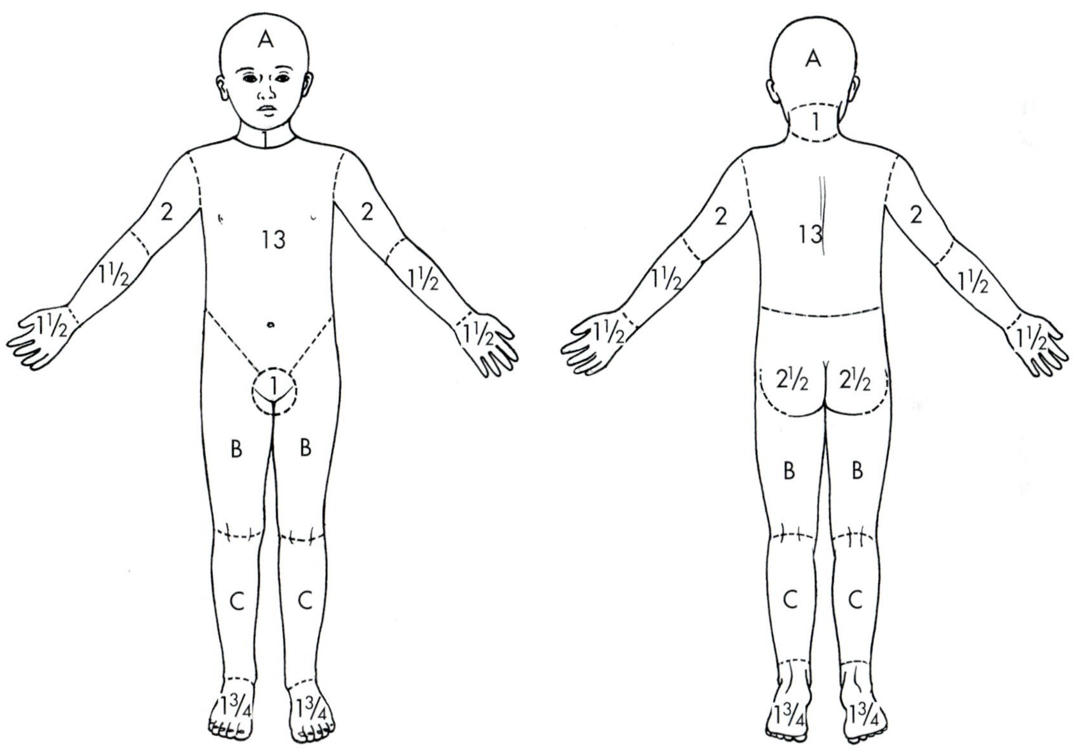

Relative percentage of areas affected by growth

	Age in Years					
	0	1	5	10	15	Adult
A—½ of head	9½	8½	6½	5½	4½	3½
B—½ of one thigh	2¾	3¼	4	4¼	4½	4¾
C—½ of one leg	2½	2½	2¾	3	3¼	3½

Total per cent burned ____________ 2° + ____________ 3° = ____________

FIGURE 34-8 Lund-Browder chart to determine relative percentage of areas of burns on body at various ages.

Rule of Nines

The body surface of an adult can be divided into areas equal to multiples of 9% of the total body surface.

1. Head and neck—9%
2. Anterior and posterior trunk—18% each
3. Upper extremities—9% each
4. Lower extremities—18% each
5. Perineum—1%

Initial Care of Burn Patient

Patients admitted to the emergency department with obvious burns may have multiple injuries and/or a pretrauma medical history that will complicate treatment. Initial care must include the following measures.

1. *Stop the burning process.* All clothing, jewelry, metal, and synthetic objects in contact with patient's skin are removed.
2. *Ensure a patent airway.* The respiratory system may be damaged from inhalation of superheated air or toxic gases. Immediate nasotracheal intubation with assisted mechanical ventilation may be necessary. Soft endotracheal tubes are preferred for prolonged intubation. Tracheotomy may be required several days later for prolonged respiratory assistance if the patient cannot be weaned from the ventilator. Bronchoscopy is performed routinely to evaluate the extent of tracheobronchial damage.
3. *Establish intravenous fluid therapy.* Blood samples are drawn for laboratory analysis and type and cross-matching when a venipuncture or cutdown is performed to establish an intravenous route for fluid and nutritional administration. Fluid and electrolyte balance must be restored as quickly as possible. Fluid, electrolytes, and protein are lost through changes in capillary permeability, causing intravascular volume shifts to interstitial tissues. Fluid shifts are directly proportional to depth and extent of the burn. Several formulas for determining fluid replacement have been developed to maintain plasma volume during the first 24 hours (Table 34-1). The calculated fluid replacement time begins at the time of injury, not when the patient arrives in the emergency department. A crystalloid solution of Ringer's lactate is infused initially because its hypertonic state decreases fluid loss from the intravascular space. Colloid-containing fluid, fresh frozen plasma, and other nutrients may be infused after the first 24 hours.
4. *Insert an indwelling Foley catheter.* Urine specimens are sent for analysis. Urine is checked for pH and specific gravity at frequent intervals. Hourly output is recorded. Adequate fluid replacement should maintain an output of at least 30 ml per hour.

TABLE 34-1

Fluid Replacement Formulas* for Burn Patients Developed at Major Burn Centers

FIRST 24 HOURS	SECOND 24 HOURS
Parkland Hospital	
Crystalloid	
4 ml Ringer's lactate/% burn/kg ½ during first 8 hr ½ during next 16 hr	Dextrose 5% in water maintenance
Colloid	
None	0.5 ml/% burn/kg
Brooke Army Hospital	
Crystalloid	
2 ml Ringer's lactate/% burn/kg ½ during first 8 hr ½ during next 16 hr	Dextrose 5% in water maintenance
Colloid	
None	0.5 ml/% burn/kg
Massachusetts General Hospital	
Crystalloid	
1.5 ml Ringer's lactate/% burn/kg ½ during first 8 hr ½ during next 16 hr	None specified
Colloid	
0.5 ml/% burn/kg None during first 4 hr ½ during second 4 hr ½ during next 16 hr	None specified

*Formula is calculated as percent of total body surface (% TBSB) × each kilogram (kg) of body weight × milliliters (ml) of fluid.

5. *Cleanse the wound.* All burns are treated aseptically. A mild cleansing agent, such as povidone-iodine, and *warm* water or saline solution are used to gently remove debris and loose devitalized tissue. Copious amounts of water, along with appropriate neutralizing agents, are used to cleanse and irrigate chemical burns. After cleansing, wet sheets under and around the patient must be removed and dry sterile ones applied. Nonwoven sheets specifically designed for burn care are commercially available.
6. *Estimate percentage and depth of burn.* Definitive treatment may be completed in the emergency department, or the patient may be transported to an immersion tank for further cleansing and debridement or to the OR for initiation of further

therapy as indicated by assessment of the burn. The burned area is covered with sterile or clean linen for transfer of the patient from the emergency department.

7. *Assess preexisting medical history and other injuries.* The patient may have a chronic illness, such as diabetes or heart disease, that must be stabilized as part of the treatment regimen. Withdrawal from alcohol or drugs may cause physiologic disturbances. The patient may have suffered other injuries in the accident causing the burn. Abuse may be suspected, as in a child or elderly person. Appropriate interventions must be taken. The burn may not be the first priority if, for example, the patient has a head injury, ruptured internal organ, or fractures.
8. *Prepare patient for transport.* The patient may go from the emergency department directly to a burn unit, the OR, or other care area. The attending physician may initiate therapy before referral to a plastic surgeon. If available, hyperbaric oxygen (HBO) therapy may be utilized. HBO produces marked vasoconstriction, decreasing loss of serum through the burn surface. This may reduce need for fluid replacement. Oxygen in cells around the burn may positively affect burn tissue to regenerate and begin healing. Partial-thickness burns may be prevented from progressing to full-thickness burns.

Methods of Surgical Treatment

Prevention of infection and promotion of healing are of utmost concern in the treatment of burned patients. The probability of infection developing increases in greater proportion to the percentage of body surface burned. Colonization may begin as early as 24 hours after the burn.

Excisional Therapy

Primary excision of necrotic tissue from deep second-degree and all full-thickness third-degree burned areas, followed immediately by skin grafting, is performed beginning as soon as possible after the injury. Debridement can be accomplished with a scalpel, freehand skin-graft knife, dermatome, electrosurgical knife, or laser beam. The surgeon selects the most appropriate instrument for the particular burned area to be excised. Layers of burned tissue are removed sequentially until capillary bleeding indicates that tissue is viable. Hypotensive anesthesia may help control massive blood loss during extensive excisions.

Mesh grafts are frequently used to expand available autografts. Microskin grafting is another alternative for maximizing a split-thickness autograft. The donor skin is cut with scissors into tiny particles. These are placed on the dermal side of a homograft. This dermal surface is placed on the recipient burn site. The skin particles grow together to resurface the area; then the homograft is rejected.

A homograft or heterograft may be applied to temporarily cover an area until regeneration proceeds or sufficient autografts can be harvested. Skin substitutes also are available to temporarily cover wounds, both recipient and donor sites. A composite silicon-nylon membrane with a chemically bonded polypeptide of collagen (Biobane) will adhere to the wound surface to inhibit infection and to control fluid loss. Another artificial material incorporates a layer of bovine hide collagen onto a layer of silicone. These biologic dressings and skin substitutes must be changed periodically (see p. 724).

Tangential Excision Burned tissue is excised until normal dermal tissue is reached below the depth of the wound. Tangential excision is usually the procedure of choice for deep partial-thickness burns of the dorsum of hands or on arms or legs. It is advantageous to minimize contractures. The wound base, containing some viable dermal structures necessary for regeneration, is covered with a split-thickness autograft. Early tangential excision and grafting in one procedure for body-surface burns can reduce mortality and septic complications and shorten hospitalization.

Escharectomy Full-thickness eschar is excised down to the fascia when viable tissues in more superficial layers are not evident, except on hands, neck, or face. All denuded areas created by excision are covered with a biologic dressing for 3 to 5 days. They are then grafted with full-thickness autografts. Frequently split-thickness mesh grafts must be used to spread over large areas and allow seepage of serous fluids. These are not placed on the face and neck or over joints. If sufficient skin is not available for autografting, homografts or heterografts continue to be used as biologic dressings for short periods. They are changed every 3 to 5 days.

Other Surgical Procedures

During the course of hospitalization a burned patient may come to the OR for one or many procedures.

Escharotomy Shrinkage of eschar may occur and cause a tourniquet effect in circumferential burns of the extremities or thorax. Bilateral incisions through the eschar, not including the fascia, are made to improve circulation to a lower extremity. Multiple incisions on the chest wall relieve respiratory distress. Sites of incisions avoid major peripheral nerves to prevent irreversible neurologic complications.

Fasciotomy If adequate decompression does not occur following escharotomy, the incision may be extended into underlying fascia. Fascia may need to be incised in the arm if compromised circulation is evident.

Amputation of Digits Amputation may be necessary to control infection in the extremity and prevent septicemia if escharotomy is unsuccessful.

Debridement Debridement of underlying tissues helps prevent extension of tissue loss. Nonviable tendons, cartilage, or bone may be excised, such as from the hand, ear, or skull.

Full-Thickness Skin Grafts With or without tarsorrhaphy, full-thickness skin grafts are used to prevent contracture of the eyelids. The cornea must be protected from exposure.

Split-Thickness Skin Grafts Autografts are applied to debrided areas as rapidly as possible. Hands and face are first priority to restore function; joints and flexion creases are second to prevent contractures; and extremities and trunk are the lowest priority. Skin from donor sites is cut thin if the site will be used again. Mesh grafts are frequently used to cover very large surfaces or irregular areas such as the perineum. Grafts are held in place with staples or sutures and dressings to achieve apposition and immobilization.

Tissue Expansion If sufficient normal skin is available, a tissue expander may be placed beneath subcutaneous tissue to broaden the width for future use as a local flap to cover an adjacent burned area following excision of scar tissue or for better closure of the donor site.

Myocutaneous Flaps Myocutaneous flaps, either on a pedicle or by free microvascular transfer, may be used in the reconstruction of burn wounds.

Biologic Dressing Changes Instead of leaving a biologic dressing in place until rejection, with attendant inflammatory reaction, a biologic dressing is usually replaced every few days until the area is ready for autograft or skin for autograft is available. Biologic dressings may be homografts of human skin from a living or cadaver donor, placental or amniotic membranes, or a heterograft of porcine skin (see Chapter 24, pp. 509-510). Porcine dressings frequently are applied initially on second-degree burns as a temporary dressing or used in conjunction with extensive excisional therapy. Synthetic skin substitutes may be preferred. A biologic dressing is used for several reasons.

1. It helps to control infection by covering denuded areas.
2. It prevents loss of serum.
3. It decreases pain.
4. It seems to stimulate formation of epithelium in dermis under it.
5. It promotes growth of granulation tissue.

Dressing Changes Occlusive dressings, if used, must be changed frequently to control infection harboring under them. An antimicrobial or chemotherapeutic agent may be applied as an integral part of the dressing.

1. *Silver sulfadiazine (Silvadene) cream* applied directly onto the burned area makes removal of a dressing less painful and does not disturb the healing process as it is removed. It is an effective topical antimicrobial and produces no metabolic side effects; some patients have developed neutropenia and delayed wound healing after its use, however. Fresh cream is applied after cleansing and debridement. A layer of fine mesh gauze is laid over it (unless the open-exposure method will be used for further healing). Then soft, absorbent material, such as fluffed gauze, and a preformed splint may be used. These are held in place by a cotton elastic bandage. An occlusive dressing may be used to hold a hand, foot, or joint in functional position.
2. *Mafenide acetate (Sulfamylon) cream* penetrates intact eschar rapidly and is quite successful in reducing bacterial counts to optimal levels for skin grafting. However, application directly on the burned area is painful for the patient after cleansing and debridement. It may cause maceration under the dressing. Absorption may result in metabolic acidosis; thus acid-base balance must be closely monitored. Prolonged use may lead to renal or pulmonary complications.
3. *Silver nitrate solution* is used infrequently. After cleansing and debridement, multiple-thickness dressings are applied to the area. These are kept saturated with 0.5% silver nitrate solution and changed every 12 hours. For a debridement, sterile distilled water is used for irrigation because saline may cause the precipitation of silver salts. It is ineffective in treating established wound infection because it does not penetrate intact eschar. Care is taken to avoid splashing silver nitrate solution on walls and floors because staining can occur. If disposable drapes and gowns are not used, stained linen must be laundered separately from other linen.

Serial Biopsy Cultures Through two linear incisions, a biopsy of tissue, including subcutaneous fat, is excised for culturing. This is done every 2 or 3 days, until the eschar begins to separate, to monitor the colonization of microorganisms in the wound. The results of serial biopsy culture enable the surgeon to make decisions specific to the therapeutic needs of the patient. An antimicrobial or chemotherapeutic topical agent is selected or changed according to these results.

Curling's Ulcer Gastrointestinal complications may occur anytime from the early postinjury period through rehabilitation. Complaints must be carefully evaluated. The patient who develops massive bleeding from a Curling's or stress ulcer in the stomach and duodenum must be operated on. Vagotomy with antrectomy is most frequently performed by a general surgeon.

Marjolin's Ulcer An ulceration caused by malignant changes can develop in the surface area of a burn scar. As long as 20 years after the burn, a prolonged ulceration can lead to squamous cell carcinoma of the skin. A Marjolin's ulcer should be excised.

Environmental Considerations for Burn Patients

1. Environmental control is perhaps the essence of burn therapy. The environment must protect the wound from further injury and microbial invasion. *A burn wound is always potentially contaminated until epithelialization occurs.* Open exposure of the wound to room air may be the choice of the plastic surgeon for selected patients. Regardless of method of treatment, the following adjuncts are used—if the equipment is available—in the care of burned patients, in addition to strict adherence to all the principles of aseptic technique.
   a. *Reverse isolation technique* may be practiced to protect the patient, whose resistance is low, from cross infection from personnel. Caps, masks, shoe covers, and sterile gowns and gloves are worn by all personnel attending the patient. This may be referred to as *protective isolation*.
   b. *Laminar,* or downward unidirectional, *airflow* away from the wound helps minimize airborne contamination.
   c. A *plastic isolator* protects the patient. Personnel do not directly enter this isolation unit. Nursing and medical care is given through clear plastic access walls. The environment around the patient inside the isolator is controlled at 90° F (32° C) and 94% relative humidity to conserve heat loss by evaporation.
2. Patients with extensive burns may be placed on a Stryker frame or a circle electric bed specially designed to facilitate handling and turning. They are transported to the OR on these frames or beds. Patients must be turned slowly and gently because they are often hypovolemic after the injury.
3. Hypothermia must be prevented. The patient's thermoregulatory mechanism is altered by the destruction of skin that normally acts as an insulator. Heat loss is the greatest single problem the burn patient faces in the OR.
   a. Room temperature should be increased to between 80° and 90° F (27° and 32° C) with low relative humidity of about 30% to 40%.
   b. OR must be ready to receive the patient directly from the burn unit. The patient should not wait in a cool holding area or corridor. Concern is for the patient's thermoregulation and potential for infection.
   c. Warm hyperthermia blanket should cover the operating table. The patient should be exposed as little as possible. Cover with warm blankets.
   d. Patient's temperature should be monitored with a rectal or esophageal probe.
   e. Solutions should be warmed before irrigation or infusion.
   f. Operating during nighttime hours is advantageous for the patient because the normal schedule for oral intake is not interrupted.
4. Hypnosis and biofeedback techniques can reduce potential postanesthetic complications when many surgical procedures are necessary to achieve acceptable functional and cosmetic results after a burn. The OR environment must be quiet to be conducive to hypnotic suggestions given to the patient.

After the initial assessment of a severely burned patient, a prolonged period of treatment begins. A multidisciplinary team must coordinate the treatment plan to achieve the best possible clinical outcomes for the patient. As with all plastic surgery patients, both physiologic and psychosocial support is essential to successful rehabilitation.

Bibliography

Alterescu V, Alterescu KB: Pressure ulcers: assessment and treatment, *Orthop Nurs* 11(2):37-49, 1992.

Anderson RD: The expanded "Bat" flap for male pattern baldness, *Ann Plast Surg* 31(5):385-391, 1993.

Brandy DA: A three step approach to punchgrafting approach, *J Dermatol Surg Oncol* 18(3):187-192, 1992.

Burgess LP et al: Wound tension in rhytidectomy: effects of skin-flap undermining and superficial musculoaponeurotic system suspension, *Arch Otolaryngol Head Neck Surg* 119(2):173-177, 1993.

Clamon J, Netscher DT: General principles of flap reconstruction: goals for aesthetic and functional outcome, *Plast Surg Nurs* 14(1):9-14, 1994.

Dinman S, Giovanne MK: The care and feeding of microvascular grafts: how nurses can help prevent flap loss, *Plast Surg Nurs* 14(3):154-164, 1994.

Duncan DJ, Driscoll DM: Burn wound management, *Crit Care Nurs Clin North Am* 3(2):199-220, 1992.

Forte R et al: Chemical peeling, *Plast Surg Nurs* 13(4):194-200, 1993.

Goodman T et al: Skin ulcers, *AORN J* 52(1):24-37, 1990.

Gu JM et al: Poor surgical technique produces more emboli after arterial anastomosis of an island flap, *Br J Plast Surg* 44(2):126-129, 1991.

Harden JT, Girard N: Breast reconstruction using an innovative flap procedure, *AORN J* 60(2):184-192, 1994.

Hom DM: The wound healing response in grafted tissues, *Otolaryngol Clin North Am* 27(1):13-24, 1994.

Houston S et al: Crafting postop care for sternal wound omentopexy, *Am J Nurs* 92(3):56-60, 1992.

Jones CE, Wellisz T: External ear reconstruction, *AORN J* 59(2):411-422, 1994.

Katez P: Reduction mammoplasty, *Plast Surg Nurs* 12(2):51-60, 1992.

Kemmy J: OR nursing law: exploring the issues concerning augmentation mammoplasty, *AORN J* 55(6):1552-1557, 1992.

Kruse BD et al: Breast imaging and the augmented breast, *Plast Surg Nurs* 12(3):109-115, 1992.

Ledford JK: Fresh tissue Mohs surgery and reconstruction of oculofacial lesions, *Surg Technol* 23(4):8-10, 1991.

Mandy SH: Intraoperative expander-assisted scalp reduction, *J Dermatol Surg Oncol* 19(12):1117-1119, 1993.

McCain L: Counseling the woman with silicone breast implants, *Plast Surg Nurs* 12(2):61-70, 1992.

McKinnon CC, Fulton JE: Facial dermabrasion, *AORN J* 51(3):739-750, 1990.

Norwood OT, Taylor BJ: Hair transplant surgery: innovative designs, *J Dermatol Surg Oncol* 16(1):50-54, 1990.

Pettis DK, Vogt PA: Complications of suction-assisted lipoplasty, *Plast Surg Nurs* 12(4):148-151, 1992.

Pruzinsky T: Psychological factors in cosmetic plastic surgery: recent developments in patient care, *Plast Surg Nurs* 13(2):64-69, 1993.

Rubayi S et al: Myocutaneous flaps: surgical treatment of severe pressure ulcers, *AORN J* 52(1):40-55, 1990.

Ruberg RL, Smith DJ Jr: *Plastic surgery: a core curriculum*, St Louis, 1994, Mosby.

Simler AG: Endoscopic augmentation mammoplasty: the umbilical approach, *Plast Surg Nurs* 14(3):149-153, 1994.

Stombler RE: Breast implants and the FDA: past, present, and future, *Plast Surg Nurs* 13(4):185-187, 1993.

Swinehart JM: Incisional slit grafting, *J Dermatol Surg Oncol* 18(3):250-252, 1992.

Swinehart JM, Griffin EI: Extensive scalp lifting: decrease in complications utilizing unilateral occipital artery ligation and other modifications, *J Dermatol Surg Oncol* 18(9):796-804, 1992.

Trevisani TP: Cosmetic surgery: a specialty worth exploring, *Surg Technol* 22(2):20-21, 1990.

Ubel CO: Micrografts and minigrafts: a new approach for baldness surgery, *Ann Plast Surg* 27(5):476-487, 1991.

Westlake C: Commitment to function: microsurgical flaps, *Plast Surg Nurs* 11(3):95-99, 1991.

Wilkes P: Rhinoplasty, *Surg Technol* 26(5):8-13, 33, 1994.

Zingg BM: Managing burns in children, *AORN J* 54(3):568-575, 1991.

CHAPTER 35

Otorhinolaryngology

EAR, NOSE, AND THROAT SURGERY

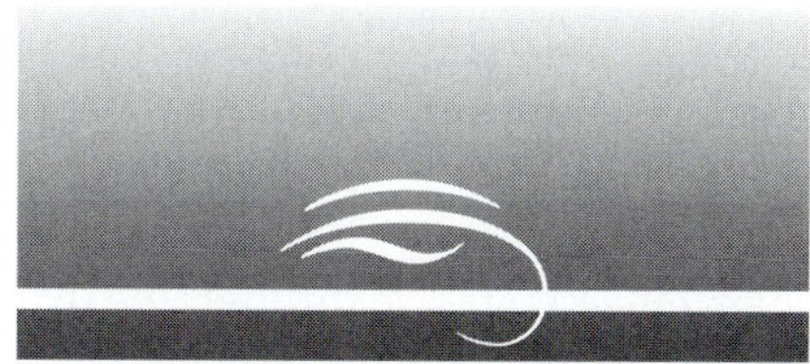

Otorhinolaryngology has traditionally been concerned with research and surgical treatment of diseases of the ear *(oto)*, nose *(rhino)*, and throat *(laryngo)*. Advances in scientific knowledge, diagnostic capabilities, and technology have broadened the scope of this field, which has led to subspecialization. General otorhinolaryngologists, commonly called *ear, nose, and throat (ENT) surgeons*, practice within the total scope of this specialty. Other surgeons confine their practice to one of the subspecialties: otology, facial surgery, or head and neck oncology. The certifying body for this specialty is the American Board of Otolaryngology, Head and Neck Surgery.

HISTORICAL BACKGROUND

Recognition of abnormal conditions of the ear, nose, and throat began in early times. Some of the first permanent records mentioning them, attributed to the Egyptians, date from 3500 BC. Breathing was thought to occur through the ears via the eustachian tubes. Therefore attempts were made to remedy deafness and ear discharges. Study of anatomy antedated the Christian era, leading to the practice of primitive procedures in India. For example, nasal fractures were splinted by insertion of a tube into the nostril.

Hippocrates realized that irregular teeth could cause various mouth and ear disorders. He also recognized otitis media, as well as the fact that congenital deafness was incurable. He advocated immediate reduction of nasal fractures.

The early centuries of the Christian era brought attempts to devise mastoid procedures. Tracheotomy, thought to have been known 2000 years ago, was described in detail by Antyllas, a surgeon of the second century. In the seventh century, physicians advocated its use to prevent suffocation in persons with laryngeal obstruction. Tracheotomies were performed frequently during a diphtheria epidemic in Europe in 1610. The lifesaving value of this procedure was further proved in later centuries when used for patients with severe croup or tuberculosis. The seventeenth century also saw removal of the tongue for tumor.

In 1855, tuning-fork tests, used in evaluating actual and residual hearing, were described by Rinne. European surgeons in the latter part of the nineteenth century attempted to restore hearing by surgical incision of the eardrum and removal of the tympanic membrane and stapes. Later, fenestration and stapes mobilization procedures were developed. Stapedectomy, devised in the 1960s, has largely replaced those procedures. Continued research in nerve deafness and transplantation may well produce a cure for many persons now consigned to a world of silence.

Research resulting in refined equipment, techniques, and prostheses has made possible the current specialization. One of the greatest advances in treatment was the development of antibiotics, which often eliminate the need for a surgical procedure.

EAR

Anatomy and Physiology

The structures of the ear (Figure 35-1) are concerned with two functions:

1. Hearing (i.e., receiving sound, amplifying it, and transmitting it to the brain for interpretation)
2. Maintaining body equilibrium

Anatomically, the ear is divided into three parts: the external, middle, and inner ear.

External Ear

The outer ear consists of the *auricle* or *pinna* composed of cartilage, except for the lobe, and skin, and the *external auditory canal.* The meatus of the auricle leads via the ear canal to the *tympanic membrane* or *eardrum.* This membrane separates the external and middle ear. Color change of the translucent eardrum, visible through a speculum, may be indicative of middle ear disease. The outermost lining of the tympanic membrane is derived from skin of the ear canal. The inner lining is continuous with the middle ear mucosa. The eardrum protects the middle ear but may be perforated by injury or pressure built up in the middle ear by infection.

Middle Ear

The middle ear consists of the *tympanic cavity,* a closed chamber that lies between the tympanic membrane and the inner ear. Within this cavity are the three smallest bones in the body, an *ossicular chain* comprised of the malleus, incus, and stapes. They resemble a hammer, anvil, and stirrups, respectively. The malleus, attached to the eardrum, joins the incus, the extremity of which articulates with the stapes, the innermost bone. The footplate of the stapes fits in the *oval* or *vestibular window,* an opening in the wall of the inner ear. The bones of the ossicular chain must be able to move mechanically to conduct sound from the eardrum to the inner ear. The *round* or *cochlear window,* also between the middle and the inner ear, equalizes pressure that enters through the oval window.

The middle ear opens into the nasopharynx by way of the *eustachian tube.* Normally closed during swallowing or yawning, the eustachian tube aerates the middle ear cavity. This mechanism is essential for adequate hearing.

Posteriorly the middle ear exits to the *mastoid process.* This inferior projection of the temporal bone is a honey-

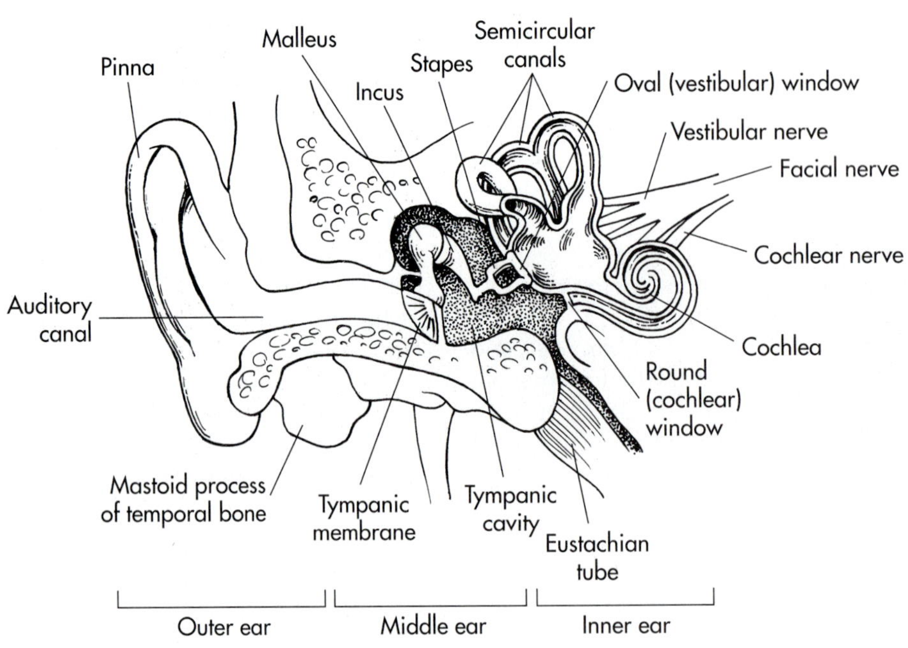

FIGURE 35-1 Anatomy of ear.

comb of air cells lined with mucous membrane. Because the antrum of the mastoid process connects with it, middle ear infection may produce mastoiditis. The middle ear is situated in the tympanic portion of the temporal bone, the inner ear in the petrous portion, which integrates with the base of the skull. The tympanic portion also forms part of the ear canal.

Inner Ear

The end organs of hearing and equilibrium are situated in the inner ear. The two main sections, cochlear and vestibular, have precise functions, although coordinated. The *cochlea,* a bony spiral, relates to hearing. The *vestibular labyrinth,* composed of three semicircular canals, relates to equilibrium. These structures house two separate fluids, *endolymph* and *perilymph,* which nourish and protect the hearing receptors. Neuroepithelium of the *organ of Corti,* the end organ of hearing, holds thousands of minute hair cells, which respond to sound waves that enter the cochlea via the oval window. Neuroepithelium of the vestibular portion also contains hair cells. Rapid head motion produces current in the endolymph that may result in nausea or vertigo. The *vestibular nerve,* a portion of the acoustic nerve, governs reflexes to muscles to maintain equilibrium.

Proximal Structures

The middle and the inner ear are adjacent to many important structures. The seventh cranial or facial nerve is enclosed in a bony canal running through the tympanic cavity and mastoid bone. The meninges of the temporal lobe of the brain are also near the middle ear and the mastoid. Facial paralysis, meningitis, and intracranial infection such as brain abscess are potential complications of ear infection.

The major blood vessels are the internal carotid artery and internal jugular vein, as well as the lateral sinus. Thrombosis and infection of the lateral sinus of the dura mater are potentially lethal complications of otitis media, with or without mastoiditis.

Auditory Process

Sound or pressure waves enter the auricle. They pass along the ear canal to the tympanic membrane. The vibration of the waves is transmitted across the middle ear sequentially by the ossicles. Amplification of sound is enhanced to some extent by mechanical action of the ossicles but mainly by aerial ratio. A large volume of sound-wave pressure from the tympanic membrane funnels to a small reactive area, the stapedial footplate, intensifying sound. At the footplate of the stapes, sound pressure is transferred to the inner ear via the oval window. The hair cells of the organ of Corti are set in motion by disturbance of the inner ear fluids as sound pressure moves from the oval to the round window. Mechanical energy is converted to electrical potential, which is delivered to the brain along auditory nerves that enter the inner ear. The brain interprets the sound as hearing.

Loss of Hearing

Hearing affects the quality and quantity of interpersonal interactions. It is a major sense for communicating within one's environment. Loss of hearing, therefore, affects social relationships. (See Chapter 8, p. 108, for discussion of hearing-impaired patients.) The type of deafness or hearing loss in varying degrees may result from:

1. Disease, such as otosclerosis, in which changes in the bony capsule of the labyrinth occur. Otosclerotic bone invades the stapedial footplate, resulting in its fixation and ultimate inability to vibrate in the oval window. Hearing loss is gradual but progressive. This type of deficiency can be surgically corrected when auditory nerve endings are not destroyed.
2. Trauma, such as perforated eardrum, requiring repair to restore function and aerial ratio.
3. Infection, usually controlled by antibiotics. Although more common in children, infection may also occur in adults. It may cause accumulation of fluid in the middle ear. Mastoiditis results from extension of otitis media.
   a. Serous otitis media may result from obstruction of the pharyngeal orifice of the eustachian tube. If blocked, for example, by hypertrophied adenoid tissue, infection, or allergic swelling, the tube is unable to equalize pressure because air cannot enter the middle ear from the pharynx. The vacuum or negative pressure thus created causes serum to be drawn into the tympanic cavity from blood vessels in the middle ear mucosa. Recurrent otitis media may require drainage of purulent exudate if conservative treatment fails.
   b. Acute otitis media may require drainage of purulent exudate if conservative treatment fails.
   c. Chronic otitis media with or without mastoiditis may follow recurrent otitis media with tympanic membrane perforation. It can produce a chronically draining ear.

Differential Diagnosis

Measurements that compare bone conduction with air conduction are important in differential diagnosis. *Bone conduction* refers to hearing as transmitted through the skull; *air conduction* refers to transmission of sound waves from the tympanic membrane to the inner ear via air. Hearing loss caused by a defect in the external or the middle ear, referred to as *conductive loss,* is a mechanical obstruction of air conduction that usually can be helped by surgical intervention. When the decrement is in the inner ear, referred to as *perceptive* or *sensorineural loss*, damage to nerve tissue and/or sensory paths to the brain is not benefited by a surgical procedure.

Auditory acuity and function are measured by various tests. The audiogram is one measurement tool. Computer-averaged tomography is used to measure and analyze electrical impulses, known as auditory brainstem responses, from the brain and cortical auditory pathway. An acoustic reflex latency test of the stapedius reflex provides information about hearing sensitivity. Auditory brainstem evoked potentials assess the patient's hearing threshold.

OTOLOGIC SURGICAL PROCEDURES

The advent of antibiotics greatly alleviated the necessity for surgical intervention prevalent in previous decades. Emphasis was on relief of infection and conversion of a draining ear to a dry one. Now infection is generally controlled pharmacologically. Attention has turned to surgical measures to improve hearing following damage from chronic infection and to restore hearing by reconstruction of sound-conduction pathways. Current techniques, instrumentation, lasers, and the operating microscope have enhanced the capability of otologists.

General Considerations in Otology

1. Local anesthesia may be used for a minor procedure on the external ear, but general anesthesia is usually used to avoid patient movement while the surgeon is manipulating delicate structures in the middle or inner ear.
   a. Inhalation anesthesia may be given by face mask for a short procedure, with the anesthesiologist seated at head of the table.
   b. Anesthesiologist sits alongside the table with the patient facing him or her when patient is intubated for a major procedure.
   c. Hypotensive anesthesia (see Chapter 17, pp. 339-340) may be employed to create a bloodless field, especially during microsurgery.
   d. Nitrous oxide diffuses into cavities, causing expansion of the middle ear. This can present a hazard in a grafting procedure, for example; nitrous oxide is discontinued before placement of a graft in the middle ear.
   e. General anesthesia may be supplemented with a local agent in some procedures, often with epinephrine to control bleeding.
2. Patient's head is turned with the affected side up and stabilized in a donut. The dependent pinna should be protected from pressure.
3. Lint-free drapes are preferred. It is mandatory that gloves be powder- and lint-free. Formation of granuloma in the oval window can cause irreversible sensorineural hearing loss.
4. Operating microscope is used for many otologic procedures.
   a. Surgeon sits at head of table to use the microscope.
   b. Microinstruments should be carefully handled before, during, and after use. See Chapters 14 and 15 for care and handling of microinstruments.
5. Compressed absorbent patties (cottonoids) moistened with normal saline solution, rather than gauze sponges, are frequently used. They must be counted.
6. Hemostasis may be achieved with epinephrine, absorbable hemostatic sponges or oxidized cellulose, laser, and bone wax.
7. Prosthetic devices should be available in an assortment of types and sizes. Tissue homografts may be used.
8. Nerve stimulator may be used to identify facial, acoustic, cochlear, and/or vestibular nerve branches. Evoked potential audiometry also may be used to monitor the seventh and eighth cranial nerves.
9. Bone instruments, including powered drills, are used for opening the temporal bone.
10. Carbon dioxide (CO_2), Nd:YAG, argon, and potassium titanyl phosphate (KTP) lasers are used during otologic procedures to control bleeding, divide nerves, and/or vaporize tissues.
11. Pressure dressings are usually applied.

External Ear

Removal of Foreign Body

Removing a foreign body from the outer canal is performed most frequently in children. The object is washed out or removed to prevent purulent infection. A plant seed or vegetable foreign body such as a pea is not irrigated because it may swell in the ear and increase the difficulty of removal. General anesthesia sometimes may be required. Trauma should be minimal during removal of a foreign body to prevent stenosis of the canal or perforation through the eardrum.

Drainage of Hematoma

Usually the result of injury, a hematoma is drained to avoid infection with subsequent chondritis and deformity of the auricle.

Excision of Tumor

Extent of the surgical procedure to excise a tumor depends on the size and type of tumor, either benign or malignant. The skin of the pinna is vulnerable to actinic (chemical) changes caused by radiant energy during exposure to the sun. Basal cell lesions do not metastasize, but squamous cell carcinoma often does. Primary cancer may be excised by a wide or wedge excision with primary closure or a wide excision with skin graft. If the lesion is extensive, partial or total pinnectomy may be necessary. The area can be skin grafted and reconstructed cosmetically with a prosthesis (see section on otoplasty, Chapter 34, p. 715). Radical temporal bone resection is indicated if the bone (canal) is involved. Neck dissection may be indicated if nodal metastases are present.

Implantation of Hearing Device

A small magnetic disk is implanted in the temporal bone behind the ear. A miniaturized external sound processor, held magnetically to the implanted disk, transforms sound into vibrations. These vibrations travel through temporal bone, bypassing external and middle ears, to stimulate the cochlea. The device helps restore hearing in a patient with moderate to severe bone conductive hearing loss but who has good acoustic nerve function.

Middle Ear

Mastoidectomy

Mastoidectomy, the eradication of mastoid air cells, may be indicated to relieve complications of acute or chronic mastoiditis. However, mastoidectomy is more commonly performed in conjunction with a reconstructive procedure (see following discussion of tympanomastoid reconstruction).

Simple Mastoidectomy The mastoid process is opened behind the ear. Air cells are removed by drilling through bone with small burrs, without involving the middle ear or external canal.

Modified Radical Mastoidectomy Simple mastoidectomy and removal of the posterior wall of the ear canal provide drainage from the mastoid into the canal. The tympanic membrane and middle ear ossicles are preserved.

Radical Mastoidectomy A radical mastoidectomy is performed for chronic mastoiditis. The middle ear cavity and mastoid antrum are combined into a single cavity for inspection and cleaning. Mastoid air cells are removed. The ossicles and tympanic membrane are partially removed. The stapes and facial nerve are preserved.

Tympanoplasty

Tympanoplasty, as a general term, refers to any procedure performed to repair defects in the eardrum and/or middle ear structures for the purpose of reconstructing sound-conduction paths. The degree of hearing improvement following tympanoplasty is related to the degree of damage. Preferably the ear should be uninfected at the time of the surgical procedure. If not, infected tissue is debrided. As microsurgical procedures, tympanoplasties are classified into five types.

1. Type I, myringoplasty, is closure of a perforation in the tympanic membrane caused by infection or trauma. The ossicular chain is normal. Autogenous fascia or vein is used to repair the perforation. A vein graft is taken from the patient's forearm or hand. Fascia, more commonly used as a patch over a perforation, is obtained from the temporalis muscle.
2. Type II is closure of a perforated tympanic membrane with erosion of the malleus. The graft is placed against the incus or remains of the malleus.
3. Type III replaces the tympanic membrane to provide protection for the stapes and round window. The tympanic membrane, malleus, and incus have been destroyed by disease. The stapes is intact and mobile. A homograft of tympanic membrane with attached malleus and incus is placed in contact with the normal stapes, permitting transmission of sound.
4. Type IV is similar to type III except that the head, neck, and crura of the stapes are missing. The mobile footplate may be left exposed with the graft placed around it. The air pocket between the graft and the round window provides sound protection for the round window. To conserve the middle ear hearing mechanism, homograft transplantation of tympanic membrane and ossicles may be used to rebuild the chain.
5. Type V is similar to type IV except that the stapedial footplate is fixed because of otosclerosis (osteospongiosis). A fenestra (small opening) is made in the horizontal semicircular canal. The homograft seals off the middle ear to provide sound protection for the round window.

Reconstruction of the middle ear may be done with a synthetic bioinert material such as high-density polyethylene sponge (Plastipore). Fibrin glue is also used. Partial and total ossicular replacement prostheses have been developed.

Tympanomastoid Reconstruction

Tympanoplasty may be combined with either simple or radical mastoidectomy. The mastoid is drained and cleaned before reconstruction of the eardrum or middle ear ossicles. Following incision behind the auricle, the tympanic membrane and tympanic cavity are inspected. The mastoid antrum is entered by drilling through mastoid bone.

Sometimes in chronic otitis media, the mucous membrane of the tympanic cavity is replaced by epithelium from the ear canal as it grows through a perforation in the eardrum. Desquamated skin cells that cannot escape form a ball or cyst, known as a *cholesteatoma.* If present in the middle ear or mastoid, a cholesteatoma is removed during mastoidectomy and/or tympanoplasty.

If left intact, a cholesteatoma can cause permanent hearing loss, balance disturbance, infection, and facial nerve paralysis.

Stapedectomy/Stapedotomy

Conductive hearing loss can result from fixation of the stapes, most often caused by otosclerosis. The surgeon aims to restore vibration from the incus to the mobile oval window membrane to transmit sound. A *stapedectomy* involves partial or total removal of the stapes. A partial stapedectomy removes only the fixed footplate (Figure 35-2); a total stapedectomy removes the entire stapes including the footplate. A *stapedotomy,* a small opening into the footplate, may be the preferred procedure. The opening is made with a handheld perforator, microsurgical power drill, or laser. An argon, CO_2, or KTP laser may be used for this purpose. A low wattage lasing beam avoids thermal damage to the perilymph and inner ear structures. Following partial or total stapedectomy or stapedotomy, the remaining superstructure is used to reconstruct the sound-conducting mechanism.

An incision is made deep in the canal near but not in the eardrum. The eardrum is folded over, giving access to the middle ear. The stapes is disconnected from the incus, fractured by fine microinstruments, and removed. The oval window is sealed by a graft of vein, perichondrium, fascia, fat, or an absorbable hemostatic sponge over the oval window. A prosthesis is inserted and connected to the incus and to the graft, thus restoring sound conduction. Prostheses are made of various inert materials such as polyethylene, stainless steel, or tantalum (Figure 35-3).

By performing the microsurgical procedure under local anesthesia with the patient awake, the surgeon can reposition the eardrum and use voice to test if hearing is improved. Otosclerosis usually involves both ears, but stapedectomy is performed on only one ear at a time.

Stapes Mobilization

The stapes is manipulated at the footplate to restore normal function. A break through an otosclerotic lesion is achieved by means of transcrural pressure or direct application of chisels and picks to the footplate. A mobile, unaffected portion of a functioning stapes remains. Various techniques are used, with or without the use of prosthetic devices. The advantage of the procedure is that the preserved stapedial footplate provides natural protection for the inner ear. The disadvantage is that frequently a continuing otosclerotic process causes the footplate to become refixed. Therefore stapedectomy is more popular because it produces long-lasting results.

Stapes procedures are performed under direct vision with the operating microscope. The procedures do not disturb the integrity or position of the eardrum.

Middle Ear Vascular Tumors

The argon laser is absorbed by red pigment. Therefore it is suited for removal of small vascular tumors in the middle ear, such as glomus tympanicum tumors. The argon laser acts by photocoagulation.

Inner Ear

Endolymphatic Sac Shunt

The endolymphatic sac is an appendage of the membranous inner ear located in the posterior fossa, anterior to the lateral sinus and posterior to the semicircular canals. An excessive accumulation of endolymph in this sac causes the episodic vertigo (dizziness), tinnitus (ear ringing), and sensorineural hearing loss of Ménière's disease. Through a simple mastoidectomy approach, the sac is opened and the inner ear drained into either the

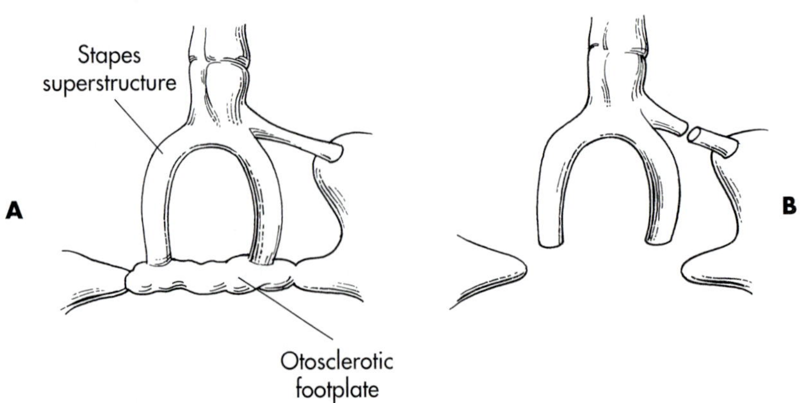

FIGURE 35-2 Partial stapedectomy. **A,** Stapes superstructure attached to fixed otosclerotic footplate. **B,** Footplate removed, superstructure remains.

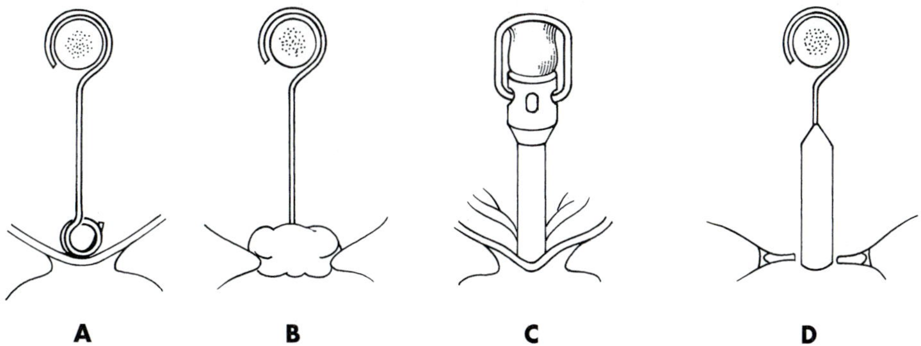

FIGURE 35-3 Stapedectomy prosthesis over incus and graft over oval window. **A,** Wire and absorbable sponge. **B,** Wire and fat. **C,** Piston-type and vein or fascia. **D,** Piston-type without graft. End of wire loop is crimped over long process of incus. Opposite end of wire or piston is on center of graft covering oval window. Grafts become covered by mucous membrane or mucoperiosteum.

subarachnoid space or the mastoid. A shunt tube is inserted to maintain drainage.

Labyrinthectomy

In labyrinthectomy the vestibular labyrinth is removed from the inner ear to correct incapacitating vertigo. This results in loss of vestibular function and hearing, however.

Vestibular Neurectomy

A middle fossa approach to the internal auditory canal for vestibular neurectomy combines otologic and neurosurgical procedures. Through a temporal bone craniotomy incision, dura of floor of the middle fossa is elevated to expose structures in superior portion of the internal auditory canal. The superior and inferior vestibular nerves, which control equilibrium, are sectioned to control intractable vertigo. The cochlear nerve, the hearing portion of the eighth cranial nerve, is not damaged, thus preserving hearing. A graft of temporalis muscle is placed over the exposed internal auditory canal to prevent leakage of cerebrospinal fluid.

Removal of Acoustic Neuroma

Acoustic neuroma resection may be performed by an otologist and/or a neurosurgeon, depending on its location and extent of neurologic involvement. An *acoustic neuroma* is a slow-growing encapsulated benign tumor of the eighth cranial, the acoustic, nerve. It originates in the neural sheath in the internal auditory canal but grows to involve nerve fibers in the posterior fossa. Initially the patient experiences unilateral hearing loss and disturbances, especially tinnitus, and equilibrium problems such as mild vertigo. The syndrome may resemble Ménière's disease or an expanding intracranial tumor. Early differential diagnosis is enhanced by brainstem evoked response audiometry, vertebral angiography, and small-volume air-contrast computed tomography.

A small neuroma, confined to the internal auditory canal, may be resected by the otologist using microsurgical technique through a middle fossa approach to preserve hearing. If a translabyrinthine approach is used to gain access to the internal auditory canal posterior to the inner ear structures, the patient will have total hearing loss after the surgical procedure. Acoustic neuromas extending into the cranial cavity are resected by the neurosurgeon (see Chapter 37, p. 773). The CO_2 laser may be used to excise acoustic neuromas through a transmastoid or craniotomy approach. Cerebrospinal fluid leak and meningitis are complications of the craniotomy approach.

For selected patients, stereotactic radiosurgery can be performed on an outpatient basis with local anesthesia. Hearing is preserved in 50% of these patients.

Implantation of Cochlear Prosthesis

A cochlear implant can restore perception of sound to patients who have profound sensorineural deafness not responsive to external amplification of a hearing aid. The implant is an electronic device that converts sound waves into electrical signals to stimulate cochlear nerve fibers in the absence of functioning hair cells. Several devices are available. All of them have external and internal components. The *external* part has a microphone/transmitter and a speech processor/receiver. The *internal* part has a receiver/stimulator and electrode/channel(s).

The internal electrode attaches to wires permanently implanted in the cochlea. Through a postauricular incision, a simple mastoidectomy is performed. Under the operating microscope, the facial recess between the posterior canal and the facial nerve is enlarged to expose the chorda tympani nerve and the middle ear. The electrode is securely seated in the mastoid cavity and placed through a recess into the middle ear. It is directed through an opening made in the round window into the scala tympani until it meets resistance. Placement is critical. A plug of fascia from temporalis muscle is placed around electrode at the round window to prevent perilymph leakage.

The internal electrode stimulates the auditory nerve to interpret sound. The single-channel model stimulates the nerve randomly so patient can discern environmental sounds but not speech. A multichannel electrode enables patient to distinguish environmental sounds and some speech by differentiating frequency, volume, and pitch of sound waves. With a single-channel electrode, a ground wire is placed under the temporalis muscle in the mastoid or middle ear. A multichannel electrode does not have a ground wire. The internal receiver is sutured in position over the temporal bone behind ear. Electromagnetic components and/or a titanium enclosure for the receiver may act as an electrical ground device. Only a bipolar active electrode should be used if electrosurgery is necessary after placement of the receiver.

The external microphone/transmitter component of the implant activates the internal receiver/stimulator. Transmission may be percutaneous or transcutaneous. In the *percutaneous model,* the transmitter is connected by a direct wire to a receiver implanted behind the ear. In the *transcutaneous model,* the transmitter converts electrical energy into magnetic currents that pass through intact skin to the receiver. In both models, sound enters the microphone and is transmitted to a speech processor, worn outside the body, where it is encoded into electrical signals or energy and amplified. The coded signals return to the transmitter and are passed to the internal receiver. The patient can adjust amplification of environmental sounds.

NOSE

Anatomy and Physiology

The supporting structures of the nose consist of two nasal bones and the nasal processes of the maxillary bones superiorly, lateral cartilages and connective tissue inferiorly, and the septum. The *septum,* composed of bone posteriorly and cartilage anteriorly, divides the nose into two chambers lined by mucous membrane. The *anterior portion* or *vestibule* holds the nasal hairs. The external anterior orifices are called *nares.*

The internal portion of the nose, the *nasal cavity* (Figure 35-4), extends to the *nasopharynx,* the space behind the *choanae* or funnellike posterior nasal orifices. The nose communicates with the ear via the eustachian tube. The hard and soft palates divide the nasal and oral cavities. The nasal and cranial cavities are separated by the ethmoid bone.

The *paranasal sinuses* are the frontal, maxillary, ethmoid, and sphenoid. *Ostia* (openings from the sinuses and nasolacrimal ducts) are located in the nasal lateral walls. The ostia provide a drainage system for the sinuses, as well as aerate them. Three turbinate bones (superior, middle, and inferior) are also situated in the lateral walls. These bones are covered with a vascular mucosa. Beneath each turbinate is a corresponding meatus. Tears drain into the nose through the nasolacrimal duct that enters the inferior meatus. Drainage from the paranasal sinuses is passed to the nose through the middle and superior meatuses.

External and internal carotid arteries and their branches supply blood to the nasal region. Because of the extensive vascularity, lymphatic supply, and proximity to the brain, infections on or about the face are potentially very dangerous. Microorganisms may readily be carried to or thrombi may form in the cavernous sinus. The sensory nerve supply of the nasal area is associated with the trigeminal or fifth cranial nerve.

The *function of the nose* is twofold:

1. It provides filtered air to the respiratory system. Fine cilia in the mucous membrane propel mucus toward the nasopharynx. Air is warmed and moistened as it passes to the trachea and lower respiratory tract.
2. It contains the end organs for smell in the olfactory epithelium, which differs from other nasal epithelium. When nasal obstruction blocks off the olfactory epithelium, loss of smell *(anosmia)* results. The senses of smell and taste are closely related.

NASAL SURGICAL PROCEDURES

Nasal procedures are concerned with two factors: adequate ventilation to accessory spaces and adequate drainage from them. Abnormalities in structure, congenital or traumatic, and disease processes hinder function. Corrective procedures are done to relieve obstruction, to ensure drainage, to resect tumors, or to control bleeding (epistaxis).

General Considerations in Rhinology

1. Computed tomography and rhinoscopy are often performed preoperatively to diagnose nature and extent of pathologic conditions, especially in the paranasal sinuses.
2. Many nasal procedures are performed with local anesthesia with or without intravenous (IV) sedation.
   a. Topical 4% cocaine may be sprayed on nasal mucosa or applied with soaked compressed absorbent patties (cottonoids) or sponges put in nos-

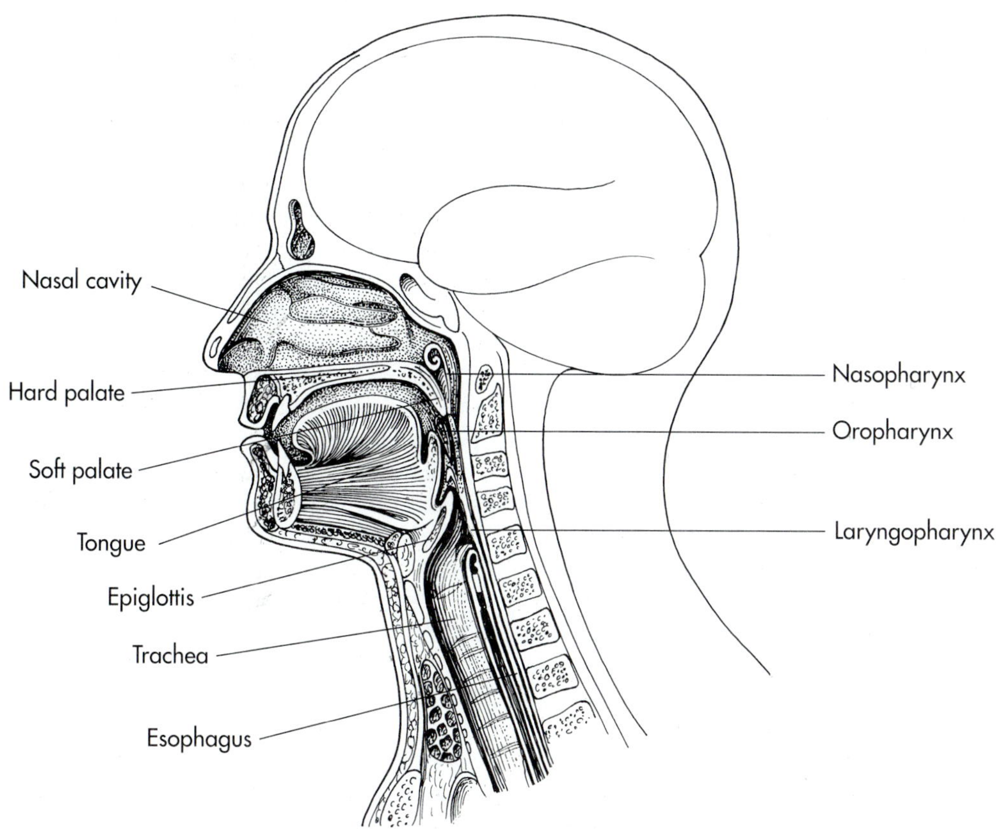

FIGURE 35-4 Cross section of nose, oral cavity, and throat.

trils. Cocaine produces vasoconstriction, as well as anesthesia.

b. Local agent, often lidocaine hydrochloride, 1% or 2%, is injected into the middle meatus. Epinephrine usually is used for vasoconstriction to control bleeding.

c. When general anesthesia is indicated, a pack is placed in the pharynx to prevent aspiration of blood after patient is intubated.

3. Paranasal sinuses and tissues underlying the mucosa are considered sterile. Therefore instrumentation must be sterile although the nasal cavity is a contaminated area.
4. CO_2, Nd:YAG, and KTP lasers may be used. Endoscopes are also used. All equipment and accessories should be checked for working order.
5. Nasal packing is inserted at end of most procedures except endoscopic sinus and laser procedures.

Nasal Cavity

The supporting structures surrounding nasal air passages can be injured or displaced. Acute or chronic disease processes can cause dysfunction or obstruction.

Epistaxis

Most nosebleeds are caused by trauma, usually at Kisselbach's plexus of arteries and veins in the anterior part of the nasal septum. Dehumidified air may cause changes in the mucosa and splitting of tiny vessels. Bleeding may be spontaneous, as in patients with arteriosclerosis, hypertension, or blood dyscrasia. Epistaxis is usually anterior and unilateral. In persons with systemic disease, such as leukemia, or with severe fracture, the bleeding is frequently posterior and more severe. Management involves locating the precise bleeding site and promptly instituting appropriate therapy. Severe hemorrhage places the patient in a precarious condition. Hypovolemia should be corrected preoperatively.

Anterior Pack Local vasoconstriction and pressure on side of the nose will control most nosebleeds. Electrocoagulation or silver nitrate is used to provide hemostasis at the bleeding point as needed. When bleeding is from the anterior ethmoid artery, inaccessible to cautery, packing is applied to the area of depression between the septum and the middle turbinate.

Posterior Pack A posterior pack may be necessary for constant pressure when bleeding is severe in the posterior part of the nose. The pack consists of rolled gauze securely tied to the middle of a length of narrow tape or strong string; commercial packs are available. To control infection and odor, gauze is lubricated with antibiotic ointment before insertion. After a catheter is passed into mouth via the nose, one end of the tape is tied to oral end of the catheter. The catheter and attached tape are then drawn back through the mouth and out one nostril, thereby pulling the pack up into the nasopharynx. Thus one end of tape comes out the nose, the other end out the mouth. These ends are secured to the patient's cheek with adhesive tape. The nasal end is taped to prevent the pack from slipping into the throat; the oral end facilitates removal of the pack. Some oozing may persist in spite of packing. The pack is left in place until bleeding is arrested, usually for at least 48 hours, but prolonged use can lead to otitis media or paranasal sinusitis.

Patients with postnasal packs are often apprehensive and uncomfortable. They must breathe through the mouth. Posterior packs tend to reduce arterial oxygen tension. All patients, especially the elderly or those with marginal pulmonary function, should be observed carefully for respiratory problems that may result from the pack dropping into the hypopharynx.

Artery Ligation A microsurgical procedure is performed to control persistent nasal hemorrhage by reducing the blood supply to the posterior portion of the nose. Some surgeons prefer artery ligation to packing, or it may be performed with a pack in place. Through an incision in oral mucosa, removal of the posterior wall exposes the maxillary sinus for transantral ligation. Terminal branches of the internal maxillary artery, a branch of the external carotid artery, are exposed, identified, and ligated with metallic clips. Electrocoagulation is employed to control intraoperative bleeding, but if it is excessive, creation of a nasoantral window establishes drainage. The replaced posterior mucosal flap is covered with absorbable gelatin sponge, and the incision is closed.

Through an incision along left side of nose, ligation of the anterior and posterior ethmoidal arteries is helpful in controlling bleeding in the superior aspect of the nose.

The argon or KTP laser may be used to control severe epistaxis. If a laser is used to control bleeding, nasal packing usually is unnecessary.

Turbinectomy

Chronic engorgement of middle and/or inferior turbinate causes nasal congestion and rhinorrhea. Rhinitis is frequently an allergic reaction. A KTP laser shrinks turbinates without removing normal mucosa. A CO_2 or Nd:YAG contact laser vaporizes superficial layer of mucosa without injuring the turbinate or ablating the turbinate. The KTP or CO_2 laser fiber handpiece is directed through a nasal endoscope. Because bleeding is minimal, nasal packing is unnecessary. Electrocoagulation and cryosurgery also have been used to treat soft tissue obstruction and refractory allergic rhinitis.

Nasal Obstruction

Surgical intervention can provide relief for certain types of nasal obstruction. For example, after the mucosa is shrunk with a vasoconstrictor and secretions are suctioned, a foreign body is removed with a forceps. An abscess or hematoma may need to be drained to relieve pressure. Accumulation of pus or blood separates the perichondrium, the connective tissue, from underlying cartilage. This may cause necrosis of cartilage with resultant deformity. Infection must be eradicated to avoid extension to the brain.

Polypectomy Polyps, soft edematous masses, projecting from nasal or sinus mucosa can obstruct the posterior choanae. Polyps usually are bilateral, but they may be unilateral, single, or multiple and frequently are infected. In addition to obstructing ventilation, they may obstruct the sense of smell if the olfactory epithelium is blocked. Some polyps may be excised with a wire-loop snare through a nasal speculum or with forceps through an endoscope. Packing is inserted to control bleeding. The KTP laser coagulates the base to debulk large, multiple polyps. The laser fiber can be directed through a straight or angled handpiece. A CO_2 laser can vaporize polyps. The laser is less invasive than other techniques. Nasal packing is rarely necessary.

Nasal Deformity

Surgical intervention can restore contour and/or improve function after an injury. A deformity in nasal structure also may be corrected to improve cosmetic appearance.

Reduction of Nasal Fracture Fracture of the septum or nasal bones often accompanies other trauma to the head. Intranasal manipulation is required to elevate depressed bone or cartilage that may be pushed into the paranasal sinuses. This should be performed as soon as possible to bring the parts in apposition. A delay of 7 to 10 days to permit edema to subside will not affect the outcome, however. Bleeding from a laceration must be immediately controlled and drained. Intranasal structure compatible with air passage must be preserved.

Septoplasty, Septal Reconstruction, Submucous Resection The terms *septoplasty, septal reconstruction,* and *submucous resection* are used interchangeably to describe correction of a deviated nasal septum. Often the result of injury, the condition interferes with breathing and drainage. Under local anesthesia, one side of the septum is incised its entire length. Membranous coverings are detached from cartilage and bone. The deformed part of the septum is removed or straightened and replaced. Bilateral nasal packing is inserted to hold tissues in place and to prevent bleeding. The procedure creates a patent airway and straight septal line, thereby reducing sinus disease and polyp formation.

Rhinoplasty Rhinoplasty, a procedure to correct deformity of the nose, may be performed by a rhinologist or a plastic surgeon (see Chapter 34, pp. 715-716). It is a major procedure involving reconstruction and molding of the bones and cartilages. Septoplasty and rhinoplasty may be performed together; *septorhinoplasty* restores both function and cosmetic appearance. Local anesthesia is usually used. The skin is taped postoperatively to maintain nasal structures in alignment. A rigid shield is applied for protection. This is not removed without a specific order from the surgeon. Temporary ecchymosis from surgical trauma surrounds the eyes postoperatively.

Repair of Perforated Septum Perforations occur most often in the anterior cartilage. If bleeding and crusting are severe, the perforation may be covered by rotated mucoperichondrial flaps. Or the mucosa of adjacent intact septum may be denuded and a skin graft applied to cover the perforation. Nasal packing is inserted.

Paranasal Sinuses

The paranasal sinuses are air-filled spaces in the skull. Because the sinus mucous membrane lining is continuous with the mucous membrane lining of the nose, nasal infection may readily spread to the sinuses. Various procedures provide drainage for patients with chronic sinusitis that may result from allergies or repeated nasopharyngeal infection. Swelling of the nasal mucosa can trap microorganisms within a sinus cavity. Ostial occlusion and abnormalities in the walls of the nasal cavity interfere with breathing, drainage, and smell. Sinus procedures are executed through an external or an intranasal approach or through an endoscope.

Maxillary Sinus Procedure

The *maxillary sinuses* are located bilaterally between the upper teeth and the eyes.

Caldwell-Luc Procedure (Antrostomy) The maxillary sinus contents are approached through an incision of the oral mucous membrane above the canine teeth. The flap is retracted. A section of maxillary bone is cut out to create a large nasoantral window for aeration and permanent drainage by gravity into the nasal fossa under the inferior turbinate. Polyps and diseased tissue are removed along with eradication of mucosa. At the completion of the surgical procedure, the sinus is packed with gauze impregnated with antibiotic ointment. One end of gauze is brought through the window and into the nose. The incision under the upper lip is sutured. The packing is eventually removed through the nose. Antrostomy is usually limited to adults because of unerupted teeth in children. A Caldwell-Luc incision is also used for removal of a tumor in the maxillary sinus.

Ethmoid Sinus Procedures

The *ethmoid sinus* cells lie bilaterally between the nose and the orbits. The maxillary sinuses are below the ethmoid bones, and the frontal sinuses are above them.

Ethmoidectomy Diseased tissue is removed from the ethmoid labyrinth, middle turbinate, and meatus. A large cavity is formed to facilitate aeration and drainage. Severe ethmoiditis can cause orbital abscess requiring drainage through an intranasal or external (Lynch) incision that extends from the inner half of the eyebrow down alongside the nose.

Turbinectomy Removal of portions of the inferior and middle turbinates increases aeration and drainage. The cavity is packed at completion of the surgical procedure.

Frontal Sinus Procedures

The *frontal sinuses* are situated above the eyes. They are usually approached through the external incision described for ethmoidectomy, or a coronal incision may be made for exposure across the scalp from ear to ear.

Osteoplastic Flap Procedure The bone covering the frontal sinus is exposed and incised. The contents of the sinus, such as a *mucocele,* a cyst lined with mucous-secreting glands, are extracted. The lining of the mucocele sac is removed and the cavity packed with fat, from the abdominal wall, to obliterate the sinus with fibrous tissue that fills in the cavity. The incised bone flap is then repositioned and the incision sutured.

Killian Procedure A frontal sinus cavity is reached by removal of the floor or anterior wall of the sinus through external incision above the eye. A large communication and drainage channel into the nose is formed.

Sphenoid Sinus Procedure

The *sphenoid sinus* is deep, almost in the center of the skull. It may be approached intranasally or via the external ethmoidectomy incision through the eyebrow.

Sphenoidotomy Sphenoidotomy involves the creation of an opening into the sphenoid sinus for drainage.

Endoscopic Sinus Surgery

Sinuscopes permit direct visualization of the paranasal sinuses and the anatomy of lateral nasal walls. The site of diseased mucosa or obstructive tissue, such as polyps, can be localized for removal, with preservation of some mucosa and restoration of drainage. The mucosa of each sinus has cilia that move air in wave forms. With an endoscopic approach, some ciliary motion may be retained for aeration. The basic principle of endoscopic sinus surgery is that most sinus mucosal disease will resolve if aeration and drainage are reestablished. Extent of the procedure depends on location of diseased mucosa and resection necessary to establish drainage. Septal deformities or inferior turbinates causing nasal obstruction may be concurrently corrected (i.e., septoplasty and turbinoplasty). Minor procedures limited to removal of disease from maxillary or ethmoid sinuses usually can be done with topical and local anesthesia. IV sedation or general anesthesia is needed for more extensive procedures, such as ethmoidectomy or sphenoethmoidectomy.

The telescopes of sinuscopes are 2.7 and 4 mm in diameter with 0-, 25- or 30-, 70-, and 120-degree viewing angles. The quartz rod telescope has a solid quartz optical cone in the light post that attaches to a halogen light source. This system provides optimum light transmission through the fiberoptics of the miniaturized scope. An attached suction/irrigation device permits unobstructed viewing. The telescope is inserted intranasally and advanced into the frontal, ethmoid, or sphenoid sinus. It is inserted through a cannula in the canine fossa to reach the maxillary sinus. Many accessory grasping and cutting instruments, including the KTP laser, are used to remove mucosa, lamina, osteum, and cells. Hemostasis is controlled with epinephrine and cautery or laser. Nasal packing usually is not required.

Functional Procedure Known as the *Messerklinger technique,* the surgeon begins at the ethmoid and works anteriorly to the frontal and maxillary sinuses to clear ethmoidal compartments of disease. If a minimal opening of the narrow osteomeatal tract at the anterior ethmoidal sinus will not achieve adequate drainage from other paranasal sinuses, a posterior ethmoidectomy and sphenoidotomy are included in the procedure.

Exenteration Known as the *Wigand procedure,* total sphenoethmoidectomy and partial middle turbinate resection are performed, beginning with a sphenoidotomy and working anteriorly to the frontal sinus. This creates a broad opening of sphenoidal, ethmoidal, frontal, and maxillary sinuses. To avoid the optic nerve, dissection does not extend beyond lateral wall of the sphenoid. Visual evoked potentials monitor optic nerve function; eyes are uncovered. The endoscopic procedure may be done bilaterally.

Resection of Tumors

Osteoma, a benign tumor, can arise from bones around the paranasal sinuses. Although rare, primary carcinoma and sarcoma do occur in the frontal, ethmoid, sphenoid, and maxillary sinuses. Most originate in the maxillary sinus. The incidence increases with age. The sinuses are proximal to the orbits, oral cavity, and base of the skull. Tumor in the maxillary sinus may be associated with oral or nasal symptoms, such as loosening of the upper teeth, bleeding from the nose, or asymmetry of the face. A malignant lesion in the ethmoid sinus may be accompanied by displacement of the eye, disturbance of smell, and nasal obstruction. Chronic sinusitis is thought to play an etiologic role because of an associated replacement of respiratory epithelium by stratified squamous cells. Most sinus tumors are squamous cell carcinomas. Often the bony walls are invaded and destroyed by the time symptoms appear because the tumor tends to extend in all directions. Exploratory surgery by Caldwell-Luc incision provides the best chance of early diagnosis. Radical craniofacial resection may be indicated (see Chapter 36, p. 746).

ORAL CAVITY AND THROAT

Anatomy and Physiology

The *oral cavity* (mouth) is lined with thick mucous membrane. This squamous mucosa connects with the nasopharynx above and the hypopharynx below. The *hard palate,* part of the maxillary bone, forms the floor of the nasal cavity and the anterior part of the roof of the mouth. The *soft palate,* a musculomembranous structure posterior to the hard palate, occludes the nasal cavity during phonation (speech) and deglutition (swallowing). These functions are aided by the *uvula,* a small conical appendage (tonguelike structure) that projects from the posterior free margin of the soft palate. It contains the uvular muscle covered by mucous membrane. The *tongue,* occupying much of the oral cavity, joins the soft palate and pharynx posteriorly by folds of mucous membrane (see Figure 35-4, p. 735).

The *throat* refers to space surrounded by the soft palate, the palatoglossal and palatopharyngeal arches, the base of the tongue, and the pharynx. The funnel-shaped *pharynx* is subdivided into the nasopharynx (above), oropharynx (middle), and hypopharynx (below). The *nasopharynx* communicates with the nasal cavity through the posterior choanae. The *oropharynx* includes the base of the tongue anteriorly, the tonsillar fossae laterally, and the oropharyngeal walls of the throat posteriorly. The *hypopharynx* leads from the oropharynx to the larynx, trachea, and esophagus. The pharynx, posterior to the larynx and the nasal and oral cavities, consists of constrictor muscles essential to swallowing. The proximity of food and air passages and the joint function of the pharynx in their passage contribute to the hazard of aspiration.

The nasopharynx and oropharynx contain masses of lymphoid tissue. The *adenoids* (pharyngeal tonsils) hang from the nasopharyngeal roof; the lingual tonsils are in mucosal crypts. The palatine tonsils lie on either side of the oropharynx. These, referred to as the *tonsils,* are supported in the tonsillar fossae by anterior and posterior pillars. A fibrous capsule adheres to each laterally.

SURGICAL PROCEDURES OF ORAL CAVITY AND THROAT

The common surgical procedures performed by ENT surgeons or laryngologists in the oral cavity and throat fall within two major classifications: those for infection and those for neoplasms or other life-threatening disorders. Small benign and early malignant tumors in oropharynx and oral cavity can be removed with CO_2 laser or local excision with primary closure. Extensive procedures for oral carcinoma are discussed in Chapter 36, pp. 751-752. Additional procedures in the oral cavity are discussed in Chapter 36. Those unique to infants and children are discussed in Chapter 42. Bleeding always is a concern in this highly vascular region.

Nasopharynx

Uvulopalatopharyngoplasty

Increasing the air space in the oropharynx corrects *obstructive sleep apnea* (OSA) caused by anatomic relationships in some patients. OSA can cause oxygen desaturation during apneic episodes that occur during sleep. This can lead to life-threatening pulmonary and systemic hypertension, cardiac dysrhythmias, and neurologic dysfunction if untreated. Upper airway obstruction may be caused by nasal obstruction, deviated nasal septum, hypertrophied adenoids and/or tonsils, or mandibular retrognathism (overbite), which may be surgically corrected. To diagnose OSA in patients who do not have obvious abnormalities, airway obstruction can be viewed during sleep with fiberoptic nasopharyngoscopy and fluoroscopy. Some of the oropharyngeal muscles may become atonic and collapse inward, and the soft palate may drop down. Patients who have a large drooping soft palate and at least moderately redundant lateral pharyngeal walls or large tonsils are good candidates for uvulopalatopharyngoplasty. These patients have moderate apnea but do not have severe cardiac dysrhythmias.

The patient is continuously monitored during induction of anesthesia. The surgeon is present and an emergency tracheotomy tray is available in case the patient's airway becomes obstructed.

The full thickness of mucosa is resected from the posterior margin of the soft palate, including the uvula, and most of the anterior tonsillar pillar. The lesser palatine artery is ligated. The tonsils or mucosa of the tonsillar fossae are resected. The remaining posterior tonsillar pillar is sutured to the resected anterior pillar. The palate is closed laterally. Extent of tissue removal varies according to width and depth of patient's oropharyngeal space.

Adenoidectomy

Adenoidectomy, the removal of hypertrophied adenoid tissue from the nasopharynx and behind the posterior choanae, may be performed in adults to relieve upper airway obstruction. This is more commonly performed in children, often to prevent recurrent otitis media. Adenoid tissue usually atrophies after adolescence.

The patient is supine. General anesthesia is administered, and patient is intubated. Adenoids can be resected with an adenotome and curette or vaporized with a CO_2 laser. Bleeding is more easily controlled with the laser. An electrocautery and/or gauze sponges soaked in epinephrine may be used following sharp dissection. Occasionally a posterior nasal pack is needed.

Oropharynx

Tonsillectomy

Chronically infected or hypertrophied tonsils are most frequently removed in childhood. However, even slightly enlarged tonsils can obstruct air flow to the lungs during sleep in an adult. Tonsillectomy may significantly improve symptoms of sleep apnea, with or without uvulopalatopharyngoplasty.

A CO_2, Nd:YAG, argon, or KTP laser may be used to excise tonsils from the tonsillar fossae. The patient is supine. General anesthesia is administered. The endotracheal tube and cuff must be protected, and other laser precautions must be taken around the oral cavity (see Chapter 36, p. 753). A smoke evacuator should be available with a CO_2 laser. A handheld laser may be used, or a beam may be directed through the microscope.

Local anesthesia is frequently used for adult tonsillectomy. The patient is positioned in semi-Fowler's or sitting position on the operating table or sits in a specially designed chair. The throat is anesthetized with a topical agent and local infiltration. With sharp and blunt dissection, each tonsil is separated from the pillars and capsule and removed from the fossa with a tonsil snare. Attention is given to hemostasis to prevent aspiration; suture ligatures, free ties, and/or absorbable lighting clips may be used. Bleeding can be difficult to control and can occur postoperatively with this technique. Less intraoperative bleeding occurs with laser tonsillectomy.

Incision and Drainage of Peritonsillar Abscess

Less common since the advent of antibiotics, incision into the anterior tonsillar pillar may be necessary to drain purulent material posterior to the tonsillar capsule following acute tonsillitis.

Resection of Tonsillar Tumor

A localized squamous cell carcinoma of the tonsil may be resected by dissection or with cryosurgery. An en bloc resection includes the primary tumor and nodes. Metastatic nodes are common. Superior progression of the tumor may reach the supratonsillar fossa, soft and hard palates, and uvula. Inferiorly, tumor may spread to posterior and lateral walls of the larynx, base of the tongue, and pyriform sinus. Neck dissection may be indicated for regional disease. Surgery may be combined with preoperative or postoperative radiation therapy. The most common complications are fistula formation and delayed healing.

Diverticulectomy

Diverticulectomy, or removal of sacs or outpocketings of lower pharyngeal mucous membrane in which food collects, may be performed in extreme cases in which regurgitation presents a hazard of aspiration. The neck of the sac is dissected from the posterior pharyngeal wall and ligated. The stump of the excised sac is inverted into the pharyngeal wall. Diverticuli may be removed endoscopically.

GENERAL CONSIDERATIONS IN EAR, NOSE, AND THROAT PROCEDURES

1. Preoperative explanations and postoperative instructions are vital to outcome. For example, following ear or nasal procedures the patient must avoid blowing the nose, which would force air up the eustachian tube potentially causing infection, force air through the incision, or dislodge a graft. To sneeze, both nose and mouth should be open.
2. Communication is a major problem for patients with loss of hearing or voice. Touch is an effective means of conveying concern and letting the patient know he or she is not abandoned. Pencil and paper or a magic slate board can be useful for the patient to communicate.
3. Care with antiseptic solutions is necessary because they are very painful and irritating if allowed to touch a perforated eardrum or get into eyes.
4. Patient may experience anxiety with drapes over the head. Air and oxygen (6 to 8 L/min) administered during the otologic procedure afford relief.
5. Although a surgical area, such as the oral cavity, is often contaminated, only sterile equipment and sterile technique are used to avoid introducing exogenous microorganisms.
6. Anesthesia is mainly local. It minimizes bleeding and postoperative discomfort in addition to affording the surgeon observation of patient response. It allows patient cooperation. Also, presence of an endotracheal tube, routine with general anesthesia, can distort features during the surgical procedure.
   a. A registered nurse observes the usual precautions for local anesthesia (i.e., monitoring vital signs and electrocardiogram [ECG]) in the absence of a stand-by anesthesiologist. He or she should record on the anesthesia record the amount of local anesthesia administered and document the patient's intraoperative responses. For example, as a result of stimulation of the vestibular labyrinth in otologic procedures, a patient may experience nausea, vertigo, or a sense of falling. The patient may be in a fairly erect position for local tonsillectomy, which may contribute to postural hypotension.
   b. Patient must be monitored for reaction to local anesthetic (see Chapter 18, pp. 355-358).
   c. Patients undergoing local anesthesia may wear pajama bottoms or underpants to the operating room (OR) in some facilities.
7. Microsurgical otologic and laryngeal procedures, endoscopies, and laser procedures require general anesthesia.
   a. Patient is intubated because aspiration of blood is a concern.
   b. Anesthesia machine may be positioned near the patient's feet. Endotracheal tube is taped, all connections must be tight, and tubes unkinked. Anesthesiologist usually sits alongside the table.
8. Various colorless solutions are on the table. Each container should be accurately and clearly labeled for foolproof distinction between, for example, cocaine, lidocaine, and epinephrine.
9. Illumination is provided by the overhead spotlight, the operating microscope, the endoscope, or the surgeon's reflective headlamp that enables him or her to see up and under surfaces. Many surgeons prefer a fiberoptic headlamp. Some want the room darkened.
10. Instrumentation is varied to suit the area. It includes very delicate, small endoscopic and microsurgical implements in addition to bone instruments because of the extensive involvement of cartilage and bone in the facial structures and skull. These areas have relatively little soft tissue. Many instruments are angulated to permit insertion into areas of difficult access and curving passages.
11. Special care with electric appliances is indicated. Electrocoagulation is used to control oozing. Compressed air or nitrogen drills with a foot-pedal control are used on bone, such as the mastoid area. A number of drills for extremely fine work, such as stapes sculpturing, are powered by small electric motors fitted into a handpiece.
12. Various types of endoscopes are used. The correct accessories must be used with each type. Light car-

riers must be suited to the scope. Diameter of aspirating tubes and forceps is small enough to pass through and length long enough to extend beyond the end of the scope. The lighting mechanism and all accessories should be checked for working order before an endoscopic procedure begins.

13. Cryosurgery may be used to destroy tumorous tissue in accessible areas, especially those that bleed profusely if incised.
14. CO_2 lasers are used to vaporize tissue. Argon lasers coagulate tissue by heat generation. KTP lasers coagulate to shrink or debulk tissues. Nd:YAG lasers cut and coagulate to minimize bleeding. Appropriate instrumentation and attachments must be available for each type of laser. Laser surgery is usually done in conjunction with the operating microscope or endoscope. All safety precautions are taken to avoid ignition and injury when a laser is used.
15. Microsurgical techniques are used for many ENT procedures because they facilitate distinction between normal and diseased tissue and allow more accurate dissection (e.g., in infinitely small areas such as the middle ear).
16. Sponges and compressed patties are relatively small and are a distinct hazard when blood-soaked because they can occlude an airway. They are more easily controlled if a string or suture is attached to them.
17. One or two drops of blood can obscure a microsurgical field. Hemostatic aids should be ready at all times. Gelfoam pledgets soaked in 1:1000 epinephrine are used frequently. Handle tissue grafts and gelatin sponges with forceps, not the hands. Gelfilm, which is brittle, may be cut while in the primary wrap.
18. Irrigation equipment and solution at body temperature should be available to remove bone dust, clean burrs, and rinse suction apparatus. Very fine suction needles or cannulas should be irrigated constantly to avoid blockage.
19. Suction should be available at all times, including several patent cannulas. The degree of suction should be variable. A foot pedal may be used to interrupt wall suction so surgeon has control of it for grasping and releasing an object (e.g., in handling a prosthetic graft). Suction-irrigators are used with sinus endoscopes.
20. Tissue grafts must be kept from drying out before use. A convenient method is to place the graft on a moist cellulose sponge in a sterile, covered Petri dish. Some surgeons intentionally dry a temporalis fascia graft to facilitate handling. This type of graft may also be flattened and thinned in a small press.
21. Many ENT procedures are done with patient in slight reverse Trendelenburg's position. This helps control bleeding.

Bibliography

Croft S: Anaesthesia for ENT surgery, *Br J Theatre Nurs* 27(3):23-24, 1990.

Fujita S: Obstructive sleep apnea syndrome: pathophysiology, upper airway evaluation, and surgical treatment, *ENT J* 72(1):67-76, 1993.

Glasscock ME et al: Preservation of hearing in surgery for acoustic neuroma, *J Neurosurg* 78(6):864-870, 1993.

Goldenberg RA et al: Laser stapedotomy, *AORN J* 55(3):759-772, 1992.

Guyuron B, Friedman A: The role of preserved autogenous cartilage grafts in septorhinoplasty, *Ann Plast Surg* 32(3):255-260, 1994.

Jones CE, Wellisz T: External ear reconstruction, *AORN J* 59(2):411-422, 1994.

Josephson GD et al: Practical management of epistaxis, *Med Clin North Am* 75(6):1311-1320, 1991.

Leach J et al: Comparison of two methods of tonsillectomy, *Laryngoscope* 103(6):619-622, 1993.

Levine HL: The potassium-titanyl phosphate laser for treatment of turbinate dysfunction, *Otolaryngology* 104(2):247-251, 1991.

Loftus BC et al: Epistaxis, medical history, and the nasopulmonary reflex: what is clinically relevant? *Otolaryngology* 110(4):363-369, 1994.

Lundsford LD, Linsky ME: Stereotactic radiosurgery in the treatment of patients with acoustic tumors, *Otolaryngol Clin North Am* 25(2):471-491, 1992.

McKennen KX: Cholesteatoma: recognition and treatment, *Am Fam Phys* 43(6):2091-2096, 1991.

Mitchell GW: Otologic devices, *Emerg Med Clin North Am* 12(3):787-792, 1994.

Parisier SC, Chute P: Cochlear implants: indications and technology, *Med Clin North Am* 75(6):1267-1276, 1991.

Randall DA, Freeman SB: Management of anterior and posterior epistaxis, *Am Fam Phys* 43(6):2007-2014, 1991.

Randall DA et al: Indications for tonsillectomy and adenoidectomy, *Am Fam Phys* 44(5):1639-1646, 1991.

Rice DH: Endoscopic sinus surgery, *Otolaryngol Clin North Am* 26(4):613-618, 1993.

Shaw CB et al: Epistaxis: a comparison of treatment, *Otolaryngology* 109(1):60-65, 1993.

Stammberger H: *Functional endoscopic nasal and paranasal sinus surgery: the Messerklinger technique,* Tuttlingen, West Germany, 1990, Karl Storz GmbH.

Teichgraeber JF, Russo RC: The management of septal perforations, *Plast Reconstr Surg* 91(2):229-235, 1993.

Tewary AK: Day-case tonsillectomy: a review of the literature, *J Laryngol Otol* 107(8):703-705, 1993.

Vleming M et al: Complications of endoscopic sinus surgery, *Arch Otolaryngol* 118(6):617-623, 1992.

Wiet RJ et al: Complications in acoustic neuroma surgery, *Otolaryngol Clin North Am* 25(2):389-412, 1992.

Yung MM: The use of rigid endoscopes in cholesteatoma surgery, *J Laryngol Otol* 108(4):307-309, 1994.

CHAPTER 36

Head and Neck Surgery

Reconstruction of the skeletal framework and all the structures of the head and neck region is not within the province of any one surgical specialty. Subspecialists from many disciplines, most notably plastic surgeons, otolaryngologists, and dentists, limit their surgical practice to specific types of problems involving areas of the head and/or neck. Training in these subspecialties is included in specialty postgraduate programs. For example, endoscopy of the head and neck area is essential for residency approval by the American Board of Plastic Surgery. The American Board of Otolaryngology added Head and Neck Surgery to its name. Oral surgery, orthodontics, prosthodontics, and periodontics are specialties within dentistry.

Dental and skeletal deformities of alignment and function coexist with aesthetic appearance. These deformities may be congenital, or they may be caused by trauma or disease. They may interfere with breathing, eating, swallowing, speaking, seeing, or hearing. A *multidisciplinary team* of surgical specialists is often required to reconstruct complex deformities. This team may be all-inclusive with a plastic surgeon, neurosurgeon, oral surgeon, orthodontist or prosthodontist, otolaryngologist, ophthalmologist, and general surgeon; or it may be limited to two or three specialists. The team may also include a radiologist, anesthesiologist, psychiatrist, speech pathologist, and social worker, plus, of course, the nursing staff. A team includes all the specialties needed for complete preoperative assessment, intraoperative care, and postoperative rehabilitation of the individual patient.

HISTORICAL BACKGROUND

Trauma has historically been a major source of facial disfigurement. Repair of mandibular fractures dates back to 600 BC. Intermaxillary wiring was documented in 1835. In 1901, René LeFort identified and classified patterns of midfacial and maxillary fractures. His classifications are still used.

Evidence of prosthetic restoration of facial disfigurement has been found in Egyptian mummies with artificial eyes, ears, and noses. Lacquered-wood nasal prostheses were made in India and China in the second century AD. Gold, silver, and metal alloy replacement parts were developed by the sixteenth century. Ceramic-like materials and rubber were fashioned into facial prostheses in the nineteenth century. After World War I, methyl methacrylate was used to make artificial eyes and dentures. Silicone elastomer has replaced other materials for nasal and ear prostheses, either implanted or affixed externally, following traumatic amputation or surgical resection. Teeth can be replaced with dental implants. Bony structures are augmented with allografts or fixated with compression devices to restore shape and function.

Head and neck oncology requires not only aggressive treatment of the cancer but innovative techniques in reconstruction and rehabilitation. Theodore Kocher performed the first upper neck dissection in the 1880s. In 1906, George Crile of the Cleveland Clinic proposed radical neck dissection with regional lymphadenectomy. But it was Hayes Martin of the Memorial Hospital for

Cancer and Allied Diseases in New York who became the undisputed father of head and neck surgery. In the 1940s he combined wide resection of the primary cancer in continuity with dissection of regional lymphatics and intervening tissues such as the mandible. Known as the *commando operation,* this procedure was made possible by the availability of antibiotics and blood transfusions and by progress in anesthesia, skin grafting, and wound drainage techniques.

During the 1960s surgeons recognized that major ablative surgery could not be successfully accomplished without regional tissue pedicle flaps. This concept was not new, however. The first regional flap recorded in the literature was a forehead myocutaneous flap reported by Shusruta, published in 700 BC. Unfortunately the concept was lost for more than 2000 years. The reintroduction of regional myocutaneous flaps in the 1970s, plus microvascularized free flaps and other types of grafts and flaps, has led to their being an important part of reconstruction for head and neck oncology and facial deformity. They reduce gross deformity, protect essential structures, improve physiologic function and appearance, and facilitate psychologic rehabilitation.

The well-established fundamentals of excisional surgery in the head and neck have increasingly become more sophisticated to include use of microvascular and microneural techniques, cryosurgery, and laser surgery. Computed tomography (CT), cephalometric tracings, radiographs, photographs, and dental models enhance diagnosis, evaluation, and planning to achieve successful outcomes of surgical intervention. The potential for altering alignment, function, and appearance is limited only by the imagination of the surgeons.

One of the most imaginative surgeons of modern times is Paul L. Tessier of Paris. In 1967 he reported his work to surgically correct gross facial and skull deformities of children with Crouzon's and Apert's syndromes. Tessier's results have had a monumental impact on the development of craniofacial surgery as a new surgical subspecialty. Surgeons are able to systematically dismantle, rearrange, and reconstruct the entire musculoskeletal system between the top of the head and the oral cavity. This requires a multidisciplinary team. Special craniofacial centers have been established for these complex procedures.

PATIENT'S SELF-IMAGE

Psychologic feelings one has about self are inherent in the behavior of a social human being. Physical appearance contributes to these feelings. Facial beauty is prized in our society. Therefore facial configuration may be perceived by the patient as a deformity and thus the source of personal discomfort, reinforced by ridicule or lack of familial or social acceptance. The psychologic trauma of a negative self-image can lead to asocial behavior.

The degree, duration, and impairment of facial disfigurement, as perceived by the patient, will influence the desire for surgical correction. Patients with recently acquired deformities as the result of trauma are usually more concerned with appearance than individuals who grew up with cosmetically displeasing facial features. Impairment of function caused by deformity or disease may offer the patient no alternative other than surgical intervention.

Patients should be psychologically prepared for and supported following ablative surgery. Extensive, or even minimal, excision of the structures and soft tissue of the face or neck can cause severe psychologic trauma. Patients should be thoroughly evaluated preoperatively. A psychiatric consultation may be advisable.

Family members should also be prepared to accept the permanent or temporary disfigurement of a loved one following ablative surgery. Reconstruction frequently is performed in stages. The patient and family must cope with the physical limitations between surgical procedures, for example, of speaking and eating, as well as physical appearance. The patient's willingness to care for the wound may be the first sign of acceptance. The home situation should be assessed to ascertain whether the patient will need home care and support after discharge.

FACE

Anatomy and Physiology

The *face* is the anterior part of the head, including the forehead, cheeks, nose, lips, and chin, but not the ears. The eyes, situated in the bony orbits, contribute to the features of the face, although they are not technically a part of the face. The structure and function of the nose, the prominent organ in the center of the face, are discussed in Chapter 35 (see p. 734 and Figure 35-4, p. 735).

The skeletal structure of the face (Figure 36-1) includes the *frontal bone* of the forehead. It forms the upper part of the orbits. Divided by sutures (i.e., lines of union between bones), the frontal bone joins the sphenoid and ethmoid, and the paired nasal, lacrimal, maxilla, and zygomatic bones. The posterior orbits are formed by the *sphenoid bone,* which is shaped like a butterfly with extended wings, and the palatal bones. The medial walls are formed by the ethmoid, lacrimal, and nasal bones and maxilla. The lateral aspect is formed by the *zygoma* (malar bone), the cheekbone. The irregularly shaped *ethmoid bone* also forms the roof and posterior lateral wall of each nasal cavity. The *nasal bones* form the bridge of the nose between the orbits.

The *maxilla,* the upper jaw that holds the palate, extends laterally to the zygoma and temporal bone, under the orbit, and along the anterior nasal cavity. The maxillary bones are paired and join in the midline between the nose and oral cavity. The alveoli that hold the teeth are along the alveolar processes of the maxillae.

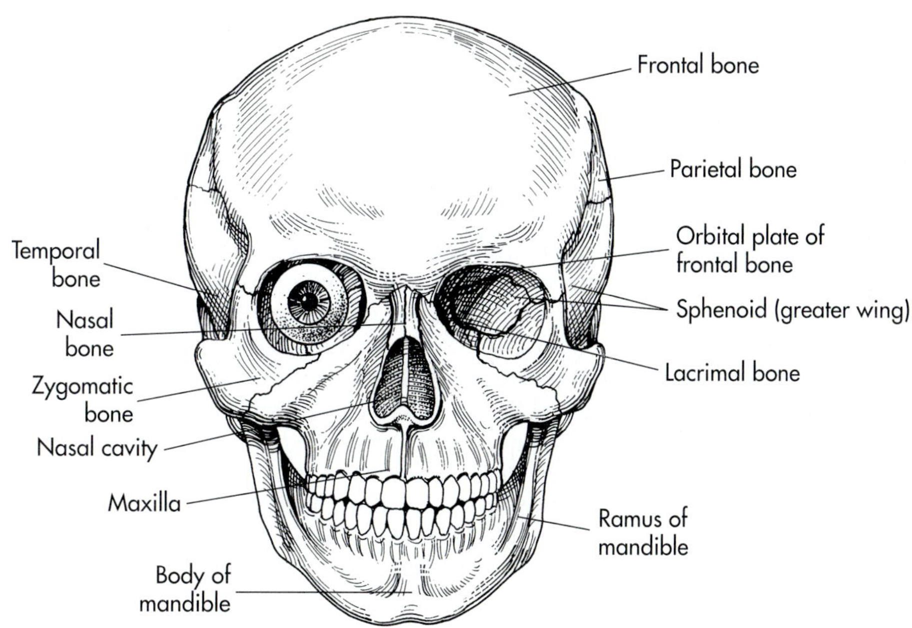

FIGURE 36-1 Anterior view of skull.

The ramus of the *mandible,* the arch-shaped bone of the lower jaw, articulates with temporal bones at the temporomandibular joints in front of the ears. The alveoli, the tooth-bearing bodies, meet at the alveolar process to form the chin (mental region).

The bony structure of the face is covered with muscles, superficial blood vessels and nerves, epidermis, and dermis. Other structures (i.e., ducts and sinuses [air spaces]) are also in the soft tissues or bony structure of the face (see discussion of paranasal sinuses in Chapter 35, pp. 734 and 737).

SURGICAL PROCEDURES OF FACE

Craniofacial Procedures

Craniofacial refers to the cranium and face. Craniofacial surgery of increasing complexity has been performed since World War II. However, the approach developed by Tessier has led to previously inaccessible anatomic areas. Exposure for dissection of soft tissues and bone to restore contour and symmetry in practically every type of facial deformity, whether congenital, neoplastic, or traumatic in origin, can be accomplished by a multidisciplinary team of surgeons. This team may include a plastic surgeon, neurosurgeon, anesthesiologist, ophthalmologist, oral surgeon, and otorhinolaryngologist. Some procedures require more than 100 separate maneuvers and may take as long as 14 to 16 hours to complete.

Many of the concepts developed for these very complex procedures are applied in the more common and less complicated procedures to reshape sections of the skull or reconstruct soft tissues. Craniofacial reconstruction should be performed as soon as indicated by the physiologic and psychologic impacts of the deformity on the patient, regardless of age. An early surgical procedure not only decreases psychologic trauma but also may prevent craniofacial distortion caused by brain and nerve damage of a disease process or traumatic injury.

Analysis of three-dimensional CT scans and cephalometric tracings accurately superimposed on transparent photographs of the patient preoperatively are essential to determine the extent of facial deformity and the plan for skeletal rearrangement. The exact size of the defects that will need bone grafts can be determined.

Many procedures involve correction of malocclusion of the mandible at the same time the orbitocranial skeleton is restructured. Dental models are cut and mounted on an articulator for reference.

Hypotensive anesthesia reduces blood loss during these extensive procedures. The patient is continuously monitored throughout the procedure to estimate blood loss. A preoperative tracheotomy may be necessary to maintain an adequate airway postoperatively.

Midface Advancement

The base of the anterior cranial fossae can be exposed through a bifrontal incision to elevate a frontal bone flap. While the neurosurgeon is raising the flap, the plastic surgeon may take donor bone from a rib and/or the iliac crest if autogenous bone grafts will be needed. Harvesting of bone graft from the calvarium, the upper domelike portion of skull, may be preferred.

The facial skeleton is separated from the cranial base. The plastic surgeon raises the periorbita, orbital contents, and soft tissue over the dorsum of the nose. The subperiosteum of the anterior maxillae is elevated. Osteotomies are cut in the supraorbital region to mobilize the lateral walls. Anterior maxillary osteotomy, through an infraorbital approach, extends across and below the frontal processes of the maxillae. Osteotomies of the anterior cranial fossae and the medial and lateral orbital walls and floors are completed. The mobilized bones can be functionally advanced in three dimensions as desired. They are then stabilized with a plating system or wired into position. To maintain stability, bone grafts also are wired into place in the resulting defects. Demineralized bone blocks, chips, or powder often are preferred to bone grafts to induce osteogenesis. The frontal bone flap is replaced, and the incision is closed.

Mandibular osteotomies may be done before closure to correct alignment of the jaws. Whether this is necessary or not, the mandible is stabilized after closure with intermaxillary wires and suspension wires to the zygomatic arch.

Depending on the deformity, variations of the intracranial and extracranial osteotomies are done to advance, align, or reposition the facial bones and reconstruct soft tissues. Many patients return to the operating room (OR) for additional corrective procedures: eyelid ptosis and/or extraocular muscle surgery performed by the ophthalmologist; dacryocystorhinostomy and/or nasal reconstruction performed by the rhinologist; and bone augmentation or resection of the maxillae and/or mandible for repositioning by the plastic surgeon or oral surgeon. During all procedures, the surgeons avoid injury to optic and facial nerves and to arteries and veins.

Orbital Procedures

An abnormally wide space between (hypertelorism) or malposition of (dystopia) the bony orbits is usually secondary to other craniofacial malformations. Only the medial orbital walls may be moved to correct minimal hypertelorism. Advancement of superior and lateral walls, rather than total orbit advancement, may suffice to correct a dystopia. A combined intracranial and extracranial approach may be necessary to change the angle of the orbits and reposition the medial canthal ligaments of the eyes.

Resection of Nasal or Paranasal Sinus Tumors

Radical craniofacial resection may be indicated to remove gigantic benign nasal dermoid tumors and malignant tumors of the paranasal sinuses. In a one-stage procedure, all involved soft tissue is excised with simultaneous correction of the underlying skeletal structure.

Basal cell carcinoma is a common type of nasal tumor. The surgical procedure may be performed alone or as combined therapy. Immediate repair by skin graft or pedicle flap accompanies excision of well-defined lesions. Reconstruction is postponed in multicentric (many-centered) cancer or doubtful extension of the tumor. More advanced lesions require replacement of the nose by prosthesis.

Erosion of a growth in one of the sinuses into an adjacent nasal wall can occlude the air passage. Resection may include partial or total maxillectomy and removal of surrounding tissues. The cavity usually is covered by skin graft. Unilateral enucleation of the eye may be necessary. A radical surgical procedure for an ethmoid tumor also may involve removal of part of the base of the skull and excision of the maxillary antrum and the palate on the affected side.

In providing maxillofacial prostheses to replace facial structure following various procedures, the prosthodontist works closely with the surgeon and radiation therapist. Splints or stents hold tissue grafts in place, seal cavities from each other, or unite bony segments. A dental prosthesis to close the defect in the upper jaw and eye prosthesis following enucleation contribute to the patient's rehabilitation following an extensive surgical procedure.

Resection of Craniofacial Tumors and Dysplasia

Malignant tumors can originate from soft tissues of the face and scalp, the oropharyngeal mucosa, the ear canal, or the lacrimal gland. They can invade the base of the skull. Fibrous dysplasia, a congenital metabolic disturbance that causes an abnormal proliferation of fibrous tissue, can result in asymmetric distortion and expansion of craniofacial bones. These conditions can collapse the paranasal sinuses, compress the optic nerve or chiasm causing loss of vision, and cause other functional disabilities. An acute epistaxis (nosebleed) can be life-threatening. A combined intracranial and extracranial approach may be used to completely remove tumor or dysplastic bone. The remaining bony structures may be reshaped or repositioned. Bone grafts and/or prosthetic implants may be used for reconstruction of the forehead, orbits, nose, maxilla, and/or mandible.

Midfacial Fractures

The facial bones provide a shield for the brain. They also protect the senses of sight, smell, hearing, and taste. Although midfacial fractures and soft tissue injuries are seldom fatal, inadequate treatment can result in disfigurement and sensory impairment. For example, virtually all blindness secondary to trauma is permanent.

Facial fractures should be suspected when the patient complains of pain, malocclusion of the jaws, or diplopia (double vision). Swelling and asymmetry of the face may be obvious. Diagnosis is confirmed by x-ray film or CT scan to identify the bone(s) involved. The LeFort classification of fractures is useful in determining the appropriate method of reduction and stabilization.

1. LeFort I is a transverse fracture of the maxilla, fragmenting the upper alveoli and palate.
2. LeFort II is a pyramidal fracture of the frontal processes of the maxillae, the nasal bones, and the orbital floor. The maxillae are freely movable.
3. LeFort III fracture includes both zygomas, maxillae, and nasal bones and the ethmoid, sphenoid, and other orbital bones. This creates a craniofacial dysjunction (separation).

Facial fractures are reduced, stabilized, and immobilized. Priorities of initial treatment following injury, however, concern airway obstruction, possible cervical spine injury, and hemorrhage. Treatment of the fracture may be delayed. The surgeon follows the principles of approaching fractures from "inside out, downward up." This means that bony structures are repaired first, then the soft tissues; the mandible or most distal fracture is reduced first before working upward toward the cranium.

The method of bony repair is determined by the complexity of the fracture(s). Intermaxillary fixation combined with interdental wiring, external pin fixation, or rigid internal fixation effect stabilization. Minifacial and midfacial plates, microplates, and mandibular plates may be combined with arch bars or bone grafts.

Reduction of Orbital Fractures The injury may involve the rim or the floor of the orbit, or both. If orbital contents are depressed into the maxillary sinus, surgical exploration through an orbital or a transsinal approach is indicated. Extent of the trauma should indicate the most appropriate surgical management.

1. *Fractures of the orbital rim,* frequently associated with fractures of the zygoma, are usually detected by deformity. The fracture is reduced by appropriate means. Fragments are wired into place as necessary.
2. *Blowout fracture of the orbit* may result from a direct blow to the eyeball, which is, in turn, transmitted to the very thin floor of the orbit. A typical fracture is in the medial third of the floor with dislocation of floor fragments into the maxillary sinus. The fracture occasionally may extend into the ethmoid plate. Consequently orbital contents, which may include the inferior extraocular muscles, are usually herniated into the antrum. This produces limitation of upward gaze and some degree of enophthalmos, a recession of the eyeball into the orbit. The herniated orbital contents are reduced from the antrum back into the orbit with special attention to freeing the entrapped muscles. Plastic or silicone sheeting may be used to close the defect in the floor. Or the fragments may be elevated by packing the antrum through a Caldwell-Luc (sinus) approach. Diagnosis may be overlooked unless a laminogram is taken.

Reduction of Nasal Fractures Fracture of the nasal bones and septum often accompanies other trauma to the head, such as a blowout fracture of the orbit (just discussed). If the zygoma or maxilla is involved, reduction may be accomplished through a small incision anterior to the ear and superior to the zygomatic arch. Periosteal elevators are used to raise depressed bone and cartilage fragments. Nasal fractures are splinted with nasal packs and an external splint.

Reduction of Zygomatic Fractures Dislocations of the zygoma are more common than fractures of the cheekbone (malar bone). Zygomatic fractures always involve the orbital bones. Those of the zygomatic arch are particularly unstable and require intraosseous or transosseous wire fixation following internal reduction with counterpressure from underneath the arch. Transantral Steinmann pinning may be necessary to maintain reduction of fragments in severely fragmented fractures.

Maxillofacial Procedures

Maxillofacial pertains to the part of face formed by the upper and lower jaws. Most maxillofacial procedures are designed to reconstruct defects in the lips, the buccal sulcus, maxilla, alveolar ridge, floor of the mouth, mandible, and/or chin. These defects may be the result of trauma or resection of tumor. Whenever feasible, intraoral incisions are used to minimize facial scarring. Soft tissue reconstructions of the lips are discussed in Chapter 34, pp. 714-715. Congenital deformities are discussed in Chapter 42, p. 864.

Intermaxillary Fixation of Fractures

Following closed or open reduction, fractures of the maxilla and mandible are usually immobilized by interdental wiring if the patient has upper and lower teeth. If the patient is edentulous (without teeth), open reduction and skeletal fixation by circumferential wiring over an intraoral splint or screws and connecting bars may be necessary.

Erich arch bars are shaped along the dental arches. Wires are passed between the teeth to anchor the splints on the upper and lower jaws. Each splint contains a series of small lugs. Tiny rubber bands, placed around opposing lugs, hold the teeth in occlusion. Splints frequently are not used for fixation of these fractures. The teeth may be held in occlusion by wires passed around opposing teeth.

NOTE Following fixation of the mandible or maxilla, wire cutters accompany the patient from the OR and remain at the bedside as long as wires or rubber bands are in place. If the patient experiences respiratory difficulty or vomiting, the wires may have to be cut to prevent aspiration. Fluids may be difficult to swallow.

If microplates can be used for rigid fixation, the interdental wiring may be released after the fixation procedure is completed.

Mandibular Fractures

Some fractures of the mandible can be immobilized by transoral placement of noncompression miniplates. This technique obviates the necessity for interdental wiring. Vitallium, titanium, or stainless steel plates and screws are used for rigid fixation.

Mandibular Reconstruction

Skeletal defects creating loss of mandibular continuity are usually the result of trauma or benign disease. Bone replacement is the most common method of restoring function and contour. The patient's own ilium provides cancellous bone that can be shaped into the configuration of the jaw. A composite graft of a freeze-dried cadaver mandible packed with autogenous cancellous bone chips also can be used. These grafts fill a bony defect but do not provide soft tissue coverage. A vascularized iliac graft is preferable to reconstruct the mandible and a large intraoral defect.

Alveolar Ridge Reconstruction

The alveolar ridge is the bony remains of the alveolar process of the maxilla or mandible that formerly contained the teeth. Some edentulous patients have atrophic maxillae and/or mandibles or bony defects caused by trauma or tumor resection that will not support artificial dentures. The alveolar ridges can be augmented or reconstructed.

Inlay Bone Grafts Bone grafts are used for augmentation of the maxillae and/or mandible. A prevascularized autogenous rib graft may be transplanted into a maxillary defect; microvascular anastomoses revascularize graft. Composite grafts of freeze-dried cadaver rib with autogenous particulate cancellous bone and marrow may be preferred in the maxilla. Iliac bone is used to augment the mandible (see previous discussion of mandibular reconstruction). Calvaria may be harvested from the frontal, parietal, or occipital cranial bones for maxillofacial bone grafts. Calvarial bone undergoes less resorption than rib and iliac bone because of its dense blood supply; graft revascularizes rapidly. Titanium osseointegration fixtures may be used to secure calvarial bone grafts in place.

Mandibular Staple The staple fastener prosthesis is implanted as an alternative to bone grafting to restore the ability of the mandible to support a denture. The titanium alloy (Tivanium) device has two transosteal pins with a set of fasteners and lock nuts between them on the curved cross-arch connecting plate. The staple is inserted with a drill guide and twist drills specifically designed for it. The staple is evenly seated in the holes drilled in the mandible to the point of contact with the inferior border.

A scratch or bend may weaken the staple and may result in a fracture of the device. A deformed staple will not fit into the drill holes properly. The prosthesis is carefully protected and handled very little before implantation.

Temporomandibular Joint Syndrome

Persistent pain and dysfunction of the temporomandibular joint (TMJ) can be associated with stress-related bruxism (tensing muscles and grinding teeth), position of teeth, malocclusion, trauma, arthritis, and other degenerative changes in one or both joints. If TMJ is unresponsive to conservative treatment, surgical intervention may be indicated.

Arthroscopy Arthroscopy, usually performed bilaterally, is used to diagnose problems such as scarring or adhesions that do not show up on CT scan or magnetic resonance imaging (MRI). Lysis of adhesions, mechanical debridement, and lavage of the TMJ may relieve symptoms. Repositioning or release of the fibrocartilaginous articular disk (meniscus) between the mandibular condyle and glenoid fossa of the temporal bone may restore function. A 1.7 or 1.9 mm arthroscope with fiberoptic camera attached is locked into a cannula sheath inserted through an inferolateral puncture wound into the joint capsule. Continuous inflow and outflow of fluid, usually iced Ringer's lactate solution, is necessary to keep joint distended for visibility and lavage. Therapeutic synovectomy and partial or complete meniscectomy may recontour the joint. A rotary shaver and/or the Ho:YAG laser may be used. The laser rapidly resects and vaporizes cartilaginous tissue and coagulates bleeding vessels.

Arthroplasty Open, direct visualization of the disk and condyle may be necessary to correct abnormal relationships. Either a preauricular or postauricular incision may be used to approach the TMJ. Condyle, fossa, and/or articular eminence may be reshaped or resurfaced. A damaged or displaced articular disk can be recontoured and repositioned. It is recontoured with a scalpel or by electrosurgical cutting and then repositioned and sutured in place. If the disk is torn or perforated, it is usually removed. A silicone elastomer implant or a titanium alloy prosthesis may be used to reconstruct the joint. The jaw may be immobilized with interdental wiring to stabilize the TMJ during healing.

Orthognathic Surgery

The jaws can be reshaped or repositioned to correct functional bite disorders and/or aesthetics. (See discussion of mentoplasty in Chapter 34, p. 716.) Occlusion (i.e., closure of teeth) depends on the anteroposterior relationship of upper and lower jaws. *Orthognathia,* derived from the Greek words *orthos* (ορθος) meaning straight and *gnathos* (γναθος) meaning jaw, relates to treatment of conditions involving malposition of maxilla or mandible, or both. Malocclusion occurs when teeth do not close together properly. It can cause difficulty in chewing and/or speaking, periodontal disease, and/or temporomandibular joint dysfunction. Psychologically debilitating facial deformity and bite disorders of genetic origin or as a result of growth disturbances or trauma include:

1. *Prognathism.* One or both jaws project forward beyond normal relationship with the cranial base. If the mandible (lower jaw) protrudes beyond the maxilla (upper jaw), it creates a prominence of chin, concave profile, and underbite. If the maxilla grows beyond the mandible, it creates an overbite.
2. *Retrognathism.* One or both jaws are positioned posterior to normal craniofacial relationship (i.e., behind frontal plane of forehead). In reference to the mandible, the condition is commonly known as a receding chin; this may create an overbite.
3. *Apertognathia.* The front teeth do not close because the back teeth come together first, creating an open bite.
4. *Micrognathia.* The dental arch, usually of the mandible, is too small to accommodate teeth. Teeth are pushed out of alignment because they are crowded together.
5. *Asymmetry.* A discrepancy in size, shape, or position of jaws creates an imbalance between right and left sides of the face.

Preoperative orthodontia may be required to align and level the teeth. The ultimate goal is to achieve functional stability of dentofacial structures with acceptable facial aesthetics. Surgical correction may include extraction of one or more teeth, maxillary and/or mandibular osteotomies with repositioning of bone segments, and/or repositioning of alveoli. Intraorally, bilateral maxillary osteotomies may be performed in conjunction with mandibular osteotomies, or either of these procedures can be done independently to change shape of facial contours.

Le Fort Osteotomy For maxillary deformities, an incision is made in mucosa of the upper lip. Osteotomies (i.e., bone cuts) are made in medial and lateral maxillary sinus walls. The vomer is cut just above the floor of the nose. Pterygoid plates are sectioned from the maxilla. The maxilla is movable for reduction, augmentation, or reposition. The maxilla can be detached from base of the skull, maintaining vascular supply via the soft palate, and cut into segments to reconstruct lower face as described for midface advancement. Usually miniplates anchored with screws bridge the osteotomy cuts.

Mandibular Osteotomy Sagittal split osteotomies through ramus and vertical osteotomies through molar region on each side allow backward or forward repositioning of the mandible. If moved posteriorly, bone on the anterior aspect is trimmed for good medullary bone contact. Rigid fixation may be obtained with miniplates or with screws placed percutaneously through stab wounds. The latter are stabilized with an external fixator. If plates and screws are used, intermaxillary fixation as described for fractures may not be necessary.

Postoperative orthodontia may be required to complete closure of spaces around the osteotomies and thus stabilize occlusal function.

Dentofacial Procedures

Just as the scope of many medical/surgical specialties, such as otolaryngology–head and neck surgery, has broadened, so has dentistry. Likewise subspecialization within dentistry, through extensive specialized postgraduate education, has given OR practice privileges to dentists who perform surgical procedures in and around the oral cavity. Among these are:

1. *Oral surgeon.* Oral surgery may be limited to exodontia (extraction of teeth) and minor surgery in the oral cavity. It may also include correction of dentofacial deformities (i.e., oral and maxillofacial surgery). A qualified oral surgeon is competent to complete a history and physical examination and thus determine the patient's ability to undergo the proposed surgical procedure.
2. *Orthodontist.* Orthodontics focuses on irregularities of the teeth, malocclusion, and associated facial problems.
3. *Prosthodontist.* Prosthodontics is concerned with artificial restoration of intraoral and external facial structures.
4. *Periodontist.* Periodontics is the treatment and prevention of disease in the gingiva (gum), underlying soft tissues, and alveoli surrounding the teeth.

Patients with medical problems admitted to the hospital by oral surgeons and all patients admitted for dental care have an admission history, physical examination, and evaluation of their overall medical risk by a physician preoperatively. This physician is responsible for the care of a preexisting condition and any medical problem that arises during hospitalization.

Just as physicians from various specialties function as members of a multidisciplinary team, so do oral surgeons and dentists, each contributing to the dental health of the patient. Frequently they also function as collegial members of the teams involved in craniofacial or maxillofacial surgery. They assist with reconstruction of the face, correction of jaw deformities, and establishment of optimum dental occlusion. For example, the orthodontist may move teeth before a maxillofacial or oral surgeon repositions jaws to correct malocclusion. Many patients undergo both preoperative and postoperative orthodontia. Prosthodontics may be necessary to replace missing teeth. Prosthodontists also may fit an artificial nose postoperatively following rhinectomy for tumor or trauma.

Patients seeking dentofacial treatment usually have functional problems. These may include difficulty with mastication (chewing), and deglutition (swallowing), speech, abnormal tongue posture, or lip incompetence. A dental surgical procedure is defined as any manipulation, cutting, or removal of oral or perioral tissues and tooth structures where bleeding occurs. These procedures are performed by oral surgeons and periodontists.

Periodontics

Diseases that affect gingiva, bone, and supporting structures such as periodontal ligaments can occur at any age. Periodontal disease is the primary cause of tooth loss in adults over 35 years of age. Treatment usually takes place in the periodontist's office. However, patients who have medical problems, such as hemophilia or other blood dyscrasia, severe diabetes, or heart disease, are admitted to the hospital. Periodontal plastic surgery encompasses resective, regenerative, and reconstructive techniques.

Gingivectomy Portions of gingiva, mucous membrane, and underlying soft tissue that covers the alveolar process and surrounds the teeth are excised to remove deep pockets of plaque, calculus, and inflamed soft tissue. The carbon dioxide (CO_2) laser may be used for this procedure.

Mucogingivoplasty Plastic surgery around the teeth and gums is done primarily to reduce inflammation, prevent accumulation of bacteria, and stop sensitivity. Another indication is to rebuild bone and soft tissue destroyed by disease or trauma. Excessive gum tissue is excised to contour or reshape gingiva for improved physiologic form or aesthetics. The alveoli may be reconstructed to change their shape and height. Gingival margins may be reshaped for site of a false tooth or fixed bridge. Gingival grafting or augmentation done before or during orthodontic treatment may reduce risk of recession of gum tissue from around roots of teeth. Autogenous mucogingival free grafts from the hard palate or pedicle flaps from adjacent tissues may be used to cover receded alveolar mucosa or exposed tooth root. Flaps or grafts are used to augment inadequate zones of masticatory gingiva. Gingival onlay grafts are also used to enhance ridges where trauma or extraction has resulted in a reduced ridge, thus correcting an aesthetic defect.

Bone Reconstruction In advanced periodontal disease, destruction of underlying alveolar bone and fibrous connective tissue can loosen teeth. Alveolar defects are rebuilt with autogenous bone grafts, mineral ceramics, polymer granulates, freeze-dried homografts, demineralized heterologous bone, or some combination of grafting material. Bone, periodontal ligaments, and cementum that covers roots have regenerative potential. *Guided tissue regeneration* involves temporary placement of a thin artificial membrane over a bony defect of a molar tooth's root surface. Adjacent cells regenerate to produce a bony framework for attachment of the root to surrounding bone.

Dental Implant Fixtures are implanted into the gingiva and attached to bone to replace or augment lost dentition. A dental implant may replace a single tooth or missing teeth. Several types are used. They are made of biocompatible metals, most commonly titanium, and may be coated with ceramic, carbon, or sapphire.

1. *Endosteal implant.* A threaded screw, cylinder, or flat blade is implanted in an alveolus in the maxilla or mandible. The number of implants placed depends on availability of bone and number of teeth to be replaced. The fixture is covered with soft tissue. By a process of *osseointegration,* a perimucosal seal and bond develops between the gingiva and surface of the implant. Some implants have small holes that allow bone to grow through them to secure the implant. After a minimum of 3 (for mandible) to 6 (for maxilla) months, a second-stage procedure is performed to connect a solid post to the implanted fixture. This extends slightly above the gingiva. The artificial tooth is attached to this post with tiny screws. Osseointegration provides firm, immobile support and distributes stress of chewing evenly within jaw.
2. *Subperiosteal implant.* The implant is placed beneath the periosteum directly onto the alveolar

bone. This type of implant is used when bone is insufficient to support an endosteal implant.

3. *Transosteal implant.* A bone plate with retaining posts, similar to mandibular staple previously described, is used when the patient has severe mandibular alveolar ridge atrophy.

ORAL CAVITY

Anatomy and Physiology

Anatomy and physiology of the oral cavity and throat are presented in Chapter 35, pp. 738-739. In addition to the hard and soft palates, pharynx, and tongue, the *salivary glands* are located in the soft tissue walls of the oral cavity. The six major paired glands are the submandibular, sublingual, and parotid. The parotid glands are the largest. The ducts of these major glands, in addition to lesser glands, secrete saliva into the mouth. Saliva functions to moisten and lubricate food to aid in swallowing, to dissolve some substances and enzymatically digest starches, and to facilitate tasting. Structures in the oral cavity are associated with both respiration and deglutition, the act of swallowing.

SURGICAL PROCEDURES OF ORAL CAVITY

Pathologic conditions may affect lips, tongue, floor of the mouth, palates, salivary glands, or pharynx. The oral region is one of the most vascular areas of the body. Hemostasis may be achieved with an electrosurgical unit, hemostatic scalpel, argon beam coagulator, or laser. Lasers are used to vaporize both benign and malignant superficial and subepithelial lesions.

Abnormalities result from congenital malformation, improper occlusion or jaggedness of teeth, and infection but most commonly from trauma and neoplasms. Adequate reconstruction restores the lining, internal structural support, soft tissue, and external coverage. Many of the craniofacial, maxillofacial, and dentofacial procedures previously described in this chapter are performed through intraoral incisions. Other procedures done orally are described in Chapters 34, 35, and 42. The following procedures may be performed by plastic surgeons, oral surgeons, laryngologists, or a multidisciplinary team through intraoral and extraoral incisions.

Excision of Salivary Gland Tumors

Benign mixed tumors of the salivary glands are more common than are malignant tumors and most frequently are located in a parotid gland. Most tumors can be removed by dissection and some by cryosurgery. The incision is of adequate size to expose the entire gland and the facial nerve. A nerve stimulator is used to identify the nerve and its branches. Injury to the nerve results in postoperative facial paralysis.

Parotidectomy

Parotidectomy, excision of a parotid gland, is performed through an incision in the neck below the angle of the mandible and extending upward to one or both sides of the ear. A swelling beneath the skin in the area in front of or below the ear is almost invariably within the substance of the parotid gland. This may be a benign, mixed, or malignant tumor. Benign lesions localized superficially may be excised by superficial subtotal parotidectomy. Lesions deep within the gland, extending under the mandible, frequently displace the soft palate in the oral cavity. Radical neck dissection or hemimandibulectomy may be indicated to remove a highly invasive malignant tumor. For most parotid tumors, the facial nerve can be isolated and preserved during total parotidectomy, unless the nerve is inextricably involved by the tumor. If the facial nerve must be sacrificed, the nerve may be primarily grafted, with the great auricular nerve as a graft, to prevent total facial nerve paralysis.

Excision of Oral Carcinoma

Primary malignant lesions may occur in the lower lip, tongue, or floor of the mouth. Because of the proximity of cervical lymph nodes, metastasis occurs early. A painful bleeding ulcer is considered a suspicious symptom. However, oral cancer in its earliest stages may be asymptomatic and painless. Small tumors may be treated with only irradiation, local excision with primary closure, or vaporization with laser beam. Larger lesions compel more extensive procedures.

Subtotal Glossectomy or Hemiglossectomy

Part (subtotal) or half (hemi-) of the tongue is removed (glossectomy). Extent of the resection will determine the type of reconstruction to resurface the oral cavity. Innervated free flaps may be used to maintain bulk and tone.

Total Glossectomy

All of the tongue and often the floor of the mouth are resected. A pectoralis major myocutaneous island flap is more advantageous than are the cervical, pectoral, or forehead flaps also used to restore the intraoral lining. Respiratory embarrassment and chronic aspiration are significant problems after glossectomy. Cricopharyngeal myotomy may be performed to facilitate swallowing and reduce aspiration. The tip of the epiglottis is often sutured to the pharyngeal wall (epiglottopexy) to decrease aspiration. Unless involved directly with tumor, the larynx is preserved. Laryngeal suspension, achieved by placing a heavy suture around the mandibular ramus, holds the larynx laterally. Extension into the larynx and cervical metastases are indications for unilateral or bilateral neck dissection, usually with laryngectomy (see pp. 754-755). A tracheotomy is always performed with a total glossectomy to maintain an airway. For postoperative alimentation a nasogastric tube is inserted before closing the pharynx.

Mandibulectomy

Partial or total removal of the lower jaw is performed for extension of tumor into bone of the floor of the mouth. It may be performed with glossectomy and radical neck dissection for wide excision. Mandibular replacement combines bone graft and synthetic materials for restoration of speech and appearance. A compound osseocutaneous flap from the iliac crest, with microvascular anastomosis of the deep circumflex iliac artery vascular pedicle, may be transferred for reconstruction. If patient is dentulous, the relationship of opposing teeth is maintained; if edentulous, patient wears a denture. Whenever possible, mandible-sparing procedures are done for carcinoma of the tongue.

NECK

Anatomy and Physiology

The *neck* connects the head and trunk of the body. It is supported by the cervical vertebrae posteriorly and muscles anteriorally and laterally. The larynx, leading to the trachea, and proximal end of the esophagus pass within the muscular structure (see Figure 35-4, p. 735). The vascular, nervous, and lymphatic systems leading to and from the head also pass through the neck. The thyroid and parathyroid glands lie along the trachea on the anterior aspect at the base of the neck.

Larynx

The *larynx,* situated anteriorly between the hypopharynx superiorly and trachea inferiorly, consists of three major cartilages supported by ligaments and muscles: the thyroid cartilage, which protects the soft inner structures, the cricoid cartilage directly beneath it, and the paired arytenoid cartilages posterior to the thyroid and joined to the cricoid. The thyroid cartilage is incomplete posteriorly, but the cricoid is a complete ring. The cricothyroid space lies between the thyroid and cricoid cartilages.

The larynx functions as an organ for speech and for closure of the glottis during swallowing to protect the respiratory passage and prevent aspiration. The *epiglottis,* an elastic cartilage covered with mucous membrane at the root of the tongue in the hypopharynx, covers the superior opening of larynx during swallowing.

Extrinsic muscles open and close the *glottis,* the space between the true vocal cords. Intrinsic muscles regulate vocal cord tension. Movement of the paired arytenoid cartilages opens and closes the glottis. Folds of mucous membrane covering muscle line the larynx. The two upper folds are the *false cords;* the two lower folds are the *true vocal cords.* The true vocal cords attach to the arytenoid cartilages posteriorly and to the thyroid cartilage anteriorly. The cords are an integral part of phonation. They vibrate to produce sounds by rhythmically moving air particles. Production of vocal sound involves coordination of musculature of the lips, tongue, soft palate, pharynx, and larynx. The mouth and pharynx are the resonating cavities.

The tenth cranial or vagus nerve innervates the larynx. Its major branch to the larynx is the recurrent laryngeal nerve. Trauma to the nerve can result in laryngeal paralysis, which is devastating if both nerves are paralyzed.

Trachea

The *trachea* is a tube composed of rings of cartilage anteriorly and membrane posteriorly. This membrane also forms the anterior wall of the *esophagus,* the musculomembranous canal between the pharynx and stomach. The trachea extends from the lower larynx to the carina in the chest, where it bifurcates to form the right and left main bronchi leading to the lungs.

SURGICAL PROCEDURES OF LARYNX

Trauma or disease involving laryngeal cartilages, mucous membrane, or the vocal cords can obstruct respiration and/or speech. Surgical procedures are directed toward diagnosis of the cause and elimination of obstruction to maintain the larynx's dual functions in respiration and phonation.

Laryngoscopy

Laryngoscopy is a visual examination of the mucous membrane lining of larynx and vocal cords with a lighted instrument, with or without the adjunct magnification of the operating microscope. Laryngoscopy is performed for diagnosis, biopsy, and/or treatment of laryngeal lesions including:

1. *Foreign body,* such as a coin or small toy.
2. *Papilloma of the vocal cords,* which prevents accurate cord approximation and normal voice.
3. *Laryngeal polyps,* with stripping of polypoid mucosa to alleviate recurrence.
4. *Juvenile papilloma,* multiple growths on the larynx, epiglottis, vocal cords, and trachea. These may be treated by cryosurgery or laser beam in lieu of excision.
5. *Leukoplakia,* a white thickening on the vocal cords, causing hoarseness. The lesion is examined histologically for differentiation from carcinoma.
6. *Laryngeal web,* adherence of the anterior aspects of the vocal cords as a result of removal of mucous membrane or following inflammation. After excision, a metal or plastic plate may be placed be-

tween the cords until normal mucous membrane regenerates. The plate is then removed.

Preoperative preparation and endoscopic technique are similar for laryngoscopy, esophagoscopy, and bronchoscopy. General anesthesia is usually used, but local topical anesthesia may be preferred for some patients. The patient is supine with the neck hyperextended and head supported. As following any anesthetization of throat, postoperative orders include nothing by mouth for a specific number of hours until throat reflexes have returned to prevent aspiration.

Indirect Laryngoscopy

In indirect laryngoscopy a laryngeal mirror is inserted through the mouth to base of the tongue. With patient in sitting position, light is reflected to the area by the surgeon's headlamp. During this simple diagnostic procedure, biopsy or polypectomy can be performed.

Direct Laryngoscopy

In direct laryngoscopy a rigid hollow tubular laryngoscope is inserted into the larynx for direct visualization. Suction tubes and grasping forceps are maneuvered through the handheld laryngoscope. Fiberoptic light carriers are connected to a light source. Endoscopic principles as discussed in Chapter 15 are applicable.

Suspension Microlaryngoscopy

For microlaryngoscopy the laryngoscope becomes self-retaining by suspension in a special appliance placed over the patient's chest. This gives the surgeon bimanual freedom in use of the operating microscope. The microscope provides binocular vision and magnification in critical inaccessible areas or areas difficult to visualize by direct laryngoscopy. A standard operating microscope with a 400 mm lens is used. Microlaryngeal instruments are added to the basic setup for direct laryngoscopy. Suspension microlaryngoscopy is used for most intralaryngeal procedures.

Laser Microlaryngoscopy

The CO_2 laser was introduced in laryngology by Doctors Jako and Strong in 1971. It was initially used for removal of recurrent laryngeal papillomas. Now CO_2 and other lasers are used to remove a variety of benign and malignant lesions in the respiratory tract, particularly in the larynx. For example, the argon laser may be used for treatment of hereditary hemorrhagic telangiectasia (dilated groups of capillaries) in the larynx.

A micromanipulator, used to direct the laser beam, is coupled to the operating microscope. The beam is focused by the microscope lens. Reflecting mirrors defocus the beam to reach into otherwise inaccessible areas. Microlaryngeal instruments are used in addition to specific laser instruments. For example, anterior commissure vocal cord retractors with suction attachments are used to clear the smoke of tissue vaporization for visibility.

Laser Safety The laser is a safe instrument around the oral cavity and neck only when safety precautions are taken.

1. Patient's eyes should be taped shut and covered with moistened sponges to prevent injury from inadvertent reflection of laser beam from a metal surface.
2. Patient's face should be covered with a moist towel so that only the oral cavity is exposed.
3. Patient's teeth should be protected from pressure of laryngoscope and from laser beam.
4. Only noncombustible anesthetic gases are used. Anesthetic gases potentially can be ignited by the laser. Nitrous oxide should not be used. Oxygen concentration may be decreased to between 21% and 30% during lasing phase of the procedure.
5. Stainless steel or laminated aluminum and silicone endotracheal tube or a ventilating bronchoscope avoids danger of ignition. Polyvinyl chloride and latex endotracheal tubes cannot be used because they are heat-labile. Red rubber and silicone tubes may be wrapped with reflecting aluminum tape, but tip is not always sufficiently protected if exposed to the laser beam. Ignition of endotracheal tubes has occurred. Moist gauze or compressed patties, attached to strings, are placed through the suspended laryngoscope to protect the balloon in cuff of the tube from rupture by stray or reflected laser beams. The balloon should be filled with sterile normal saline solution, which may be tinted with methylene blue dye, so that it will not ignite if ruptured. If a cuff does rupture, immediate replacement of the tube is necessary. A tracheotomy tray should be available for emergency use.
6. Combustible materials, such as sponges and drapes, are kept moist. Water effectively inhibits penetration of laser energy into surrounding tissue and materials.
7. Division of a blood vessel larger than 0.5 mm requires ligation or electrocoagulation.
8. All other precautions for laser surgery are taken (see Chapter 15, pp. 274-278).

Laryngeal Injuries

Patients with abnormal laryngeal conditions bear close watching for respiratory distress. The anterior, unprotected location of the larynx predisposes it to trauma, such as crushing injury. Treatment is concerned primarily with maintenance of the airway, which may be occluded by edema, hematoma, torn mucosa, or cartilaginous fragments.

Cricothyrotomy, an emergency incision into the larynx, and/or *tracheotomy*, an incision into the trachea, may be necessary to open the airway or to prevent asphyxia. An intraluminal stent inserted into the larynx superiorly to the tracheotomy tube and fixed to it for stabilization may be worn for several months until the laryngeal laceration heals and an intralaryngeal airway re-forms. The stent is used to mold the tissues.

Preservation of voice is also a major concern. Severe laryngeal injury may result in permanent voice impairment. In unilateral vocal cord paralysis, because of muscle atrophy and muscle imbalance, a weak, hoarse ("air-spilling") voice is present. Inadequate glottic closure can be treated by injection of Teflon (Polytef) paste into the affected cord to augment its size and thus help to bring the two cords into apposition. The injected material becomes firm and retains its shape. A functioning cord and marked improvement in voice quality result. This modality is used commonly when the recurrent laryngeal nerve is affected. It is not indicated, however, for acute glottic incompetence. A suspension of Gelfoam powder in saline can be used for temporary augmentation until compensation or need for permanent augmentation occurs.

Procedures for Carcinoma of Larynx

Procedures vary depending on size and location of the lesion, extent of invasion, and presence of regional or distant metastasis, as well as the patient's age, general condition, and rehabilitative capacity. Classification of malignant lesions by location includes *glottic* (true cords), *supraglottic* (above true cords), and *infraglottic* (below true cords). In the early stages, cancer of the larynx is one of the most curable of all malignant tumors because of the sparse lymphatic supply in the region of the vocal cords. Radiologic study of the lesion by various methods, such as contrast laryngography, is a valuable adjunct in selecting an appropriate therapeutic modality. Laryngograms can identify mucosal irregularity, vocal cord thickening or tumor, and outline the lesion, as well as portray functional alteration of laryngeal structures.

Symptoms vary as well. Hoarseness for more than 2 weeks' duration often is a result of cord fixation by a malignant glottic lesion. Dysphagia is suggestive of a tumor at the esophageal opening. Dyspnea from airway obstruction is a late manifestation.

Whenever possible the surgeon will perform a conservative laryngectomy to retain some natural voice. These procedures yield the same rate of cure of selected cancers as a radical procedure, total laryngectomy, without sacrificing phonation, deglutition, and respiratory function. A neck stoma is usually necessary, however, for breathing.

Laryngofissure With Partial Laryngectomy

Laryngofissure, division of or opening into the larynx, may be necessary to remove a foreign body or tumor. Laryngofissure with partial laryngectomy through an incision in the thyroid cartilage is performed to remove a large tumor confined to one vocal cord. A tracheotomy (see pp. 755-757) is performed to maintain the airway. Postoperative hoarseness may diminish as scar tissue forms to replace excised vocal cord.

Supraglottic Laryngectomy

The epiglottis, false cords, and hyoid bone are removed in a supraglottic laryngectomy when a tumor is located in the epiglottis (i.e., is supraglottic). A horizontal incision is made above the true vocal cords, thus preserving voice and normal airway. Neck dissection may be done simultaneously. A temporary tracheotomy is always part of the procedure because of danger of aspiration and postoperative edema. With the epiglottis removed, liquids in particular can easily spill into the trachea. A cuffed tracheotomy tube (see p. 757) is a necessary precaution postoperatively.

Vertical Hemilaryngectomy

In hemilaryngectomy through a vertical incision, one true cord, false cord, arytenoid, and half the thyroid cartilage are removed. The epiglottis, cricoid, and opposing cords are preserved. Following healing, scar tissue fills in the surgical defect, almost approximating the remaining vocal cord. Thus the patient has a usable although hoarse voice and satisfactory airway and can eat normally. Sometimes a muscle flap is used for glottic reconstruction to improve voice quality. A prophylactic tracheotomy usually is done to protect the airway. Subcutaneous emphysema (i.e., infiltration of air under skin) is a potential complication.

Total Laryngectomy With or Without Neck Dissection

A radical procedure, total laryngectomy is performed for advanced lesions involving the larynx and/or hypopharyngeal area, with or without neck dissection. The entire larynx, hyoid bone, cricoid cartilage, two or three tracheal rings, and strap muscles are removed. This resection destroys connection between the pharynx and the trachea. Pharyngeal walls and lower trachea are preserved. The pharyngeal opening to trachea is closed, thus leaving the pharynx open only to the esophagus. The patient breathes and expels bronchial secretions through a permanent stoma at base of anterior neck. This is created by suturing tracheal stump to the skin *(tracheostomy)*. Size of the stoma should be recorded on the patient's record in the event of emergency need for a tube at a later time. In patients with a permanent stoma, resuscitation is always via the stoma.

The nose no longer humidifies the air to the lungs. Sense of smell is also lost because the nasal olfactory epithelium is not stimulated by inhalation. Acclimatization to air intake through the neck constitutes a major adjustment for the patient.

A nasogastric tube is inserted during the surgical procedure for temporary feeding. Although the patient no longer has a normal voice, normal eating is resumed after healing takes place.

Formation of a salivary fistula is one complication of laryngectomy. Swallowed saliva leaks out through a weakness in the pharyngeal suture line and through the skin. Rupture of the carotid artery, especially in preirradiated patients, is another complication. This may occur if radical neck dissection was performed also, which places the artery in the surgical area.

Rehabilitation should begin preoperatively at the time of diagnosis and include the family. It incorporates input from many professional disciplines because major disability results from the surgical procedure. In working with a speech pathologist, some patients learn to develop esophageal speech. By intake of a bolus of air into the esophagus and vibration by cricopharyngeal muscles, sound is produced to articulate speech. Persons unable to perfect the technique may use an artificial larynx, an electronic device that includes pitch and volume.

Many patients are unable to acquire usable esophageal speech, with or without the artificial larynx. Some of these patients have undergone surgical procedures to rebuild a functioning glottis or to create a permanent tracheoesophageal fistula to shunt pulmonary airflow to the pharynx for phonation. Aspiration pneumonia caused by leakage of saliva and food is a major problem following these procedures. Also, pharyngeal constrictor muscle spasms or stenosis may inhibit speech rehabilitation. *Voice restoration* for these aphonic patients may be enhanced by a valved prosthesis. This is inserted through a tracheoesophageal fistula to allow free flow of air into the esophagus for phonation, to prevent aspiration, and to maintain patency of the fistula. Three types of one-way valve *voice prostheses* are used.

1. *Blom-Singer duck bill prosthesis,* so named from shape of the slit valve, is a silicone tube with retention flanges (collarlike projections). The fistula for the prosthesis is created through an esophagoscope inserted into the cervical esophagus. A needle is introduced to puncture posterior tracheal wall and anterior esophagus at the superior aspect of the laryngectomy stoma. A rubber catheter stent is inserted through the puncture to maintain patency during healing. When the prosthesis is fitted, the flanges are taped to the peristomal skin. The patient occludes the stoma to produce a voice.
2. *Blom-Singer tracheostoma valve and low-pressure prosthesis* has a diaphragm that opens during normal respiration and closes in response to expiratory airflow for speech. The circular valve is recessed slightly into the tracheostoma, with the housing fixed to the peristomal skin with a hypoallergenic adhesive. The patient does not manually occlude the stoma during speech.
3. *Panje voice prosthesis,* commonly known as the voice button, is a biflanged silicone valve inserted into a simple tracheoesophageal stab wound. An insertion guide is used to place the prosthesis through the tracheostoma into the created fistula. The patient occludes the stoma to speak.

Practical help and moral support are offered to the newly laryngectomized patient by others who are members of support groups, such as the International Association of Laryngectomees and the Lost Chord Club. The American Cancer Society is also a resource for assistance.

SURGICAL PROCEDURES OF TRACHEA

Upper respiratory tract obstruction and ventilatory failure may require surgical intervention when the need for intubation or positive-pressure ventilation would be long-term or of indefinite duration or when severe laryngeal obstruction is present. The obstruction is bypassed or resected.

Tracheotomy/Tracheostomy

Tracheotomy is an incision into the trachea below the larynx. *Tracheostomy* is the formation of an opening into the trachea into which a tube is inserted through which the patient breathes. Performed in any age group to improve or maintain patency of the airway or relieve obstruction, the opening in the trachea provides easy accessibility for suctioning secretions from the tracheobronchial tree or administering anesthesia to patients with facial trauma or burns. A tracheotomy is commonly a controlled prophylactic procedure but can be an acute emergency. An endotracheal tube may give temporary relief before and during tracheotomy.

A transverse incision above the cricoid cartilage into the larynx (cricothyrotomy) may be necessary to establish an airway in an emergency.

Airway crisis may result from mechanical obstruction by a tumor, foreign body, infection, or secretions. It also results from congenital, neurologic, or traumatic conditions. Some of the many indications for tracheotomy are a foreign body in the hypopharynx or larynx, acute laryngotracheal bronchitis or epiglottitis in infants and children, layrngeal edema, or any other condition that obstructs respiration.

Tracheotomy is often done under local anesthesia. The patient is supine with support under the shoulders to hyperextend the neck. A transverse incision is made, producing a better cosmetic result, or a midline vertical incision is made between the cricoid cartilage and the suprasternal notch. The overlying isthmus of the thyroid gland is retracted or divided, and the exposed third and fourth tracheal rings are incised through a midline vertical incision (Figure 36-2). After tracheal aspiration to remove blood and secretions, a tracheotomy tube is inserted with the obturator in place. Immediately after insertion the obturator is removed to open the airway. (This remains with the patient constantly in case of future need.) The outer cannula is suctioned and the inner cannula fixed in place. The wound is closed with a few sutures, or superficial edges of the area above the tube may be sutured and the area below left with natural tissue approximation to facilitate drainage. A smooth-edged dressing split around the tube protects the skin. Commercial tracheotomy dressings are available. Tapes tied to the ends of the outer cannula are secured around the neck. Proper tension allows insertion of one finger between the tape and skin. If tied too tightly, the tapes may compress the jugular vein; if too loosely, the tube can obtrude with coughing. The tube should not be removed in the first 24 to 48 hours by any person unable to perform a tracheotomy because the tract to the trachea may occlude and not be immediately located.

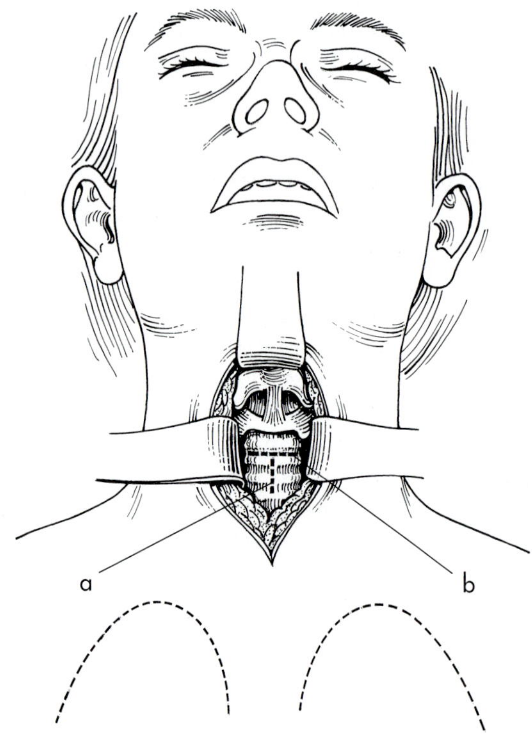

FIGURE 36-2 Tracheotomy incisions. Midline vertical incision *(a)* is made between cricoid cartilage and suprasternal notch. Transverse incision *(b)* is used for emergency tracheotomy and cricothyrotomy.

A sterile tube identical to the one inserted and a tracheotomy set accompany the patient from the OR and constantly remain with him or her until they are released by the surgeon's order.

A tracheotomy is an open wound. Although rigid asepsis is not possible, every effort is made to keep contamination to a minimum. Only sterile equipment, with minimal handling, is used to prevent infection. Suctioning through a tracheotomy tube is done as a sterile procedure, with sterile catheter and gloves. Careful suctioning prevents trauma. Insert the catheter without application of suction, which could injure tracheal walls and suction out oxygen in the borderline patient. Apply suction as the catheter is withdrawn. Run sterile solution through catheter after use to clean it and maintain patency. Disposable catheters are recommended; use once and dispose.

Some patients who have undergone tracheotomy come to the OR for a change of the tube or other procedure. These patients may require suctioning while waiting in the holding area. Knowledge of and preparation for each patient is a prime responsibility of the circulator. These patients require humidified air, which can be delivered by various devices, to keep secretions liquefied and to prevent drying of tissues. Other needs are constant observation and special communication (e.g., pencil and paper).

Tracheotomy Tubes

Although an endotracheal tube may provide ventilation for short-term therapy, a tracheotomy tube is easier to suction and immobilize for extended use. It also reduces the possibility of laryngeal injury.

Various materials such as plastic, nylon, and silicone have largely replaced sterling silver and stainless steel tubes. The plastic tubes have certain advantages:

1. They can be left in situ during radiation therapy.
2. They are lighter in weight, softer, more pliable, and less traumatic.
3. They can be cut to the desired length.
4. They are bonded to the inflatable cuff.

The inside and outside diameters of some tubes are labeled in millimeters. French or Jackson scale is stated on others. All hospitals keep a variety of sizes and types of sterile tracheotomy tubes available in the OR suite, in the emergency department, and on emergency arrest/crash carts.

Most tubes have three parts—the outer cannula, inner cannula, and obturator (Figure 36-3). The inner can-

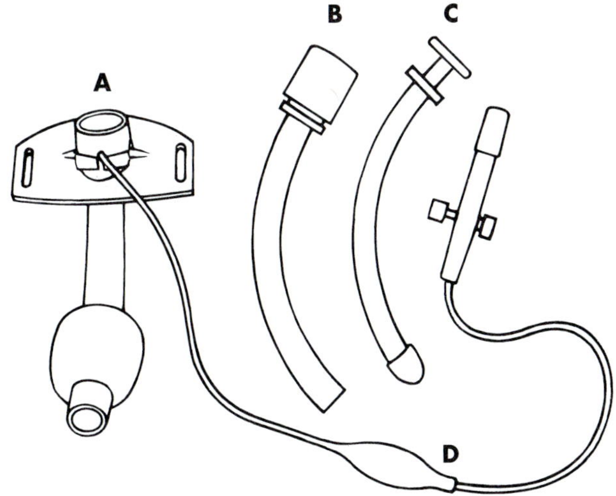

FIGURE 36-3 Tracheotomy tube. **A,** Outer cuffed cannula. **B,** Inner cannula. **C,** Obturator. **D,** Pilot balloon in inflation line.

nula is periodically removed and cleaned to prevent blockage by crusting of secretions. *It always must be replaced immediately within the outer cannula* so that the latter remains free of crusting. The obturator provides a smooth tip during tube insertion to prevent trauma to the tracheal wall. Some plastic tubes do not require an inner cannula because they remain relatively free of crust. If crusts do form, the tube must be changed.

Some tubes have a built-in soft cuff that is inflated to eliminate any free space between the tube and the tracheal wall, thus preventing aspiration of drainage down the trachea. Cuffed tubes also facilitate function of any ventilatory apparatus. A pilot balloon in the inflation line, attached to the outer cannula, indicates cuff inflation or deflation (Figure 36-3, *D*). *Proper cuff inflation-deflation is highly important.* Irritation and pressure of the cuff against the tracheal wall can cause damage such as ulceration and necrosis of the mucosa, which can lead to infection, tracheobronchial fistula, erosion into the innominate artery, or stenosis from scarring. Precautionary measures include deflation at regular intervals, by physician's written order, to increase blood flow to the cuff site; use of low-pressure or controlled-pressure cuff; constant monitoring of intracuff pressure; and minimum inflation to ensure a leak-free system. Overinflation can reduce tube diameter, as well as cause the cuff to extend over the tip of the tube, thus obstructing ventilation. Or the tracheal wall may herniate over the tube end. Underinflation may cause subcutaneous emphysema. Cuffs also should inflate symmetrically. The amount of air needed for inflation varies with the size of the trachea and the tube. Understandably, less air is needed for larger tubes. Usually 2 to 5 ml of air provide a closed system.

Specific tubes have special variations, such as an opening in the wall opposite the bevel to permit ventilation in case of bevel occlusion. Others have a radiopaque tip that allows radiologic visualization of tube position. Many have connectors, some of which are a built-in swivel type permitting lightweight, flexible, easy connection to a ventilating system. These connectors reduce the hazard of accidental disconnection. Still others have a fenestration in the outer cannula permitting air to flow through the larynx. These tubes are used to allow assessment of spontaneous breathing and coughing in preparation for decannulation in patients no longer requiring mechanical ventilation. With air passing through the larynx, the patient can speak with the proximal end of the cannula plugged. A so-called speaking tube permits introduction of humidified air and oxygen through a special line and, with upward flow of the gas through the larynx, the patient can speak.

Tracheotomy Set

A tracheotomy set, with all essential equipment for performing a tracheotomy, should be in the OR during any extensive procedure on the face or neck, thyroidectomy, or radical neck dissection. If a tracheotomy tube is inserted during the surgical procedure, the obturator must accompany the patient at all times. If a tube is not needed, the tracheotomy set accompanies the patient and remains at the bedside for a few days postoperatively, in case a respiratory obstruction caused by edema develops. A set is kept at the bedside of a patient on a respirator. Sterile sets must *always* be available. Tubes are wrapped and sterilized individually. Sterile disposable tracheotomy tubes are commercially available.

Tracheal Resection

Tracheal obstruction can result from trauma or tumor, thus occluding the patient's airway. Localized erosion and scarring, causing narrowing of trachea, can develop from prolonged endotracheal intubation or tracheotomy. An obstructive or stenotic lesion can be resected and the trachea reconstructed by end-to-end anastomosis. Through a cervical, low-collar skin incision, the upper trachea and subglottis are mobilized. A right posterolateral thoracotomy incision is used for lesions in the distal trachea near the carina, where the trachea bifurcates into the right and left bronchi. A longitudinal incision is made in stenotic area, and an anode tube, a flexible wire-reinforced endotracheal tube, is inserted into distal trachea to maintain respiration. The trachea is transected circumferentially above and below the obstructed segment. The laryngeal attachments to the trachea are released. The neck is flexed so edges of the trachea can be approximated without tension. The neck may be kept flexed during postoperative healing by a heavy suture from chin to chest. The patient remains intubated, with end of the tube located beyond the anastomosis for 1 or 2 days.

SURGICAL PROCEDURES OF NECK

Many laryngologists and plastic surgeons, as well as some oral and general surgeons, perform neck dissect when cervical lymph nodes are involved in cancer of the head and neck. A multidisciplinary team, including a thoracic and/or general surgeon, may perform some complex resections and reconstructive procedures.

The patient may be positioned with neck extended, usually over thyroid elevator (see Chapter 21, p. 443). Arms are secured at sides of the body and not on armboards, thus preventing distortion of body contour in the neck region. The table may be tilted into a reverse Trendelenburg's position.

Thyroid Procedures

The *thyroid gland,* located in the anterior aspect of the neck, is composed of two lobes that lie on either side of the trachea and are united by a narrow band, the isthmus. The *thyroid hormone* controls the rate of body metabolism and may influence physical and mental growth.

Hyperthyroidism (Graves' disease), hypothyroidism, and an enlarged gland (goiter) are the main disorders of the thyroid gland. Drugs, radioactive iodine, and/or surgical resection are used to treat hyperthyroidism. This disease, rare in elderly patients or the very young, affects women more frequently than it does men. Replacement of the thyroid hormone with drug therapy is the specific treatment for hypothyroidism. Oral administration of thyroid extract or iodine may reduce glandular size, but surgical excision is frequently necessary to remove benign or malignant tumors.

Thyroid Biopsy

A needle biopsy or an excisional biopsy may be performed to aid in establishing a diagnosis of thyroiditis or differentiating between nodular goiter and carcinoma.

Thyroidectomy

During all thyroidectomy procedures, care is exercised not to damage the laryngeal nerves and parathyroid glands. A transverse collar incision is made in a natural skin crease about 2 cm (1 inch) above the clavicle. The cervical fascia is incised vertically in the midline. Throughout the surgical procedure, meticulous hemostasis is maintained. Blood supply arises from external carotid arteries to upper poles of the thyroid gland and from subclavian arteries to lower poles. The superior laryngeal nerves, which innervate the cricothyroid muscles, and recurrent laryngeal nerves, which innervate the vocal cords, are identified. Trauma to these nerves can result in temporary or permanent laryngeal paralysis. Voice disturbances with hoarseness occur with paralysis of one vocal cord.

Postoperative complications of thyroidectomy include hematoma, edema of the glottis, injury to recurrent laryngeal nerve, muscle rigidity and spasm (tetany), and acute thyrotoxicosis. A tracheotomy set should remain at the patient's bedside postoperatively for at least 24 hours, in the event of respiratory obstruction.

Thyroidectomy is usually performed by a general surgeon. Depending on the pathologic diagnosis, the surgeon chooses the most appropriate procedure for removal of a part of or the entire thyroid gland.

Thyroid Lobectomy An entire lobe is removed, especially for toxic diffuse goiter, which is usually benign. In case of malignant growth, the lobe and lymph nodes in the neck that drain into the involved area may be dissected.

Subtotal Thyroidectomy The usual procedure for hyperthyroidism is removal of approximately five sixths of the thyroid gland. This procedure generally relieves symptoms permanently because the remaining thyroid tissue secretes sufficient hormone for normal function.

Total Thyroidectomy Excision of both lobes plus the isthmus may be the procedure of choice for palpable disease in both lobes.

Substernal Intrathoracic Thyroidectomy Invasion of the gland into substernal and intrathoracic regions can cause tracheal obstruction. The sternum may have to be split to remove a large adherent intrathoracic goiter.

Parathyroid Gland Procedures

The *parathyroid glands* are small endocrine glands that regulate metabolism of calcium and phosphorus. Four or more glands are located within or attached to substance of the thyroid gland, two on each side, or they may migrate into the neck or mediastinum. Primary hyperparathyroidism is associated with hypercalcemia, which may be secondary to renal, skeletal, or gastrointestinal disease. A single or multiple glands may be diseased and surgically excised. The incision and exposure are the same as described for thyroidectomy.

Subtotal Parathyroidectomy

A single diseased gland, confirmed by frozen section, is excised. Up to three and a half glands may be removed if all glands appear to be involved as in diffuse hyperplastic disease. Parathyroid glands are handled by their pedicles to avoid crushing, suturing, or violating the capsule. Inadvertently implanted parathyroid tissue may cause recurrence of disease or persistent or recurrent hypercalcemia. A remnant of normal tissue is left, however, to avoid hypoparathyroidism, which may cause severe tetany. Removed normal tissue may be cryopreserved for autotransplantation in muscle, usually in forearm, if hypoparathyroidism develops or reoperation is necessary for recurrent or persistent hyperparathyroidism.

Total Parathyroidectomy With Autotransplantation

All parathyroid tissue is removed when all glands are abnormal. First described by Halsted in 1907, a portion of a gland is immediately transplanted into a vascularized muscle, usually the sternocleidomastoid, which is in the surgical field. Some surgeons prefer to put the transplant in a forearm muscle. This procedure may be done when embedded parathyroid glands are removed in conjunction with a total thyroidectomy. Postoperative supplemental calcium and vitamin D should be considered for treatment of hypoparathyroidism.

Thyroglossal Duct Cystectomy

During fetal development, the thyroid gland descends through the thyroglossal duct from the foramen cecum near the base of the tongue to the neck below the larynx. In adulthood, remnants of this embryonic duct may form a cyst in the anterior midline of the neck. Excision requires removal of the entire cystic sac and a portion of hyoid bone that surrounds the duct.

Cervical and Scalene Lymph Node Biopsy

Cervical and/or scalene nodes are biopsied for diagnosis of metastatic extension of cancer or tuberculosis into these lymphatic nodes. The procedure may be performed by a thoracic surgeon.

Neck Dissections

Tumors, benign and malignant, occur in the head and neck regions. Although the origin of many of these neoplasms is technically in the head, the cervical lymph nodes frequently are involved secondarily by metastases from a primary head or neck malignant tumor. Treatment is directed toward definitive management for eradication of the tumor and metastases, with consideration for rehabilitation. In an attempt to eradicate all cancer foci, neck dissection may be performed at a time later than removal of a primary lesion of, for example, the parotid gland or tongue, or simultaneously as a one-stage procedure. This composite resection removes primary tumor and metastatic lesions at the same time en masse. Sometimes, however, metastasis occurs before a primary lesion is discovered.

Various reconstructive techniques provide immediate restoration to improve speech, reestablish oral function, or prevent airway obstruction. Others involve delayed reconstruction. The method of repair depends on the type of defect resulting from excision of the lesion. Preoperatively, the patient's emotional stability is analyzed if the surgical procedure will result in cosmetic deformity. Reconstruction is planned so that local tissue can be used whenever feasible and normal function is preserved whenever possible. The aim of reconstruction is to restore function and appearance.

Radical Neck Dissection

Malignant tumors of the oral or pharyngeal cavities, cutaneous malignant melanoma, and skin cancer in the head and neck region often require wide resection of the primary lesion and excision of all the cervical lymph nodes on one or both sides of the neck. This procedure gives the patient with cancer of the cervical lymphatic chain a chance for cure and arrest of spread. When metastasis is known to be present or is highly suspected because of location or stage of the malignancy, the surgical procedure is predicated on the assumption that metastases are regional and not distant.

The head and neck surgeon plans the surgical procedure with reconstruction in mind, so that the incisions will allow good exposure but provide as much local flap tissue as possible for reconstruction. Incisions used for the tumor resection will necessarily vary according to the type of reconstruction planned. Thus no single surgical procedure can be used to treat all lesions. However, certain basic features remain common to all neck dissections.

All lymph-bearing tissue from the midline anteriorly to the trapezius muscle posteriorly and from the mandible superiorly to the clavicle inferiorly is removed. All tissue between the deep cervical fascia and the platysma muscle externally is removed except the carotid artery system; the vagus, phrenic, and hypoglossal nerves; and the brachial plexus.

The massive tissue resection, removal en bloc, includes the jugular vein, eleventh cranial (spinal accessory) nerve, sternocleidomastoid muscle, and submandibular salivary gland. Elimination of the motor nerve to the trapezius muscle contributes to muscular atrophy, subsequent shoulder drop on the affected side, and possibly decreased strength in raising the arm.

Various techniques are used to close the large defect in the anterior neck. When the occipital, posterior auricular, facial, and superior thyroid arteries can be preserved, arterialized skin flaps designed to incorporate branches from these vessels can be constructed with the length up to three or four times the width. Otherwise the length of a flap should not exceed twice the width. A deltopectoral pedicle flap or a pectoralis major myocutaneous free flap may be needed (Figure 36-4). An exposed carotid artery must be covered. Cervical flaps carrying their own blood supply may be used for this and to restore the oropharyngeal lining intraorally. A pedicle flap of sternocleidomastoid muscle from the clavicle may be an alternative.

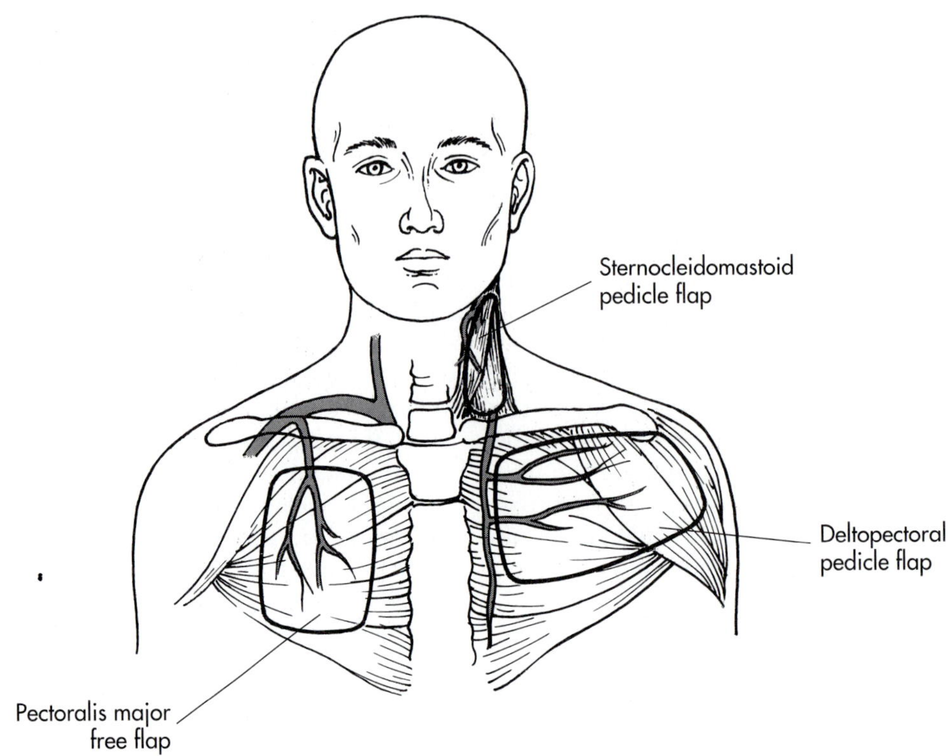

FIGURE 36-4 Myocutaneous flap to close defect following radical neck dissection may be a deltopectoral pedicle flap, a pectoralis major free flap, or a sternocleidomastoid pedicle flap.

The mandible is preserved unless involved by direct extension of tumor into the bone. Access through a mandibular osteotomy or partial mandibulectomy is usually required for effective resection in the posterior oral cavity. Solid bony continuity and realignment of the dental arches are established for functional restoration of speech and chewing. A revascularized free fibular graft, a bone graft from the rib or iliac crest, cancellous bone chips, or a composite graft may be used to stabilize the mandible.

Effective drainage of the wound is important to healing. This is accomplished by application of continuous negative pressure to catheters inserted through stab wounds below the clavicle. Drainage protects the viability of the thin skin flaps and facilitates approximation of wound surfaces.

A prophylactic tracheotomy may be performed to protect the patient from respiratory distress in neck dissection alone. A tracheostomy is always done in a composite radical neck resection.

A feeding esophagostomy tube or cervical pharyngostomy tube is inserted for anticipated extended extraoral feeding. This permits suction to avoid aspiration and gastric distention in addition to providing a feeding route. The tube is usually inserted in the OR.

Potential complications of neck dissection are numerous, depending on the tumor itself, irradiation therapy, or necessary sacrifice of vital structures. Intraoperatively, hemorrhage may occur from injury to a major vessel or the thoracic duct. Postoperatively, invasion of overlying skin necrosis into a major vessel wall, such as the carotid artery, can cause an often fatal blowout of the vessel. Slight previous bleeding may be a forewarning. Balloon occlusion of the carotid artery may be used to prevent hemorrhage.

Although reconstruction begins at the time of primary neck dissection, the patient usually requires considerable postoperative rehabilitation psychologically and staged procedures before cosmetic and functional reconstruction is complete.

SURGICAL PROCEDURES OF ESOPHAGUS

Esophageal disorders may be acquired or congenital (see Chapter 42 for discussion of congenital disorders). Abnormalities result from trauma, inflammation, or neoplasm. They may be studied by a gastroenterologist and/or laryngologist.

Esophagoscopy

Endoscopic direct visualization of the interior of the esophagus is performed to remove foreign bodies; to obtain biopsy, brush cytologic, or secretion specimens for diagnosis; and to examine the esophagus and esophageal orifice of the stomach for organic disease.

Inspection is made for diverticula, varices, strictures, lesions, or hiatal hernia, which may manifest as symptoms of obstruction, regurgitation, or bleeding.

Esophagoscopes are either rigid hollow metal tubes or the flexible fiberoptic type of scope that reduces discomfort and trauma. Accessory instruments, such as aspiration tubes and biopsy forceps, are similar for all endoscopes. Removal of an obstructing mass such as a steak bolus in the esophagus is better accomplished with the rigid metal scope. Various sizes of scopes are available to suit the individual patient's situation.

Patient is positioned with shoulders even with, or a little over, edge of body section of the operating table. The head section is lowered. The patient's head is held by an assistant. The patient is encouraged to relax by breathing deeply if the procedure is done with local topical anesthesia. The head is raised or lowered slowly, at the direction of the endoscopist as the esophagoscope is passed, until the neck is hyperextended. The esophagoscope is passed through the mouth and cricopharyngeal lumen to the cardiac sphincter at the esophagogastric junction. The entire area is carefully scrutinized. The esophagus may be distended by insufflation of air to assist in viewing in presence of stenosis, or a lumen finder may be necessary. The scrub person introduces tips of aspirating tubes, grasping forceps, bougies, and other long accessories into a rigid esophagoscope for the endoscopist.

Removal of Foreign Bodies

Removal of foreign bodies from the pharynx and/or esophagus is relatively common. Persons who wear upper dentures are especially prone to swallowing sharp bones that cannot be felt against the covered palate. Pieces of meat or dental bridgework may lodge or become impacted in the food passage, occluding the airway by pressure. This is an emergency situation necessitating provision of a patent airway by endotracheal intubation or tracheotomy and endoscopic removal of the bolus or foreign object. Acute esophageal obstruction increases salivation, creating the danger of tracheopulmonary aspiration.

Children frequently swallow objects such as coins, buttons, parts of toys, or safety pins that may remain in the throat. Metallic objects are visible on roentgenograms, but many others are not.

It is dangerous to attempt to push an object toward the stomach because esophageal perforation can result. Esophagoscopy is the method of choice for removal, although the procedure is often difficult and painstaking. All effort is made to prevent trauma, with resultant mediastinitis.

Dilatation of Stricture

The esophageal lumen can narrow because of the formation of scar tissue resulting from inflammation or a burn at any level. Treatment consists of regular dilatation with mercury-filled bougies of graduated sizes. Steroid administration is adjunctive therapy.

When an individual suffers a severe burn as from swallowing a caustic material, gastrostomy may be indicated to bypass the esophagus until it heals. Dilatation of such strictures utilizes retrograde fusiform bougies with spindle-shaped shafts that are linked together. They are carried through the gastrostomy, up the esophagus, and out the mouth. The treatment is continued for an extended period.

Dilatation of stricture at the cardioesophageal junction may be necessary in patients with cardiospasm *(achalasia)*. Gross dilatation above the stricture, often the result of muscular atrophy, leads to regurgitation. Diagnosis is made by roentgenography, esophagoscopy, or gastroscopy. If dilatation is unsuccessful, a myotomy at the esophagogastric junction (Heller's procedure) is performed to enlarge the opening into the stomach. Severe unyielding strictures may necessitate resection or esophageal replacement.

Neoplasms of Esophagus

Most often malignant, neoplasms of the esophagus are treated by resection, photodynamic therapy, or irradiation. Dysphagia or obstruction demands immediate investigation. Surgical procedures fall under the classification of gastrointestinal surgery (see Chapter 29, p. 591).

Cervical Esophageal Reconstruction

Restoration of continuity of the alimentary tract is a major challenge following ablative surgery of the neck, particularly after cervical esophagectomy or circumferential pharyngectomy. Location of the primary tumor and its extension and the extent of resection are contributing factors in determining the most satisfactory reconstruction. A pectoralis major myocutaneous flap or a free revascularized intestinal autograft (see Chapter 34, p. 713) will satisfactorily restore continuity in some situations.

Transposition of the mobilized stomach, jejunum, or colon into the neck may be performed when the entire esophagus is resected. Two teams working simultaneously perform this pull-up procedure. The team of general surgeons performs the abdominal dissection to mobilize the stomach or intestine while the other team resects the primary tumor in the neck. The tumor may arise from the hypopharynx, cervical esophagus, or thyroid gland. Radical neck dissection is carried out for extension into the cervical lymph nodes. Anastomosis of the stomach or intestine to an esophageal remnant may be accomplished with a circular intraluminal stapler if the primary esophageal tumor is above the level of the thoracic inlet. Primary pharyngogastric anastomosis may be required for high transsection of the pharynx.

GENERAL CONSIDERATIONS IN HEAD AND NECK SURGERY

1. Eyes should be protected during skin preparation to prevent solution from getting into eyes and to prevent corneal abrasion after patient is draped.
2. Eyelid edema caused by facial trauma may expose the conjunctiva. Lubricate with ophthalmic ointment or artificial tears to minimize corneal damage.
3. Monitoring during extensive procedures includes at least arterial and venous pressure lines, an indwelling Foley catheter for keeping accurate output record, and a rectal temperature probe.
4. Instrumentation may include bone and dental power saws and drills, bone instruments, nasal instruments, oral retractors, and soft tissue instruments.
5. Electrosurgical and cryosurgical units, hemostatic scalpel, argon beam coagulator, laser beam, and the operating microscope may be used. All equipment is checked for proper working order and used correctly.
6. Surgeon often wears headlight to supplement overhead lighting.
7. Wire cutter must accompany patient who has had intermaxillary wiring of the jaws. Nursing personnel in the postanesthesia care unit (PACU) and on the nursing units must know which wires to cut in an emergency.
8. If the patient did not have a tracheotomy in the OR, a sterile tracheotomy tray should accompany any patient who has a potential risk of airway obstruction postoperatively.

BIBLIOGRAPHY

Bronheim H et al: Psychiatric aspects of head and neck surgery, *Gen Hosp Psychiatry* 13(3):165-176, 1991.

Bruno BJ, Gustafson PA: Cranial bone harvest, grafting: a choice for maxillofacial reconstruction, *AORN J* 59(1):242-251, 1994.

Byers RM: Neck dissection: concepts, controversies, and technique, *Semin Surg Oncol* 7(1):9-13, 1991.

Carlile F: Laser removal of warts in the throat, *Surg Technol* 25(8):8-11, 1993.

Colman JJ: Osseous reconstruction of the midface and orbits, *Clin Plast Surg* 21(1):113-124, 1994.

Csendes A, Braghetto I: Surgical management of esophageal strictures, *Hepatogastroenterology* 39(6):502-510, 1992.

Diz Dios P et al: Functional consequences of partial glossectomy, *J Oral Maxillofac Surg* 52(1):12-14, 1994.

Donald PJ: Combined middle fossa/infratemporal fossa surgery, *AORN J* 55(2):480-489, 1992.

Esposito BW et al: Facial trauma, *AORN J* 55(6):1467-1480, 1992.

Hinderer UT: Nasal base, maxillary, and infraorbital implants, *Clin Plast Surg* 18(1):87-105, 1991.

Kennedy M: Type I thyroplasty for voice improvement, *Surg Technol* 26(6):8-11, 1994.

Krasner PR: Avulsed teeth, *AORN J* 53(4):998-1004, 1991.

LaMuraglia MV et al: Tracheal resection and reconstruction: indications, surgical procedure, and postoperative care, *Heart Lung* 20(3):245-252, 1991.

Leung SF et al: Pretreatment neck node biopsy, distant metastasis, and survival in nasopharyngeal carcinoma, *Head Neck Surg* 15(4):296-299, 1993.

Lockhart JS et al: Total laryngectomy and radical neck dissection, *AORN J* 55(2):458-479, 1992.

McHenry A, Piotrowski JJ: Thyroidectomy in patients with marked thyroid enlargement: airway management, morbidity, and outcome, *Am Surg* 60(8):586-591, 1994.

McKennis AT, Waddington C: Thyroplasty type I for unilateral vocal cord paralysis, *AORN J* 60(1):38-42, 1994.

McQuarrie DG: Head and neck cancer, *AORN J* 56(1):79-97, 1992.

Milner SM, Bennett JD: Emergency cricothyrotomy, *J Laryngol Otol* 105(11):883-885, 1991.

Mioduski TE, Guinn NJ: Dental implants, *AORN J* 51(3):729-737, 1990.

Neville WE et al: Tracheal reconstruction, *AORN J* 54(3):470-482, 1991.

Omura K et al: Composite reconstruction of the esophagus, *J Surg Oncol* 52(1):18-20, 1993.

Panje WR, Hetherington HE: Jejunal graft reconstruction of pharyngoesophageal defects without microvascular anastomosis, *Ann Otol Rhinol Laryngol* 103(9):693-698, 1994.

Radkowski D et al: Thyroglossal duct remnants, *Arch Otolaryngol* 117(12):1378-1381, 1991.

Reisser JK: Laryngotracheal reconstruction with rib graft, *Surg Technol* 26(10):8-10, 1994.

Rodau SK et al: Arthroscopic temporomandibular joint surgery: a new approach to temporomandibular joint disorders, *AORN J* 58(5):931-943, 1993.

Rohrich RJ et al: Optimizing the management of orbitozygomatic fractures, *Clin Plast Surg* 19(1):149-165, 1992.

Sargent LA: Craniofacial surgery: advances in surgical technique, *Surg Technol* 23(3):15-17, 1991.

Sloan ES: Face value: trends and advances in craniofacial surgery, *Today's OR Nurse* 12(9):17-22, 1990.

Steuer K: Facial fractures, *AORN J* 54(4):774-792, 1991.

Stieg PE, Mulliken JB: Neurosurgical complications in craniofacial surgery, *Neurosurg Clin North Am* 2(3):703-708, 1991.

Stone CD, Heitmiller RF: Simplified, standardized technique for cervical esophagogastric anastomosis, *Ann Thorac Surg* 58(1):259-261, 1994.

Swarts NK: Vocal cord paralysis, *AORN J* 53(1):62-68, 1991.

Takaku S, Toyoda T: Long-term evaluation of discectomy of the temporomandibular joint, *J Oral Maxillofac Surg* 52(7):722-726, 1994.

Tarabichi M: Transsinus reduction and one-point fixation of malar fractures, *Arch Otolaryngol* 120(6):620-625, 1994.

Tiwari R et al: Total glossectomy with laryngeal preservation, *Arch Otolaryngol* 119(9):945-949, 1993.

Weilitz PB, Dettenmeier PA: Back to basics: test your knowledge of tracheostomy tubes, *Am J Nurs* 94(2):46-50, 1994.

CHAPTER 37

Neurosurgery

Neurosurgeons specialize in surgery associated with dysfunction, disease, or injury of the nervous system. The nervous system includes the brain and spinal cord (*central nervous system*, CNS) and the cranial, spinal, and autonomic peripheral nerves (*peripheral nervous system*, PNS). Neural tissues control motor and sensory functions throughout the body. Generalized cerebral function is manifested in overall behavior, level of consciousness, orientation, and intellectual performance. These functions may be altered by a metabolic disorder, a chromosomal defect, a disease process, or a traumatic injury. Assessment of neurologic deficits or changes in functional activity establishes the indications for neurosurgical intervention. The scope of neurosurgery is broad and includes removal of pathologic lesions; relief of pain, spasm, or other neurophysiologic conditions; and repair of nerve injuries and tissue defects.

HISTORICAL BACKGROUND

The earliest time when surgical procedures were done is not known, but evidence exists in trephined skulls from prehistoric burial sites. It is possible that these trephines were done to let out evil spirits. This may be considered the forerunner of psychosurgery to treat mental illness by frontal lobotomy or topectomy, procedures rarely performed since the advent of tranquilizing drugs.

The Smith Papyrus from Egypt, from the sixteenth century BC, describes the brain and treatment of head and vertebral column injuries. Marinus of Alexandria described in the first century AD seven cranial nerves numbered in pairs. Their functions were further elaborated by Galen. In the seventeenth and eighteenth centuries, Thomas Willis and Samuel Soemmering identified the other five pairs of cranial nerves.

Ancient Greeks and Romans used cranial instruments. Hippocrates described the use of a trephine to treat headache. He also treated skull fractures, epilepsy, and blindness. However, surgery of the nervous system advanced slowly through the centuries. Cranial surgery, for example, was limited until the 1880s to treating trauma or trephining to evacuate pus or blood. The first brain tumor was removed in England in 1884 by Sir Rickman Goodlee. In 1887, William W. Keen of Philadelphia was the first surgeon in the United States to excise a tumor from the brain.

Sir Charles Sherrington (1857-1952) was a pioneer in the study of the physiology of the spinal cord. In 1887 Sir Victor Horsley (1857-1916) removed a spinal cord tumor. Subsequently Horsley attempted surgical procedures on the brain. He was the first to approach the pituitary gland. He may be considered the first neurosurgeon.

The recognized father of modern neurosurgery is Harvey W. Cushing (1869-1939). Among his many accomplishments, Cushing described the relation of intracranial pressure to blood pressure in 1900 and, in 1932, pituitary basophilism, commonly known as *Cushing's disease.* He established at Harvard the first school of neurosurgery, which led to development of a discipline recognized throughout the world.

Application of increasing knowledge of neurophysiology and advances in diagnostic methods, such as those of Walter E. Dandy and A. Egas Moniz, led to the success of intracranial and intraspinal procedures. Stereotaxis led to development of less destructive techniques to replace some extensive invasive procedures and to treatment of some otherwise inoperable lesions. Use of lasers has further enhanced neurosurgery. The operating microscope opened up a new field of microneurosurgery that has created interest in cerebral revascularization techniques previously unattempted and offers advantages in surgical management of many other pathologic lesions. The sophistication of physiologic monitoring techniques has facilitated these therapeutic modalities.

DIAGNOSTIC PROCEDURES

Computed tomography (CT) scanning provides safe and accurate diagnoses of many disorders in the CNS. Several forms of scanning are used. Water-soluble contrast agents are injected into the subarachnoid space to define intracranial and intraspinal cerebrospinal fluid pathways. *Positron emission tomography* (PET) assists with the morphologic study of brain metabolism and cerebral blood flow. *Single photon emission computed tomography* (SPECT) provides a simple study of cerebral biochemistry. Developments in technology of CT scanning have obviated the need in some patients for invasive x-ray studies, such as pneumoencephalogram, ventriculogram, myelogram, and arteriogram.

CT-guided stereotactic biopsy allows the neurosurgeon to obtain diagnosis from lesions that are either inaccessible or too small to be otherwise approached. Stereotaxis orients anatomic relationships on three intersecting geometric coordinates (see p. 774). Information from the CT scan is fed into a computer to calculate the angle of approach and the depth of the lesion. In the operating room (OR), a biopsy probe or endoscope is introduced into the target area through a burr hole in the skull (see p. 770) to obtain a tissue sample.

Magnetic resonance imaging (MRI) provides views of the brain and skull similar to CT scans but without radiation. MRI is also valuable in evaluating acute spine and spinal cord injury.

MRI-guided stereotactic surgery is an adaptation of method described for CT-guided stereotactic biopsy.

Cerebral angiography has been an important diagnostic tool since its introduction in 1927. Newer techniques include digital subtraction angiography for visualizing and evaluating vascular disorders. *Transcranial Doppler ultrasonography* is used to measure the velocity of cerebral blood flow. This noninvasive technique is useful in the diagnosis of intracranial vascular lesions. Ultrasonography also is used to distinguish between cystic and solid brain and spinal tumors. Ultrasonic probes can be placed on exposed dura mater to localize small intracranial tumors.

Evoked potential techniques are used to evaluate somatosensory, visual, and auditory pathways in the brainstem, spinal cord, and peripheral nerves. See Chapter 28 for discussion of all these diagnostic procedures.

SPECIAL CONSIDERATIONS IN NEUROSURGERY

Neurosurgical procedures are classified according to anatomic location in the nervous system: brain and cranial nerves, spinal cord and nerve roots, and autonomic and somatic peripheral nerves. Regardless of location of surgical site, neural tissue is handled gently to minimize functional disability from surgical trauma. Hemostasis is a critical factor to sustain the vital functions of circulation and respiration. Visibility of structures in the surgical site also should be ensured.

Hemostatic Agents

The hemostatic agents commonly used by the neurosurgeon for most procedures include the following.

Scalp Clips

The scalp is highly vascular. Bleeding is controlled by Leroy, Raney, or Michel temporary clips placed over the edges of the wound with a special clip applier as the primary incision is made. The clips are removed during closure of the wound.

Bone Wax

Victor Horsley discovered the value of beeswax to seal bleeders in bone during his animal experiments in 1885. Now supplied as a refined blend of beeswax and a synthetic ester, bone wax is used on cranial and vertebral bones. The wax is rolled into small 4 to 5 mm balls and placed on a smooth surface within reach of the neurosurgeon.

Compressed Absorbent Patties (Cottonoids)

Compressed absorbent patties, made of rayon, cotton, or polyester, rather than gauze sponges are used on fragile, delicate neural tissues to absorb blood and fluids. They also are used for protection of wound edges and for hemostasis. Assorted sizes are moistened with normal saline solution and pressed out flat on a smooth surface easily accessible to the neurosurgeon. Although they have no loose fibers, they could pick up lint if placed on a towel.

The policy for sponge counts should include counting these patties. They are retrieved before the surgical site is closed. Some neurosurgeons use only patties with a thread securely attached to each one. This reminds the surgeon that they are in the wound and facilitates their removal. They should be x-ray detectable.

Chemical Agents

Chemical hemostatic agents may be used following resection to control bleeding from large vessels, sinuses, or the surface of a tumor bed. The scrub person moistens gelatin sponge with normal saline or topical thrombin before handing it to the neurosurgeon. Microfibrillar collagen, supplied in fibers or knitted sheet form, is applied dry. The tips of tissue forceps should be dry to prevent this substance from adhering to them. Oxidized cellulose also is applied dry but is removed after hemostasis has been attained.

Ligating Clips

Clips are applied on larger vessels where electrocoagulation would be insufficient or its thermal effect would be hazardous. Some permanent clips, such as intracranial aneurysm clips, are specifically designed only for neurosurgical use. Each type and size clip requires a specific applier.

Electrosurgery

Monopolar current is used to cut and coagulate tissue and small vessels. Current is conducted through hemostatic forceps, fine smooth-tipped tissue forceps, or metal suction tip to bleeding vessels. A combination suction-fulguration tip also may be used. Bipolar current is frequently used for more precision in coagulation of tiny vessels without damage to surrounding tissue.

Lasers

Argon, carbon dioxide (CO_2), potassium-titanyl-phosphate (KTP), Nd:YAG, and tunable dye lasers are selectively used in neurosurgery in conjunction with the operating microscope, endoscopes, and stereotaxis. Each type has benefits, but all have definite limitations. Depending on the type of laser and the location and type of tumor or vascular lesion, the laser may vaporize, shrink, or coagulate tissue. Precise hemostasis, minimal damage to contiguous structures, and visualization of effects are definite advantages of laser surgery for removal of brain and spinal cord tumors. Lasers are also used to assist in microvascular anastomoses.

Cryosurgery

Some brain tumors may be frozen with a cryoprobe and then removed by dissection, although this is done infrequently. Cryohypophysectomy is the most common cryosurgical procedure (see p. 775). A lesion may be created with a cryoprobe for psychosurgery.

Ultrasonic Aspirator

Although not technically a method of hemostasis, ultrasonic emulsification and aspiration devices fragment and remove tissue with minimal bleeding. The emulsification process assists in hemostasis of small vessels. The technique can be used to debulk or remove benign tumors in relatively inaccessible areas of the brain and intramedullary spinal cord. The high-frequency sound waves of the ultrasonic probe fragment the tumor while sparing adjacent structures, such as nerves and blood vessels. The tumor is emulsified and removed by suction. Various settings on the instrument allow the surgeon to adjust for removal of firm or calcified tumor or soft masses.

Interventional Neuroradiology

With fluoroscopy, a team consisting of a neurosurgeon and a neuroradiologist may insert a percutaneous transfemoral catheter into a strategic point in the intracranial circulation feeding an arteriovenous malformation, an aneurysm, or a vascular occlusion. A substance, such as silicone or isobutyl 2-cyanoacrylate, or a detachable microballoon is injected to effectively embolize the lesion or its major deep-feeding arteries. This facilitates surgical resection of the lesion by minimizing potential hemorrhage. The intravascular procedure may be done preoperatively or intraoperatively.

Adjuncts to Visibility

Neural tissues should be as clean, dry, and visible as possible without damaging them. Visibility is enhanced by the following procedures.

Irrigation

Most wounds are irrigated frequently with normal saline or Ringer's lactate solution. The scrub person should keep a bulb syringe filled ready for use. The solution should be maintained at 105° to 110° F (40.5° to 57° C). A sterile thermometer in the basin of solution helps provide a safety check.

Suction

Suction is necessary to evacuate blood, cerebrospinal fluid, and irrigating fluid from the surgical site so the neurosurgeon can identify structures. Necrotic tissue, pus, or cystic matter may also be aspirated. Usually a Frazier tip is used. Caution is taken to avoid applying vacuum directly on normal neural tissue, especially brain tissue. This tissue is protected by compressed absorbent patties. Suction should be available for all neurosurgical procedures.

Retractors

A variety of self-retaining retractors, such as Leyla or Greenberg, are used to retract scalp or skin and muscles. Dura mater is usually retracted with traction sutures. Blunt malleable flat and spoon-shaped spatulas are used to retract brain tissue. Because visibility of structures is critical, retractors with a fiberoptic lighting system incorporated into them may be used, especially for intracranial procedures.

Headlight

A fiberoptic headlight is used by some neurosurgeons for supplemental lighting in the surgical site.

Endoscope

A side-viewing fiberoptic endoscope may be used to enhance visibility at obscure angles in otherwise visually inaccessible areas. This endoscope is particularly useful to identify lesions in the sella turcica, cerebral aneurysms, and intervertebral disks, for example. An endoscope may be used for placement of electrodes for stimulators or a catheter for radioisotopes. The argon laser can be used through a ventriculoscope for intraventricular obliteration of the choroid plexus and intravascular treatment of lesions and neoplasms. The Nd:YAG laser can be used through a flexible or rigid neuroscope to vaporize a cyst. A straightforward rigid 0-degree scope may be used for electrocoagulation or laser obliteration of tissue and to obtain a CT-assisted stereotactic biopsy.

Neuroguide Intraoperative Viewing System

The neuroguide intraoperative viewing system provides capabilities for viewing structures through a tiny opening in the brain for diagnostic and therapeutic procedures with minimal trauma to tissues.

Operating Microscope

The operating microscope provides an intense light, as well as magnification for visualization of intracranial structures. Microsurgery permits removal of tumors and vascular lesions that are otherwise inaccessible or inoperable. The CO_2 laser may be used through a micromanipulator. The microscope also is used for some spinal procedures and peripheral nerve repair. A fiberoptic camera attached to a microscope projects the surgical site onto a video monitor screen. This provides a clear view for the assistant and scrub person. In lieu of using the microscope, the surgeon may wear binocular loupes to magnify the surgical site.

CRANIAL SURGERY

Anatomy and Physiology

An understanding of basic anatomy and physiology is essential for preparing for the approach the neurosurgeon will use to reach intracranial structures. The brain is approached through the *cranium,* the portion of the skull that encloses the brain. Eight bones form the cranium: the single frontal, sphenoid, and ethmoid bones anteriorly; the paired temporal and parietal bones forming the middle fossa; and the occipital bone posteriorly. Although these bones are fused together to protect and support the brain, the *cranium* is described as being divided into three areas: the anterior, middle, and posterior fossae. *Galea,* tough fascia-like tissue over the cranium, connects muscles of the temples, forehead, and base of the skull. The *scalp* (skin) covers the muscles and extracranial vessels and nerves in subcutaneous tissue.

The *meninges,* fibrous membranes lying between the cranium and brain, are the dura mater, arachnoid, and pia mater. Cranial *dura mater,* firmly attached to the cranium, has two layers that separate in planes to form venous sinuses. The *arachnoid,* which lies next to the dura mater, has threadlike connections with the *pia mater,* which closely adheres to the brain. The *subarachnoid space* is formed between the arachnoid and pia mater. The pia mater follows the convolutions of the surface of the brain. The *cortex* is the superficial outer layer of gray matter of the brain, often referred to as *cerebral cortex* or *cerebellar cortex,* depending on location. The *brain* has three distinct anatomic units that consist of several subdivisions, as shown in Figure 37-1.

Cerebrum

The right and left hemispheres of the cerebrum are connected centrally by the corpus callosum, a broad band of nerve fibers. The cerebrum occupies most of the area within the cranium and is arranged into superficial folds called *gyri* and furrows called *sulci,* which are surgical anatomic landmarks. The outer cerebral cortex is the gray matter (substance) of the brain; the inner tissue is the white matter. The brain in each hemisphere is divided into four lobes.

1. *Frontal lobe* lies within the anterior fossa.
2. *Parietal lobe* lies in the superior and anterior portion of the middle fossa.
3. *Temporal lobe* lies inferior to the frontal and parietal lobes within the middle fossa.
4. *Occipital lobe* lies posteriorly within the middle fossa.

The *hypothalamus* and *thalamus* also lie within the cerebrum. Although it lies in the sella turcica outside the cerebrum, the pituitary body attaches to the hypothalamus.

Cerebellum

Also consisting of two hemispheres, the cerebellum lies below the occipital lobes, posterior to the brainstem, within the posterior fossa. It is about one fifth the size of the cerebrum.

Brainstem

Including the midbrain, pons, and medulla oblongata, the brainstem lies anteriorly within the posterior fossa. It extends from the cerebral hemisphere to the base of the skull, where it merges with the spinal cord. It also contains the nuclei of 10 of the 12 pairs of cranial nerves, all except the olfactory (I) and optic (II) nerves.

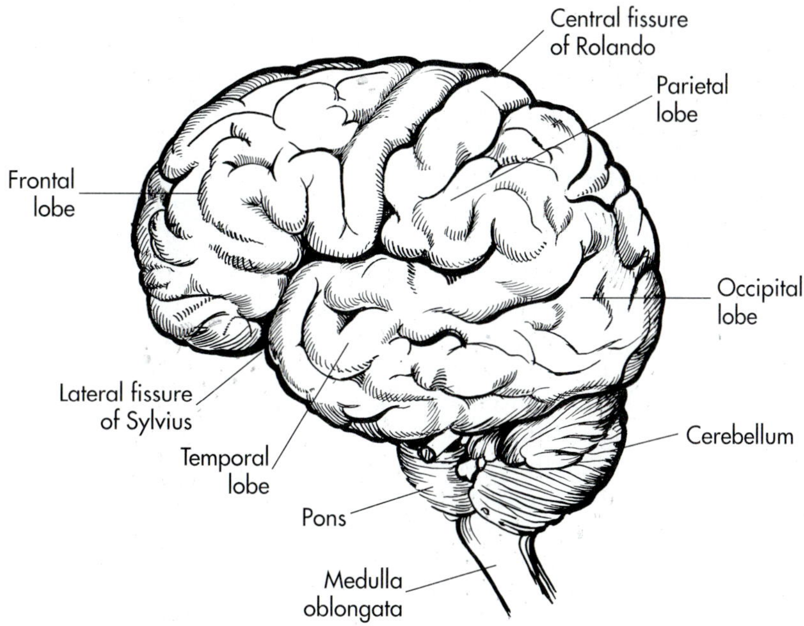

FIGURE 37-1 Left lateral view of cerebral hemisphere.

Ventricles

The lateral ventricles, one lying in each hemisphere, are within the cerebrum. These open into a central cavity, the third ventricle, which is connected by the aqueduct of Sylvius with the fourth ventricle lying anterior to the cerebellum and posterior to the brainstem. *Cerebrospinal fluid* (CSF) produced in choroid plexuses, which are vascular extensions of the pia mater lining the ventricles, circulates through the subarachnoid space around the meninges covering the brain and spinal cord to cushion these structures. The normal adult volume of circulating CSF is 125 to 150 ml. Obstruction to the flow of CSF causes increased intracranial pressure.

General Considerations

The patient's fear of an inability to function independently as a result of intracranial surgery is paramount, either consciously or subconsciously. The brain is the core of one's being. Many neurosurgical patients are not premedicated, which allows neurologic assessment before induction of anesthesia or during a procedure performed under local anesthesia. The circulator should be sensitive to the patient's fears and offer reassurance. Psychologic support is especially significant for an awake patient. Explanation of what to expect is critical.

1. Preparation of the patient in the OR usually begins with clipping hair. Hair usually can be removed from a male patient with electric clippers. A female head is shaved after initial hair removal with clippers. The neurosurgeon or assistant usually removes it. Hair on the head is considered the patient's personal property. When all of it is removed, it is saved unless permission is granted by the patient to destroy it.
2. Location of the intended line of incision and the type of procedure determine the head holder that will be needed to position the patient. The basic unit of a neurosurgical headrest attaches in place of the head piece on the standard operating table. The head holder, either a headrest or a skull clamp, stabilizes and supports the head. The circulator must be familiar with the desired neurosurgical positions and the headrests, skull clamps, and attachments for each.
   a. *For supine position,* the configuration of the headrest contours to the back of the head. The supine position is used most commonly for approaches to the frontal, parietal, and temporal lobes within the anterior and middle fossae. *Lateral position* may be preferred for some of these surgical procedures, such as a unilateral approach to the right or left temporal lobe.
   b. *For prone position,* a padded circular or horseshoe-shaped headrest equalizes weight distribution around the face. Eyes are lubricated and taped closed for protection. The prone position is used to reach the occipital lobe. It may also be used for a suboccipital approach, but most neurosurgeons prefer the sitting position to approach the posterior fossa.

c. *For sitting position,* the headrest is attached at the head end of the operating table to support the back of the head for a unilateral or nasal approach. For a posterior approach, a head holder supports the forehead. The frame of the head holder is attached to siderails of the back section of the table (Figure 37-2) so patient's head can be lowered in the event of an air embolus. The sitting position allows greater torsion and flexion of the neck than either a lateral or prone position and a more accessible approach to the cerebellopontine angle.

d. *For rigid fixation of skull,* a skull clamp provides stability that is necessary for microsurgical procedures and is desirable during lengthy procedures. This eliminates risk of pressure-related complications around the face or eyes in prone or lateral positions and minimizes risk of air embolism in sitting position. Three pins on the clamp partially penetrate the outer table of the skull. Pins on one side may be spring loaded, as on the Mayfield skull clamp (Figure 37-3), to join the skull and the clamp into one rigid mechanical unit. The skull clamp is attached to the operating table with a frame that accommodates the desired position.

3. Infiltration of a local anesthetic agent beneath the scalp is desirable for many intracranial procedures. The scalp, extracranial arteries, and portions of the dura mater are the only structures covering the brain that are sensitive to pain. Epinephrine may be added to the agent to prolong its effectiveness and to constrict superficial blood vessels. The anesthetic may be injected before the patient is prepped and draped.

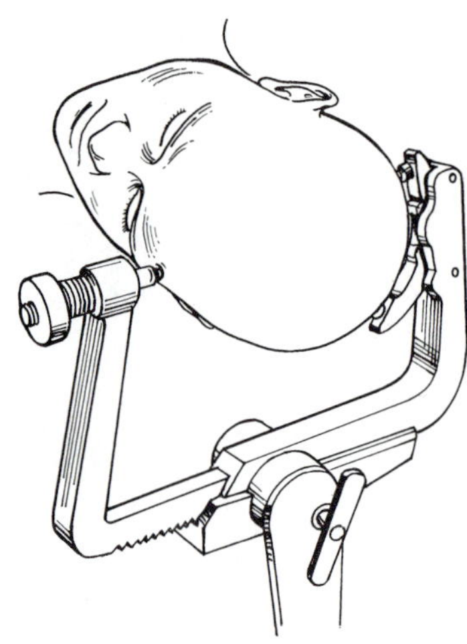

FIGURE 37-3 Mayfield skull clamp stabilizes head for a right frontotemporal craniotomy. Single pin on left and two spring-loaded pins on right penetrate outer table of skull.

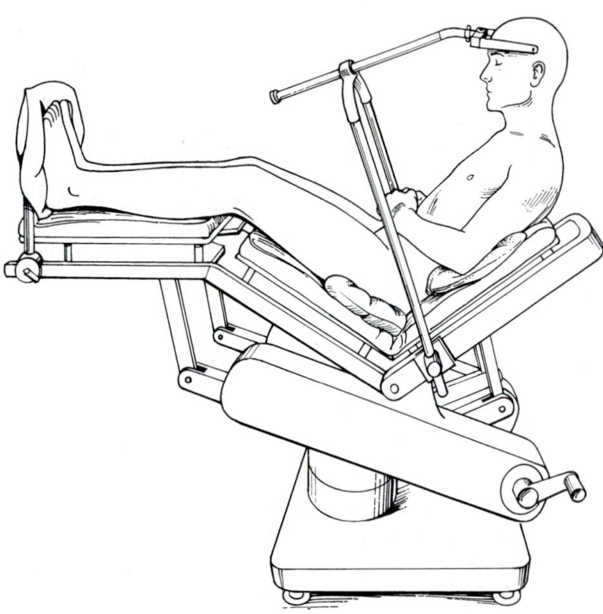

FIGURE 37-2 Neurosurgical sitting position for posterior approach. Frame of head holder is attached to siderails of back section of operating table. Note that legs are flexed at thighs and are approximately at level of heart. Feet are padded at right angles to legs. Subgluteal padding protects sciatic nerves.

4. Administration of general anesthetic agents via endotracheal tube may be preferred for extensive intracranial procedures, although the skull and brain are insensitive to pain. The patient is positioned after he or she is anesthetized and before prepping and draping.
5. Anticipation of difficulty in achieving hemostasis by the methods previously discussed is not unusual for some procedures to remove vascular intracranial lesions. Controlled hypotension may be initiated by the anesthesiologist, with the concurrence of the neurosurgeon, to lower blood pressure (see Chapter 17, pp. 339-340).
6. Prevention of cerebral edema during repair of cranial injuries may be accomplished with hypothermia. Hypothermia may also be used to decrease cerebral blood flow and venous pressure and to decrease brain volume and intracranial pressure. Patients are cooled to a core temperature between 57° and 68° F (14° to 20° C) either by surface-induced hypothermia, bloodstream cooling, or a combination of both. Core body temperature can be monitored via a thermal probe placed in the esophagus, rectum, or contained within the indwelling Foley catheter.

Hypothermia with elective circulatory arrest and extracorporeal cardiopulmonary bypass is an alternative when conventional approaches to control of blood loss would be unsatisfactory. The desired core temperature before beginning extracorporeal cardiopulmonary bypass is 64° F (18° C). The body cooling process may take 1 hour. An 18- to 24-French arterial perfusion cannula is placed in the right femoral artery for oxygenated blood return, and a 28- or 32-French venous return cannula is placed in the left femoral vein for venous drainage. Normally the brain cannot tolerate ischemia for more than a few minutes. This time is extended with lowering of body temperature. The average circulatory arrest time is between 12 and 45 minutes at 64° F (18° C). Hypothermia decreases cellular metabolism and therefore decreases oxygen consumption of the brain and heart during interruption of circulation. Intermittent administration of cold crystalloid cerebroplegia solution also may help protect the brain during cardiopulmonary bypass and profound hypothermia.

Blood viscosity increases as body temperature decreases. Two or three units of the patient's blood may be withdrawn and replaced with chilled normal saline solution. (See hemodilution, Chapter 17, p. 340.) During rewarming, this blood is autotransfused. Crystalloid priming solution from the cardiopulmonary bypass machine also causes hemodilution.

7. Prevention of potential air embolism in patients in Fowler's or sitting position must be considered. The brain is higher than the heart in these positions. Venous pressure may be lower than atmospheric and can allow for entry of air into the heart via an open venous channel. A pneumatic counterpressure device may be used (see Chapter 23, pp. 473-474). An antishock garment extends from the patient's rib margin to the ankles and is inflated if the patient becomes hypotensive. In lieu of an antishock garment, antiembolic stockings or sequential compression stockings are worn. If a Gardner-Wells frame with pin fixation is used, antibiotic ointment is applied around each fixation pin to form an airtight seal. This reduces risk of air embolism and infection.
8. Reduction of intracranial pressure and brain volume may be accomplished by withdrawing spinal fluid. An intrathecal catheter or Tuohy needle is inserted, before prepping and draping, for the anesthesiologist to remove CSF during the surgical procedure as desired by the neurosurgeon.
9. Demarcation of the desired outline for the incision may be made on the scalp after the skin prep and before draping. A sterile disposable skin marker is available.
10. Instrumentation is usually arranged on a Mayfield or Phalen table or on a double Mayo stand setup over the patient in supine or prone position. The scrub person stands on a tiered platform to easily set up and reach the instruments as they are needed. The instrument table surface can be raised or lowered. The drapes over the head are attached to the table drapes (see Chapter 22, p. 462, for procedure). A one-piece sheet that provides a combined sterile table cover and the patient's cranial drape with a self-adhering incise area is available.

    If the patient will be in Fowler's or sitting position, the instrument table is placed above and lateral to drapes over the patient. The drapes form a tent on the side of the anesthesiologist so he or she can have access to the patient throughout the procedure.
11. Prevention of sudden movement around the surgeon and bumping the operating table or microscope is crucial. A slip of the surgeon's hand under the operating microscope or in the cranial cavity could be fatal for the patient.
12. Prevention of peripheral nerve and circulatory damage requires that the circulator check pressure points on the patient's body during prolonged procedures. Some microneurosurgical procedures take 10 hours or longer to complete. An egg-crate or foam mattress or gel pads should be used if the patient is supine or prone on the operating table.

Physiologic Monitoring

Cerebral edema (brain swelling), cerebral arterial perfusion, and intracranial pressure can be safely controlled before, during, and after the surgical procedure. These parameters are continuously monitored, however. An intraarterial catheter is often inserted for continuous direct arterial blood pressure monitoring and for drawing samples for arterial blood gas analyses. A central venous pressure line may be established also. A pulmonary artery catheter may be inserted to measure fluid volume and to diagnose air embolism. Capnography is used routinely. Mass spectrometry is the most sensitive method of monitoring concentrations of inspired and expired gases. This sensitive device detects any type of gas, including nitrogen.

Doppler Ultrasound

A *precordial Doppler ultrasound* transducer is secured over the precordium (i.e., over right side of heart to the right of the sternum between third and sixth intercostal spaces). This is used primarily for continuous monitoring for gas entrapment or air embolism in patient in sitting position. An altered ultrasound response results if air is present in the right atrium. A catheter can be passed transarterially to evacuate air from the right atrium.

A sterile *transcranial Doppler ultrasound* transducer monitors changes in redistribution of cerebral blood flow, as following obliteration of a large intracranial vascular malformation. This technique is also used to monitor cerebral vasospasm. Elevation of transcranial Doppler velocities precedes clinical signs of cerebral ischemia. The transducer can also be placed over the cerebral cortex to verify location and depth of a tumor or cyst.

Evoked Potentials

Somatosensory evoked potentials guide the anesthesiologist in handling arterial blood pressure, ventilation, inspired oxygen concentration, or patient positioning. Changes in cortical evoked potentials can indicate cerebral ischemia and systemic hypoxia. Both cortical and subcortical sensory evoked potentials can record surgical invasion of the spinal cord, peripheral nerve, nerve plexus, brainstem, or midbrain. To avert permanent injury to the patient, the surgeon may adjust retractors, alter approach to a tumor, or perform a subtotal tumor resection on the basis of changes in evoked potentials. The anesthesiologist may adjust the depth of anesthesia.

Auditory brainstem evoked potentials, with stimulus to the ear, may be used to monitor the eighth cranial nerve and brainstem during surgical procedures in the posterior fossa, if performed under local anesthesia.

Visual evoked potentials may be used during the surgical procedure for pituitary tumors, optic nerve decompression, aneurysms, and some other types of lesions. A strobe light flash is used to elicit responses. The light-emitting diodes are placed over closed eyelids and secured before the patient is prepped and draped.

Intracranial Pressure

Intracranial pressure (ICP) rises with an increase in volume of the brain, CSF, and/or cerebral blood supply, or with decompensation, the inability to compensate for pressure changes. In adults, normal ICP ranges from 10 to 20 mm Hg (or 13 to 27 cm H_2O). When an abnormal elevation is sustained, ICP prevents adequate perfusion of the cerebral cortex. The brain is deprived of blood supply. Pressure monitoring is the only exact method to determine a rise in ICP and impending neurologic crisis during cranial procedures or following head injury. ICP monitoring is accomplished by implanting a ventricular catheter, subarachnoid screw, or epidural sensor.

A ventricular catheter is an invasive but the most accurate method of *ICP monitoring*. The cannula and reservoir are inserted into the ventricle through a burr hole or twist drill hole in the skull. Proper positioning of stopcocks is important because incorrect placement may result in excessive CSF drainage with a sudden drop in ICP and possible brain herniation. This method evaluates volume/pressure responses and permits drainage of large amounts of CSF and installation of contrast media and antibiotics. Catheter patency should be checked frequently. Postoperatively the patient is observed for signs of infection, such as meningitis or ventriculitis.

A hollow steel subarachnoid screw is placed in subdural space via a twist drill hole in the skull and a small incision in dura mater. Although this method measures ICP accurately and directly from CSF, it cannot be used to drain large amounts of fluid; it can provide access for CSF sampling. The screw may become occluded with blood or tissue. It should be checked frequently for patency.

A small epidural sensor is implanted in the epidural space of the brain through a small burr hole in the skull. The sensor is attached to a transducer, which converts CSF pressure to electrical impulses. The sensor cable is plugged into a monitor that produces a continuous readout. This is the least invasive method of ICP monitoring, but its accuracy is questionable.

Electroencephalogram

The function or organic activity of the brain may be monitored periodically throughout the surgical procedure by electroencephalogram (see Chapter 19, pp. 377-378). Sterile subdermal needle electrodes may be used if surface scalp electrodes cannot be used.

Craniectomy

Craniectomy is removal *(-ectomy)* of a portion of the bones of the skull *(cranium)*. The bone is perforated or removed to approach the brain. This may be accomplished through one or more burr holes or twist drill holes. Each hole is drilled manually with a Hudson brace and burr or with an electric or air-powered instrument. *Burr holes* are approximately ½ inch (13 mm) in diameter. Some diagnostic and therapeutic procedures are performed through them. Additional bone may be removed with a rongeur to increase exposure of the brain for more extensive procedures, such as an approach to the cranial nerves or tumors in the posterior fossa or suboccipital region.

The bone may be cut between the burr holes with a flexible multifilament wire (Gigli saw) or air-powered craniotome. A dura guard attachment protects the dura mater. A large area of bone is raised for temporary or permanent removal. Attached to the muscle, which acts as a hinge, the bone may be turned back to expose the underlying dura. This is referred to as raising a *bone flap*.

Burr holes may be plugged with a soft, pliable silicone, disk-shaped cover, with or without a channel for introduction of a hypodermic needle. The cover may be used to eliminate a cosmetically undesirable indentation of the scalp into the created bone defect. Postoperative access to the cranial cavity through the hole or channel in the cover can be used for drainage of fluid or instillation of chemotherapeutic drugs. Intracranial pressure monitoring devices can also be attached. Other types of implantable infusion pumps also are inserted through a craniectomy.

Brain Pacemaker

Electrode plates of a brain pacemaker or cerebellar stimulator are implanted through small occipital and suboccipital craniectomies. Silicone-coated polyester fiber mesh plates, each with four pairs of platinum-disk electrodes, are applied to the anterior and posterior surfaces of the cerebellum. One or two receivers, implanted just below the clavicle, are attached to the electrodes on the cerebellum by subcutaneously placed leads. Stimulation of the pacemaker electrodes is controlled by an external transmitter through an antenna placed on the skin over the subdermal receiver. This device is used to control muscular hypertonia and seizures related to cerebral palsy, epilepsy, stroke, or brain injury.

Craniotomy

Scalp, bone, and dural flaps are raised to expose a large area of the cerebrum for exploration, definitive treatment, or excision of lesions within the brain. The three semicircular or U-shaped flaps are turned in opposite directions. Hemostatic forceps or compression clips designed to control bleeding from the scalp are applied to the galea and over the edge of the skin flap. The bone flap is turned as described for craniectomy. Moistened sponges protect both the scalp and bone flaps. The dural flap is protected with large compressed patties. For wound closure, the thin but tough fibrous dural flap is laid over the brain. Usually it is sutured with many interrupted stitches to provide a tight seal that prevents leakage of CSF. The bone flap may be anchored with stainless steel sutures or silicone burr hole buttons. The galea is closed with interrupted sutures before the scalp is sutured or approximated with staples.

A silicone rubber suction drain may be placed in the subdural space to drain residual fluid from a subdural hematoma or the bed of a brain tumor or to remove red blood cells in CSF after craniotomy.

Intracranial tumors can originate from the neural tissues of the brain itself, the meninges, glandular tissue, choroid plexuses, cranial nerves, blood vessels, embryonal defects, or metastatic lesions (Table 37-1). A craniotomy may be performed to remove a circumscribed, encapsulated, slow-growing, benign brain tumor. Some of these tumors, such as a meningioma, are highly vascular. Primary or metastatic malignant tumors are broadly classified as *gliomas*. These have an unregulated cellular proliferation of rapidly growing cells, which invade surrounding brain tissue. *Glioblastoma multiforme*, one of the most common, is the most malignant type of brain tumor. Hemorrhagic and edematous effects of a rapidly growing tumor may be an indication for a lobectomy to give the brain area for expansion and to impede mortality. The rigid characteristics of the skull prevent its expansion or contraction; however, the brain can expand or contract. Subdural decompression by craniectomy to reduce ICP and papilledema may be the palliative procedure of choice. By anatomic location, some benign tumors are considered malignant because they cannot be safely removed without severe neurologic deficits or a threat to life-sustaining functions. Microneurosurgery and stereotaxis (see p. 774) provide access to tumors in some anatomic locations that are otherwise impossible to reach, such as in third ventricle and pineal regions.

Cranioplasty

Traumatic or surgically created skull defects are corrected with autogenous bone grafts or a synthetic or titanium prosthesis. Large defects in the anterior or middle fossae are covered for protection of the brain and for cosmetic effect. The bone flap may be removed following an intracranial procedure to allow cerebral decompression postoperatively. It is stored under sterile conditions in the bone bank until it can be positioned in the skull.

Bone removed because of an extensively comminuted fracture or bone disease may be replaced with methyl methacrylate. This material contours better than preformed titanium plates. The resin powder is mixed with the liquid polymer to form a doughy mass. This is placed in a sterile plastic bag and rolled to the thickness of the skull with a roller. While still pliable, it is molded to the contour of the head and the size of the defect. When hardened, it can be trimmed with a rongeur and the edges smoothed with a special small emery wheel mounted on the electric bone saw. The prosthesis is wired to the skull in several places. The brain expands to meet it and leaves no dead space between it and the dura.

NOTE The outside of the ampules of resin powder and liquid polymer and the mixing bag must be sterile. They can be sterilized in ethylene oxide gas or immersed for 10 hours in glutaraldehyde solution. The roller and emery wheel can be steam sterilized.

Dural defects can be closed with autogenous fascia graft, fibrin film, polyethylene film, synthetic absorbable mesh, or freeze-dried human cadaver dura mater grafts. (See Chapter 24.)

Intracranial Microneurosurgery

The magnification and lighting afforded by the operating microscope have refined intracranial microneurosurgical techniques and made possible approaches to many neurologic problems. (See Chapter 15 for discussion of the operating microscope.) A CO_2 laser may be adapted to the microscope for ablation of benign or malignant intracranial tumors. Some other microneurosurgical procedures include the following.

Excision of Acoustic Neuroma

Middle fossa or translabyrinthine approaches may be used by otologists for removal of small acoustic neuromas confined in the internal auditory canal (see Chapter 35, p. 733). A neurosurgeon resects an acoustic neuroma that more commonly extends into the posterior fossa of the cranial cavity. An acoustic neuroma can grow pro-

TABLE 37-1

Intracranial Neoplasms

CELL OF ORIGIN	SITE	AGE AND GENDER	DEGREE OF MALIGNANCY
Astrocytoma—grades I and II			
Astrocyte	Cerebrum	Young adults Equal between genders	Low malignancy, slow growing, becomes cystic, well-differentiated cell structure; average survival is 6 yr
Astrocytoma—grades III and IV			
Astrocyte	Cerebrum and white matter	Middle age Male > female	Highly malignant, slow growing, poorly differentiated cell structure; 20% of all brain tumors are this type; average survival is 6 yr
Ependyoma			
Cells lining ventricular system of brain; most common in fourth ventricle	Fourth ventricle and distal spinal cord	Children and young adults Equal between genders	Low malignancy, slow growing, variable differentiation of cell structure; may calcify; 10% of all brain tumors are this type; survival is measured in months according to location of tumor
Glioblastoma multiforme			
Glial cells	Cerebral hemispheres and corpus callosum	Middle age Equal between genders	Highly malignant; infiltrative, rapidly growing; highly cellular with many necrotic foci; 50% of all brain tumors are this type; average survival is 1 yr
Medulloblastoma			
Uncertain, primitive bipotential cells	Cerebellum, fourth ventricle, and subarachnoid space	Children Male > female	Moderate malignancy, rapidly growing, moderate differentiation of cell structure; 10% of all brain tumors are this type; average survival is 15 mo
Meningioma			
Arachnoid cell	Parasagittal and lateral convexities, sphenoidal ridge, and thoracic spinal cord	Middle age Female > male	Usually benign; encapsulated and easily separated from nervous tissue
Neurilemoma (schwannoma)			
Schwann cells of cranial nerves and spinal nerve roots	Cranial nerve VIII in cerebellopontine angle and thoracic spinal cord	Middle age Equal between genders	Usually benign; pain and parasthesia are common
Oligodendroglioma			
Oligodendrocyte	Cerebrum, white matter	Middle age Equal between genders	Low malignancy, slow growing, moderate differentiation of cells; 5% of all brain tumors are this type; average survival is 5 yr

gressively into the trigeminal, facial, and abducens nerves and into the cerebellopontine angle (the area between the pons, medulla oblongata, and cerebellum). Potentially life-threatening, symptoms of these involvements are manifested by facial weakness, paresthesia, and dysphagia.

The suboccipital retrolabyrinthine approach is preferred by most neurosurgeons. The patient is placed in semi-Fowler's or sitting position, with pin fixation in the Gardner-Wells frame. This position provides good exposure but has the potential risk of air embolism. The operating microscope offers the potential for preservation of functional hearing. Particular caution must be taken to obtain meticulous hemostasis, to spare the auditory artery if hearing is to be preserved, and to avoid trauma to or resection of the facial nerve. It is impossible, however, to salvage facial nerve function in a percentage of patients. If the facial nerve is sacrificed, the patient may return for a facial-hypoglossal or facial-accessory nerve anastomosis 4 to 6 weeks postoperatively.

A retromastoid, transtemporal approach with the patient in lateral position or a subtemporal, transtentorial approach with the patient supine may be preferred. The surgeon's decision to preserve or sacrifice the facial nerve and/or hearing will influence the approach to an acoustic neuroma. The ultrasonic aspirator and/or CO_2 laser may be used to remove the tumor.

Decompression of Cranial Nerves

Microvascular decompression relieves the severe and disabling symptoms of some cranial nerve disorders such as trigeminal neuralgia (tic douloureux), glossopharyngeal neuralgia, acoustic nerve dysfunction, and hemifacial spasm. Initial symptoms of hyperactivity in a cranial nerve can progress to loss of function. Some disorders are caused by mechanical cross-compression, usually vascular, of the nerve root at the brainstem. Symptoms depend on sensory and/or motor functions of the nerve.

With patient in sitting position, a retromastoid craniectomy is performed to explore the cerebellopontine angle. A supracerebellar exposure is used for the trigeminal nerve and an infracerebellar exposure for the remainder of the cranial nerves. An artery or vein compressing the nerve root may be mobilized away from the nerve. A tiny piece of Silastic sponge may be placed between the vessel and nerve to relieve the pulsating pressure on the nerve. A tissue sling may be created to lift the vessel off the nerve. Preoperatively undiagnosed tumors are excised. If vascular decompression or another pathologic condition is not evident, the nerve may be sectioned to relieve pain.

Cerebral Revascularization

For cerebral revascularization, an extracranial artery is anastomosed to an intracranial artery for bypass of stenotic or occlusive vascular disease distal to bifurcation of the common carotid artery. This provides an additional and significant source of blood to the cerebral circulation. An artery in the scalp, such as the superficial temporal, occipital, or another branch of the external carotid artery, is anastomosed to a branch of the middle cerebral artery or a cortical branch of the cerebral artery. Vessels must be 1 mm in diameter or larger. The procedure is primarily prophylactic to prevent development of a major brain attack (stroke) in patients who have had transient ischemic attacks or minor strokes with temporary disruption of brain function caused by blockage of the cerebrovascular system.

The patient is positioned supine with head turned or laterally with head stabilized flat on the operating table for an approach through a temporal craniectomy. The anastomosis is made on the surface of the brain, either end-to-end, side-to-side, or end-to-side of the arteries.

In some patients, plaque can be removed from the middle cerebral artery rather than bypassing the occlusion. Cerebral embolectomy with a detachable balloon or other intravascular technique may be done to obliterate carotid-cavernous fistula or arteriovenous malformation in conjunction with extracranial-intracranial arterial bypass. Cranial bypass is procedure of choice for cerebral revascularization in a patient who has a vascular lesion that cannot be treated by carotid endarterectomy.

Excision of Arteriovenous Malformation

An arteriovenous malformation (AVM) is an abnormal communication between the arterial and venous systems involving many dilated blood vessels. As the fistulous connections gradually enlarge under pressure, blood is diverted from surrounding brain tissue, causing scarring and compression as a result of poor perfusion. This process is accelerated by multiple small hemorrhages from the thin, engorged vessels. Progressive neurologic deficits can cause seizures and life-threatening subarachnoid, intraventricular, or intraparenchymal hemorrhage.

A large, diffuse AVM involving multiple vessels and high-flow shunts can be difficult to excise. The strategy of the neurosurgeon may be to perform a staged resection with intraoperative embolization initially to reduce the number of fistulous arteries and size of shunts. For embolization, small Silastic beads may be introduced into an AVM via a catheter placed into the internal carotid artery. This procedure usually is done a month before surgical resection.

Using the operating microscope, the surgeon carefully coagulates or clips the arteries as close to the AVM as possible. Normal arteries that perfuse the brain beyond the AVM must be preserved. At least one vein must remain patent to drain the AVM until other vessels are occluded. Then this is occluded and the AVM is removed.

Occlusion of Aneurysms

Aneurysms of the cerebral and vertebral arteries vary from the size of a pea to the size of an orange. Most intracranial aneurysms are located near the basilar surface of the skull and arise from the internal carotid or middle cerebral arteries. Cerebral artery (berry) aneurysms are usually located on the circle of Willis at the base of the brain between the hemispheres of the cerebrum. Most aneurysms are associated with a congenital defect of the media of the intracranial vessel wall. Hemodynamic forces of pulsatile pressure cause enlargement, outpouching, and thinning of the arterial wall, which eventually ruptures. This is the most common source of subarachnoid hemorrhage. Most aneurysms seal spontaneously, but a surgical procedure may be indicated to prevent rebleeding. If diagnosed, an unruptured asymptomatic aneurysm may be occluded before rupture.

With patient in sitting position for suboccipital or subfrontal craniectomy, the aneurysm is exposed for occlusion. The neck (base) is occluded with a low-pressure aneurysm clip or ligated if it can be isolated. If it cannot be isolated, the aneurysm and parent vessel may be wrapped in fine mesh gauze and coated with methyl methacrylate, isobutyl 2-cyanoacrylate, or other epoxy resin to reinforce the wall. More commonly the aneurysm is coagulated with bipolar electrosurgery or laser. Induced hypotension may be used to decrease blood flow in the artery feeding the aneurysm. This aids in dissection and occlusion. The operating microscope is used for delicate dissection of the arteries at the base of the brain.

Stereotaxis

Stereotaxis is the accurate location of a definite circumscribed area within the brain from external points or landmarks on the skull. It defines three-dimensional coordinates (planes) by which to approach deep structures without damaging overlying structures. The technique is used to create or ablate a lesion in otherwise inaccessible parts of the brain. By determination of specific reference points on CT scan or PET scan and MRI, the exact area for target site of the lesion is calculated by computer. The computer, especially designed for stereotactic surgery, provides measurements for correct alignment of instrumentation and calculation of depth of target tissue within the brain.

A *stereoencephalotome,* a specially designed mechanical apparatus, is attached to the skull. After this is in place, computerized data show localizers of the apparatus in relation to intracranial structures. The ventricular system provides the internal landmarks. Of the many models available, three basic types of stereoencephalotomes are used.

1. *Semicircle arc system.* Steel screws are tapped through each of four burr holes for fixation of the head to a ring supported from a table attachment or a pedestal on the floor. The ring is secured to arc plates. The head rather than the apparatus is moved.
2. *Rectilinear system.* The apparatus can be moved back and forth and side to side around the head to make adjustments.
3. *Single arc system.* An arc over the head allows angular adjustments.

Nursing personnel must know how to sterilize and assemble the apparatus and must prepare necessary instrumentation. The patient is in a sitting position for fixation of the stereoencephalotome into burr holes.

The stereoencephalotome can obstruct the surgeon's access for an intracranial procedure. A frameless stereotaxic system enables the neurosurgeon to continually interact with CT scans and MRI displays via a computer linkage throughout an intracranial procedure. Known as an *interactive image-guided stereotactic neurosurgery system,* the system incorporates three-dimensional images from cameras mounted over the operating table, position-sensing probes and forceps, and a computer system.

With a stereoencephalotome in place, stereotactic surgery can be performed through a burr hole, rigid or flexible endoscope, or open craniotomy. A lesion may be made or removed by laser, high-frequency or radiofrequency electrocoagulation, cryosurgery, ultrasound, radiation, hyperthermia, or mechanical curettage. Procedures are performed under local anesthesia when patient cooperation to test motor or sensory function may be needed during the surgical procedure. Various types of intracranial procedures are performed with computer-assisted stereotaxis.

Aspiration

A needle or cannula is placed into target tissue to aspirate a cyst, abscess, or hematoma. Tissue may be obtained for biopsy.

Functional Neurosurgery

For functional neurosurgery, lesions are created in the brain to reduce intractable pain or to control tremors or psychotic behavior.

Electrostimulation Intermittent electrostimulation of the brain by stereotactically implanted electrodes can control a variety of benign intractable pain problems. One electrode is placed in the somatosensory system to evaluate pain of central origin and another in the paraventricular gray matter for pain of peripheral origin. Following postoperative evaluation of the effectiveness of electric stimulation of each electrode, the patient returns to the OR to have a receiver placed under the skin on the anterior chest wall. A connecting wire is tunneled from the receiver to the electrode. An external transmitter and antenna placed over the receiver stimulate the electrode as desired by patient.

Radio-Frequency Retrogasserian Rhizotomy Radio-frequency retrogasserian rhizotomy relieves the pain of trigeminal neuralgia, also known as *tic douloureux*. The fifth cranial nerve, the trigeminal nerve, carries sensory impulses for touch, pain, and external temperature from the face, scalp, and mucous membranes in the head. Trigeminal neuralgia is an intense paroxysmal pain in one side of the face. It can be controlled by damaging the gasserian (trigeminal) ganglion.

An insulated cannula with an uninsulated tip is placed through the cheek and foramen ovale and is advanced to the gasserian ganglion. The ganglion is coagulated when a radiofrequency generator activates the tip of the cannula. Several lesions can be made to achieve the desired extent of paresthesia.

Thalamotomy The forerunner of other stereotactic procedures, thalamotomy destroys a selected portion of thalamus for relief of pain, epileptic seizures, involuntary tremor or rigidity of muscles as in Parkinson's disease, and occasionally for emotional disturbances. Functionally the thalamus, located in midbrain, is the principal relay point in the cerebrum for sensory impulses passing from lower parts of the nervous system to the cerebral cortex.

Cingulotomy Bilateral symmetric radiofrequency electrolytic lesions are placed to disrupt pathways of cingulum. The *cingulum* is a bundle of connecting fibers in the medial aspect of each cerebral hemisphere between frontal and temporal lobes. Cingulotomies are performed for severe chronic pain, addiction, or some intractable psychoses that have not responded to other methods of treatment.

Psychosurgery

Intractable depression, obsessive-compulsive disorders, or chronic anxiety may be treated by cingulotomy as described or by *frontal lobotomy*. Under stereotaxic control, a probe is inserted into the white matter of the frontal lobe of brain to create a lesion by cryosurgery or electrocoagulation. The lesion disrupts neural cortical/subcortical connections in the frontal lobe anterior to the lateral ventricles that control emotions. Some surgeons implant fine electrodes that remain indwelling for weeks to months. These can be used for chronic stimulation of surrounding tissue or to create additional electrocoagulative lesions. Complications include epilepsy, indecisiveness, and altered personality. Studies have shown that memory and intellect are not impaired. Psychosurgery is performed only if other treatments, such as medication or psychotherapy, have failed to provide relief.

Intracranial Vascular Lesions

Some cerebral aneurysms or AVMs can be electrocoagulated, coagulated with argon laser, vaporized with CO_2 laser, or clipped through stereotactic instrumentation. Thrombosis of an aneurysm or embolization of an AVM may be performed for lesions that are otherwise inoperable or before a microneurosurgical procedure to control bleeding.

Intracranial Neoplasms

Computer-assisted stereotaxis helps locate and reach the margin of a deep-seated intracranial tumor either by open craniotomy or through an endoscope. Then a CO_2 or KTP laser beam or other agent can be directed to destroy the tumor while preserving normal cerebral tissue.

Cryohypophysectomy Creation of cryogenic lesions may be the procedure of choice for treating growth-hormone–producing pituitary adenomas with no suprasellar extension. The cryosurgical probe is introduced into the sella turcica through a frontal burr hole. During creation of the lesion, ocular movements and visual acuity are carefully monitored.

Interstitial Radiation Radioactive substances may be stereotactically implanted into malignant brain tumors. Multiple catheters can be placed throughout the target volume. The catheters are afterloaded with radioactive iridium-192 or iodine-125 seeds (see Chapter 45, p. 924). The catheters are inserted percutaneously through twist drill holes. For photoradiation therapy, a hematoporphyrin derivative may be injected preoperatively and activated by argon or tunable dye laser to create a cytotoxic photochemical reaction in tumor cells.

Interstitial Hyperthermia Catheters and remote sensors are implanted into the tumor volume. Sufficient heat is conducted through sensors to raise the temperature within the tumor to a degree that destroys its cells. This is effective against radioresistant hypoxic cells and poorly vascularized and metabolically inactive tumors.

Stereotactic Radiosurgery Intense beams of high-energy gamma radiation or microwave-generated energy photons from a linear accelerator are directed to specific targets within the brain, while sparing normal brain tissue. *Gamma knife stereotactic radiosurgery* does not actually use a knife and is technically not surgery as the name implies. This noninvasive procedure utilizes stereotaxis to identify the location of an intracranial tumor or AVM. A specially designed helmet fits over the patient's head and stereoencephalotome frame. A single high dose of cobalt-generated gamma radiation is directed through holes in the helmet. The beams are collimated and focused on the lesion. The gamma unit is a specific installation for this procedure. The treatment takes 5 to 30 minutes. It does not remove the lesion, but it can stop its growth and reduce its size.

Control of Epilepsy

Epilepsy, caused by erratic electrical rhythms in the brain, manifests in a variety of intermittent disabling behaviors, most commonly convulsive seizures. Epilepsy may result from a congenital anomaly within the brain or can develop following trauma, meningitis, or acute febrile illness. Patients with intractable seizures uncontrolled with medication may be candidates for surgery to remove the focal point of the seizures.

Electroencephalogram (EEG) monitoring, CT scans, PET scans, and MRI help identify the specific location of abnormal brain tissue causing seizures. One of two invasive procedures may be necessary if these tests are inconclusive:

1. *Subdural grid implantation.* Via a frontotemporoparietal craniectomy, a Silastic grid with metal disks attached to stainless steel or platinum electrodes is placed on cortex of the brain. Grid size varies depending on area to be monitored. The grid is anchored to dura mater. The electrodes are tunneled under the skin to an area outside the incision before dura, bone, and skin flaps are closed. Subsequently, seizure activity coming from surface of the brain is monitored for several days by an EEG connected to the electrodes. The grid also maps the brain to locate areas of motor, sensory, visual, speech, and memory control. The patient returns to the OR for removal of the grid. Cortical resection also may be performed at this time.
2. *Stereotaxic depth electrode implantation.* By correlating CT, PET, and/or MRI images with reference points on the stereotactic frame, electrodes are implanted directly into the brain. These are connected to an EEG to determine the focus of seizures within specific areas of the brain. After weeks of monitoring, the patient returns to the OR for removal of the electrodes. The epileptic focus may be destroyed by creating a stereotactic lesion at this time (see stereotactic thalamotomy, p. 775).

Surgical Procedures

After an epileptic focus is identified, a definitive procedure can be performed to stop or reduce seizure activity. The objective, however, is to maintain cerebral capabilities for language, speech, memory, vision, movement, and other sensory and motor neurologic functions.

Cortical Resection Epileptogenic tissue is resected from the cerebral cortex where the epileptic focus is localized. An anterior temporal lobectomy is most commonly performed. Frontal and other extratemporal sites may be resected if the epileptic focus does not interfere with neurologic functions.

Corpus Callosotomy The corpus callosum, a fibrous band of neurons, or anterior commissure connecting the two hemispheres in midline of the brain is severed. This prevents passage of neuronal discharges from a focal seizure between hemispheres, thereby preventing secondary generalized seizures.

Hemispherectomy A hemisphere severely damaged by widespread, persistent, multifocal seizures may be removed. This radical procedure is usually performed only on children with unilateral pathologic foci, including infantile hemiplegia (palsy), hemiparesis (paralysis), and hemianopia (loss of vision). The hemisphere (i.e., half of brain) is resected with preservation of basal ganglia. If an abnormal hemisphere is removed at an early age, the normal half of the brain can take over much of the missing function.

Extracranial Procedures

The cranial procedures previously discussed include access to the surgical site through the skull. A few cranial neurosurgical procedures do not require craniectomy or intracranial incision.

External Occlusion of Carotid Artery

When an internal carotid or middle cerebral artery aneurysm cannot be reached or controlled by other surgical techniques, a carotid clamp can be applied extracranially in the neck. Progressive turns on the clamp over several days cause it to occlude the carotid artery gradually until complete occlusion of blood supply to the aneurysm is accomplished.

Endovascular Procedures

A thin catheter with a very fine guidewire can be advanced into a cerebral vessel to fix a problem within the brain. For example, a thrombotic material may be injected to seal off a cerebral aneurysm. *Cerebral angioplasty* utilizes a tiny balloon catheter to reopen the clogged or narrow lumen of a cerebral blood vessel.

Transsphenoidal Procedures

As a palliative surgical procedure, *hypophysectomy,* the enucleation of the pituitary gland, may be performed for pain relief and endocrine ablation in patients with disseminated metastatic carcinoma of the breast or prostate gland or to relieve intractable pain from other types of disseminated carcinoma. The microsurgical transsphenoidal approach also is used for removal of intrapituitary tumors or other lesions within the region of the sella turcica, a cavity of the sphenoid bone. Visual loss and endocrinopathy are the main symptoms of pituitary tumor. Tumor tissue in the sella turcica is distinguished both by color and texture from the normal firm, yellowish anterior and red-gray posterior lobes of the pituitary.

Patient is placed in semi-Fowler's position with head slightly flexed and tilted so that the patient's body is out of the way when the neurosurgeon sits in front of the face to work in the midsagittal plane. The image intensifier is positioned lateral to patient's head with horizontal beam centered on the sella turcica. A television monitor is placed behind and just above patient's head so surgeon can look at the screen in line with the binocular of the microscope. Televised radiofluoroscopy is used as an aid in placing instruments and resecting tissue. The image intensifier is switched on and off, as needed, to minimize exposure to radiation.

Floor of the sella turcica is exposed through the sphenoid sinus. A horizontal incision is made under upper lip, at junction of gingiva, and carried deep to the maxilla. Soft tissues are elevated; bone and nasal cartilage are resected. The resected nasal cartilage is preserved on the instrument table for possible replacement. A specially designed nasal speculum is inserted in the oral incision to visualize the sphenoid sinus. This is opened wide until floor of sella turcica can be identified. The floor is opened with an air-powered drill. The microscope is brought into position for visualization of pituitary and other structures and lesions inside and around the sella turcica.

Head Injuries

A patient with severe head injury requires *first* a patent airway. A relaxed jaw and tongue should be raised; if necessary, suction through the mouth. An endotracheal tube may be inserted. Ultimately a tracheotomy may be necessary.

Vital signs, blood pressure, dilatation of pupils, and level of consciousness are checked frequently. An intravenous osmotic dehydrating solution, such as mannitol, may be ordered to reduce cerebral edema if there is no evidence of intracranial hemorrhage. After these supportive measures have been carried out, definitive treatments are initiated.

1. Scalp lacerations are thoroughly cleansed, debrided, and sutured. Because scalp is highly vascular, lacerations bleed profusely. Hypovolemic shock is rare but possible.
2. Simple linear or comminuted fractures usually require no treatment. A depressed skull fracture must be elevated when bone is pressed 5 mm or more into any part of the brain.
3. Compound fracture requires debridement. Extent of the surgical procedure depends on the specific extent of injury. Dura may need to be sutured. Some macerated brain tissue may have to be excised.
4. Intracranial hematoma may be present. Depending on location, intracranial hemorrhage may require an immediate emergency surgical procedure.
   a. *Epidural hematoma.* Bleeding caused by rupture or tear of the middle meningeal artery, or its branches, forms a hematoma between the skull and dura. Usually associated with a skull fracture, symptoms of increased ICP caused by rapid compression of the brain may occur immediately or within a few hours. An arterial hemorrhage presents an extreme surgical emergency to evacuate the clot and clip or electrocoagulate the bleeding vessel through a burr hole or small craniectomy.
   b. *Subdural hematoma.* Bleeding between dura mater and arachnoid is usually caused by laceration of veins that cross the subdural space. A large encapsulated collection of blood over one or both cerebral hemispheres produces increased ICP and other neurologic changes. The onset and extent of these changes depend on cause, size, and rapidity of growth of the hematoma. Treatment may necessitate a burr hole. A bone flap may be raised if more extensive exploration is indicated. Subdural hematoma may be:
      (1) Acute. Usually caused by arterial bleeding, symptoms occur rapidly. The vessel must be ligated with clips or electrocoagulated.
      (2) Subacute. Usually caused by venous bleeding, symptoms appear within 24 to 48 hours to 5 days after the injury.
      (3) Chronic. Symptoms do not appear until 6 or more months after the injury.
   c. *Intracerebral hematoma.* Tears in the brain substance at the point of greatest impact most commonly occur in the anterior temporal and frontal lobes. Although usually absorbed, hematoma may require evacuation and debridement of necrotic tissue.

Complications of Cranial Surgery

All cranial procedures present risks of postoperative seizures and neurologic deficits. Paralysis, muscle weakness, gait disturbances, and ataxia may be temporary or permanent. Neurologic damage can follow hemorrhage, occlusion of cerebral circulation, and increased ICP. Any sudden, sustained rise in ICP raises blood pressure to maintain cerebral blood flow and elevates pulmonary vascular pressure. This can lead to acute neurogenic pulmonary edema. This is also a complication of venous air embolism. Both venous and arterial air embolism can result in ventricular dysrhythmias and fibrillation. Infection is always a potential complication.

SPINAL SURGERY

The vertebral column extends from the foramen magnum at the base of the skull to the coccyx. (See description of vertebrae in Chapter 32, p. 677.) The spinal cord passes through a canal in the cervical and thoracic vertebrae to a level of the second or third lumbar vertebra. It terminates in a fibrous band that extends through the lumbar vertebrae and sacrum and attaches to the coccyx. Pairs of spinal nerve roots branch off to each side of the body from 31 segments of the spinal cord as it passes through the vertebrae. They carry sensory and motor impulses between the CNS and the PNS.

Because of proximity of the vertebral column to the spinal cord, both neurosurgeons and orthopaedic surgeons perform surgical procedures in this area. They may work together as a multidisciplinary team. For example, the neurosurgeon may remove a herniated lumbar intervertebral disk and the orthopaedist will do the spinal fusion or stabilization (see Chapter 32, pp. 678-679). Only the most common surgical procedures for spinal lesions performed by the neurosurgeon are described here.

Laminectomy

Removal of the spinous process(es) and lamina from one or more vertebrae is performed to expose an intervertebral or spinal cord lesion. A laminectomy is usually carried out through a vertical midline skin incision with patient in prone or lateral position. However, some neurosurgeons prefer a transverse skin incision with the patient in a modified prone position. The patient may be positioned on a Hastings, Wilson, or Andrews frame to hyperextend the spine, to reduce epidural blood loss by lowering blood pressure in vena cava, and to relieve pressure on the abdomen.

Extent of the incision depends on the number of laminae to be removed. Fascia and muscles are retracted to expose the spinous processes and laminae. These are cut off with a rongeur, as necessary, for exposure of the spinal cord dura, spinal nerve roots, or interlaminar lesion. An intervertebral disk, spinal cord tumor, bone fragments, and extradural or intradural foreign bodies may be removed after the laminectomy is completed.

Diskectomy

Herniated or ruptured intervertebral disks are the most common spinal problems seen by neurosurgeons. Most of these occur in the lower lumbar and lumbosacral regions and are traumatic in origin. Displaced intervertebral disks are rare in the thoracic area but do occur in the cervical spine. During the surgical procedure, a ruptured portion of the annulus fibrosus or herniated nucleus pulposus may be excised. Herniated lumbar nucleus pulposus may be removed by microdiskectomy or percutaneous diskectomy. See description of herniated and ruptured disks and diskectomies in Chapter 32, p. 678.

Excision of Spinal Cord Tumor

Primary tumors of the spinal cord include ependymoma, lipoma, meningioma, and neurofibroma. The posterior segment of the vertebral arch must be removed to expose the dura over the involved section of the spinal cord. The dura is incised and retracted with sutures. The tumor is excised and the dura closed tightly to prevent leakage of CSF. Both intrinsic and extrinsic spinal cord tumors can be removed by laser with decreased tissue trauma. The laser is especially useful in areas difficult to reach by dissection, such as the foramen magnum or anterior spinal cord.

Rhizotomy

Anterior motor roots of spinal nerves can be divided to control the involuntary muscle contractions associated with torticollis and spastic paralysis. Cutting roots of cervical spinal nerves controlling the neck muscles, for example, relieves the muscular imbalance that causes the head to rotate intermittently and tilt significantly in patients with torticollis.

Treatment of Spinal Injuries

Vertebral fractures, with or without dislocation, can cause spinal cord compression that denervates nerve tracts below the injury. Spinal cord injury also may be caused by penetrating or stretching trauma or by damage to blood vessels that supply the cord. Spinal cord injuries are classified as:

1. *Complete.* The patient lacks sensation, proprioception (position sense), and voluntary motor function below level of spinal cord damage. Lesions above the fifth cervical vertebra (C5) will cause partial to complete diaphragmatic paralysis. Injury in the cervical region will result in quadriplegia (i.e., functional impairment from the neck down). Lumbar cord injuries lead to paraplegia (i.e., excluding paralysis of the upper extremities).
2. *Incomplete.* Some sensory, proprioceptive, and motor impulses are present. Loss of function depends on extent and location of injury.

Spinal cord edema or hematoma can cause a cord lesion to ascend and worsen the neurologic deficit. Resultant paralysis may be relieved if the surgical procedure to remove bone fragments or to drain a hematoma compressing the spinal cord is done within a very short time after injury. Results are frequently discouraging. Damage to the cord may be too extensive for return of function or, at best, only an incomplete return. Care must be taken in moving and positioning the patient to avoid further paralysis. The patient should be log rolled (i.e., turned or lifted without flexing the vertebral column).

A lumbar puncture with pressure readings may be done. If a block in the flow of spinal fluid is present, a laminectomy is done to decompress the spinal cord in a patient with complete paralysis or partial paralysis that is becoming progressively worse. A laminectomy may also be done to remove bone fragments. Internal fixation may be combined with decompression for thoracolumbar fractures.

Temperature control and monitoring of fluid and electrolyte balance are essential to the outcome for the patient with spinal cord injury. The patient loses thermoregulatory ability after injury and tends to assume the temperature of the environment. Lack of vascular adaptation affects fluid balance. Pulmonary edema and left ventricular failure can occur. Pulmonary embolus also is a potential complication.

Anterior Cervical and Thoracic Procedures

The anterior cervical spine can be exposed through a transverse skin incision in the neck and dissection through the cleavage plane between the carotid artery and esophagus. The spinous processes and laminae remain intact. A ruptured intervertebral disk and/or a fracture-dislocation with bone fragments compressing the cervical spinal cord or nerve roots can be completely explored. Removal of the posterior margins of the vertebral bodies may be indicated to decompress the nerve root. The operating microscope is a valuable adjunct to anterior cervical intervertebral diskectomy and for an anterior approach to other cervical spinal lesions. A bone graft may be placed between the vertebral bodies for interbody fusion, usually by an orthopaedic surgeon.

An anterior approach is also the procedure of choice for thoracic vertebral disk herniations, spinal cord tumors, or fractures. A thoracic surgeon assists with a transthoracic approach. Fractured bone fragments can be stabilized by anterior spinal fusion or placement of posterior rods by costotransversectomy in the thoracic region.

Cervical Traction

To stabilize the head and neck of a patient with a cervical spine injury, traction is applied by means of a Sayre sling as an emergency measure. A Sayre sling is a canvas or leather halter that buckles around the neck and chin. The patient lies with head at foot of the bed. Traction appliances are attached to the footboard. Countertraction is accomplished by the weight of the patient, who rests in bed in semi-Fowler's position.

If the patient has a cervical fracture and/or dislocation, the Sayre sling may be replaced in the OR by an appliance, such as Gardner-Wells, Vinke, or Crutchfield tongs, for skeletal traction. A sterile table setup with a dissecting set of instruments and a drill is necessary. Through a small incision over lateral parietal bones on each side of the head, holes are drilled in the skull for positioning the mechanical apparatus. Pins of Crutchfield tongs, when tightened, are controlled by a locking and positioning mechanism that forces points medially and upward away from the inner table of the skull. Traction is then transferred from the Sayre sling to the tongs, giving the patient free movement of the jaw. The amount of weight applied to the tongs depends on extent of injury and weight of the patient. Halo traction allows the patient to be ambulatory.

Relief of Intractable Pain

Many patients suffer intractable pain in advanced stages of some illnesses such as cancer, occlusive arterial disease, demyelinating or degenerative diseases, or from some benign lesions. Intractable pain cannot be relieved satisfactorily by drugs without hazard of narcotic addiction or incapacitating sedation. Implantation of a continuous infusion pump for intraspinal administration of low doses of morphine may be the procedure of choice, however, for chronic pain of malignant tumor origin. Other surgical techniques may be indicated to interrupt the sensory fibers carrying pain sensations through the spinal cord to the brain.

Anterior Cervical Cordotomy

Cervical cordotomy is performed by exposing cervical portion of the spinal cord through an anterior incision. A microsurgical technique may be used to sever sensory fibers at base of the brainstem to relieve intractable pain of advanced carcinoma. This procedure provides good relief from severe pain for some patients.

Commissural Myelotomy

Commissural or sagittal midline myelotomy may be preferred to relieve intractable midline or bilateral pain in the lower half of the body. The sensory nerve fibers of the cervical or thoracic spinal cord are exposed and severed. The operating microscope is a valuable aid to the neurosurgeon in identifying the nerve tracts to be cut or resected.

Percutaneous Cervical Cordotomy

To avoid an open surgical procedure, a percutaneous approach to cervical cordotomy may be used to destroy sensory fibers. With local anesthesia, a spinal needle is introduced just below the ear into a cervical interspace. The neurosurgeon avoids the pyramidal tract that carries motor impulses. The position of the needle is checked on x-ray film or image intensifier. An electrode wire, inserted through the needle, is connected to a radiofrequency lesion generator. The fibers are destroyed when the positive charge is activated through the electrode. The patient retains the sense of touch but not pain.

Electrostimulation

Chronic intractable pain of organic origin may be relieved by electrostimulation in some selected patients. Fibers of the peripheral nerves conduct pain impulses to the spinal cord. These pain impulses can be blocked by induced electrostimulation that modifies the impulses transmitted from peripheral nerve receptors through the spinal cord to the brain. Electrodes to transmit an electric current to the spinal cord or peripheral nerve are placed transcutaneously or percutaneously or implanted.

Transcutaneous Electric Nerve Stimulation (TENS) TENS is applied to the surface of the skin over the spinal cord or a peripheral nerve. These devices are used for many types of chronic pain problems.

Percutaneous Stimulation An electrode is inserted under local anesthesia into the spinal canal or subcutaneous tissue adjacent to a peripheral nerve. This procedure is performed in the OR or radiology department with fluoroscopic control and sterile conditions. The patient is prepped and draped as for an invasive procedure. For spinal cord stimulation, two platinum-tipped electrodes are threaded cephalad through needles placed in the epidural space. After the electrodes are connected to a percutaneous transmitter, they are manipulated until the patient feels paresthesia in the desired area. When the electrodes are in the correct position, they are secured to the lumbodorsal fascia by Silastic patches. The distal ends are attached to a lead wire brought through the skin. This connects to an external transmitter for temporary stimulation. When conversion is to be made from temporary to permanent stimulation, the electrodes are attached to a receiver implanted in the lateral chest wall, usually on the left side midway between the axilla and waistline. An antenna, placed on the skin over the implanted receiver, connects to the external transmitter.

Dorsal Column Stimulation The dorsal column stimulator operates on the same principle as the percutaneous stimulator. However, a laminectomy is performed to suture the electrode over the dorsal column of the spinal cord. For permanent peripheral nerve stimulation, the electrode is attached to a major sensory nerve. The receivers for these stimulators are implanted in subcutaneous tissues.

PERIPHERAL NERVE SURGERY

The PNS includes the cranial nerves, spinal nerves, and autonomic nervous system located outside the CNS. *Ganglions,* a group of nerve cell bodies also located outside the CNS, can transmit either *autonomic* (involuntary) or *somatic* (both reflex and voluntary) impulses. *Somatic nerves* supply voluntary muscles, skin, tendons, joints, and other structures controlling the musculoskeletal system. *Afferent nerve fibers* carry sensory impulses from the organs and muscles to the CNS. *Efferent fibers* transmit motor impulses from the CNS back to them. Peripheral nerve procedures are performed on both the autonomic and somatic nervous systems. The neurosurgeon may identify nerves and test function with a nerve stimulator before or after dissection or repair.

Autonomic Nervous System

The autonomic nervous system is an aggregation of ganglions, nerves, and plexuses through which the viscera, heart, blood vessels, smooth muscles, and glands receive motor innervation to function involuntarily. This system is divided into:

1. *Sympathetic nervous system.* This thoracolumbar division arising from the thoracic and first three lumbar segments of the spinal cord includes the ganglionated trunk near the spinal cord, plexuses, and the associated preganglionic and postganglionic nerve fibers. The efferent fibers transmit impulses that stimulate involuntary activity in the heart, blood vessels, smooth muscle of the viscera, and all the glands in the body.
2. *Parasympathetic nervous system.* This craniosacral division includes the preganglionic fibers that leave the CNS with cranial nerves III (oculomotor), VII (facial), IX (glossopharyngeal), and X (vagus) and the first three sacral nerves, outlying ganglions near the viscera, and postganglionic fibers. In general, this system innervates the same structures but has a regulatory function opposite to that of the sympathetic nervous system. These efferent fibers act to restore stability for quieter activity.

Surgical procedures most frequently performed on the autonomic nervous system are discussed, but other surgeons perform some of them.

Sympathectomy

Resection or division of the sympathetic ganglions and nerve fibers of the autonomic nervous system is performed in an attempt to increase peripheral circulation or to decrease the pain of peripheral vascular disease or intractable pain of other organic origin. It may be an emergency procedure to relieve severe vasospasm following arterial embolism or freezing of an extremity. The paravertebral ganglionic chains and/or nerve fibers that innervate the affected area are resected or divided. The procedure may be termed *sympathetic ganglionectomy* or *splanchnicectomy,* but usually the surgical procedure is specified by the location of the ganglions and nerves. (General and vascular surgeons also perform some of the following surgical procedures.)

Upper Cervical Sympathectomy Upper cervical sympathectomy is done to increase the blood supply in the internal carotid arteries. Through an anterior cervical approach in the neck, the superior cervical ganglion is resected. Ptosis of the eyelid may occur postoperatively because this ganglion innervates eyelid retraction.

Cervicothoracic Sympathectomy Cervicothoracic sympathectomy may be performed to treat Raynaud's phenomenon of the upper extremities by relieving the chronic vasoconstrictive process or to relieve angina pectoris or causalgia. Through a transaxillary-transpleural incision, the stellate ganglion of the middle cervical ganglionic chain is hemisected and the lower half resected along with the second through fifth thoracic nerve ganglions. In selected patients, video-assisted thoracoscopy is used to perform sympathectomy to treat Raynaud's phenomenon, thoracic outlet syndrome, reflex sympathetic dystrophy, and hyperhidrosis of the upper limbs.

Thoracic Sympathectomy Thoracic sympathectomy is usually done for the relief of chronic intractable pain of biliary and pancreatic disease. Through a posterior paravertebral incision over the transverse processes of the thoracic vertebrae, the ganglions of the sixth through twelfth thoracic nerves are resected and the splanchnic nerves divided.

Thoracolumbar Sympathectomy Thoracolumbar sympathectomy is performed for the treatment of essential hypertension. Usually done in two stages, bilateral resection is necessary to reduce blood pressure by altering vascular tone and denervating the viscera. With patient in prone or lateral position, a paravertebral incision parallel to the vertebral column extends from the ninth rib downward and then curves anteriorly toward the iliac crest. The lower half of the thoracic and the first through third lumbar chains with the ganglions and splanchnic nerves are resected.

Lumbar Sympathectomy Lumbar sympathectomy may be of some value in the treatment of lower extremity vasospastic disease, such as Raynaud's phenomenon and Buerger's disease, ischemic ulcers as a result of vasospasm of the peripheral vessels, and some types of causalgia. Usually through a flank incision, the lumbar chain and ganglions located in the retroperitoneal space between the vertebral column and the psoas muscle are resected from above the second to below the third ganglions.

Presacral Neurectomy

The hypogastric nerve plexus may be resected for relief of idiopathic intractable dysmenorrhea and pelvic pain.

Vagotomy

Truncal vagotomy is total vagal denervation of all structures below the diaphragm. Selective vagotomy is performed more frequently to denervate a specific branch of the vagal nerve. (See Chapter 29, p. 593.)

Somatic Nervous System

As cranial and spinal nerves extend out from the CNS into plexuses and peripheral nerve branches throughout the body, the *somatic nervous system* provides involuntary control over sensations and both voluntary and involuntary control over muscles. Loss of sensation and muscular control occurs distal to the site of severed or compressed nerve fibers. Sensation and function will be restored only if regeneration of nerve axons takes place distally from an unobstructed axis cylinder proximal to the site of disruption.

Nerve injuries in the lower extremity tend to be the result of a major impact, such as an automobile accident; upper extremity injuries are more often associated with industrial accidents. Nerve injuries usually are associated with multisystem trauma such as fractures and lacerations. An injury may occur at any point along a peripheral nerve as from penetrating trauma that severs the nerve or blunt trauma that produces contusions or traction to the nerve. Lower extremity nerves do not recover as rapidly as upper extremity nerves.

Most peripheral nerve surgery is performed to repair traumatic nerve injury in an extremity. However, dissection is also done to remove tumors or relieve pain. Etiologic factors determine location and length of the skin incision.

Neurorrhaphy

Neurorrhaphy, the suturing of a divided nerve, must provide precise approximation of the nerve ends if function is to be restored. Primary repair may be accomplished by suturing the *epineurium,* the outer sheath. Under magnification of the operating microscope, accurate fascicular alignment and epineural end-to-end suturing of larger nerve bundles are the desired technique to enhance regeneration of function. For a successful result, however, nerves are not repaired under tension. Primary repair soon after injury may be advantageous to align the fascicles.

A tumor, such as a neurofibroma or posttraumatic neuroma, is excised. If the nerve ends can be brought together without tension, they are anastomosed. Silastic membrane may be wrapped around the anastomosis to prevent adhesions with the surrounding tissue.

Neurolysis

Neurolysis, freeing of a nerve from adhesions, relieves pain and restores function. Release of the transverse carpal ligament overriding the median nerve in the wrist affords relief of carpal tunnel syndrome, for example. (See discussion of tunnel syndromes in Chapter 32, pp. 675-676.)

Neurotomy, Neurectomy, and Neurexeresis

Neurotomy is division or dissection of nerve fibers. *Neurectomy* is excision of part of a nerve. *Neurexeresis* is extraction or avulsion of a nerve. These procedures may be performed to relieve localized peripheral pain.

BIBLIOGRAPHY

Bernstein M, Parrent AG: Complications of CT-guided stereotactic biopsy intra-axial brain lesions, *J Neurosurg* 81(2):165-168, 1994.

Blomstedt GC: Craniotomy infections, *Neurosurg Clin North Am* 3(2):375-385, 1992.

De LaPorte C et al: Spinal cord stimulation in failed back sugery, *Pain* 52(1):55-61, 1993.

Diering SL, Bell WO: Functional neurosurgery for psychiatric disorders: a historical perspective, *Stereotactic Functional Neurosurg* 57(4):175-194, 1991.

Donald PJ: Combined middle fossa/intratemporal fossa surgery: the challenge of skull base tumor resection, *AORN J* 55(2):480-489, 1992.

Dzwierzynski WW, Sanger JR: Reflex sympathetic dystrophy, *Hand Clin* 10(1):29-44, 1994.

Hay P et al: Treatment of obsessive-compulsive disorder by psychosurgery, *Acta Psychiatr Scand* 87(3):197-207, 1993.

Hodges K, Root L: Surgical management of intractable seizure disorders, *J Neurosurg Nurs* 23(2):93-100, 1991.

Jenike MA et al: Cingulotomy for refractory obessive-compulsive disorder: a long-term follow up of 33 patients, *Arch Gen Psychiatry* 48(6):548-555, 1991.

Kawakami N et al: Intraoperative ultrasonographic evaluation of the spinal cord in cervical myelopathy, *Spine* 19(1):34-41, 1994.

Koch F et al: Giant cerebral aneurysm repair: incorporating cardiopulmonary bypass and neurosurgery, *AORN J* 54(2):224-241, 1991.

Kubo Y et al: Microsurgical anatomy of the lower cervical spine and cord, *Neurosurgery* 34(5):890-895, 1994.

Laskowski-Jones L: Acute spinal cord injury: how to minimize the damage, *Am J Nurs* 93(12):23-31, 1993.

League D: Interactive, image-guided, stereotactic neurosurgery systems, *AORN J* 61(2):360-370, 1995.

Mangum S, Sunderland PM: A comprehensive guide to the halo brace, *AORN J* 58(3):534-546, 1993.

McEwen DR: Transsphenoidal adenomyectomy, *AORN J* (61)2:321-337, 1995.

Nestos A et al: The gamma knife: neurosurgery without an incision, *AORN J* 51(4):968-981, 1990.

North RB et al: Spinal cord stimulation for chronic, intractable pain: experience over two decades, *Neurosurgery* 32(3):384-394, 1993.

Popovic EA, Kelly PJ: Stereotactic procedures for lesions of the pineal region, *Mayo Clinic Proc* 68(10):965-970, 1993.

Reynolds B: Stereotactic-guided craniotomy for resection of a cerebral AVM, *Surg Technol* 27(2):8-13, 1995.

Robinson KS: Early signs of epidural hematoma, *Am J Nurs* 94(4):37, 1994.

Rose DD et al: Cervical spine injury: perioperative patient care, *AORN J* 57(4):830-850, 1993.

Rutkowski KL: Grid implantation in seizure patients, *AORN J* 52(5):953-975, 1990.

Schott GD: Visceral afferents: their contribution to sympathetic dependent pain, *Brain* 117(4):397-413, 1994.

Schram J et al: Intraoperative SEP monitoring in aneurysm surgery, *Neurolog Res* 16(1):20-22, 1994.

Sekhar LN et al: Surgical resection of cranial base meningiomas, *Neurosurg Clin North Am* 5(2):299-330, 1994.

Sloan PA: Neuropathic cancer-related pain, *J Palliative Care* 7(2):44-46, 1991.

Soloman RA et al: Surgical management of unruptured intracranial aneurysms, *J Neurosurg* 80(3):440-446, 1994.

Tatum SR, Wang A: Hemispherectomy: a radical solution, *Today's OR Nurse* 12(3):9-12, 1990.

Thomas DG, Kitchen ND: Minimally invasive surgery: neurosurgery, *Br Med J* 308(6921):126-128, 1994.

Walker MJ: Selective dorsal rhizotomy: reducing spasticity in patients with cerebral palsy, *AORN J* 54(4):759-772, 1991.

Wilberger J, Chen DA: Management of head injury: the skull and meninges, *Neurosurg Clin North Am* 2(2):341-350, 1991.

Williams EM et al: Neuroendoscopic laser-assisted ventriculostomy of the third ventricle, *AORN J* 61(2):345-359, 1995.

Winston KR: Hair and neurosurgery, *Neurosurgery* 31(2):320-329, 1992.

Yamasaki T et al: Intraoperative use of the doppler ultrasound and endoscopic monitoring in the stereotactic biopsy of malignant brain tumors, *J Neurosurg* 80(3):570-574, 1994.

CHAPTER 38

Thoracic Surgery

Thoracic surgery concerns disorders of the lungs, mediastinum, thoracic esophagus, diaphragm, and chest wall. Surgical intervention is most frequently indicated for neoplasms, traumatic injuries, and disease processes such as tuberculosis. Inclusion of vital organs of respiration and circulation within the thoracic cavity mandates special attention to sustaining an oxygenated blood supply to body tissues, especially the brain, during and after the surgical procedure.

HISTORICAL BACKGROUND

Interest in the thorax and lungs dates back to ancient times. The brutal practice of dissecting live criminals was related by Celsus who noted that when the *diaphragma*, or transverse septum, was cut, the thorax was widely opened and the person died. Vesalius used animals to demonstrate to his students the transparent pleura and motion of the lungs beneath it. As exposure was widened and the pleural cavity entered, the lung was seen to collapse. Experimental animals were revived by tracheotomy with a reed pipe used as a tracheotomy tube. Invention of the stethoscope by René Laënnec in the eighteenth century facilitated the study of thoracic disease.

Learning safe access to the pleural cavity and lungs was a difficult step in the development of thoracic surgery. Thoracentesis with needle and trocar, for open drainage of acute empyema, was performed in the United States in the mid-nineteenth century. Sporadic attempts at thoracic surgery (e.g., pulmonary resection) in the nineteenth century were accompanied by unacceptable mortality.

In 1913 Franz Torek, a pioneer in chest surgery, successfully removed a carcinoma of the esophagus by resecting the ribs. Sucking wounds of the chest, created by shell fragments during World War I, drew new interest in thoracic problems. In 1920 Evarts Graham brought attention to the significance of the relaxation of vital capacity to the size of an opening in the thorax and in 1923 presented a staged procedure: cautery pneumonotomy and partial excision of the lung. The first successful pneumonectomy, using exposure by rib resection, took place in 1931.

Development of thoracic surgery paralleled advances in endoscopy, endotracheal anesthesia, mechanical ventilation, closed chest-drainage systems, and respiratory care techniques.

CHEST AND THORACIC CAVITY

An essential balance must be maintained between atmospheric pressure outside the chest and internal pressures within the thoracic cavity to sustain the vital function of respiration. Knowledge of the anatomy and physiology of the chest and thoracic cavity is necessary for an understanding of thoracic surgery.

Chest (Thorax)

The thorax, or chest, is the part of the trunk between the neck and abdomen. It holds the chief organs of respiration and circulation—the lungs and heart—and the great vessels. These vital organs function under the protection of a bony framework consisting of the sternum, 12 pairs of ribs, and 12 thoracic vertebrae, all encased within soft tissue. The framework is bounded superiorly by structures of the lower part of the neck and inferiorly by the diaphragm. Eleven external and internal intercostal muscles, which lie between the ribs, have a corresponding artery, vein, and nerve, which require meticulous dissection to avoid inadvertent injury.

The ribs articulate posteriorly with the thoracic vertebrae. The first seven ribs articulate anteriorly in the midline with the *sternum* composed of three parts: manubrium, gladiolus, and xiphoid process. The eighth, ninth, and tenth ribs are joined anteriorly to the cartilage of the rib above each; the eleventh and twelfth ribs have no anterior fixation. The esophagus, trachea, and great vessels leading to and from the neck and arms pass through the small space between the manubrium and vertebrae. Any structure pushing into this narrow opening (e.g., a mediastinal tumor) may obstruct breathing, venous return from the neck and arms, and swallowing.

Thoracic Cavity

The thoracic cavity is divided into right and left compartments by the *mediastinum,* the space and vertical loose connective tissue wall between the two pleural cavities. The mediastinum has superior, anterior, middle, and posterior sections, each containing structures: the thymus lies within the anterior and superior sections, the thoracic aorta within the posterior, the heart and great vessels in the middle, and the esophagus and trachea in the superior section. Organs are surrounded and suspended by the loose tissue diffused throughout the mediastinum. Division of the pleural cavities is flexible, and alterations in pressure affecting one cavity are felt in the other.

Lungs

The lungs lie in the right and left pleural cavities (Figure 38-1). The main function of these porous, spongy, conical organs is oxygenation of the blood with inspired air and expiration of carbon dioxide. The apex of each extends to the neck; the base rests on the diaphragm. The lungs are enveloped by serous membrane, the visceral or pulmonary *pleura.* Parietal pleura lines the internal surface of the thoracic cavity.

The trachea divides at the *carina* into two main branches, the *bronchi,* leading to the right and left lungs. The right lung, with three lobes, is larger than the left lung, which has only two lobes. The left lung is narrower and shares the space in the left chest with the heart.

The *bronchopulmonary segments* within each lung are wedges of tissue separated by veins and thin connective membrane. Although configuration of the segments differs and variations in the bronchi and blood vessels exist between the right and left lungs, it is generally accepted that both lungs normally have 10 bronchopulmonary segments. (Some nomenclatures refer only to eight or nine segments in the left lung.) Although not demarcated by surface fissures as are the lobes, these segments represent zones of distribution of the secondary bronchi and may be excised individually when the segment contains a small lesion, thus preserving the uninvolved portion. Each segmental bronchus subdivides into numerous increasingly

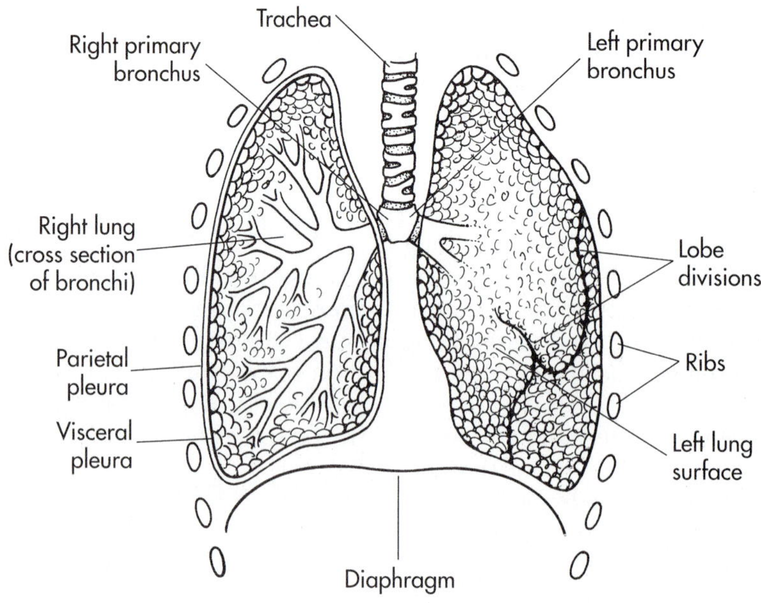

FIGURE 38-1 Respiratory system within thoracic cavity.

smaller branches that eventually end in terminal *bronchioles.* These fine tubules invested by smooth muscles can constrict to close off the air passage, as in asthma. The terminal bronchioles give rise to respiratory bronchioles from which arise the *alveoli.* The approximately 300,000,000 alveoli are the functional units wherein oxygenation takes place at the capillary level.

The *hilus* of the lung, on the mediastinal surface, is the point of entry for the primary bronchus, nerves, and vessels. The right primary bronchus is a more direct continuation of the trachea. The pulmonary veins and arteries to and from the heart provide pulmonary circulation. Organs of respiration are innervated by the autonomic nervous system.

Physiology

The size of the thorax varies with the bellows action of the thoracic wall and diaphragm, increasing with inspiration and decreasing with expiration. A partial vacuum between parietal and visceral pleurae expands the lungs. A negative (subatmospheric) pressure normally within the thorax is essential to life. Alterations of intrapleural pressure are of major concern because an uncontrolled opening in the thoracic wall and pressure change can be fatal. Uncontrolled increased positive pressure in one side causes a collapse of the lung on the other side. Referred to as *mediastinal shift,* this reaction attends entrance of either air or fluid into the pleural cavity, compressing the opposite lung and causing dyspnea. When the mediastinum has moved its limit, it can no longer accommodate a great pressure change; the lung on the affected side collapses. Air in the pleural space between parietal and visceral pleura constitutes *pneumothorax.* Blood in pleural space is *hemothorax.*

A mediastinal shift disturbs heart action and circulation. Changes in pressure balance within the thorax reduce *vital capacity,* the greatest amount of air that can be exchanged in one breath. Many diseases and conditions alter vital capacity, for example, anesthesia, thoracic tumors, or chest trauma.

ENDOSCOPY

Elective surgery depends on accurate diagnosis by radiologic and physiologic pulmonary function studies and by biochemical, cytologic, and histologic determinations and evaluations. Frequently endoscopic procedures are performed to obtain secretions and tissue biopsies. Some lesions can be treated endoscopically.

Bronchoscopy

Disorders of the bronchus are most commonly infection, presence of foreign body, trauma, or neoplasms. Diagnosis is made by radiologic study and endoscopy. *Bronchography,* a radiologic study of the tracheobronchial tree, is frequently done in conjunction with bronchoscopy. *Bronchoscopy,* direct visualization of the tracheobronchial tree through a bronchoscope, is done for:

1. Diagnosis: securing an uncontaminated secretion for culture, taking a biopsy, or finding the cause of cough or hemoptysis
2. Treatment: removing a foreign body, excising a small tumor, applying medication, aspirating the bronchi, or providing an airway during performance of a tracheotomy

Foreign bodies in the trachea and bronchi are very serious, requiring careful history and immediate bronchoscopy with preparation for potential tracheotomy. Maintaining a safe airway during extraction is a major risk. If the airway is not seriously obstructed, the aspirated foreign body may remain in the bronchus for months without producing symptoms until suppuration develops. Coughing and hemoptysis bring the patient to the physician.

Bronchoscopes are of two types: a rigid hollow metal tube or a flexible fiberoptic type. The rigid bronchoscope commonly uses a fiberoptic light carrier to allow visualization of trachea and primary bronchi. It is the scope of choice for foreign body retrieval. It has a side channel incorporated into the length of the instrument and perforations along the sides of the tube to allow oxygenation of bronchi and administration of anesthetic gases if used. Aspirating tubes, foreign body or biopsy forceps, and carbon dioxide (CO_2) laser beams are manipulated through the rigid bronchoscope. Both rigid and flexible fiberoptic bronchoscopes are used for diagnostic and therapeutic procedures. Flexible bronchoscopy is used frequently for the patient with decreased range of neck motion. Tiny forceps can be inserted through the working channel of the flexible fiberoptic bronchoscope to obtain a tissue biopsy. Because the diameter is smaller, the flexible fiberoptic scope reaches into bronchi of upper, middle, and lower lobes for examination and/or biopsy. Diagnostic needle aspiration, forceps biopsy, and bronchial brushings and washings are performed in accessible areas. Mediastinal lymph nodes can be aspirated through flexible bronchoscope. Various types and lengths of aspirating tubes, forceps, and brushes are used to remove tissue and secretions. The Nd:YAG or argon laser can be used with either a rigid or a flexible bronchoscope.

If the gag reflex can be controlled, bronchoscopy can be performed under local anesthesia and intravenous sedation. General anesthesia may be necessary. The bronchoscope is inserted over tongue and through vocal cords to the trachea. Patient's head is turned to right to visualize left bronchi with a rigid scope and to left for right bronchi. Bronchi may be examined to ascertain patency of the tracheobronchial tree or to locate source of an obstruction or bleeding. The person who assists the bronchoscopist introduces tips of instruments into scope.

All persons involved with bronchoscopy should wear gowns, gloves, masks, and eye protection to protect themselves from bronchial secretions and blood.

Some pulmonary lesions are treated by laser. The CO_2 laser is used for stenosis, granulation tissue, or other obstructive lesions that are not highly vascular. Video-assisted flexible fiberoptic laser bronchoscopy is more commonly performed using the Nd:YAG laser. This laser is preferred for vascular lesions, such as neoplasms, to produce hemostasis as it cuts. The argon laser is used for photodynamic therapy to shrink or destroy bronchial tumors (see Chapter 45, pp. 921-922). Everyone in the room, including the patient, is required to wear appropriate eye protection of the correct optical density for the type of laser in use. All other precautions for the use of a laser also are observed (see Chapter 15, pp. 276-278).

Airway obstruction can be relieved by insertion of silicone rubber stents. These may be either a T-tube or T-Y bifurcation prosthesis.

Ideally a sterile bronchoscope should be used for each patient; however, when mucous membranes are intact, the bronchoscope is considered a semicritical item and may be high-level disinfected. Thorough cleaning of the bronchoscope and instrumentation is necessary immediately following the procedure. Terminal sterilization is recommended before storage.

Mediastinoscopy

Mediastinoscopy may immediately follow bronchoscopy. To prevent needless thoracotomy it is performed for assessment of resectability in patients with suspected bronchogenic carcinoma and for diagnosis of mediastinal lesions. Mediastinoscopy uncovers mediastinal lymph nodes for direct visualization and biopsy. Subaortic nodes draining the left lobe of the lung may be out of reach for biopsy with this technique. With the scope, the mediastinoscopist can see down to the carina and about 4 cm distal to it along each bronchus. If more than one biopsy is obtained, each specimen should be placed in a separate container and identified by location. The procedure gives a high percentage of accurate diagnoses and information in staging the extent of a lesion and determining operability for curative resection. Sometimes a frozen section is done while the patient is in the operating room (OR), and resection is performed immediately following a report from the pathologist.

General endotracheal anesthesia is used. Patient is supine with neck hyperextended and head turned slightly to the right. A small transverse incision is made in or about 2 cm above the suprasternal notch between borders of the sternocleidomastoid muscle. Dissection is carried down to pretracheal fascia. After blunt dissection the sterile mediastinoscope is passed behind the suprasternal notch and advanced behind the aortic arch into superior mediastinum to level of the carina. Care is exercised because of proximity to the great vessels. Bleeding is controlled by coagulation with an insulated electrosurgical suction tip. Although mediastinoscopy usually is performed without complication, major bleeding may require immediate thoracotomy. A chest x-ray film frequently is obtained after mediastinoscopy.

Thoracoscopy

Thoracoscopy provides visualization of the pleural space, parietal and visceral pleura, mediastinum, pericardium, and thoracic wall. Evaluating pleural effusion (i.e., the accumulation of fluid, pus, or blood in the pleural space) and obtaining biopsies of pleural or lung tumors are the most common indications for thoracoscopy. Definitive treatment of spontaneous pneumothorax, as in patients with cystic fibrosis, with a sclerosing agent such as antibiotic powder or talc poudrage may be performed under thoracoscopic guidance. A laser may be used to vaporize thickened tissues.

General anesthesia with endotracheal anesthesia is necessary. Patient is positioned in a partial or full lateral position, depending on insertion site the surgeon selects. A small skin incision 2 to 4 cm (1 to 2 inches) is made over and carried through the intercostal space. The surgeon incises parietal pleura to enter the pleural cavity. It may be necessary to resect a portion of rib for access to the pleural space. After anesthesiologist deflates the lung, the sterile thoracoscope is inserted into the pleural cavity. When the scope is removed, a chest tube is inserted and connected to a sterile closed water-seal drainage system (see p. 788) to remove residual air and fluid.

SPECIAL FEATURES OF THORACIC SURGERY

Entry into the thoracic cavity can be accompanied by pulmonary distress. Team members especially skilled in meeting emergency situations are essential. Patients require close observation and monitoring because changes may occur rapidly. A pulmonary artery catheter (Swan-Ganz, see Chapter 19, pp. 373-374) is inserted to monitor pulmonary capillary wedge pressures and arterial blood gases. Equipment for bronchoscopy, esophagoscopy, and mediastinoscopy must be readily available. Other preparations are routinely completed for entry into the chest for intrathoracic procedures.

1. Endotracheal anesthesia permits the lungs to expand and function even when subjected to atmospheric pressure. Administration of anesthesia under controlled positive pressure prevents physiologic imbalance and lung collapse in the presence of controlled pneumothorax. Use of a double-lumen endotracheal tube permits expansion of unaffected lung and collapse of lung on the surgical side. At

conclusion of the surgical procedure, the affected lung is reexpanded by the anesthesiologist and negative pressure in chest is restored. Portable chest x-ray films may be taken immediately to assess status of the surgical area, pleural cavities, and lung reexpansion.

2. Instrumentation includes a basic laparotomy setup with the addition of thoracic instruments. These include bone instruments and power saw (Figure 38-2 shows rib strippers/raspatories, shears, and approximator/contractor), large self-retaining chest retractor/rib spreader (Figure 38-3), bronchus clamps and lung forceps (Figure 38-4), and long instruments for work in a deep incision.
3. Large variety of sutures may be used for soft tissues, vessels, and bone. The bronchus usually is closed with staples.
4. Sponges for hemostasis or blunt dissection are placed on long ring-handled forceps. Periosteal bleeding may be controlled by electrocoagulation. Bone wax may be needed to control bone marrow oozing.
5. Blood for transfusion should be available at all times. Hemorrhage is a major threat intraoperatively and postoperatively. Blood may be salvaged for autotransfusion (see Chapter 23, p. 486).
6. Surgical field is potentially contaminated by secretions and contact with open air passages when a bronchus is opened and sutured. Used items and instruments are isolated in a discard basin. Maintenance of a dry field is important to prevent aspiration of blood and fluid, which predisposes the patient to postoperative pneumonia.
7. Airtight pleural cavity must be restored and negative pressure maintained for maximum pulmonary func-

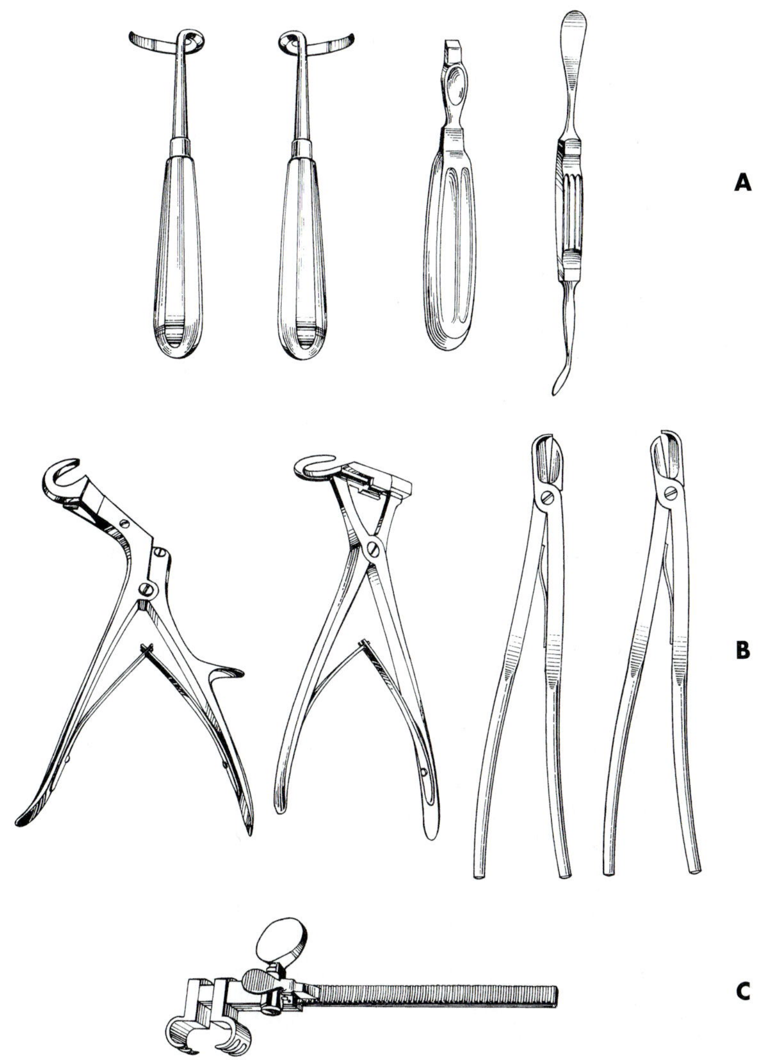

FIGURE 38-2 Rib instruments. **A,** Strippers/raspatories. **B,** Shears. **C,** Approximator/contractor.

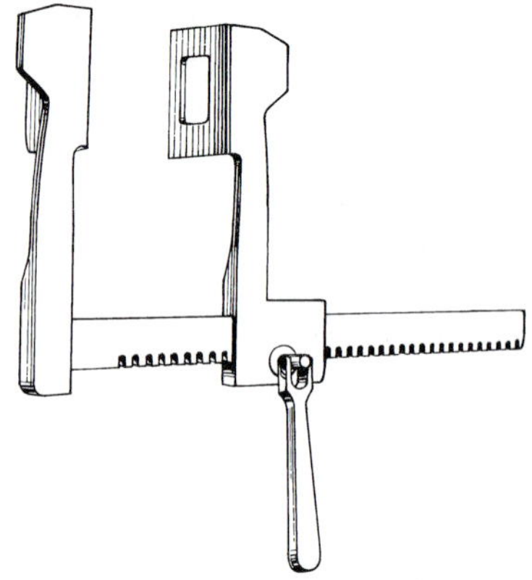

FIGURE 38-3 Self-retaining chest retractor/rib spreader.

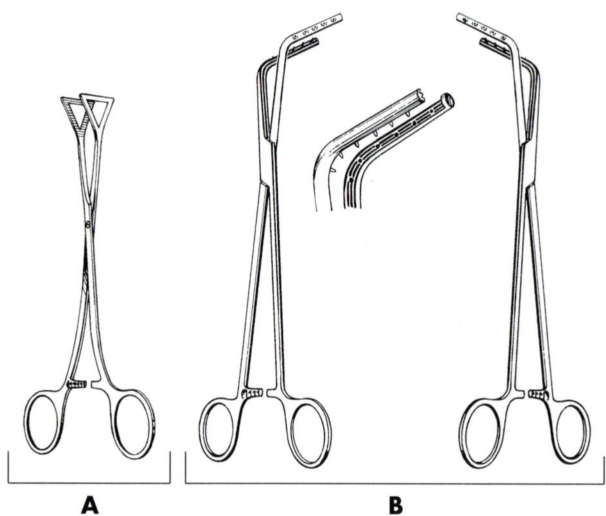

FIGURE 38-4 Thoracic tissue forceps. **A,** Bronchus clamps. **B,** Lung forceps.

tion postoperatively. Except after a few specific procedures, a sterile closed water-seal drainage system is essential. (Review discussion of chest drainage in Chapter 25, p. 529.) Chest tubes are inserted through a stab wound and anchored to the chest wall with suture and tape. Two or three tubes are sometimes inserted into the pleural space and connected to separate drainage systems. The tube at base of the pleural space is usually inserted at the seventh costal interspace, near anterior axillary line, to evacuate fluid. An upper tube, if indicated, is inserted at apex through the anterior chest wall at the third costal interspace to evacuate air leaking from the lung. Key points to remember include:

a. Connections must be physically tight and securely taped at the time of dressing application. The connections should not be obscured from observation of drainage, however.
b. System components must be kept below the level of the patient's body to prevent reentry of air or fluid from the drainage collection system into the pleural cavity.
c. Tubes may be clamped before insertion and connection to the drainage system depending on the surgeon's preference. Tubes are not routinely clamped at other times unless specifically directed by the surgeon.

THORACIC INCISIONS AND CLOSURES

Factors Influencing Choice of Incision

The following factors determine the surgeon's choice of incision:

1. Adequate exposure into the thoracic cavity
2. Physiologic intrapleural pressure changes and constant movement of the chest
3. Maintenance of integrity of the chest wall and diaphragm

Because of continuity with neck and abdominal structures, the thoracic cavity may be entered for neck and upper abdominal procedures as well as for thoracic procedures.

Access to Thorax

Surgeon preference and the procedure determine the method of entrance into the thorax. Access may be gained by anterior, lateral, or posterior approaches or a combination of these. Entrance through the rib cage may be intercostal between the ribs, through the periosteal bed of an unresected rib, or by rib resection. By incising near the top of a rib, the surgeon protects nerves and vessels that lie in the intercostal spaces. An intercostal approach may be used to drain an empyema pocket or mediastinal abscess or to biopsy lymph nodes or a lung. To enter via the periosteal bed, periosteum of rib is incised and removed from the unresected rib, and an incision is made through the bed. For entrance via a rib resection, periosteum is incised and removed superiorly and inferiorly with a periosteal elevator, and the rib is divided. Rib spreaders increase exposure, but if it is still inadequate, the rib above or below the incision also may be resected.

Commonly Used Thoracic Incisions

Posterolateral Thoracotomy

With patient in lateral chest position, a posterolateral incision permits maximum exposure to lung, esophagus, diaphragm, and descending aorta for exploration of the thoracic cavity. Beginning anteriorly in the submammary fold, about at nipple level, a curved incision is made, extending below the scapular tip, following course of underlying ribs. Then curving upward and posteriorly, it may be carried as high as the spine of the scapula. Subcutaneous tissue is incised; latissimus dorsi, lower margin of trapezius, rhomboideus, and serratus muscles are divided; and bleeders are ligated. In dividing the serratus muscle, special precaution is taken to avoid the neurovascular bundle on the surface.

In closure, ribs are reapproximated with a rib approximator/contractor and sutures, intercostal muscles are sutured, and incision in the periosteal bed and pleura is closed. Muscles are reapproximated anatomically and sutured; subcutaneous tissue and skin are closed.

Posterolateral thoracotomy is used for pulmonary resections, for repair of a hiatal hernia, and for procedures on the thoracic esophagus or posterior mediastinum.

Anterolateral Thoracotomy

For anterolateral incision patient is supine. Supports are placed under affected side to tilt the shoulder 20 to 45 degrees for extension of the incision posteriorly. A pad behind the buttocks may rotate the hips slightly. A submammary incision, immediately below the breast but above the costal margin, extends from anterior midline to midaxillary or posterior axillary line. To avoid the axillary apex and a painful scar, the posterior end of the incision is curved downward. Superiorly, access is desired at about the fourth interspace. Further anterior exposure can be gained if desired by transecting the sternum and continuing incision to the contralateral interspace. Pectoralis muscles are divided, serratus anterior fibers separated, intercostal muscles divided, and the thorax entered through an intercostal space. When an anterior incision extends to the sternal border, internal mammary arteries and veins are ligated and divided. If the incision is carried far laterally or posteriorly, injury to the long thoracic nerve must be avoided to prevent a "winged" scapula.

In closure, sternum is reapproximated with heavy suture, ribs are approximated with pericostal sutures, and muscles, subcutaneous tissue, and skin are closed.

Anterolateral thoracotomy is used for resection of pulmonary cyst or a local lesion or for open lung biopsy.

Thoracoabdominal Incision

With patient in lateral position, the thoracoabdominal incision extends from posterior axillary line to abdominal midline, paralleling the selected interspace (usually the seventh or eighth). Following insertion of a rib spreader, incision in intercostal muscles and pleura may be extended posteriorly from within for added exposure. The diaphragm may be divided peripherally. This incision exposes upper abdomen, retroperitoneal area, and lower aspect of the chest (Figure 38-5).

In closure, diaphragm is closed with interrupted sutures. Costal margin is secured by approximating the margins of divided costal cartilages with suture. Tissue layers are closed in reverse order of incision.

Thoracoabdominal incision is used for repair of hiatal hernia, and esophagectomy, and in general surgery for retroperitoneal tumor and cardioesophageal lesions.

Median Sternotomy

Patient is supine for a median sternotomy. A vertical incision extends through the midline from suprasternal notch to below the xiphoid process, which is removed. A power saw is used to split the sternum. In closure, heavy-gauge stainless steel sutures are used to close the sternum.

Median sternotomy incision is used for simultaneous bilateral pulmonary surgical procedures; for mediastinal neoplasms or trauma; for pulmonary embolectomy and cardiac and aortic procedures; and for access to lower cervical and upper thoracic vertebrae. This incision may be preferred for resection of peripheral neoplasms in patients with impaired pulmonary function, particularly in upper and middle lobes of the lungs.

Other Less Common Incisions

Alternative incisions may be used, such as:

1. *Transaxillary* approach, for lung biopsy or wedge resection, particularly in lower lobe; for thoracic sympathectomy or exposure of second to fifth tho-

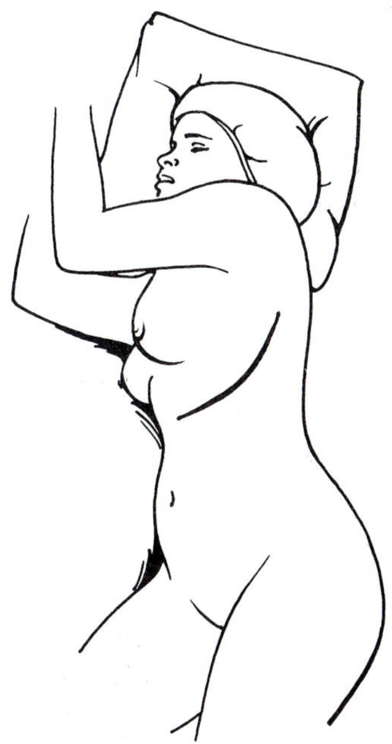

FIGURE 38-5 Left thoracoabdominal incision with patient in lateral position.

racic ganglia; or for exposure for thoracic outlet syndrome. This vertical incision causes minimal injury to muscles of the chest wall and preserves muscles of the shoulder.

2. *Supraclavicular,* scalene approach, for phrenic nerve section, cervicothoracic sympathectomy, axillary vein thrombosis, or thoracic outlet syndrome. The incision is parallel to the clavicle. The first rib may be resected.
3. *Cervical mediastinotomy,* for drainage high in the mediastinum, such as following esophageal perforation.
4. *Anterior* approach, for upper dorsal sympathectomy, exposing upper thoracic ganglia.

THORACIC SURGICAL PROCEDURES

Pulmonary resection often is the procedure of choice for malignant tumors and benign diseases such as bullous emphysema and tuberculosis. Bronchopleural fistula and pulmonary fibrosis are also among concerns of the thoracic surgeon.

Mediastinotomy

Anterior mediastinotomy may be indicated when x-ray studies show hilar or mediastinal nodal involvement inaccessible to mediastinoscopy. With patient supine under general anesthesia, an incision is made over the right or left third costal cartilage. The cartilage bed is incised. Extrapleural dissection is carried toward hilus of the lung, and a biopsy is taken. If desired nodes are deep, a mediastinoscope may be inserted through the incision to obtain the biopsy. Alternatively, the pleural space may be entered for a lung biopsy. If this space is entered, closed water-seal chest drainage is required. If it is not entered, the incision is closed in layers without drainage. Mediastinotomy allows assessment of extent of a lesion or a deformity.

Excision of Lesions

A median sternotomy (i.e., a vertical sternal splitting procedure) may be necessary to resect a cyst or a benign or malignant tumor in the upper anterior mediastinum. Through a posterolateral thoracotomy incision, a tumor may be resected or an abscess drained in the posterior mediastinum.

Correction of Pectus Excavatum

Congenital deformities of the chest wall are usually corrected in childhood. See discussion of pectus excavatum, a depression deformity of chest wall in Chapter 42, p. 866. *Pectus carinatum* (pigeon chest) is forward projection of sternum resembling the keel of a boat. *Pectus excavatum* (funnel chest), which is more common, is caused by elongation of costal cartilages, which pushes sternum back toward the spine.

Surgical correction of pectus excavatum, sometimes delayed until adolescence or adulthood, is performed to relieve respiratory distress or pressure on the heart from mechanical compression, or for cosmetic improvement. Various techniques may be employed. Usually, with the patient supine and upper chest slightly hyperextended, costal cartilages are exposed by muscle splitting and/or division through an anterior midline or horizontal inframammary incision. Involved costal cartilages and deformed rib ends are freed from sternal attachments and resected or straightened. The sternum is mobilized and restored to normal position, and its corrected position is maintained by fixation. An alternative method corrects the contour deformity with a silicone prosthesis introduced through an inframammary incision. Dacron patches on the posterior surface stabilize the prosthesis.

Thoracotomy

Incision through the thoracic wall (i.e., thoracotomy) is indicated for drainage of pleural spaces, exploration of the thoracic cavity, or cardiac and pulmonary procedures. Thoracic surgical procedures, exclusive of cardiac procedures, include the following.

Closed Thoracostomy

Closed thoracostomy is performed to establish continuous drainage of fluid from the chest (usually purulent from sepsis) or to aid in restoring negative pressure in the thoracic cavity. It involves insertion of a tube through an intercostal space via a trocar and cannula.

Open Thoracotomy

Open thoracotomy may be employed for spontaneous pneumothorax, for large air leaks that prevent reexpansion of the lung, or for persistent leaks and incomplete lung reexpansion. This type of pneumothorax usually occurs from rupture of a bleb on the lung surface. By posterolateral incision through the fourth interspace, an apical bleb may be ligated or the involved segmental area of the lung resected. Abrasion or cauterization of the parietal pleura effects adhesion to the visceral pleura, thereby eliminating future rupture of blebs. Open chest drainage also is used to eliminate an empyemic cavity, which accompanies chronic disease and lung adherence to the chest wall. With this procedure, portions of one or two ribs are removed to aid in the establishment of drainage.

Exploratory Thoracotomy

Exploratory thoracotomy is usually performed to confirm diagnosis and extent of involvement of bronchogenic carcinoma or other chest disease, such as a mediastinal lesion, when the pathologic process cannot be confirmed by endoscopy. A biopsy is taken, most often from lower margin of upper lobe for disseminated lung disease. This may be done under local anesthesia through an anterior thoracotomy. Mediastinal lymph nodes usually are biopsied also. Through a posterolateral incision, lungs and hemithorax are exposed after ribs are spread and pleura is opened. Interstitial bleeding or chest trauma are other indications for exploration.

Lung Resection

All or part of a diseased or traumatized lung may be resected. Generally, the indications are neoplasms; emphysematous blebs; and fungal infection, localized residual lung abscess, tuberculosis and/or bronchiectasis resistant to nonsurgical treatment. Neoplasms are the predominant indication. An anterior intercostal incision with division of costal cartilages above and below the incision may be used for excision of pulmonary nodules or lung biopsy. Posterolateral incision is commonly employed for lobectomy and pneumonectomy. Endotracheal anesthesia is used. Special precautions in pulmonary resection include meticulous hemostasis and closure of the bronchus, as well as continual attention to cardiopulmonary function preoperatively, intraoperatively, and postoperatively. Particular hazards are hemorrhage, which is difficult to control because of the size and friability of major pulmonary vessels and proximity to the heart; cardiopulmonary insufficiency; and risk of injury to other intrathoracic structures such as the vagus, phrenic, and left recurrent nerves and the esophagus. Specific resections include the following.

Segmental Resection Removal of individual bronchovascular segments of a lobe is preferred when wide excision is not necessary, as for a pathologic process confined to a segment or for acute hemorrhage. Arteries, veins, and bronchus to the involved segment are ligated and divided. The segment is separated from surrounding lung tissue and removed. The proximal bronchial stump is closed with sutures or staples.

Wedge Resection Wedge resection is a conservative procedure performed when a lesion is thought to be benign. Along with an adequate margin of normal lung tissue, the diseased peripheral portion of a lobe is removed and the lung tissue is sutured. A stapler may expedite removal and closure. A frozen section is done. If a benign diagnosis is confirmed, the wound is closed in layers, and a chest tube for closed water-seal drainage is inserted. If the lesion proves to be malignant, lobectomy or other appropriate procedure may be done. The advantage of wedge resection is its simplicity with minimal blood loss and procedural time.

Lobectomy One or more lobes of a lung are excised when disease or neoplasm is confined to the lobe. The remaining portion of the lung expands to fill the space formerly occupied by the removed lobe. Through a posterolateral incision, entrance to the chest may be intercostal or by rib resection. The pulmonary pleura is incised and freed from the hilus of the lobe. Arteries and veins to the pulmonary tissue being resected are ligated and divided. The bronchus of the lobe is identified by lung inflation while the bronchus to be resected is clamped. Suction of blood and secretions from the open bronchus may precede closure of the bronchus by sutures or staples. A suture line in the bronchus is covered with a flap of parietal pleura to prevent leakage. Dissection is completed, the specimen is removed, and the chest is closed.

Bronchoplastic Reconstruction Extensive partial pulmonary resection may be followed by bronchoplastic reconstruction to ensure maximum preservation of residual pulmonary tissue. These techniques require successful bronchial anastomoses to retain a patent airway to the bronchioles.

Pneumonectomy Major indications for excision of an entire lung are malignant neoplasms or extensive unilateral pulmonary disease. The chest wall is opened by posterolateral incision, pleura incised, lung exposed, and pleural cavity examined. Following immobilization of the lung, hilus is dissected free on all sides. The pulmonary artery and veins are ligated and divided. The bronchus is clamped, divided, and closed with sutures or staples. Bronchus is checked for air leaks by instillation of normal saline solution, and the bronchial stump is covered with surrounding pleura. After wound closure, intrathoracic pressure is measured and residual air aspirated from the hemithorax until desired pressure is reached. Use of chest drainage is governed by surgeon preference, but usually no chest tube is inserted.

Sacrifice of one lung places entire respiratory and circulatory function on the remaining lung. Potential complications are respiratory insufficiency, cardiac dysrhythmia, and a predisposition for infection because of dead space. The empty hemithorax gradually fills with fluid and eventually consolidates, thus preventing mediastinal shift. Dehiscence of the bronchial closure may produce bronchopleural fistula.

Thoracoplasty

Thoracoplasty is usually done extrapleurally. The chest wall is mobilized to obliterate the pleural cavity or reduce thoracic space by resection of one or more ribs. Indications are inadequate expansion of lung to fill pleural space after resection, persistent shift of mediastinum to the empty space after pneumonectomy, or chronic empyema. Tissue fibroses, contracts, and eventually obliterates the space. Thoracoplasty is reserved for patients in whom excessive space in the chest cannot be eliminated satisfactorily by other means to maintain mediastinum in the midline.

Pulmonary Decortication

In patients with empyema, a fibrinous thickening or peel on the visceral pleura may restrict pulmonary ventilation. Pulmonary decortication, a pleural procedure, removes restrictive layer or membrane over the lung to reexpand the entrapped lung and fill space remaining after drainage of an empyemic cavity. Minimum damage to the rib cage by thoracotomy incision is desired to permit motion of the chest wall that is as normal as possible. An intercostal incision is usually preferred, but in some patients resection of a rib may facilitate access to the intrapleural space. Adequate postoperative drainage via chest tube(s) is essential.

Transplantation

Transplantation of either a single lung or both lungs may be an option for the patient with end-stage pulmonary fibrosis, obstructive lung disease, or cystic fibrosis. In a patient with a single-lung transplant for pulmonary fibrosis, omentum may be wrapped around the anastomosis of the bronchus. This helps seal off the area and promotes vascular growth at the site of anastomosis. Lung allografts and combined heart-lung transplants are discussed in Chapter 44, pp. 910-911.

Repair of Hiatal Hernia

Repair of herniation of the stomach through the diaphragm may be performed by a general surgeon (see Chapter 29, p. 602) or by a thoracic surgeon using thoracic routines, such as chest tube insertion with closed water-seal drainage. The thoracic approach is preferred when:

1. Exposure from an abdominal approach would be difficult, as with an obese patient
2. Hernia is incarcerated into the thoracic cavity and would be difficult to reduce through diaphragm into the abdomen
3. Hernia is recurrent and direct visualization will facilitate the procedure
4. Herniation is caused by blunt trauma or a penetrating abdominothoracic wound

Thymectomy

The thymus gland lies on the pericardium in the anterior mediastinum from its origin in the cervical region around the trachea. The lobes are separated from the arch of the aorta and great vessels by a layer of fascia. Thymectomy is usually performed through a median sternotomy, but the gland may be excised through a transcervical incision. The pericardium, innominate vein, a portion of the superior vena cava, and a portion of the lung are removed en bloc to resect a thymoma. The phrenic nerve is spared to prevent diaphragmatic paralysis. Thymectomy without en bloc resection may be done to relieve symptoms of myasthenia gravis.

Thoracic Outlet Syndrome

The thoracic outlet is area bordered by the manubrium anteriorly, first rib anterolaterally, and first thoracic vertebra posteriorly. The major blood vessels and nerves of the head and upper extremities pass through this space. Following a neck injury, changes can occur in the anterior and/or middle scalene muscles, causing pressure on these nerves and vessels. Symptoms include pain and parasthesia of the upper extremities extending into the finger tips. When conservative treatment fails to relieve pain, scalenectomy or scalenotomy is performed. A supraclavicular incision with resection of the first rib or a transaxillary incision is used. In extreme circumstances bilateral resection of the first rib may be necessary.

CHEST TRAUMA

Trauma to the chest varies in severity and may result in injury to the thoracic wall or intrathoracic organs such as the heart and lungs. If severe, the patient is plunged into critical condition. Rapid initial evaluation of the extent of injury is necessary to preserve life, with priority needs met first. These include resuscitation with relief of airway obstruction, treatment of shock and blood loss, and restoration of normal cardiorespiratory dynamics to the extent possible. Impairment of these dynamics may be caused by various factors such as disturbance of lung expansion or cardiac tamponade.

Trauma is categorized as *blunt* or *penetrating*. Blunt trauma usually results from a fall, blow, severe cough, blast, or deceleration injury. The patient may have little overt evidence of chest injury, even though he or she may be bleeding internally from pulmonary contusion. Penetrating wounds are usually caused by a low- or high-velocity missile, such as a knife stab or bullet. Surgical exploration may be required to control bleeding and/or air leak. Open thoracotomy may be performed in the emergency department and the patient brought to the OR with the chest open for further exploration of the wound and for closure.

Blunt Trauma

Fractured Ribs

Rib fracture is the most common injury to the chest wall, the fourth to the eighth ribs being the ones mainly involved. Pain may be relieved by intercostal nerve block. Surgical treatment is usually not required unless sharp edges or displaced bone fragments puncture the pleura or lung. Extensive pneumothorax requires immediate reexpansion of the lungs.

Multiple rib or sternal fractures often produce an unstable chest wall, resulting in *flail chest.* Normal respiration changes to paradoxic motion of the chest wall. The chest wall collapses on inspiration and expands on expiration. This results in ineffective respiration and coughing. As the chest wall expands, the free-floating sternum is sucked inward, thus impairing ventilation and producing hypoxia. The following measures are used to stabilize the chest wall.

1. *Internal stabilization* is achieved by controlled mechanical ventilation. An endotracheal tube or tracheotomy tube may be necessary to decrease pulmonary resistance and increase perfusion. Frequent suctioning maintains a clear airway; thus paradoxic motion and dead air space decrease.
2. *Surgical stabilization* is achieved by inserting pins or wiring fractures together. Fracture of the sternum, scapulae, and clavicles also may be involved in the injury.

Ruptured Organs

Blunt trauma can cause rupture of the diaphragm, aorta, or thoracic tracheobronchial tree necessitating emergency thoracotomy. Contusions of the lung and pericardium may cause hemorrhage.

Penetrating Wounds

Anatomic visualization of the path of the projectile or instrument producing injury is important. A knife, for example, should not be removed except under direction of a physician because it may be penetrating the heart or a major vessel.

An open chest wound must be converted to a closed chest wound. Air rushes into an open wound, building up atmospheric positive pressure inside the pleural space. Pneumothorax followed by mediastinal shift ensues.

Thoracentesis

Air or blood in the pleural cavity may be detected and aspirated by needle and syringe. A chest tube may be inserted into the pleural space percutaneously for closed thoracostomy drainage. If bleeding persists, the chest is opened and vessels are ligated or repaired.

Closure of Sucking Wound

Pneumothorax is relieved and further air prevented from entering the chest during respiration by suturing the wound and inserting chest tube(s).

LUNG-ASSIST DEVICE

A lung-assist device such as intravascular oxygenator (IVOX) may be used temporarily to assist the patient with acute respiratory failure or adult respiratory distress syndrome. The IVOX allows the patient's damaged lungs to heal. The device is inserted into the common femoral vein and advanced into the vena cava. It has hundreds of thin-walled, hollow fibers made of polypropylene coated with gas-permeable membranes. The gas conduit that exits from the skin has two tubes: one delivers oxygen, and one removes carbon dioxide. The oxygen inlet tube is connected to a pump to produce a flow of oxygen through the lumina of the fibers into venous blood. Carbon dioxide transfers through the outflow membrane, controlled by a vacuum pump. The device can be used for up to 7 days. It can provide up to 50% of the patient's gas exchange requirements.

INTRATHORACIC ESOPHAGEAL PROCEDURES

Esophageal disorders may be congenital or they may be acquired by trauma or disease, as discussed in Chapters 29, 36, and 42. Thoracic surgeons may perform esophageal resections for a benign tumor, such as a leiomyoma, or for relief of obstruction in the thoracic esophagus, such as a stricture, stenosis, or achalasia. Esophageal myotomy with or without fundoplication may relieve obstruction in lower segment. Resections are performed for malignant tumors. Early detection of esophageal carcinoma increases the rate of cure by surgical resection. Unfortunately, symptoms are not usually apparent in the early stages, so that carcinoma of the esophagus generally presents a poor prognosis. Most surgical procedures provide palliation rather than cure. Radical en bloc mediastinectomy may become the procedure of choice, but esophagectomy is more commonly performed.

Esophagectomy

For esophagectomy patient is in lateral position. A posterolateral thoracotomy or thoracoabdominal incision is extended across the chest wall to expose the affected segment of the esophagus (i.e., upper, middle, or lower third). The thoracic cavity is opened and the mediastinal pleura is incised. The esophagus is dissected away from the aorta and transected above and below the lesion.

For combined thoracoabdominal exposure of a lesion in the lower third of the esophagus, the diaphragm is opened and the stomach mobilized for transection and intrathoracic esophagogastrostomy. In some patients, resection and anastomosis may be performed without thoracotomy by means of a substernal resection to avoid morbidity associated with thoracoabdominal exposure.

High esophageal resection followed by hypopharyngeal reconstruction may be the procedure of choice for tumors in the upper third of the esophagus. Reconstruction of the cervical esophagus is discussed in Chapter 36, p. 761. Total esophagectomy for tumors in the middle third may be carried out through abdominal and cervical incisions, without thoracotomy. The stomach is mobilized for esophagogastric anastomosis in the neck.

COMPLICATIONS OF THORACIC SURGERY

Continuous movement of the chest causes postoperative pain. The patient is likely to breathe shallowly and not adequately raise secretions that accumulate as a result of inhaled anesthetics and sedation. Obstruction in the bronchi from retained secretions can lead to pneumonia and/or atelectasis. The plan of care should include preoperative teaching of breathing techniques to assist the patient in clearing airway secretions.

Development of one pulmonary complication frequently predisposes the patient to development of another. Other potential complications are pneumothorax from an air leak, hemothorax from hemorrhage, and pleural effusion. Empyema and persistent undrained fluid or air pockets can develop in intrathoracic spaces. A bronchopleural fistula may necessitate closure. Pulmonary shunting is also a major complication.

Chylothorax is a potential complication of thoracic surgery. *Chylothorax* is the leakage of chyle from the thoracic duct of the lymphatic system into the pleural space. This complication may occur in response to trauma or after a surgical procedure in the chest cavity. Surgical repair is performed.

Adult respiratory distress syndrome (ARDS), also known as *progressive pulmonary insufficiency* or *shock lung,* may develop in the first 24 to 48 hours following a traumatic injury such as pulmonary contusion or from diffuse or aspiration pneumonia. Beginning with dyspnea, grunting respirations, and tachycardia, signs progress to cyanosis, hypoxemia, and alveolar infiltration. Mortality is high. An intravascular oxygenator/intravenacaval blood gas exchanger may be used as a temporary booster lung (see p. 793) for a patient with ARDS or acute respiratory failure.

BIBLIOGRAPHY

Andrews CO, Gora ML: Pleural effusions: pathophysiology and management, *Ann Pharm* 28(7-8):894-903, 1994.

Arroliga AC, Matthay RA: The role of bronchoscopy in lung cancer, *Clin Chest Med* 14(1):87-98, 1993.

Blossom GB et al: Thymectomy for myasthenia gravis, *Arch Surg* 128(8):855-862, 1993.

Cina C et al: Treatment of thoracic outlet syndrome with combined scalenectomy and transaxillary first rib resection, *Cardiovasc Surg* 2(4):514-518, 1994.

Cybulsky IJ, Bennett WF: Mediastinoscopy as routine outpatient procedure, *Ann Thorac Surg* 58(1):176-178, 1994.

DeFilippi VJ et al: Transcervical thymectomy for myasthenia gravis, *Ann Thorac Surg* 57(1):194-197, 1994.

Dial L: The IVOX: a booster lung device, *Surg Technol* 22(6):13-15, 1990.

Dichter JR et al: Approach to the immunocompromised host with pulmonary symptoms, *Hematol Oncol Clin North Am* 7(4):887-912, 1993.

Elfeldt RJ et al: Long-term follow-up of different therapy procedures in spontaneous pneumothorax, *J Cardiovasc Surg* 35(3):229-233, 1994.

Ellis FH, Gibb SP: Esophageal reconstruction for complex benign esophageal disease, *J Thorac Cardiovasc Surg* 99(2):192-199, 1990.

Ellison DW, Wood VE: Trauma-related thoracic outlet syndrome, *J Hand Surg* 19(4):424-426, 1994.

Fosse E et al: Thoracoscopic pleurodesis, *Scand J Thorac Cardiovasc Surg* 27(3-4):117-119, 1993.

Gross SB: Current challenges, concepts, and controversies in chest tube management, *AACN Clin Issues Crit Care Nurs* 4(2):260-275, 1993.

Hayward RH et al: Access to the thorax by incision, *J Am Coll Surg* 179(2):202-208, 1994.

Kaiser LR: Thymoma: the use of minimally invasive resection techniques, *Chest Surg Clin North Am* 4(1):185-194, 1994.

Kitzrow C: Photodynamic therapy for bronchial and esophageal tumors: perioperative implications, *AORN J* 55(6):1483-1492, 1992.

Lechin AE, Varon J: Adult respiratory distress syndrome (ARDS): the basics, *J Emerg Med* 12(1):63-68, 1994.

Lodenkemper R, Schoenfeld N: Role of endoscopy in the preoperative assessment of bronchial carcinoma, *Arch Chest* Dis 49(2):138-143, 1994.

Lynch TJ: Management of malignant pleural effusions, *Chest* 103 (suppl 4):385s-389s, 1993.

Milanz JR et al: Intrapleural talc for the prevention of recurrent pneumothorax, *Chest* 106(4):1162-1165, 1994.

Molko TA, Pairolero PC: Management of bronchopleural fistula, *Surg Technol* 24(3):10-13, 1992.

Moser NJ et al: Management of postpneumonectomy syndrome with a bronchoscopically placed endobronchial stent, *South Med J* 87(11):1156-1159, 1994.

Nakanishi R et al: Combined thoracoscopy and mediastinoscopy for the evaluation of mediastinal lymph node metastasis in left upper lobe cancer, *J Cardiovasc Surg* 35(4):347-349, 1994.

Nicholson C et al: Are you ready for video thoracoscopy? *Am J Nurs* 93(3):54-57, 1993.

Roviaro G et al: Videothorascopic excision of mediastinal masses: indications and techniques, *Ann Thorac Surg* 58(6):1679-1683, 1994.

Sarsam MA et al: Postpneumonectomy chylothorax, *Ann Thorac Surg* 57(3):689-690, 1994.

Spach DH et al: Transmission of infection by gastrointestinal endoscopy and bronchoscopy, *Ann Intern Med* 118(2):117-128, 1993.

Sutedja G, Postmus PE: Bronchoscopic treatment of lung tumors, *Lung Cancer* 11(1-2):1-17, 1994.

Tampinco-Golos I: Endoscopic thoracotomy: a new approach to thoracic surgery, *AORN J* 55(5):1167-1180, 1992.

Thomson IA, Simms MH: Postoperative chylothorax, *Cardiovasc Surg* 1(4):384-385, 1993.

Urschel JD, Horan TA: Mediastinoscopic treatment of mediastinal cysts, *Ann Thorac Surg* 58(6):1698-1700, 1994.

Waller DA et al: Video-assisted thoracoscopic surgery versus thoracotomy for spontaneous pneumothorax, *Ann Thorac Surg* 58(2):372-376, 1994.

Windsor PG et al: Sclerotherapy for malignant pleural effusions: alternatives to tetracycline, *South Med J* 87(7):709-714, 1994.

CHAPTER 39

Cardiac Surgery

Cardiovascular surgery encompasses the spectrum of clinical pathologic processes associated with congenital anomalies and acquired diseases of the circulatory system. The often complex surgical procedures involving the heart, great vessels, and peripheral blood vessels mandate the need for experienced operating room teams with special education and training. The goal of cardiovascular surgeons is to restore or preserve adequate cardiac output and circulation of blood to the brain and tissues throughout the body. Technologic advancements in diagnosis, anesthesia, hemodynamic monitoring, extracorporeal circulation, myocardial preservation, prosthetic devices, and transplantation have made possible the correction of many defects and the treatment of cardiovascular diseases.

HISTORICAL BACKGROUND

The Smith Papyrus from the sixteenth century BC contains observations on the heartbeat. Hippocrates counted the pulse. Hemophilus (circa 300 BC) described frequency, rhythm, size, and strength as the principal properties of the pulse. But the treatise on the pulse by Me Ching of China in 280 AD became a hallmark in medicine. The circulation of blood was not understood, however, until William Harvey (1578-1657) demonstrated that blood makes a complete circuit in the body. Harvey, an English physician, derived knowledge of comparative anatomy from dissections and experiments on the heart chambers, arteries, and veins. Then in 1791 Galvani, a physiologist and surgeon, discovered the fundamentals of electrical stimulation of the heart.

From these early descriptions, little progress was made in understanding and treating problems associated with the heart or blood vessels until the twentieth century. Stephen Paget published the first textbook of thoracic surgery in 1896. In the chapter on the heart he stated, "Surgery of the heart has probably reached the limits set by nature to all surgery; no new method, and no new discovery, can overcome the natural difficulties that attend a wound of the heart." His successors in the twentieth century have expunged this contention. The advances in cardiac surgery are to medicine what aerospace is to aviation.

Elliott Cutler, in 1924, used a sternum-splitting incision to open the chest for exposure of the heart. Early procedures on the heart and vessels included correction of coarctation of the aorta and patent ductus arteriosus, both congenital anomalies. In the late 1940s Charles Bailey placed his finger into the heart to open a mitral valve stenosis. This *closed* mitral commissurotomy began the evolution of modern cardiovascular surgery, which has accelerated rapidly since about 1950.

Development of the heart-lung machine, which permits safe direct vision for *open heart* procedures, is credited to John Gibbon. In 1953 at Jefferson Medical College in Philadelphia he performed intracardiac surgery using the first successful pump oxygenator. Since then many complex surgical procedures have been developed, such as heart valve replacement, made possible only with the aid of cardiopulmonary bypass.

Heart catheterization and angiography provide evaluation of hemodynamics in intracardiac and intravascular function. Revascularization of an ischemic myocardium to increase blood supply has progressed from abrasion of the epicardium with talcum powder in the 1950s to internal mammary artery implantation and coronary bypass procedures developed in the 1960s. Electronic devices provide cardiac pacing for an irregular heartbeat. Care of cardiac patients immediately following a surgical procedure has improved markedly, reducing mortality, due in no small measure to sophisticated monitoring modalities.

The greatest challenge to cardiac surgeons continues to be the physiologic problems associated with cardiac transplantation and development of mechanical devices as substitutes for organs beyond repair. Since the first successful heart transplant by Christian Barnard in South Africa in 1967, cardiac transplantation has become an accepted modality in some medical centers. The advent in 1981 of a combined heart-lung transplant and the implantation of a mechanical artificial heart in 1982 may provide hope in the future for patients with end-stage cardiopulmonary diseases.

Cardiac surgery, more than any other surgical specialty, owes its successes to teams of experts in chemistry, biology, immunology, biomedical engineering, and electronics working cooperatively with courageous surgeons and cardiologists.

HEART AND GREAT VESSELS

Cardiac procedures involve the heart and associated great vessels. Congenital malformations corrected in infancy or early childhood are discussed in Chapter 42. This chapter focuses on surgical procedures performed for acquired heart diseases. To understand diagnostic procedures, hemodynamic monitoring, myocardial preservation techniques, and cardiopulmonary bypass used in conjunction with cardiac surgery requires knowledge of the normal anatomy and physiology of the heart.

Anatomy and Physiology

The cardiovascular system supplies oxygen and nutrients to body cells and carries waste away from cells by the flow of blood through the system. The heart, blood, and lymph vessels constitute this circulatory system. The heart, the hollow muscular organ located in the thorax, maintains the circulation of blood throughout the body.

Heart

The *heart* is located in the middle mediastinum slightly left of midline. The heart is a muscular "pump" enveloped by a closed, double-walled, fibroserous sac, the *pericardium*. The outer parietal layer forms the sac that contains a small amount of clear serous fluid that lubricates the heart's moving surfaces. The base of the pericardium is attached to the diaphragm; the apex surrounds the great vessels arising from the base of the heart (Figures 39-1 and 39-2).

The layers of the heart are the *epicardium* (outer visceral pericardium), *myocardium* (muscle fibers), and *endocardium* (inner membrane lining). Divided into right and left halves by an oblique longitudinal septum, each half of the heart has two chambers, a thin-walled upper *atrium* and a thick-walled lower *ventricle*. The atria receive blood from veins; the ventricles pump blood into and along the arteries. The heart's rounded apex, formed by the left ventricle, is behind the sixth rib slightly to the left of the sternum. The base is formed by the atria and great vessels. The atria, lying mainly behind the ventricles, continue anteriorly on each side of the aorta to form the auricular appendages. The long axis of the heart extends from base to apex (i.e., from behind forward, downward, and to the left).

Four *heart valves* promote unobstructed unidirectional blood flow through the chambers (see Figure 39-4). These valves are of two types:

1. *Atrioventricular (AV) valves.* Bases of the cusps, the endocardial leaflets, of these valves attach to the fibrous ring that surrounds their opening between the atrium and ventricle on each side of the heart.
   a. *Right tricuspid valve* has three cusps.
   b. *Left mitral valve* has two cusps.
2. *Semilunar valves.* These valves open to allow blood to flow from the heart chambers into the great vessels.
   a. *Pulmonary valve* between right ventricle and pulmonary trunk has three cusps.
   b. *Aortic valve* between left ventricle and aorta has three cusps.

When the ventricle begins to contract, the AV cusps float up to close the opening, preventing a backflow of blood, as the semilunar valves open. Sequential heart sounds (S_1 and S_2) are heard by stethoscope as the valves open and close.

Coronary circulation is predominantly right or predominantly left. The coronary arteries arise from the aorta and, with their branches, supply oxygen and nutrients to the heart muscle. The left coronary artery divides shortly after its origin into two main trunks:

1. The anterior descending or interventricular branch courses toward the apex of the heart. Its branches distribute over the anterolateral wall of the left ventricle. Septal branches supply the anterior interventricular septum.
2. The circumflex branch passes posteriorly. Following the atrioventricular groove and passing under the left atrial appendage, it meets the right coronary artery at the base of the junction of both ventricles. The right coronary artery is directed to the right, passing to the posterior aspect of the heart

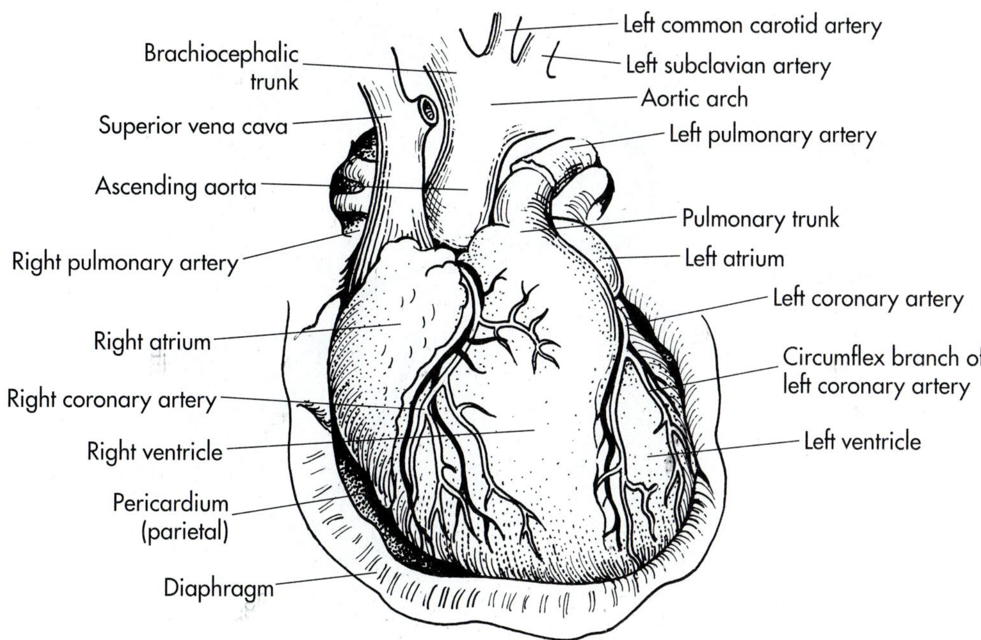

FIGURE 39-1 Anterior view of heart and great vessels.

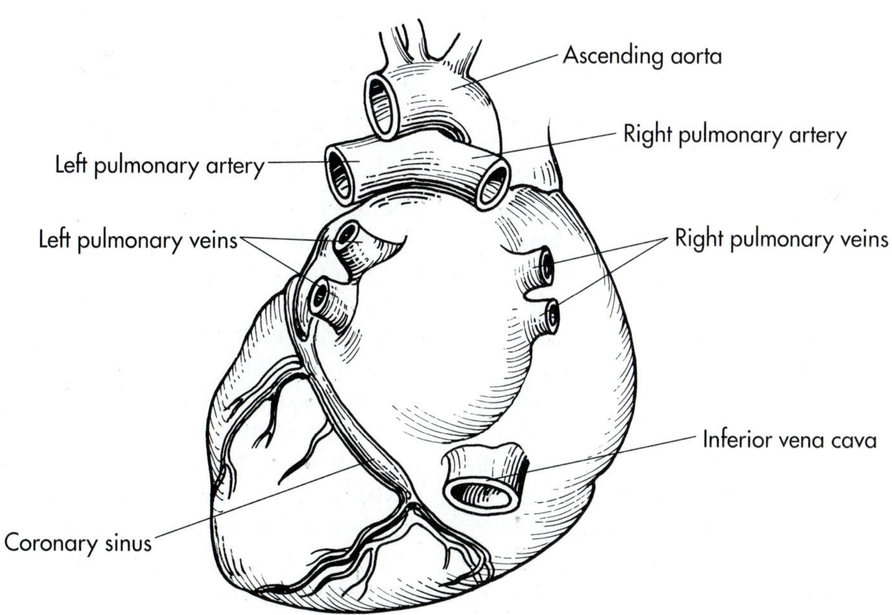

FIGURE 39-2 Posterior view of heart and great vessels.

and eventually running between the two ventricles. Its branches supply the posterior interventricular septum.

The vagus nerve (parasympathetic) and cardiac branches of the cervical and upper thoracic ganglia (sympathetic) innervate the heart.

Conduction System

The heart's conduction system (Figure 39-3) permits synchronous contraction of the atria followed by contraction of the ventricles. The right and left sides of the heart function simultaneously but independently. Muscular contractions of the atria and ventricles are controlled by an electrical impulse that originates in the

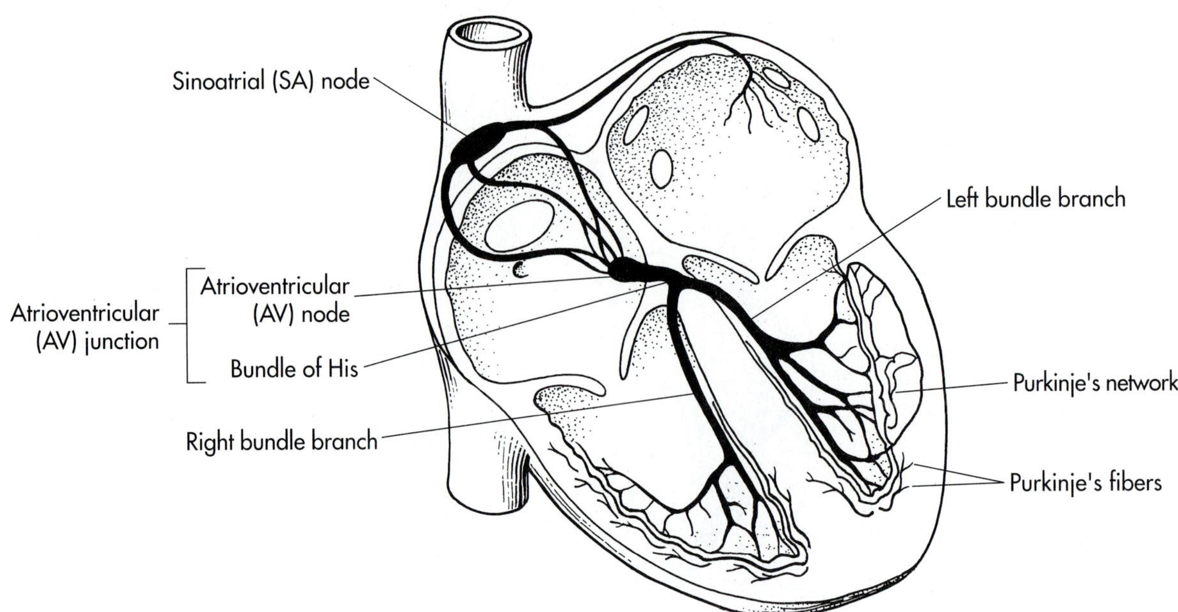

FIGURE 39-3 Conducting system within heart. Electrical system is composed of sinoatrial (SA) node, atrioventricular (AV) node, and bundle of His, at atrioventricular junction; left bundle branch; right bundle branch; Purkinje's network of Purkinje's fibers.

sinoatrial (SA) node. This "pacemaker" is a dense network of specialized Purkinje's fibers that begin at the junction of the right atrium and superior vena cava. These fibers become continuous with muscle fibers of the atrium at the node's periphery. The stimulus is passed to the *smaller atrioventricular (AV)* node beneath the endocardium in the interatrial septum. A mass of interwoven conductive tissue, this node's specialized fibers are continuous with atrial muscle fibers and the atrioventricular bundle of His. The *bundle of His* provides conduction relay between atria and ventricles. Arising from the AV node, the band of conducting tissue passes on both sides of the interventricular septum, its branches dividing and subdividing to penetrate every area of ventricular muscle and to transmit contraction impulses to the ventricles. Thus expansions of conducting tissue, providing coordinated excitation of muscle areas, spread through both atria and ventricles. Each atrial contraction (depolarization) is followed by a period of recharging (repolarization) during which the ventricles contract. Ventricular contraction is followed by a period of recovery while the chambers fill with blood as the atria contract.

Cardiac Cycle (Circulation)

Myocardial contraction is referred to as *systole*, relaxation as *diastole*. Venous blood from the entire body enters the right atrium via the *vena cava* and passes through the tricuspid valve to the right ventricle from which it is ejected through the pulmonary valve into the pulmonary arterial trunk. Right and left *pulmonary arteries* originating from the trunk carry the blood to the lungs, where it takes up oxygen and gives off carbon dioxide. Oxygenated blood is transported from the lungs to the left atrium by the *pulmonary veins* and enters the left ventricle through the mitral valve. Contraction of the left ventricle propels blood through the aortic valve into the *aorta* from which it is carried to all parts of body by arterial branches (Figure 39-4). The highest pressure reached during left ventricular systole is the *systolic blood pressure.* Following contraction the ventricle relaxes, during which time systemic intraarterial pressure falls to its lowest level, *diastolic blood pressure.* Each contraction of the right ventricle forces blood through the pulmonary valve into the pulmonary arteries to the lungs. In summary, there are two circulations:

1. *Pulmonary,* from right ventricle to lungs and back to left atrium
2. *Systemic,* from left ventricle to aorta, to body tissues and organs, and back to right atrium

Diagnostic Procedures

Interference in any part of the circulatory system can jeopardize survival. A surgical procedure is preceded by extensive cardiovascular assessment on the basis of noninvasive and invasive studies that dictate subsequent treatment.

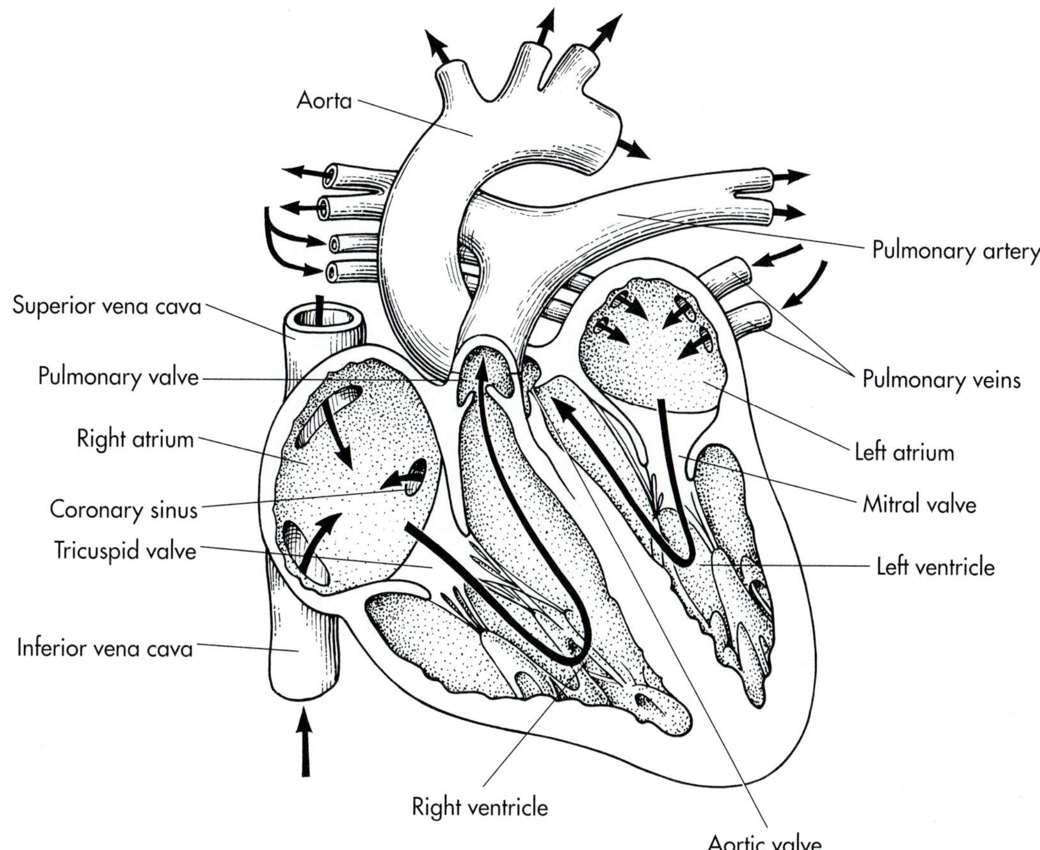

FIGURE 39-4 Circulation of blood through heart. *Arrows* indicate direction of flow from superior vena cava and inferior vena cava into right atrium, through tricuspid valve into right ventricle, and through pulmonary valve into pulmonary artery. Blood flows from pulmonary veins into left atrium, through mitral valve into left ventricle, and through aortic valve into aorta.

Noninvasive Procedures

Routine examination and electrocardiography are augmented by determination of venous pressure, cardiac output, circulation time, and blood chemistry studies. Chest x-ray film reveals heart size, position, and outline. Screening or functional capacity testing, such as stress testing, is informative. Pulmonary function tests may detect left ventricular failure. Echocardiography with ultrasonic waves reveals the heart structure and gives information pertinent to congenital heart disease and valvular disease. Radionuclide imaging may be used to detect regional reductions in myocardial blood flow and thus help to confirm or deny the diagnosis of myocardial infarction (i.e., necrosis of a portion of the myocardium caused by obstruction in a coronary artery).

Invasive Procedures

Radiographic visualization following injection of a nontoxic radiopaque substance permits study of the heart chambers, great vessels, and coronary circulation.

Angiography *Angiocardiography,* with intravascular injection of a radiopaque substance, permits radiographs of the heart chambers, thoracic vessels, and coronary arteries. Rapid serial radiographs or motion pictures on an enlarged fluoroscopic screen show the heart outline and passage of contrast materials in the great vessels. *Selective angiocardiography* or *coronary angiography* is done in association with cardiac catheterization to evaluate coronary artery disease and to determine the extent of obstructive disease in the coronary vessels. Aneurysms also may be diagnosed by angiography. (See Chapter 28, pp. 568-569, for a more complete discussion of angiography.)

Cardiac Catheterization Under image-intensification fluoroscopy, a sterile catheter is introduced through a cutdown into a brachial vessel in the arm or percutaneously into a femoral vessel in the groin and is passed into the heart or a coronary artery. The procedure permits precise:

1. Evaluation of heart function
2. Measurements of intracardiac pressure
3. Visualization of heart chambers

Catheterization is used to diagnose coronary artery disease, valvular heart disease, or congenital anomalies. It is the ultimate tool for diagnosis of ischemic heart disease.

For study of the coronary arteries, a single catheter is passed and its tip inserted into the ostia of the arteries for injection of dye and trace of solution flow. Cinefluorograms record findings. After catheter removal, the incision is closed and pressure dressings are applied.

For right-sided heart catheterization, a pulmonary artery catheter is inserted through the vein to obtain pressures in the right atrium and ventricle, pulmonary artery, and pulmonary artery wedge. Measurements of thermodilution, cardiac output, and oxygen saturation also may be obtained. The right internal jugular vein may be cannulated and a bioptome, a specially designed biopsy forceps, advanced to obtain a right endomyocardial biopsy. For left-sided heart catheterization, a catheter is inserted into an artery and advanced through the aortic valve into the left ventricle.

Physiologic monitoring with a multichannel recorder is continuous during the procedure. Potential complications include dysrhythmias, air embolus, thrombosis, and vascular and/or cardiac perforation.

SPECIAL FEATURES OF CARDIAC SURGERY

The principles of general and thoracic surgery apply to cardiac surgery, but several factors require emphasis:

1. Extra minutes are not available; seconds save lives.
2. Team concept is of utmost importance. An experienced team working together can handle emergencies expeditiously.
3. Comprehensive physical and psychologic preparation of the patient precedes a surgical procedure. Postoperatively the patient is taken to an intensive care unit. The patient is monitored constantly intraoperatively and postoperatively.

General Considerations

1. Operating room (OR) for cardiovascular surgery should be equipped with:
   a. Cardiac defibrillator, pacemaker, and intraaortic counterpulsation devices
   b. Cardioplegic (to induce cardiac arrest) and inotropic (to modify cardiac muscle contractility) drugs, to include but not limited to:
      (1) Calcium channel-blocking agents
      (2) Dopamine hydrochloride (Intropin)
      (3) Dobutamine hydrochloride (Dobutrex)
      (4) Epinephrine hydrochloride (Adrenalin)
      (5) Intravenous nitroglycerin
   c. Laboratory facilities for blood gas and acid-base balance determinations. Modern analyzers have microprocessors to determine values.
2. Basic thoracic setup is used with the addition of cardiovascular instruments (i.e., various noncrushing vascular and anastomosis clamps, cardiotomy suction tips and sump tubes, and cardiovascular sutures).
3. Prosthetic devices should be properly sterilized. Many types of valves, patches, grafts, and catheters are available. They should be biocompatible, nonthrombogenic, and nonbiodegradable.
4. Local and/or systemic hypothermia may be used intraoperatively to reduce the body's need for oxygen and to preserve myocardial function (see pp. 804-805). Commercial preparations of sterile slush for local hypothermia are convenient.
5. Intraoperative autotransfusion is often used for blood volume replacement (see Chapter 23, p. 486). Blood substitutes such as hetastarch, an albumin substitute for plasma expansion, may be administered. Properly cross-matched blood should be available for transfusion in the event of excessive blood loss. Platelets, stored at room temperature, may be given after cardiopulmonary bypass to enhance clotting. Often little or no blood is needed for transfusion in many procedures when cardiopulmonary bypass is used (see p. 803).
6. Closed water-seal drainage or suction drainage is used postoperatively to drain the chest or mediastinum.

Invasive Hemodynamic Monitoring

Although placement of invasive pressure monitoring lines is not their responsibility, perioperative nurses should be aware of the implications of data and the potential for complications (e.g., infection or thrombus). For assessment of tissue perfusion, invasive hemodynamic monitoring is used to determine blood pressures in major arteries, veins, and heart chambers. Indwelling catheter lines are inserted to measure:

1. Radial and femoral artery pressures.
2. Central venous pressure (CVP).
3. Pulmonary artery pressures. The Swan-Ganz catheter line also determines right atrial, right ventricular, and pulmonary capillary wedge pressures of left ventricular function.

These invasive monitoring techniques are discussed in detail in Chapter 19, pp. 371-375. Indwelling intravascular catheters are inserted preoperatively. During a surgical procedure they provide information relative to the effects of anesthetic agents, surgical manipulation of the heart, hypothermia, extracorporeal circulation, induced ischemia, and cardiac arrest. A registered nurse may draw blood samples from the pressure lines at intervals during cardiopulmonary bypass perfusion for blood gas analysis (see discussion of technique in Chapter 19, pp. 365-366). Catheter patency is maintained with heparinized flush solutions.

In addition to artery and CVP pressure lines, during an open heart procedure the surgeon may insert a small plastic catheter directly into the left atrium to assess *left atrial pressure.* Postoperatively this catheter is connected to a transducer and monitor. The transducer balancing port must be level with the right atrium. The catheter is flushed with heparinized 5% dextrose in water because inadvertent overload with this solution is less dangerous than is overload with normal saline. Also, an air filter is attached to the end of pressure tubing as a precaution against fatal air embolism. Every part of the line and filter must be flushed and free of air, or the pressure bag could force a bubble into the left atrium, causing an embolus. In absence of mitral valve disease, left atrial pressure at end of atrial diastole, just before the mitral valve opens, indicates left ventricular end-diastolic pressure and, therefore, left ventricular filling pressure and function.

Postoperatively, hemodynamic monitoring detects dysrhythmias caused by impaired myocardial perfusion, transient reduction in cardiac output with subsequent hypotension, hypovolemia secondary to hemorrhage, and tamponade. Circulating blood volume, pulmonary volume overload leading to pulmonary edema, and reactions to titrated vasopressor drugs can also be identified.

Noninvasive Intraoperative Monitoring

Noninvasive technologies are used intraoperatively to evaluate the effectiveness of some repairs and/or tissue perfusion. These devices include:

1. *Echocardiography.* A transesophageal ultrasound probe is used for assessment of graft patency, myocardial perfusion, adequacy of valve replacement, or ventricular function. A Doppler color flow probe also may be useful to quantitatively assess other repairs.
2. *Electrophysiologic measurements.* A computerized mapping system is used to identify the focus of dysrhythmias.
3. *Near-infrared reflectance spectroscopy.* A device equipped with a sensor is attached to the patient's head. Light transmitted through the skin and skull to the brain is reflected to light detectors in the sensor. Changes in oxygen levels in the brain change light absorption. These changes may alert the anesthesiologist and surgeon to a developing oxygen deficit.

Cardiopulmonary Bypass

Cardiopulmonary bypass is the technique of oxygenating and perfusing blood by means of a mechanical pump-oxygenator system. Referred to as the *heart-lung machine,* this apparatus temporarily substitutes for the function of the patient's heart and lungs during cardiac surgery. Cardiopulmonary bypass is used for most intracardiac (open heart) and coronary artery procedures. Venous blood is diverted from the body to the machine for oxygenation *(extracorporeal circulation)* and is pumped back to the patient.

During bypass the lungs are kept deflated and immobilized. In preparation for bypass, the patient is heparinized to prevent clot formation. Cannulae are inserted, for venous diversion, into the inferior and superior vena cavae through small incisions in the right atrium. A cannula for return of oxygenated blood to arterial circulation is placed in the ascending aorta or femoral artery. Cannulae are connected to the machine by sterile tubing before institution of bypass.

The perfusionist who operates the cardiopulmonary bypass machine, often called the *pump technician,* must be familiar with its function, care, and operation. The perfusionist may be employed by the cardiac surgeon or by the hospital.

Components of Bypass System

Oxygenator Oxygen is taken up and carbon dioxide is removed from the blood. Types of oxygenators include:

1. *Bubble.* Bubbles of oxygen are supplied to the blood by direct blood/gas contact.
2. *Membrane.* Oxygen and carbon dioxide diffuse through a permeable Teflon or polyethylene membrane that contains the blood. This method diminishes blood/gas interface. Several types of disposable membrane oxygenators are available.
3. *Microporous membrane.* Blood film is separated from ventilating gas by a microporous polypropylene membrane folded like an accordion and operated like a bubble oxygenator. Blood pressure in this oxygenator exceeds gas pressure at all times, thus precluding gas bubbles passing through the microporous membrane.

Heat Exchanger Incorporated in the circuit, a heat exchanger regulates blood temperature. Water at thermostatically controlled temperature circulates through the exchanger, which can rapidly produce, control, or correct systemic hypothermia. Hypothermia is often used in conjunction with bypass to reduce oxygen demands of tissues and to protect the myocardium during arrest.

Pump Rollers turning over sterile plastic tubing propel reheated oxygenated blood in a relatively nonpulsatile flow through a blood filter and bubble trap to the arterial cannula for recirculation through the body. Rate of flow can be varied. It is calculated according to patient weight or body surface area. Reduced flow accompanies hypothermia.

Perfusion

Immediately before the surgical procedure the machine is primed (filled) with a combination of crystalloid and colloid solutions, a balanced electrolyte component, and a cardiopreservative solution including sodium bicarbonate and heparinized plasma volume expander. Some circuits are heparin-coated by the manufacturer. For a hemodilution technique of priming, the system is filled with fluid that will replace blood diverted to the pump-oxygenator system and is recirculated through the circuit to remove air bubbles. The priming solution should be of sufficient volume and of a suitable hematocrit level so that when mixed with the patient's blood the resultant buffered plasma will be capable of achieving adequate perfusion and preventing myocardial acidosis. Blood is added as needed to maintain an adequate oxygen-carrying capacity and perfusion rate.

Bypass may be partial or total. In *partial*, only a portion of venous return is routed to the pump-oxygenator circuitry, the remaining portion following normal systemic circulation. In *total* bypass, all venous return is diverted to the machine for total body perfusion. Purse-string sutures in the vena cava are tightened around the caval cannulae inserted to drain all venous return to the machine. The heart is arrested.

During perfusion the patient is monitored intensely (i.e., arterial and venous pressures, body and blood temperatures, blood gases and electrolytes, and urinary output). General anesthesia may be maintained by an anesthetic vaporizer that adds vapor to the oxygenating mixture or by intravenous anesthesia.

At conclusion of the defect repair, air is removed from heart, the patient is rewarmed, heartbeat is restored, ventilation is reestablished by respirator, and perfusion is gradually decreased to wean patient from the machine. After discontinuance of bypass, cannula are removed and purse-string sutures around insertion sites are tied. Protamine sulfate is injected to reverse the effect of the heparin previously administered.

Cardiopulmonary bypass may also be employed in conjunction with deep hypothermia during neurosurgical procedures, in major organ transplantation, and for pulmonary embolectomy. It is also used to assist in the event of ventricular failure, to treat some types of pulmonary dysfunction, and to perfuse an isolated segment of the body for cancer chemotherapy.

Myocardial Preservation

A bloodless, motionless field allows direct vision of the heart and its interior for repair of coronary circulation or intracardiac defects. Cardiopulmonary bypass isolates the heart while the body is perfused with oxygenated blood. Cardiac arrest is purposely induced. During bypass, the perfusionist is in control of the patient's body temperature and preservation of body and brain. The surgeon assumes responsibility for preservation of the heart. Bypass time is kept to a minimum because ischemia causes myocardial injury of time-related severity. Deliberate arrest may be effected by one or a combination of methods.

Aortic Cross-Clamping The aorta is occluded with a vascular clamp to block systemic circulation. Ischemic (anoxic) cardiac arrest occurs as the blocked systemic blood within the heart becomes deoxygenated and cardiac metabolic needs are depleted. This technique can be maintained for only a limited period, however, because myocardial damage and necrosis will occur when the oxygen supply and energy required to maintain the subcellular system are depleted. Cerebrospinal fluid pressure may increase.

Cardioplegia Modern, safe cardiac surgery is based on the use of cardioplegic solutions used alone or in combination with other techniques discussed. These are preparations of a small amount of potassium in crystalloid, blood, or other solution. When injected into the coronary artery system, hyperkalemia immediately induces complete electromechanical cardiac arrest. The composition and temperature of the solution and infusion techniques can be determined for each patient's disease process. Some solutions have a calcium antagonist, such as verapamil or nifedipine, to help prevent myocardial ischemia. Some are infused warm, others cold. Infusion may be continuous or intermittent. Most commonly, a cold potassium cardioplegic solution is introduced into the coronary arteries retrograde; antegrade cardioplegia is sometimes indicated in selected patients. Coronary perfusion pressure during administration of the cardioplegic solution may influence regional delivery. When the solution is flushed out of the collateral circulation at the end of the surgical procedure, the heartbeat may resume spontaneously. If not, ventricular fibrillation is treated with countershock.

Hypothermia Hypothermia reduces systemic metabolic needs and oxygen requirements. It exerts a protective effect during cardiopulmonary bypass through a temperature-related decrease of intracellular metabolism, thus allowing tissues to tolerate a prolonged period of decreased perfusion. Hypothermia is an essential component to ischemic myocardial preservation, but because of its calcium-loading effect, cardioplegic arrest precedes initiation of hypothermia. Local hypothermia can be induced by topical application of iced saline slush around heart or iced Ringer's lactate solution to heart externally and/or internally. Cardiac arrest also can be induced by deliberately lowering systemic body temperature moderately to 78.8° to 89.6° F (26° to 32° C) or deeply to below 78.8° F (26° C). This is achieved by a cooling perfusate in the heart-lung machine.

Complications

Although excellent results are obtained with most procedures, significant derangements can occur following cardiopulmonary bypass. These are most obvious in infants or after prolonged surgical procedures in adults. Alterations in clotting may occur as a result of heparinization of blood, mechanical damage to platelets and clotting factors, and direct exposure of blood to oxygen. If trauma or transfusion reaction hemolyzes red blood cells, viscosity in renal tubules may cause tubular necrosis and renal failure.

Inadequate or extended perfusion and oxygenation may promote tissue anoxia and metabolic acidosis. Fluid and electrolyte balance merit close watching, particularly for hypervolemia. When nonblood fluids are used to prime the pump, they may diffuse into interstitial spaces. As this fluid returns to circulation postoperatively, hypervolemia may result. Furthermore, increased levels of aldosterone and antidiuretic hormone induced by the stress of surgery cause retention of sodium and water. Fluids are restricted for 24 hours postoperatively. Cerebral edema and brain damage at times ensue, for unknown reasons. However, these developments are generally temporary.

"Post-pump psychosis" consists of visual and auditory hallucinations and paranoid delusions. This often terminates when the patient is transferred from the intensive care unit.

The most severe pulmonary complication of extracorporeal circulation is *postperfusion lung syndrome.* Its cause is unknown. It is often fatal because of the development of atelectasis, pulmonary edema, and hemorrhage. Metabolic acidosis during bypass may lead to *low cardiac output syndrome* postoperatively. This occurs most frequently in patients with long histories of cardiac disease. Finally, cardiac tamponade is another potential complication, reflected by a drop of more than 10 mm Hg in systolic blood pressure during the patient's inspiration *(pulsus paradoxus).*

CARDIAC SURGICAL PROCEDURES

The purposes of heart surgery are to correct acquired or congenital anatomic abnormalities (see discussion of pediatric procedures in Chapter 42, pp. 866-868), repair or replace defective heart valves, revascularize ischemic myocardium, and improve or assist ventricular function. The hours immediately before the surgical procedure can be a highly stressful period for the patient. Mental stress can cause myocardial ischemia (i.e., inadequate blood supply to the heart) without symptoms of chest pain. Therefore the patient should be monitored from arrival in the OR suite, through induction of anesthesia, and throughout the surgical procedure. Administration of oxygen before induction of anesthesia may be indicated to help reduce stress. Procedures may be performed with or without cardiopulmonary bypass.

Commonly Used Thoracic Incisions

Median Sternotomy

For median sternotomy patient is supine. A vertical incision extends through the midline from the suprasternal notch to approximately 2 inches below the xiphoid process. Retrosternal tissue is dissected. The sternum is split (divided) with a powered sternal saw. Caution is used to avoid injury to underlying mediastinal structures. The blade has a safety guard to prevent penetration into the mediastinum.

At closure, heavy-gauge stainless steel sutures are placed around or through the sternum, tightly pulled together, and twisted. The ends are buried in the sternum. Other nonabsorbable sutures may be used to provide firm fixation. The linea alba, subcutaneous tissue, and skin are sutured. Complications are brachial plexus injury, costochondral separation from too vigorous sternal retraction during the surgical procedure, and keloid formation.

Median sternotomy incision is used for open heart procedures and pericardiectomy.

Transsternal Bilateral Thoracotomy

A bilateral submammary incision is made with patient supine for transsternal bilateral thoracotomy. In the midline the incision curves superiorly to cross sternum at the fourth intercostal space level. Lateral extension is to the midaxillary line. The pleural cavity is entered via the interspace after division of pectoralis muscles. The internal mammary arteries and veins are ligated and divided. Sternum is divided horizontally.

At closure, the sternum is reapproximated securely, ribs are approximated with pericostal sutures, and remaining tissue layers are closed.

This incision is used for resection of ventricular aneurysm, aortic arch grafts, and complicated pericardiectomies. This incision is less commonly used and causes more discomfort for the patient.

Other Thoracotomy Incisions

Left anterolateral or posterolateral thoracotomy incisions may be preferred for some cardiac procedures. See descriptions of these incisions in Chapter 38, pp. 788-789.

Valvular Heart Disease

Valvular heart disease may arise from a congenital abnormality or can be acquired. Abnormal vibrations or heart murmurs may be congenital or the end result of disease such as rheumatic fever or degenerative change. Valves can become thickened and calcified, resulting in loss of valve substance, narrowing of the orifice, and immobility. They then develop *insufficiency,* failure to close completely, and permit blood leakage or regurgitation. Failure to open completely is caused by *stenosis,* which impedes flow. A defective valve is reconstructed if possible. To prevent heart failure, prosthetic valves are inserted in patients who have a return of symptoms after reconstruction or have a valve that cannot be reconstructed.

Closed Mitral Commissurotomy

Closed mitral commissurotomy is an example of closed heart surgery. The breaking apart of fused stenosed leaflets of the mitral (left AV) valve reduces left atrial and right ventricular pressures that decrease lung function. The thorax is entered by left anterolateral incision. To provide hemostasis, purse string sutures are placed around the left auricular appendage before opening it. The surgeon frees fused leaflets by inserting a finger, valvulotome (knife), or transventricular dilator into the valve. After this is accomplished, purse string sutures are tied, and the auricular appendage is sutured. Lungs are reexpanded, a chest tube is inserted, the incision is closed, and the tube is connected to closed water-seal chest drainage.

Open Mitral Commissurotomy

Fused leaflet commissures in a mitral valve that have not become thickened and calcified may be incised under direct vision (i.e., open mitral commissurotomy) during cardiopulmonary bypass. This improves leaflet function and protects against thromboembolism. A potential hazard of the open method is air embolism by expulsion of air from left ventricle into aorta. Residual air must be vented to avoid this complication.

Valve Replacement

A diseased mitral or aortic valve may be excised and replaced. Several types of prosthetic heart valves are available. They may be mechanical or biologic. With disk- or ball-type synthetic mechanical valves, the disk or ball freely opens and closes according to the flow of blood. One type consists of a cage in which a spherical ball is enclosed. Other models are constructed with disks resembling leaflets of human valves. The disks of some are tilted. The metal ring at the base of the cage may be covered with polyester fabric to facilitate suturing. It also encourages tissue ingrowth, an aid to long-term fixation. Biologic valves also have been developed from homograft or heterograft (porcine bioprosthesis or bovine pericardial xenograft) donor material. Glutaraldehyde storage solution is rinsed thoroughly from heterografts before use. An effective prosthesis is nontoxic, nonthrombogenic, and nondeteriorating. The surgeon selects the most suitable type and size for the defect to be repaired. Contamination of a valve can cause a serious postoperative endocarditis. Sterility is maintained before and during insertion.

Mitral Valve Replacement Cardiopulmonary bypass is used for mitral valve replacement, an open heart procedure. Through a median sternotomy or left thoracotomy incision, the pericardium is incised and retracted. When bypass cannulae are placed, the left ventricle may be vented with a plastic tube to decompress the heart and prevent overdistention of the ventricle during unclamping of the aorta after anoxic arrest. The left atrium is opened. The mitral valve is exposed, inspected, and removed by circumferential excision and severance of muscular attachments to the ventricular wall. The surgeon usually prefers to leave the chordae tendineae and papillary muscles intact. The fibrous ring or annulus surrounding the valvular opening remains intact. A sterile prosthetic valve is inserted and sutured in place, and the atrium is sutured. Teflon felt pledgets are commonly used as a buttress under the sutures to prevent the annulus from tearing when the prosthetic valve is seated and the sutures are tied.

The probability of thromboembolic complications is sufficient in a patient with chronic atrial fibrillation and an enlarged left atrium to warrant postoperative anticoagulant therapy. Therefore a durable synthetic mechanical prosthetic device may be the valve of choice for this procedure.

Postoperatively, temporary pacing may be required (see p. 810). Pacing wires are implanted in the wall of the right or left ventricle during the surgical procedure. If sequential pacing will be necessary, additional wires are placed in the right atrium. Then the pericardium is closed. Blood is returned to the heart, and air is removed from it. Partial cardiopulmonary bypass is resumed as the patient is being weaned from the machine. Cannula incisions are closed. Thoracic wound closure is carried out, and closed water-seal chest drainage is used.

Aortic Valve Replacement The surgical procedure for aortic valve replacement is basically the same as that described for mitral valve replacement except that the aortic valve is exposed through a transverse incision in the aorta. Either a mechanical valve or bioprosthesis may be used. Biologic prostheses offer the advantage of low embolic rate and obviate the need for prolonged anticoagulation therapy. Cryopreserved fresh aortic valve homografts, either from a homograft bank or commercially available allograft, may be preferred.

The aortic valve may be replaced with the patient's own pulmonary valve (i.e., an autograft).

Valve Reconstruction

Reconstruction of the patient's own valve may restore normal mitral valve function, particularly in children and young adults. *Valvuloplasty* and *annuloplasty* are valve-sparing procedures to maintain integrity of mitral structure and ventricular function. An annuloplasty ring, either flexible or nonflexible, may be used for support and to provide continuity and permanence of repair. Thromboembolism is less of a threat than following valve replacement; thus anticoagulant therapy is not indicated postoperatively.

Percutaneous Transluminal Balloon Valvuloplasty

An interventional cardiac catheterization procedure (see pp. 801-802), balloon valvuloplasty may be an option to treat valvular stenosis in high-risk patient who cannot tolerate valve replacement. A catheter with a deflated balloon is inserted under fluoroscopy across a stenosed aortic, pulmonary, tricuspid, or mitral valve. The balloon is repeatedly inflated until the valve is opened.

Coronary Artery Disease

Coronary arteries supplying the myocardium (heart muscle) may become stenosed or obstructed, which is referred to as *occlusive coronary artery disease* or *ischemic heart disease*. Resultant myocardial ischemia may result in angina (pain) or myocardial infarction (necrosis). Occlusive disease of the coronary arteries characteristically affects vessels in their proximal segments and at the origin of major branches. Significant obstructions occur most frequently in the right coronary, right posterior descending, left anterior descending, and circumflex arteries. More than one artery can be occluded. Revascularization to improve blood supply to the myocardium is possible by surgical intervention in selected patients.

Coronary Artery Bypass Graft

Single or multiple arterial bypasses are done depending on the number of vessels affected and degree of obstruction present. The internal mammary (thoracic) artery and segments of saphenous and cephalic veins are used to bypass coronary artery obstruction. The gastroepiploic, inferior epigastric, splenic, and radial arteries also may be used as free grafts. Cryopreserved saphenous vein and umbilical vein allografts also are used. Most cardiac surgeons wear loupes for magnification while constructing an anastomosis between the graft and the coronary artery. Some surgeons prefer to use the operating microscope during this part of the procedure.

The chest is opened by median sternotomy, and the pericardium is incised. Cardiopulmonary bypass is established; techniques are influenced by the surgeon's preferred procedure and the extent of grafting. After the conduit or graft is anastomosed, cardiopulmonary bypass is discontinued; all incisions are closed and checked for leaks. The patient is hemodynamically stabilized. The wound is closed in the usual manner for sternotomy with closed water-seal chest drainage.

A patient with a heavily calcified aorta is at risk for embolization and/or rupture of the great vessels. In extreme circumstances, bypass to the right coronary or left anterior descending artery can be performed without arresting the heart or using cardiopulmonary bypass. Bleeding is controlled with small clamps and occlusion with vessel loops. The heart is closely monitored for ischemia. Cardiopulmonary bypass is instituted as an emergency measure if the heart tissue fails to perfuse adequately during the procedure.

An argon laser may be used to weld or fuse tissues together, a technique known as *laser-assisted vascular anastomosis* or *arterial welding*.

Internal Mammary Artery Conduit Because of its long-term patency rate, at least one internal mammary artery is used as a conduit for myocardial revascularization. The left internal mammary artery is dissected up to its origin from the subclavian artery, freeing it from the retrosternal aspect of the chest wall. After mobilization, the pericardium is notched to minimize the distance to the coronary artery. Side-to-side or end-to-side anastomosis is performed primarily between the internal mammary artery and the left anterior descending coronary artery, distal to the obstruction. The right internal mammary artery will reach vessels supplying all but the posterolateral wall of the left ventricle. To provide adequate drainage without tension on the arterial conduit, the pericardium is not sutured. Segments of either right, left, or both internal mammary arteries also are used as free grafts to bypass other diseased coronary arteries.

Saphenous Vein Bypass Graft The procedure for saphenous vein bypass graft is expedited by two teams: one harvests the saphenous vein for graft while the other opens the chest and prepares for cardiopulmonary bypass. An adequate length of vein is removed to obtain sufficient graft material. The distal end of each vein segment is identified, and the graft is placed in heparinized normal saline solution after harvest. It is handled gently to avoid trauma to the intima. The vein is reversed to permit a normal direction of blood flow through venous valves into the aorta. The affected coronary artery is opened distal to the obstruction; the proximal end of the saphenous vein is anastomosed end-to-side to the artery, creating the distal anastomosis, thus bypassing the obstruction. Usually a fine 6-0 or 7-0 monofilament nonabsorbable suture is used. The proximal anastomosis is established by creating a small opening in the aorta with a punch and suturing the distal end of the vein to the aperture. Saphenous or other vein or artery bypass grafts are completed before the internal mammary artery is anastomosed to form a vascular conduit. Manipulation of the heart could stress the anastomosis.

Coronary Artery Angioplasty

Restoration of perfusion from the left coronary system is possible by direct enlargement of the left main coronary artery lumen in selected patients in whom clinical circumstances preclude bypass grafting. A curved incision is made in the lateral aortic wall. Either the posterior or anterior aspect of the left main coronary artery is incised across the stenosis. An autologous onlay pericardial or onlay saphenous vein patch is sutured between the artery and the aortic wall.

Endarterectomy, removal of an organized thrombus and attached endothelium or atherosclerotic fatty plaques from the arterial wall, may be performed in conjunction with left coronary angioplasty or right coronary bypass grafting. Small spatulas, wire loops, miniature abrasive drills, or ultrasonic devices may be used to remove plaque.

Laser angioplasty removes plaque in coronary arteries distal to a site for an anastomosis. A hand-held excimer or a CO_2 laser may be used. The CO_2 laser may also be used for canalization of the myocardium. Tiny channels are created through the wall of the left ventricle into the myocardium. Blood seeps into sinusoids to revascularize the myocardium.

Percutaneous Transluminal Coronary Angioplasty

Percutaneous transluminal coronary angioplasty is performed under fluoroscopy with image intensification. Balloon dilation of coronary arteries may be the procedure of choice for selected patients with significant atherosclerotic narrowing in a major coronary artery. The coronary arteries are approached by either percutaneous femoral artery entry or brachial artery cutdown. A balloon-tipped catheter is passed through a guiding catheter into area of coronary artery with atherosclerotic material (plaque). The balloon is inflated by a hydraulic pump to compress plaque against the arterial lining and dilate the arterial wall, thus enlarging the lumen. During time the balloon is inflated, normal flow of oxygen supplied by the artery to the myocardium is interrupted. Oxygenation distal to the balloon may be maintained with oxygenated perfluorochemical emulsion (Fluosol) flowing through the catheter.

Catheters with ultrasonic devices or tiny drill heads may be used to pulverize atherosclerotic plaque before balloon dilation. Other procedures may be performed as an alternative to or in conjunction with balloon angioplasty.

Laser Angioplasty An argon laser probe, an Nd:YAG optical fiber, or a pulsed excimer laser may be used for laser angioplasty. An integrated system combines direct laser energy and fiberoptics with a balloon angioplasty catheter. The catheter positions the laser fiber, which then vaporizes the plaque or thrombus obstructing the coronary vessels.

Intracoronary Stent A stent may be inserted to act as a buttress to keep an artery open. The coronary artery to be stented should be at least 3 mm in diameter. The stent permanently implanted at the site of the stenosis widens the arterial lumen by compressing atherosclerotic plaque against the arterial wall. The stainless steel mesh or springlike coil stent is tightly wrapped around a balloon catheter. As the balloon is inflated, the stent expands. After the balloon is deflated and removed, the stent remains in place to provide structural support and keep the artery from collapsing.

Coronary artery angioplasty procedures usually are performed in the cardiac catheterization laboratory or special procedures room in the radiology department. However, a standby OR team should be available for emergency coronary artery bypass in the event that acute coronary obstruction or perforation occurs.

Cardiac Dysrhythmias

Some cardiac rhythm disorders are unresponsive to drug therapy. Normally the electrical cardiac impulse begins at the SA node, thus controlling the rhythm of the heart rate. Fibers from the SA node conduct the impulse through the atria into the AV node and then transmit it along the bundle of His into the ventricles, ending in the Purkinje's fibers. Occasionally some other part of the heart develops a rhythmic discharge with a rate more rapid than the SA node. This causes tachycardia (i.e., rapid heartbeat). The impulse also may repeatedly reenter the system, most often at the AV node–bundle of His junction (atrioventricular junction), causing overstimulation of the heart. With *epicardial* and *endocardial mapping* techniques, the surgeon is able to pinpoint electrical activity causing dysrhythmia. Preoperatively the mapping procedure is done under fluoroscopy. Electrical impulses from electrode catheters, placed in the heart via a femoral vein, activate sites in the heart to reproduce the abnormal rhythm and to obtain a direct electrocardiogram. Premature cycles, the origin of electrical signals, and accessory pathways can be pinpointed. Intraoperative mapping may be needed to correlate preoperative studies or to identify other sites or pathways masked by antiarrhythmic drugs. The origin and site of a dysrhythmia determine the surgical procedure.

Endocardial Resection

Severe ventricular dysrhythmias associated with ischemic heart disease and malignant ventricular tachydysrhythmias can be treated by ablating areas of endocardial damage (i.e., endocardial resection). The specific site or focus of the ventricular dysrhythmia is excised or the reentry pathway is interrupted. Atrial incisions may be made to channel electrical impulse from the SA node to the AV node to treat atrial focal tachycardia.

Cryoablation

When location of a ventricular tachycardia makes excision difficult, cryosurgery can be used to ablate the site. Cryoablation is also used to fuse the ends of fibers causing reentrant dysrhythmias from accessory pathways, as in Wolff-Parkinson-White syndrome. This syndrome is characterized by premature atrial beats that initiate supraventricular tachycardia or atrial fibrillation that can cause ventricular fibrillation. Many patients with this syndrome require cardioversion intraoperatively; thus external defibrillator pads are placed before the patient is draped. Partial cardiopulmonary bypass also is used as a precaution against hypotension and coronary damage from induced tachycardia during mapping and cardiac manipulation. Temporary pacing wires are sewn onto the heart (see p. 810) before the chest is closed.

Balloon Electric Shock Ablation

For balloon electric shock ablation, cardiopulmonary bypass is established and a small incision is made in the left atrium. A deflated balloon is passed through this incision and across the mitral valve into the left ventricle. The balloon is inflated to make contact with the endocardium for mapping with the electrodes inside the balloon. Electrical currents are passed through these electrodes to deliver electric shock to specific locations selected for ablation. Endocardial resection or cryoablation may be preferred when the focus of ventricular tachycardia is mapped intraoperatively using the balloon.

Ventricular Aneurysm

Atherosclerotic coronary disease predisposes an individual to myocardial infarction. Ventricular aneurysm, a segmental dilation of the ventricular wall, may develop any time from a few weeks to years after infarction. Predominantly occurring in the left ventricular wall, the aneurysm results from ventricular force on an area of nonfunctioning scar tissue. The thin-walled fibrous aneurysm often contains clots within it. A left ventricular aneurysm usually produces hemodynamic instability manifested by congestive heart failure and ventricular dysrhythmia. The surgeon can excise the aneurysm and reconstruct the ventricle.

The chest is opened by median sternotomy. Cardiopulmonary bypass is established before the adhesion between the aneurysm and pericardium is detached. The ascending aorta is cross-clamped. The aneurysmal sac is opened with a vertical incision. Fibrotic myocardium is excised circumferentially, leaving a rim of fibrous tissue to hold the sutures used to close the ventricle. Before completion of closure, air is removed from the ventricle by suction. The heartbeat is restored, decannulation is performed, and all incisions are closed.

Aneurysmectomy may be done as a single procedure or in conjunction with cardiomyoplasty, valve replacement, coronary artery bypass, or endocardial resection.

Cardiomyoplasty

Skeletal muscle flap can be used to reinforce the damaged heart muscle (i.e., cardiomyoplasty) in patients who are not candidates for cardiac transplantation because of medical contraindications or other exclusionary problems. Structurally, skeletal muscle is different from myocardial muscle and is more easily fatigued. After conditioning by electrical stimulation for several weeks preoperatively, the skeletal muscle is less prone to fatigue and endures repeated contraction at a normal heart rate caused by an implanted stimulator.

The two-step cardiomyoplasty procedure can be performed in a single surgical procedure or in two stages for patients who are unable to withstand long periods under general anesthesia. In step one, with the patient in left thoracotomy position, a muscle flap of latissimus dorsi, rectus abdominis, pectoralis, psoas, or diaphragm is dissected free. A small segment of the second or third rib is resected to form a window through which the flap is rotated upward into the mediastinum. Intramuscular pacing wires are woven into the musculature of the flap. In step two, with patient in supine position, a sternotomy is performed. The flap is wrapped around the damaged portion of myocardium and secured around the heart. The pericardium is not sutured closed. A small pocket is made in the skin of the upper abdomen, and a generator is implanted and attached subcutaneously to the ends of the pacing wires.

Cardiopulmonary bypass is not routinely used during the procedure, but it is available on a stand-by basis, if needed. Postoperatively some patients require ventricular counterpulsation with an intraaortic balloon pump until the muscle flap is fully functional. Postoperatively the stimuli for contraction is started at week 2 and gradually increased over a 4- to 6-week period so that the newly attached flap is not disrupted before proper healing has occurred. After 4 to 6 months, the flap to myocardial contraction ratio can reach 1:1 or 1:2. Contraindications to cardiomyoplasty include hypertrophic myocardium and end-stage cardiac disease because the muscle flap is unable to contract sufficiently over the thickened cardiac wall.

Cardiac Transplantation

Cardiac transplantation may be an acceptable option for the patient with limited life expectancy who is incapacitated by end-stage myocardial disease secondary to:

1. Valvular disease with cardiomyopathy
2. Coronary artery disease
3. Postmyocardial aneurysm
4. Idiopathic cardiomyopathy
5. Congenital heart disease
6. Cardiac tumor

See Chapter 44, p. 910, for discussion of heart allotransplantation.

Mechanical Devices

Mechanical assist devices may be indicated for patients with cardiac dysfunction. These devices may be implanted in conjunction with other cardiac surgical procedures or to provide long-term assistance for life-sustaining cardiac function.

Cardiac Pacemaker

The conducting system of the heart may be altered or interrupted at any point by degenerative disease, drugs, or surgical trauma. This may cause syncope, diminished cardiac output, hypotension, dysrhythmias, partial or complete heart block, or sinus bradycardia (sick sinus syndrome). Patients with these conditions may be treated by artificial pacing (i.e., delivery of electric impulse by a pacemaker) to correct atrial and ventricular dysrhythmias and to interrupt chronic atrial fibrillation.

A pacemaker consists of a pulse generator, which produces electrical impulses, and leads to carry impulses to stimulating electrodes placed in contact with the heart. A pacing system includes electromyocardial conduction. Lithium batteries supply power for years to the microprocessor of the pulse generator. Platinum alloy or stainless steel electrodes, with leads encased in plastic, may be unipolar or bipolar. With bipolar systems, electric current flows between two electrodes during pacing; it flows between the electrode tip and pulse generator in unipolar systems.

A pacemaker may be either a stand-by *ventricular demand* type or a *physiologic* type. Both types are intermittent and noncompetitive with the patient's own pacing system. They monitor the heart's normal activity. The impulse to stimulate the heart is not emitted unless the rate of heartbeat falls below a preset level. Also known as the R-wave–inhibited or QRS-inhibited pacemaker, electrodes of the ventricular demand pacemaker are placed in the ventricle. Stimulating electrodes are placed in the atrium or ventricle, or both, depending on the type of physiologic pacemaker to be used.

Effective external pacing for ventricular standstill led to the development of partially implanted electrode leads connected to an external stimulator for long-term pacing for other conditions. Fully implantable pacemaker systems for long-term use have been available since 1960. An implantable microprocessor generator is hermetically sealed in a metallic container impermeable to body fluids. Selection of a system depends on the specific pacing requirements of the individual patient. Pacemakers may be temporary or permanent. Endocardial (transvenous) or epicardial (myocardial) electrode leads may be used. Most of these units are programmable to alter pacing function. Temporary pacing is often necessary before and during permanent-system implantation. Systemic complete heart block and sinus bradycardia are the most frequent indications for permanent implantation. A single-chamber ventricular pacemaker may be implanted. The dual-chamber pacemaker, most commonly in the DDD mode (Table 39-1), senses and synchronously paces both chambers and triggers or inhibits response to vary the ventricular rate with the atrial rate. Permanent pacing may be initiated by the following devices.

Endocardial Pacemaker A transvenous electrode lead is placed in the endocardium and attached to a pulse generator. With local anesthesia, an incision is made just beneath the clavicle or in the deltopectoral groove, preferably on the side of the chest opposite the patient's dominant hand. The subcutaneous tissue is opened to underlying fascia to create a pocket for the pulse generator. The lead may be inserted through the cephalic, subclavian, or internal or external jugular vein. Under fluoroscopy the endocardial electrode catheter (lead) is advanced via the superior vena cava into the apex of the right ventricle, where it is wedged against the endocardium. Atrial leads are directed into the right atrial appendage. The lead is connected to the pulse generator, which in turn is placed into a previously prepared subcutaneous pocket. The incision is closed with or without suction drainage.

Epicardial Electrodes With the patient under general anesthesia, epicardial electrodes are placed via a transthoracic approach to the myocardium. For an extrapleural parasternal approach, the pericardium is entered by subperichondrial resection of the fifth costal cartilage. Two sew-on or screw-in type electrodes are implanted 1 cm apart in the myocardium of the right or left ventricle and/or atrium. After the pacing thresholds are measured from an external source, electrode leads are tunneled under the costal margin to the pulse generator implanted in a subcutaneous pocket in the left

TABLE 39-1

Identification Code for Cardiac Pacemakers*

FIRST LETTER (CHAMBER PACED)	SECOND LETTER (CHAMBER SENSED)	THIRD LETTER (MODE OF RESPONSE TO SENSING OF PATIENT'S HEART RATE)	FOURTH LETTER (PROGRAMMABLE FUNCTIONS)	FIFTH LETTER (TACHY-ARRHYTHMIA FUNCTION)
A = Atrium	A = Atrium	I = Inhibited response	P = Programmable rate and output only	N = Normal rate
V = Ventricle	V = Ventricle	T = Triggered response	M = Multiprogrammable	B = Bursts
D = Dual/both chambers	D = Dual/both chambers	D = Dual function/ inhibited and triggered response	C = Communicating noninvasive program	S = Scanning
	O = No sensing	R = Reverse response	O = Nonprogrammable	E = External
		O = No response		

*Sequence of letters describes parameters and functions.

upper quadrant of the abdominal wall. Water-seal chest drainage is necessary only if the pleura has been opened.

Precautions With Pacemakers Use of an electrosurgical unit is usually avoided during placement of a pacemaker or when a surgical procedure is performed on a patient with a pacemaker. Electromagnetic interference may affect the pulse generator, depending on the type of pacemaker. If it is necessary to use the electrosurgical unit, it should be kept as far away from the pulse generator as possible. The dispersive electrode should be placed on thigh area, not near chest.

A pacing system analyzer measures the amount of energy in milliamperes (mA) needed to stimulate the heart. It is used to locate area of myocardium where least amount of energy will be needed, generally 0.4 to 0.8 mA, and to test functioning of the electrode and pulse generator before placement. Telemetric communication capabilities of some pacemakers allow the surgeon to obtain direct evidence of battery output.

The patient with a pacemaker requires adequate follow-up care. He or she should carry identification containing the serial number, model, rate, manufacturer's name, and date of insertion. *The circulator records this information in the patient's chart, along with the time of insertion.* Patients with demand or radio-frequency units should be warned to avoid proximity to electromagnetic devices, such as microwave ovens, because electrical interference may stimulate heart activity. Newer models have metallic shielding to minimize this concern.

Battery depletion is the most common indication for replacement of the pulse generator. The old generator is removed from the subcutaneous pocket. A new one is connected to the electrode and inserted into the pocket. Occasionally electrode problems and/or erosion of or infection around the generator require surgical intervention.

Cardioverter-Defibrillator

The automatic implantable cardioverter-defibrillator (ICD) has the capability of recognizing potential life-threatening episodes of ventricular tachycardia or fibrillation. The system has a pair of sensing electrodes to monitor changes in heart rate, cycle length, and waveform. After the onset of ventricular tachycardia, two defibrillating electrodes deliver a synchronized shock to terminate it. The electrical conduction pattern of the heart is converted to a more normal pattern. Newer models are capable of pacing as well as defibrillating. Supplied sterile, the pulse generator of the device is powered by lithium batteries hermetically sealed in a titanium case. The device may be implanted in addition to endocardial resection or other ablation, or instead of a surgical procedure for dysrhythmia. Placement of this device is similar to procedures described for implantation of cardiac pacemakers.

The wavelength of the electrosurgical unit or magnetic field of magnetic resonance imaging (MRI) can deprogram the ICD and cause the device to discharge aberrant electrical current into the myocardium. A specialized electromagnetic wand can be placed over the chest to deactivate the device for subsequent surgical procedures requiring the use of electrosurgery. The same electromagnetic wand can be used to reactivate and reprogram the ICD. ICDs are not affected by household appliances, such as microwave ovens, computer terminals, or television sets.

Intraaortic Balloon Pump

An intraaortic balloon pump (IABP) is a left ventricular supportive device used to assist a patient with prolonged myocardial ischemia, reversible left ventricular failure, or cardiogenic shock. It often is inserted in the OR in conjunction with an open heart procedure for circulatory support during weaning from cardiopulmonary bypass. An IABP reduces left ventricular workload and increases delivery of oxygen to the myocardium, thereby increasing cardiac output and systemic perfusion. An IABP cannot be effective without partial ventricular function.

The cylinder-shaped balloon is inserted into the descending thoracic aorta, just below the left subclavian artery, by way of a femoral artery (Figure 39-5). The balloon catheter may be inserted percutaneously or by direct vision, or it can be inserted via a prosthetic arterial graft anastomosed end-to-side to the femoral artery. After insertion, the balloon catheter is connected to a pump console.

The IABP uses principles of *counterpulsation*. In contrast to systemic arteries, coronary arteries are constricted during systole and fill during diastole. Therefore, inflating the balloon during diastole increases coronary perfusion, aiding contractility and oxygen transport. When the balloon is inflated, the blood volume displaced increases coronary arterial pressure. When the balloon deflates during systole, the resistance against which the ventricle pumps is decreased. Balloons vary in size to provide 20, 30, or 40 ml volume displacement, thus giving a maximum assist without total aortic occlusion. When the balloon is placed and the position is verified by chest x-ray film, the complete system is vented of air and filled with either helium or carbon dioxide, for balloon inflation, depending on the type of counterpulsator. The ratio of ventricular assist is determined by the individual patient's hemodynamic status. The pump can be regulated automatically, triggered by an electrocardiogram signal, or operated manually. To prevent potential thrombi, pumping should be continuous. Intraaortic balloons are made of antithrombic material. The manufacturer's instructions for use should be followed. Pumps are equipped with sensors (e.g., alarm and automatic shut-off) to minimize danger.

Weaning from the IABP is usually gradual, as tolerated by the patient. Lower-extremity pulses are checked during and periodically after balloon catheter removal to assess circulation in foot on side of catheter insertion and to check for the presence of clots. Complications associated with an IABP include distal extremity ischemia, thrombus or emboli, gas embolism, arterial or aortic perforation, bleeding, and infection.

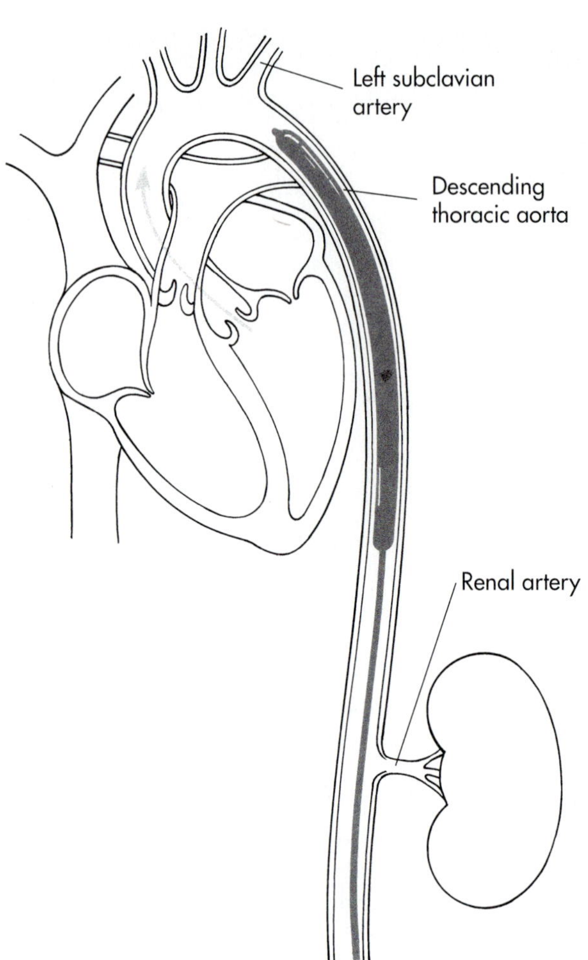

FIGURE 39-5 Intraaortic balloon catheter positioned in descending thoracic aorta, above renal artery and below left subclavian artery, via femoral artery.

Extracorporeal Membrane Oxygenator

An extracorporeal membrane oxygenator (ECMO) is used as a resuscitative device for patients who have potentially reversible respiratory and/or cardiac failure. It also is commonly used to prolong extracorporeal circulation when the patient is in distress after removal from cardiopulmonary bypass. ECMO also can be used for a short interim period to sustain the patient's life while waiting for an organ transplant or after major trauma.

Two methods of extracorporeal membrane oxygenation include:

1. *Venoarterial bypass.* The common carotid artery and the internal jugular vein are common sites for cannulation. Venoarterial bypass supports both heart and lungs by removing deoxygenated venous blood via a vein, removing carbon dioxide, adding oxygen, and returning the oxygenated blood to the body via an artery. The device is used for patients of all ages. It is the method of choice for cardiopulmonary assist in the preterm neonate because other appropriately sized assistive devices are unavailable.
2. *Venovenous bypass.* The right atrium and the femoral vein are common sites for cannulation.

Venovenous bypass supports pulmonary function by oxygenating venous blood and decreasing the circulating venous carbon dioxide level. The advantages are lower mechanical flow rates and decreased risk of arterial emboli. The patient receives ventilatory assist, which supplements the oxygenation process.

Ventricular Assist Device

A powered ventricular assist device (VAD) can be used to wean patients from cardiopulmonary bypass when the IABP, drugs, and/or cardiac pacing are ineffective, to support circulation following postinfarction cardiogenic shock or traumatic myocardial contusion, and to provide a temporary bridge for support before transplantation. The mechanical device maintains systemic and myocardial perfusion while promoting metabolic and hemodynamic recovery of a reversibly damaged myocardium. The VAD does not depend on cardiac contractility or electrical conduction. It acts as an artificial ventricle. The VAD consists of a flexible polyurethane blood sac, a flexible diaphragm, and a pump assembly enclosed within a rigid polysulfone housing. Inlet and outlet valves maintain unidirectional blood flow. The VAD is attached to the patient via inflow and outflow cannulas. Support can be to the left, right, or both ventricles.

1. *Left ventricular assistance (LVA).* Blood is withdrawn from left atrium into a left ventricular assist device (LVAD) and returned to ascending aorta. The polyurethane inflow cannula can be inserted into either left atrium or left ventricle. The outflow cannula has a segment of woven polyester that is anastomosed end-to-side to the thoracic aorta.
2. *Right ventricular assistance (RVA).* Blood is withdrawn from right atrium into right ventricular assist device (RVAD) and is returned to the pulmonary artery. The inflow cannula is placed in right atrium. The outflow cannula is anastomosed end-to-side to the main pulmonary artery.
3. *Biventricular assistance (BVA).* Both LVA and RVA devices are used to support both ventricles simultaneously.

The cannulas exit the pericardial sac below the costal margin. They are connected to parts of the VAD after removal of all air. Depending on intended duration of support, the housing is exteriorized or implanted.

1. *Extracorporeal* VAD, used for short-term ventricular assistance, is externally powered pneumatically with compressed air or electrically with centrifugal force. The housing rests on the patient's chest with the inflow and outflow cannulas passing through the chest wall. The power source is attached to the air-inlet port or pumphead. The skin is approximated or the chest is left open and covered with sterile material sutured to wound edges. Then the chest is covered with a sterile occlusive dressing. The patient returns to the OR for removal of the device and chest closure or heart transplantation, usually within 10 days.
2. *Implantable* VAD, for long-term use, is an electrically activated pump implanted in left upper quadrant of the abdomen. The internal battery pack and control unit in the housing are connected to an external battery pack. The cannulas pass through the diaphragm.

The rate of pumping and movement of the diaphragm inside the VAD are programmed by the power console. Another type of LVAD is mounted on a catheter connected to a pump and external motor. The catheter, inserted via femoral artery or by transthoracic or retroperitoneal approach, draws blood out of left ventricle and returns it to descending aorta.

Total Artificial Heart

Clinical trials are in process to test an artificial heart that can be permanently implanted to maintain circulation in the patient with irreparable myocardial damage or end-stage cardiac disease who does not meet the criteria for cardiac transplantation. A total artificial heart also could be used as temporary support while the patient is awaiting a transplant.

In 1982 William DeVries implanted the first total artificial heart. The Jarvik-7 was an air-driven, double-chambered device that replaced the ventricles. Connector cuffs were sutured to the atria, pulmonary artery, and aorta. These cuffs attached to rims of openings on the device. Power was supplied to the pumping chamber through percutaneous tubes to an external source of compressed air. The patient was essentially tethered to a machine. Many complications, such as emboli, hemorrhage, and infection, were associated with the device.

A newer, totally contained artificial heart is powered electrically with the addition of a hydraulic actuator that will increase cardiac output during exercise and decrease the potential for hematologic complications. A double diaphragm type of pump is implanted in the chest to work in place of the ventricles. The power source is smaller and quieter than the Jarvik-7 and connects to the device via cables through the skin. The efficiency and compactness of the unit permit limited activity.

General Considerations

Many devices are available for cardiac pacing, ventricular support, and treatment of cardiogenic shock. A portable cardiopulmonary support system, external pulsatile pump, and other devices are used. It is critical that these devices be properly sterilized and handled. *Read package labels and inserts for specific manufacturer's instructions.* The circulator should affix labels and record serial numbers and identifying data in the patient's chart. In the event of a mechanical failure, this information becomes important.

The scrub person should set a separate table for assembling devices. Check to be certain all parts are available. A missing component could be catastrophic.

COMPLICATIONS OF CARDIAC SURGERY

Cardiogenic shock may be precipitated by coronary air embolism, pulmonary embolism, myocardial contusion, mechanical venous obstruction, or hypothermia. Precautions are taken intraoperatively to avoid postoperative cardiogenic and/or hemorrhagic shock. Excessive bleeding can result from stress to the clotting mechanism. Cardiac tamponade (i.e., the filling of pericardial sac with blood, thus compressing the heart) is potentially fatal. Sinus bradycardia, supraventricular tachycardia, ventricular tachycardia, and other dysrhythmias are common in the immediate postoperative period following open heart surgery. Infections of the sternum and/or mediastinum may require additional surgical intervention, such as muscle grafting and debridement. Infection of the cardiac suture line can be a fatal complication. Infection of a prosthetic valve or implanted device can cause endocarditis, malfunction, hemodynamic abnormalities, or embolus. Attention to sterile technique and patient monitoring is especially critical during cardiac surgery.

BIBLIOGRAPHY

Abou-Awdi N et al: New support for the failing heart, *Am J Nurs* 91(1):38-41, 1991.

Ainsworth W: ECMO: some infants' last chance, *Can Nurs* 89(9):27-30, 1993.

Anderson H et al: Extracorporeal life support for adult cardiorespiratory failure, *Surgery* 114(2):161-172, 1993.

Anderson JR et al: Comparison of two strategies for myocardial management during coronary artery operations, *Ann Thorac Surg* 58(3):768-772, 1994.

Antonioli LC, Bennett HC: Vein harvesting for coronary bypass surgery: the RN first assistant's role, *AORN J* 59(5):969-982, 1994.

Bavin TK, Self MA: Weaning from intra-aortic balloon pump support, *Am J Nurs* 91(10):54-59, 1991.

Beattie S: CABG surgery: the second time around, *Am J Nurs* 93(8):42-45, 1993.

Bell PE, Diffee GT Jr: Cardiopulmonary bypass, *AORN J* 53(6):1480-1496, 1991.

Borst HG et al: Tactics and techniques of aortic arch replacement, *J Cardiovasc Surg* 9(5):538-547, 1994.

Bower JO: New therapy for ventricular arrhythmias: implantable cardioverter/defibrillators with pacing therapies, *AORN J* 59(5):985-996, 1994.

Brunet F et al: Extracorporeal carbon dioxide removal technique improves oxygenation without causing overinflation, *Am J Respir Crit Care Med* 149(6):1557-1562, 1994.

Bubien RS et al: What you need to know about radiofrequency ablation, *Am J Nurs* 93(7):30-36, 1993.

Collins MA: When your patient has an implantable cardioverter defibrillator, *Am J Nurs* 94(3):34-38, 1994.

del Nindo PJ et al: Extracorporeal membrane oxygenation support as bridge to pediatric heart transplantation, *Circulation* 90(5):66-69, 1994.

Donn SM: Alternatives to ECMO, *Arch Dis Child* 70(2):81-83, 1994.

Dougherty KG et al: Laser ablation of coronary arteries: preliminary findings, *AORN J* 54(2):244-261, 1991.

Ergin MA et al: Hypothermic circulatory arrest and other methods of cerebral protection during operations on the thoracic aorta, *J Cardiovasc Surg* 9(5):525-527, 1994.

Gallegos-Alvarez M, O'Brien M: Right gastroepiploic artery conduit use in myocardial revascularization, *AORN J* 60(5):763-777, 1994.

Glynn L et al: Extracorporeal membrane oxygenation in pediatric patients, *Surg Technol* 24(5):8-12, 1992.

Good LP, Gentzler RD: Coronary atherectomy, *AORN J* 53(1):32-39, 1991.

Hages N, Jabr K: Continuous warm blood cardioplegia, *Surg Technol* 25(6):8-12, 1993.

Hayashida N et al: The optimal cardioplegic temperature, *Ann Thorac Surg* 58(4):961-971, 1994.

Jameson N, Bates JD: Practical innovations: protecting the phrenic nerve during open heart surgery, *AORN J* 58(2):325-328, 1993.

Kater KM et al: Corralling atrial fibrillation with "Maze" surgery, *Am J Nurs* 92(7):34-38, 1992.

Kato NS et al: Inaccuracies and variability of indirect pressure measurements during cardioplegia administration, *Ann Thorac Surg* 58(4):1188-1191, 1994.

Koroteyev A et al: Skeletal muscle: new techniques for treating heart failure, *AORN J* 53(4):1005-1020, 1991.

Kouchoukos NT et al: Management of the severely atherosclerotic aorta during cardiac operations, *J Cardiovasc Surg* 9(5):490-494, 1994.

Kurose M et al: Emergency and long-term extracorporeal life support following acute myocardial infarction: rescue from severe cardiogenic shock related to stunned myocardium, *Clin Cardiol* 17(10): 552-557, 1994.

Magovern GJ Jr et al: Extracorporeal membrane oxygenation: preliminary results in patients with postcardiotomy cardiogenic shock, *Ann Thorac Surg* 57(6):1462-1468, 1994.

Martella AT et al: Continuous normothermic retrograde cardioplegia for valve surgery, *J Heart Valve Dis* 3(4):404-409, 1994.

May D, Daley K: Percutaneous transluminal coronary angioplasty: study of open heart surgical standby: effective patient, OR management, *AORN J* 59(4):811-819, 1994.

McEwen DR: Postoperative complications related to coronary artery bypass grafting, *AORN J* 60(6):982-988, 1994.

McLean RF et al: Cardiopulmonary bypass, temperature, and central nervous system dysfunction, *Circulation* 90(5):250-255, 1994.

Mickleborough LL et al: Transatrial balloon technique for activation mapping during operations for recurrent ventricular tachycardia, *J Thorac Cardiovasc Surg* 99(2):227-233, 1990.

Phillips SJ: Resuscitation for cardiogenic shock with extracorporeal membrane oxygenation systems, *Semin Thorac Cardiovasc Surg* 6(3):131-135, 1994.

Plotkin JS et al: Extracorporeal membrane oxygenation in the successful treatment of traumatic adult respiratory distress syndrome: case report and review, *J Trauma* 37(1):127-130, 1994.

Quaal SJ: *Comprehensive intra-aortic balloon counterpulsation,* ed 2, St Louis, 1993, Mosby.

Regas ML: Reoperative cardiac surgery, *AORN J* 57(5):1131-1148, 1993.

Seifert PC: *Mosby's perioperative nursing series: cardiac surgery,* St Louis, 1994, Mosby.

Strimike CL: Caring for a patient with an intracoronary stent, *Am J Nurs* 95(1):40-45, 1995.

Vargo RL: Bridging to transplant: mechanical support for heart failure, *Crit Care Nurs Clin North Am* 5(4):649-659, 1993.

Witherell CL: Questions nurses ask about pacemakers, *Am J Nurs* 90(12):20-26, 1990.

Wouters R: Sternitis and mediastinitis after coronary artery bypass grafting: analysis of risk factors, *Tex Heart Inst J* 21(3):183-188, 1994.

Wright PA, Elkins RC: Pulmonary autograft: an aortic valve replacement alternative, *AORN J* 56(4):639-656, 1992.

CHAPTER 40

Peripheral Vascular Surgery

Circulation within the peripheral vascular system affects the brain, internal organs, and the extremities. An expanding body of knowledge relating to vascular physiology and development of the art of vascular surgery has improved the quality of life for many patients with peripheral vascular diseases.

HISTORICAL BACKGROUND

For centuries human beings have been plagued with peripheral vascular disease and its complications, such as pain or loss of an extremity or life. However, little was understood about diseases of the vascular system that cause arterial stenosis or occlusion until the contributions of the Scottish brothers William and John Hunter. Their studies of aneurysm formation, pathology, and treatment provided the foundation for concepts of modern vascular surgery. William Hunter (1718-1783) was the first to describe an arteriovenous fistula and aneurysm. Then John Hunter (1728-1793) performed a successful surgical procedure for popliteal aneurysm. Others subsequently experimented with vascular anastomoses. Alexis Carrel (1873-1944) received the Nobel prize in 1912 for his work at the University of Chicago with blood vessel anastomoses and organ transplantation. Suturing of blood vessels was the vital link necessary for the development of successful vascular surgery.

An endarterectomy to remove a localized vascular occlusion was first performed in 1946. In 1948 the first bypass graft was implanted to treat diffuse vascular disease. In the following decades many surgical procedures have become feasible with use of improved diagnostic techniques and instrumentation, sutures, synthetic grafts, and microvascular techniques.

In 1983 the American Board of Surgery began a certification program in general vascular surgery. To qualify, candidates must have specialized training and practice in peripheral vascular surgery and be a Diplomate of the American Board of Surgery or the American Board of Thoracic Surgery.

PERIPHERAL VASCULAR SYSTEM

Circulatory problems may affect any part of the body, but this discussion focuses on the most common pathologic conditions amenable to vascular procedures performed by vascular surgeons.

Anatomy and Physiology

Vessels in the thorax, abdomen, extremities, and extracranial cerebrovascular area constitute the *circulatory system* (Figure 40-1). The ascending aorta, originating from the left ventricle, carries oxygenated blood from the heart to the arteries. The major arteries leading to the head and upper extremities branch off from the aortic arch in the middle mediastinum above the heart. These are the brachiocephalic trunk, left common carotid, and subclavian arteries. The thoracic aorta then descends through the posterior mediastinum at the left side of the vertebral column. Passing through the diaphragm, the abdominal aorta descends to the level of

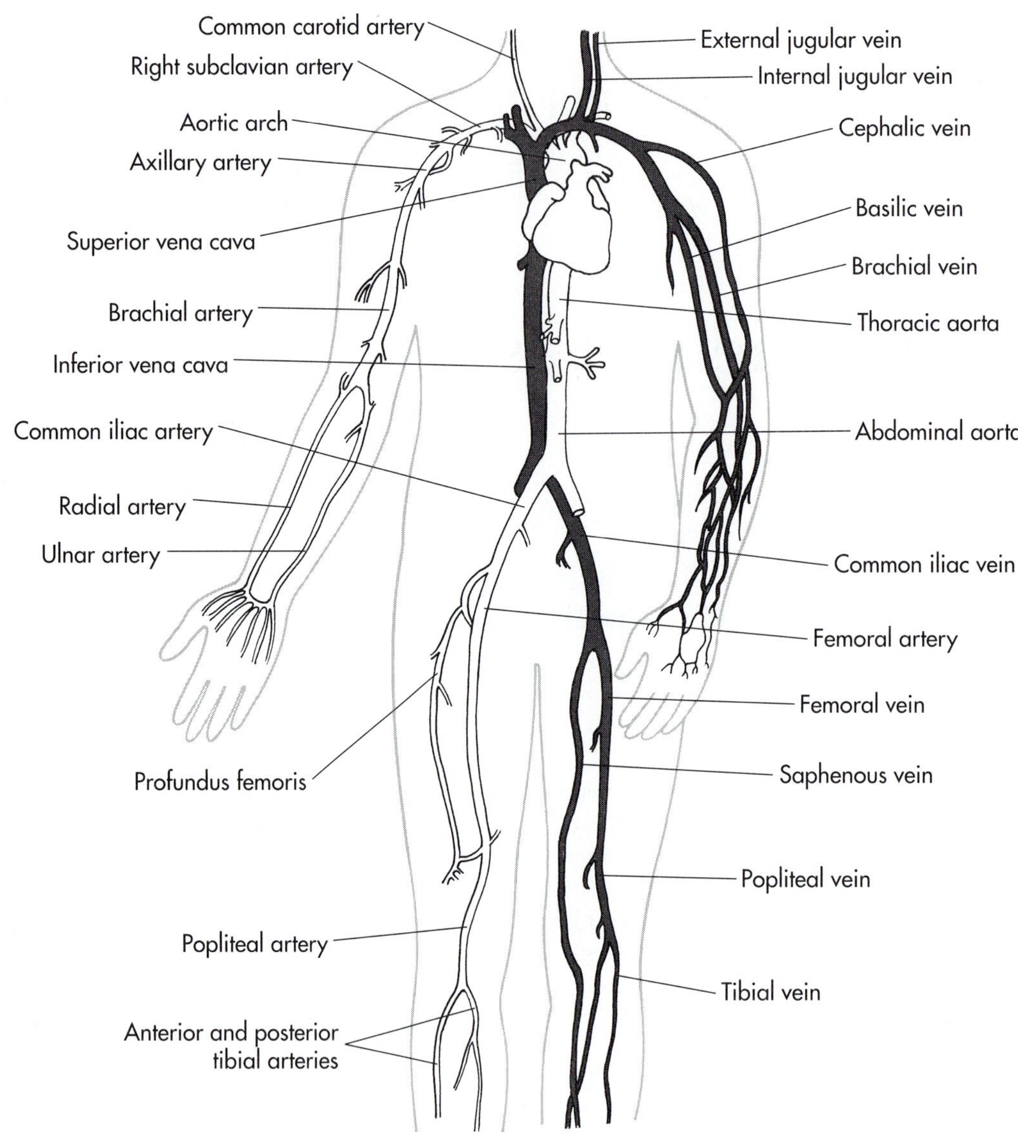

FIGURE 40-1 Circulatory system. Arteries are shown as white vessels. Veins are shown as black vessels.

the fourth lumbar vertebra where it bifurcates (i.e., divides) to form the common iliac arteries leading to the lower extremities. Arteries from the abdominal aorta carry blood to the kidneys and the abdominal and pelvic organs. The femoral artery, originating from the iliac, is the main artery in each leg.

Blood flows from the arterial system through the capillary network and returns to the heart via the venous system. The venae cavae enter the right atrium. The superior vena cava, formed by the union of the two brachiocephalic veins, returns unoxygenated venous blood from the head, neck, upper extremities, and chest. The inferior vena cava, which begins at the level of the fifth lumbar vertebra, returns blood from the lower extremities, pelvis, and abdominal organs.

The walls of the blood vessels have three layers: the *intima,* the innermost smooth endothelial layer in contact with the blood; the *media,* the middle muscular layer; and the *adventitia,* the outer layer of connective tissue.

Vascular Disease

Vascular diseases that cause occlusion or stenosis are usually acquired. *Atherosclerosis* is the most common arterial disease. It is a diffuse disease, beginning as a disruption of the intima of a large artery. Cholesterol enters the media to stimulate muscle growth, and platelets accumulate around the disruption of the intima to form plaque or a thrombus. Often this process becomes localized around vessel orifices and branches (i.e., at bifurcations). The disease may produce stenosis (narrowing) and subsequent occlusion or ectasia (dilation) and aneurysm. Atherosclerosis is the principal factor in transient ischemic attacks (TIAs), cerebrovascular accident (stroke), myocardial infarction (heart attack), and aortic stenosis. Risk factors include familial history, a high serum cholesterol level, smoking, and hypertension (Box 40-1).

Inadequate blood supply causes ischemia in tissues. If untreated, this can lead to thrombus, embolus, ulceration, necrosis, or gangrene. Obstruction to venous return, venous stasis disease, can cause hemodynamic imbalances. Through vascular surgery, vessels are repaired, reconstructed, or replaced to improve peripheral (systemic) circulation. The most frequently performed procedures are done to revascularize a lower extremity for limb salvage, to repair an aortoiliac aneurysm, and to improve cerebral blood flow through the carotid arteries.

Diagnostic Procedures

Preoperative assessment of cardiac risk is critically important in planning the care of a patient who requires major vascular surgery. Then peripheral arterial and venous diseases are assessed. Table 40-1 compares assessment factors of peripheral arterial and venous obstructive diseases in an extremity. Peripheral vascular laboratories, similar to cardiac catheterization laboratories, have been established in many health care facilities to perform noninvasive studies before and following surgical intervention.

Noninvasive Procedures

Computed tomography (CT) and *magnetic resonance imaging* (MRI) are noninvasive techniques of choice to confirm a diagnosis of aortic aneurysm, thrombus, or

BOX 40-1

Risk Factors for Development of Peripheral Vascular Disease

- Advanced age
- Diabetes
- Familial predisposition
- Habitual long periods of standing
- High-fat diet causing high serum cholesterol
- Hypertension
- Obesity
- Repeated pregnancies
- Sedentary lifestyle
- Smoking
- Stress

TABLE 40-1

Comparison of Peripheral Arterial and Venous Obstructive Diseases in an Extremity

ASSESSMENT OF EXTREMITY	ARTERIAL OBSTRUCTIVE DISEASE	VENOUS OBSTRUCTIVE DISEASE
Color	Dusky, blue, gray, pallor distal to obstruction	Red, purple, brown hemosiderin spots
Temperature	Cool, cold	Warm, hot
Visual and palpable	Dry, shiny, flaking; vessels not obvious; lack of hair on affected part	Moist, peeling; vessels may be tortuous and inflamed; thickened tissue
Sensation	Numbness, tingling, pain during exercise (intermittent claudication); pain at rest in severe disease; increased pain when exposed to cold	Aching, throbbing, tightness, feeling of heaviness; muscles feel fatigued
Mobility	Painful range of motion, limited flexion and extension caused by avascular necrosis at the tissue level; elasticity is diminished	Painful range of motion, limited flexion and extension caused by congestive edema in joints
Size	Not enlarged, average for body build	Swollen, edematous
Integrity of surface layer	Peeling, infarcted, serous oozing ulcers	Stasis ulceration, open draining ulcers
Pulses	Weak or absent	Usually present
Condition of digits	Mottled, blackened, fragile, painful; can become gangrenous	Edematous, reddened, painful; can become gangrenous

atherosclerotic plaque in arterial walls, especially in the abdominal and carotid circulation. *Carotid phonoangiography* and *oculoplethysmography* are techniques to obtain blood-flow measurements to localize obstructions in vessels of the head and neck. A *pulse volume recorder* can also be used to localize segmental obstructions in the vascular system. *Photoplethysmography* is used to measure systolic pressure in digital arterial systems. Diagnosis of deep vein thrombosis may be made by *phleborheography,* a plethysmographic technique in which recordings are obtained of rhythmic changes in venous volume in the legs associated with respiration.

Ultrasonography, which is a major diagnostic tool to measure segmental arterial pressures and venous patency in extremities, may be used for abdominal circulation as well. Doppler color-coded flow imaging and transcranial Doppler imaging are replacing carotid phonoangiography and ocular plethysmography for evaluation of carotid circulation. High-resolution, B-mode ultrasound provides real-time images of venous systems in the upper and lower extremities. Saphenous and cephalic vein mapping accurately measures vein diameter, location, and quality for preoperative determination of suitability of the vein for use as an arterial conduit in arterial reconstruction. Ultrasound also detects venous thrombosis. With a pulse Doppler blood-flow detector, longitudinal and/or transverse cross-sectional scans are obtained. The images are produced on the screen of storage oscilloscope. A photograph of the screen provides a permanent record of the arteriograph or venograph.

Invasive Procedures

Selective *angiography* permits radiographic study of a particular segment of the vascular system. *Aortography* visualizes the aorta. *Arteriography* shows patency of an artery or a branch of the aorta and its collateral circulation. *Phlebography* detects deep vein thrombosis; a venogram visualizes veins. Angiography requires injection of a nontoxic radiopaque substance. The pain associated with injection of intraarterial contrast material can be so intense that the procedure may be done under continuous epidural anesthesia or general anesthesia.

Angioscopy is an endoscopic technique to visualize the interior of vessels. A small (ranging from 1.5 to 3 mm) flexible fiberoptic angioscope has a coupling for magnification of the view onto a television monitor. The lining and structures within the blood vessels are visualized as the scope is advanced within each vessel. Angioscopy is an alternative preoperative diagnostic technique to angiography for many patients and may be used to evaluate the effectiveness of therapy intraoperatively. It can reveal retained atherosclerotic plaque or thrombus and suture lines.

Intravascular ultrasonic scanning employs a miniaturized ultrasonic probe at the end of a 5 to 9 French catheter. The probe is introduced into the vessel percutaneously. Images are obtained of the entire circumference to determine thickness of vessel wall and distribution of plaque within the wall. This technique may be used intraoperatively as well as percutaneously.

SPECIAL FEATURES OF PERIPHERAL VASCULAR SURGERY

Vascular injury can occur during invasive diagnostic, monitoring, or therapeutic procedures. Iatrogenic arterial injuries, those resulting from an unexpected outcome of a procedure, can cause loss of function or even death from ischemia, hemorrhage, or embolus. The patient must be carefully observed and monitored for signs of complications during and following vascular procedures. Infection is a devastating postoperative complication that must be avoided through strict adherence to aseptic and sterile techniques. Other considerations include the following:

1. Thorough understanding of principles of general surgery should be combined with special training in vascular surgical techniques. An experienced operating team is essential because of the tendency of blood to clot. Speed and accuracy are imperative.
2. Hypothermia/hyperthermia blanket or mattress is put on the operating table before patient arrives, in the event that it is needed. Temperature regulation may be a problem during long procedures or when multiple blood transfusions are given.
3. Local or monitored anesthesia care (MAC) is usually preferred for most conservative interventional procedures (see pp. 822-823). General anesthesia or regional block is used for surgical procedures.
4. Meticulous care is exercised in anastomosing vessels to avoid danger of postoperative thrombosis and stenosis.
5. To prevent undue trauma to vessels, an assortment of scissors, noncrushing vascular clamps, and forceps specifically designed for vascular surgery is included in the instrument setup. Umbilical tape or synthetic vessel loops are used for retraction and vascular control.
6. Operating microscope may be used for anastomosing vessels. Appropriate instrumentation for microsurgery must be available.
7. Synthetic nonabsorbable suture materials are preferred because they are strong and pass through vessel walls and grafts easily with minimal trauma and tissue reaction. Swaged needles also minimize trauma. A larger swaged suture-to-needle ratio is

advantageous to avoid leakage. Holes made in graft materials by needle are occluded by the larger suture. Double-armed needle sutures are frequently used for vessel anastomosis.

8. Heparinized solution must be available for use as an anticoagulant. If given intravenously for immediate systemic effect, the optimal dose is 70 to 100 units per kilogram of body weight. Thromboelastography may be used intraoperatively to monitor effects of heparin administration. At end of procedure, before closure, protamine sulfate in an equivalent dose may be given to reverse the anticoagulant effect.
9. Hemostatic agents can be used independently or in combination. An absorbable gelatin sponge, microfibrillar collagen, oxidized cellulose, and topical thrombin should be available. Vasodilators and vasopressors must be available.
10. Blood must be available for replacement if the hematocrit level falls below 26%. Blood is lost by the flushing of clots and debris. Blood loss should be calculated. Blood may be salvaged from the thoracic or abdominal cavity during procedures on great vessels for autotransfusion (see Chapter 23, p. 486). A cell-saver device may be used to salvage only red blood cells for platelet transfusion. Blood may be warmed before transfusion to help prevent inadvertent hypothermia.
11. Antiembolic stockings should be worn by the patient during and following the surgical procedure.
12. Doppler ultrasound, pulse volume recorder, and/or intravascular imaging techniques are used intraoperatively to monitor hemodynamic changes and to assess blood flow following peripheral vascular reconstruction. A pulmonary artery catheter (Swan-Ganz) is usually inserted to monitor pulmonary artery pressures during and following the procedure.

The most serious immediate postoperative complications are thrombus and hemorrhage. The patient may need to return to the operating room (OR) for *immediate* correction of these problems.

Vascular Prostheses

Biologic or synthetic prosthetic grafts are required to bypass vascular obstruction or to reconstruct vessels. These substitute conduits for blood flow vary in length, diameter, and configuration to meet requirements of each situation. A graft may be straight or bifurcated into a Y shape. Pieces of synthetic material may be cut to size for use as patch grafts.

The American National Standards Institute has established requirements for product characteristics and labeling of textile and nontextile synthetic grafts, vascular homografts, and vascular heterografts. Grafts sterilized in see-through containers or packages permit the surgeon to select the appropriate size after exposure of the surgical site. Manufacturer's instructions for sterilizing and handling must be strictly followed.

Biologic Vascular Grafts

Autografts, homografts, and heterografts may be used for arterial or venous grafting.

Saphenous Vein An autogenous vein is an ideal graft because it is lined with endothelial cells, which inhibit clotting. These cells produce fibrinolytic substances and plasminogen factor essential to maintain patency. The saphenous vein is most commonly used for an autogenous arterial bypass or vein graft. It is used in one of two ways:

1. *In situ conduit/bypass.* To revascularize a lower extremity, the saphenous vein is exposed but left in place. Using microscissors, a valvulotome, and/or a disposable valve cutter, the surgeon cuts the valves to allow reversal of blood flow. The artery to be bypassed is anastomosed proximally and distally to the saphenous vein. This technique minimizes trauma to the vein and preserves endothelial structure and antithrombogenic properties. Renal and mesenteric revascularization also can be accomplished by grafting nonreversed segments of saphenous vein.
2. *Reversed vein graft.* When a segment of saphenous vein is harvested for placement in the arterial system, the vein is reversed from its normal anatomic position so that the valves will not obstruct arterial blood flow. The endothelial integrity must be maintained by gentle dissection and handling. Two surgeons may work simultaneously, one exposing the surgical site while the other prepares the vein for grafting. A separate sterile table, supplied with fine vascular instruments, is used for vein preparation. The surgeon may wear magnification loupes to check for imperfections in the vein. The valves may be cut, especially in small-diameter segments. The vein is flushed with cold solution, usually heparinized plasmalyte with papaverine hydrochloride, and immersed in this solution until the recipient site is prepared.

Synthetic Vascular Prostheses

Various forms of synthetic materials are used to construct arterial vascular prostheses. Some materials are more suitable for specific applications than are others. The surgeon selects the most appropriate graft for each patient.

Knitted Polyester Knitted polyester (Dacron) grafts are porous enough to allow ingrowth of fibrous tissue into interstices. However, they are also porous enough to allow seepage of blood through the material. Therefore they must be preclotted before insertion. For the *preclotting process,* the surgeon withdraws blood from the patient at the surgical site before anticoagulation therapy. The blood is transferred to the scrub person, who may inject it into lumen of the graft and/or soak the graft in blood in a sterile basin. The prime goal in preclotting is to make the wall of the graft impervious to blood by filling interstices with fibrin. The fabric-fibrin conduit later becomes firmly placed in tissue and provides a hypothrombogenic flow surface.

Filamentous Velour Knitted velour construction of polyester grafts has uniform porosity for easy preclotting and ensures rapid tissue ingrowth. They may be crimped or noncrimped, with velour inside and/or outside. One type, the exoskeleton (EXS) prosthesis, has a spiral polypropylene support fused to the outer surface of noncrimped velour. This graft was developed specifically for use across the knee joint. Another type, with amikacin bonded to knitted filamentous velour polyester with a collagen matrix, provides an antibiotic in the prosthetic wall. This construction also renders the porous graft impervious to leaks, obviating the need for preclotting. Bonded albumin also reduces porosity and potential thrombosis. This can be achieved by "baking on" autologous plasma. The graft is soaked in the patient's plasma and then steam sterilized. This thermal process alters the fibrin and protein elements in plasma.

Woven Polyester The weave of woven polyester (Dacron) grafts is tight enough to be leakproof. Therefore these grafts do not require preclotting. The more inflexible construction limits their use, however, to aortic replacement or bypass of large caliber arteries.

Polytetrafluorethylene The microporous wall of polytetrafluoroethylene (PTFE) serves as a lattice framework into which cells grow to become a microthin lining for contact with blood. These prostheses (Gore-Tex, Impra) do not require preclotting. Vascular grafts, constructed of expanded and reinforced PTFE, maintain dimensional stability. Configuration may be straight, tapered, or bifurcated. It may be supported by external rings to resist compression.

The inside lumen of the graft may be seeded during the surgical procedure with the patient's own endothelial cells to sustain patency. The graft may be bonded with an antibiotic before implantation to prevent infection.

Composite Vein Graft

A composite graft of autogenous vein and synthetic, usually PTFE, may be the surgeon's choice as a substitute for an insufficient length of saphenous vein. The prosthetic graft is anastomosed to a segment of reversed or in situ autogenous vein, usually the saphenous. A cephalic vein may be used for a graft. The prosthetic graft must be cut to match the diameter of the vein.

CONSERVATIVE INTERVENTIONAL THERAPY

Peripheral vascular disease is often managed by a team of collaborating vascular surgeons, cardiologists, and radiologists. Multifaceted care encompasses invasive interventional procedures to treat occlusive disease conservatively.

Percutaneous Transluminal Angioplasty

Severe ischemia or incapacitating claudication resulting from localized or segmental stenosis or occlusive disease can be conservatively treated by recanalization to restore the lumen in the obstructed vessel. Atherosclerosis in the iliac, femoral, and popliteal arteries is the most common indication for *percutaneous transluminal angioplasty* (PTA). Stenosis in renal arteries also can be treated.

PTA is performed under local anesthesia and fluoroscopy, frequently in the radiology department by a radiologist or in the angiography or cardiac catheterization laboratory by a cardiologist. The artery is punctured percutaneously, and a guidewire is advanced through the stenosis or occlusion. Various techniques are used to dilate a stenotic lesion or to displace or ablate plaque.

Balloon Angioplasty

A Gruntzig or other type of balloon dilation catheter is passed over the guidewire and positioned across the lesion. Catheters of several diameters with balloons of various widths and lengths are available. Determination of appropriate balloon size and length is made on the basis of angiogram findings. When the balloon is inflated, atheromatous material is compressed against the arterial wall. It remolds and cracks, splitting the plaque and intima (inner lining) and stretching the media (middle layer) and adventitia (outer layer), thus dilating the lumen of a stenosis or recanalizing an occlusion. The balloon is repeatedly inflated and deflated until the lumen is dilated.

Intraluminal Stent A prosthetic stent may be placed along the vessel wall to maintain patency following dilation. The Palmaz stent, for example, is a stainless steel mesh tube mounted coaxially on a balloon angioplasty catheter. After the stent is positioned in the artery, the balloon is inflated to expand the stent. The stent remains in place when the balloon is deflated and removed. Stents made of titanium, polypropylene, or other materials either operate in a similar manner or are self-expanding, such as the Gianturco stent.

Laser Angioplasty

For laser angioplasty a laser fiber is introduced into an occluded artery to destroy plaque or thrombi. The laser usually is used to supplement balloon angioplasty. The procedure may be done percutaneously or as an open surgical procedure via an angioscope. Several different types of laser probes are available. The physician selects the most appropriate probe on the basis of location and size of the artery and determination of the degree of calcification in plaque or other cause of obstruction. The delivery system determines the mechanism of action.

1. *Thermal laser* uses argon or Nd:YAG laser energy to heat the tip of a metal probe to a temperature between 392° and 752° F (200° and 400° C). The probe is at end of a fiberoptic catheter. Plaque is vaporized as the tip is moved through the obstruction. This "hot-tip" technique may cause some damage to vessel walls. The laser fiber may be positioned within a balloon to destroy thrombus selectively or to seal arterial wall while vessel is dilated. Temperature between 203° and 230° F (95° and 110° C) in surrounding tissues dries and disintegrates thrombus. The combination of pressure from inflated balloon and diffuse laser energy adheres loose flaps of arterial tissue back onto the arterial wall, a process known as *arterial welding*.
2. *Photothermal laser* uses contact Nd:YAG laser energy. A sapphire-tipped probe or catheter heats plaque by photooptical effect at the point of contact for vaporization of plaque, followed by rapid cooling to prevent damage to intima.
3. *Photochemical laser* uses an excimer laser with pulsed energy or a tunable dye laser to destroy plaque with minimal generation of heat. With the athermal action of a "cold laser," the intima is not damaged. However, heavily calcified plaque cannot be ablated by excimer laser.

Intravascular Ultrasonic Energy

An ultrasonic probe on the tip of a catheter can be used to recanalize occluded or stenosed peripheral vessels.

Atherectomy

In atherectomy catheter-mounted instruments are used for transluminal removal of atherosclerotic plaque. A high-speed rotating cam, burr, and/or side cutter are positioned under fluoroscopic guidance. The plaque is pulverized and retrieved to restore patency of the vessel. These instruments may be used intraoperatively.

Thrombectomy and Embolectomy

For thrombectomy and embolectomy a local anesthetic is infiltrated percutaneously. A Fogarty catheter is inserted proximally and advanced into a vessel distally beyond an obstruction. The balloon on the tip is inflated. As the catheter is withdrawn, thrombotic or embolic material is removed to restore blood flow, usually to an extremity. This procedure may be done with fluoroscopy to selectively cannulate vessels.

Fibrinolytic Therapy

In fibrinolytic therapy streptokinase or urokinase may be given by local bolus infusion into the occluded vessel or directly injected into the thrombus. These drugs activate plasminogen and cause liquefaction of fibrin, thus dissolving the clot or loosening it for removal by balloon catheter. This therapy may be used in conjunction with angioplasty (thrombolysoangioplasty) or infused intraoperatively, especially in tibial vessels, for lower limb salvage.

NOTE Vascular instruments and supplies for an open surgical procedure must be immediately available in the event a vessel is perforated or injured during any of the conservative interventional techniques. A perforation may be closed with sutures; a patch graft, in situ conduit, or synthetic prosthesis may be necessary.

PERIPHERAL VASCULAR SURGICAL PROCEDURES

If conservative therapy is unsuccessful or contraindicated, a surgical procedure may be indicated.

Arterial Bypass

Occlusive disease or trauma may cause blockage of an artery. Arterial injury may indirectly occur near site of fractures. The vessel lumina above and below the lesion is usually normal. Vascular reconstruction is performed in an attempt to restore normal circulation. The surgeon selects an appropriate method to bypass the obstruction.

1. Involved segment may be excised and the ends anastomosed if they can be approximated without tension.
2. If direct suture is impossible, the involved segment is excised and an autograft or synthetic prosthetic graft is used as replacement.
3. Lesion can be bypassed using the long saphenous vein from one thigh as a vein graft, or a synthetic prosthetic graft may be used. Ends of the graft are anastomosed to the artery proximal and distal to the lesion. The obstructed segment of the artery is not resected.
4. Lesion can be bypassed by interposing a prosthetic graft between a patent artery and the artery

distal to lesion, an *extraanatomic bypass*. The graft is placed in subcutaneous tissues. For example, in femoral-femoral bypass, graft is placed from femoral artery of the unaffected leg to the femoral artery of the ischemic leg. In axillofemoral bypass, graft is placed from axillary artery to femoral artery of the ischemic leg.

Femoropopliteal Bypass

The femoral artery is most prone to obstruction by occlusive vascular disease in a lower extremity. A femoropopliteal bypass may be procedure of choice for severe ischemic disease and limb salvage. It is the most frequently performed bypass procedure in an extremity. The patient is positioned supine on the operating table with thigh of affected leg slightly abducted and knee flexed and supported. The entire extremity is prepped and draped to allow adequate exposure. Incisions are made over the femoral and popliteal arteries to expose arteries and explore area before bypassing the obstruction in the femoral artery. An autogenous in situ saphenous vein graft, PTFE or noncrimped velour graft, or composite graft may be used. Anastomoses may be visualized with an angioscope. During the surgical procedure, pulsations of the proximal and distal popliteal artery are checked, as well as pulsations in the foot, with a sterile Doppler pulse detector.

Endarterectomy

Atherosclerotic plaque may cause localized stenosis in major peripheral arteries. *Endarterectomy* is excision of the diseased endothelial lining of artery and the occluding atheromatous deposits so as to leave a smooth lining. Loosely attached plaque may be removed by dissection in the media with wire-loop strippers, spatulas, and/or catheters. Long-segment endarterectomy may be facilitated in the iliac, femoral, and popliteal arteries with a powered Hall oscillating endarterectomy valvulotome or other high-speed drill to pulverize plaque as described for atherectomy (see p. 823). A saphenous vein or patch graft may be used to close arteriotomy site. Plaque also can be vaporized with a laser beam (see discussion of laser angioplasty, p. 823) from femoral and carotid arteries. Subsequent inflammation and fibrosis are minimal; healing is rapid.

Carotid Endarterectomy

One of the most commonly performed vascular procedures, carotid endarterectomy is done to prevent brain attack (stroke) in the patient with severe carotid artery insufficiency. Atherosclerotic plaque in the common carotid, at the bifurcation, and/or in internal and external carotid arteries causes localized stenosis or ulceration that impedes cerebral blood flow. Endarterectomy is indicated when stenosis causes TIAs. The procedure often is done under superficial and deep regional cervical block; general anesthesia may be preferred. The patient is continuously monitored by electroencephalogram (EEG) or computerized EEG topographic brain mapping (CETBM) to assess cerebral circulation and neurologic deficits.

Patient is positioned supine with head turned away from affected side. Care must be taken not to place undue extension on neck because this may occlude vertebral blood flow. An oblique incision about 4 inches (10 cm) long in the neck is carried through subcutaneous tissue, platysma muscle, and anterior border of the sternocleidomastoid muscle. Retraction of the sternocleidomastoid muscle and jugular vein allows exposure of common carotid artery and its branches. After systemic heparinization, special vascular instruments are used to clamp above and below the occluded area. In certain instances an intraluminal shunt is inserted in the artery to maintain blood flow to the brain while plaque is removed. Many surgeons use a shunt routinely; others use alternative means of cerebral protection, such as deliberately producing mild to moderate hypertension or hypercapnia. Cerebral protection during carotid cross-clamping is a primary concern to prevent serious neurologic complications.

Arteriotomy, incision in an artery, is made in the common carotid artery below the plaque and is extended upward; in internal and external carotid arteries it begins above the plaque and extends downward. The plaque is dissected free and removed in its entirety. Most of the underlying media also is removed. A headlight and magnifying loupes are worn by the surgeon to enhance visibility during dissection and closure of the arteriotomy. To check blood flow, a Doppler pulse detector is used after the artery is closed. Occasionally, if an adequate lumen cannot be established, a PTFE or saphenous vein patch graft angioplasty or bypass grafting is necessary. Bilateral endarterectomies may be indicated for severe bilateral occlusion, but the surgical procedures are performed at least a week apart.

Aneurysmectomy

An aneurysm is a localized abnormal dilation in an artery resulting from mechanical pressure of blood on a vessel wall weakened by biochemical alterations. Loss of structural integrity is implicit as the aneurysm forms in the media. A *fusiform aneurysm* is a uniform circumferential dilation. Less common is a *saccular aneurysm*, which is a saclike outpouching in the media of the vessel wall (Figure 40-2). Cystic medial necrosis causes a *dissecting aneurysm*, usually in the thoracic aorta, in which the media separates from the intima. Atherosclerosis is the most common cause, but trauma may be a factor in formation of an aneurysm. The abdominal aorta, thoracic aorta, aortic arch, and popliteal arteries are vessels most often affected. Diagnostic evaluation

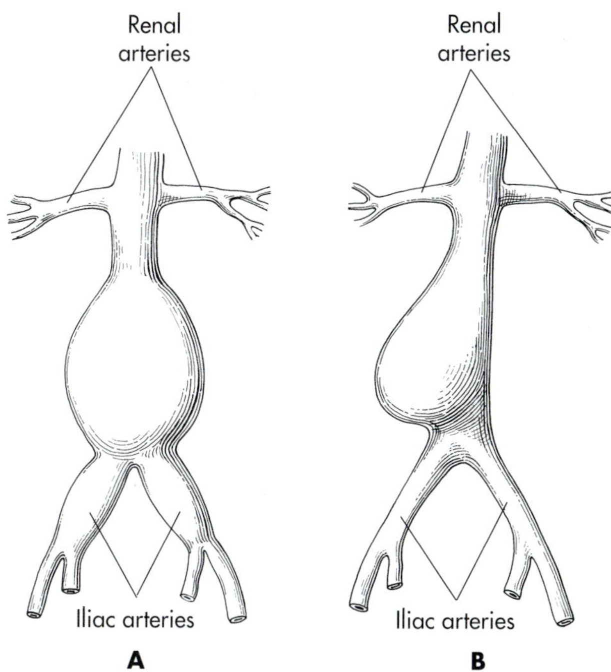

FIGURE 40-2 Abdominal aortic aneurysm between renal and iliac arteries. **A,** Fusiform (circumferential) type. **B,** Saccular (saclike) type.

combines physical examination, laboratory findings, and results of ultrasonography, CAT, MRI, and aortography and/or angiography. Location and extent of the lesion determine operability and the type of reconstruction. For example, cross-clamping of descending thoracic aorta to remove an aneurysm will impair blood supply to the spinal cord. Repair in the arch or ascending aorta can impair cerebral and coronary perfusion. Flow through visceral, mesenteric, and renal arteries may be affected by abdominal aortic aneurysmectomy or aortoiliac reconstruction. Vital structures must be protected during aneurysmectomy.

A ruptured aneurysm precludes further evaluation. This is a surgical emergency. A transbrachial or transfemoral occluding balloon catheter may be placed in the aorta to prevent exsanguinating hemorrhage. The surgical procedure must be performed *immediately*.

Resection of Abdominal Aortic Aneurysm

An abdominal aortic aneurysm usually develops between the renal and iliac arteries (Figure 40-2). Abdominal aneurysmectomy may be a lifesaving procedure. However, serious hazards, including massive hemorrhage and injury to ureters and other nearby structures, are associated with it. Renal failure is a potential complication. Modern techniques have greatly reduced mortality. Survivors of the procedure enjoy the same life expectancy as do other patients with comparable atherosclerotic disease.

Constant monitoring of cardiac function with a Swan-Ganz pulmonary artery catheter (see Chapter 19, pp. 373-374) is used in these high-risk patients. Patients whose condition is unstable may require frequent blood gas determinations. Central venous pressure monitoring is a guide for regulating fluid replacement. Blood must be available for transfusion. Autotransfusion may be used if massive hemorrhage is encountered, as with a ruptured aortic aneurysm. Urinary output must be recorded. An indwelling Foley catheter is inserted preoperatively. Mannitol can be infused to prevent ischemic renal failure. Blood flow in extremities should be checked immediately preoperatively and postoperatively to detect embolic problems. A Doppler device usually is used.

A long midline incision from the xiphoid process to the pubis usually is used. The abdomen is thoroughly explored, the small intestinal mesentery mobilized, and the posterior peritoneum overlying the aorta incised to expose the aneurysm. A self-retaining abdominal wall retractor helps give needed exposure. The small intestine and ascending colon are delivered outside the abdomen to increase exposure and to prevent injury. Warm moist tapes, plastic sheeting, or a Lahey (bowel) bag may be used to protect these structures.

An extended posterior retroperitoneal approach may be preferred, especially in the patient who has had previous abdominal surgery or who is obese. Patient is placed in lateral position with left side up. An oblique flank incision is extended along superior margin of the twelfth rib, which may be resected. The entire abdominal aorta and left renal artery are exposed without need to enter the pleural or peritoneal cavities. The kidney, ureter, and peritoneal sac are reflected anteromedially and packed with moist tapes. Exposure is maintained with self-retaining and handheld retractors. If access to iliac or femoral arteries is required, the patient's hips are rotated to a prone position and longitudinal incisions are made in the groin.

Before occlusion of the aorta, blood is withdrawn if needed for preclotting in the graft. Heparin is injected for anticoagulation. Aortic clamps are placed proximal to the aneurysm, and the iliac arteries are clamped distally. The distal aortic stump or iliac arteries may be closed with staples. If the aneurysmal wall is opened, clot and loose intraluminal debris are removed. A tube graft is used if the aneurysm is confined to the aorta (Figure 40-3, *A*). More commonly, a bifurcated graft is sutured in place above the aneurysm and to the common iliac or femoral arteries distally (Figure 40-3, *B*). Branches of other arteries are anastomosed to the graft as necessary, depending on segment of aorta being replaced. The graft may be placed inside the aneurysm, the *open inclusion method*, and the sac is closed over the graft. With the *closed exclusion method*, the graft is placed beside the unopened aneurysm sac. Living tissue, either

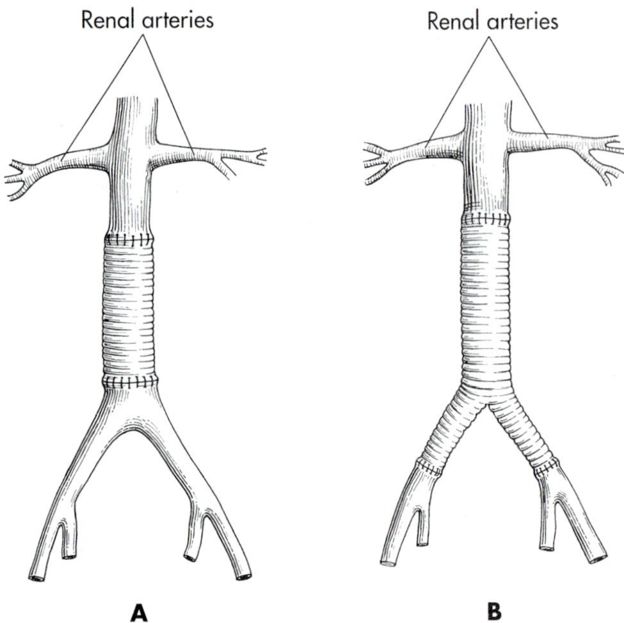

FIGURE 40-3 Resected abdominal aneurysm replaced with tube graft **(A)** or bifurcated graft **(B)**.

the aneurysm sac or mesentery, must cover the prosthesis to prevent contact of prosthesis with the intestines. Failure to accomplish this may result in fistula formation. After the aortic clamps are released, anastomoses are checked for leakage. The incision is usually closed with nonabsorbable sutures. Retention sutures frequently are used for a long abdominal incision.

Embolectomy

An *embolus* is a mass of undissolved matter carried by the bloodstream until it lodges in a blood vessel and occludes it. An embolus may be an air bubble, a fat globule, a clump of bacteria, a piece of tissue, or a foreign body. The occlusion of a blood vessel by an embolus causes various symptoms, depending on the size and location of the occluded vessel. Occlusion of a vessel in the brain, lungs, or heart can cause rapid and sudden death. Surgical intervention is the primary treatment for an embolus unless the surgical procedure is contraindicated. Selected patients may be treated with heparin, vasodilators, and perhaps sympathetic blocks. Renal or mesenteric emboli are usually treated by embolectomy or bypass grafting. For an embolectomy, the affected blood vessel is incised and the embolus is removed.

Pulmonary Embolus

Occlusion of a pulmonary artery or one of its branches usually occurs from emboli originating from veins in the lower extremities or pelvis. Emboli pass up the inferior vena cava to the right side of the heart and are ejected from the right ventricle into the pulmonary artery. Pulmonary embolism may be diagnosed by lung scans, pulmonary angiograms, and phlebograms.

Pulmonary Embolectomy Massive pulmonary embolism can cause irreversible cardiac arrest or profound refractory hypotension and hypoxemia. If portable cardiopulmonary bypass equipment is available, cannulae can be inserted at the patient's bedside or in the emergency department or intensive care unit. Then the patient is transported to the OR. Median sternotomy is performed to establish total cardiopulmonary bypass (see Chapter 39, pp. 803-805) and for access to the pulmonary artery. Pulmonary emboli are removed by manual extraction; by passage of forceps into both right and left pulmonary arteries; by passage of balloon catheters into pulmonary arterial segments; and by squeezing both lungs to force peripheral thrombi through a pulmonary arteriotomy. The incision can be extended for vena caval ligation to prevent recurrent embolization.

Pulmonary Thromboendarterectomy Chronic pulmonary thromboembolic disease may develop from failure to resolve a massive pulmonary embolus, from repeated embolic episodes, or from a combination of both. Removal of obstructions in the main pulmonary arteries by thromboendarterectomy improves hemodynamics. The procedure is performed with the patient under induced hypothermia and cardiopulmonary bypass; thrombi are removed from the upper, middle, and lower lobes of the right pulmonary artery and then from the left pulmonary artery.

Vena Caval Devices A surgical procedure may be indicated when anticoagulant therapy fails or is contraindicated *to prevent* passage of emboli to the lungs from the deep veins in the lower extremities and pelvis. Blood flow within the vena cava may be partially interrupted with clips or filter devices. This allows blood to return to the right ventricle of the heart without passage of the emboli. Vena caval ligation or plication may be performed by an abdominal approach. A Moretz clip is placed via a retroperitoneal approach.

Under fluoroscopic control, the applicator of a Mobin-Udden umbrella filter or Greenfield filter is inserted through a right internal jugular venotomy. It is advanced through the right atrium into the inferior vena cava. The cone-shaped filter is ejected and fixed in position below the renal veins and above the point of juncture of the iliac veins. A filter may be placed at completion of a diagnostic angiogram to avoid a second procedure, especially for a high-risk patient. The filter does not interfere with MRI, but the radiologist should be informed of its presence before any imaging procedure.

The Greenfield filter is a permanent implant. It can be placed from a femoral vein route, if preferred. Natural body processes dissolve clots that become lodged in the device. Postoperatively the patient usually is placed on anticoagulant therapy. Complications include lower extremity edema, which may indicate an obstruction in the filter that requires prompt medical attention.

Venous Stasis Disease

When valves of the veins fail to function normally, increased back pressure of blood causes the veins to become dilated, tortuous, or elongated. These are known as *varicose veins*. Pain and secondary complications, such as thrombophlebitis and varicose ulcers from venous stasis, may follow. It is believed that there is a familial tendency toward varicosities, which afflict both men and women. Habitual long periods of standing, repeated pregnancies, and obesity are other predisposing factors.

A procedure may be performed to bypass a venous obstruction, such as iliac-venous occlusion or femoropopliteal occlusion. Venous valve repair, a *valvuloplasty*, or venous valve transposition may be performed to correct femoral valvular incompetence and severe venous stasis and to salvage the saphenous vein. The perforator or superficial femoral veins may be ligated for severe venous stasis with marked fibrosis and ulcerations. Injection-compression sclerotherapy to treat varicose veins may be preferred to surgical treatment.

Ligation and Stripping of Varicose Veins

For ligation and stripping of varicose veins in a leg, the saphenous vein is excised in toto with the aid of a semiflexible stripping device beginning at the ankle. Additional incisions are made along the course of the vein to ligate branches as the stripper is moved upward toward the groin. Branches are occluded with ligating clips and are transected. At the groin, an incision is made over the palpated stripper. The vein is ligated at the saphenofemoral junction. Preoperatively, the surgeon may mark areas of varicosity for incision. Following closure of incisions and application of dressings, full length of the leg is wrapped in cotton elastic bandages for compression.

Fasciotomy

Decompression by fasciotomy is the treatment of choice for prevention of compartment syndromes following acute ischemia in the upper or lower extremity. Vascular compromise can occur following a penetrating or crush injury. Release of the overlying fascia may be indicated for clinical evidence of increased pressure, such as pain, edema, pallor, and diminished sensation.

Epidural Spinal Electrical Stimulation

Epidural spinal electrical stimulation (ESES) may be used to improve nutritional blood flow in patients with severe lower limb ischemia. This can lead to the healing of ischemic ulcers. Intravital capillary microscopy is performed before and after ESES to measure red blood cell velocity in skin capillaries. This procedure uses a microscope connected to a television camera, television monitor, and video recorder. With patient in sitting position, dorsum of the foot is placed over the microscope. Fluorescein dye is injected intravenously. Time for perfusion of the capillaries is measured. Under local anesthesia and x-ray control, an epidural electrode is placed parallel to the spinal column. After stimulation of the electrode, perfusion in the foot is tested again.

Vascular Shunts

Normal circulation can be altered to increase or decrease blood flow to a specific organ, either temporarily or permanently. A vascular anastomosis or prosthetic device may be used to establish a route for the diversion of blood flow. For example, vascular isolation of the liver can be achieved with an *atrial caval shunt*. This shunt permits continuous venous return to the ventricle to sustain cardiac output during repair of traumatized suprahepatic or retrohepatic vena cava and/or hepatic veins. A straight tube or inflatable balloon catheter may be inserted to establish the shunt.

Portosystemic Shunts

A shunt between portal and systemic venous systems is definitive treatment for esophageal varices complicated by portal hypertension. However, the surgical procedure may be only palliative. Many patients have progressive liver disease leading to liver failure. Shunting does not repair an already damaged liver, but it can prevent further hemorrhage. Portal hypertension, increase in portal venous pressure, is caused by obstruction to intrahepatic blood flow as a result of cirrhosis, hepatitis, or thrombosis. The increased pressure thus produced results in venous dilation that causes varices. The patient also may have ascites. The purpose of the surgical procedure is to reduce portal hypertension and/or portal venous blood flow. The surgeon selects the most appropriate type of shunt to achieve the purpose.

Distal Splenorenal Shunt Known as the Warren shunt, this procedure involves anastomosis between the splenic vein and left renal vein. The hilum of the spleen and tail of the pancreas are exposed through a left subcostal incision. The splenic vein is completely dissected from the pancreas to its bifurcation at the splenic hilum. This technical maneuver preserves portal profusion but eliminates collateral circulation to control bleeding from gastric and esophageal varices by decompression. The splenoportal system must be patent and have adequate distance between splenic and renal veins for the anastomosis. An autogenous jugular or external iliac vein graft may be interposed to ensure a tension-free splenorenal anastomosis. A splenectomy may be performed. Other modifications may be made to meet specific patient circumstances.

Mesocaval Shunt The side of the superior mesenteric vein may be anastomosed to the proximal end of the divided inferior vena cava. Or an interposition autologous vein or synthetic H-graft creates a shunt between the inferior vena cava and superior mesenteric vein. A mesocaval shunt is an option if a splenic vein is too small for a successful splenorenal shunt. A superior mesenteric–inferior vena caval shunt is well tolerated by young patients.

Portacaval Shunt A portacaval shunt may be performed with end-to-side or side-to-side anastomosis between the portal vein and inferior vena cava or with an interposition H-graft inserted between the portal vein and inferior vena cava. A ringed PTFE graft may be used, or an autologous graft may be obtained from an internal jugular or saphenous vein. The shunt relieves hypertension by bypassing obstruction and diverting the return flow of blood to the liver from the portal vein, thus decompressing esophageal varices.

Depending on the type of portosystemic shunt the surgeon plans, a subcostal or transabdominal incision may be used. Two suction setups should be available to evacuate the copious amounts of ascitic fluid that may be anticipated when the peritoneum is opened. Abdominal and vascular setups are prepared. Pressure within the portal vein is measured with a manometer, via a cannulated branch of the superior mesenteric vein, at the beginning and conclusion of the surgical procedure. Because of venous distention and the vascularity of the surgical area, hemorrhage is a major intraoperative hazard. Care is taken to avoid injury to adjacent structures, including the hepatic artery and common bile duct.

Arteriovenous Shunts and Fistulas

With arteriovenous shunts and fistulas, blood flow is established directly from an artery to a vein without going through the capillary network. Access to the vascular system through an arteriovenous shunt or fistula is necessary for the patient suffering from end-stage renal disease who is being maintained on long-term chronic hemodialysis (see Chapter 31, p. 639). The endogenous Cimino-Brescio arteriovenous fistula is established internally at the wrist, under local anesthesia by anastomosis between the radial artery and cephalic vein. If vessels are inadequate, a synthetic PTFE graft may be interposed between the artery and vein. A loop fistula may be created with a graft from brachial artery to cephalic or basilic vein in the antecubital fossa or brachial artery to axillary vein in the upper arm. Enzymatically treated bovine carotid artery heterografts are used occasionally to create arteriovenous shunts or fistulas. Thrombosis and infection are the most frequent complications. A thrombectomy, using a Fogarty balloon catheter, may reestablish patency. Total excision of the graft is necessary in the event of generalized infection.

Vascular Anastomosis

The operating microscope is needed for *microvascular anastomosis* of small vessels to revascularize tissue. Patency of the anastomosis depends on factors related to blood flow, coagulation, and vessel spasm. Vessels must be approximated without trapping adventitia in the lumen. Collagen fibers, tissue thromboplastin, and other thrombogenic factors in adventitia predispose the patient to rapid platelet aggregation that may cause thrombus formation. Interrupted sutures are placed through full thickness of vessel wall (i.e., adventitia, media, and intima). Veins are technically more difficult to anastomose than arteries because their walls are thinner and have less substantial muscularis. Anastomoses may be end-to-end or side-to-side. An interpositional vein graft may be needed to add length or to bridge gap between ends of either an artery or a vein. A patent artery should pulsate distal to the anastomosis. Although this procedure is used most frequently for tissue transplantation (e.g., vascularized free flaps or replants such as severed digits) the peripheral vascular surgeon may be needed to assist with vascular problems that require microvascular techniques.

Laser-assisted vascular anastomosis, also referred to as *vascular tissue welding,* fuses medium-sized (6 to 8 mm) vessels together to form an anastomosis. The adventitial surface is less thrombogenic than following suturing and heals faster with less scar tissue. The argon laser is used for this technique. It may be used to create an arteriovenous shunt at the wrist for hemodialysis, to reattach severed limbs, and to repair damaged vessels.

Limb Salvage

Amputation of a lower extremity may be required for peripheral vascular disease or lymphedema with lymphangitis. All efforts are made to salvage the limb; amputation is the last resort. Ischemia can cause debilitating pain, skin ulcers, and gangrene, often secondary to smoking or diabetes. Revascularization by the techniques described may save the patient from the emotional trauma of amputation. This is a prime objective of the peripheral vascular surgeon.

Bibliography

Allen SL: Perioperative nursing interventions for intravascular stent placements, *AORN J* 61(4):689-698, 1995.

Belkin M et al: Abdominal aortic aneurysms, *Curr Opin Cardiol* 9(5):581-590, 1994.

Bensen JL, McClellan W: Retroperitoneal approach to abdominal aortic aneurysm, *AORN J* 53(1):42-59, 1991.

Berengoltz-Zlochin SN et al: Subintimal versus intraluminal laser-assisted recanalization of occluded femoropopliteal arteries, *J Vasc Interven Radiol* 5(5):689-696, 1994.

Borgini L, Almgren CC: Peripheral vascular angioscopy, *AORN J* 52(3):543-550, 1990.

Chuter TA et al: Bifurcated stent-grafts for endovascular repair of abdominal aortic aneurysm, *Surg Endosc* 8(7):800-802, 1994.

Cruz LD: Use of lasers in vascular disease discussed at international congress, *AORN J* 51(5):1160-1172, 1990.

Fahey VA: *Vascular nursing,* ed 2, Philadelphia, 1994, Saunders.

Fellows E: Abdominal aortic aneurysm: warning flags to watch for, *Am J Nurs* 95(5):26-32, 1995.

Fogarty AM: Angioscopy, *AORN J* 53(3):725-728, 1991.

Gulli B, Templeman D: Compartment syndrome of the lower extremity, *Orthop Clin North Am* 25(4):677-684, 1994.

Henderson LJ, Kirkland JS: Angioplasty with stent placement in peripheral arterial occlusive disease, *AORN J* 61(4):671-685, 1995.

Kaufman JA et al: MR angiography in the preoperative evaluation of abdominal aortic aneurysms, *J Vasc Interven Radiol* 5(3):489-496, 1994.

Kellar SJ: Upper extremity revascularization: axillary-brachial bypass for temporary arteritis, *AORN J* 56(3):435-441, 1992.

Kupeli IA: Factors affecting outcome in patients undergoing peripheral vascular surgery, *Anesthesiology* 80(2):483-485, 1994.

Long J et al: Pulmonary thromboendarterectomy: clinical profile, surgical treatment, *AORN J* 59(4):801-810, 1994.

MacSweeny ST et al: Pathogenesis of abdominal aortic aneurysm, *Br J Surg* 81(7):935-941, 1994.

McEwen DR: Arteriovenous fistula: vascular access for long-term hemodialysis, *AORN J* 59(1):225-232, 1994.

Mills JL et al: The utility and durability of vein bypass grafts originating from the popliteal artery for limb salvage, *Am J Surg* 168(6):646-650, 1994.

Petrone S: Laser assisted balloon angioplasty: bypassing traditional methods, *Today's OR Nurse* 12(6):22-27, 1990.

Sapienza P et al: Comparative long-term results of laser-assisted balloon angioplasty and atherectomy in the treatment of peripheral vascular disease, *Am J Surg* 168(6):640-644, 1994.

Soong CV et al: Bowel ischemia and organ impairment in elective abdominal aortic aneurysm repair, *Br J Surg* 81(7):965-968, 1994.

Yamamoto N et al: Monitoring for spinal cord ischemia by use of the evoked spinal cord potentials during aortic aneurysm surgery, *J Vasc Surg* 20(5):826-833, 1994.

Zelinskas EJ: Abdominal aortic aneurysmectomy with graft bypass, *Surg Technol* 25(12):8-13, 23, 1993.

SECTION ELEVEN

Multidisciplinary Perioperative Considerations

CHAPTER 41

Ambulatory Surgery

The concept of ambulatory surgery is not new. Its history can be traced back to Egypt in 3000 BC. Simple surgical procedures have been done in physicians' offices for years. However, changes in reimbursement policies by the federal government and other third-party payers in the 1970s motivated surgeons in all specialties to consider operating in ambulatory settings from which the patient goes home, after a short recovery period, on the same day as the surgical procedure. Many surgical procedures curtail physiologic functions only minimally. Immediate ambulation is possible. Rapid-acting anesthetic agents and sophisticated but minimally invasive technology make many relatively complex surgical procedures amenable to ambulatory surgery.

Ambulatory surgery may be defined as surgical patient care performed under general, regional, or local anesthesia without overnight hospitalization. It is cost effective and convenient, but it must be efficient and consistent with standards, policies, and procedures followed for hospitalized surgical patients. Patients have a right to expect comprehensive perioperative care from an ambulatory care facility. The risks, anxiety, and fears associated with a surgical procedure are not eliminated just because the setting is different.

AMBULATORY SURGICAL CARE FACILITY

Various terms are used to describe ambulatory care facilities, including outpatient surgery, same day surgical unit, one day surgery, or ambulatory surgery center. Irrespective of its name or location, an ambulatory care facility must provide an admitting room, an area for patients to change clothes, a preoperative holding/preparation area, an operating room (OR), areas for preparation and storage of supplies, a recovery room with patient lavatory, and a family waiting room. The decor should be pleasing to enhance patient and family relaxation. Parking areas should be conveniently located near the entrance or exit. Space requirements are determined by the number and types of surgical procedures to be performed and types of equipment necessary to perform them, as well as the type of facility. Office space may be needed for administrative and business functions. An ambulatory care facility may be:

1. *Hospital-based dedicated unit.* Patients come to an autonomous, independent, self-contained unit within or attached to the hospital but physically separated from the inpatient OR suite.
2. *Hospital-based integrated unit.* Patients share the same OR suite and other hospital facilities with inpatients. Separate preoperative holding areas usually are provided.
3. *Hospital-affiliated satellite surgery center.* Patients come to an ambulatory surgery center owned and operated by the hospital but physically separated from it.
4. *Freestanding ambulatory surgery center.* Patients come to a totally independent facility that is privately owned and operated, often by physicians, for the purpose of providing surgical care.

5. *Office-based center.* Patients come to a physician's office that is equipped for surgery. Many surgeons, dermatologists, periodontists, and podiatrists perform surgical procedures in their offices. This office-based center may accommodate one or more surgeons in the same specialty or may be a multiphysician, interdisciplinary clinic.

In addition to obtaining a state license and certificate of approval, an ambulatory care facility should comply with standards set by the Accreditation Association for Ambulatory Health Care and/or the Joint Commission on Accreditation of Healthcare Organizations. Freestanding centers and offices must have a patient transfer/admission agreement with a nearby hospital. If complications develop, such as adverse reactions to anesthesia or postoperative bleeding, or if an unexpected finding necessitates further surgery, the patient may need to be admitted to a hospital. Freestanding recovery care centers have been developed to accommodate a 24- to 48-hour uncomplicated postanesthesia recovery period. Although infrequent, the most common reasons for admission to a freestanding recovery care center or hospital after ambulatory surgery are pain, nausea and vomiting, urinary retention, and concern for wound integrity.

Approximately 65% of all surgical procedures are performed safely on an ambulatory basis without compromising the quality of care. However, some facilities limit their use only to those surgical procedures that can be performed with local or regional block anesthesia. Other facilities allow surgeons to perform surgical procedures with the patient under general anesthesia. Although procedures performed in an ambulatory care facility usually are of short duration, 15 to 90 minutes, appropriate selection and evaluation of patients are essential. Nursing care and anesthesia management also are crucial factors in the ambulatory surgical patient's experience.

AMBULATORY SURGICAL PATIENT

Many persons prefer to recuperate at home after a surgical procedure rather than in the hospital. These patients may be candidates for ambulatory surgery, depending on the nature and extent of the surgical procedure and on the ability to follow instructions or to receive adequate care at home. Consideration must be given to the duration and complexity of the surgical procedure, risk of anesthesia, degree and duration of postoperative pain and discomfort, and probability of postoperative complications. Either surgeon or patient may request to have nursing care provided through a home health agency or in a recovery center. Several types of home/hotel-like facilities provide care for up to 72 hours postoperatively. A hospital short-stay unit may provide postoperative as well as preoperative care for nursing observation and pain control.

Patient Selection

Patients eligible for ambulatory surgery are carefully selected. Criteria considered include:

1. General health status. Acceptable patients are in class I, II, or stable III of the physical status classification of the American Society of Anesthesiologists (see Chapter 16, p. 308). Patients are evaluated physically and emotionally to determine possibility of complications developing during or after the surgical procedure. This includes a complete medical history, physical examination, and a preanesthesia evaluation.
2. Results of preoperative tests. Patients may have tests on admission the morning of the surgical procedure, but preferably tests are performed before scheduled date of the surgical procedure so that results can be evaluated. This avoids cancellation on day the surgical procedure is scheduled if unsatisfactory results so warrant. The results must be on the chart that accompanies the patient to the OR.
   a. Laboratory tests usually include a complete blood count and urinalysis. The less costly spun hematocrit and dipstick urinalysis may be acceptable for some patients.
   b. Multichemistry profile and chest x-ray film may be required for adults scheduled for general anesthesia, if clinically indicated.
   c. Electrocardiogram (ECG) may be required before general anesthesia for patients over 35 or 40 years of age.
3. Willingness and psychologic acceptance by patient and family. The patient must be willing and able to recuperate at home. Some persons will feel more secure in a hospital if they lack adequate home care. Each patient is individually assessed. Provision is made for competent care at home. Compliance with preoperative and postoperative instructions by the patient and availability of a responsible family member or support person are essential.
4. Recovery period. The surgeon should anticipate minimal or no postoperative complications. Patients in whom a prolonged period of nausea and vomiting is anticipated or in whom pain will not be relieved by oral analgesics are not ideal candidates for ambulatory surgery.
5. Reimbursement sources. Most third-party payers prefer less costly ambulatory surgery whenever a procedure can be safely performed in this setting. Patient safety and quality of care depend on patient screening and support systems.

Patient Instructions

Written instructions are given to the patient by the surgeon during an office visit or by the nurse during a preadmission visit to the ambulatory care facility. These describe admission, preoperative, intraoperative, recovery, and discharge procedures. Instructions should be written in a language that the patient can understand. To protect both the surgeon and the facility, the patient should sign for receipt of these instructions as well as sign an informed consent for the surgical procedure. Instructions include:

1. Preoperative preparations
   a. Make an appointment for preadmission testing and teaching session, unless these instructions are given at this time.
   b. Take nothing by mouth after midnight, or other specified hour, before admission unless ordered to do so by the surgeon.
   c. Arrive at the facility by ___ AM/PM. (Time will depend on time surgical procedure is scheduled.)
   d. Notify surgeon immediately of a change in physical condition, such as a cold or fever.
   e. Wear loose, comfortable clothing, leave jewelry and valuables at home, and remove makeup and nail polish.
2. Postoperative discharge
   a. Arrange for a responsible support person to accompany you home. You may not be permitted to drive or leave unattended.
   b. Do not ingest alcoholic beverages, drive a car, cook, or operate machinery for 24 hours if sedation or general anesthesia has been administered.
   c. Delay important decision making until a full recovery is made.
   d. Take medications only as prescribed and maintain as regular a diet as tolerated.
   e. Shower or bathe daily unless instructed otherwise. This helps relieve muscle tension and discomfort and keeps the wound clean.
   f. Call surgeon if postoperative problems arise.
   g. Keep follow-up appointment with the surgeon.

The patient's level of understanding of these instructions and concept of what is to happen must be assessed preoperatively. A telephone call from the perioperative nurse to the patient the day or within the week before the surgical procedure helps clarify any misunderstandings. Preoperative teaching and discharge instructions can be reinforced at this time. The time the patient should arrive on the day of the procedure is verified. Admission time varies according to the surgical schedule. A minimal wait at the facility helps reduce preoperative anxiety. Patients are usually admitted at least an hour before the scheduled time of their surgical procedures.

NOTE The perioperative nurse's phone call reminds the patient of the date and time an elective surgical procedure is scheduled. This helps minimize cancellations.

PATIENT-NURSE RELATIONSHIP

Good patient-nurse rapport is essential in an ambulatory care facility. The positive aspects of the patient-nurse relationship must develop quickly because the time spent together is brief. Patients are alert and often anxious. Preoperative medication usually is kept to a minimum. Patients need continual reassurance throughout surgical procedures. This demands qualified personnel with maturity, proficiency, and an ability to convey empathy. Staff members, more than environment, contribute to the warm caring atmosphere essential in dealing with alert patients and their families.

The patient-nurse relationship begins with the preoperative interview. The patient is assessed to determine a nursing diagnosis based on health status data. The nurse verifies information about past medical/surgical history; if the patient sees a physician or takes medication on a regular basis; and if the patient wears glasses, contact lenses, false teeth, dental caps, or a prosthesis of any kind. Particular attention is given to medications and allergies. Many patients are vague regarding medications they take and what allergic responses they have to them. If comprehension of the questions is doubtful or a language barrier exists, access to a family member, friend, or interpreter is essential.

Following the interview, the patient changes from street clothes into a patient gown. The nurse escorts the patient into the preoperative holding area where the patient is prepared as necessary for the specific surgical procedure. Baseline vital signs and blood pressure are taken. Unless sedation is given, the patient may walk from this area into the OR. This helps minimize the patient's feeling of dependency. Conversation with the nurse reinforces the patient-nurse relationship and helps the nurse assess the patient's psychologic responses.

INTRAOPERATIVE PATIENT CARE

Anesthesia management is rarely difficult if careful selection of patients, preoperative evaluation, and instructions are adhered to. Premedication, if given, is minimal. The surgical procedure should be less than 90 minutes in duration for general anesthesia and less than 3 hours for regional block. Local anesthesia or regional block is preferable if appropriate. Spinal anesthesia seldom is used.

Patients who receive general anesthesia are scheduled early in the day to allow maximum recovery time. Rapidly dissipating agents are administered. Intravenous (IV) agents associated with prolonged recovery are avoided unless there is specific indication for their use. Doses of IV agents, such as narcotics and barbiturates, may be reduced to avoid delayed recovery. Indications for endotracheal intubation are the same as for inpatients. (See Section Seven for an in-depth discussion of all anesthetic agents and their administration.) Anesthetic techniques should provide adequate depth of anesthesia but with minimal cardiorespiratory changes and side effects. Various combinations of agents and drugs are used.

NOTE Some anesthesiologists permit a parent to stay with an infant or child during induction of general anesthesia.

The patient is monitored continuously for reaction to drugs and for behavioral and physiologic changes (see Chapters 18 and 19). If an anesthesiologist is not in attendance, a perioperative nurse should be assigned to monitor the patient. This nurse takes and records vital signs before the injection of a local or regional block anesthetic agent or analgesic and every 15 minutes thereafter, monitors physiologic status according to written policy and procedure, and institutes emergency measures if an adverse reaction occurs. Therefore the perioperative nurse must have a basic knowledge of the function and use of monitoring equipment that includes attaching a pulse oximeter and electrocardiograph leads. This nurse may be responsible for interpreting, identifying, and reporting abnormal readings. Additional functions, if requested by the surgeon and permitted by policy, may include starting oxygen therapy when clinically indicated, administering IV therapy, or giving medications. Cardiopulmonary resuscitation (CPR) equipment and nurses certified in CPR must be available. All pertinent data and therapy are documented.

NOTE

1. Policies and procedures related to nurses monitoring patients receiving local anesthesia should include patient risk criteria, the type of monitoring to be used, and interventions within the scope of nursing practice.
2. Administration and monitoring of IV sedation must comply with state statutes. Nurses must follow the manufacturer's instructions and indications for dosage and use of all medications.

The awake and alert patient must receive physical and emotional comfort throughout the surgical procedure. This patient should be told what is about to take place, for example, "You will feel a needle sting"; what to expect, for example, "You will have a burning sensation"; and what is expected of him or her, for example, "Tell us if you feel pain." The patient's questions should be answered truthfully and realistically. The patient should be reassured that appropriate amounts of anesthesia will be administered as needed. However, conversation by team members must be appropriate and kept to a minimum. Hand signals between the surgeon and scrub person are more useful than a verbal request for instruments. However, the surgeon may request a No. 10 or 15 rather than a knife, a Mayo or Metz rather than scissors. Strange noises should be explained to the patient (e.g., suction to remove irrigating solution or the sound of electrosurgical unit). Background music *of the patient's choice* may help relax and distract the patient. Headsets and earphones are useful for this purpose and help to block out other noises. Traffic in and out of the room should be kept to a minimum. A sign should be placed on the door to indicate the type of anesthesia being used (e.g., "patient awake," "local anesthesia").

Intraoperatively the same precautions are observed by all team members as for any surgical procedure. These include strict adherence to the principles of aseptic and sterile techniques (see Chapter 12) and other OR routines (see Chapter 20).

RECOVERY, DISCHARGE, AND FOLLOW-UP

Postoperatively, management of pain, nausea, and vomiting, plus monitoring vital signs and maintaining fluid and electrolyte balance, are responsibilities of the postanesthesia nurse. Medications usually are given intravenously in small dosages because oral medications on an empty stomach tend to increase nausea and vomiting. Routine orders may be established by policy for these analgesics and antiemetics.

Consciousness, rational behavior, and ambulation do not imply full recovery. Blood pressure and pulse rate may return to the normal range while residual myocardial depression continues. Patients may lapse back into sleep or drowsiness as the drugs used for general anesthesia are metabolized. Most complications occur within the first 48 hours. Patients must never be left unattended. Discharge must be contingent on the ability to walk safely and readiness for self-care at home under the supervision of a responsible support person. Patients are not allowed to drive home if general or regional anesthesia has been administered. Select patients who have had local anesthesia without sedation may be permitted to drive home if an order is written by the surgeon.

Patients are discharged on written order of the anesthesiologist and/or surgeon as per policy, in company of a responsible support person, when all discharge criteria are met. These criteria include:

1. Alert and oriented
2. Stable vital signs
3. No respiratory distress, hoarseness, or croupy cough following endotracheal intubation
4. Gag reflex present; able to swallow and cough
5. No dizziness, nausea, or vomiting
6. No bleeding and no or minimal swelling or drainage on dressings

7. Able to tolerate fluids and has voided
8. No excessive pain that will not be alleviated with oral medications at home
9. Able to ambulate, per developmental age, or per physical limitations
10. Clear vision, with glasses if normally worn

Written discharge instructions are verbally reviewed with the patient and family member and/or significant other. If problems occur after discharge, the patient is encouraged to contact the surgeon or the ambulatory care facility. Many patients feel comfortable using the nursing staff as a resource agent to answer questions. Patient education is an essential element of ambulatory surgical care.

The following day or at most within 2 days of discharge, a nurse should call to check on the patient's progress and to reiterate postoperative instructions. The nurse reminds the patient to keep the follow-up appointment with the surgeon. Patients who plan to return to work within a day or two may be asked to phone the nurse because they may not be home when the nurse makes routine calls during the day.

DOCUMENTATION

Development, implementation, and evaluation of the plan of care should be documented in the patient's medical record. Documentation should include but is not limited to:

1. Preoperative care
   a. Preanesthetic evaluation by the anesthesiologist if general, regional, or local anesthesia with sedation is to be given
   b. Nursing assessment data, nursing diagnoses, expected outcomes, plan of care, and preoperative teaching by perioperative nurse
   c. Medical history and physical examination
   d. Laboratory reports and results of other tests
   e. Informed consent for the surgical procedure
2. Intraoperative care
   a. Anesthesia and medications administered
   b. Vital signs and intraoperative monitoring data
   c. Intraoperative implementation of the plan of care
   d. Surgical procedure note by the surgeon
   e. Any unexpected outcomes
3. Postoperative care
   a. Postanesthesia care, including monitoring patient responses and medications
   b. Discharge instructions, including follow-up appointment with the surgeon and signs and/or symptoms of potential complications that require immediate medical attention
   c. Radiology, pathology, and any other medical reports
   d. Physical and psychologic status at the time of discharge
   e. Mode of transport from the facility and destination, including relationship to the accompanying support person
4. Remote postoperative care
   a. Follow-up phone call within 24 to 48 hours to assess the patient's progress
   b. Follow-up phone call within 6 weeks to assess the patient's satisfaction with outcomes and services for continuous quality improvement data

ADVANTAGES AND DISADVANTAGES OF AMBULATORY SURGERY

Advantages

The development of rapid-acting anesthetics that have minimal prolonged side effects and the availability of short-acting narcotics to control pain and antiemetics to reduce nausea allow the surgeon to perform many surgical procedures in an ambulatory care facility. The advantages of ambulatory surgery are that it:

1. Lowers cost for patient
2. Returns patient immediately to familiar surroundings that are less stressful than a hospital environment
3. Reduces period of patient's dependency and lifestyle disruption
4. Eliminates psychologic trauma of hospitalization and separation from family or significant other or from parents for infants and children
5. Frees hospital bed space without increasing hospital bed capacity for patients who require more extensive care
6. Frees hospital staff and resources for patients with more serious problems
7. Reduces risk of nosocomial (hospital-acquired) infection that is inherent in hospitalization

The concept of ambulatory health care services is expanding to community emergency care centers, rather than hospital-based emergency departments, for the treatment of minor trauma and illness. Some ambulatory centers provide short-stay care for invasive diagnostic and/or radiologic studies.

Disadvantages

Ambulatory surgery is not suitable for every patient. Although most patients who receive their care in an ambulatory setting benefit from the experience, the following disadvantages have been identified.

1. Some patients have unrealistic expectations of their physical capabilities postoperatively. They

tend to feel fine until the anesthetic wears off. They may overextend the use of an anesthetized body part while still under the influence of local anesthesia.
2. Patient's anxiety level may increase if enough time is not allotted for preoperative preparation. This gives the impression of being rushed through the system as if on a production line.
3. Unforeseen complications may arise in a patient who has never had an anesthetic before. A young child having general anesthesia for an inguinal hernia repair may experience a metabolic crisis such as malignant hyperthermia (MH). Allergic responses to drugs and local anesthetics are potential adverse reactions. (See Chapters 18 and 19 for details of anesthetic complications.)
4. Unexpected secondary diagnosis may be discovered during a surgical procedure that will necessitate a more extensive procedure than anticipated or a second surgical procedure in an inpatient facility. Prolonged procedures will increase the waiting period for patients scheduled to follow the unexpected extended procedure. The patient will have to be discharged at a later time. This may impose a hardship on the family (e.g., child care).
5. Emergency transport to an inpatient facility may be necessary in the event of a surgical accident. For example, inadvertent penetration of a major artery or organ during a laparoscopic procedure may induce life-threatening hemorrhage. Instrumentation, supplies, blood volume replacement, and blood salvage equipment may not be readily available in the freestanding ambulatory setting.
6. Time or space constraints may cause patients to feel they are being discharged too soon.
7. Patients may experience pain, nausea, vomiting, bleeding, swelling, and other complications that may necessitate overnight admission to the hospital for treatment and/or observation.

CONTINUOUS QUALITY IMPROVEMENT

Patient satisfaction is a key indicator of quality. Did the care received meet the patient's expectations? What are the patient's perceptions of care? In addition to the postdischarge telephone call, the patient may be asked to complete a questionnaire a week or more after discharge. Questions relate to physical facilities, waiting periods, preoperative teaching, anesthesia or surgical complications, discharge instructions, and overall satisfaction with the nursing care.

Supplemental questionnaires sent to surgeons are useful to obtain information for compiling statistics related to postoperative infections and complications (i.e., patient outcomes).

A total quality improvement program includes monitoring of patient care and the environment, evaluation of patient outcomes and services, and identification and resolution of problems. It focuses on outcomes (i.e., results in accordance with standards for professional practice, ethical conduct, and legal requirements). Quality improvement in an ambulatory care facility must include evaluation of policies and procedures regarding appropriateness of patient selection, surgical procedures performed, and services provided.

Most ambulatory surgery patients are satisfied with their care. Studies have shown that most patients will choose to have a surgical procedure performed in an ambulatory setting again if further surgery is indicated. Lower incidents of postoperative complications have been documented, as well as lower costs of treatment for the patient. The preoperative teaching is beneficial in helping patients attain the expected outcomes. Careful patient evaluation and planning can make the surgical intervention performed in the ambulatory setting a successful and positive experience for the patient, family, significant others, and the caregiver.

BIBLIOGRAPHY

Bales SG: Integrating operating room suites and adjusting to outpatient demand, *Min Invas Surg Nurs* 7(4):133-134, 1993.

Burden N: *Ambulatory surgical nursing*, Philadelphia, 1993, Saunders.

Caldwell LM: Surgical outpatient concerns, *AORN J* 53(3):761-767, 1991.

Carr T, Webster CS: Recovery care centers: an innovative approach to caring for healthy surgical patients, *AORN J* 53(4):986-991, 1991.

Fondiller SH: New frontiers in ambulatory care, *Am J Nurs* 91(2):73-78, 1991.

Hawshaw D: A day surgery patient follow-up survey, *Br J Nurs* 3(7):348-350, 1994.

Henderson JA: Implications of outpatient surgery growth, *OR Manager* 9(9):24-26, 1993.

Hylka SC: Comparative cost analysis of surgical procedures in an ambulatory eye center, *Nurs Econ* 12(1):51-55, 1994.

Llewellyn JG: Short stay surgery: present practices, future trends, *AORN J* 53(5):1179-1191, 1991.

Mathias JM: Cross-training prepares ASC nursing staff for flexibility, *OR Manager* 8(12):14-15, 1992.

Murphy EK: OR nursing law: liability exposure in ambulatory settings, *AORN J* 54(6):1287-1289, 1991.

Oberle K et al: Follow-up of same day sugery patients: a study of patient concerns, *AORN J* 59(5):1016-1025, 1994.

Parnass SM: Ambulatory surgery patient priorities, *Nurs Clin North Am* 28(3):531-545, 1993.

Patterson P: ASCs accepting older, higher risk patients, *OR Manager* 7(7):14-15, 1991.

Pica-Furey W: Ambulatory surgery—hospital-based vs freestanding: a comparative study of patient satisfaction, *AORN J* 57(5):1119-1127, 1993.

Poss C: Outpatient surgery documentation, *AORN J* 53(1):81-92, 1991.

Schwanitz L: Top surgery center consolidates services, *OR Manager* 9(4):17, 1993.

Singer HK: Then and now: a historical development of ambulatory surgery, *J Post Anesth Nurs* 8(4):276-279, 1993.

Smith I, White PF: Anesthesia for ambulatory surgery, *Curr Rev Nurs Anesth* 16(20):171-180, 1994.

Spry C et al: Ambulatory surgery: RN staff in an ambulatory surgery center, *AORN J* 59(3):601-602, 1994.

Study identifies best practices in ambulatory surgery centers, *OR Manager* 9(1):1, 8-9, 1993.

Swan BA: A collaborative ambulatory preoperative evaluation model: implementation, implications, evaluation, *AORN J* 59(2):430-437, 1994.

White PF, Smith I: Ambulatory anesthesia: past, present, and future, *Int Anesthesiol Clin* 32(3):1-16, 1994.

CHAPTER 42

Perioperative Pediatrics

The surgical problems peculiar to children from birth to maturity are not limited to any one area of the body or to any one surgical specialty. Malformations and diseases affect all body parts and therefore may require the skills of any of the surgical specialists. However, pediatric surgery is a specialty in itself and is not adult surgery scaled down to infant or child size. Skill is required in performing pediatric surgical procedures. Specialists in all fields develop these skills as a refinement of their specialties. Surgeons who perform pediatric surgery should have knowledge of the physiologic, embryologic, and pathologic problems peculiar to the newborn, infant, and child.

DEVELOPING A PEDIATRIC PLAN OF CARE

The nursing process is tailored to meet the unique needs of each pediatric patient. Assessment and nursing diagnosis are based on chronologic, physiologic, and psychologic factors specific to each patient. The plan of care should reflect consideration for age but should also include interventions modified according to developmental stage. Developmental theorists emphasize that although the child has reached a certain age or physical size, psychologic growth is the key parameter by which communication is measured. Understanding individual differences related to age, size, and developmental stage enables the operating room (OR) team to develop a positive rapport with the patient and family, which facilitates attainment of expected outcomes.

Considerations in Perioperative Pediatrics

Factors related to age, physical size and development, and psychologic adaptation makes each pediatric patient unique. Not every patient of a particular age group will meet standardized height and weight criteria; a child may be short or tall or thin or heavy for his or her age. A child's psychologic adaptation depends on developmental variables. Although norms have been established by age groups, the plan of care should reflect consideration for individual differences. Therefore an individualized plan of care is essential for each pediatric patient.

Chronologic Development

The chronologic age of the patient is a primary consideration in the development of the plan of care. An age-related baseline is a useful beginning for assessing pediatric patients effectively. Terminology used to categorize ages of pediatric patients includes:

1. Fetus: in utero.
2. Newborn infant, referred to as a *neonate:*
   a. Potentially viable. Gestational age more than 24 weeks; birth weight more than 500 g and capable of sustaining life outside of the uterus
   b. True preterm (premature). Gestational age less than 37 weeks; birth weight 2500 g or less
   c. Large preterm (premature). Gestational age less than 37 weeks; birth weight more than 2500 g

d. Term neonate. Gestational age 38 to 40 weeks; birth weight usually between 3402 to 3629 g (if less than 2500 g, the neonate is considered small for gestational age [SGA])
e. Postterm (postmature). Gestational age more than 42 weeks

Neonatal period is first 28 days of extrauterine life

3. Infant: 28 days to 18 months
4. Toddler: 18 to 30 months
5. Preschool: 2½ to 5 years
6. School age: 6 to 12 years
7. Adolescent: 12 through 16 years

Physiologic Development

The physiologic development of pediatric patients is compared with national averages when establishing baseline norms. Physiologic development is influenced by genetics, nutrition, health status, and environmental factors. Comparison of the patient's age, size, and psychologic development with established norms may enable the caregiver to assess for deficiencies in size or weight that may indicate a health problem. A small, frail child may have a congenital cardiac deformity or a malabsorption syndrome. An extremely thin, malnourished adolescent may be intentionally bulimic or anorexic in response to a body-image psychologic problem. An obese child may have an endocrine disease or a psychologic disturbance that causes overeating. Most dosages of medications are based on body weight.

Psychologic Development

Assessment of psychologic development is based on age-related criteria (Table 42-1) but includes assessment of individual differences. Comparison of established norms and assessment data is helpful in developing the plan of care. Environmental and parental influences can cause variance in affect, attitude, and social skills. Environmental influences on psychologic development include ethnic, cultural, and socioeconomic factors. The age of the patient may indicate his or her level of involvement with the environment. For example, an infant may have exposure only to immediate family members for external stimuli, but a preschool child may have experience with nursery school and other children on a daily basis.

Parenting practices may directly influence the way the patient responds to caregivers and the perioperative environment. Pediatric patients respond differently in the presence of parents or guardians. Infants may be more cooperative if a parent is present. Conversely, an adolescent may want to demonstrate independence by asking the parent to leave the room. These actions may be completely opposite if the child has been abused or neglected. Lack of parental nurturing can cause a global deficit, including poor development of language and cognitive skills. Understanding the patient's level of psychologic development can help the caregiver communicate more effectively with the pediatric patient throughout the perioperative experience. Interaction should be according to his or her individual developmental level regardless of chronologic age.

CLASSIFICATIONS OF PEDIATRIC SURGERY

Pediatric surgery in all specialties can be divided into three classifications: congenital anomalies, acquired disease processes, and trauma.

Congenital Anomalies

A congenital anomaly is a deviation from normal structure or location in any organ or part of the body. It can alter function or appearance. Multiple anomalies are often present at birth. If the anomaly does not involve sustaining life functions, surgical intervention may be postponed until the results can be maximized and the risks of the surgical procedure are minimized by growth and development of body systems. If the newborn has a poor chance of survival without a surgical procedure, the risk is taken within hours or days after birth. Defects in the alimentary tract are the most common indication for an emergency surgical procedure during the newborn period, followed in frequency by cardiac and respiratory system defects. Mortality in the newborn is influenced by three uncontrollable factors: the multiplicity of anomalies, prematurity, and birth weight. The presence of three or more anomalies is referred to as the VACTERL association or syndrome:

V Vertebral defect, such as spina bifida
A Anal malformation, such as imperforate anus
C Cardiac anomaly, such as patent ductus arteriosus and ventricular and atrial septal defects
T Tracheoesophageal fistula
E Esophageal atresia
R Renal anomaly, such as horseshoe kidney and renal dysplasia
L Limb defect, such as syndactylism

Acquired Disease Processes

Among acquired disease processes, appendicitis is the most common surgically corrected childhood disease. Malignant tumors occur in infants and children, but with minimal frequency when compared with occurrence rate for adults. Benign lesions are surgically excised, usually without further difficulty to the child.

Trauma

Accidental injury is the leading cause of death in children. Injury can occur during the birth process and any

TABLE 42-1

Psychologic Developmental Stage Theories

CHRONOLOGIC AGE RANGES (APPROXIMATE)	DEVELOPMENTAL STAGE BY THEORIST			CHARACTERISTICS OF PSYCHOLOGIC DEVELOPMENT
	ERIKSON	PIAGET	LOEVINGER	
Birth-18 mo	Trust vs. mistrust	Sensorimotor	Presocial	Learns to view self as being separate from the environment; begins to develop the concept of hope; learns to develop attachments to others; is dependent on caregiver for warmth, security, nourishment, nurturing, and stimulation; begins to use sounds and short words to communicate ideas; may view hospitalization as abandonment
19 mo-3 yr	Autonomy vs. shame/doubt	Preoperational	Symbiotic	Develops a two-way relationship with primary caregiver; suffers separation anxiety when isolated from established relationships; has short trials of independence; personality becomes introverted or extroverted; establishes a sense of will; uses sentences for communication; has fear of immediate threats; does not project thoughts beyond the present situation
4-6 yr	Initiative vs. guilt	Preoperational	Impulsive	Asserts a separate identity; begins to have fear of real and imagined situations; senses peer acceptance and/or rejection; is concerned about disfigurement; may act out feelings; believes that every action has a purpose, either reward or punishment; learns to be self-protective; fears death or nonexistence; death is not always understood as being permanent; develops short-term self-control; uses compound sentences to communicate; mimics terminology used by fantasy characters
7-11 yr	Industry vs. inferiority	Concrete operational	Conformist	Imitates actions and attitudes of peers and heroes; is aware of the differences of others and identifies with a particular social group; fears loss of self-control; understands the world in moderate detail; prefers honest explanations and reassurance of safety; does not want to be treated like a baby; strives for competency in daily tasks; can distinguish between fact and fantasy; has a greater understanding of death and its permanence; wants to be accepted as an individual; communicates well verbally and with basic writing skill

Continued

TABLE 42-1

Psychologic Developmental Stage Theories—cont'd

CHRONOLOGIC AGE RANGES (APPROXIMATE)	DEVELOPMENTAL STAGE BY THEORIST			CHARACTERISTICS OF PSYCHOLOGIC DEVELOPMENT
	ERIKSON	PIAGET	LOEVINGER	
12-16 yr	Identity vs. role confusion	Formal operational	Self-aware Conscientious	May change opinion in response to stereotypes; develops close personal relationships; understands values, rules, and ideals; begins to feel more important as an individual; fears alienation; body image is extremely important; is capable of abstract thought and reasoning; has a sense of aesthetic beauty; can merge sensory information and logic to derive a conclusion; prefers privacy and confidentiality; may question authority; is aware of opposite sex; may explore sexual activity; dreams about future lifestyle; wants to prove self-worth; globally communicates verbally and in writing
17 yr-adulthood	Intimacy vs. isolation	Formal operational	Individualistic	Becomes aware of and accepts the interdependence of mankind; may feel some hostility toward authority; sometimes torn between the desire to be totally independent and dependent; seeks companionship of opposite sex; may be sexually active; refines interpersonal skills; demands privacy and confidentiality; plans for independent lifestyle as approach; refines verbal and written communication skill

time thereafter to any part of the body. Children are prone to lacerations, fractures, or crushing injuries of hands and arms, resulting in nerve, vessel, tendon, bone, and/or soft tissue damage. Trauma can be the cause of physical deformity, prolonged hospitalization with multiple surgical procedures, and emotional problems. The margin for error in diagnosis and treatment of a child is less than that for an adult with a similar injury. A child's blood volume is small, and even a small loss of blood can be critical. The comparatively large skin area causes rapid heat loss. Because the child's chest cavity is small, an abdominal or chest injury can be critical. Fatal collapse can result rapidly. It is imperative that a diagnosis be made quickly, that the patient be sent to the operating room (OR) if indicated, and that lifesaving measures be taken immediately.

GENERAL CONSIDERATIONS

Many anomalies, diseases, and traumatic injuries formerly considered fatal or inoperable now yield to successful surgical intervention. Knowledge has advanced pediatric surgery through:

1. Recognition of differences in needs of newborns, infants, and children from those of adults
2. Accurate diagnosis, especially in the fetus and the preterm and term neonate: many defects can be corrected if diagnosis is made early; neonatology has become a subspecialty of pediatrics
3. Understanding of preoperative preparation of the patient and family
4. Availability of total parenteral alimentation for management of many neonatal surgical problems
5. Advances in anesthesiology: new agents, perfection of techniques of administration, and an understanding of the responses of infants and children to anesthetic agents
6. Refinements in surgical procedures and instrumentation
7. Understanding of postoperative care; some facilities have neonatal and pediatric intensive care units

Physiologic Differences by Age Factor

Newborns, infants, and children through adolescence differ from each other according to age, body weight, and physiologic development. All differ from adults. Infants, for example, have great vitality beyond that indicated by their size, but their reactions are different from those of adults.

Metabolism

Infants have relatively greater nutritional requirements than do adults for minimizing loss of body protein; thus disturbances develop more rapidly in infants than in adults. The resting metabolic rate of an infant is two to three times that of an adult. Complications increase proportionately with increase in time of fluid restriction because infants are prone to hypovolemia and dehydration. Procedures on infants and toddlers should have priority on the surgical schedule so that these pediatric patients may return to a normal feeding and fluid intake routine as quickly as possible.

1. Infants are given regular formula or a varied diet up to 6 hours before anesthesia and clear liquids, usually dextrose in water, up to 2 hours before the surgical procedure. A satisfactory state of hydration is thus maintained and milk curds are absent from the stomach. Infants may be breast-fed up to 4 hours before the surgical procedure. Breast milk has less or no curd and empties faster from the stomach than formula. Infants should not miss more than one or two feedings. Oral intake is resumed promptly after the infant recovers from anesthesia, except following an abdominal surgical procedure.
2. Toddlers and preschool children usually are permitted clear liquids up to 2 to 4 hours preoperatively. Intake of clear oral fluids in small amounts decreases the level of gastric acid contents by stimulating gastric emptying and diminishes the hunger-deprivation response.
3. Children over 5 years of age may have nothing by mouth (NPO) after midnight or 6 hours before induction of anesthesia. Exceptions may be necessary for children with fever, diabetes, or other special problems. For these children, clear liquids with supplemental glucose may be ordered to be given orally up to 2 hours preoperatively.
4. Older children may require slower progression of oral dietary intake postoperatively and are maintained with supplemental intravenous therapy that includes protein and vitamins. Vitamins K and C may be given to patients of any age group.

Fluid and Electrolyte Balance

The newborn is not dehydrated and withstands major surgical procedures within the first 4 days of life without extensive fluid and electrolyte replacement. The renal system is easily overloaded by the administration of intravenous fluids. The newborn has a lower glomerular filtration rate and less efficient renal tubular function than does an adult. (Renal function improves during the first 2 months of life and approaches adult levels by age 2 years.) During the time of an average surgical procedure on a newborn, 10 to 30 ml of fluid may be administered. Usually 5% dextrose in half-strength normal saline solution is infused.

Administration of excessive intravenous dextrose solution is avoided in infants younger than 1 year of age because they maintain lower glycogen stores. During physiologic stress the patient easily becomes hyperglycemic. Hyperglycemia acts as an osmotic diuretic, causing increased urinary output and dilutional hyponatremia. The increased urine volume can be a false indicator of renal and hemodynamic status. Seizures and neurologic damage may result. Seizures may be clinically undetected while the infant is under general anesthesia because the pharmacologic agents act as anticonvulsants.

Infants have a relatively larger body-surface area to body-mass ratio than do adults. When they become dehydrated, which can occur rapidly, bodily functions are disturbed, as is the acid-base balance. Plasma proteins differ in concentration from those of an adult. Fluid and electrolyte replacements are necessary. In children older than 1 year of age, isotonic solutions, such as normal saline or Ringer's lactate, are given intravenously per kilogram of body weight.

The hemoglobin level is lowest at 2 to 3 months of age (Table 42-2). The blood volume of the average newborn is 250 ml, approximately 75 to 80 ml per kilogram of body weight (Table 42-3). Significant blood loss re-

TABLE 42-2

Pediatric Hematologic Value Ranges

AGE	HEMOGLOBIN (g/dl)	HEMATOCRIT (%)	LEUKOCYTES (mm^3)	PLATELETS (mm^2)
Cord blood	13.7-20.1	45-65	9000-30,000	350
2 wk	13.0-20.0	42-46	5000-21,000	260
3 mo	9.5-14.5	31-41	6000-18,000	250
6 mo-6 yr	10.5-14.0	33-42	6000-15,000	250
7-12 yr	11.0-16.0	34-40	4500-13,500	250

TABLE 42-3

Pediatric Blood Volume

AGE	BLOOD VOLUME (ml/kg)
Newborn	75 to 80
6 wk-2 yr	75
2 yr-puberty	72

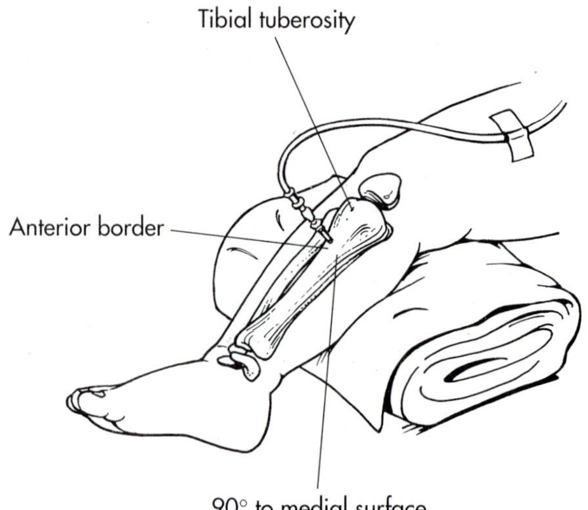

FIGURE 42-1 Intraosseous infusion into tibia. Insertion site for needle placement is in anterior midline 1 to 3 cm below tibial tuberosity. Note that needle is perpendicular to medial surface and tubing is secured on thigh.

quires replacement. Blood is typed and cross-matched in readiness. Although blood loss is small in most cases, loss of 30 ml may represent 10% to 20% of circulating blood volume in an infant. The small margin of safety indicates the need for replacement of blood loss exceeding 10% of circulating blood volume. When replacement exceeds 50% of the estimated blood volume, sodium bicarbonate is infused to minimize metabolic acidosis.

Hypotension in an infant is not apparent until 50% of the circulating volume is lost. Hypotension is usually caused by myocardial depression from anesthetic agents, primarily inhalation anesthesia. The infant's myocardium has fewer contractile muscle fibers and more noncontractile connective tissue than present in an older child or adult and therefore lacks myocardial force to maintain cardiac output. The cardiac output is dependent on the heart rate. Any decrease in heart rate directly affects blood pressure and body tissue perfusion.

Intravenous infusions should be administered with precautions.

1. Dehydration is avoided. Therapy for metabolic acidosis, should it develop, is guided by measurement of pH, blood gases, and serum electrolytes.
2. Blood-volume loss is measured as accurately as possible and promptly replaced. In an infant, rapid transfusion of blood may produce transient but severe metabolic acidosis because of citrate added as a preservative.
3. Intravenous fluids and blood are infused through pediatric-size cannulated needles or catheters connected to drip-chamber adapters and small solution containers. Umbilical vessels may be used for arterial or venous access in newborns less than 24 hours after birth. In extreme circumstances, the umbilical vein can be accessed through a small infraumbilical incision and cannulated from inside the peritoneal cavity for rapid infusion. Scalp veins are used frequently on infants. If venous access cannot be quickly established, intraosseous infusion may be indicated for fluid replacement (Figure 42-1). A cutdown on an extremity vein, usually the saphenous vein, may be necessary for toddlers and older children. An extremity should be splinted to immobilize it.
4. An extra length of tubing may be needed between the cannula and solution container so that tubing will reach under the drapes and the container can be elevated high enough for the solution to drip. Remember that the tubing lies on the operating table under the drapes. Take care that instruments are not placed on the tubing to obstruct flow. A plastic basin cut in half can be placed over the tubing as a protection. A 250 ml solution container is used to help avoid danger of overhydration. Adapters are set for accurate control of the desired flow rate.

Body Temperature

Newborns (especially preterm), infants, and children have wider average body temperature variations than do adults. This can vary with environmental changes. Body temperature in the newborn tends to range from as low as 97° to 100° F (36° to 37.7° C). Temperature begins to stabilize within this range 12 to 24 hours after birth if the environment is controlled. The relatively high rate of heat loss in proportion to heat production in the infant results from an incompletely developed thermoregulatory mechanism and from body-mass ratio with only a thin layer of subcutaneous fat for insulation. Extensive superficial circulation also causes rapid dissipation of heat from the body. A hypothermic newborn or infant metabolizes anesthetic agents more slowly and is susceptible to postoperative respiratory depression and delayed emergence from anesthesia. The first sign of hypothermia in a child younger than 1 year of age is a heart rate below 100 beats per minute.

Oxygen consumption is at a minimum when abdominal skin temperature is 97° F (36° C). A room temperature 5° F (9° C) cooler than that of abdominal skin produces a 50% increase in oxygen consumption, creating the hazard of acidosis. These factors account for the infant's susceptibility to environmental changes. Heat loss can occur in infants by:

1. *Evaporation.* When skin becomes wet, evaporative heat loss can occur.
2. *Radiation.* When heat transfers from body surface to surfaces such as walls of the room that are not in direct contact with the body, radiation heat loss can result.
3. *Conduction.* When air currents pass over skin, heat loss by convection results; cold diapers and blankets can cause heat loss by conduction.

Newborns, infants, and children are kept warm during the surgical procedure to minimize heat loss and to prevent undesired hypothermia. Body temperature tends to decrease in the OR because of cooling from air conditioning and open body cavities. Room temperature should be maintained as warm as 85° F (29° C). Other precautions should also be taken.

1. Hyperthermia blanket or water mattress is placed on the operating table and warmed before the infant or child is laid on it. It is covered with a double thickness of fabric. Temperature is maintained at 95° to 100° F (35° to 37.7° C) to prevent skin burns and elevation of temperature above the normal range. Excessive hyperthermia can cause dehydration and convulsions in the anesthetized patient.
2. Radiant heat lamp should be placed over newborn to prevent heat loss through radiation. Warming lights with infrared bulbs may be used if a radiant warmer is not available. These lights should be about 27 inches from the infant to prevent burns; the distance should be measured. A plastic bubble pack also provides insulation around the newborn to prevent heat loss by conduction.
3. Wrapping head (except face) and extremities in plastic, such as Saran wrap, or Webril helps prevent heat loss in infants and small children. An aluminum warming suit or blanket may be used for toddlers and older children. Forced-air warming blankets also are effective in maintaining core temperature.
4. Telethermometer monitors body temperature throughout the surgical procedure. This electronic instrument provides direct temperature readouts on a screen from a heat-sensing probe. Rectal, esophageal, axillary, or tympanic probes are used. A probe placed into the rectum should not be inserted more than 2 or 3 cm (an inch) because severe trauma to an infant through perforation of the rectum or colon can occur.
5. Drapes should permit some evaporative heat loss to maintain equalization of body temperature. An excessive number of drapes, which can retain heat and put a weight on the body, is avoided.
6. Solutions should be warm when applied to tissues to minimize heat loss by evaporation and conduction. The circulator should pour warm skin preparation solutions immediately before use. (Check manufacturer's recommendations for warming solutions. Some iodine-based solutions become unstable when heated.) The scrub person dampens sponges in warm saline before handing them to the surgeon.
7. Blood can be warmed before transfusion by running tubing through a blood warmer or a basin of warm water. Intravenous solutions should also be warmed.
8. Blankets should be warmed to place over the infant or child immediately after dressings are applied and drapes are removed. Keep the infant covered whenever possible before and after the surgical procedure to prevent chilling from the air conditioning.

Hyperthermia (i.e., core temperature of the body over 104° F [40° C]) during the surgical procedure presents a hazard. Causes are fever, dehydration, decrease in sweating from atropine administration, excessive drapes, and drugs that disturb temperature regulation such as general anesthetics and barbiturates. Dire consequences ensue. If the patient is febrile preoperatively, the surgical procedure should be delayed to allow reduction in temperature and to permit fluid administration. If an immediate surgical procedure is necessary and fever persists, anesthesia is induced and external cooling is employed.

Cardiopulmonary Response

The heart rate fluctuates widely among infants, toddlers, and preschool children and varies during activity vs. at rest (Table 42-4). Infants younger than 1 year of age tolerate a heart rate between 200 and 250 beats per minute without hemodynamic consequence. Heart rhythm disturbance is uncommon unless a cardiac anomaly is present. Cardiopulmonary complications manifest as respiratory compromise more frequently than as cardiac dysfunction. After age 5 years, cardiopulmonary response to stress resembles that of a young adult.

Cardiac and respiratory rates and sounds are continuously monitored in all age groups by precordial or esophageal stethoscopy. Blood pressure, vital signs,

TABLE 42-4

Pediatric Vital Sign Ranges

AGE	HEART RATE/MIN	RESPIRATIONS/MIN	BLOOD PRESSURE
Newborn	100-170	30-60	40 systolic
Infant			
1 mo	110-150	26-34	80/54
6 mo	115-130	26-40	90/60
1 yr	110-150	26-34	96/65
Toddler			
18-30 mo	110-130	24-28	98/65
Preschool			
4 yr	80-120	20-30	99/65
School-age			
6-9 yr	70-115	20-30	100/60
10 yr	70-110	18-26	110/60
Adolescent			
14 yr	60-110	16-24	118/60

electrocardiogram (ECG), and other parameters as indicated are also monitored throughout the surgical procedure (Table 42-4). A pulse oximeter can be placed on the palm of the hand or on the midfoot of a newborn or small infant. Smaller patients suffer oxygen desaturation easily. A pulse oximeter reading of 80% is clinically diagnostic of central cyanosis. Hypoxemia can cause bradycardia to decrease oxygen consumption of the myocardium.

Infants and toddlers are particularly susceptible to respiratory obstruction because of their anatomic structure. They are obligate nasal breathers. They have small nares, a relatively large tongue, presence of lymphoid tissue, and small diameter of trachea, causing disproportionate narrowing of the airway. A cylindric thorax, poorly developed accessory respiratory muscles, and increased volume of abdominal contents limit diaphragmatic movement. The chest is more compliant and collapses easily.

Infection

Newborns and infants are susceptible to nosocomial infection and show less resistance to overcoming it than do adults. Many preterm infants who have respiratory distress and circulatory problems survive because of advances in perinatal medicine. This has increased the population of high-risk and debilitated infants with reduced humoral and cellular defenses to infection. Aseptic technique is essential in handling neonates and all other pediatric patients.

An elective surgical procedure should be delayed in the presence of respiratory infection because of the risk of airway obstruction. Intubation of inflamed tissues may cause laryngeal edema. *Coryza,* inflammation of mucous membranes of the nose, is often a premonitory sign of an infectious respiratory disease.

Pain

Infants and children are sensitive to pain. Their pain may be intense, but infants, toddlers, and preschool children are unable to describe its location and nature. School-age children may refer pain to a part of the body not involved in the disease process. Insecurity and fear in an older child may be more traumatic than is the pain itself. Children should be observed for signs of pain (i.e., vocalizations, facial expressions, body movements, and physiologic parameters). Children also differ from adults in their response to pharmacologic agents; their tolerance to analgesic drugs is altered (Table 42-5).

Preparation of Pediatric Patient

The pediatric surgical patient should be considered as a whole person with individual physical and psychosocial needs assessed in relation to the natural stages of development. Equally important are the adjustment and attitude of the parents toward the child, the illness, and the surgical experience. Parents' anxiety about the impending surgical procedure may be transferred to the child. Emotional support of both the patient and parents, as well as parent and child teaching, are important

TABLE 42-5

Pediatric Sedation and Pain Management

DRUG AND DOSAGE	DURATION	CONSIDERATIONS IN ADMINISTRATION
Acetaminophen 10 mg/kg PO 20-25 mg/kg rectally	3-4 hr	Analgesia for minor procedures; antipyretic; absorption is delayed in infants so dose should not be repeated for 6 hr; no effect on coagulopathy; no respiratory depression; may be combined with narcotic for major procedures
Codeine 0.5-1 mg/kg IM or PO	3-4 hr	Moderate pain relief; not given IV; can be given with acetaminophen
Diazepam 0.04-0.02 mg/kg IM or IV 0.12-0.8 mg/kg PO Not used for continuous infusion	1-3 hr 3-4 hr	Sedation and seizure control; can cause respiratory depression, jaundice, and vein irritation at IV site
Fentanyl citrate 1-2 μg/kg IM or IV Continuous infusion: 0.5-2 μg/kg/hr PO lozenge is available	30-60 min	Excellent pain and anxiety relief; metabolized slowly in smaller children and infants; reversible with naloxone; short half-life; can cause respiratory depression, nausea, and vomiting; PO lozenge provides sedation but causes high incidence of preoperative nausea and vomiting
Hydromorphone hydrochloride 1-4 mg per dose every 4 hr IM, IV, PO	4-5 hr	Not used for infants and young children; used for adolescents; side effect include CNS and respiratory depression, hypotension, bradycardia, increased intracranial pressure, and peripheral vascular dilation
Ibuprofen 5-10 mg/kg PO or rectally	3-4 hr	Can cause gastrointestinal bleeding; may affect platelet aggregation
Lorazepam 0.1 mg/kg IV	6-8 hr	Long half-life; sedation and seizure control; can cause respiratory depression, nausea, vomiting, and vein irritation at IV site; used for adolescents
Meperidine hydrochloride 1-1.5 mg/kg IM, IV, or subcutaneous Can be given PO, but less effective	3-4 hr	Excellent pain relief; reversible with naloxone; can cause respiratory depression, suppression of intestinal motility, and hypotension; may cause nausea and vomiting; not used in increased intracranial pressure; poor sedation; not a good premedicant
Midazolam hydrochloride 0.1 mg/kg IV 0.08 mg/kg IM 0.5-0.75 mg/kg PO 0.3 mg/kg rectally in 5 ml normal saline Continuous infusion: 0.1 mg/kg/hr	30-60 min	Short half-life; may cause respiratory depression; excellent amnesic; sedation of choice for most pediatric patients

PO, By mouth; *IM,* intramuscularly; *IV,* intravenously; *CNS,* central nervous system.

Continued

TABLE 42-5

Pediatric Sedation and Pain Management—cont'd

DRUG AND DOSAGE	DURATION	CONSIDERATIONS IN ADMINISTRATION
Morphine sulfate		
0.1-0.2 mg/kg IM, IV, or subcutaneous Not well absorbed PO Continuous infusion: 0.25-2 mg/kg/hr; average dose 0.06 mg/kg/hr	4-5 hr	Excellent pain relief; reversible with naloxone; can cause respiratory depression, suppression of intestinal motility, and hypotension; may cause nausea and vomiting; not a good premedicant
Pentobarbital		
2-4 mg/kg IM, PO, or rectal	3-4 hr	Causes sedation and hypnosis; short-acting
Sufentanil citrate		
1-2 μg/kg IV Nasal spray	1-2 hr	Is 10 times more potent than fentanyl; very short half-life

aspects of preoperative preparation to help them cope. When an event is threatening, a person changes cognitive and behavioral responses to deal with the specific demands of the situation. Most adults face stress with more control when fear of the unknown is eliminated. Therefore, parents need to be forewarned of events that will occur and to be taught how to care for their child preoperatively and postoperatively. If children are forewarned of sensations to be experienced, cognitive control of the event may occur. Children do not differ from adults in this respect. However, understanding varies with age.

1. Psychologically it is better for both the infant and the parents if a congenital anomaly is corrected as soon after birth as possible. The infant younger than 1 year of age will not remember the experience. Parents will gain confidence in learning to cope with a residual deformity as the infant learns to compensate for it.
2. Separation from parent(s) or a trusted guardian is traumatic for infants over 6 months of age, toddlers, and preschool children. Infants require cuddling and bonding. Toddlers are only reaching the autonomy stage when hospitalization forces them into passive behavior, and thus their separation anxiety is greatest. Young children may fear strangers. The parent's presence is necessary for the toddler, and he or she should be encouraged to stay with the hospitalized child as much as possible. The child should be permitted to bring a toy or other security object to the OR suite if a parent cannot be present. In some facilities a parent is permitted to stay with the child through induction and to rejoin the child in the postanesthesia care unit (PACU) if the patient's condition permits.

NOTE
- Ambulatory surgery, if feasible, is an advantage because the child enters the facility an hour or two before the surgical procedure and returns home following recovery from anesthesia. This minimizes the trauma of separation.
- Many anesthesiologists encourage parents to accompany an infant or child to the OR and to stay through induction if they wish to do so. The presence of a parent can significantly reduce anxiety and ease induction. Some facilities allow parents to accompany the child to the holding area but restrict entrance into the OR. Highly anxious parents who have difficulty coping with stress may upset the child more than if they are not present.

3. Fear of body mutilation or punishment may be of paramount importance to a preschool or young school-age child. Children from 2 to 5 years of age have great sensitivity and a tenuous sense of reality. They live in a world of magic, monsters, and retribution, yet they are aggressive. School-age children, who have an enhanced sense of reality, value honesty and fairness. Their natural interest and curiosity aid communication. These children need reassurances and explanations in vocabulary compatible with their developmental level. Choose words wisely. Avoid negative connotations. Stress positive aspects. Talk on the child's level about his or her interests and concerns.
4. Anxiety in the school-age child may be stimulated by remembrance of a previous experience. Many children undergo two or more staged surgical procedures before the deformity of a congenital anomaly or traumatic injury is cosmetically reconstructed or functionally restored. Familiarity with the nursing staff reassures the child. Ideally the same circu-

lator who was present for the first surgical procedure should visit preoperatively and be with the child during subsequent surgical procedures.
5. Fear of the unknown about general anesthesia may become exaggerated into extreme anxiety with fantasies of death. The school-age child and adolescent need facts and reassurances. Do not refer to general anesthesia as "putting you to sleep." The child may equate this phrase with the euthanasia of a former pet who never returned home. Rather say, "You will sleep for a little while," or "you will take a nap." Tell the child about the "nice nurses" who will be in the "wake-up room after your nap." Encourage parents to also display confidence and cheerfulness to avoid transmitting anxiety. Parents should be honest with their child but maintain a confident manner. The perioperative nurse should do the same. However, do not give a school-age child information not asked for; answer questions and correct misunderstandings. Be especially alert to silent, stoic, noncommunicative children, many of whom have difficult induction and emergence from anesthesia.

NOTE

- Some facilities hold "parties" for children and their parents before or after admission to explain routines and procedures before the surgical experience. At other facilities, personnel take children to the OR suite so they can see the different attire, lights, tables, anesthesia machine, and other equipment that might interest them. A child-sized anesthesia mask becomes a play toy and not something to be feared. A plastic mask, like those that pilots wear in an airplane, is less psychologically traumatic to a child than is an opaque black rubber mask. An effective method of explaining procedures to children is to use a doll and dress it as the child will look postoperatively. For example, put a cast on the doll if the child will have one postoperatively.
- A preoperative visit by a perioperative nurse should be planned to get to know the child and provide emotional support to the family. Parents should be taught to provide care, especially before and after an ambulatory procedure. Verbal instructions may be supplemented with a videotape or storybook to reinforce understanding for both child and parents.
- Children who have lost a sibling frequently fear hospitalization.

PEDIATRIC ANESTHESIA

Pediatric anesthesia has become increasingly specialized as the many variables in the management of infants and children have become better understood. The anesthesiologist recognizes and respects the small margin for error and the uniqueness of the physiology and responses to drugs of pediatric patients. For example, the high metabolic rate of children causes rapid oxygen consumption. Changes occur rapidly in infants and children.

Preoperative Assessment

A preoperative visit by the anesthesiologist to establish rapport and assess the patient is also a vital part of preparation of the pediatric patient. This visit is preferably made with the parents present so the child will consider the anesthesiologist a trustworthy and caring friend. During physical assessment, special attention is given to heart, lungs, and upper airways. Loose teeth are noted. Possible difficulties are anticipated. Preoperative care includes correction of dehydration, reduction of excessive fever, compensation for acidosis, and restoration of depleted blood volume. An American Society of Anesthesiologists (ASA) physical status classification is assigned to the pediatric patient (see Chapter 16, p. 308). Consideration is given to age, developmental stage, psychologic characteristics, and past history to determine the patient's probable response to the anesthesia experience.

Premedication

Psychologic preparation of the child over 7 years of age can decrease the need for an anxiolytic (i.e., a sedative or minor tranquilizer to reduce anxiety). Crying greatly increases mucus in the respiratory tract. At discretion of anesthesiologist, premedication may be ordered to produce serenity. Some anesthesiologists prefer children to be well medicated; others favor minimal or no sedation. Infants younger than 1 year of age usually do not require premedication. Premedication, which is tailored to the individual, varies considerably by age, weight, and health status. Preanesthetic sedation should allow the patient to be taken to the OR lightly asleep and should facilitate induction of anesthesia without awakening the child. It should also provide some analgesia during the recovery period.

Timing of administration is extremely important. To be effective, drugs should be given at least 45 to 60 minutes before the surgical procedure. *The circulator should check with the anesthesiologist and surgeon before sending for the patient.* If ample time is not available for the appropriate effect of premedication, the anesthesiologist may prefer to omit the medication to avoid precipitation of psychologic trauma. Fast-acting drugs are available and may be useful for rapid sedation preoperatively. Narcotics, such as morphine sulfate and meperidine hydrochloride (Demerol), are rarely indicated for routine premedication in healthy pediatric patients.

No ideal premedicant exists, but the following drugs are commonly used. (Also see the comparison of sedatives in Table 42-5.)

1. *Sufentanil citrate (Sufenta)* given nasally (i.e., sprayed onto nasal mucosa) facilitates separation from parents by causing relaxation and drowsiness. The child becomes calm and cooperative.

2. *Fentanyl citrate (Sublimaze)* can be incorporated into a lozenge or a flavored hard candy mounted on a stick (i.e., an "anesthetic lollipop"). When child licks the candy, the drug is absorbed into the bloodstream through oral mucosa and produces sedation for 30 to 60 minutes.
3. *Diazepam (Valium)* 0.04 to 0.02 mg/kg intramuscularly (IM) or 0.12 to 0.8 mg/kg given orally (PO) causes relaxation for 3 to 4 hours.
4. *Midazolam hydrochloride (Versed)* 0.08 mg/kg administered IM 15 minutes before induction greatly reduces anxiety.
5. *Scopolamine hydrobromide* 0.006 mg/kg may be added to an IM injection of midazolam hydrochloride for further sedation and amnesic effect.
6. *Atropine sulfate* 0.01 to 0.02 mg/kg may be administered IM, intravenously (IV), or subcutaneously to inhibit secretions, especially in a child with a severe airway problem, or to counteract bradycardia. Cardiac effects last about 1 hour. Dosage is decreased to 0.04 mg/kg for infants under 5 kg. It is not given in presence of fever or glaucoma.
7. *Glycopyrrolate (Robinul)* 0.004 to 0.01 mg/kg administered IM lowers gastric acidity. It may be given as an alternative to atropine sulfate to reduce secretions. It is contraindicated in presence of paralytic ileus, urinary tract obstruction, and glaucoma.

Anesthesia Equipment

Simple lightweight anesthesia equipment is used. Disposable equipment is popular. Face masks, designed for minimal dead space, are available to closely fit a child's relatively flat face. Nonrebreathing circuits provide less resistance and valves for fresh flow of gas at higher flow rates relative to a child's metabolism and ventilation. High gas flows require scavenging equipment. To avoid hypothermia, anesthetic gases are warmed and humidified. Neonates are especially at risk for fluctuations in temperature regulation.

Induction

Induction is facilitated by a quiet atmosphere, a soft voice, and a reassuring touch. Children should be told what to expect without precipitating fear. The induction experience can be described as "getting on a merry-go-round. Noises will seem louder." To avoid confusion it is best for the child to listen to one person speak at this time. The circulator should remain at the patient's side, maintain a gentle touch, and be alert to the patient's needs and condition.

1. Restraints should be loose. Minimal pressure should be applied. If the patient is a newborn, infant, or toddler, restraint straps are omitted while the circulator holds the patient during induction. A toddler or preschool-age child is less frightened when holding onto someone's hands. Restraints can be applied after the patient is asleep.
2. A few drops of food extract of the child's choosing (e.g., mint, banana, or strawberry) can be placed in the face mask. This makes the anesthetic gas more acceptable and gives the patient a sense of control. The scent of anesthetic gas may be compared to "special jet fuel" used for the trip in an airplane or spaceship.
3. If the child is awake, crying, or struggling, apprehension during induction can be avoided by distraction and rapport. It is not easy to establish rapport with young children. Their cooperation may be solicited by counting out loud, singing the alphabet song, blowing up a balloon, taking a "space trip," or discussing a favorite plaything or television character. The face mask can be held slightly above the face, permitting anesthetic gas to flow by gravity, and lowered gently as the child becomes drowsy. Some anesthesiologists permit the child to hold the mask.
4. Induction may be accompanied by regurgitation and aspiration of gastric contents in infants with pyloric stenosis, tracheoesophageal fistula, intestinal obstruction, or food in the stomach. The hazard is minimized by aspirating gastric contents with a sterile catheter before induction and leaving the tube in place for drainage during the surgical procedure. *Rapid-sequence induction* may also be used. This consists of thiopental sodium, muscle relaxant, and intubation with cricoid pressure (Sellick maneuver) applied to close the esophagus and avoid silent regurgitation of food from the stomach.

Types of Induction

Inhalation If asleep from premedication on arrival in the OR, the child can be anesthetized quickly. If the child is awake, induction may be initiated with high-flow nitrous oxide and oxygen, with the gradual addition of halothane.

Nitrous oxide may increase peripheral vascular resistance if it is used to maintain general anesthesia for cardiovascular procedures. It may also increase the risk of air embolus because it combines with smaller air bubbles that may enter the system during repair of congenital heart defects. Potent inhalants may cause myocardial depression and decrease cardiac output in very young children. Atropine may minimize this effect.

Rectal Given by enema, methohexital sodium (Brevital), 15 mg/kg of 1% solution, produces sleep in 6 to 8 minutes and lasts 45 to 60 minutes. This is a painless method used in the presence of parents for preschoolers or toddlers. The parent may hold the child. It is a good method for short diagnostic procedures. The anesthesiologist remains with the patient. Once the child is asleep, the anesthetic state may be maintained with an inhalant. Gentle assisted ventilation may be needed.

Intravenous IV infusion is often preferred for patients over 9 or 10 years of age. Induction with a small dosage of barbiturate or ketamine hydrochloride is rapid. Studies have shown that IV induction causes less psychologic trauma than inhalant methods. A mixture of lidocaine hydrochloride and prilocaine hydrochloride in a cream base is commercially available for application to site to decrease pain associated with venipuncture.

Ketamine hydrochloride, 1 to 2 mg/kg IV, is useful in a combative, burned, or hypovolemic patient. If given IM to a healthier child who weighs less than 10 kg, the usual dose is 5 to 10 mg/kg.

TABLE 42-6

Recommended Endotracheal Tube Sizes

AGE	DIAMETER (mm)
Preterm	2.5-3.0
Newborn	3.0
Newborn-6 mo	3.5
6-12 mo	3.5-4.0
12 mo-2 yr	4.0-4.5
3-4 yr	4.5-5.0
5-6 yr	5.0-5.5
7-8 yr	5.5-6.0
9-10 yr	6.0-6.5
11-12 yr	6.5-7.0
13-14 yr (and older)	7.0-7.5

Intubation

Airway obstruction in infants and children usually occurs early during anesthesia administration. When anesthesia deepens, airway insertion is essential after prior assisted ventilation. Assisted or controlled ventilation reduces the labor of breathing and therefore reduces metabolism. Placement of an endotracheal tube in the trachea of a newborn or infant differs from placement in a child or adolescent. Regardless of age, the airway must remain patent. Sterile equipment and gentle manipulation to avoid soft tissue injury are essential for intubating and suctioning. Other considerations include the following:

1. Endotracheal intubation is used by some anesthesiologists for all procedures in infants younger than 1 year of age. It is necessary for intraabdominal, intrathoracic, and neurosurgical procedures and for those about the head or neck areas, as well as for emergency procedures when contents of the stomach are uncertain. Intubation while the patient is awake may be used in neonates.
2. Size of endotracheal tube is selected according to the width and length of the trachea. (See Table 42-6 for endotracheal tubes sizes.) Endotracheal tubes for children under 8 years of age are not cuffed. The tube allows for a slight space around the exterior circumference. Soft tissue at the narrowest level of the cricoid cartilage, located just below the vocal cords, forms a loose seal around the tube.
3. Nasotracheal tube may inadvertently dislodge adenoid tissue and carry it into the trachea.
4. Head of a newborn or infant is elevated slightly and not hyperextended during placement of the endotracheal tube. A toddler also has a larger occiput and therefore needs little posterior extension of the head. A child with Down's syndrome is predisposed to instability of the odontoid articulation at the first cervical vertebra (C1) and is at risk of dislocation if the head is placed in extreme hyperextension.
5. Straight blade is usually used on the laryngoscope because the epiglottis must be raised to visualize the glottis during intubation (Figure 42-2). In an infant the epiglottis is long and stiff and projects posteriorly at an angle of 45 degrees above the glottis. The epiglottis of a toddler and a preschool child is short and easily traumatized.
6. Intubation and suctioning are preceded and followed by oxygen administration. If the process of introducing the endotracheal tube takes longer than 30 seconds, the patient should be ventilated with 100% oxygen before additional attempts at intubation ensue.
7. Length and diameter of suction catheter should be considered when suctioning oropharyngeal secretions. An oversized catheter may perforate the oropharynx, trachea, bronchus, or esophagus.
8. Newborn's head is maintained in a neutral position, midway between full extension and full flexion, while an endotracheal tube is in place. The tip of the tube should be placed at the midtrachea position. The average distance between the vocal cords and the carina, where the trachea separates into two branches, is only 4 or 5 cm (about 2 inches) in a term neonate and much less in a preterm neonate. If the head shifts, the tube can slip up or down and lead to disastrous consequences.

Anesthetic Agents and Maintenance

The following characteristics of anesthetic agents and maintenance of anesthesia are considered:

1. Topical agents are not frequently used because of the hazard of overdose.
2. Inhalation anesthesia, especially with halothane, is popular. Nitrous oxide–oxygen-halothane is fre-

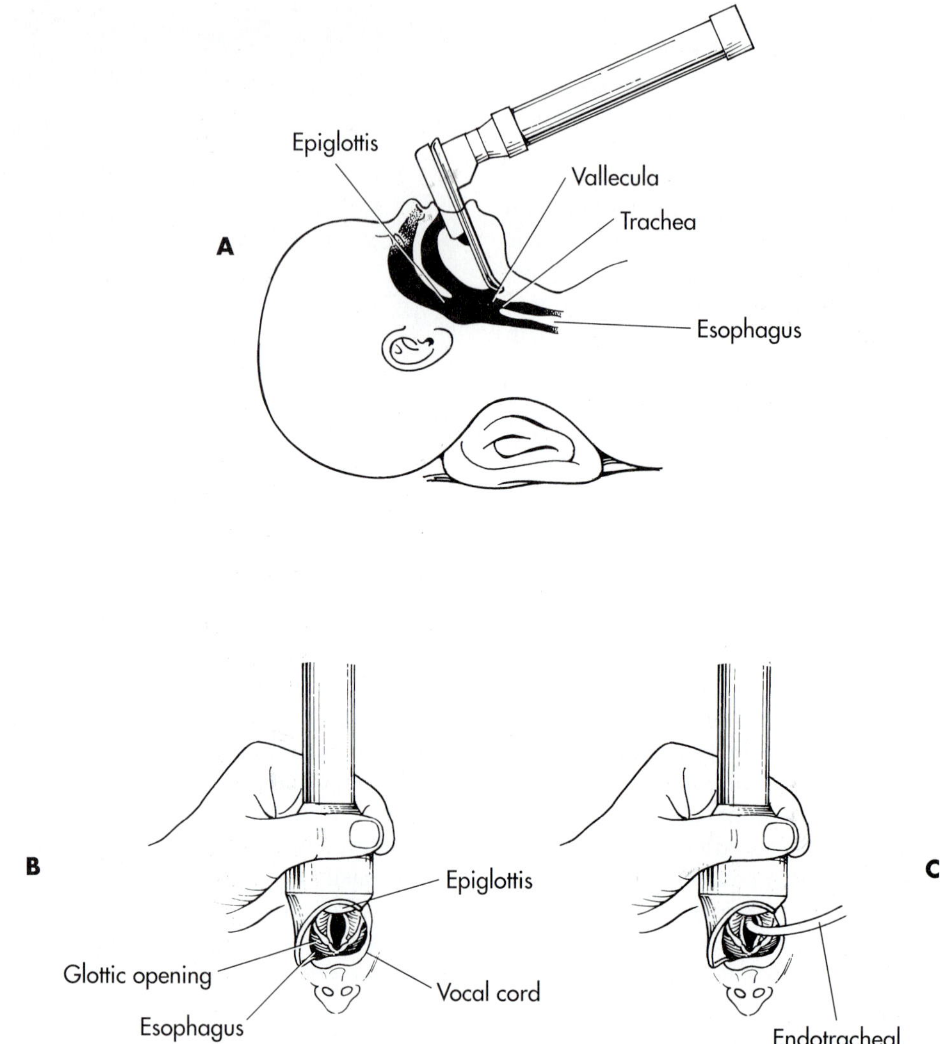

FIGURE 42-2 Intubation of infant, toddler, or preschool child. **A,** Straight blade on laryngoscope is advanced to vallecula, space between base of tongue and epiglottis. **B,** Gentle elevation of tip of blade lifts epiglottis to visualize glottic opening between vocal cords. **C,** Endotracheal tube is advanced below blade into trachea.

quently used in combination with intravenous agents. Halothane and succinylcholine are contraindicated if there is a family history of malignant hyperthermia. Nitrous oxide is used with caution in patients with congenital cardiac defects, particularly in cyanotic conditions. Isoflurane (Forane) is irritating, necessitating slow and more difficult induction to prevent laryngospasm, but it offers the advantage of circulatory support. It is not useful in short procedures.

Alveolar concentrations of inhaled anesthetics rise much more rapidly in pediatric patients than in adults because of relatively greater blood flow and smaller functional residual capacity. Children therefore have higher anesthetic requirements than do adults. To produce the same level of anesthesia, neonates require about 40% more halothane than do adults. Increased anesthetic requirement and more rapid induction can cause hypotension and reduced cardiac output in infants and children.

3. Ketamine provides sedation for preschool children during invasive diagnostic procedures. It is a short-acting general anesthetic for short procedures, such as burn debridement, tonsillectomy, or circumcision. Because it does not alter pharyngolaryngeal reflexes or skeletal tone, intubation is unnecessary. Cardio-

vascular and respiratory stimulation is minimal; ketamine may be useful in asthmatic and other poor-risk patients. It is contraindicated in the patient who has increased intracranial pressure. It is not advised for teenagers. Premedication with diazepam counteracts possible emergence delirium.

4. Local anesthesia is commonly used as a supplement to light general anesthesia. Long-acting agents, such as bupivacaine hydrochloride (Marcaine), prolong postoperative analgesia, thus reducing or eliminating the need for narcotics (Table 42-7).
5. Epidural anesthesia can be administered for sensory blockade intraoperatively. The epidural catheter may be left in place for prolonged postoperative analgesia. A continuous infusion of narcotics provides uninterrupted pain management, as administered to adults (see Chapter 18, pp. 351-352), to attenuate postoperative stress response.
6. Narcotics are used in situations similar to adult indications (see Chapter 17, pp. 333-334, and Table 42-5). Nitrous oxide–narcotic-relaxant provides stable anesthesia for the very ill patient. Fentanyl has minimal cardiovascular effect.
7. Critically ill neonate does not tolerate anesthesia well. Adequate ventilation and oxygenation are vital, but care is taken to avoid oxygen toxicity with resultant retrolental fibroplasia; neovascularization of the retina can produce blindness. Neonates and preterm infants under 34 weeks' gestational age and 1500 g or less body weight are at risk. Adequate blood-gas tension is ensured only by intraoperative invasive measurement.
8. Neuromuscular blockers are used judiciously. Infants younger than 1 year of age exhibit a lesser degree of blockade from succinylcholine than do older children. Bradycardia and intraocular tension rise are more conspicuous in infants. Response decreases with age. Dosage varies. A peripheral nerve stimulator should be used to assess blockade to avoid overdosage. Blockers seldom are required in infants because of their poorly developed abdominal musculature.
9. Consideration is given for postoperative analgesia. When halothane is reduced near the end of the surgical procedure, a narcotic may be given. Regional or local infiltration will also provide relief of pain, for example, following circumcision or cleft lip repair.
10. *Malignant hyperthermia* is a potentially severe intraoperative complication (see Chapter 19, pp. 383-386). Placing surgical gloves filled with ice directly over major arteries, including the femoral, carotid, and axillary, is a rapid method to cool infants and small children.

TABLE 42-7

Local Anesthesia for Pediatric Patients

AGENT	MAXIMUM PEDIATRIC DOSE
Lidocaine hydrochloride	
Without epinephrine	4.5-5 mg/kg
With epinephrine (epinephrine should not exceed 10 μg/kg)	7-10 mg/kg
Bupivacaine hydrochloride	3 mg/kg
Tetracaine hydrochloride	2 mg/kg
Procaine hydrochloride	15 mg/kg
Chloroprocaine hydrochloride	15 mg/kg
Cocaine hydrochoride	1 mg/kg

Emergence and Extubation

Airway problems are the most common concern on emergence from anesthesia and immediately postoperatively. At conclusion of the surgical procedure, the oropharynx is suctioned. Some anesthesiologists also suction the stomach. All monitors are left in place until the patient is fully awake and extubated.

Extubation of an infant or child is a treacherous time. It is preceded and followed by oxygen administration and performed either under deep anesthesia or on return of spontaneous respiration because laryngospasm is possible between these periods. Heart and breath sounds are monitored following extubation. If spasm occurs, oxygen is given by positive pressure. Airway obstruction, aspiration, and hypothermia are hazards of the recovery period. Children, particularly in the 2- to 5-year age group, may develop hoarseness and a croupy cough following removal of an endotracheal tube. Racemic epinephrine (Vapanefrin) provides relief; 0.5 ml of 2.25% diluted in 3 ml of sterile water can be delivered through a face mask and nebulizer. Constant observation following extubation is required.

Postoperative Care

The patient should not be taken from the OR with a body temperature below 95° F (35°C). Below this crucial level, the risk of acidosis, hypoglycemia, bradycardia, hypotension, and apnea increases. This metabolic depression and delayed return of activity set the stage for possible sudden cardiac arrest. Dehydration and low humidity increase viscosity of secretions. Pediatric patients require *close* watching for development of laryngeal edema noted by croupy cough, sobbing inspiration, intercostal retraction, tachypnea, or tachycardia. Laryngeal edema greatly reduces the small diameter of the airway of an infant or toddler. Controlled humidity and oxygen are vital.

PEDIATRIC PATIENT CARE CONSIDERATIONS

Basic principles of patient care and OR techniques discussed in preceding chapters apply to pediatric surgery. A few points specific to pediatric surgery are mentioned to differentiate this specialty from care of adult patients.

1. Hair is not removed with a depilatory or shaved, except for cranial procedures and as ordered by the surgeon for an adolescent.
2. Diagnostic studies may be done in the OR under local anesthesia before induction of general anesthesia for an open surgical procedure. An infant may be swaddled on a padded board to restrain him or her from moving while x-ray films are taken and to permit easy change of position. A sugar nipple or pacifier will help comfort and keep the infant quiet.
3. Patient is protected from injury. An infant or child should never be left alone anywhere in the OR suite, including the holding area. Preparation for induction should be made before the child's arrival.
   a. Guard against a fall from a crib or stretcher. Siderails should remain up at all times. An overbed cage on a crib helps confine a toddler without restraint. Children are restrained at all times while on a stretcher or in a specially designed pediatric cart.
   b. Do not place a crib where the patient can reach an electric outlet or near any article that can be picked up and cause injury.
   c. Pad wrists and ankles after infant is asleep with several layers of sheet wadding. Restrain with muslin or roller gauze and pin straps to sheet on the operating table. Sheet wadding prevents possible abrasion of delicate skin by the restraint straps. Care is taken not to restrict circulation.
   d. Safety pins, open or closed, are not left within reach of an infant or child.
4. Catheters as small as size 8 French are available for use as needed in newborns and infants. A plain tip or whistle tip catheter is used for a stomach tube. An indwelling Foley catheter with a 3 ml balloon may be used for urinary drainage. Small, calibrated drainage containers are connected to permit accurate determination of output.
5. Positioning principles are essentially the same as those described in Chapter 21. Correspondingly smaller towel rolls, pillows, gel pads, and bead bags are used to protect pressure points and to stabilize anesthetized infants and children. Size of child or adolescent determines the appropriate supports to maintain desired position. A small towel roll at each side of body takes weight of drapes off the small body of an infant or keeps the patient in a lateral position.
6. Disposable drape sheet without a fenestration is often advantageous: the surgeon can cut an opening of desired size to expose site of intended incision. Small towels and nonpiercing towel clips are used with a laparotomy sheet if self-adhering and disposable drapes are not available. A standard opening 3 × 5 inches (7.6 × 12.7 cm) in a pediatric laparotomy sheet is frequently too large for a newborn or infant. Part of the fenestration may be covered with a towel.
7. Sponges are weighed while still wet; blood loss through suction is measured and estimated in drapes. The surgeon and anesthesiologist will determine if blood replacement is necessary, volume for volume, as it is lost.
8. Adhesive tape is abrasive to tender skin and should be avoided when possible. An adhesive spray or collodion is adequate over a small incision with a subcuticular closure and is especially desirable under diapers, unless dressings are needed to absorb drainage. Care is taken that clothing or blanket does not touch this substance until it is dry. Skin closure strips may be used instead of a liquid adhesive.
9. Dressings on the face or neck should be protected from vomitus and food particles, as well as from an infant's or toddler's hands. Elbows should be splinted when the patient potentially may disturb the incision, dressings, or a tube. This is particularly important following eye surgery or cleft lip or palate surgery and when a tracheotomy tube is inserted (Figure 42-3).
10. Stockinette pulled over dressings on an extremity protects them from becoming dirty and helps keep them in place. This can be changed easily as needed, leaving the dressings in place.

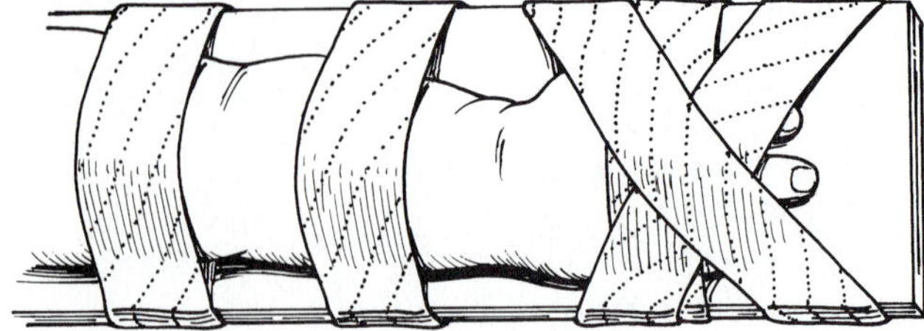

FIGURE 42-3 Upper extremity restraint to splint elbow and hand of infant or toddler. Hand is pronated on armboard.

Instrumentation

Gentleness and precision in handling small structures and fragile tissues are essential. Basic or standard instrument sets, sutures, needles, and other items used for surgical procedures on adults are duplicated in miniature to take care of infants and children in each surgical specialty. The perioperative nurse and surgical technologist should be informed about their patient and then use good judgment in preparing supplies for pediatric surgery.

1. Size and weight are more critical factors than age in the selection of instruments, sutures, needles, and equipment.
2. Small instruments are used on the delicate tissues of a newborn, infant, or small child.
3. Hemostats should have fine points. A mosquito hemostat will clamp a superficial vessel but not a major artery.
4. Noncrushing vascular clamps permit occlusion of major blood vessels. They also can be placed across the intestine of a newborn or infant rather than a large, heavy intestinal clamp.
5. Lightweight instruments will not inhibit respiration. Instruments not in use on tissues are *never* laid on the patient, especially not on the chest. An instrument's weight could restrict respiration or circulation or cause bruises. Return instruments to the Mayo stand or instrument table immediately after use.
6. Umbilical tape or vessel loops are used frequently to retract blood vessels and small structures, thereby giving the surgeon greater visibility in a small surgical site and eliminating the weight of retractors.
7. Needleholders have fine-pointed jaws to hold small, delicate needles.
8. Surgical procedure on an adolescent will require adult-sized instruments.
9. Scrub person closely watches the tissue being dissected and selects the instruments to hand to the surgeon accordingly.

COMMON SURGICAL PROCEDURES

General Surgery

Endoscopic Procedures

Gastroscopy, colonoscopy, and laparoscopy are performed for diagnosis of complaints of abdominal pain or symptoms of intestinal obstruction or inflammation. Procedures such as insertion of a gastrostomy tube; polypectomy, sphincterotomy, and appendectomy can be done in lieu of laparotomy. Endoscopic injection of sodium morrhuate is an alternative to portosystemic shunt in children with bleeding esophageal varices.

Anastomosis Within Alimentary Tract

Alimentary tract obstruction in a newborn or young infant is the most frequent cause for an emergency surgical procedure. The common sites of obstruction are in the esophagus, duodenum, ileum, colon, and anus. *Atresia,* an imperforation or closure of a normal opening, and *stenosis,* a constriction or narrowing, are the common causes of obstruction. The obstructive lesion is usually resected, and the viable segments of the viscera are anastomosed. A temporary gastrostomy, ileostomy, or colostomy may be necessary. Intestinal obstruction can develop in infants and children months to years after the newborn period from a predisposing or associated congenital anomaly or acquired disease process. Inflammatory diseases such as necrotizing enterocolitis, ulcerative colitis, Meckel's diverticulitis, or Crohn's disease, as well as other intestinal conditions such as Hirschsprung's disease or familial polyposis, require intestinal resection and anastomosis. An endorectal pull-through may be the procedure of choice to preserve the rectum.

Biliary Atresia A form of intrauterine cholangitis that results in progressive fibrotic obliteration of bile ducts, biliary atresia may cause jaundice in the newborn. Excision of extrahepatic ducts or hilar dissection with a hepatic portoenterostomy procedure, such as portal hepatojejunostomy, is performed before the infant is 2 months old to relieve jaundice by improving bile drainage. If liver function becomes progressively impaired, liver transplantation may ultimately be necessary for survival.

Esophageal Atresia Esophageal atresia, with or without *tracheoesophageal fistula,* is an acute congenital anomaly characterized by esophageal obstruction, accumulation of secretions, gastric reflux, and respiratory complications. The goal of repair is to obtain an end-to-end esophageal anastomosis. The timing and technique to accomplish this goal depend on the specific type of anomaly, degree of prematurity, birth weight, and extent of other associated anomalies. Repair may be either primary or staged. A gastrostomy is performed initially to establish a conduit for feeding the newborn. Repair includes division of the tracheoesophageal fistula, if present, and anastomosis of the esophageal pouches. Submucosal myotomies and lengthening of the upper pouch permit primary anastomosis to establish alimentary tract continuity. This may be delayed to allow the esophagus to grow as the infant grows so that the gap between the pouches shortens. A transthoracic or retrosternal interposition colon graft may be necessary for esophageal replacement if the gap between the proximal and distal segments is too large for a primary esophageal anastomosis. Usually an extrapleural approach is used for these procedures.

Imperforate Anus

If the anus remains closed (i.e., imperforate) during fetal development, the intestinal tract is opened surgically soon after birth. A posterior sagittal anorectoplasty or an abdominoperineal pull-through procedure may be done for primary management. Many children endure fecal incontinence or chronic constipation as they grow into their teens following these procedures in infancy. Various secondary procedures are performed, most frequently an endorectal pull-through procedure or gracilis muscle transplant for reconstruction of the rectal sphincter.

Pyloromyotomy

Pyloric stenosis is a congenital obstructive lesion in the pylorus of the stomach. Onset of symptoms usually occurs between the third and eighth weeks of life. The stenosis is relieved by pyloromyotomy. After cutting through serosa, muscle layers of the pylorus are divided.

Herniorrhaphy

Herniorrhaphy (i.e., hernia repair) is the most frequently performed elective surgical procedure in infants and children by general surgeons. Of the four types of hernias seen in pediatric patients, indirect inguinal hernia is the most common; it occurs much more frequently in male patients than in female patients and appears during the first 10 years of life. Female patients who have an inguinal hernia also may have a prolapsed ovary in the hernial sac. Although frequently seen, most umbilical hernias do not require surgical intervention. Hiatal (diaphragmatic) hernias and femoral hernias require surgical correction but are rarely acute problems in childhood. A hiatal hernia is a surgical emergency in the newborn if abdominal contents are in the chest, causing acute respiratory distress. Hernias in infants and children are caused by congenital weakness in the fascia, abdominal wall, or diaphragm.

Omphalocele

Failure of abdominal viscera to become encapsulated within the peritoneal cavity during fetal development results in herniation through a midline defect in the abdominal wall at the base of the umbilicus (i.e., omphalocele). Contents in the omphalocele sac are surgically reduced back into the peritoneal cavity. The method of closure depends on the extent of the defect. Skin may be closed primarily if the defect is small. More commonly, primary closure of the abdominal wall is facilitated by vigorous stretching of the wall and emptying of intestinal contents from the sac. Closure is performed without undue tension. Synthetic mesh or sheeting may be used. For large defects, closure of the abdominal wall usually is staged with implantation of a silicone silo or pneumatic prosthesis to reduce intestines at the first stage, followed by removal of the device and abdominal wall closure at the second stage. Similar techniques are used for closure of *gastroschisis,* a full-thickness abdominal wall defect lateral to and separate from the umbilicus, with herniation of abdominal viscera.

Appendectomy

Appendicitis, an acute inflammation of the appendix, is the most common cause for an abdominal surgical procedure in the school-age child. Gangrene or rupture may occur before diagnosis or surgical intervention. A questionable diagnosis may be confirmed by laparoscopy. Appendectomy may be performed by laparoscopy (see Chapter 29, p. 598).

Splenectomy

Removal of the spleen may be indicated to correct hypersplenic disease, either congenital or acquired. Emergency splenectomy is necessary following rupture of the spleen, usually from blunt trauma. An attempt is made to salvage as much of the organ as is possible to minimize future susceptibility to infection.

Urology

Pediatric urology concerns itself basically with the diagnosis and treatment of infections and congenital anomalies within the genitourinary tract. Some type of anomaly of the genitourinary system may be found in 10% to 15% of newborns. Secondary infections are frequently associated with congenital anomalies; chronic diseases are frequently associated with infections. The following surgical procedures include those most commonly performed by pediatric urologists.

Cystoscopy

Diagnostic evaluation and therapeutic removal of obstructions within the structures of the genitourinary tract may be performed through an infant- or child-sized cystoscope. Cystoscopes from 9.5 through 16 French are used for infants and children. A size 3 French ureteral catheter can be introduced through the smallest-size cystoscope.

Nephrectomy, Nephrostomy, or Pyeloureteroplasty

Hydronephrosis, congenital or acquired, may necessitate surgical intervention. Nephrectomy is indicated only if severe disease is unilateral with a contralateral kidney capable of life-sustaining function. More conservative nephrostomy or pyeloureteroplasty is indicated for bilateral or moderate to mild kidney disease.

Wilms' Tumor

Wilms' tumor is a malignant solid renal tumor that develops rapidly in a child usually under 5 years of age. Nephrectomy is necessary to resect tumor. If the adrenal gland is intimately connected to tumor in upper pole of the kidney, the gland is resected en bloc with the renal mass. Vascular extension of the tumor into suprahepatic vena cava may necessitate cardiopulmonary bypass to ligate all tumor vessels. Ipsilateral periaortic lymph node dissection often is performed.

Neurogenic Bladder

Defective bladder function may be the result of a central nervous system lesion such as myelomeningocele or spinal cord trauma. To preserve renal function and to achieve urinary continence in presence of neurogenic bladder, an enterocystoplasty may be performed. This procedure retains an intact urinary tract. An artificial urinary sphincter can be implanted to achieve dryness in the child who has sufficient dexterity to operate the pump.

Exstrophy of Bladder

In exstrophy of the bladder, a congenital anomaly, the bladder herniates through the lower abdominal wall in the suprapubic region. Repair requires reconstruction of lower abdominal wall and external genitalia, as well as provision for passage of urine. This can usually be accomplished in one surgical procedure on a female infant but requires two or more staged procedures in a male infant. A gastrocystoplasty may be the procedure of choice. If urinary continence cannot be established, urinary diversion through ureteral reimplantation may become necessary.

Ureteral Reimplantation

Repositioning of the ureters (i.e., ureteral reimplantation) may be performed to correct either congenital or acquired total urinary incontinence or vesicoureteral reflux.

Incontinence, involuntary leakage of urine from the bladder, causes parents to seek help for an infant or child. Incontinence is usually not caused by a single factor. The urologist plans the procedure on the basis of an accurate assessment of anatomic and physiologic causes. Creation of a tubularized trigonal muscle, when reconstructed into a new bladder neck, acts as a sphincter to maintain continence. With ureters in the normal position, this muscular tube in the bladder wall cannot be constructed. Therefore the ureters are reimplanted superiorly into the bladder through a created tunnel. Care is taken that the ureters are not hooked or angled but follow a smooth curve into the bladder.

Vesicoureteral reflux is the most common reason for reimplanting ureters in pediatric patients. Chronic reflux, regurgitation of urine from the bladder into the ureters, can lead to pyelonephritis and hydronephrosis. Ureteral reimplantation may be required to prevent kidney damage. The objective of the surgical procedure is to position a segment of the ureters at a higher level within the bladder wall so that urine lies below orifices and intravesical pressure prevents reflux.

When ureters cannot be reimplanted in the bladder, a urinary diversion procedure may be necessary. Ureters are usually anastomosed to a nonrefluxing colon conduit.

Urethral Repair

The external opening of the urethra may be displaced at birth. *Hypospadias* is an anomaly in the male in which the urethra terminates on the underside of the penis or on the perineum; in the female, the urethra opens into the vagina. With *epispadias* in the male, the urethra terminates on the dorsum of the penis; in the female, it terminates above the clitoris. Multistage procedures are usually necessary to correct these anomalies. The goal is to center the meatus at tip of glans penis of the male. This may be accomplished in a one-stage procedure by a transverse island flap derived from prepuce or by a vertical-incision/horizontal-closure technique for distal coronal or subglandular hypospadias. This procedure is usually performed between ages 1 and 4 years.

Orchiopexy

One or both testicles that failed to descend during fetal development can be brought into the scrotum and stabilized with a traction suture until healing takes place. Frequently done as a two-stage Torek orchiopexy, the testicle and supporting structures are dissected free from the inguinal region. An adequate length of spermatic vessels is released to permit the testicle to reach the scrotal sac. After it is pulled down through the scrotum, the testicle is sutured to fascia of the thigh. Two to three months later at the second-stage procedure, the testicle is freed from the fascia and embedded into the scrotum.

If one or both testicles are absent, silicone prostheses may be inserted into the scrotum for cosmetic appearance. Psychologically for child and parents, undescended testicles *(cryptorchism)* or absence *(agenesis)* of testicles is usually repaired at age 5 or 6 years, before the boy begins school.

Circumcision

Excision of the foreskin of the penis (circumcision) may be done to prevent *phimosis,* in which the foreskin becomes tightly wrapped around the tip of the glans penis, or to remove redundant foreskin. Circumcision is the most commonly performed pediatric surgical procedure. It should be done under local anesthesia on newborns. Circumcision, as an elective procedure, is contraindicated if an abnormality of the glans penis or urethral meatus is present. Urethral repair usually utilizes the foreskin as graft tissue.

Orthopaedic Surgery

Pediatric orthopaedic surgery is principally elective and reconstructive in nature to correct deformities of the musculoskeletal system. These deformities may be congenital, idiopathic, pathologic, or traumatic in origin. The extensiveness of the anomalies and functional disorders often involve prolonged immobilization and hospitalization. Many patients require a series of corrective procedures. Some of the conditions most commonly seen in the OR include the following.

Fractures

Fractures that occur in infants and children generally are treated as they are in adults, as described in Chapter 32. However, fixation devices are not well tolerated by children and often prevent uniting of the fracture. Closed reduction of long bone fractures is preferable.

Tendon Repair

Tendons may be lengthened, shortened, or transferred to correct congenital deformities of the hand or foot. Lacerated tendons are repaired to restore function. A tourniquet is always used to control bleeding. The tourniquet cuff size should be appropriate for size of infant or child. Padding under cuff is applied smoothly. Sheet wadding may be used under an infant cuff to protect delicate skin. The cuff should be tight but without restricting circulation before inflation. Time of inflation is closely watched to prevent ischemia. The surgeon may ask the circulator to release the pressure every 30 minutes on an infant or up to 1 to 2 hours for an older child, depending on age. Tendon procedures are often lengthy.

Congenital Dislocated Hip

Displacement (dysplasia) of the femoral head from its normal position in the acetabulum can be present at birth, either unilaterally or bilaterally. If diagnosed early in infancy, closed reduction with immobilization usually corrects the dislocation without residual deformity. If not diagnosed until after the child has begun to walk, open reduction of the hip with an osteotomy to stabilize the joint may be necessary.

Leg-Length Discrepancies

The epiphyseal cartilaginous growth lines progressively close as the child matures. Bones lengthen from the activity of the epiphyses. The absolute physiologic criterion for completion of childhood is when this cartilage becomes a part of bone. A discrepancy in activity of an epiphyseal line may retard or overstimulate growth of a bone in one extremity and not its contralateral counterpart. When this occurs in one femur, legs become unequal in length. The orthopaedic surgeon may correct leg-length discrepancies, usually in excess of 1 inch (2.5 cm), by epiphyseal arrest (i.e., stopping growth of the bone). This is done in the contralateral leg to let the shorter extremity catch up. The longer leg may be shortened by a closed intramedullary procedure. Under fluoroscopy, a reamer is inserted into the medullary canal of the femur through a small incision high on the hip. After the reamer widens the canal, a rotating saw is manipulated to cut a section from the bone. The bone ends are aligned and fixed with a flexible intramedullary rod.

Slipping of the upper femoral epiphysis causes displacement of the femoral head, which can occur as a result of traumatic injury or as a chronic disability usually seen in obese adolescents. Fusion of the epiphysis to the femoral neck may be necessary to prevent slipping and shortening of the leg.

Many limb deformities in children are a complex combination of angulation and shortening as a result of trauma, infection, metabolic bone disease, congenital deformity, and developmental problems. The Ilizarov external fixator technique (see Chapter 32, pp. 666-667) provides an alternative treatment option. Thin, strong wires are transfixed through bones and attached to rings under tension. The rings, which encircle a leg or arm, are held firmly in place with threaded rods. Bolts on the rods are turned several times a day to pull cut ends of bone apart. Corticotomy, performed through a small skin incision after wires are inserted, preserves periosteal and endosteal blood supply to bone. This promotes rapid healing to regenerate new bone that fills in the gap.

Talipes Deformities

Combinations of various types of deformities of the foot, especially those of congenital origin, are referred to as *talipes* plus the medical term to describe whether the forefoot is inverted *(varus)* or everted *(valgus)* and whether the calcaneal tendon is shortened or lengthened.

Talipes varus, the condition known as *clubfoot,* is the most common of these deformities. Either unilateral or bilateral, the forefoot is inverted and rotated, accompanied by shortening of the calcaneal tendon and contracture of the plantar fascia. Conservative treatment by casting during infancy usually corrects a mild postural deformity before the infant bears weight on the foot. A wedge cast with turnbuckles may be applied to an older child to allow gradual manipulation. If conservative treatment is unsuccessful, an open surgical procedure may be necessary.

Talipes equinovarus, an idiopathic true clubfoot deformity, almost always requires surgical intervention for correction. In varying degrees, talipes equinovarus includes an incomplete dislocation (subluxation) of the talocalcaneonavicular joint with deformed talus and calcaneous bones, a shortened calcaneal tendon, and soft tissue contractures. As a result, the forefoot curls toward the heel (adduction, supination), the midfoot points downward (equinus), and the hindfoot turns inward (varus). The orthopedic surgeon uses a sequential release approach to obtain maximum correction of all contractures and realigns bones in the ankle joint. Pins are inserted, and the extremity is casted to maintain alignment of the foot and ankle.

Scoliosis

Scoliosis is a lateral curvature and rotation of the spine, most frequently seen in rapidly growing school-age (over age 10) or adolescent females. Treatment depends on degree and flexibility of the curvature, chronologic and skeletal age of the child, and preference of the surgeon. The child may be fitted with a Milwaukee brace, immobilized in a cast, or stretched by traction. As an alternative to these techniques, an electrical device may be applied with an underarm brace to stimulate muscle contraction on convex side of curvature. If untreated at an early stage, scoliosis produces secondary changes in vertebral bodies and in the rib cage. Spinal fusion is ultimately performed if the curvature has become severe (50% or more) or must be stabilized following corrections. Government-mandated screening programs in schools have reduced the need for surgical correction in many children.

1. Wedge body jacket or Minerva jacket (see Chapter 32, pp. 680-681) may be applied. Turnbuckles may be incorporated. Turnbuckles are adjustable metal rods placed along the edges of the wedge of the cast. Gradual opening of the turnbuckles by the surgeon as tolerated by the patient corrects the lateral curvature of the spine.

   Sayre sling, an appliance used for head traction, is sometimes used when applying a body jacket to correct slight scoliosis. Traction is obtained by means of pulleys and a rope suspended from the ceiling or an arm of the fracture table.
2. Halo traction is used to stretch the spine in some patients in whom the spine is too rigid to be straightened in a cast. A metal band is applied to the skull by means of four pins inserted into the cortex of the skull. A Steinmann pin is inserted into the distal end of each femur. A traction bow is put on each pin. Weights, usually equal, are put on the halo and Steinmann pins and gradually increased as tolerated. When x-ray films show maximum correction, a spinal fusion is done. Traction may be continued until healing has taken place to the degree that there will be no loss of correction; a plaster jacket is then applied.
3. Risser jacket is applied a few days preceding posterior spinal fusion to gain as much correction as possible. The orthopaedic table is used. Traction is applied by a chin strap, similar to a Sayre sling, and countertraction is applied by a pelvic girdle. The spine is straightened as much as possible and the body and head are encased in plaster.

   Posterior spinal fusion may be performed as a two-stage procedure: vertebral body wedge resection at the first stage and insertion of Cotrel-Dubousset or Harrington rods with fusion at second stage. Bone fragments removed during the first stage may be saved for the second-stage fusion or sent to the bone bank. Rods and hooks are stainless steel; appropriate instruments are required to insert them. Two rods are inserted, one on either side of the curvature. These rods are secured to the spine and force it into a more nearly normal position. Implanted on outside of vertebral column, the rods apply a longitudinal force on the spine. The spine is then fused.

   The procedure may be done through a window in the Risser jacket, but usually the cast is bivalved and the patient lies in the anterior section. If the procedure is done through a window, an electric cast cutter should be at hand to bivalve the cast if the patient has any respiratory difficulties. After the procedure the bivalved posterior part is put in place and the jacket is fastened together by several rounds of plaster or by webbing straps with buckles. The patient is in the Risser jacket for a year. Progress is checked by x-ray films.
4. Segmental spinal fixation with Luque rods may be the procedure of choice to stabilize the spine following fusion. Two L-shaped rods are placed next to the spinous processes and held by wires threaded under the lamina of each vertebra to be fused. Transverse traction internally on each vertebra stabilizes the spine without need for a postoperative cast.
5. Anterior spinal fusion through a transthoracic approach is performed as a one-stage procedure to correct severe curvatures in patients who have malformed vertebral bodies. With Dwyer instruments, titanium staples are fitted over vertebral bodies on convex side of the curve. Each staple is held in place by two titanium screws. A multistrand titanium cable, threaded through the heads of the screws, is tightened to compress the vertebrae and straighten the curve. Staples and screws are secured the full extent of the curvature. A plaster body jacket may be applied after the procedure to immobilize the back until the fusion is healed. The patient is then ambulatory.

Ophthalmology

Congenital Obstruction of Nasolacrimal Duct

An obstruction, usually at lower end of nasolacrimal duct, that enters the inferior meatus of the nose often results in dilatation and infection of the lacrimal sac. Treatment consists of passing a malleable probe from the lid punctum through the nasolacrimal passages to push out the obstructing plug of tissue.

Oculoplastic Procedures on Eyelids

Congenital malformations such as *ptosis* (drooping of upper or lower eyelid) are corrected by extraocular procedures. Ptosis repair is indicated when the levator is inadequate. In the levator resection procedure, which shortens the muscle and gives a more physiologic result, the levator muscle may be approached through the skin (Berke method) or the conjunctiva (Iliff method). A fascial sling procedure to support the lid consists of attaching the upper lid margin to the frontalis muscle. Materials used include autogenous fascia from the thigh, homograft fascia, or synthetic nonabsorbable suture material. The Fasanello-Servat is a simpler procedure for obtaining only a small amount of lid elevation.

Extraocular Muscle Procedures

Surgical procedures on extraocular muscles to correct strabismus or squint are the third most commonly performed pediatric procedures between ages 6 months and 6 years. The trend is to correct the congenital type during infancy and the acquired type in preschool years. Patterns of using two eyes together are more flexible and adaptable in a young child. These procedures on extraocular muscles are done to correct muscle imbalance and promote coordination either by strengthening a weak muscle or by weakening an overactive one. The mechanical strength of a weak muscle can be increased by:

1. *Tucking.* Tuck is sutured in muscle to shorten it, thereby increasing its effective power.
2. *Advancement.* Attachment point of muscle is freed and reattached closer to the cornea, thereby increasing its leverage.
3. *Resection.* Part of muscle is removed to shorten it, and cut ends are sutured together.

An overactive muscle can be weakened by:

1. *Tenotomy.* Point of attachment of the muscle is severed and muscle is dropped back, held by ligaments only.
2. *Recession.* Muscle is detached from the eyeball and reattached farther back to decrease its action.
3. *Myotomy.* Fibers of a section of muscle are divided to diminish muscle action.
4. *Myectomy.* A section of muscle belly is excised.
5. *Fadin procedure.* Muscle belly is sutured to posterior sclera, thereby restricting muscle action considerably, producing a super-weakening effect.

Intraocular Procedures

Congenital Cataract Extraction Under the operating microscope, with use of irrigation-aspiration and cutting instruments, the cataract and often the posterior capsule and a portion of the anterior vitreous are removed at one time. This procedure obtains a clear optical zone so that a contact lens can be fitted on the infant's eye within a few days postoperatively. The goal is to avoid intractable amblyopia (lazy eye) by correcting the defect during the first few weeks of life. An intraocular lens may be implanted. More commonly, epikeratophakia is performed to reshape the cornea or an epi lens is made from a donor cornea.

Goniotomy Although rare, early surgical intervention for congenital glaucoma is urgent to prevent blindness. Goniotomy is a microsurgical procedure that involves dividing a congenital layer of abnormal tissue covering the drainage angle of anterior chamber. It is performed by use of a special operative contact lens placed on the eye that permits visualization of the angle. An incision is made through an opening in the contact lens.

Otorhinolaryngology

Myringotomy

Secretory otitis media is the most common chronic condition of childhood. Fluid accumulates in the middle ear from eustachian tube obstruction. This condition is corrected by myringotomy, an incision in the tympanic membrane (eardrum) for drainage. By aspiration of fluid and pus, pressure is released, pain is relieved, and hearing is restored and preserved. Myringotomy is done to prevent perforation of the eardrum and possible erosion of middle ear ossicles. When exudate is especially viscid, the patient has "glue ear" or mucoid otitis media.

Tympanostomy is commonly performed bilaterally in association with myringotomy. A self-cleaning plastic pressure-equalizing tube is placed through incision in the tympanic membrane, bypassing eustachian tube, to facilitate aeration of middle ear space and to prevent re-formation of serous otitis media. The tube usually extrudes spontaneously. Premature extrusion before normal eustachian tube function resumes may necessitate replacement of the tube.

Middle Ear Tympanoplasty

Congenital fused ossicles in the middle ear often are associated with stenosis or absence of an external auditory canal. Depending on the deformity, tympanoplasty may be performed with a temporalis fascia graft. If mobilization or ossiculoplasty is impossible, a total or partial ossicular prosthesis may be implanted to replace one or more ossicles. Congenital or acquired conductive deafness may be helped by tympanoplastic surgical techniques. Single-channel cochlear implants, approved for children, may be helpful for the profoundly deaf child (see Chapter 35, pp. 733-734).

Correction of Choanal Atresia

Newborns are obligate nose breathers and may die at birth if choanal atresia, congenital closure of nasal passages, is undiagnosed. They are unable to breathe and feed properly without an adequate nasal airway. Excision of bone or fibrous tissue blocking the posterior choanae usually is performed via a transseptal approach to create an opening into the nasopharynx. A carbon dioxide (CO_2) laser may be used to develop appropriate apertures.

Adenoidectomy

Abnormally enlarged lymphoid tissue or infected adenoids can obstruct breathing. A child usually is at least 2 years old before having adenoid tissue in the nasopharynx removed, but adenoidectomy can be done at an earlier age. Removal of adenoids can positively influence the outcome of otitis media with effusion in childhood. An adenoidectomy is usually done in conjunction with a tonsillectomy.

Tonsillectomy

Tonsillectomy, the excision of hypertrophied or chronically infected tonsils, is not generally advised before the child is 3 years of age. General anesthesia is used for patients up to about 14 years of age. Tonsillectomy and adenoidectomy are frequently performed together, appearing on the surgical schedule as T&A. Sterile technique is carried out throughout the procedure. Precautions during the surgical procedure include control of bleeding and prevention of aspiration of blood or tissue.

Esophageal Dilatation

Children, usually of preschool age, may ingest caustic agents that cause chemical burns of the mouth, lips, and pharynx and corrosive esophagitis. Long-term gradual esophageal dilatation with balloon catheters or bougies may be necessary to restore adequate oral intake of food after the acute phase of traumatic injury. When all attempts at dilatation fail, the esophagus is replaced. The most satisfactory source of esophageal replacement is the colon.

Laryngeal Papillomas

Recurrent respiratory papillomatosis is localized in the larynx of children. Laryngeal papillomas are benign, wartlike lesions caused by human papilloma virus. Hoarseness is an early symptom; airway obstruction is a later life-threatening sign. Ablation with the CO_2 laser, manipulated through the operating microscope, preserves underlying laryngeal muscles and ligaments while vaporizing papillomas located on vocal cords. Laser ablation is not a cure; recurrence often necessitates repeated procedures to maintain a patent airway.

Tracheal or Laryngeal Stenosis

Some accidental injuries result in a narrowing (i.e., stenosis) of the trachea or larynx. Of greater concern are the injuries that result from therapy for respiratory problems, especially in newborns. Prolonged endotracheal intubation can lead to injury from tubes that are too large for the lumen, are too long, or move too much. These injuries may require balloon dilatation and/or endoscopic resection of the stenotic area. Most infants then require an intraluminal stent to maintain patency of their airways.

In the presence of severe circumferential intraluminal scarring with involvement of the cartilages, surgical reconstruction becomes necessary. *Laryngotracheoplasty* widens the stenosed cartilaginous framework of the airway in the midline anteriorly and posteriorly and reconstructs the mucosal lining. Free or composite rib cartilage grafts are taken with mucosal tissue of the perichondrium for lining the airway. A stent assembly with a tracheotomy tube supports the reconstructed airway during healing. It can then be removed and the tracheostomy closed.

Tracheotomy

Tracheotomy, incision into the trachea and insertion of a tracheotomy tube, is advisable in cases of severe inflammatory glottic diseases, when endotracheal intubation would be required for longer than 72 hours, and when respiratory support is necessary for longer than 24 to 48 hours to treat respiratory problems. Appropriate sizes and types of tracheotomy tubes for infants and children should be available. Tubes that are too large, too rigid, or too long or that have an improper curve can produce ulceration and scarring at pressure points. Strictures that develop at the site of the tracheotomy may require resection to relieve airway obstruction after decannulation. Infants have a shorter neck and are prone to distal displacement of the tracheotomy tube from the intratracheal insertion point. Head motion will cause the tube to shift superiorly if it is not secured in position by ties.

Plastic and Reconstructive Surgery

With the exception of burns and other traumatic tissue injuries, most plastic and reconstructive surgery performed on infants and children is done to correct congenital anomalies. The most common of these include the following.

Cleft Lip

Lack of fusion of the soft tissues of the upper lip creates a cleft or fissure. Cleft lips vary in degree from simple notching of lip to extension into the floor of the nose. They may be unilateral or bilateral. The number of procedures required for correction depends on severity of the deformity. Some plastic surgeons do a primary *cheiloplasty*, closure of cleft lip, within the first few days after birth to facilitate feeding and to minimize psychologic trauma of parents. Surgeons who prefer to wait until the infant is older follow the "rule of 10": 10 weeks, 10 g of hemoglobin, 10 lb of body weight. Regardless of preferred timing, infiltration of local anesthetic agent with epinephrine is usually the anesthetic of choice.

To relieve tension on the incision postoperatively, a Logan bow (a small curved metal frame) may be applied over area of the incision and held in place by narrow adhesive strips to splint the lip. Skin closure strips may be used. Arm or elbow restraints are used to prevent infant from removing the bow or strips and injuring the repaired lip. These restraints are applied in the OR.

Cleft Palate

Failure of tissues of the palate to fuse creates a fissure through the roof of the mouth. Palatal clefts may be a defect only in the soft palate or may extend through both hard and soft palates into the nose and include the alveolar ridge of the maxilla. Cleft palate is often associated with cleft lip; however, the two deformities are closed separately. *Palatoplasty*, closure of the soft palate, is done before speech begins to avoid speech defects. A mouth gag is used during the surgical procedure to permit access to the palate without obstructing the airway. General anesthesia is administered via an endotracheal tube. This may be supplemented by infiltration of a local anesthetic agent. When epinephrine is used by the surgeon to minimize bleeding, the anesthesiologist is informed.

In patients with bilateral and, frequently, unilateral clefts, an additional surgical procedure will be performed to elevate the tip of the nose and correct asymmetry before the child is 4 years of age.

Hemangioma

Hemangiomas are the most common of all human congenital anomalies. A hemangioma is a benign tumor (angioma) made up of blood vessels that may pigment or appear as a growth on the skin. All hemangiomas have abnormal patterns of hemodynamics, which is the effect of blood flow through tissues. Variations in vessel size distinguish the different types of these tumors. Argon or tunable dye laser or surgical excision in combination with skin graft or pedicle flap repair are treatments of choice for intradermal capillary hemangiomas (port-wine stain). Cryosurgery, surgical excision, or steroid therapy may be used for some other cavernous-type tumors.

Otoplasty

Abnormally small or absent external ears can be reconstructed in several surgical stages. Autogenous rib cartilage graft with perichondrium intact or a silicone or a porous polyethylene prosthesis is used for the supporting framework to produce anatomic contour. Usually necessitated by microtia, a congenital anomaly, reconstruction of the external ear can follow traumatic injury with loss of all or part of the pinna. Free flaps of temporoparietal fascia are used to secure a prosthesis or may be used to cover a carved cartilage armature for secondary reconstruction.

Otoplasty procedures to correct protruding or excessively large ears are performed more frequently than are procedures for microtia. These procedures often are done on preschool-age children, usually boys, to prevent psychologic harm from teasing.

Syndactyly

Syndactyly is a congenital anomaly characterized by fusion of two or more fingers or toes. Webbing between fingers is the most common congenital hand deformity. Tissue holding digits together is cut to separate fingers. Separation of webbed digits almost always requires skin grafts to achieve good functional results.

Polydactyly

Polydactyly is a congenital anomaly characterized by presence of more than normal number of fingers or toes. A supernumerary digit may be alongside thumb or little finger on one or both hands. Extra digits on the feet are less common. Skin and tissue resemble a rudimentary digit. Some supernumerary digits contain bone, ligament, and tendon. Excision is recommended at an early age. If the excised digit contains rudimentary bone, multistage procedures may be required to enhance function of the remaining digits of the affected extremity.

Neurosurgery

Children of all ages sustain head injuries with hematomas that must be evacuated (see Chapter 37, p. 777). Although brain tumors occur in children, the more frequently performed pediatric neurosurgical procedures are related to correction of congenital anomalies.

Craniosynostosis

If one or more of the suture lines in the skull, normally open in infancy, fuses prematurely (craniosynostosis), the skull cannot expand during normal brain growth. A newborn with multiple suture involvement may require surgical intervention because of increased intracranial pressure. Even fusion of a single suture puts a newborn at risk for altered cranial capacity and brain damage. The surgeon performs a craniectomy to remove the fused bone and to reopen the suture line(s). A strip of polyethylene or Silastic film may be inserted to cover bone edges on each side, or newly formed suture lines may be cauterized with Zenker's solution to prevent refusion. In an older infant or child, more extensive freeing of other bones may be necessary to achieve decompression of frontal lobes and orbital contents.

Craniofacial microsomia with severe facial asymmetry and the dysostosis of Apert's syndrome and Crouzon's disease also are associated with multiple skull and facial deformities. Craniofacial surgery, performed by a multidisciplinary team (see Chapter 36, pp. 745-746), involves repositioning and reshaping of skull and facial bones and a variety of soft tissue reconstructive techniques. Microplating systems may be used for rigid fixation of bones. The skull may provide a donor site without creating a deformity if bone grafts are required. Demineralized cadaver bone powder may be used to stimulate bone growth.

Encephalocele

Encephalocele is the herniation of brain and neural tissue through a defect in the skull. This is present at birth as a sac of tissue on the head. Usually these lesions can be removed 6 to 12 weeks after birth, unless complicated by hydrocephalus.

Hydrocephalus

Usually congenital, dilatation of the ventricles by obstruction, excessive formation of cerebrospinal fluid, or failure of the absorptive mechanisms produces impairment in the normal circulation of cerebrospinal fluid. Fluid accumulates in the ventricles (i.e., hydrocephalus). Intracranial pressure thus created causes enlargement of the infant's head if it develops before fusion of cranial bones and often causes brain damage. Hydrocephalus may be diagnosed in utero by cephalocentesis, and a ventriculoamniotic shunt may be inserted to drain the ventricles. After birth, surgical treatment involves establishment of a mechanism for transporting excess fluid from the ventricles to maintain a close-to-normal intracranial pressure. This may be done by implantation of a shunt, which carries fluid from the lateral ventricle to the peritoneal cavity *(ventriculoperitoneal shunt)* or to right atrium of the heart *(ventriculoatrial shunt)*. Other types of shunts are used, but less commonly, to bypass localized obstructions.

One end of the shunt catheter is put into the ventricle; the other end may connect to a one-way valve, which in turn is connected to the catheter that drains fluid distally from the head. An endoscopic technique may be used for catheter placement in the ventricle. Shunt malformation is usually caused by obstruction by the choroid plexus or debris. This complication can be reduced by positioning the shunt catheter tip opposite the foramen of Monro visually via a miniature fiberoptic pediatric neuroendoscope.

Catheters are made of silicone rubber. An antithrombotic coating may be incorporated into the distal end. Some valves are regulated to open for drainage when predetermined pressure in the ventricle is reached. Other valves are designed as flushing devices to keep the distal catheter patent; skin over the device is manually depressed to flush the system. For each patient the surgeon chooses the shunt mechanism that will be safest for the particular type of hydrocephalus being treated. Follow-up minor revisions are sometimes necessary, generally because of growth of the child.

As an alternative to a shunt procedure, a ventriculostomy can relieve intracranial pressure. A rigid neuroendoscope in introduced into the third ventricle. The contact fiber of a Nd:YAG laser, inserted through the scope, blanches and perforates the floor of the third ventricle at several points to establish circulation of cerebrospinal fluid into the subarachnoid space.

Myelomeningocele

A saclike protrusion may bulge through a defect in a portion of the vertebral column that failed to fuse in fetal development. If the nerves of the spinal cord remain within the vertebral column and only the meninges protrude into the sac, the congenital anomaly is a *meningocele*. However, if sac also contains a portion of the spinal cord, it is a *myelomeningocele*, with associated permanent nerve damage. Degree of impairment depends on level and extent of the defect. Clubfeet, dislocated hips, hydrocephalus, neurogenic bladder, paralysis, and other congenital disorders often accompany myelomeningocele. Each patient is evaluated and treated individually according to priorities of his or her needs. In general, it is best to delay the surgical procedure to repair a myelomeningocele until danger of development of hydrocephalus has passed or cerebrospinal fluid has been shunted. If sac is covered with a thin membrane, *meningitis* (infection of meninges) is an imminent danger unless the defect is repaired soon after birth, usually within the first 48 hours, to close cutaneous, muscular, and dural defects.

Spina Bifida

Spina bifida, incomplete closure of the paired vertebral arches in the midline of the vertebral column, may occur without herniation of the meninges. A spina bifida may be covered by intact skin. Laminectomy may be indicated to repair the underlying defect.

Spastic Cerebral Palsy

Selective posterior rhizotomy can improve muscle tone and function of school-age children with spastic cerebral palsy. The procedure involves division of lumbar and sacral posterior nerve roots associated with abnormal motor response as identified by nerve stimulation.

Thoracic Surgery

Aspiration of a foreign body can seriously compromise a child's respiratory status. Bronchoscopy may be necessary, with the child under general anesthesia, to remove the object. Bronchoscopy is also performed to diagnose tracheobronchial compression by an innominate artery, a vascular ring, or other pathologic condition causing obstruction, stridor, or apnea. Thoracoscopy provides visualization of the chest wall and visceral pleura for diagnosis of diffuse or localized pulmonary disease. An intrathoracic biopsy can be obtained via a thoracoscope.

Pectus Excavatum

Pectus excavatum, a congenital malformation of the chest wall, is characterized by a pronounced funnel-shaped depression over lower end of the sternum. Cardiopulmonary impairment can result from pectus excavatum. The deformity is corrected by resecting lower intercostal cartilages and substernal ligaments to free up the sternum. The sternum is elevated and the cartilages are fitted to the sides of the sternum. The surgical procedure is done primarily for cosmetic purposes, but occasionally it is necessary to establish normal respiratory and circulatory function.

Cardiovascular Surgery

Congenital cardiovascular defects are the result of abnormal embryologic development of the heart or major vessels. Most are diagnosed in infancy, often when symptoms of congestive heart failure develop within the first few days or months after birth. Corrective or palliative procedures are necessary to sustain or prolong the life of these infants. Many of these cardiovascular procedures are enhanced by or possible with the use of profound hypothermia and cardiopulmonary bypass (see Chapter 39). However, significant brain damage may be associated with cardiovascular bypass in infants. Bypass perfusion time should not exceed 40 minutes between periods of temporary normal circulatory perfusion. Congenital defects in infants or children that are amenable to surgical intervention include the following.

Anomalous Venous Return

Failure of any one pulmonary vein or a combination of these veins to return blood to the left atrium precludes the full complement of oxygenated blood from entering the systemic circulation. The anomalous pulmonary vein or veins are transferred and anastomosed to the left atrium.

Coarctation of Aorta

A *coarctation* is a narrowing or stricture in a vessel. This is one of the more common congenital cardiovascular defects, usually occurring in the aortic arch. It may cause hypertension in the upper extremities above the obstruction and hypotension in the lower extremities from slowed circulation below the coarctation. To correct the defect, the coarctation is resected and the aorta may be anastomosed end-to-end. An aortic patch graft may be necessary when the length of the coarctation prevents anastomosis. A subclavian flap angioplasty capable of growth in length and width is the surgical procedure of choice in infants.

Patent Ductus Arteriosus

During fetal life the ductus arteriosus carries blood from the pulmonary artery to the aorta to bypass the lungs. Normally this vessel closes in the first hours after birth to prevent recirculation of arterial blood through the body. If closure does not occur, blood flow may be reversed by aortic pressure, causing respiratory distress. Surgical intervention is indicated, in lieu of prolonged ventilatory support, to prevent development of chronic pulmonary changes. The patent ductus arteriosus is clamped and ligated with ligating clips or suture.

Septal Defects

An open heart procedure with cardiopulmonary bypass is necessary to close abnormal openings in the walls (septa) separating the chambers within the heart.

Atrial Septal Defect An opening in the septum between right and left atria may be sufficiently large to allow oxygenated blood to shunt from left to right and return to the lungs. This can increase pulmonary blood flow, with resultant pulmonary hypertension if the defect is not closed. If defect cannot be closed with sutures, a patch graft is inserted.

Ventricular Septal Defect The ventricular septal defect is usually located in the membranous portion of the septum between the right and left ventricles. It is the most common of the congenital heart anomalies. Patients with small defects are relatively asymptomatic, and repair may be unnecessary. Large defects with left-to-right shunting of oxygenated blood back to the lungs, thus increasing pulmonary hypertension, are closed. A patch graft may be required to close the defect.

Atrioventricular Canal Defect An atrioventricular canal defect is present if the atrioventricular canal of connective tissue that normally divides the heart into four chambers has failed to develop. Deficiencies are present in lower portion of interatrial septum, upper portion of interventricular septum, and tricuspid and mitral valves. The result is a large central canal that permits blood flow between any of the four chambers of the heart. Corrective procedure involves repair of mitral and tricuspid valves and patch grafts to close septal defects. Creation of a competent mitral valve is of utmost importance to relieve pulmonary hypertension.

Tetralogy of Fallot

Tetralogy of Fallot is a combination of four defects:

1. Ventricular septal defect
2. Stenosis or atresia of pulmonary valve and/or outflow tract into pulmonary artery
3. Hypertrophy of right ventricle
4. Dextroposition (displacement) of aorta to right so that it receives blood from both ventricles

Often referred to as "blue babies," infants with tetralogy of Fallot are cyanotic because insufficient oxygen circulates to body tissues. Total correction of the multiple anomalies is difficult. Assessment of the technical ease of correction is generally the dominant consideration. If cyanosis is severe, a palliative shunt procedure may be performed during infancy to increase pulmonary blood flow.

1. *Blalock-Taussig procedure:* end-to-side anastomosis of right subclavian artery to corresponding pulmonary artery. Mixed arterial-venous blood from aorta flows through shunt to pulmonary artery and into lungs for oxygenation.
2. *Potts-Smith-Gibson procedure:* side-to-side anastomosis of aorta and left pulmonary artery. The shunt enlarges as child grows but is more difficult to reconstruct than is a Blalock shunt at a later time when a corrective procedure is performed.
3. *Waterston procedure:* anastomosis of aorta and right pulmonary artery. The anastomosis is placed on posterior aspect of aorta to provide perfusion to both pulmonary arteries.

With cardiopulmonary bypass and hypothermia, the ventricular septal defect is closed with a patch graft that also corrects the abnormal communication between the right ventricle and aorta. Then the obstruction to pulmonary blood flow is relieved. This may include enlarging the pulmonary valve and/or widening the outflow tract. Resection of obstructing cardiac muscle may be necessary with insertion of a prosthetic outflow patch. An aortic allograft containing the aortic valve with the septal leaflet of the mitral valve and the ascending aorta attached may be inserted. The septal leaflet of the mitral valve is used as a portion of the right ventricular outflow patch. All or part of the aortic valve and ascending aorta is used as a new conduit with the pulmonary artery or as a patch graft.

Transposition of Great Vessels

In a transposition, the aorta rises from the right ventricle and the pulmonary artery from the left ventricle. This creates essentially two separate circulatory systems, one systemic and the other pulmonary, but they are not interconnected as in normal anatomy. Life depends on presence or creation of associated defects to permit exchange of blood between the two systems. A palliative procedure is performed in the newborn to sustain life until the infant grows enough to tolerate a corrective procedure. Oxygenation is improved by the *palliative procedure.*

1. *Rashkind procedure:* balloon atrial septostomy. A balloon-tipped catheter is advanced into right atrium, through foramen ovale, and into left atrium. The inflated balloon is pulled across the atrial septum to enlarge the foramen ovale, thus creating an atrial septal defect.
2. *Blalock-Hanlon procedure:* atrial septectomy to create an atrial septal defect. A segment of right atrium is excised.
3. *Pulmonary artery banding:* pulmonary artery is constricted in presence of a large ventricular septal defect to prevent irreversible pulmonary vascular obstructive changes from developing.

A *corrective procedure* usually is done when the child is between 18 and 36 months of age.

1. *Mustard procedure:* intraatrial baffle, made of pericardial tissue, is sutured between pulmonary veins and mitral valve and between mitral and tricuspid valves. The baffle directs systemic venous return into the left ventricle and lungs and allows pulmonary venous return to enter the right ventricle and aorta.
2. *Senning procedure:* flaps of intraatrial septum and right atrial wall form new venous channels to divert pulmonary venous blood flow. Any atrial and/or septal defects are closed.
3. *Jatene procedure:* aorta and pulmonary artery are anatomically switched (i.e., transposed). This procedure is useful in infants with a ventricular septal defect or a large patent ductus arteriosus in addition to transposition of the great arteries.

Tricuspid Atresia

The absence (atresia) of a tricuspid valve between the right atrium and ventricle prevents normal blood flow through the chambers of the heart. Blood flows through an atrial septal defect, into an enlarged left ventricle, and through a small right ventricle to the pulmonary artery. Anastomosis of superior vena cava to right pulmonary artery or an aorticopulmonic artery shunt may be created as a palliative procedure to increase pulmonary blood flow in infancy. When the child is 3 or 4 years old, a corrective reconstructive Fontan procedure is performed. This procedure involves direct anastomosis of pulmonary artery to right atrium to create a connection between pulmonary and systemic venous circulation.

Truncus Arteriosus

In truncus arteriosus a single artery carries blood directly from heart with a large associated ventricular septal defect to coronary, pulmonary, and systemic circulatory systems. Initial palliative banding of the pulmonary arteries, as close to their origins off the truncus as possible, decreases pulmonary blood flow in an infant in congestive heart failure. At a later stage a corrective procedure can be performed to close the ventricular septal defect and insert a conduit with an ascending aortic graft and aortic valve. Correction in infancy requires replacement of the conduit as the child grows.

Valvular Stenosis

Congenital aortic and/or pulmonary valve stenosis requires valvotomy, an incision into the valve to open the narrowed or constrictive area obstructing blood flow.

FETAL SURGERY

Maternal prenatal testing after 9 weeks of gestation (see Chapter 30, pp. 627-628) makes possible prenatal diagnosis of some malformations in the fetus. An abnormal amount of fluid in cystic structures, such as myelomeningocele, is detected, as are some congenital anomalies in the abdomen and intestinal tract. Diagnosis of cleft lip and palate is possible. Obstructive uropathy, including renal parenchymal loss and obstructive hydronephrosis, is most commonly diagnosed. Prenatal diagnosis allows a choice of elective cesarean section by the mother to avoid further compromise during delivery and to promote immediate postnatal care of the neonate.

Some selective lesions are amenable to surgery in utero (i.e., fetal surgery). Among these lesions are hydronephrosis, hydrocephalus, severe hiatal (diaphragmatic) hernia, cystic adenomatoid malformation, sacrococcygeal teratoma, and urethral obstruction. The procedure may be performed by an open technique (i.e., uterus is opened and part of fetus is lifted out as necessary to correct defect) or by a closed technique performed percutaneously with ultrasonography or laparoscopic endoscopy. The latter technique does not correct the anomaly, but it decompresses the obstruction to reduce anticipated mortality.

When fetal surgery is considered, the following criteria are used:

1. Pregnancy has a single fetus.
2. Prognosis is poor for the fetus without surgical intervention.
3. Fetus is viable with low mortality risk to mother and potential benefit to fetus.
4. Parents are fully counseled about risks and benefits to mother and fetus and give consent.
5. Multidisciplinary team experienced in fetal diagnosis and anomalies will manage the infant after birth. This team includes an obstetrician, neonatalogist, and pediatric surgeon.
6. High-risk obstetric unit and neonatal intensive care unit are available.

In Utero Transfusion

Erythroblastosis fetalis is a disease of the fetus and newborn characterized by hemolytic anemia as a result of incompatibility of blood groups between the mother and fetus. During pregnancy, maternal antibodies cause destruction of fetal red blood cells. In utero blood transfusion via placental vessels may alter the degree of red blood cell destruction and production. The blood transfused is of the mother's blood type. If subsequent exchange transfusions are needed after birth, the blood type of the donor must match that of the newborn.

The incidence of Rh isoimmunization has been decreased since the advent of Rh immune globulin (RhoGAM) in 1968. Prenatal care is important in all pregnancies to enhance the viability of the newborn.

BIBLIOGRAPHY

Andrews SE: Laser ablation of recurrent laryngeal papillomas in children, *AORN J* 61(3):532-544, 1995.

Davis JL, Klein RW: Perioperative care of the pediatric trauma patient, *AORN J* 60(4):561-570, 1994.

Derkay CS et al: Retrieving foreign bodies from upper aerodigestive tracts in children, *AORN J* 60(1):53-61, 1994.

Ellerton M, Merriam C: Preparing children and families psychologically for day surgery, *J Adv Nurs* 19(6):1057-1062, 1994.

Fina DK: A chance to say goodbye, *Am J Nurs* 94(5):42-45, 1994.

Heiney SP: Helping children through painful procedures, *Am J Nurs* 91(11):20-24, 1991.

Hendricks-Ferguson VL, Ortman MR: Selective dorsal rhizotomy to decrease spasticity in cerebral palsy, *AORN J* 61(3):514-525, 1995.

Holt L, Maxwell B: Pediatric orientation program, *AORN J* 54(3):530-540, 1991.

Huddleston KR: Patent ductus arteriosus ligation, *AORN J* 53(1):69-80, 1991.

Huddleston KR: Strabismus repair in the pediatric patient, *AORN J* 60(5):754-760, 1994.

Joy S, Grosfeld JL: Wilms' tumor, *AORN J* 53(2):437-448, 1991.

Kyzer SP, Stark SL: Congenital idiopathic clubfoot deformities, *AORN J* 61(3):492-506, 1995.

LaRosa-Nash PA et al: Implementing a parent-present induction program, *AORN J* 61(3):526-531, 1995.

Levine AH: Fetal surgery, *AORN J* 54(1):16-32, 1991.

Murphy EK: Issues regarding parents in the operating room during their children's care, *AORN J* 56(1):120-124, 1992.

O'Malley ME, McNamara ST: Children's drawings: a preoperative assessment tool, *AORN J* 57(5):1074-1089, 1993.

Pierce LA: Safety and care of children during surgery, *Plast Surg Nurs* 14(2):99-100, 1994.

Schmidt K et al: How to apply the AHCPR's pediatric pain guideline, *Am J Nurs* 94(3):69-74, 1994.

Schweer L, Ose MB: Implementation of a regional pediatric trauma center, *AORN J* 61(3):558-571, 1995.

Steward DJ: *Manual of pediatric anesthesia,* ed 4, New York, 1995, Churchill Livingstone.

Thompson SW: *Emergency care of children,* Boston, 1990, Jones Barlett.

Vegunta RK et al: Surgical management of abdominal wall defects in infants, *AORN J* 58(1):53-63, 1993.

Wells MP, Hanes NA: Tonsillectomy, adenoidectomy in the day surgery unit, *AORN J* 58(1):64-71, 1993.

Williams EM et al: Neuroendoscopic laser-assisted ventriculostomy of the third ventricle, *AORN J* 61(2):345-359, 1995.

Wong DL: *Wong and Whaley's clinical manual of pediatric nursing,* ed 4, St Louis, 1996, Mosby.

CHAPTER 43

Perioperative Geriatrics

PERSPECTIVES ON AGING

The process of aging is an orderly transformation of the body and mind that begins with birth and concludes with death. The term *geriatric* is taken from the Greek word *yeros* (γεροs), which means old. Persons over 65 years of age often are considered old or elderly. In actuality, however, a person with advanced age may maintain functional capabilities throughout his or her lifetime until adaptation to biologic, psychologic, and/or social influences is no longer sufficient to sustain the independent activities of daily living. The main influences on the aging process are genetics, environment, and lifestyle. The medical discipline of geriatrics is related to the clinical implications of the physiology of aging and the diagnosis and treatment of diseases affecting the aged. *Gerontology* is the comprehensive scientific study of all aspects of the aging process, including physiologic, psychologic, economic, and sociologic problems and considerations of the aging person. These factors are studied from the standpoint of the impact they have on the aging individual and the elderly population within society.

Data about the changes that take place as the result of natural processes and those changes that take place as the result of environmental exposure are inconclusive because the only data available are derived from comparisons between existing generations. Experiences and exposures have been vastly different and widely influenced by the time period of their life spans. No normal measurements are available on which to base the parameters of the aging process.

Life expectancy has increased steadily as science has made major advances in the study of disease processes, prevention, and treatment. The United States Department of Health and Human Services indicates that a person born in 1954 can expect to live to the age of 68 years. A person born in 1988 can expect to live 74 years. By the year 2030, 1 in every 10 persons will be older than 85 years of age. Only 41% of the population will be below the age of 35 years. The median age will be 40 years. The increase in life expectancy and the decrease in mortality mean that the largest patient population will be geriatric patients, the fastest growing segment of the population.

As the life expectancy of the geriatric population increases, the incidence of *comorbidity* increases. Comorbidity is the existence of two or more disease processes in a single individual. For example, coronary artery disease may also be present in a patient with osteoporosis. This same patient may be hypertensive and diabetic. All of these medical diagnoses should be taken into account in the development of the plan of care. Comorbidity is the most frequent negative influence on the health status and functional ability of the geriatric patient. It is also a major consideration in the attainment of expected outcomes. A chronic condition affects recovery following surgical intervention. Many geriatric patients have multiple chronic or debilitating health problems.

Aging is viewed from many perspectives; some are positive and some are negative. Positive aspects involve respect for maturity and the wealth of knowledge gleaned from experiences. The negative aspects are the debilitation, pervading weaknesses, and dependence that can occur during the closure of life. Philosophers tend to focus on the positive, inner peace derived from wisdom acquired over many years. The view of aging adopted by an individual is based in part on the view of aging created by the individual's cultural background. Geographic, financial, educational, and subjective influences shape the prototype of the aged individual's place in society.

Cultural Considerations

Many cultures that can trace their heritage back for many generations have positive views of aging. Repetitious story telling and historical accounts support the cultural growth of an individual from youth to old age. Many cultures appreciate, honor, and respect their older members for their experience and maturity. Growing old with dignity is not feared or deemed repulsive. A positive view of aging may be observed in the geriatric patient who is a first-generation immigrant to a new land. This individual may not have assimilated the value systems of the new environment and may have retained many time-honored beliefs. The values held dear are deeply ingrained. However, negative views of aging may be generated by cultures that are primarily youth-oriented. Most members of these societies are second- and third-generation descendants of immigrants. They have developed value systems that do not reflect their country of origin. In a close community values are supported within the belief structure of the group as a whole.

Culture is a set of structured social behaviors and personal beliefs that enable an individual to respond to social situations and relationships within a close community. The foundation of human relationships in a culture is more than ethnicity or race. Specific cultural practices such as dietary habits, lifestyle, or hygiene should be of concern to the perioperative nurse. The patient's physical condition may be a direct result of a traditional activity such as fasting, for example. The geriatric patient who has been fasting may appear dehydrated, malnourished, or confused. This should be taken into consideration before the patient has a surgical procedure. The psychologic assessment may reflect a high risk for an alteration in self-image because, although the patient may feel comfortable in his or her culture, he or she may have had a negative interaction with societal influences. For example, the media glorify young bodies and degrade the natural aging process. Advertisers use models that reflect the desirable aspects of youth and beauty. Cultural climate has a direct effect on the geriatric patient. The expected outcomes of the geriatric patient undergoing surgical intervention will be influenced by his or her cultural views of aging and those of society as a whole.

Theories of Aging

Biologic, psychologic, and ethnocultural factors influence the manner in which the individual ages. Each aged individual is unique and distinct. The *extrinsic* influences surrounding the physical and psychosocial components depend on the interaction of the person with the environment and his or her view of health and wellness. Many older persons tend to optimistically overstate their actual health status and minimize or dismiss symptoms as age related. The *intrinsic* influences on the aging process are also interdependent, but to a less controllable degree. Some inherited traits, such as pathologic conditions, are continued through the generations. Perioperative nurses should understand the unique aspects of the individual geriatric patient before developing a perioperative plan of care. Generic care plans do not address the specific problems, needs, and health considerations of the individual. Understanding the theories of the aging process enable the perioperative nurse to provide care throughout the surgical experience in a way that will optimize the possible attainment of identified expected outcomes. The following theories explain aging as it is defined by science and research.

Wear and Tear Theory

The wear and tear theory suggests that the body loses its ability to keep pace with the maintenance of life processes. The sustenance of life suffers because the body begins to deteriorate in a natural, wearing-down process. The body continually tries to maintain homeostasis and life processes, but because of cellular loss and destruction caused by interactions with the environment, the body degenerates over time. During this process the body becomes increasingly vulnerable to injury and disease. If a disease state occurs, the body is less able to cope with normal homeostasis and even less able to tolerate the assault of illness. Eventually the body is not able to support life and ceases to function. Examples of wear and tear include, but are not limited to the following.

1. Prolonged exposure to the sun and other external sources can cause breakdown of the skin. Thinning of the skin makes bedridden or inactive persons vulnerable to pressure sores.
2. Turbulent blood flow in the areas of bifurcation of blood vessels may cause rupture if the vessels are weakened by arteriosclerosis.
3. Abuse of chemical substances and alcohol can cause damage to liver and brain cells. Nicotine is responsible for many effects of smoking. Although these are self-induced effects rather than natural wear and tear, abuses affect health status.

Genetic Mutation Theory

Deoxyribonucleic acid (DNA) has been a target for age-related changes because it preserves the ongoing genetic message for the replication of cells and the maintenance of the organism. DNA is a form of a template, or coding mechanism, for the preservation of the life processes of cellular structures. Various agents damage the DNA codes through physical, chemical, or biologic interactions. An alteration in the structure of DNA can cause the organism to change in a manner that is different from the original design. The alteration can take place within the cell itself or be caused by a force in the environment. Mutated DNA cannot perform the processes necessary for the normal activities of the cell. A cell containing wrongly coded DNA will replicate itself in the wrong patterns and continue to do so. It does not return to normal.

In the aging process, DNA may have mutated for a variety of reasons and will continue to produce the wrong type of cells during replication. For example, skin cells may be deficient in collagen or in elastic properties associated with supple tissue. As a result, the skin replication process may yield drier, less elastic skin. This is characteristic of the skin of an older person. In certain circumstances, the mutated DNA could cause tumor production or other pathologic conditions, such as skin cancers.

Major organ systems affected by these changes are the central nervous system, the musculoskeletal system, and the cardiovascular system. Other systems affected include the gastrointestinal, genitourinary, endocrine, and integumentary systems. Essentially, no body system is exempt from the genetic changes that take place during the aging process.

Viral Theory

Researchers have approached the concept that viruses may invade human cells and remain inactive until the body loses its ability to suppress them. This theory is closely linked to the genetic mutation theory because the virus can hide undetected in the DNA for many years. The replication process of the virus is similar to the replication of DNA. Some viruses are able to use genetic materials as a disguise to fool the body's immune system. The body does not recognize the virus as an invader or foreign substance.

The mechanism of viral activation is unknown but is very injurious to the body. Major target systems include the endocrine, nervous, and immune systems. The incubation period may be several decades. Because there is no proof of the viral theory, treatment or cure is unknown.

Environmental Theory

Exposure to natural and man-made elements in the environment may accelerate the aging process. Climate is often blamed for an increased rate of aging, yet when specific geographic regions are studied, the natural flow of the aging process is comparable. Tropical climates are cited most often as areas of premature aging. Studies of tropical populations show that aging is not accelerated by the temperature, but mortality is affected by poor nutrition, parasites, and tropical diseases. Both tropical and desert groups tested did not show any mean blood pressure elevations diagnostic of hypertension, arteriosclerosis, or coronary artery disease between the ages of 20 and 83 years. The most astounding finding was the absence of angina pectoris and sudden heart attack deaths. This may be due in part to a physically strenuous lifestyle and consistency in diet that is low in animal fat.

Extremes of climate do not seem to accelerate the aging process either. Studies involving Eskimo populations have shown that, despite the difficult conditions of their lifestyles, blood pressure or cholesterol measurements do not vary significantly between the ages of 20 and 54 years. Mortality is affected by the harshness of the cold climate and the risk of physical injury or death associated with hunting and lifestyle practices.

Neither has altitude been shown to accelerate the aging processes. Studies performed among Peruvian Indians have shown stable blood pressures in a range lower than that of persons living at sea level. Ischemic heart disease is very low at higher altitudes. In several documented communities of mountain-dwelling people, many residents were over age of 100 years.

Ionizing radiation has been targeted as a cause of environmentally accelerated aging. Studies have not shown this to be true. Relevant evidence has shown that exposure to ionizing radiation accelerates disease processes and pathologic conditions such as skin cancer, blood dyscrasias, and reproductive anomalies. Populations living in areas where frequent nuclear tests took place have not shown signs of rapid aging when compared with control groups in nuclear-free areas. The most significant finding was an increase in leukemia and skin tumors.

Pollution causes many physiologic changes in the body. Chemicals in air, food chain, and water supply have been shown to increase the incidence of health decline and disability. Exposure to pollutants throughout the life span dramatically shortens life expectancy through pathologic processes such as chronic lead poisoning and lung cancer.

Physical Factor Theory

Free radicals are being investigated as a potential cause of premature aging. These are imbalances between the production and the elimination of unstable chemical compounds in the body. More research is needed to prove or disprove this theory.

Low-caloric diets do not alter the aging process in human beings. In populations studied for dietary habits, no increase in the life span is evident between those who have a low caloric intake and the control groups. The most remarkable factor is the lack of increase in body weight after the age of 30 years. A low-caloric diet may range between 1800 and 2500 kilogram calories (kcal) per day depending on body size and gender. Notably, low-caloric diets are usually deficient in animal protein. Aged individuals who have low-caloric diets generally have lower blood pressure and lower serum cholesterol levels with no significant change throughout the aging process. Subcutaneous fat deposits do not increase with age.

High-caloric diets ranging in excess of 3200 kcal per day for men and 2200 kcal per day for women have the opposite effect on aging. With the increase in caloric intake comes the increase in body mass that causes the individual to decrease body mobility. This is particularly evident in Euro-American populations, which frequently show a steady increase in weight up to the age of 60 years. Women, especially, experience a thickening in fat deposits as they mature. Blood pressure and serum cholesterol levels steadily increase. The most significant elevations begin at age 50, with the development of coronary artery heart disease and atherosclerosis.

Animal fat content and excess calories are not the only considerations in the dietary aspect of aging and health. Vegetarians do not always follow a low-caloric pattern. They too can have a diet rich in fats, particularly if they consume saturated fat in the form of coconut oil. Salt is another consideration in the aging of the cardiovascular system. Diets high in sodium tend to increase the circulating blood volume, thereby increasing the systolic blood pressure. Studies have shown that the increase of systolic blood pressure significantly increases the risk of heart disease and stroke.

Exercise plays an important role in the health of the aging individual. Most of the world's populations that have been studied have an exercise regimen that is linked to their activities of daily living. Persons in cultures characterized by many intrinsic diseases, parasites, malnutrition, poor hygiene, and harsh living conditions have remarkable physical fitness because of the amount of exercise they perform to sustain life. Those in affluent societies, in which the inhabitants are overfed and underexercised, do not enjoy good health in the same manner as the moderately fed and highly exercised residents of less advantaged societies.

The endocrine system declines and the hormones responsible for the regulation of many interrelated body systems decrease in volume. Beta cells of the pancreas, thyroid, and ovaries in female and testes in male exhibit less activity and affect many other organ systems. For example:

1. Decrease in estrogen production can increase risk for osteoporosis and heart disease in women.
2. Decrease in thyroid activity will decrease basal metabolic rate and increase weight gain.
3. Decrease in efficiency of insulin production will decrease efficiency of glucose metabolism.
4. Decrease in testosterone production may decrease libido in men.

Myths About Aging

Many misconceptions surround the process of aging. *Myths*, from the Greek *meethos* (μυθος), are stories created to explain practices or beliefs of unknown origin about a person, place, or event. The creation of a myth about aging may be based on an isolated incident or a single observation and may not apply to all elderly persons. Some myths have a small basis in fact, but most are unfounded and have a harmful effect on social policy and interpersonal relationships. The creation of myths about the aging process may result in negative stereotypes. Belief in negative stereotypes results in discrimination and improper treatment of the aging individual. Abnormal signs, symptoms, or behaviors exhibited by a geriatric patient usually indicate the presence of a pathologic process and should not be discounted as normal expectations of the aging process. Some of the myths about aging are as follows.

1. *Old people are senile.* This is not true. If mental processes are in decline, usually a contributing factor such as stroke, carotid insufficiency, or Alzheimer's disease is the cause.
2. *Old people do not engage in sexual behavior.* Sexual desire remains throughout the life span. Sexual activity may decline because of decreased physical mobility, circulatory impairment, or the unavailability of a partner. Self-gratification may be the only outlet.
3. *Old people always decline in health after a surgical procedure.* This is false. The identification of problems, needs, and health considerations during the assessment phase of the nursing process decreases the probability of unmet expected outcomes.

Myths and stereotypes must not be allowed to influence the assessment of geriatric patients. Every aspect of the physical, psychosocial, and ethnocultural data should be assessed as unique to each individual and not as a generic group expectation. Reaching the age of 65 years does not instantly transform individuals into being old and debilitated. As persons grow older, they may experience more developmental aging before they experience physical aging. Some persons become more frail as they age, but this is not true of everyone. Age alone does not make individuals less productive members of society. Limitations and disabilities may be decreased by the twenty-first century because of scientific advances and a better understanding of the aging process and health promotion activities.

PERIOPERATIVE ASSESSMENT OF GERIATRIC PATIENT

The patient's ability to adapt to aging should be assessed by the perioperative nurse as part of the nursing process. With the exception of nursing diagnoses directly associated with the anticipated surgical procedure, specific nursing diagnoses should be associated with the patient's adaptation to the aging process. If positive adaptation has not been met, the risk is high for an augmentation of existing health conditions, such as a cardiovascular incident (i.e., stroke, myocardial infarction, or hypertensive crisis). Recognition of potential problems in the attainment of expected outcomes is as important as identifying actual problems. Comorbidity is a leading cause of death among the elderly. Over 73% of all geriatric patients have more than one medical diagnosis capable of causing death.

The postoperative phase of care is very important to the well-being of the geriatric patient. Maintaining or improving the preoperative level of wellness should be considered a primary expected outcome. A preoperative functional assessment is the foundation of the plan of care. Baseline parameters vary to a high degree between individuals. All patients do not age at the same rate. Some are very "young" or very "old" at 70 years. The difference should be assessed, and the optimal outcomes should be identified for each geriatric patient according to the individual's level. Influences on the level of function include physical ability, psychosocial support and resources, and environmental interactions.

Functional Assessment

Functional assessment can serve multiple purposes. In the preoperative phase, the plan of care includes the patient's unique differences, family involvement, resources, and level of independence. Much of this data is obtained by observation, interview, and lifestyle questionnaires. The information may be obtained from the patient, family, or significant other. Many aspects of the patient's unique nature will be easily discerned during the preoperative interview. Allow adequate time for the interview, at least 30 minutes, so that the patient has time to reflect and respond. Reaction time slows with age. Listen for subtle modifications or inconsistencies in information the patient gives about his or her health status. Consider sensory deficits and modify the environment as needed during the interview. Establish rapport with respect for the dignity of the geriatric patient.

During the intraoperative phase, the functional assessment may allow for anticipation of needed supplies or additional help to accommodate the needs of the patient. The physical motion parameters allow the patient to experience some independence in self-care. Patients tend to regress when they are not permitted to do things for themselves. A self-care deficit takes place when a patient feels the loss of independence while restrained on an operating table. The freedom to assist with the transfer from the transport stretcher to the operating table gives the patient a sense of participation in his or her own care. Maintaining a high level of self-esteem and value will enable the patient to prevent emotional regression or loss of control.

Activities of Daily Living

During the course of a normal day, the individual performs self-maintenance tasks and interacts with the environment. The ability to perform these activities of daily living is influenced by health status, emotions, mental clarity, and mobility. Limitations may be permanent or temporary. Many of the temporary limitations can be eliminated by medical or surgical treatment. The perioperative nurse should assess for the activity level of the geriatric patient. Advance preparations may need to be considered before the patient can undergo a surgical procedure. Because of identified physical limitations, special positioning or additional padding may be needed in combination with some form of communication assistance at the time the surgical procedure is performed. The functional baseline is the patient's capacity to perform self-care (i.e., feeding, bathing, toileting). Any deviation from the baseline assessment in the postoperative phase should be recorded and should be reported to the patient's physician.

Functional Activities The activity patterns of geriatric patients reflect many aspects of their daily lives. The ability to feed, bathe, and toilet themselves is one way to measure physical and psychologic wellness. Basic daily activities, such as grooming and dressing, may be indicators of the level of the patient's involvement with his or her own care. The range of self-care activities will depend on whether the patient is active and mobile enough to shop for food and prepare meals, for example, or is living in assistive housing where these services are provided. The ability to provide self-care should be assessed preoperatively to evaluate the outcome in the postoperative phase (i.e., resumption of activity level).

Functional Capacity A basic assessment of physical strength and endurance will indicate whether the patient will be able to move from the transport stretcher to the operating table. A patient who is weak or disabled by arthritis will need assistance or a total lift device. A patient who is visually impaired also may need assistance.

Communication through speech and hearing is vital to establishing the cognitive baseline. A hearing deficit or aphasia could be mistaken for a cognitive impairment. The patient who uses a hearing assist device should be permitted to wear it to the operating room (OR) and, if possible, throughout the surgical procedure. It should be in place during emergence from anesthesia so patient can hear requests to deep breathe or to move extremities.

Tactile sensation dulls with age. Inability to feel external stimuli may lead to an inadvertent injury. Sensory ability should be assessed. Any sensory deficit, including visual and hearing impairment, should be documented in the plan of care. The administration of general anesthesia will alter the tactile assessment parameter during the intraoperative phase of care. As the patient emerges from anesthesia, the postanesthesia recovery nurses use the baseline assessment to measure the progress of the patient in the postoperative phase. The evaluation of expected outcomes should include a sensory assessment because of the interdependent aspects of the central nervous system with other vital physiologic systems.

Cognitive ability should be assessed. The patient may be required to comprehend a command that may be vital to the perioperative experience. A cognitive deficit may be of organic origin or a language barrier. Inability to understand, regardless of the reason, can cause anxiety for the patient and the caregiver. Psychologic impact should be assessed preoperatively because a change in mood or temperament may indicate an unexpected outcome caused by an injury or physical problem resulting from the surgical procedure. Dementia, delirium, and emotional depression are common in the elderly. Sudden withdrawal or change in affect should be investigated promptly.

Alertness, short-term memory, capabilities to concentrate and problem solve, and motivation toward self-care are areas of cognition that influence the geriatric patient's ability to adapt to illness and recovery. The cognitively impaired person experiences disorientation and responds inappropriately to the environment. The impairment may be temporary but often is prolonged following anesthesia. It may also be a permanent or chronic condition.

External Interactions

The manner in which the individual experiences illness depends on external forces and the number of barriers that may interfere with the attainment of outcomes. The nursing diagnoses may include a self-care deficit or an alteration in mobility status. These diagnoses factor significantly in the postoperative phase and should be taken into consideration and placed in the plan of care. The reaction of the patient to either one of the aforementioned nursing diagnoses will depend on his or her interactions with the external environment, the availability of resources, and the presence of barriers.

Resources The level of independence exercised by the geriatric patient may be contingent on the resources available. The type of housing may depend on self-care ability and financial security. In developing the plan of care, the perioperative nurse should consider how the patient will manage to meet his or her postoperative needs at home. Will help be available or will arrangements for a visiting nurse or a family caregiver be needed? Transportation to and from the surgeon's office for postoperative checkups should be considered.

Barriers The type of housing may be a problem for the postoperative geriatric patient. If he or she lives alone in a multilevel dwelling, going up and down stairs may pose a significant problem. The location of the bathroom or kitchen may complicate the self-care process. Financial constraints may limit the availability for home health care visits by an independent agency. The unavailability of family members may necessitate planning for institutionalization. This may be temporary, but it may become permanent.

Psychosocial Assessment

Gathering data about a geriatric patient should begin with the assessment of how this individual views other aged people and own progression through the aging process. The assessment of self-concept may be an important indicator of a decline in psychologic health status. A patient's views of health and normative activity are influenced by his or her culture and will affect the attainment of outcomes. If the patient believes that older people are helpless, he or she may see the role of the aging process as one of helplessness. Although capable of many independent activities, this individual may adapt to an illness by becoming helpless. Even temporary periods of needing help may cause an older patient to believe that the condition is permanent. The perioperative nurse should be aware that the geriatric patient may temporarily experience a period of helplessness. By establishing a functional baseline and by stressing the temporary nature of postoperative recovery, the nurse can help the patient return to his or her routine.

The elderly patient may feel rejected, unsupported, and worthless. Between 10% and 65% of elderly patients suffer depression and self-image alteration. Physical decline may be rapid when psychologic well-being is threatened. The perioperative nurse should be aware that the geriatric patient who is depressed and lonely needs additional emotional support throughout the surgical experience.

The perioperative nurse should be aware of his or her own subjective views of aging and cultural attitudes and not allow personal feelings to influence the assessment process. Assessment of a geriatric patient should take into consideration the culture of origin, the cultural influence of current residence, and the individual's subjective perception of wellness and illness. Self-perception has a great influence on how well the geriatric patient adapts to aging. The nursing diagnoses should reflect the patient's adaptation because adaptation will affect the attainment of the expected outcomes. The perioperative plan of care should reflect the need for ongoing evaluation by postoperative caregivers.

Adaptation to Aging Process

Many adjustments should be made by the individual during the aging process. Adaptation to aging is unique to the individual and is influenced by physical condition, psychologic strengths and weaknesses, family and significant others, social support system, financial resources, and functional ability. The geriatric patient develops a belief system about his or her life expectations primarily based on subjective feelings. If the patient is in decline, the outlook is usually negative, based on how he or she feels at that particular period in time. If the patient is feeling well and able-bodied, the outlook is usually positive, which helps delay fear of health decline outside the expected parameters of aging.

Prevention of decline not related to normative aging is a key factor in the avoidance of health deficits. The patient who can postpone health problems caused by factors that include avoidable health considerations, such as accidents, poor nutrition, inactivity, depression, and the effects of loneliness, smoking, substance abuse, and obesity, will enjoy a higher quality of life in the geriatric years.

Self-Perception of Health

The patient's view of his or her health figures highly in the actual status of health. If his or her perception of health is regarded as important, then good health preventive maintenance will be a priority. The patient who feels well will perform the activities of daily living to the best of his or her ability. Minor interruptions in health status will not cause a major problem in the long-term prognosis of his or her return to baseline parameters.

Physical Assessment

Physical assessment of the geriatric patient begins with his or her general appearance. The perioperative nurse should first observe the patient from head to toe. The basic picture or image the patient creates can give information about his or her health status. The patient should be assessed for posture, mobility, gait, rising or sitting, dexterity, body height and weight, body odors, psychologic affect, communication, and comprehension of surroundings. The perioperative nurse should perform an assessment of the total patient by each body system. Refer to Table 43-1 for a summary of physiologic changes associated with the normal aging process.

Any medications the patient takes on a routine or periodic basis should be listed on the chart with the last dosages of all drugs itemized. The patient should be encouraged to discuss all drugs, such as vitamins or topical ointments. Recreational drugs (i. e., street drugs, narcotics) should not be excluded from consideration just because the patient is elderly. Many drugs can alter the results of blood work and physical assessment findings. Drugs such as aspirin can alter blood tests for clotting times. Pain medication can alter sensorium. Smoking and alcohol use are important to assess because they can affect many body systems. All assessment data should be recorded in the chart. The perioperative nurse should read the physician's medical history and physical examination report and review laboratory reports (Table 43-2) to discern medical diagnoses. Any additional abnormal findings should be reported to the surgeon and the anesthesiologist.

Integumentary System

Assessment of the integument includes the skin, fingernails and toenails, and all hair patterns of the body, face, and scalp. The nurse should ask the patient if any skin changes have taken place within the past several months. The skin is inspected for color, temperature, sensation, texture, turgor, thickness, and the amount of subcutaneous tissue. The geriatric patient has a decreased number of sweat glands and an increased sensitivity to external temperature. The patient may complain of skin dryness, itching, and flaking. The surface of the body should be inspected for sores, ulcers, and moles that have exhibited change over time. Presence of broken or injured skin areas may indicate a pathologic condition, such as skin cancer or diabetes. Skin rashes may indicate an allergy. Color of skin can indicate problems with other body systems, such as cardiovascular or respiratory, and liver disease. Bruises or abrasions may indicate a recent fall or possible elder abuse. Careful assessment of the body surface can reveal pertinent data about the patient's health status, but differentiating normal from abnormal skin condition may be difficult. Skin is often wrinkled as a result of connective tissue changes. Pigmentation and skin tags can be normal lesions in the aging process. Establishing a preoperative baseline for the condition of the skin will facilitate evaluation of the expected outcome (i.e., no injury to the skin as a result of surgical intervention).

The nails and nail beds of the fingers and toes should be observed for their presence or absence, texture, growth pattern, cleanliness, infection, and color. Clubbing and cyanosis of the fingertips and nail beds may indicate cardiovascular disease. Extreme overgrowth and deformity of toenails may indicate decreased circulation to the feet and legs. Accumulation of soil and debris under the nails may indicate the inability to wash properly. Twisted and gnarled digits may be painful to the touch. Positioning plans for the surgical procedure should take this into consideration. The nurse should be aware that even the surgical drapes may create enough pressure to cause discomfort.

TABLE 43-1

Physiologic Changes Associated With Normal Aging Process in Geriatric Patient

AGE-RELATED FACTORS	ASSESSMENT FACTORS
Integumentary system	
Decreased subcutaneous fat, decreased turgor (elasticity)	Thin, dry skin, wrinkles
Diminished sweat glands, tactile sensation dulls	Poor thermoregulation, heat and cold sensitivity
Thickened connective tissue	Keratosis (patchy overgrowths of dermis), warts, skin tags especially on face and neck
Increased fat deposits over abdomen and hips	Poor excretion of fat-soluble drugs
Diminished capillary blood flow, reduced vascularity, capillary fragility	Pressure sores, delayed wound healing, purpura or lentigo (liver spots), bruises
Dry mucous membranes, decreased salivation and secretions	Dry mouth and vagina
Musculoskeletal system	
Diminished protein synthesis in muscle cells, decreased muscle mass and tone	Muscle weakness, reduced strength, muscle wasting
Erosion of cartilage, thickened synovial fluid, fibrosed synovial membranes	Joint pain, swelling, stiffness, diminished range of motion
Diminished mobility, flexibility, and balance	Poor gait, poor posture, risk of falling
Increased porosity and demineralization of bone, thinning of intervertebral disks, decreased height	Anklylosing spondylosis, kyphosis, osteoporosis
Respiratory system	
Atrophied respiratory muscles, kyphosis or other postural changes, rib cage rigidity	Chest wall limitations
Reduced vital capacity	Dyspnea
Risk of pneumonia	Ineffective cough, and above respiratory factors
Cardiovascular system	
Decreased cardiac output and stroke volume	Chronic fatigue and dyspnea, orthostatic hypotension
Myocardial irritability and stiffness, decreased size of sinoatrial and atrioventricular nodes	Slow heart rate and circulation, dysrhythmias and murmurs
Increased vascular resistance, rigidity in arteries	Hypertension
Thickening and dilation of veins	Venous insufficiency, varicosities
Decline in renal blood flow	Edema in tissues
Gastrointestinal system	
Decreased esophageal peristalsis, slowed emptying of stomach	Indigestion, frequent antacid use
Diminished saliva production slows breakdown of carbohydrates, reduced gastric secretion of hydrochloric acid impairs absorption of vitamins and minerals, hepatic insufficiency affects absorption of fats	Malnutrition
Loss of perineal and anal sphincter tone	Diarrhea, fecal incontinence
Decreased intestinal peristalsis, loss of abdominal muscle turgor, reduced mucosal secretions in intestines	Constipation, frequent laxative use
Endocrine system	
Reduced hormonal activity, decreased physical activity	Slowed basal metabolic rate, subnormal temperature
Slowed release of insulin from the pancreas	Impaired glucose metabolism
Reduced thyroid hormone production	Dry skin, temperature intolerance, poor appetite, lethargy, memory lapse
Disturbed fluid and electrolyte balance	Hydration status

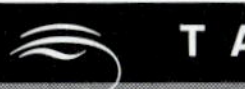

TABLE 43-1

Physiologic Changes Associated With Normal Aging Process in Geriatric Patient—cont'd

AGE-RELATED FACTORS	ASSESSMENT FACTORS
Genitourinary system	
Decreased renal blood flow, reduced number of glomeruli, reduced glomerular filtration rate, decreased excretory ability	Renal function diminished, risk of acid-base imbalance and drug toxicity
Loss of elasticity and muscle tone in ureters, bladder, and urethra	Urinary frequency, urgency, and nocturia
Decreased bladder muscle and sphincter tone, estrogen deficiency in female, enlarged prostate in male	Stress incontinence
Enlarged prostate in male	Urinary retention
Reduced testosterone, hypertrophied prostate, sclerosis of penile arteries and veins	Male: slow erection and ejaculation
Reduced estrogen, atrophied vulva, clitoris, and vagina	Female: sagging breasts, painful intercourse
Nervous system	
Decreased number of brain cells, reduced cerebral blood flow, reduced oxygen supply to brain	Cognitive deficits: delirium, temporary state of confusion, forgetfulness, disorientation, irritability, and/or insomnia; dementia, a permanent state of cognitive impairment
Decreased neurons	Paresthesia, akinesia, diminished pain perception
Diminished neurotransmitters, decreased neurons	Tremors, head nodding, or other repetitive movements
Degeneration of myelin sheath lessens motor neuron conduction	Reflexes and reaction time slowed
Reduced sound transmission as eardrum thickens, decreased hair cells and neurons, reduced blood supply to cochlea	Auditory impairment
Weakened lens muscles, hardening of lens, flattening of cornea, reduced blood supply leads to macular deterioration, increased rigidity of iris, reduced size of pupil	Visual impairment: decreased acuity, poor perception of light and color, poor peripheral vision

Scalp hair patterns may show areas of thinning or loss. The nurse should note the condition of the hair, such as cleanliness, hair dye, and grooming. The condition of the hair may show the level of interest or ability the patient has in self-care. A lack of care may be caused by inability or disinterest caused by depression. The patient who suffers from dementia may be unaware that the hair is dirty or uncombed.

Body hair patterns may be sparsely distributed with areas of thinning or absence. For this reason, hair removal from the surgical site is not routinely indicated. The extremities should be observed for patterns of hair growth or absence. The lower legs may not have much hair because of circulatory changes. The color of the legs should be observed at this time; duskiness and mottling may indicate a problem with arterial blood flow, whereas ruddiness may indicate a venous blood flow problem. The shape and size of the lower leg should be checked for edema or ulceration. The condition of the extremities may have implications for positioning for the surgical procedure and may indicate the need for further systemic testing.

Musculoskeletal System

Assessment of the musculoskeletal system includes muscles, bones, posture, and gait. Muscle mass is usually decreased because muscle fibers atrophy, decrease in strength, and are fewer in number. Fibrous tissue replaces the lost mass. With less exercise and motion, the strength of the muscle is compromised. Tendons become hardened and the range of motion decreases. Muscle cramps are common.

The patient may report a decrease in height. This is caused by demineralization of the bones, kyphosis, and narrowing of disk spaces in the vertebral column. The long bones do not decrease in length but become thin

Text continued on p. 889

TABLE 43-2

Geriatric Laboratory Values in Normal Aging Process

LABORATORY TEST	REFERENCE VALUE FOR PATIENT OVER AGE 65	CLINICAL IMPLICATION OF INCREASED VALUE	CLINICAL IMPLICATION OF DECREASED VALUE	NOTES
Hematology				
Hemoglobin (slightly decreased in both sexes; larger decrease in male)	M: 11.5-14.9 g/dl F: 11.7-13.8 g/dl	CHF, advanced COPD, dehydration, severe burns, polycythemia, high altitude	Anemia, cancer, chronic renal failure, fluid overload	Measures for anemia
Hematocrit (slight decrease in male)	M: 40%-50% F: 36%-46%	Dehydration, trauma, surgery, burns, polycythemia, diabetic acidosis, emphysema	Hemorrhage, anemia, leukemia, lymphoma, liver disease, kidney disease, malnutrition, lymphoma, collagen disease	Calculates red blood cell indices and hydration status
Red blood cells (RBCs) (number unchanged)	M: 4.6-6.0 F: 4.0-5.0	Dehydration, polycythemia, high altitude, advanced COPD	Fluid overload, anemia, hemorrhage, chronic infection, leukemia, kidney disease	Abnormal clotting conditions may cause decreased count
Reticulocyte (unchanged with normal aging)	0.5%-1.5% of total RBC	Bone marrow response to anemia, incompatible transfusion, hemolytic anemia	Hypoplastic or pernicious anemia	Indicates number of immature RBCs
Mean corpuscular volume (MCV) (slightly increased in both sexes)	80-98 μm³	Macrocytic anemia, chronic liver disease, anticonvulsant drugs, antimetabolites	Microcytic anemia, malignancy, rheumatoid arthritis, lead poisoning, radiation	Helps differentiate among the anemias
Mean corpuscular hemoglobin (MCH) (unchanged)	27-31 pg	Macrocytic anemia	Microcytic or hypochromic anemia, iron deficiency	Helps differentiate among the anemias
Mean corpuscular hemoglobin concentration (MCHC) (unchanged)	32-36 g/dl	Spherocytosis	Hypochromic anemia, thalassemia	Helps differentiate among the anemias
Erythrocyte sedimentation rate (ESR) (increases in both sexes)	(age 50-85) M: <20 mm/hr F: <30 mm/hr (> age 85) M: <30 mm/hr F: <42 mm/hr	Acute MI, lupus, gout, rheumatoid arthritis, burns, surgery, bacterial infections, TB, some malignancies	Polycythemia, CHF, sickle cell anemia, degenerative arthritis, factor V deficiency, low plasma protein	Can be used to monitor inflammatory processes or occult conditions such as tuberculosis or tissue necrosis
White blood cells (WBCs) (number unchanged but function decreases)	4500-10,000/cm³	Acute infections, acute MI, tissue necrosis, parasites, stress, collagen disease	Hemopoietic disease, viral infection, lupus, alcoholism, rheumatoid arthritis	Determine whether production has decreased in the presence of organ system decline

CHF, Congestive heart failure; *CNS,* central nervous system; *COPD,* chronic obstructive pulmonary disease; *DIC,* disseminated intravascular coagulopathy; *GI,* gastrointestinal; *IM,* intramuscular; *MI,* myocardial infarction; *MS,* multiple sclerosis; *TB,* tuberculosis.

TABLE 43-2

Geriatric Laboratory Values in Normal Aging Process—cont'd

LABORATORY TEST	REFERENCE VALUE FOR PATIENT OVER AGE 65	CLINICAL IMPLICATION OF INCREASED VALUE	CLINICAL IMPLICATION OF DECREASED VALUE	NOTES
Neutrophils (amount unchanged, but they become less effective)	Total 50%-70%	Acute infection, inflammatory disease, tissue damage, Hodgkin's disease	Bone marrow depression, viral disease, leukemia	Helps differentiate type of leukocytes
Lymphocytes (amount unchanged, but B and T cell function decrease; increase in autoantibody production)	25%-35% (mean)	Acute viral infections, chronic bacterial infections, lymphocytic leukemia, Hodgkin's disease, multiple myeloma, adrenocortical hypofunction	Cancer, leukemia, MS, kidney disease, bone marrow depression, lupus, adrenocortical hyperfunction	Decreased level indicates immunosuppression; highest values measured at approximately 8:00 PM (2000 hr)
Monocytes (slight increase in both sexes)	4%-6% (mean)	Viral disease, parasites, cancer, monocytic leukemia, collagen disease	Lymphocytic leukemia, aplastic anemia	Value may peak at noon, 12:00 PM (1200 hr)
Eosinophils (unchanged)	1%-3% (mean)	Parasites, cancer, allergies, thrombophlebitis	Cushing's syndrome, stress, skin disease, burns, shock	Value may peak at midnight, 12:00 AM (0000 hr)
Basophils (unchanged)	0.4%-1.0% (mean)	Healing stage of infection/inflammation, leukemia	Stress, hypersensitivity reaction, hyperthyroid	Measures this type of leukocyte
Platelets (unchanged)	150,000-400,000/µL	Hemorrhage, infection, malignancy, recent surgery, splenectomy, inflammatory disease, pulmonary embolism, cirrhosis, TB, cardiac disease, pancreatitis, fracture	Bone marrow disease, defective thrombopoiesis caused by folic acid or B_{12} deficiency, immune disease, DIC, severe burns, massive blood transfusions, kidney or liver disease	If <100,000, bleeding is likely; <50,000 spontaneous bleeding can take place; <5,000 can be fatal Many drugs can alter the results
Iron (decreases to 50%-75% of the normal young adult value by age 70)	M: 73-143 µg/dl F: 76-122 µg/dl	Pernicious hemolytic anemia, folic acid deficiency, liver damage, thalassemia, lead toxicity	Iron deficiency anemia, chronic blood loss, GI malignancy, peptic ulcer, rheumatoid arthritis, chronic renal failure	Helps differentiate cause of anemias
Total iron-binding capacity (TIBC) (decreases)	M: 291-387 µg/dl F: 293-355 µg/dl	Iron deficiency anemia, acute/chronic blood loss, polycythemia	Hemolytic anemias, sickle cell, renal failure, liver disease, rheumatoid arthritis, GI malignancy	Helps differentiate cause of anemias

Continued

TABLE 43-2

Geriatric Laboratory Values in Normal Aging Process—cont'd

LABORATORY TEST	REFERENCE VALUE FOR PATIENT OVER AGE 65	CLINICAL IMPLICATION OF INCREASED VALUE	CLINICAL IMPLICATION OF DECREASED VALUE	NOTES
Ferritin (unchanged, more sensitive indicator than serum iron value)	M: 20-300 ng/ml F: 20-120 ng/ml	Hemochromatosis, iron overload, acute or chronic infection, chronic renal failure, malignancies	Iron deficiency anemia, malnutrition, liver disease, nephrotic syndrome, malignancy	Reflects iron stores; recent transfusions can alter results
Transferrin (65-170 µg/dl are bound to iron; decreases with age)	250-390 µg/dl	Severe iron deficiency anemia	Liver damage, acute or chronic infection, cancer, anemia	Used to evaluate iron transport ability of blood
Bilirubin	Indirect 1.1 mg/dl Direct <0.5 mg/dl	*Indirect:* liver damage, fasting *Direct:* biliary duct obstruction *Direct and indirect:* hemolysis, biliary obstruction causing liver damage		Helps determine liver function; breaks down in presence of light
Activated partial thromboplastin time (APTT) (unchanged by age)	Clot 25-36 sec	Presence of heparin or other anticoagulants		Monitor anticoagulant therapy; measures intrinsic coagulation (except factor VII and XIII)
Partial thromboplastin time (PTT)	60-85 sec (Platelin) 25-35 sec (differs with method used to run test)			Less sensitive than APTT
Prothrombin time (PT) (unaffected by age)	M: 9.6-11.8 sec F: 9.5-11.3 sec	Deficient fibrinogen, prothrombin, or factors V, VII, X, vitamin K deficiency, liver disease		Measures extrinsic coagulation factors
Glucose (increase 2 mg/dl per decade after age 35)	70-110 mg/dl	Diabetes mellitus, hyperadrenalism, stress, infection, burns, pancreatitis, thiazide use, recent surgery, acromegaly, pheochromocytoma	Alcoholism, malnutrition, physical exercise, hypoglycemia, stomach, liver or lung cancer, hypothalamic lesions, hypoadrenalism, cirrhosis of liver	Two fasting blood sugar readings of ≥140 mg/dl confirms diabetes; hyperglycemia of aging may be caused by decreased insulin biosynthesis and changes in body composition associated with aging
Low-density lipoprotein (LDL)	<130 mg/dl desirable 130-159 mg/dl borderline	Increased risk for coronary artery disease		Condition is treated if value is >160 mg/dl, coronary artery disease, and two risk factors are present

TABLE 43-2

Geriatric Laboratory Values in Normal Aging Process—cont'd

LABORATORY TEST	REFERENCE VALUE FOR PATIENT OVER AGE 65	CLINICAL IMPLICATION OF INCREASED VALUE	CLINICAL IMPLICATION OF DECREASED VALUE	NOTES
High-density lipoprotein (HDL) (female may be higher than male until 70 years of age)	>35-40 mg/dl	Exercise, weight loss, alcohol intake	Coronary heart disease, diabetes, uremia, obesity, smoking, high-fat diet	Elevations desirable
Cholesterol (increased in male to age 50; decreased in female to age 50, then increases to age 70 and decreases again after age 70)	<200 mg/dl desirable level	Uncontrolled diabetes, hypothyroidism, cirrhosis of liver, hyperlipidemia, nephrotic syndrome	Malabsorption, starvation, hyperthyroidism	Helps determine function of liver, nervous and cardiovascular systems, and metabolism
Triglycerides (values increase with age for female)	10-190 mg/dl 250-500 mg/dl = borderline risk	Biliary obstruction, diabetes, nephrotic syndrome, alcoholism	Malnutrition	In combination with increased cholesterol helps determine increased risk of coronary artery disease
Uric acid (male values are higher throughout life span, but female values elevate at age 40-50 yr)	M: 2.6-9.2 mg/dl F: 1.9-8.5 mg/dl	Gout, alcoholism, metastasis, leukemia, glomerulonephritis, CHF, hemolytic anemia, polycythemia, psoriasis	Tubular acidosis, folic acid deficiency, burns, pernicious anemia	Thiazide diuretics can cause an increase in the elderly
Blood urea nitrogen (BUN) (increases slightly with age)	M: 7.6-35.5 mg/dl F: 5.9-31.6 mg/dl	Acute MI, high protein intake, prerenal failure, renal disease, GI bleeding, sepsis, diabetes, high licorice ingestion, urinary tract obstruction	Low protein diet, severe liver damage, overhydration, malnutrition	May overestimate renal function in the elderly; should be interpreted in combination with creatinine to assess hydration status
Albumin (decreases with age because of decreased liver function by age 65 yr)	M: 3.5-4.7 g/dl F: 3.7-4.6 g/dl	Multiple myeloma	Malnutrition, anemia, burns, liver disease, gallbladder disease, kidney disease, lupus, colitis, essential hypertension, metastasis	Less than 52%-68% of total protein may indicate kidney or liver disease
Total protein (slight decrease with age)	6.0-7.8 g/dl	Dehydration, vomiting, diarrhea, diabetes, acidosis, fulminating infection, leukemia, myeloma	Malnutrition, uncontrolled diabetes, malabsorption, GI disease, essential hypertension, blood dyscrasia	Used in diagnosis of liver and kidney disease

Continued

TABLE 43-2

Geriatric Laboratory Values in Normal Aging Process—cont'd

LABORATORY TEST	REFERENCE VALUE FOR PATIENT OVER AGE 65	CLINICAL IMPLICATION OF INCREASED VALUE	CLINICAL IMPLICATION OF DECREASED VALUE	NOTES
Creatinine (female values may be decreased due to lower muscle mass)	M: 0.8-1.2 mg/dl F: 0.6-0.9 mg/dl	High meat or fish intake, renal failure, shock, acute MI, lupus, cancer, diabetic nephropathy, acromegaly, large muscle mass	Decreased amounts not clinically significant	May increase with age and should be measured before giving prolonged administration of medication excreted by kidneys
Potassium (slight increase after age 60 yr)	M: 3.7-5.6 mmol/L F: 3.5-5.3 mmol/L	Renal failure, hyperadrenalism, metabolic acidosis	Vomiting, diarrhea, laxative abuse, dehydration, starvation, stress, trauma, recent surgery, metabolic alkalosis, burns, hyperaldosteronism	Cardiac arrest can result if values are <2.5 or >7 mmol/L
Sodium	135-146 mmol/L	Excess sodium intake, inadequte fluid intake, diabetes insipidus, prolonged hyperventilation, impaired renal function, aldosteronism	Excess sodium loss by GI suctioning, prolonged sweating, diuretics, diarrhea, vomiting, adrenal insufficiency, burns, chronic renal insufficiency with acidosis	Assess with hydration status
Chloride	100-108 mEq/L	Severe dehydration, renal shutdown, hyperventilation, primary aldosteronism	Vomiting, gastric suctioning, intestinal fistula, CHF, edema	Hypochloremia may develop into tetany and depressed respirations; hyperchloremia may develop into rapid breathing, stupor, and coma
Calcium (age-related renal changes may decrease the baseline level)	8.0-10.2 mg/dl	Hyperparathyroidism, Paget's disease, metastasis, bone fractures, immobility, ingestion of calcium carbonate antacids, bone demineralization	Hypoparathyroidism, malabsorption, Cushing's syndrome, peritonitis, renal failure, obstructive jaundice	Hypercalcemia can cause stupor, coma, and cardiac arrest
Phosphate	2.5-4.5 mg/dl	Bone disease, acromegaly, intestinal obstruction, diabetic acidosis, renal failure	Alcoholism, diabetes, hyperalimentation, gram-negative bacteremia, alkalosis, acute gout, aspirin poisoning, prolonged diarrhea and vomiting	Measured to assess renal function and acid-base balance; evaluated in combination with serum calcium

TABLE 43-2

Geriatric Laboratory Values in Normal Aging Process—cont'd

LABORATORY TEST	REFERENCE VALUE FOR PATIENT OVER AGE 65	CLINICAL IMPLICATION OF INCREASED VALUE	CLINICAL IMPLICATION OF DECREASED VALUE	NOTES
Lactic dehydrogenase (LDH)	M: 61-200 ImU/ml F: 71-206 ImU/ml	Acute MI, placement of intracardiac prosthetic valve, cardiac surgery, hepatitis, pernicious anemia, malignancy, pulmonary embolus, any hemolytic condition	Irradiation	Evaluated in combination with cardiac studies
Amylase	60-180 Somogyi units/ml	Acute pancreatitis, perforating peptic ulcer, upper GI surgery, acute alcohol poisoning, salivary gland disease, strangulated hernia, mesenteric thrombus, lung cancer	Pancreatic failure, liver damage, hepatitis	Results are more accurate in an early AM sample; helps differentiate acute pancreatitis from other cause of abdominal pain
Alkaline phosphatase (ALP) (increases in women after age 45 yr)	M: 90-239 U/L F: 87-250 U/L	Healing fractures, bone tumors, liver disease, biliary obstruction	Vitamin D toxicity, hypothyroidism, pernicious anemia, malnutrition, vitamin C deficiency, magnesium deficiency	Usually performed in combination with other liver enzyme tests to assess liver condition
Creatinine kinase (CK) Creatinine phosphokinase (CPK)	18-392 IU/L M: 55-170 IU/L F: 30-135 IU/L	Hypokalemia, MI, postconvulsion status, carbon monoxide poisoning, malignancy, hyperthermia, embolism after defibrillation	Sedentary lifestyle	Immobility causes a low baseline and makes the diagnosis of acute MI difficult
CPK isoenzymes	CPK-MM 94%-100%	Continuous tremors, hypokalemia, skeletal muscle damage		Multiple IM injections can influence, as can strenuous exercise
	CPK-MB 0%-6%	Acute MI, hypokalemia, cardiac ischemia, cardiac surgery, muscular dystrophy, polymyositis		Rise 4-8 hr after MI, peaks 18-24 hr and is present in 100% by 48 hr; return to normal in 3-4 days
	CPK-BB 0%	Brain tissue injury, malignancy, shock, pulmonary infarction, renal failure, necrosis of large intestine, uremia, malignant hyperthermia		

Continued

TABLE 43-2

Geriatric Laboratory Values in Normal Aging Process—cont'd

LABORATORY TEST	REFERENCE VALUE FOR PATIENT OVER AGE 65	CLINICAL IMPLICATION OF INCREASED VALUE	CLINICAL IMPLICATION OF DECREASED VALUE	NOTES
Serum glutamic-oxaloacetic transaminase (SGOT); also known as asparate aminotransferase (AST)	8-20 IU/L	Acute MI, liver disease, trauma, IM injections, irradiation injury, pulmonary infarction		May falsely elevate after administration of opiates; progressively decreasing value indicates improvement of acute condition
Acid phosphatase	0-1.6 IU/L	Prostate cancer, Paget's disease, multiple myeloma	Decrease following an increase may indicate successful treatment of prostate cancer	Prostate manipulation 48 hr before test may alter the value
Serum glutamic-pyruvic transaminase (SGPT); also known as alanine aminotransferase (ALT) (in male, peak at age 50, then decreases to lowest point after age 65)	M: 0-45 IU/L F: 20-37 IU/L	Hepatitis, mononucleosis, cholecystitis	Vitamin B_6 deficiency	Distinguish between hepatic and cardiac tissue damage
Prostate-specific antigen (PSA)	0.1-2.6 mg/ml	Prostatic cancer		Not present in all types of prostate cancer; prostate manipulation may alter results; cystoscopy or sigmoidoscopy may cause prostate manipulation
Triiodothyronine T_3 (decrease in male after age 60, decrease in female after age 70 or 80)	80-200 ng/dl	Hyperthyroidism, thyrotoxicosis, toxic thryoid adenoma	Severe trauma or illness, malnutrition	Measures level of thyroid function
Thyroxine T_4 (small decrease up to 25% with age)	4.5-11.5 μg/dl	Hyperthyroidism, viral hepatitis, myasthenia gravis	Hypothyroidism, strenuous exercise, renal failure, protein malnutrition	Measures level of thyroid function
Thyroid stimulating hormone (TSH) (increases in both sexes after age 60 yr)	2-5.4 μU/ml	Goiter, thyroiditis, iodine deficiency, neck radiation, subtotal thyroidectomy	Hyperthyroidism, pituitary or hypothalamic related hypothyroidism	Measures level of thyroid function
Estrogen (male gradually increase, female markedly decrease)	M: 40-115 pg/ml F: <30 pg/ml	Ovarian cancer, adrenocortical tumor, some testicular tumors	Ovarian failure, pituitary insufficiency, psychogenic stress	Female sex hormone

TABLE 43-2

Geriatric Laboratory Values in Normal Aging Process—cont'd

LABORATORY TEST	REFERENCE VALUE FOR PATIENT OVER AGE 65	CLINICAL IMPLICATION OF INCREASED VALUE	CLINICAL IMPLICATION OF DECREASED VALUE	NOTES
Luteinizing hormone (LH)	M: 5-20 mIU/ml F: >75 mIU/ml	Ovarian failure	Hypothalamic or pituitary hypofunction, testicular tumors, testicular failure	May be evaluated in combination with other sex hormone levels to determine the effectiveness of replacement therapy
Follicle stimulating hormone (FSH)	M: 10-15 mIU/ml F: 40-250 mIU/ml	Testicular failure, end stage acromegaly, seminoma, ovarian failure	Anorexia nervosa, panhypopituitarism, hypothalamic lesions	May be evaluated in combination with other sex hormone levels to determine effectiveness of replacement therapy
Prolactin (male increase, female may decrease slightly)	M: 1-20 ng/ml F: 1-20 ng/ml	Hypoglycemia, stress, postoperative pituitary surgery, dopamine depletion	Primary hypothyroidism, pituitary adenomas, lung or kidney tumors, increased estrogen levels	In the presence of pituitary tumor, value may exceed 100 ng/ml
Testosterone (male gradual decrease until age 70 yr, then marked drop; female decrease with age)	M: 3.9-7.9 ng/ml F: 0.21-0.37 ng/ml	Testicular tumors	Testicular failure, hypopituitarism	Male sex hormone
Total carbon dioxide (CO_2)	22-34 mEq/L	Metabolic alkalosis, respiratory acidosis	Metabolic acidosis, respiratory alkalosis	Consider the value in relation to pH and arterial blood gas values
Arterial pH (unchanged)	7.35-7.45	Respiratory or metabolic alkalosis	Respiratory or metabolic acidosis, narcotics	Acid-base level of the blood
Arterial oxygen (PaO_2) (gradual decrease)	75-100 mm Hg		Respiratory or cardiac disease	Measures the amount of oxygen (O_2) the lungs are delivering to the blood
Arterial carbon dioxide ($PaCO_2$) (unchanged or may increase with age)	35-45 mm Hg	Impaired respiratory function, respiratory acidosis	Hyperventilation, respiratory alkalosis	Value compared in combination with bicarbonate (HCO_3) and pH to determine whether respiratory efforts are compensating for abnormal metabolic state
Oxygen (O_2) content	15%-23%		Impaired respiratory function	Measures the amount of O_2 carried by hemoglobin

Continued

TABLE 43-2

Geriatric Laboratory Values in Normal Aging Process—cont'd

LABORATORY TEST	REFERENCE VALUE FOR PATIENT OVER AGE 65	CLINICAL IMPLICATION OF INCREASED VALUE	CLINICAL IMPLICATION OF DECREASED VALUE	NOTES
Oxygen (O_2) saturation	94%-100%		Impaired respiratory function	Measures how much hemoglobin is carrying O_2
Bicarbonate content (HCO_3)	21-28 mEq/L	Metabolic alkalosis	Metabolic acidosis	Measures how the pH is influenced by metabolism
Urinalysis				
Bacteria	None	Urinary tract infection		10%-50% of all elderly have asymptomatic bacteruria that returns after treatment and rarely causes renal damage or becomes a septic illness
Bilirubin	None	Liver disease		Not a reliable monitor of glycemic status because the aged kidney has altered physical and reabsorptive properties
Glucose	None	Diabetes, renal disease, thyroid disorders, liver disease, some CNS disorders, heavy metal poisoning, hyperalimentation		
Ketones	None	Uncontrolled type I diabetes, starvation, metabolic complications of hyperalimentation		
pH	4.5-8.0	Alkalotic: urinary tract infection, metabolic or respiratory acidosis	Acidotic: renal tuberculosis, pyrexia, phenylketonuria, acidosis	
White blood cells (WBC)	0-4	Urinary tract or kidney infection		Treatment recommended only in the presence of additional symptoms
Red blood cells (RBC)	0-3	Urinary tract disease, renal failure		Increased amount indicates the need for further evaluation
Protein	0-1, not to exceed 150 mg/24 hr	Renal disease, CHF, diabetes		Common in elderly and can be caused by subclinical urinary tract infection
Specific gravity (lower maximum in elderly)	1.005-1.020	Dehydration, acute glomerulonephritis, shock, CHF, liver failure	Diabetes insipidus, fluid excess, tubular necrosis	Severe renal damage usually present if specific gravity does not change with changes in fluid intake

and brittle (osteoporosis), especially in elderly women; 78% of all patients over 70 years of age have some degree of osteoporosis. Estrogen supplements after menopause may decrease the occurrence of brittle bones. However, fractures in the ends of long bones, hips, vertebrae, and wrists are common in elderly persons. Assistance or total lifting may be necessary to help the geriatric patient move from the transport stretcher to the operating table for the surgical procedure. The plan of care should include lifting help or devices and adequate positioning supplies. Care must be taken not to injure bony structures that may be weakened by osteoporosis.

Ankylosing spondylosis, a chronic inflammatory disease characterized by fixation or fusion of a vertebral joint, often causes age-related postures. The geriatric patient's body assumes an altered shape with increased forward thoracic curvature (kyphosis) and flattening of the lumbar curvature. The patient may not be able to lie flat on the operating table. Supine positioning may be painful unless the upper back and neck are supported. Fractures or subluxation of the cervical spine are possible if the ankylosed neck is allowed to fall back with the weight of the head. Twisting and forceful flexion can cause permanent damage to the vertebral column. Anteroposterior angles of the chest may be increased because of respiratory disease. Respiratory effort and chest excursion should be taken into consideration in planning positioning. In the preoperative assessment, the flexibility of the patient's spine and the presence of any deformity or associated disease should be noted. Flexion at the hip may be painful when the legs are maintained in a straight position. Placement of the safety strap over the thighs may exert counterpressure on the thighs, causing the legs to forcefully straighten against the flattened lumbar curvature. Modified positioning may include a small pillow under the knees and thighs to allow the age-related flexion angle of the hips to assume a natural position. Care in the placement of the safety strap should include circulatory checks throughout the surgical procedure.

The hands and feet may have painful deformities that should be considered when moving the patient to the operating table and during positioning. Joints may be affected by arthritis, thickened synovium, and crystalloid formation in the synovial fluid. Arthritic joints are painful. The patient may have a long history of taking nonsteroidal antiinflammatory medications, corticosteroids, salicylates, and analgesics. The preoperative assessment should include evaluation for the side effects associated with long-term use of these medications. Gastrointestinal bleeding, prolonged clotting times, renal insufficiency, liver changes, loss of appetite, and alteration in mental status are common side effects. These could adversely affect the desired outcomes of the surgical procedure.

The patient's center of gravity is altered by multiple body-shape changes. Postural imbalance caused by impaired mobility is frequently the cause of falls that result in fractures. Some geriatric patients limit attempts at ambulation because they fear the possibility of falling. Risk of falls is further increased by complicating conditions such as sedation, electrolyte imbalance, impaired vision, and altered proprioception (muscular stimulation). Orthostatic hypotension contributes to the potential for falling when the elderly patient rises from a sitting position and experiences a sudden drop in blood pressure. A fall may be symptomatic of a health problem or a systemic illness.

Cardiopulmonary System

Assessment of the lungs, heart, and circulation is a good source of information about the general health condition of the patient. The cardiovascular and respiratory systems are closely interrelated. To assess the lungs, the nurse should ask the patient to describe how his or her breathing is affected by exertion. By observing the patient's physical activity, respiratory effort, shape of the chest, and color of the lips, the nurse can assess difficulty or inefficiency in breathing. The nurse should palpate the trachea to determine if it is in midline. A deviation to the right or left may indicate the presence of a tumor. Tracheal position is an important consideration in the maintenance of an airway during a surgical procedure. By listening to lung sounds with a stethoscope over the intercostal spaces, the nurse can refine the assessment to include specific sounds found in identified areas of each lobe. Percussion of the posterior chest wall tends to produce resonance except in very thin elderly persons in whom tone is very hyperresonant. The normal sound is hollow, moderately loud with a low pitch and long duration. Sound flattens over rib bones. If the patient slumps forward and rounds the shoulders, the intercostal spaces widen for better percussion.

Establishment of a preoperative respiratory system baseline is important. Intraoperative breathing difficulty may be avoided by adapting a position to accommodate the needs of the patient. Postoperative problems may be diagnosed and treated more efficiently if the patient's original respiratory condition has been assessed. Lung disease may affect the ability to clear secretions from the bronchial tree by coughing. Pneumonia is a common postoperative complication in elderly patients. Coughing and deep breathing exercises should be taught preoperatively.

The heart and systemic circulation are assessed as separate units and together as a system. The patient should be asked whether he or she experiences dizziness, fainting, palpitations, or other abnormal subjective symptoms. The perioperative nurse should listen to heart sounds with a stethoscope. Dysrhythmias, unrelated to heart disease, are not uncommon in the elderly patient. The sinoatrial and the atrioventricular nodes decrease in size with age. Signal interruption may take place. Clicks, murmurs, and abnormal sounds should be recorded in the assessment data. Many geriatric patients have systolic murmurs caused by aortic stenosis. The apical pulse should be counted and compared with the peripheral pulses of the radial, popliteal, posterior tibial, and dorsalis pedis arteries. The difference between the apical and the peripheral pulse may indicate an obstruction in a major artery. The jugular veins should be observed for distention. Veins in the lower extremities should be inspected for varicosities. Leg pain caused by circulatory impairment is common in the elderly.

The carotid arteries should be auscultated with a stethoscope. Bruits and systolic murmurs, which are abnormal sounds, may indicate an evolving blockage. Dizziness or cognitive impairment may be caused by carotid insufficiency. Care must be taken not to exert pressure over the carotid area because manipulation of a plaque could cause an embolus to break loose and travel to the brain. Sudden changes in mental status during a surgical procedure performed under local anesthesia could be caused by an arterial occlusion.

The geriatric patient usually has decreased or slowed circulation to all areas of the body. This should be taken into consideration during the administration of local anesthetics. Absorption of the medication will take longer and the effects will be delayed. The surgical site should be tested for the effects of anesthesia before the incision is made. Vasoconstrictive additives, such as epinephrine, may have an exaggerated effect. Postoperative dressings should not be applied too tightly because healing is affected by circulatory efficiency.

Blood pressure should be assessed in the sitting and lying positions. Both arms should be tested. Elevated systolic and diastolic blood pressures are a common finding in 40% of the geriatric patient population.

Assessment of laboratory blood values is important (see Table 43-2). Anemia is common among the elderly and is frequently overlooked as a potential cause for cerebral ischemia. Men (21%) and women (34%) both have slight normal decreases in hemoglobin and hematocrit levels because the blood-forming mechanisms lose efficiency with age. In men the decrease in androgen production may cause a noticeable decrease in hemoglobin. Extreme decreases in hemoglobin and hematocrit values are significant in the diagnosis of pathologic conditions in major organ systems, especially the gastrointestinal or genitourinary systems. Nutritional deficit may cause anemic conditions also. In the absence of any other confirmed pathologic condition, a hemoglobin level below 12 g/dl or a hematocrit below 35% may signal anemia caused by malnutrition.

The white blood cells do not decrease in volume, but they decrease in effectiveness. Inflammatory responses may be decreased or absent in the geriatric patient. This natural body response to injury may leave the patient more vulnerable to infection. The febrile response to infection may be diminished and may not be a good indicator of a disease process. Often the baseline temperature of the elderly is subnormal.

Gastrointestinal System

Assessment of the gastrointestinal system should begin by observing for visual signs of nutritional status, such as body weight, muscle wasting, bloating, and generalized weakness. Postoperative healing is profoundly affected by the ability of the cells to repair themselves. Adequate nutrition and the ability to handle the necessary nutrients in the gastrointestinal system are essential for tissue restoration. Many socioeconomic, psychologic, and physiologic factors influence the nutritional status of the geriatric patient. Living on a fixed income may limit amount of nutritious food the patient is able to purchase. An adequate diet should include at least 1 g of protein per kilogram of desirable body weight, with an emphasis on a decreased number of calories. The average daily caloric intake of an elderly woman should range between 1280 and 1900 calories and of an elderly man between 1530 and 2300 calories. The perioperative nurse should keep in mind that the actual caloric needs are unique to the individual patient and may vary in the presence of diabetes or other disease processes. Rapid weight gain or loss may indicate a serious pathologic condition. Dietary control should focus on the quality of food, not the quantity of food. Weight should be considered a vital sign in the elderly and should be recorded in both pounds and kilograms. Many medications are prescribed according to body weight in kilograms.

Psychologically, the patient may feel that food does not taste right and may refuse to eat. Many psychologic reasons for malnutrition have their roots in a physiologic cause. The patient's appetite may be decreased because taste receptors in the mouth are fewer. The sense of smell also may be diminished. The patient's teeth may be in disrepair. Some patients are totally edentulous (toothless). Loose or missing teeth must be assessed because of the danger of aspirating a tooth during the surgical procedure. The inability to taste, chew, and swallow discourages eating. Saliva production decreases and makes swallowing more difficult. During the preoperative assessment, the perioperative nurse may find that decreased ability to taste salty and sweet foods may cause an increase in the addition of salt and sugar to the diet. Increased salt intake may predispose the patient to congestive heart failure. Added sugar may cause an increase in unwanted body fat in proportion to muscle mass. The geriatric patient undergoing general anesthesia may receive stimulants and depressants; many of these are fat soluble. The fat-soluble drugs will absorb faster but will be excreted more slowly because of lower levels of intracellular fluid. Medications are unevenly distributed in the body, and the anticipated actions are unpredictable because fewer receptor sites react to the presence of the drug.

Digestion can be assessed by questioning the patient about food intake and the effects of the presence of food in the stomach. Elderly patients have decreased stomach motility, less gastric secretions, and slower stomach emptying time. The esophagus loses muscular tone and dilates slightly. Food may remain in the esophagus for longer periods of time. The perioperative nurse should ask the patient about the use of antacids and laxatives. Frequent use of antacids may indicate swallowing or stomach problems that should be investigated. Esophageal reflux in the presence of a hiatal hernia may need to be assessed preoperatively to prevent aspiration of gastric secretions. The inability to lie flat with food in the stomach may be the first symptom of a high-risk situation. Positioning and rapid sequence induction of anesthesia may be a consideration. Cricoid pressure may be necessary for intubation and prevention of aspiration.

The elderly patient may use laxatives to maintain bowel regularity. Decreased motility, less intake of bulk and fluids, and inactivity cause constipation. Oil-based laxatives can lead to malabsorption of the fat-soluble vitamins A, D, E, and K, which further impairs nutritional and general health status. Absorption of nutrients is impaired naturally in the elderly as a process of aging because intestinal blood flow is reduced and absorptive cells lining the intestines are decreased. Fiber is an important dietary additive but should be used with caution inasmuch as it can cause bowel obstruction or diarrhea. Diarrhea in the geriatric patient causes a serious threat to well-being because the hydration status becomes perilously imbalanced.

Minimum oral fluid intake should be 1500 ml daily. Some geriatric patients have limited fluid intake. The patient may fear incontinence, have altered sensorium and cognition, be unable to drink fluid independently, or have decreased thirst sensation as part of the aging process. The serious nature of fluid balance in the elderly is reflected in the unstable electrolyte values and the direct impact this has on cardiac status. Preoperative assessment of hydration should be performed by the perioperative nurse. Signs of dehydration are dry tongue, sunken cheeks and eyes, severe loss of skin turgor, concentrated urine, and, in some instances, mental confusion. Blood tests may show an elevated urea level above 60 mg/dl. The dehydrated geriatric patient should have preoperative intravenous fluids to prevent complications.

Endocrine System

The endocrine system interfaces with all major systems of the body. The normal age-related changes in other body systems complicate the assessment of endocrine functioning. The endocrine system consists of the thyroid, parathyroid, pancreas, adrenal, pituitary, and pineal glands and the ovaries or testes.

The thyroid gland reduces thyroid hormone production 50% by the age of 80 years. The effects of this decreased production may cause dry skin, memory lapse, temperature intolerance, lethargy, and appetite disturbance. Many signs and symptoms of thyroid disease may be confused with the normal aging process. Comorbidity may cause a patient with normal thyroid function to have abnormal laboratory test results. Men have decreased thyroid hormone production by age 60, whereas women have decreased production by age 70.

Insulin, produced by the beta cells in the pancreas, affects glucose metabolism and storage. In healthy patients, glucose levels in the blood cause the release of insulin by the pancreas. In the elderly, the response of the pancreas is slowed and the release of insulin may not be triggered by the same stimulus. Many elderly patients are diabetic and have impaired glucose metabolism. Diabetes may be caused by deficient insulin production, insensitive insulin receptors, altered insulin release mechanisms, or inactivation of circulating insulin. An imbalance in blood glucose levels during the surgical procedure may predispose the patient to an unwanted outcome. Diabetic patients frequently experience more postoperative infections and complications. Uncontrolled blood glucose metabolism has negative implications for all major body systems. Ongoing assessment is important for the attainment of expected outcomes.

Genitourinary System

Assessment of the genitourinary system includes the bladder, urethra, ureters, kidneys, reproductive history, and genitalia. The first noticeable sign of a problem with the genitourinary system may be the odor of urine. The odor may be caused by lack of cleanliness but usually is caused by incontinence. More than 30% of the elderly population experience some form of urinary incontinence, but many are reluctant to discuss this problem and may try to avoid it. The problem may stem from stress incontinence, confusion, neurologic disorders, urinary tract infection, or immobility that prevents ability to get to the bathroom quickly. The elderly patient may fear loss of bladder control during the surgical procedure. Previous bladder or prostate gland surgery may predispose the patient to involuntary urine release. The perioperative nurse should include this situation in the plan of care because if the patient has the opportunity to empty the bladder preoperatively, the problem may be minimized during the surgical procedure. Nursing diagnoses should reflect not only urinary incontinence but the associated anxiety level of the patient. Assessment of the genital area should include observation of the perineum for redness and excoriation. The bladder should be palpated while the patient is supine. A distended bladder after the patient has voided may indicate urinary retention with an overflow condition. This should be checked preoperatively before the patient is catheterized in the OR. The urethra could be inadvertently traumatized if an obstruction, such as a tumor or an enlarged prostate gland, is present.

The kidneys decrease in effectiveness as the patient ages. Renal blood flow and glomerular filtration rate decrease by as much as 50% by age 50. Although no overt signs of a disease process are present, the perioperative nurse should be aware that the older patient is at increased risk for renal insufficiency and is highly susceptible to fluid overload, dehydration, or renal failure.

A baseline assessment of intake and output should be made. During the surgical procedure urinary output may be used to monitor the renal status of the patient. Renal impairment may delay the excretion of drugs by the kidneys and further complicates fluid balance. The urine should be assessed for color, concentration, presence of particulate matter, and odor. Minimum urinary output during the procedure should be at least 30 ml per hour. More urine may be produced if the patient is taking diuretics or medication for blood pressure or cardiac control. Monitoring urinary output is difficult if the patient does not have an indwelling catheter or if he or she should experience urinary incontinence during the procedure. Postoperative care should include emptying the bladder to evaluate the expected outcome of adequate urinary output.

Reproductive assessment consists of the number of pregnancies a woman had during her childbearing years. Data about the method of birth should be included. Childbirth by cesarean section or previous gynecologic surgery may indicate the possibility of pelvic adhesions that may be encountered if the planned surgical procedure includes entering the peritoneal cavity. Multiple vaginal births may cause uterine and bladder prolapse. The presence of a pessary for uterine elevation should be noted. Estrogen replacement should be noted. The possibility of osteoporosis and heart disease is greater in elderly women who have not had estrogen replacement after menopause.

The breasts of both male and female patients should be palpated for masses. The male patient may exhibit gynecomastia, which is an increase of breast tissue caused by decreased testosterone production. Previous mammograms should be available if breast surgery is planned. Any hormonal therapy should be noted in the assessment. If the breast is biopsied, the specimen may be tested for estrogen receptor sites. The loss of fibrous breast tissue in the woman is normal. The main palpable finding will be the terminal milk ducts, which feel like strands or spindles. Masses are not a common finding and should be investigated. Nulliparous women may be predisposed to breast cancer. Nipple discharge or retraction may indicate a serious condition. The breasts of the elderly woman may be pendulous and flaccid. Prepping and draping may be slightly more difficult because of the sagging skin and lack of muscle tone.

The male genitalia may be diminished in size. The penis may be smaller. The testes descend lower into the scrotum because the rugae are decreased or absent. Pubic hair may be sparse, pale, and coarse. The ability to achieve erection may be decreased or absent, and the ability to ejaculate may be diminished. Orgasm may still be possible without the presence of an erection. The prostate may be enlarged. The incidence of prostatic cancer increases with age. The elderly male patient may experience embarrassment during a prostate examination. All efforts should be made to preserve his dignity. Positioning may be difficult because of inflexible joints. The patient can be positioned in a lateral, modified jackknife or modified dorsal recumbent position. The presence of stool may hinder the palpation. Rectal sphincter tone should be assessed in the patient who may be undergoing a transrectal procedure. Many prostate biopsies utilize transrectal ultrasound and needle aspiration and sampling of the gland. Anal tears, hemorrhoids, fissures, and defects in the musculature should be documented in the assessment data. Postoperative bleeding could be wrongly assessed as a problem caused by the surgical procedure. Baseline data may help to resolve the situation.

The female genitalia should be assessed externally and internally. The patient should be placed supine in a modified lithotomy position. Spinal curvature or respiratory difficulty may prevent the patient from lying flat. Arthritic joints make lithotomy positioning a painful effort. Care should be exercised not to create embarrassment during the examination. The vulvar area should be inspected. The mons and labia will appear smaller and looser because of the loss of subcutaneous fat pads and the decrease in estrogen production. Lesions and discolorations should be noted. The skin of the perineum may be shiny, atrophic, and dry. The prepuce and clitoris may be atrophied. Orgasm is still possible. The vaginal opening may appear small, dry, and inelastic. Previous history of hysterectomy or oophorectomy should be obtained. The absence of the uterus or ovaries does not preclude the examination of the vaginal vault. The anus should be inspected for tears, fissures, and hemorrhoids.

The internal assessment includes a very gentle examination by insertion of a gloved, well-lubricated finger into the vagina. The vagina may feel shortened. The position of the bladder, rectum, and cervix should be ascertained. Protrusion of the bladder, rectum, or cervix may be present inasmuch as the patient experiences a loss of muscle tone with age. The abdomen is palpated as the uterus is carefully elevated. The uterus atrophies as part of the aging process. Enlargement is caused by disease. The endometrium will still respond to stimulation of hormonal therapy. The adnexa are identified, and no masses should be felt. The use of a smaller, prewarmed, well-lubricated speculum is usually necessary for visualization of the cervix and obtaining a Papanicolaou (Pap) smear. The vaginal lining will look thin, smooth, dry, and atrophied. Care is essential to prevent trauma when inserting fingers or instruments into the vagina. Discharge and foul odors are abnormal and should be reported. Vaginal bleeding is a sign of a pathologic condition in the elderly woman.

Sexuality in the elderly is an often overlooked and ignored reality. The activity between geriatric sex partners may vary in performance, but sexual pleasure is not abandoned because of advancing age. Intercourse may not take place in the same way as when the partners were young, but sexual contact and mutual gratification remains pleasurable. Many elderly patients have been forced to deny their sexuality because of the loss of their sexual partner. Self-gratification may be practiced, but not openly discussed because of the personal nature of the act. The subject of sexuality should be approached gently, without jokes or condemnation. A surgical procedure that may alter sexual habits can be devastating. Empathy is critical to the patient's adjustment to a change of lifestyle. Counseling may be necessary to assist the patient and the sexual partner to express concerns. The perioperative nurse should be prepared to answer questions and listen to the patient as he or she expresses a sense of loss. The plan of care should reflect the nursing diagnosis of alteration in sexuality and sexual expression.

Nervous System

Assessment of the nervous system includes the brain, spinal cord, peripheral nerves, and sensory organs. The nervous system is uniquely interdependent with every system of the body. Age-related changes in the brain consist of a decreased number of neurons, decreased impulse transmission rate, increased reflex response time, and decreased brain mass. The perioperative nurse should assess the elderly patient and establish a baseline of neurologic function. Any deviation from the baseline during the surgical procedure may indicate the presence of an additional or new pathologic condition involving the brain (e. g., stroke). Postoperatively the ongoing assessment monitors the risk for postprocedural deficit caused by medication or a pathologic condition.

The spinal cord and peripheral nerves are assessed together. During the functional assessment, the patient is observed ambulating, sitting, standing, maintaining posture, making intentional hand motions, and performing cooperative purposeful actions such as writing. The perioperative nurse is able to observe for tremor, gait disturbance, shuffling of feet, unilateral weakness, or an alteration in mobility caused by a neurologic deficit. Assessment of medications taken at home is important to determine the presence of transient nervous system side effects such as shaking and intention tremor. Smoking can cause a temporary decrease in cerebral blood flow, resulting in dizziness that may mimic a neurologic problem.

Sensory changes associated with aging involve decreased pressure and pain perception, difficulty differentiating between hot and cold, hearing loss, decreased visual acuity, and alteration in the senses of smell and taste and in spatial perception during locomotion. Preoperative assessment of tactile sensory conditions will enable the plan of care to reflect the need for caution during the use of heat- or cold-producing equipment such as hypothermia/hyperthermia mattress, and protection of bony pressure points.

If a patient has sensory impairments such as visual disturbance, hearing loss, and altered spatial perception, he or she is at high risk for injury caused by falls. Allowing the patient to wear hearing aids and eyeglasses to the OR is beneficial to his or her adaptation to the surgical environment. Unexpected outcomes caused by sensory alteration can be prevented by developing a plan of care that takes into consideration the combined baseline abilities and sensory needs of the patient. For example, assessment of hearing ability will dictate the need to facilitate communication.

INTRAOPERATIVE CONSIDERATIONS

Special precautions are indicated in caring for geriatric patients in the operating room. The following factors should be taken into account:

1. *Hypothermia.* Geriatric patients are at risk when core body temperature falls below 96.8º F (36º C). A decreased basal metabolic rate, limited cardiovascular reserve, thinning of the skin, and reduced muscle mass affect the production and conservation of body heat. Measures must be taken to prevent inadvertent hypothermia caused by environmental factors. Raising the room temperature; using warm blankets and hyperthermia mattress; warming anesthetic gases, solutions, and intravenous fluids; and covering the patient's head are precautionary measures. (Refer to precautions to prevent hypothermia in Chapter 19, p. 383.)
2. *Positioning.* Patients should be lifted, not pulled, during transfer to and from and during positioning on the operating table. Skin is sensitive to abrasion because of decreased dermal thickness and turgor (elasticity). Joints may be stiff or

painful due to calcification or degenerative osteoarthritis. Support of the back and neck prevents discomfort from osteoporosis, kyphosis, or rheumatoid arthritis. Padding and air supports protect pressure points and bony prominences. Circulation and respiration must not be further compromised. Decreased cardiac output, arteriosclerosis, venous stasis, reduced vital lung capacity, and reduced tissue oxygenation are characteristic changes in elderly persons.

3. *Antiembolic measures.* Slow circulation and hypotension predispose elderly persons to thrombus formation and emboli. Antiembolic stockings or a sequential compression device on the legs helps decrease this risk.
4. *Monitoring.* A decrease in renal circulation and excretory ability affects electrolyte balance and excretion of drugs. Fluid and blood loss are not well tolerated. Hypovolemia can progress rapidly. Blood loss and urinary output must be monitored. Monitoring of blood gases and electrolytes also may be indicated, depending on the type of surgical procedure and the patient's preoperative condition. Reaction to anesthetic agents and drugs is closely monitored in all patients. Fluctuations in cardiac rate and rhythm may portend an impending crisis.

Anesthesia Considerations

Geriatric patients present a special challenge to the anesthesiologist. Physiologic function gradually deteriorates with age but not in a predictable manner or progression. The aging process is not a disease but a fundamental biologic alteration. Disease in the elderly is superimposed on senescent changes. The aged are more prone to multiple organ system failure. Central nervous system changes produce effects on other systems' performance.

Characteristics of some aged persons include memory loss and confusion, which are exaggerated in an institutional environment, malnutrition, anemia, osteoporosis, low blood volume, poor liver or renal function, arteriosclerosis, diminished autonomic tone and reflexes, instability of circulation, and diabetes. Reactivity to stimuli decreases with advancing years. These patients therefore experience an altered response to stress exemplified in a high pain threshold. They are more susceptible to the action of all drugs. Abnormal sleeping and breathing patterns, with production of apnea by hyperventilation, are accentuated by opioids. These phenomena translate to lower doses of opioids for analgesia and less anesthetic needed because the minimum anesthetic concentration required declines progressively with advanced age.

In the elderly, oxygen mask fit may be difficult because of loss of teeth and/or jaw substance. Induction may be prolonged and ventilation difficult because of chronic obstructive pulmonary disease or emphysema. With rapid fall in blood pressure, patients are susceptible to hypoxia, stroke, renal failure, and development of myocardial infarction. Anesthetization problems are augmented because surgical procedures tend to be major and take longer; many procedures pertain to malignant tumors, with reoperation necessary.

A decrease in muscle mass, including the myocardium, with a corresponding increase in body fat takes place in the aging process. Most anesthetics are fat soluble. Cardiac output and pulmonary capacity diminish with age, with a decline in maximal oxygen uptake. These fundamental physiologic changes necessitate reduction of anesthetic dosages in geriatric patients. Anesthesia may reduce oxygen to the heart, kidneys, and brain. Geriatric patients are prone to hypotension, hypothermia, cerebral edema, and hypoxemia postoperatively.

Surgical mortality is higher in the aged than in the general population, especially if the surgical procedure is an emergency one that does not allow sufficient time for thorough preoperative evaluation and preparation. Complications related to the cardiovascular system and cerebral circulation frequently are followed by respiratory problems, aspiration, and infection. Surgical morbidity can be reduced, however, by skillful anesthesia management.

POSTOPERATIVE CONSIDERATIONS

Geriatric patients' health status will be compromised by the interaction of drugs, anesthesia, and the surgical procedure. Postoperatively the following must be monitored:

1. *Drug interactions.* Tolerance may be poor and detoxification is slow. Drugs metabolize slowly in the liver and are excreted slowly by the kidneys. Fat-soluble drugs have a prolonged duration because they are absorbed by body fat, which increases with aging. Many anesthetic agents are fat soluble and also are myocardial and respiratory depressants. Narcotics and sedatives interact with anesthetics. Patients must be monitored for hypoxia. Oxygenation to the heart, kidneys, and brain will be less efficient. General anesthesia and some drugs cause transient mental dysfunction.
2. *Aspiration.* Elderly persons may have difficulty swallowing because of dry mucous membranes, reduced salivation, and reduced esophageal peristalsis. Cough is less productive because of muscular atrophy in the chest and rigidity of the rib cage. Patients must be watched for aspiration.
3. *Infection.* Respiratory, urinary, or gastrointestinal tract infections may develop as a result of immunodeficiency. Pneumonia can be fatal. Poor dental

hygiene may be the source of systemic infection. Healing will be further retarded if an infection develops in a wound that is already compromised by a reduced vascular supply. Fever associated with infection in younger patients may not be as obvious in geriatric patients. Elevation of white blood cell count may be a better indicator.

Geriatric patients require a thorough preoperative assessment, an experienced anesthesiologist, considerate and knowledgeable nursing care, meticulous aseptic and sterile techniques, and careful postoperative management.

The patient and his or her family and/or significant others should be included in the development of the postoperative discharge plan. Planning should incorporate follow-up care with the surgeon.

Bibliography

Bender P: Deceptive distress in the elderly, *Am J Nurs* 92(10):28-32, 1992.

Berger S, King EC: Elder care: designing services for the elderly, *AORN J* 51(2):448-454, 1990.

Burke MM, Walsh MB: *Gerontological nursing: care of the frail elderly,* St Louis, 1992, Mosby.

Bush HA, Job SA: Elder care: stressors of providing care to the elderly, *AORN J* 57(4):938-946, 1993.

Carnevali DL, Patrick M: *Nursing management for the elderly,* ed 3, Philadelphia, 1993, Lippincott.

Collinsworth R: Elder care: determining nutritional status of the elderly surgical patient: steps in the assessment process, *AORN J* 54(3):622-631, 1991.

Dellasega C, Shellenbarger T: Discharge planning for cognitively impaired adults, *Nurs Health Care* 13(10):526-531, 1992.

Gawlinski A, Jensen GA: The complications of cardiovascular aging, *Am J Nurs* 91(11):26-30, 1991.

Holt J: How to help confused patients, *Am J Nurs* 93(8):32-36, 1993.

Mezey DM et al: *Health assessment of the older individual,* New York, 1993, Springer.

Moddeman G: The elderly surgical patient—a high risk for hypothermia, *AORN J* 53(5):1270-1272, 1991.

Moore LW, Proffitt C: Elder care: communicating effectively with elderly surgical patients, *AORN J* 58(2):345-355, 1993.

Newbern VB: Is it really Alzheimer's? *Am J Nurs* 91(2):50-54, 1991.

Potts S et al: A quality-of-care analysis of cascade iatrogenesis in frail hospital patients, *QRB* 19(6):199-205, 1993.

Schaie KW, Willis SL: *Adult development and aging,* ed 3, New York, 1991, Harper Collins.

Selman SW, Mistretta, EF: Elder care: perioperative concerns of the older adult undergoing total joint replacement, *AORN J* 55(2):618-622, 1992.

Sullivan EM et al: Elder care: nursing assessment, management of delirium in the elderly, *AORN J* 53(3):820-828, 1991.

Tappen RM: Elder care: Alzheimer's disease: communication techniques to facilitate perioperative care, *AORN J* 54(6):1279-1286, 1991.

Theis SL, Merritt SL: A learning model to guide research and practice for teaching elder clients, *Nurs Health Care* 15(9):464-468, 1994.

Thomas BL: Elder care: pain management for the elderly: alternative interventions. Part I. *AORN J* 52(6):1268-1272, 1990, Part II. *AORN J* 53(1):126-132, 1991.

Urrows ST et al: Profiles in osteoporosis, *Am J Nurs* 91(12):32-37, 1991.

Valente SM: Recognizing depression in elderly patients, *Am J Nurs* 94(12):18-24, 1994.

Williams TF, Katzman B: Elder care: aging research and its influences on health care, *AORN J* 54(1):118-120, 1991.

CHAPTER 44

Organ Procurement, Transplantation, and Replantation

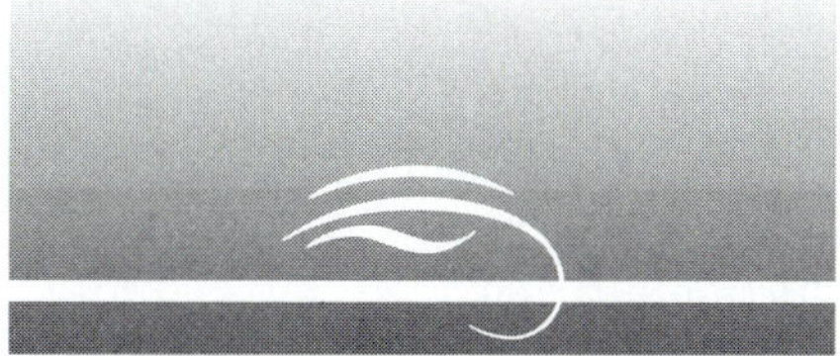

Transplantation is transfer of an organ or tissue from one person to another or from one body part to another. Concentrated efforts continue in search of compensation for or suitable replacement for deficient tissues and organs. The indication for organ transplant is irreversible functional failure of the organ. Goals of transplantation include changing appearance, restoring function, and/or improving quality of life.

HISTORICAL BACKGROUND

Interest in transplantation is many centuries old. Celsus wrote that tissues could survive after grafting from one part of the body to another. Galen attempted reconstruction of facial defects. Centuries later it was observed that full-thickness autografts survived whereas allografts failed, although the reason was not understood.

Darwin's theory of evolution and Mendel's laws of heredity shed new light in the nineteenth century, spurring researchers to pursue the study of regenerative capacity in animals. In the early twentieth century, Alexis Carrel and Charles Guthrie performed blood vessel anastomoses, an essential component of organ transplantation. Performing heterotopic heart transplantation in animals, they demonstrated that a heart could be removed, transplanted, and resume beating.

In the 1930s the maintenance of organs in vitro opened the way to organ preservation. Expanded information concerning patient response to surgical procedure during the decade of the 1940s marked advances in surgical therapy. Open heart surgery, as well as acquisition of basic knowledge required for clinical transplantation, evolved in the 1950s. Pioneers in transplantation biology, Peter Medawar and Frank M. Burnet, received the Nobel prize in 1960 for their work on immunologic tolerance in tissue transplantation in animals.

Many scientific disciplines contribute to and integrate information to aid progress in clinical transplantation. Foremost among these areas are physiology, genetics, immunology, and pathology. Practical application of clinical transplantation became possible in the 1960s after investigative efforts led to the development of supportive techniques such as cardiopulmonary bypass and immunosuppressive drug therapy.

Kidney transplantation, begun in 1954, preceded heart transplantation by more than a decade. However, the first successful heart transplant, performed by Dr. Christian Barnard in 1967 in South Africa, expanded the era of clinical organ transplantation. Although survival rates vary, most body tissues and organs can be transplanted or grafted. Availability of donor organs remains a problem.

TYPES OF TRANSPLANTS

Some tissues and whole organs can be transplanted and grafted to restore bodily function. The type of transplant selected will depend on the purpose of the graft, anatomic function, and availability of the tissue or organ. The types of biologic transplants are listed in Box 44-1.

TISSUE TRANSPLANTATION

Some tissues can function normally even though they are moved from one area of the body to another or are obtained from a donor.

1. *Skin grafts* provide a protective surface covering, initially acquiring then eventually losing vascular connection with the host.
2. *Corneal grafts* replace nonfunctioning corneal tissue.
3. *Bone grafts* afford temporary structural supports and a pattern for regrowth of the host's bone, the graft then being resorbed.
4. *Ossicles and tympanic membrane* in the ear can be transplanted to restore bone-conduction hearing loss.
5. *Cartilage* restores contour in a defect of cartilaginous facial structures.
6. *Blood vessel grafts* bypass or replace diseased or obstructed segments of vessels.
7. *Bone marrow* restores hematologic and immunologic functions.
8. *Heart valves* replace stenosed or diseased valves.

Tissue transplants can be either autografts or allografts. The American Association of Tissue Banks sets standards for retrieving, processing, storing, and labeling tissues and for donor criteria for allografts (Box 44-2). Tissue for transplantation is procured from suitable cadaver (nonliving) donors, either heartbeating or nonheartbeating (see p. 902), or from living donor of bone or bone marrow. Table 44-1 details procurement parameters for tissue allografts.

Potential donors are screened to avoid transmission of infection or disease. Cultures are taken at the time of procurement for microbiologic and serologic testing. Tissue is not transplanted until negative test results are obtained; tissue is discarded if the test result is positive. Living bone donors are tested for human immunodeficiency virus (HIV) immediately after donation and again after 90 days because seroconversion can be delayed. Recipients also should be tested and should be negative for HIV and hepatitis B virus (HBV). Incidences of graft failure and superinfection are high in immunocompromised patients with HIV. A baseline is essential to establish that the patient was not infected by the act of grafting. Patients with HIV or HBV are not barred from receiving an allograft, but baseline data can help rule out cause for rejection or infection.

BOX 44-1

Types of Biologic Transplants

allografts (homografts) Tissue grafted between different or genetically dissimilar individuals of the same species.

autografts Tissues grafted in the same person from one part of the body to another. Donor is also the recipient.

isografts Tissues grafted between genetically identical donor and recipient, as between identical twins.

heterografts (xenografts) Tissues grafted between two dissimilar species. Heterografts may be used when allograft material is unavailable or temporary replacement is necessary.

orthotopic transplant Transplant to an anatomically natural or normal recipient site.

heterotopic transplant Transplant to an anatomically abnormal location in the host. Heterotopic grafts may function normally in the unnatural site.

BOX 44-2

Donor Selection Criteria for Tissue Allografts

Negative for viral, bacterial, or fungal infection or disease
Negative for sexually transmitted disease
Negative for neurologic disease
Negative for autoimmune disease
Negative for metabolic bone disease
Negative for malignancy or suspected malignant neoplasm
Negative for disease of unknown origin
Negative for death of unknown origin
Negative for use of systemic medication
Negative for parenteral drug use
Negative for exposure to toxic substances
Not ventilator-dependent for more than 7 days before brain death
Not immobile or bedfast for more than 7 days before brain death
Normothermic 98.6° F (37° C) for more than 7 days before brain death

Banked tissues are labeled with the donor's name and/or identification number, pertinent medical history, pathology report of the donor, final culture and serology reports of donors, type and site of donation, date and time of procurement, and method of procurement and preservation.

TABLE 44-1

Tissue Allograft Procurement Parameters

AGE OF DONOR	PHYSIOLOGIC STATUS OF DONOR	TIME BETWEEN PROCUREMENT AND GRAFTING	OTHER CONSIDERATIONS
Cornea			
Both sexes: 3 mo-80 yr	Nonheartbeating cadaver donor	Procured 6-8 hr postmortem at room temperature Procured 48 hr postmortem if donor has been refrigerated at 39.2° F (4° C)	Corneas are not perfused tissue. Heartbeating status is unimportant. Tissue may be procured in morgue or setting other than OR, under sterile conditions.
		Transplanted fresh 7-10 days after procurement	Corneas are usually used fresh rather than in cryopreserved state.
		Cryopreserved cornea may be stored for 1 yr	Cryopreservation of corneal tissue is not commonly done.
Skin			
Both sexes: 14-75 yr	Nonheartbeating cadaver donor	Procured 6-8 hr postmortem at room temperature Procured within 24 hr postmortem if refrigerated at 39.2° F (4° C) Cryopreserved skin can be stored for 5 yr at −238° F (−150° C)	At least 75% of skin surface should be free of abrasion, scars, or deformities to qualify as donor. Skin is procured before bone and is taken only from below nipples to knees on ventral surface and scapulae to popliteal area on dorsal surface. Tissue is taken to the depth of dermal layer (split thickness). 70 kg donor can provide 7-8 square feet of skin. Newly procured skin is stored at 39.2° F (4° C) in preservation medium for maximum of 24 hr. Cryopreserved skin is thawed at temperatures not to exceed 59° F (15° C) for use on recipient. Allograft skin is frequently used as a biologic dressing in combination with autograft skin. The recipient autograft is meshed 6:1 then covered by allograft that has been meshed 2:1. Allograft skin is temporary and is replaced on the recipient every 48-72 hr until natural reepithelialization at the autograft site begins.
Iliac crest			
Female: 18-50 yr Male: 18-70 yr	Nonheartbeating cadaver donor	Procured within 12 hr postmortem at room temperature Procured within 24 hr postmortem if refrigerated at 39.2° F (4° C) Cryopreserved bone can be stored for 3 yr at −112° F (−80° C)	Bone is procured after the recovery of any other internal organs and skin. Preferably, bone is procured under sterile conditions; however, it may be procured under clean conditions in a setting such as the morgue and secondarily sterilized by ethylene oxide followed by aeration. Sterile bone can be freeze-dried and stored at room temperature.

Continued

TABLE 44-1

Tissue Allograft Procurement Parameters—cont'd

AGE OF DONOR	PHYSIOLOGIC STATUS OF DONOR	TIME BETWEEN PROCUREMENT AND GRAFTING	OTHER CONSIDERATIONS
Joints and long bone			
Female: 18-50 yr Males: 18-55 yr	Nonheartbeating cadaver donor	Procured within 12 hr postmortem at room temperature Procured within 24 hr postmortem if refrigerated at 39.2° F (4° C) Cryopreserved bone can be stored for 3 yr at −112° F (−80° C)	Bone is procured after the recovery of any other internal organs and skin. Preferably, bone is procured under sterile conditions; however, it may be procured under clean conditions in a setting such as the morgue and secondarily sterilized by ethylene oxide followed by aeration. Sterile bone can be freeze-dried and stored at room temperature. Joints are not used as joints per se but are cut into pieces to fit a defect.
Both sexes: femoral head not age dependent; usually acceptable to age 75	Living nonrelated donor (femoral head or rib)		Living nonrelated donor femoral head can be salvaged during total joints arthroplasty procedure and processed for use as bone plug or ground bone grafting tissue.
Heart valves			
Female: 0-40 yr Male: 0-35 yr	Nonheartbeating cadaver donor	Cryopreserved valves can be used within 1-2 yr	Size match is important.

Bone Marrow Transplantation

Bone marrow is procured and transplanted using a similar protocol as organ procurement and transplantation because it is also fraught with hazards of rejection. However, it is essentially a tissue transplant. Bone marrow is transplanted only after conventional methods of treatment have failed to replenish depleted bone marrow cells. The marrow given by infusion restores hematologic and immunologic functions. Indications for treatment are acute lymphoblastic leukemia, myelogenous leukemia, aplastic anemia, and some other blood diseases. Bone marrow transplantation is the only cure for severe combined immunodeficiency disease, a genetic disorder in which a child lacks adequate immune defenses to fight infections. Bone marrow transplants also are given to victims of severe radiation exposure. Contraindications are renal or cardiac disease.

Blood type and human leukocyte antigen (HLA) compatibility are essential. A bone marrow transplant may be one of three types.

1. *Autologous:* donor is the recipient. Stem cells are collected from the leukemic patient in remission, cryopreserved, and stored to be infused during a subsequent relapse.
2. *Allogeneic:* donor is HLA compatible with recipient. Marrow is harvested for immediate infusion into the recipient.
   a. Syngeneic donor, an identical twin, is preferred.
   b. Genotypically compatible sibling or parent has identical tissue type.
   c. Unrelated allogeneic donor must be HLA compatible. Graft-versus-host disease (GVHD) is unique to allogeneic bone marrow transplantation. Donor T cells immunologically attach to recipient cells, causing tissue damage at the site of antigen localization.
3. *T cell–depleted marrow:* mature T lymphocytes are removed from donor marrow before infusion into the recipient to prevent GVHD.

Before transplantation, the recipient is given a high-dose regimen of immunosuppressive chemotherapy to eradicate leukemic, lymphoid, and bone marrow cells, thereby inducing marrow depression. The recipient also receives total body irradiation (TBI) to penetrate areas resistant to the drugs. During this period of pretransplant preparation, the patient is placed in reverse isolation, preferably in a laminar airflow clean or sterile (germ-free) environment. The patient is closely monitored for side effects of immunosuppressive chemotherapy and TBI.

When pretransplant protocols are completed, the donor is hospitalized before the scheduled transplantation. In the operating room (OR) under general or spinal anesthesia, 500 to 700 ml of bone marrow is aspirated at multiple sites from the iliac crests; the sternum may also be used. The marrow is filtered, heparinized, and placed in sterile containers for infusion. The donor is watched for bleeding and may need blood and fluid replacement.

Marrow is infused into the recipient intravenously or via a Hickman or Broviac catheter over several hours. The patient is constantly attended and closely monitored for adverse reactions during this time. By an unknown process, the marrow migrates into the marrow cavities of the bones. For 10 to 30 days after transplantation, the recipient may receive daily transfusions of lymphocytes, platelets, and granulocytes, preferably taken from the donor, to counteract the predictable side effects (mainly hemorrhage and infection) of pretransplant immunosuppressive therapy. If it is not from an identical twin, blood is irradiated to destroy lymphocytes before transfusion. Mature blood cells and platelets are unaffected. Daily marrow aspirations and complete blood counts are done on the host. Success or failure of transplantation is usually decided 10 to 20 days afterward when the new marrow begins to function.

ORGAN TRANSPLANTATION

Transplantation can be a lifesaving treatment for some end-stage diseases. Although tissue grafts are commonplace, transplantation of functional, whole, vital organs presents physiologic, philosophic, and ethical dilemmas. A biologically related donor makes a real sacrifice to become an organ donor. Therefore cadaver sources are used primarily. Transplantation can potentially restore the recipient to near-normal physiologic status.

Kidney transplantation was initially the most successful and principal clinical application of organ transplantation. If the graft fails, the patient may survive by returning to hemodialysis indefinitely before receiving another transplant. Transplant of a heart, liver, pancreas, or the lungs, if rejected, does not afford the same option as kidneys, however. No practical prolonged artificial support exists for these organs in the event of allograft failure.

Transplantation of each organ involves unique technical and physiologic problems, but the major barriers and causes of failure of transplants are immunologic rejection and infection. Immunodeficiency varies depending on the amount of immunosuppression the patient receives to prevent rejection. Defense mechanisms are depressed by immunosuppressive agents, making the patient prone to opportunistic pathogens. Reverse protective isolation may be advisable if the patient develops leukopenia, a decrease in white blood cells. In other aspects of care, transplant recipients are similar to other critical surgical patients with severe chronic illnesses who require measures that minimize the risk of infection.

The American Society of Transplant Surgeons and the International Society of Transplantation meet regularly to exchange ideas and information among persons of different scientific backgrounds. The aim is to achieve the best possible patient survival rather than merely transplant survival.

The Organ Transplant Registry of the American College of Surgeons in conjunction with the National Institutes of Health collects data on transplantation procedures and approves and funds various registries. The Federal Organ Transplantation and Procurement Act of 1983 provided financial grants for initial development of regional organ procurement centers and a transplant registry. A national task force has also been established to analyze medical, legal, ethical, economic, and social issues of concern in organ procurement and transplantation.

Organ banks collect organs and tissues from donors, exchange organs geographically, and register patients in need of a transplant. The register includes information about the patient's blood grouping and tissue typing. Computer lists of patients waiting for donor organs are maintained by the United Network for Organ Sharing and the North American Transplant Coordinator Organization 24-Hour Alert. Regional organ procurement organizations coordinate with these registries to match donated organs with compatible recipients nationwide. The position of the recipient on the waiting list is determined by the severity of the illness. Other countries have similar mechanisms. The United Kingdom (UK) Transplant Register, for example, has membership in the Euro Transplant Register. Organs procured within the UK can be transported by air to another country in Europe, and vice versa, for a histocompatible recipient. The number of patients awaiting transplants exceeds the supply of available donor organs. Many patients die waiting for a suitable organ to become available.

Many persons carry a signed "Uniform Donor Card" or other identification stating that in case of death certain or all organs and tissues may be removed for transplantation. This donor card or a living will is legal written consent under the Uniform Anatomical Gift Act enacted by all 50 states. However, written or telephone consent must be obtained from a potential donor's family before procurement may commence. Federal and state laws mandate *required-request* or *routine-inquiry*. These laws require that the family of every medically suitable potential donor be asked to consider donation of organs and tissues. As a result of these laws, organs and tissues are procured in many hospitals and then are transported to organ banks or transplantation centers. Procurement teams from these centers may go to the community hospital (host facility) to procure organs and tissues.

Time is paramount when critical organs are involved because their value depends on preserving maximum functional viability. The time factor is less urgent with less critical tissue. A transplantation coordinator contacts the regional registry and procurement team(s) when a potential donor has been identified.

Organ Procurement

Immunologic rejection and shortage of donor organs remain the principal deterrents to transplantation. The goal is selection of a donor-recipient match with adequate histocompatibility to permit an organ to function without complications. Organs and tissues come from two primary sources: cadaver (heartbeating and nonheartbeating) and living related donors (Table 44-2). Tissue donors may be ages newborn to 80 years. All vital organ donors must be without sepsis or malignant processes, ages newborn to 65 years, and with good function of the donor organ(s). Technical aspects of the procedure must ensure viability of organs throughout the procurement period. Organ donation is the ultimate gift of life the donor gives the recipient.

Cadaver Donors

Death is confirmed by irreversible cessation of all functions of the brain and brain stem. (See criteria for brain death in Table 44-3.) To be suitable for organ or tissue donation following death, cadaver donors are classified as *heartbeating* or *nonheartbeating.*

Heartbeating donors are persons with confirmed brain death in whom vital organs can be preserved in vivo. Brain death usually resulted from severe neurologic trauma as from head or spinal cord injury, hemorrhage, or anoxia. Death must occur in a location where a cardiopulmonary support system is immediately available (i.e., in the emergency department, OR, or other critical care unit). To be a potential organ donor, a brain-dead individual is maintained on mechanical ventilation and/or cardiopulmonary bypass to prevent ischemic damage to vital organs. Maintenance of a heartbeating donor before and during procurement includes:

1. Systolic blood pressure above 90 mm Hg
2. Central venous pressure of 5 to 10 mm Hg
3. Hydration with crystalloids and colloids
4. Urine output minimum 100 ml per hour, ideally 200 to 300 ml per hour
5. Ventilation with 100% oxygen
6. Core body temperature of 98.6° F (37° C)

Nonheartbeating donors are not suitable for parenchymal organ procurement. Because cardiopulmonary or ventilatory support was not provided after brain death, the major organs have suffered thrombosed vascularity and ischemia. Skin, bone, heart valves, blood vessels, and cornea may be acceptable for procurement from selected nonheartbeating donors (see Table 44-1).

Multiple Cadaveric Organ Procurement The heartbeating donor is brought to the OR and treated with the same respect and care given to any other patient. Organs and tissues are removed under sterile conditions by a procurement team and preserved and transported to the recipient(s). The procurement team includes two surgeons, two assistants, and a scrub person. A circulator and a scrub person from the host facility assist with the procedure. An anesthesiologist also is necessary to maintain vital functions until the aorta is cross-clamped and cardiopulmonary support is no longer needed. A procurement coordinator from an affiliated organ procurement agency or organ bank usually accompanies the team and assists wherever needed throughout the procurement process. The procurement team brings necessary supplies to package the organ(s) and tissue(s) for transport.

The procurement process includes the following functions.

1. Procurement coordinator facilitates procurement process by:
   a. Obtaining blood samples and arranging tissue typing to assist the organ bank with potential placement of procured organs
   b. Documenting necessary information, making any needed phone calls, and coordinating host facility personnel with the procurement team
   c. Assisting the physician with communications with the donor family.
   d. Calling the procurement team
   e. Assisting the circulator and scrub person with setup of the procurement room.
2. Circulator and scrub person assist procurement process by:
   a. Gathering sterile supplies, to include
      (1) Laparotomy drape pack and extra medium drapes
      (2) Nonabsorbable sutures for ligating ties (usually 0, 2-0, 3-0, 4-0 silk) and for closure (usually a size 2 monofilament suture on a large cutting needle) as requested by surgeon
      (3) Umbilical tapes, at least 30 inches long
      (4) Suction tubings with tips
      (5) Electrosurgical handpieces with blades
      (6) Scalpel blades, no. 10
      (7) Bone wax
      (8) Bulb syringes
      (9) Laparotomy sponges
      (10) Cold normal saline solution for irrigation
   b. Setting up sterile instrumentation, to include
      (1) Chest tray with sternal saw and self-retaining chest retractor
      (2) Major abdominal laparotomy tray and large self-retaining abdominal retractor

TABLE 44-2

Organ Procurement Parameters

AGE OF DONOR	PHYSIOLOGIC STATUS OF DONOR	TIME BETWEEN PROCUREMENT AND TRANSPLANTATION	OTHER CONSIDERATIONS
Heart			
Female: 0-40 yr Male: 0-35 yr	Heartbeating cadaver donor	3-6 hr, fresh tissue	Heartbeating cadaver donor: total heart and segments of great vessels.
	Nonheartbeating cadaver donor	Cryopreserved valves can be used within 1-2 yr	Nonheartbeating cadaver donor: heart valves only. Size match is important. Donor criteria include no cardiac disease and normal cardiac enzymes.
Lung			
Both sexes: 0-45 yr	Heartbeating cadaver donor	1-4 hr	Heartbeating cadaver donor lung(s) may be given en bloc to one recipient. The lungs may be separated and/or divided into segments (lobes) for several recipients.
	Living related donor		One lobe from living related donor is transplanted into recipient. Size match is important. Donor criteria include no evidence of trauma, negative sputum culture, normal chest x-ray film.
Heart-lung en bloc			
Both sexes: 0-50 yr Younger ages preferred	Heartbeating cadaver donor	1-4 hr	Heartbeating cadaver donor heart and lungs are transplanted en bloc into recipient. Size match is important. Donor criteria same as for individual heart or lung donation.
Liver			
Both sexes: 0-45 yr	Heartbeating cadaver donor	8-24 hr	Heartbeating cadaver donor liver may be divided into two segments for two separate recipient patients.
	Living related donor		Small segment of living related donor's liver is transplanted into recipient. Size match is important. Donor criteria include normal liver function, normal liver enzymes and bilirubin, no evidence of trauma.
Kidney			
Both sexes: 6 mo-60 yr	Heartbeating cadaver donor	48-72 hr Ideally, should be transplanted within 12 hr	Heartbeating and nonheartbeating cadaver donor kidneys are given to two separate recipients.
	Nonheartbeating cadaver donor in highly selected circumstances	Procured within 45 min of cardiac arrest, with immediate in situ cooling	
	Living related donor		One kidney from living related donor is transplanted into recipient. Donor criteria include normal renal function, normal serum creatinine, no evidence of trauma.

Continued

TABLE 44-2

Organ Procurement Parameters—cont'd

AGE OF DONOR	PHYSIOLOGIC STATUS OF DONOR	TIME BETWEEN PROCUREMENT AND TRANSPLANTATION	OTHER CONSIDERATIONS
Pancreas			
Both sexes: 3 mo-60 yr	Heartbeating cadaver donor	12-24 hr	Heartbeating cadaver donor pancreas is transplanted as a whole or partial organ for one recipient.
	Living related donor		Tail segment of pancreas from living related donor may be transplanted into recipient. Donor criteria include normal pancreatic function, normal blood glucose regulation, normal serum amylase, no evidence of diabetes mellitus, no evidence of trauma.
Kidney-pancreas			
Both sexes: 3 mo-60 yr	Heartbeating cadaver donor	12-24 hr	Heartbeating cadaver donor kidneys and pancreas are simultaneously transplanted into recipient. Usually performed for diabetic nephropathy. Donor criteria is the same as for individual kidney or pancreas donation.

TABLE 44-3

Brain Death Criteria

CRITERIA	CLINICAL ASSESSMENT
Irreversible coma not caused by pharmacologic agent, hypothermia, or unknown cause	No response to external stimuli. No cerebral brain activity on EEG over a period of 10 min. EEG activity has no prognostic value for estimation of cerebellar and brainstem activity.
Absence of spontaneous movement, decerebrate, and decorticate posturing	Spinal nerve reflexes may be unaffected because these reflexes do not require cortical (brain) activity.
Apnea with no spontaneous respiration not influenced by hypothermia or pharmacologic agent	Elevated carbon dioxide in the blood is not a stimulus for breathing. No spontaneous respiratory effort for 3 min when removed from ventilatory assist device. $Paco_2$ greater than 55.
No cranial nerve reflexes	Fixed and dilated pupils. Pupils are unreactive to light. No corneal reflex (no blinking when cornea is touched). No oculocephalic reflex (doll's eyes). No oculovestibular reflex (no response to ice water instilled in ear). No response to pain on face and head (pin prick, supraorbital pressure). No response to upper or lower airway stimulation (no gag or cough reflex when suctioned or stimulated by endotracheal tube).

(3) Vascular tray
(4) Minor tray for organ preparation table (benching table)
(5) Basin sets

c. Providing nonsterile equipment, to include
(1) Electrosurgical units
(2) Suction containers to accommodate at least 24 L of fluid
(3) Power source for sternal saw
(4) Extra intravenous (IV) poles
(5) Hyperthermia/hypothermia blanket
(6) Defibrillator
(7) Skin preparation solution
(8) Isopropyl alcohol, 70%, to make slush or slush machine, if available
(9) Crushed ice; dry ice is not used for organ preservation

4. Anesthesiologist assists procurement process by:
   a. Ventilating the donor with 100% oxygen
   b. Monitoring electrocardiogram (ECG), blood pressure, urinary output, and fluid and electrolyte balance
   c. Administering drugs as necessary (e.g., dopamine or dobutamine for vasomotor regulation, muscle relaxants to neutralize spinal reflexes and relax the abdomen, osmotic diuretics for renal function, and heparin for anticoagulation)
   d. Monitoring and replacing blood as appropriate
   e. Monitoring and maintaining core body temperature and initiating cooling: cold fluids, usually Ringer's lactate or Collins' solution with 30,000 U of heparin, are infused intravascularly 10 minutes before aorta and vena cava are cross-clamped for removal of heart.
5. Incisions are made by the procurement surgeon to provide maximum access to organs and tissues.
   a. Midline, sternal splitting incision is made from suprasternal notch to pubis to remove vital thoracic and abdominal organs (Figure 44-1). Parenchymal organs take between 2 and 3 hours to procure.
   b. Eyeballs are enucleated to procure corneas. Glass balls may be put in the sockets.
   c. Skin is taken with a dermatome from flat body surfaces, excluding upper chest, neck, face, arms, lower legs, and feet (Figure 44-2). Skin procurement may take 1 to 1½ hours to perform.
   d. Skin is excised and the muscles are separated. Long bones and iliac crests are removed in toto (Figure 44-3) and replaced with wooden, fiberglass, or metal dowels to maintain structural integrity. Bone procurement may take 5 to 6 hours to complete.
   e. Multiple incisional closures may take 1 to 1½ hours.

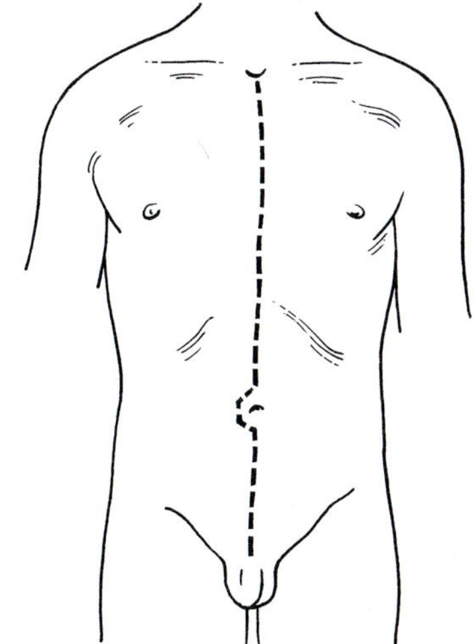

FIGURE 44-1 Midline, sternal splitting incision from suprasternal notch to pubis is made for procurement of thoracic and abdominal organs from heartbeating cadaver donor.

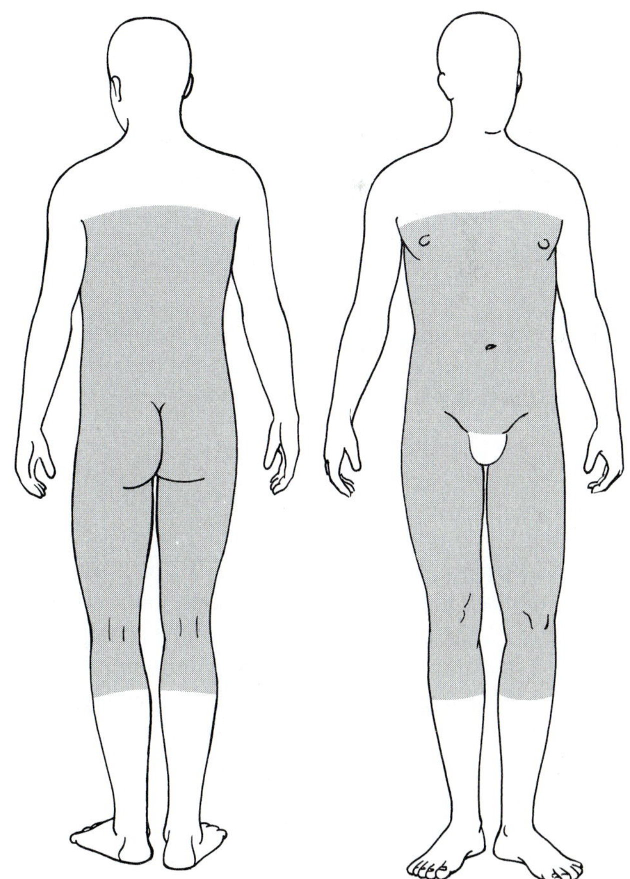

FIGURE 44-2 Skin is removed with dermatome from anterior and posterior flat surfaces between midchest and knees for cadaveric allografts.

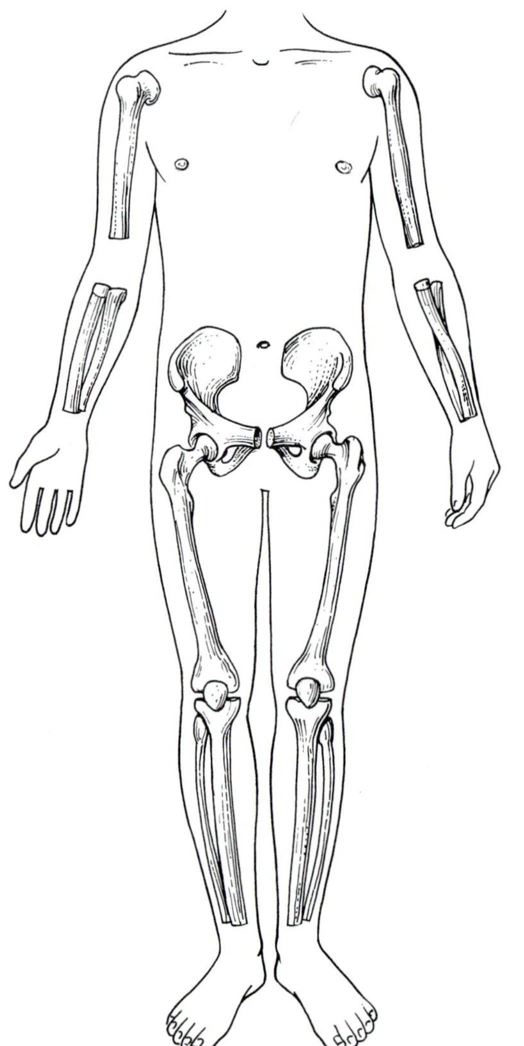

FIGURE 44-3 Long bones and iliac crests are procured for bone allografts. Humerus, tibia, and fibula are cut distally. Radius, ulna, and femur are disarticulated at both ends. Pelvis is cut at pubic and sacroiliac joints.

6. Sequence of organ removal is coordinated to maintain their viability. Kidneys and liver are mobilized and cannulated for in situ cooling. The aorta is cross-clamped, and the heart is removed first, followed by the liver, then the kidneys, pancreas, and intestines. A combined heart-lung procurement may be performed after other organs are removed. Enucleation of the eyes for corneal procurement usually follows retrieval of the parenchymal organs. Then skin is taken, followed by bone.
   a. A small sterile table should be set up so that organ and tissue packaging for transport can be completed away from the main sterile field.
   b. Closure should be as aesthetic as possible for later viewing at funeral services, if desired.

Additional Considerations in Cadaveric Organ Procurement The procurement coordinator remains at the host facility after the procurement team has departed. The coordinator's role extends into the aftercare given to the donor's body and the psychologic support and debriefing of the OR team. After closure and dressing of all incisional wounds, the donor's body should be bathed, and all drainage tubes and IV access lines removed. The body should be labeled with identification tags and placed on a clean transport cart. The head of the stretcher should be elevated 20 to 30 degrees. Ice packs should be placed over the eye sockets to decrease serous pooling. This will be of benefit to the mortician who will prepare the body for viewing. The donor's body is prepared as aesthetically as possible for the benefit of the family and loved ones.

The OR team may experience a sense of sadness and loss. This is normal and to be expected. Death is not a common event in the OR. Although the patient is technically brain dead before arriving in the OR, the patient gives the outward appearance of being sustained on life support as in general anesthesia. After the aorta and vena cava are cross-clamped, there is no further need of ventilatory support and the ventilator is turned off by the anesthesiologist. The sudden silence can feel overwhelming. The OR team may need the added support given by the procurement coordinator, who has experienced the same feelings and understands the psychologic impact of each stage of the procurement process. Personnel who specialize in procurement state that they feel the same sense of loss despite years of experience and exposure. An understanding of the outcome is important in the grieving process. Participation in the aftercare of the body helps to provide the OR team with a sense of closure and completion of patient care. Some of the same sadness may be shared by the critical care nursing staff members who helped monitor and maintain the donor's vital signs before transfer to the OR. Although the urge to be emotionally strong may exist, it is therapeutic to shed tears of sorrow.

The donor's family also will need support and communication from the procurement coordinator. The coordinator makes himself or herself known to the family and maintains communication with them for several months or longer as needed and provides referrals for follow-up counseling if the need arises. The coordinator informs the family of the progress of the recipients. In select situations, donor and recipient families may be brought together, thus forming lasting friendships.

The financial aspects of donor maintenance and subsequent organ procurement are paid by the procurement agency and are not the responsibility of the donor's family. Medical bills accumulated before the patient was identified as a potential donor are paid by the family.

Living Related Donors

Kidney, lobe of liver or lung, tail segment of pancreas, or marrow transplant from a biologically living related donor has distinct advantages: the results are better than are those with cadaver organs because donor-recipient matches are usually good (identical twin sources are ideal for compatibility); waiting time is reduced; and the procedure is planned and performed under controlled circumstances. The use of living donors involves a special protocol.

1. Adults, preferred over adolescents or children, must be able to give informed consent voluntarily without coercion. Children are used as donors only for a twin or for a patient with predictable results. If the donor is a minor, court (legal) and parental or guardian consents are required to avoid bias. The donor must fully comprehend the sacrifice; if the physician deems it advisable, psychiatric examination is included along with intelligence testing.
2. Donor must be in excellent health. The *donor's* physician confers with him or her and performs the preoperative physical examination to permit a rational decision. Renal arteriograms are done to confirm bilateral kidneys and identify renal vasculature before a nephrectomy.
3. Donor should have no psychiatric complications. Donor reactive depression may follow organ removal if adequate gratitude is not shown by all concerned.

Preservation of Organ Allografts

Successful use of donor tissue depends on rapid organ resection and cooling because the period of ischemia must be kept to a minimum. Long-term preservation of tissue remains a problem; current techniques utilize a variety of cryoprotective agents. Uncontrolled freezing may produce lethal cell injury. This technique is used for skin, bone, semen, and blood suspensions but not for whole organs. Hypothermia above freezing at 39.2° F (4° C) with or without perfusion with cold solutions reduces general metabolic demands, thereby providing a safety margin. Methods of hypothermia include the following.

1. Simple flush techniques with cold electrolyte solutions and storage by immersion in an electrolyte or flush-out solution in a plastic container kept at a hypothermic temperature
2. Hypothermic continuous pulsatile perfusion with an oxygenated electrolyte solution.

A potassium-based preservation solution, developed at the University of Wisconsin (known as UW or Belzer's solution) extends preservation time of the liver to 24 hours and of the kidney and pancreas up to 72 hours. A total organ perfusion system (TOPS) consists of a machine that pumps artificial blood through the donor organ during transport. Minicomputers and microsensors regulate pH levels, blood pressure, and nutrient levels. This system also extends preservation for 24 to 72 hours. The potential for altering immunogenicity of an organ and improving its regenerative processes are the focus of research in perfusion techniques.

The organ is placed in a sterile container filled with perfusate. This container is placed in sterile double-plastic bags and packed in ice. Dry ice is not used. If the organ will be transported to another facility, a Styrofoam ice cooler usually is used as the outer container.

Immunologic Rejection

The technical aspects of transplantation have been largely solved. However, the body possesses an innate tendency to reject and destroy any foreign material introduced into it except tissue from an identical twin. Transplanted cells from donors even slightly dissimilar to the recipient may be rejected.

Organ rejection involves the patient's immunologic system. Both cellular and humoral immune systems seem to be involved in responses to transplanted cells. Activation of the immune system is a response to antigens introduced by donor graft. An immunologic reaction usually is accompanied by a febrile systemic reaction, local inflammation, and deteriorating function of the graft. A knowledge of antigens, individual-specific and species-specific, and their genetic transmission is important for avoidance of violent reactions. Many factors influence the strength and rate of a rejection reaction. Some of these are acquired immunologic tolerance, lymphatic depression, or previous sensitization by blood transfusions, pregnancies, or transplants. Rejection may be reversible with intensive therapy or progressive with cessation of transplant function.

Combating Rejection

Attempts must be made to find compatible donors and to minimize rejection.

Preoperative Matching of Donor to Recipient

Tissue typing and matching determine genetic disparity between donor and recipient. Histocompatibility implies acceptability by an individual of tissue from another. Histocompatibility tests, although not infallible, result in improved organ survival from both living and cadaver sources. They assist in donor-recipient selection. The better the histocompatibility match and degree of genetic similarity between the donor and the recipient, the less serious is the rejection. Histocompatibility testing, *tissue typing,* is based on detection of cell-surface antigens known to affect rejection. Favorable results are expected when few histocompatibility antigens are detected. Preformed antibodies appear to have a harmful effect on graft survival. Testing employs serologic techniques, which include in vitro analysis for study of cell-to-cell interaction and identification of the mediator of the interaction, and also cell-culture techniques. Complex assay techniques measure effects of antibodies and lymphocytes against donor tissue in a culture setup. *Cross-matching* between recipient's serum and donor's peripheral blood target cells is accomplished by multiple serologic reagents or flow cytometry using fluorescent-labeled monoclonal antibodies.

Immunosuppressive Therapy in Recipient Specific alterations in immune responses are produced by inactivating or destroying lymphoid cells potentially capable of responding to the antigens. The goal is to selectively suppress antigenic reactions to the transplant without impairing the body's defense against pathogenic organisms. An attempt is made to neutralize or modify the body's protective antigenic mechanisms by use of various immunosuppressive agents to allow the transplant to remain and function. This barrier can be pierced at least temporarily by creating an increase in transplant tolerance or by paralyzing the recipient's immunologic system. Because lymphocytes and globulins seem to be mainly responsible for rejection, an attempt is made to vary their synthesis. Antibody formation and immune reaction can be suppressed by certain factors. Protocol is fairly standard in all transplantation centers.

1. Cyclosporine (Sandimmune), a soil fungus derivative, is a potent immunosuppressant that acts mainly on thymus-derived lymphocytes (T cells), the cells primarily responsible for rejection. This drug reduces rejection, especially in the early or inductive phase, without suppressing the entire immune system. It may be given orally or intravenously. It is always used with low doses of adrenal corticosteroids but usually not with other immunosuppressive agents. Its absorption rate is variable. Toxic effects on the kidneys must be monitored. Verapamil, a calcium-channel blocker, may be given to reduce renal toxicity.
2. Immunosuppressive agents, such as FK 506 or 5R-506, may be preferred to cyclosporine to prevent rejection.
3. Monoclonal antilymphocyte globulin, muromonab-CD3 (Orthoclone OKT3), derived from mouse antibodies is used to successfully treat established allograft rejection without affecting the entire immune system. Monoclonal antibodies have the ability to reverse the initial episode of rejection by binding to specific targeted surface antigens on mature T cells. They suppress only the activity of T cells that cause acute rejection.
4. Polyclonal antilymphocyte globulin, antibodies derived from horse serum, may be used for induction of immunosuppression or for reversal of rejection. It usually is given with other immunosuppressive agents.
5. Corticosteroids, such as prednisone, have an anti-inflammatory effect useful in reversing early rejection reaction. There is an inverse relationship between steroids and lymphocytes. T cells migrate from the circulation to lymphoid tissue.
6. Agents cytostatic or cytotoxic to lymphatic tissue, such as azathioprine (Imuran), suppress the entire immune system and have serious side effects on other systems. They interfere with DNA synthesis. Extracorporeal perfusion with these drugs and localized radiation to the transplant may be used, either separately or concurrently.
7. Heterologous horse or rabbit antithymocyte globulin or antilymphocytic globulin or serum acts against circulating T cells and induces suppressor cells.

Employment of immunosuppressive measures is not without complication. Leukopenia and susceptibility to infection are common sequelae. Therapy may not totally abolish rejection by the host but may delay the onset and decrease the incidence of rejection episodes during the crucial first month or two following transplantation.

Pretransplantation Transfusions Blood transfusions from a living related donor expose the recipient to a limited number of leukocyte antigens that seem to reduce the risk of sensitization to the prospective donor transplant and to increase graft survival. Different blood products, including platelets, and pharmacologic conditioning may be part of a pretransplantation transfusion protocol to induce specific immune modification in the recipient. However, random preoperative blood transfusions before a cadaveric organ transplantation may increase the risk of sensitization, although this may improve allograft survival.

Kidney Transplantation

Kidney transplantation has significantly improved the quality of life for many patients with chronic renal disease. Patients may choose to accept transplantation rather than remain on hemodialysis for the rest of their lives. Indication for transplantation is end-stage renal disease, most often glomerulonephritis, pyelonephritis, polycystic disease, or nephrosclerosis. Recipients may be infants (at least 8 to 12 months with body weight of

6 to 8 kg) to adults 70 years of age without severe extrarenal disease, malignancy, or active sepsis. Nephrectomy is not performed before transplantation unless the patient has uncontrollable hypertension. Patients with detected presensitization states may have to wait longer for a suitably matched cadaver donor and statistically have a lower 1-year graft survival rate than do unsensitized patients.

Recipients are carefully prepared preoperatively with kidney dialysis, fluid and electrolyte intake regulation, pretransplantation transfusions, and control of hypertension. Proper donor-recipient matching is performed.

Donor preparation is equally important. Removal of a kidney is associated with low morbidity, although a living related donor must guard against injuring the remaining kidney for the rest of his or her life. The donor is therefore advised to avoid body-contact sports.

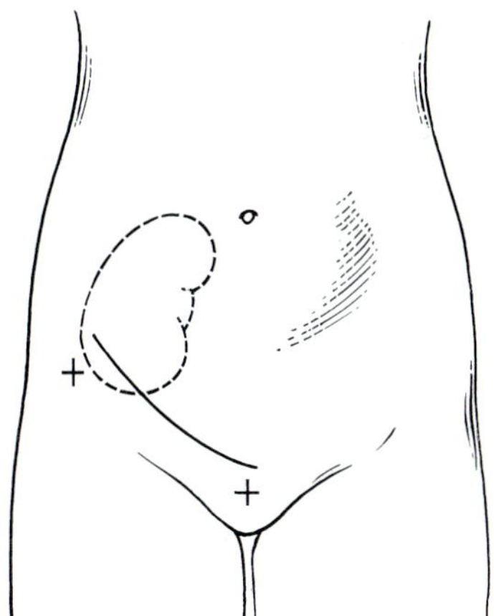

FIGURE 44-4 Kidney transplant is placed in the iliac fossa through a lower oblique abdominal incision.

Transplantation Procedure

Unless a cadaver donor organ is used, two adjoining ORs and teams are employed. One team procures and preserves the donor kidney while the other prepares the recipient site and transplants the kidney.

Donor Nephrectomy In a living related donor the kidney is removed through a flank incision. Adequate renal perfusion and urinary output, maintenance of adequate blood pressure and ureteral blood supply, and gentleness in manipulation are extremely important intraoperatively. As soon as it is excised, the kidney is flushed with cold heparinized solution to remove red blood cells. Total ischemia time is usually less than an hour. The donor's incision is closed per routine technique. (See Chapter 31, p. 637.)

Recipient Procedure The iliac fossa is the standard site for transplantation in an adult patient (Figure 44-4). The hypogastric artery is anastomosed to the renal artery and the common iliac vein to the renal vein. Reconstruction of the urinary tract is the main technical problem. Implantation of a donor ureter into the bladder, ureteroneocystostomy, is the preferred technique for urinary drainage. Alternative methods include ureteroureterostomy and ureteropyelostomy.

Complications of Renal Allotransplantation

Complications may be renal-related or extrarenal. The most common renal-related complications include rejection (the dominant cause of graft failure), recurrent nephritis, acute tubular necrosis, and technical failure from genitourinary or vascular problems. Postoperative management is similar to that of other surgical patients, with emphasis on initial adequacy of renal function, prevention of hazardous effects of immunosuppressive therapy, and observation for allograft rejection. Possible *types of rejection* are:

1. *Hyperacute,* caused by presensitization. This is an immediate acute rejection that occurs right after anastomosis of blood vessels or within 24 hours. It includes thrombosis and extensive destruction of allograft vasculature.
2. *Accelerated,* caused by presensitization. The graft may function for up to 5 days, followed by rapid loss of renal function. Treatment for both hyperacute and accelerated rejection is immediate removal of the transplant.
3. *Acute.* This usually occurs 1 week to 4 months following transplantation and is often reversible unless immune response is severe. Systemic and local symptoms, as well as reduced urinary output and abnormal laboratory findings, are present.
4. *Chronic.* Antibodies developing long after transplantation produce insidious onset with mild hypertension and diminishing renal function. This rejection is not reversible. Acute and chronic rejection may be diagnosed by renal biopsy.

Extrarenal complications, usually caused by immunosuppressive or corticosteroid therapy, include infection (the leading cause of death on a long-term basis), pneumonitis, hepatitis, gastrointestinal bleeding, and psychologic problems from perpetual fear of rejection. Immunosuppressive therapy must be used with caution.

Results of kidney transplantation are gratifying; life can be significantly prolonged. Causes for concern are chronic liver failure and vascular disease, a major cause of death in dialysis patients, which may occur in long-term transplant recipient. The incidence of malignant neoplasm in patients surviving renal transplantation more than a year exceeds that expected in the general population.

Heart Transplantation

Heart transplantation may be performed in selected patients with end-stage cardiac disease such as irreversible extensive myocardial failure, widespread atherosclerotic deterioration, or ischemic disease with symptoms at rest. Transplant recipients usually are under 55 years of age with a life expectancy of less than 1 year. Patients may be on a dopamine infusion regimen while waiting for a suitable donor.

A suitable heartbeating cadaver donor must have a blood type compatible with the recipient, be approximately the same weight and size as the recipient, and not have evidence of cardiac disease. Donors are usually younger than 40 years of age.

Optimum preservation of the donor heart is crucial so that it will resume full activity after transplantation. Ischemia time must be less than 6 hours. After removal, the donor heart is rapidly cooled to 39.2° F (4° C) and transported to the recipient.

While the donor heart is being procured in another OR or transported from another hospital, the transplantation team prepares the recipient. The recipient is brought to the OR. When the procurement team has inspected the donor heart and deemed it suitable, the transplantation team is notified by the procurement coordinator. After induction of anesthesia, a pulmonary artery catheter and transesophageal echocardiography probe are placed. A median sternotomy is performed. Most recipients have had previous sternotomies, and many adhesions may be present. Careful dissection is necessary to avoid potential embolization from a dilated left ventricle. The myocardium is not manipulated until the aorta is cross-clamped. The recipient's heart is not mobilized until the donor heart is ready for transplantation. The surgical procedure is similar to routine open heart procedures utilizing cardiopulmonary bypass. Two surgical modalities are used for cardiac transplantation.

1. *Total orthotopic heart replacement.* Ventricles, atrial appendages, and most of the coronary sinus are excised from the donor heart. The opened atria, aorta, and pulmonary artery of recipient heart are anastomosed to the donor heart. Both donor and recipient sinoatrial nodes are left intact.
2. *Heterotopic implantation.* The donor heart is inserted in an abnormal position in the right side of the chest as an assist device to enhance cardiac function. The recipient's heart is not removed. This less desirable alternative procedure may be indicated when increased pulmonary vascular resistance is a result of left ventricular failure in the recipient's heart. The donor's right atrium is anastomosed to recipient's right atrium. Anastomoses are completed between aorta and pulmonary veins of donor to left atrium of recipient.

Most deaths occur in the first 2 postoperative months, the crucial period of immunologic rejection. Electrocardiogram changes such as drop in voltage, reduced cardiac output, arteritis, myocardial ischemia, and myocardial necrosis occur during rejection. Diagnosis and monitoring of acute rejection may be facilitated by serial transvenous endomyocardial biopsies, which also may confirm effectiveness of therapy. Under fluoroscopy, a forceps is passed through a catheter into the apex of the right ventricle via the right internal jugular vein. A small sample of myocardium is removed for histologic study. A major obstacle to long-term survival is the development of obliterative coronary artery disease in the transplanted heart. The rejection process accelerates atherosclerosis. Improvement in survival rates is attributed to more accurate early diagnosis of rejection and vigorous measures to prevent atherosclerosis, thought to result from immunologic injury to the intima of the coronary vessels. An increase in malignant neoplasms in heart transplant patients has been observed. These patients need psychologic support to maintain a will to live and to adjust to problems that may arise at any time.

Combined Heart-Lung Transplantation

The organs of the cardiopulmonary system can be transplanted as a unit. Patients with primary pulmonary hypertension or pulmonary vascular disease secondary to congenital heart disease may be candidates for heart-lung transplantation. Patients with cystic or pulmonary fibrosis and chronic end-stage pulmonary disease also may receive combined transplants. If cardiac function in these patients has not been affected by the disease, their hearts may be used as heartbeating donor cardiac transplants.

In both the donor and recipient, the trachea is transected above the carina and the heart and lungs are removed en bloc. The surgical technique preserves the recipient's phrenic, vagus, and recurrent laryngeal nerves on pedicles, a portion of the right atrium and vena cava, and the aortic arch. The donor heart and lungs must fit without compression within the recipient's thoracic cavity. The donor trachea, right atrium, and aorta are anastomosed to corresponding structures in the recipient. Cyclosporine given preoperatively and postoperatively enhances healing of the tracheal anastomosis and combats cellular-mediated rejection. Bacterial pneumonia from subclinical bacterial contamination in the donor tracheobronchial tree is the most common cause of morbidity and mortality after heart-lung transplantation.

Lung Transplantation

Transplantation of a single lung, usually the left one, may be performed in a patient with end-stage pulmonary fibrosis who is dependent on oxygen therapy.

Both lungs may be replaced sequentially, as two single lung transplants, rather than as an en bloc combined heart-lung transplant. Children suffering from bronchopulmonary dysplasia, primary pulmonary hypertension, or congenital hiatal (diaphragmatic) hernia may benefit from a partial lung transplant. A lobe from a living relative may be transplanted rather than a whole lung from a cadaver source.

Optimum preservation of the donor organ is vitally important and timing is critical. Ischemic time must be less than 4 hours; results improve as ischemic time decreases. Recipient preparation usually occurs simultaneously with donor procurement.

Single lung transplantation involves bronchus to bronchus, pulmonary artery to pulmonary artery, and recipient pulmonary veins to donor atrial cuff anastomoses. Omentum is wrapped around the bronchus to provide additional blood supply and to support the anastomosis.

Many special problems affect the success of clinical lung transplantation.

1. Recipients usually have some degree of pulmonary infection at the time of the surgical procedure. The recipient's remaining lung, if diseased, may be a source of infection.
2. Ventilation-perfusion imbalance between the transplanted lung and the remaining lung may result in reduced function in the transplant.
3. Imminent rejection is not recognized easily.
4. Vascular and fibrotic changes produced by rejection create ischemia and anoxia.
5. Healing at site of bronchial anastomosis is a problem, but less so with cyclosporine and an omental wrap.
6. Procedure is technically difficult. Size of donor lung, hilar structures, and bronchus must approximate those of recipient.

Liver Transplantation

Hepatic transplantation may be performed in selected patients with nonmalignant end-stage liver disease. Ideal recipients are patients with primary liver disease. Successful liver transplantation is performed on infants and children with biliary atresia who develop chronic liver failure or those with other liver or biliary problems. Preexisting infection in any part of the body is a distinct contraindication because patients' preoperative status is poor and they lack protective proteins normally produced by the liver. Postoperative infection is always a marked danger.

The liver is susceptible to damage from ischemia. However, a donor liver can be preserved for up to 24 hours with infusion of cold Belzer's solution. A portion of the donor liver can be used for a child in urgent need of a transplant. The right or left lobe, or left lateral segmental graft may be transplanted. For this *reduced-size liver transplantation* (RSLT) procedure, one team divides the donor organ while another team performs a hepatectomy on the recipient(s). (A segmented liver may be used for two recipients.) A lobe from a living related donor also can be transplanted.

Anatomic complexity, friability of tissue, and vascularity of the liver contribute to the technical hazards of liver transplantation. The surgical procedure may take up to 20 hours to complete. Extensive dissection is required, as well as ligation of vessels to avoid postoperative hemorrhage. The vena cava must be mobilized. After it is divided, the liver is removed and the donor organ anastomosed to upper then lower vena cava as quickly as possible. During this critical period, venous return from lower half of the body must be decompressed via a venovenous extracorporeal membrane oxygenation (ECMO) pump from iliac to axillary arteries. Following anastomoses of portal vein and hepatic artery, any bleeding must be controlled before bile duct reconstruction.

Rejection may be noted by changes in laboratory findings, such as alterations in serum enzyme levels and elevated serum bilirubin. Cellular infiltration of the graft causes impairment of clotting factors, liver-cell necrosis, and impaired function. Complications from reconstruction of the biliary tract may lead to graft failure.

Pancreas Transplantation

A variety of techniques have been used in clinical pancreatic transplantation in the treatment of patients with severe diabetes and associated systemic complications. The goal is to provide physiologic islet function to achieve more satisfactory carbohydrate metabolism, to restore normal glucose homeostasis, and to prevent or halt secondary complications associated with diabetes mellitus. The whole pancreas, the distal segment, or isolated islets may be transplanted. The whole organ is obtained from a cadaver source. A kidney may be transplanted along with the pancreas. A composite splanchnic organ graft may be obtained, which includes the entire pancreas, spleen, and a segment of the duodenum. A segment of pancreas, usually the tail and body, can be obtained from a living related donor and placed into the extraperitoneal space in the iliac fossa. Splenic artery and vein of the donor segment are anastomosed to external iliac artery and vein of the recipient. Islet cells or beta cells may be isolated for transplantation; beta cells are injected into the liver.

The transplantation procedure must allow drainage of exocrine secretions from the pancreatic ducts. This is most commonly accomplished by pancreaticocystostomy for urinary drainage or pancreaticojejunostomy for enteric drainage. Insulin is secreted into the systemic circulation via arterial anastomoses between the donor organ and the recipient vessels.

Small Intestine Transplantation

Small bowel can be procured from a living related or cadaveric donor. From a living related donor, a minimal segment of 100 to 150 cm of small intestine with a branch of the superior mesenteric artery and vein may be transplanted to correct short-bowel syndrome, genetic enzyme deficiencies, or malabsorption disorders in children. The whole small bowel can be utilized from a cadaver donor. Because the body reacts to lymphoid tissue transplanted with intestine, the transplant may be irradiated to kill lymph cells but not mucosal cells.

REPLANTATION OF AMPUTATED PARTS

Replantation may be attempted to salvage a traumatically amputated digit, hand, or entire upper extremity. A severed foot or lower extremity presents more formidable problems because of the functional necessity for weight bearing. The victim of amputation of the scalp, nose, external ear, or penis also is a candidate for replantation. Using microsurgical techniques, replanted parts can survive with varying degrees of effectiveness. Functional recovery, up to 80% of normal in some patients, may take up to a year or longer because it takes time for nerves to regenerate (approximately 2 inches [5 cm] per month). A team of specialists in hand surgery or plastic and orthopaedic surgeons with microvascular skill is vital to success in these arduous procedures. Experienced teams are on call in replantation centers.

Correct care and preservation of the severed part for transport with the patient are also vital to success. The amputated part should be placed dry into a plastic bag, which is then sealed and immersed in crushed ice inside an insulated container (e.g., Styrofoam) to retard melting of the ice during travel. *The part should not be warmed, frozen, or packed in dry ice.* Rapid transport and cooling with ice buy time.

Initial treatment involves assessment of the total patient. The patient and family should be supported emotionally but not given definitive promises in regard to outcome. In judging whether to perform replantation, the surgeon considers numerous factors: the need for the part, associated disease and injuries, economic and psychologic factors, and age. Two criteria are of special significance.

1. Replanted part should have potential for being useful.
2. There should be no undue risk to the general safety of the patient if the procedure is performed.

Replantation is more successful in young patients than in older patients. Also, incomplete amputations are more successful because they have intact subcutaneous venous circulation in the skin bridges. Restoration is much more difficult in crush injuries than in sharp, clean amputations. Contraindications to replantation include prolonged warm ischemia, severe bruising or crushing injury, multiple fractures or injury at different levels in the same digit, or associated injuries that preclude the effort.

Supportive therapy following injury includes tetanus toxoid, intravenous antibiotics and fluids or blood products, and judicious administration of anticoagulants.

Preoperative patient preparation is in anticipation of a long procedure. The surgical procedure may take from 4 to 16 hours. The patient is placed on an air or water mattress. The head, scapulae, sacrum, and heels are padded. A footboard may be used and antiembolic stockings or sequential compression devices applied. An indwelling Foley catheter is inserted. Most replants of the hand are done under IV conscious sedation and axillary or supraclavicular block with a long-acting agent, such as bupivacaine hydrochloride (Marcaine) without epinephrine. General anesthesia is used for children and may be needed for adults for a long procedure.

These surgical procedures usually involve a two-team approach; one team prepares the recipient site and the other prepares the severed or distal part. In the OR the part is cleansed with Ringer's lactate or normal saline solution; water will lyse cells. Debridement of crushed tissue is carried out. Vessels are isolated for repair, and vessel patency is ensured. The basic steps of replantation of digits or extremities include:

1. Identifying proximal and distal tendons, nerves, and vessels.
2. Shortening bone within an acceptable limit necessary for tension-free repair of blood vessels, nerves, and soft tissues.
3. Stabilizing skeletal structure such as with internal wire-fixation techniques to maintain joint continuity and fusion in functional position.
4. Suturing tendons and ligaments, both extensors and flexors, appropriately to lessen the junctional scar process that can inhibit motion.
5. Anastomosing veins. A general rule is that more veins are anastomosed than are arteries to provide sufficient venous return and thereby minimize edema. Swelling creates pressure that impedes circulation, leading to necrosis.
6. Anastomosing arteries. The vessels may be flushed with heparin solution, and systemic anticoagulants may be given. Antispasmodic agents may be needed.
7. Repairing nerves and soft tissues.
8. Skin grafting or tissue flap or transfer if necessary.

NOTE

- Microsurgical techniques are necessary for nerve, artery, and vein repairs of structures that have an external diameter of 1 mm or less.

- Backup replantation teams should be available for lengthy procedures. This is especially important when the patient has multiple amputations or requires repeat of replantation soon after the initial procedure.

To avoid constriction, a circular bandage is not applied. Instead, a foam bandage is used and the extremity is suspended from a bedside IV pole with stockinette wrapped around the arm. The dressing is padded to prevent pressure sores and nerve damage. The original dressing is not changed for 10 days unless indicated.

Postoperative care is extremely important. Dressings must be checked carefully because even slight manipulation can cause great damage. Checking only the tip of the digit for circulation is not adequate. Circulation is verified by *cautiously* looking into the dressing to check capillary refill, color, temperature, and drainage. A Doppler flowmeter and a temperature probe may be used to evaluate circulation. Patients are not permitted to smoke because nicotine is a vasoconstrictor. Constriction of vessels may reduce circulation.

The many hours expended by the OR team initially to achieve a successful repair of all structures can relieve the patient of subsequent procedures. The objective is to obtain maximal return of function by minimizing permanent disability. Physical and occupational therapies are important in rehabilitation.

Bibliography

Bandelow LR et al: Living related liver transplants: a solution to donor shortage in pediatric patients, *AORN J* 58(2):258-279, 1993.

Chabalewski F, Norris MKG: The gift of life: talking to families about organ and tissue donation, *Am J Nurs* 94(6):28-33, 1994.

Curry J: Concerns raised about the quality of banked bone, *OR Manager* 10(2):1, 6, 9, 1994.

Dimond B: Transplants and donor cards: the legal significance, *Accid Emerg Nurs* 1(1):49-52, 1993.

Flye MW: *Atlas of organ transplantation,* Philadelphia, 1995, Saunders.

Grover LK: The potential role of accident and emergency departments in cadaveric organ donation, *Accid Emerg Nurs* 1(1):8-13, 1993.

Kawamoto KL: Organ procurement in the operating room: implications for perioperative nurses, *AORN J* 55(6):1541-1546, 1992.

Kirchner SA: Living related lung transplantation: a new dimension in single lung transplantation, *AORN J* 54(4):703-714, 1991.

Martinelli AM: Organ donation: barriers, religious aspects, *AORN J* 58(2):236-252, 1993.

McCullagh P: *Brain dead, brain absent, brain donors: human subjects or human objects,* New York, 1993, John Wiley & Sons.

Pezze JL, Whiteman K: Transplantation's newest weapon FK 506, *Am J Nurs* 91(10):40-42, 1991.

Proposed recommended practices: surgical tissue banking, *AORN J* 59(2):515-520, 1994. (Adopted by AORN in 1995.)

Russel S, Jacob RG: Living-related organ donation: the donor's dilemma, *Patient Educ Couns* 21(2):89-99, 1993.

Samartan K: Organ procurement surgery: what perioperative nurses can expect, *AORN J* 58(2):217-233, 1993.

Smith JC: Organ donation in intensive care: a look at the ethical issues, *Intensive Crit Care Nurs* 8(4):227-233, 1992.

Smith KA: Demystifying organ procurement: initiating the protocols, understanding the sequence of events, *AORN J* 55(6):1530-1540, 1992.

Trusler LA: Management of the patient receiving simultaneous kidney-pancreas transplantation, *Crit Care Nurs Clin North Am* 4(1):89-95, 1992.

Welte K: Matched unrelated transplants, *Semin Oncol Nurs* 10(1):20-27, 1994.

Wolf ZR: Nurses' experiences giving postmortem care to patients who have donated organs: a phenomenological study, *Schol Inquir Nurs Prac* 5(2):73-93, 1991.

Wolf ZR: Nurses' responses to organ procurement from nonheart-beating cadaver donors, *AORN J* 60(6):968-981, 1994.

Wujcik D, Downs S: Bone marrow transplantation, *Crit Care Nurs Clin North Am* 4(1):149-166, 1992.

CHAPTER 45

Surgical Oncology

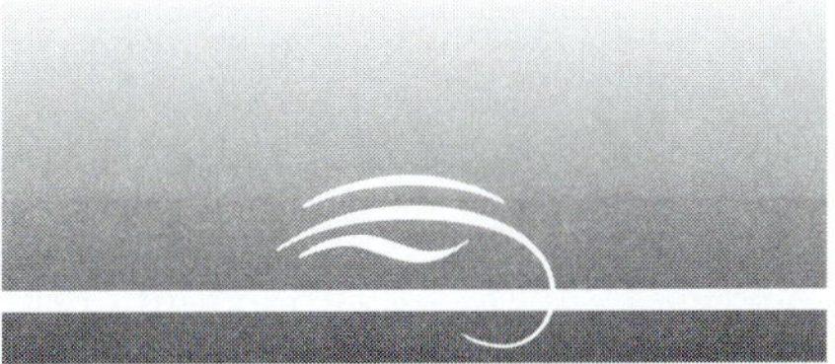

Oncology is the study of scientific control over neoplastic growth. It concerns the etiology, diagnosis, treatment, and rehabilitation of patients with known or potential neoplasms.

DEFINITIONS

A neoplasm is an atypical growth of abnormal cells or tissues that may be a *benign* or *malignant* tumor. Table 45-1 compares characteristics of benign and malignant tumors and their effects on patients. Four characteristics differentiate malignant from benign tumors. A malignant tumor:

1. Is anaplastic. Cells, resembling cell forms, are morphologically and functionally differentiated from normal tissue of origin. They vary in size, shape, and texture.
2. Infiltrates and destroys adjacent normal tissue.
3. Grows in a disorganized, uncontrolled, and irregular manner, usually rapidly and perceptibly increasing in size within weeks or months.
4. Has power to metastasize. Tumor cells migrate from the primary focus to another single focus or multiple foci in distant tissues or organs via lymphatic or vascular channels.

Clarification of terminology is essential to an understanding of oncology (Box 45-1).

POTENTIAL CAUSES OF CANCER

Cancer is a broad term that encompasses any malignant tumor. The exact cause of cancer is unknown. Cancerous tumors can be caused by exposure to chemical toxins, ionizing radiation, chronic tissue irritation, cigarette smoke, ultraviolet rays, viral invasion, and genetic predisposition. Studies have shown that immunosuppression may contribute to the incidence of cancer by altering biochemical metabolism and cellular enzyme production. Other research has shown that dietary influences, such as nitrates and high-fat diets, may contribute to cancer in certain individuals. Whether malignant or benign, neoplasms consist of cells that divide and grow uncontrollably at varied rates. The stimulus for growth can be intrinsic, such as hormonal, or extrinsic, such as exposure to external elements. Neoplastic overgrowth or invasion of surrounding tissue causes dysfunction and may eventually cause the death of the patient.

Early detection of cancer influences morbidity and mortality. A screening examination may identify a neoplasm before clinical symptoms develop. Table 45-2 includes recommended cancer screening examinations.

TABLE 45-1

Comparison of Benign and Malignant Tumors

BENIGN	MALIGNANT
Characteristics	
Expansive	Invasive
Localized	Spread to distant sites
Encapsulated	No capsule
Slow growth	Rapid growth
Resembles parent tissue	Varied differentiation
Normal cell reproduction	Disorganized cell reproduction
Organized mitoses	Abnormal mitoses
Effect on patient	
Pain uncommon	Severe pain common
Little nutritional effect unless mechanical obstruction involved	Cachexia, nausea, and vomiting

High-Risk Related Factors

With respect to cancer the high-risk factors are:

1. Age, gender, or racial, genetic, or hereditary predisposition (Table 45-3 identifies neoplasms associated with familial cancer syndromes)
2. Exposure to *carcinogens*—cancer-producing agents such as cigarette smoke, coal tar, ionizing radiation, ultraviolet rays, and chemicals (Table 45-4 lists examples of chemical carcinogens)
3. Predisposition from specific environmental conditions or acquired conditions or diseases (Table 45-5 gives examples of viral-mediated carcinogens)

TREATMENT AND PROGNOSIS OF CANCER

Treatment and prognosis are based on type of cancer and extent of the disease. Each type differs in its symptoms, behavior, and response to treatment. Cancer is a potentially curable disease, but it is the second leading cause of disease-related death in the United States.

BOX 45-1

Glossary of Terms Used in Oncology

anaplasia Change in cellular differentiation and orientation causing a more primitive structural appearance and function. Anaplastic cell changes are characteristic of malignancy.

cancer Broad term that describes any malignant tumor within a large class of diseases. More than 100 different forms of cancer are known, each with histologic variations. Cancerous tumors are divided into two broad groups:

1. *Carcinoma* is a malignant tumor of epithelial origin affecting glandular organs, viscera, and skin.
2. *Sarcoma* is a malignant tumor of mesenchymal origin affecting bones and muscles.

chemotherapy Use of chemical or pharmacologic agents to treat infections and other diseases, such as cancer.

cytoreductive surgery Mechanical reduction in cell volume at the tumor site by sharp or blunt tissue dissection. Vessel- and nerve-sparing procedures include the use of an ultrasonic aspirator and/or hydrostatic pulsed lavage.

cytotoxin Chemical or pharmacologic agent that causes cell damage or death. Some cytotoxic agents alter cellular metabolism or physical characteristics, making the cell vulnerable to destruction by other means, such as a laser.

immunotherapy Use of agents that stimulate or activate the body's own host defense immune system to combat disease.

neoplasm Atypical new growth of abnormal cells or tissues, which may be malignant or benign.

-oma Suffix denoting a tumor or neoplasm.

oncogene Potentially cancer-inducing genetic material derived from viral or host DNA. Rapidly dividing cells may be transformed to malignant state by viral invasion, radiation, chemical exposure, or other mutagenic agent.

oncologist Specialist in the study and treatment of neoplastic growths. A *surgical oncologist* has been trained to perform specialized surgical procedures.

radiation therapy Localized use of ionizing radiation to injure or destroy malignant cells.

tumor Any neoplasm in which cells are permanently altered but have the capability of growth and reproduction. A tumor consists of two elements—the tumor cells themselves and a supporting framework of connective tissue and vascular supply.

- **benign tumor** Aggregation of cells closely resembling those of the parent tissue of origin. Tumor usually grows slowly by expansion, is localized, and is surrounded by a capsule of fibrous tissue.
- **malignant tumor** Progressively growing tumor originating from a specialized organ such as the lung, breast, or brain, or a tumor localized to a specific body system such as bone, skin, lymph nodes, or blood vessels.

TABLE 45-2

Cancer-Screening Examinations

GENDER	AGE	FREQUENCY OF EXAMINATION
Pelvic examination by palpation and inspection		
Female	18-40 years	Every 1-3 years
	Over 40	Every year
Pelvic examination by palpation and inspection, including Pap smear		
Female	Start at age 18 or at age of onset of sexual activity if younger	Yearly; may be performed less frequently on advice of physician if patient has had three negative Pap smears in 3 consecutive years
Endometrial tissue sample		
Female	At menopause or sooner at recommendation of physician	Sample for baseline in high-risk patient
Breast self-examination		
Female and male	Start at age 18 and throughout life span	Female: monthly after menses or at same time each month after menopause Male: monthly
Clinical breast examination		
Female	Start at age 18 and throughout life span	Corresponds with pelvic examination sequence unless previous history of breast disease or high-risk for breast disease
Mammography		
Female	Baseline at age 35; every 1-2 years ages 40-49; yearly after age 50	Frequency after baseline is individualized according to age, health, and risk-factor analysis by physician; mammography, when performed, should precede clinical breast examination so that data analysis will be complete
Testicular self-examination by palpation and inspection		
Male	Start at age 16 and throughout life span	Monthly
Prostate		
Male	Over age 50; start at age 40 for men at high risk	Yearly, prostate-specific antigen (PSA) blood test
Digital rectal examination		
Male and female	Over age 40	Yearly; frequency may vary according to individual risk factors or at the recommendation of physician
Stool guaiac examination		
Male and female	Over age 50	Yearly; age and frequency may vary according to symptoms and the recommendation of physician
Sigmoidoscopy or colonoscopy		
Male and female	Over age 50	Every 3-5 years or according to the advice of physician; age and frequency may vary in the presence of risk factors or individual symptoms; colonoscopy may be advised according to risk factors
Generalized physical with health counseling		
Includes palpation of thyroid, gonads, lymphatics and inspection of oral mucosa		
Male and female	Over age 20	Every 3 years
Male and female	Over age 40	Every year

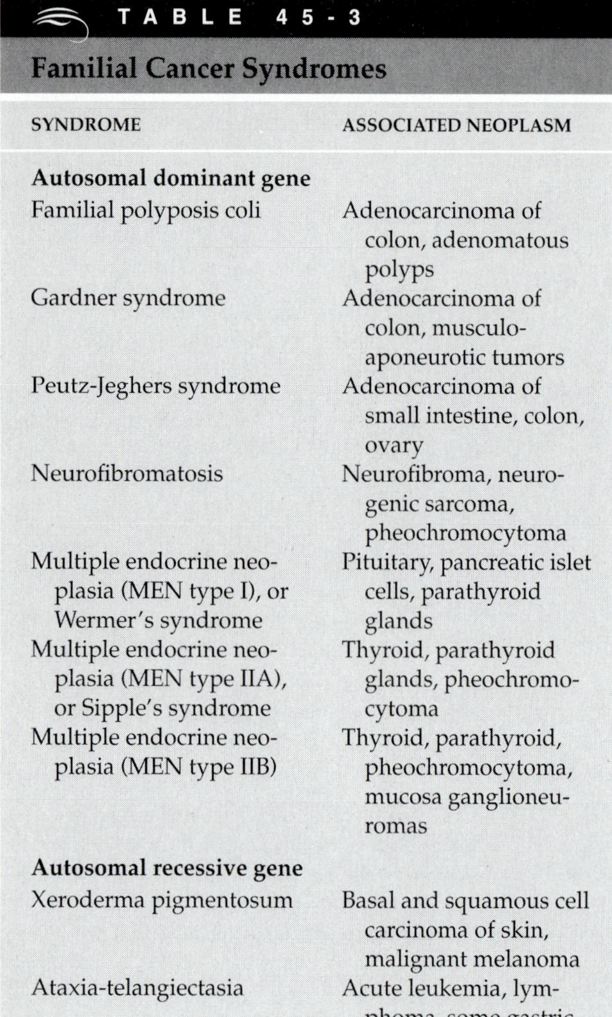

TABLE 45-3

Familial Cancer Syndromes

SYNDROME	ASSOCIATED NEOPLASM
Autosomal dominant gene	
Familial polyposis coli	Adenocarcinoma of colon, adenomatous polyps
Gardner syndrome	Adenocarcinoma of colon, musculo-aponeurotic tumors
Peutz-Jeghers syndrome	Adenocarcinoma of small intestine, colon, ovary
Neurofibromatosis	Neurofibroma, neurogenic sarcoma, pheochromocytoma
Multiple endocrine neoplasia (MEN type I), or Wermer's syndrome	Pituitary, pancreatic islet cells, parathyroid glands
Multiple endocrine neoplasia (MEN type IIA), or Sipple's syndrome	Thyroid, parathyroid glands, pheochromocytoma
Multiple endocrine neoplasia (MEN type IIB)	Thyroid, parathyroid, pheochromocytoma, mucosa ganglioneuromas
Autosomal recessive gene	
Xeroderma pigmentosum	Basal and squamous cell carcinoma of skin, malignant melanoma
Ataxia-telangiectasia	Acute leukemia, lymphoma, some gastric cancers

TABLE 45-4

Examples of Chemical Carcinogenesis

CHEMICAL	SITE OF NEOPLASM
Alkylating agents	
Nitrogen mustard, cyclophosphamide, chlorambucil	Leukemia, urinary bladder
Vinyl chloride	Angiosarcoma of liver
Polycyclic hydrocarbons	
Tar, soot, oils	Skin, lung
Aromatic amines and azo dyes	
β-Naphthylamine, benzidine	Urinary bladder
Food products	
Saccharin	Urinary bladder
Aflatoxin (mold on peanuts)	Liver
Betel nuts	Oral mucosa
Medication	
Androgenic metabolic steroids	Liver
Diethylstilbestrol	Vagina
Phenacetin	Renal pelvis
Inorganic compounds	
Chromium	Lung
Nickel	Lung, nasal sinuses
Asbestos	Serosal membranes, lung
Arsenic	Skin

Clinical Signs and Symptoms

The clinical signs and symptoms of cancer are:

1. Palpable tumor or abnormal thickening of tissue
2. Abnormal bleeding or discharge
3. Obvious change in wart or mole
4. Lesion that does not heal
5. Steady decrease in weight, appetite, and energy
6. Chronic cough
7. Change in bowel or bladder habits

Extent of Disease

Carcinoma in Situ

In carcinoma in situ, normal cells are replaced by anaplastic cells but the growth disturbance of epithelial surfaces shows no behavioral evidence of invasion and metastasis. This cellular change is noted most frequently in stratified squamous and glandular epithelium. Car-

TABLE 45-5

Viral-Mediated Carcinogenesis

VIRAL FAMILY	TYPE OF NEOPLASM
DNA-associated	
Papilloma (condyloma)	Squamous papilloma and squamous cell carcinoma
Hepatitis B	Hepatocellular carcinoma
Herpesvirus	
Epstein-Barr	Burkitt's lymphoma, nasopharyngeal carcinoma
Cytomegalovirus	Kaposi's sarcoma
Herpes simplex type II	Uterine cervical carcinoma
RNA-dependent	
Human T-cell lymphotrophic type I (retrovirus C)	T-cell leukemia, lymphoma

cinoma in situ also is referred to as intraepithelial or preinvasive cancer. Common sites include:

1. Uterine cervix
2. Uterine endometrium
3. Vagina
4. Anus
5. Penis
6. Lip
7. Buccal mucosa
8. Bronchi
9. Esophagus
10. Eye

Localized Cancer

Localized cancer is contained within the organ of its origin.

Regional Cancer

The invaded area of regional cancer extends from the periphery of the organ or tissue of origin to include tumor cells in adjacent organs or tissues (e.g., the regional lymph nodes).

Metastatic Cancer

In metastatic cancer the tumor has extended, by way of lymphatic or vascular channels, to tissues or organs beyond the regional area.

Disseminated Cancer

In disseminated cancer, multiple foci of tumor cells are dispersed throughout the body.

Curative vs. Palliative Therapy

Cancer is basically a systemic disease. Therapy is *curative* if the disease process can be totally eradicated, but success depends largely on early diagnosis. When a cure is not possible, *palliative* therapy relieves symptoms and improves quality of life but does not cure the disease. Tumors are classified to determine the most effective therapy.

Tumor Identification System

A standardized tumor identification system, which includes classification and staging, is essential for establishing treatment protocols and evaluating the end result of therapy. Hospitals maintain a tumor registry of patients to evaluate therapeutic approaches to specific types of tumors.

Classification includes the anatomic and histologic description of a tumor. *Staging* refers to the extent of tumor. Three basic categories of the system are:

T—primary tumor
N—regional nodes
M—distant metastases

The TNM categories are identified by pretherapy clinical diagnosis, tissue biopsy, and/or histopathologic examination following surgical resection of the tumor. Numeric subscripts are used to describe the findings; for example, bronchogenic carcinoma $T_1\ N_0\ M_0$ means primary tumor in the lung without positive regional nodes or distant metastases. If a positive lymph node is identified in the area, it is indicated in a subscript, (e.g., $T_1\ N_1\ M_0$). If a metastatic site also is diagnosed, it is indicated in the subscript (e.g., $T_1\ N_1\ M_1$). The subscripts correspond to the number of histiologically different tumors at the primary site, positive lymph nodes, or metastatic sites identified (Box 45-2). Older staging systems are referred to in literature as stages I, II, III, and IV.

After treatment, the estimation of residual tumor volume is indicated by *R*.

Adjunctive Therapy

Surgical resection, endocrine therapy, radiation therapy, chemotherapy, immunotherapy, hyperthermia, or combinations of these procedures are used in the treatment of cancer. The surgeon or oncologist must determine the most appropriate therapy for each patient. Consideration is given to:

BOX 45-2

Tumor Identification Scale

Primary tumor

TX	Primary tumor is discovered by the detection of malignant cells in secretions or cell washings but not directly visualized
T0	No evidence of primary tumor
Tis	Tumor (carcinoma) in situ
T1	Tumor is 3 cm or less at largest dimension
T2	Tumor is larger than 3 cm at largest dimension
T3	Tumor directly invades surrounding tissue
T4	Tumor invades surrounding tissue and adjacent structures, such as blood vessels or bone

Regional lymph nodes

NX	Unable to assess nodes
N0	No regional lymph node metastasis
N1	Metastasis to ipsilateral nodes or direct extension to nodes
N2	Metastasis to contralateral nodes

Distant metastasis

MX	Distant metastasis cannot be assessed
M0	No distant metastasis
M1	Distant metastasis is confirmed

Posttreatment residual tumor

RX	Unable to assess residual tumor
R0	No residual tumor
R1	Microscopic residual tumor
R2	Macroscopic residual tumor

1. Type, site, and extent of tumor and whether lymph nodes are involved
2. Type of surrounding normal tissue
3. Age and general condition of patient, including nutritional status and whether other diseases are present
4. Whether curative or palliative therapy is possible

Pretreatment workup is extensive for all modes of therapy. Each form of therapy for cancer has certain advantages and limitations. Factors affecting response to treatment are host factors, clinical stage of malignancy, and therapy employed.

SURGICAL RESECTION

Surgical resection is the modality of choice to remove solid tumors. Resection of a malignant tumor is, however, localized therapy for what may be a systemic disease. Each patient must be evaluated and treated individually. The surgical procedure must be planned appropriately for the identified stage of disease. The surgeon selects either a radical curative surgical procedure or a salvage palliative surgical procedure, depending on localization, regionalization, and dissemination of tumor. Surgical *debulking* may be the procedure of choice for some types of surgically incurable malignant neoplasms. The tumor is partially removed without curative intent to make subsequent therapy with radiation, drugs, or other adjunctive measures more effective and thereby extend survival. In planning the surgical procedure, the surgeon considers length of expected survival, prognosis of surgical intervention, and effect of concurrent diseases on the postoperative result.

Accessible, well-differentiated primary tumors are frequently treated by excision. Extremely wide resection may be necessary to avoid recurrence of the tumor. The pathologist is able to make judgments about questionable margins by evaluating frozen sections while the surgical procedure is in progress. The pathologist's findings guide the surgeon during resection so that residual tumor is not left in the patient.

Many of the surgical procedures described in previous chapters are performed for ablation of tumors by primary resection. In addition, *lymphadenectomy* may be performed as a prophylactic measure to inhibit metastatic spread of tumor cells via lymphatic channels. Other modalities of therapy may be administered preoperatively, intraoperatively, and/or postoperatively to reduce or prevent recurrence or metastases.

Specific Considerations

Malignant tumor cells can be disseminated by manipulation of tissue. Because of their altered nutritional and physiologic status, patients with cancer may be highly susceptible to the complications of postoperative infection. To minimize these risks, specific precautions are taken in the surgical management of these patients.

1. Skin over the site of a soft tissue tumor should be handled gently during hair removal and antisepsis. Vigorous scrubbing could dislodge underlying tumor cells. In vascular tumors, manipulation during positioning or skin preparation could cause vascular complications such as emboli or hemorrhage.
2. Gowns, gloves, drapes, and instruments are changed following a biopsy (e.g., a breast biopsy) before incision for a radical resection (e.g., a mastectomy). The tumor is deliberately incised to obtain a biopsy for diagnosis. However, margins of healthy tissue surrounding a radical resection must not be inoculated with tumor cells.
3. Instruments placed in direct contact with tumor cells are discarded immediately after use. Even when the tumor appears to be localized, most cancers have disseminated to some degree. Therefore some surgeons prefer to use each instrument once and then discard it.
4. Some surgeons prefer to irrigate the surgical site with sterile water instead of sterile normal saline solution to cause destruction of cancerous cells by crenation.
5. Antibiotics are administered preoperatively, intraoperatively, and postoperatively as a prophylactic measure to provide an adequate antibacterial level to prevent wound infection.
6. Time-honored precautions such as handling tissue gently, keeping blood loss to a minimum, and avoiding an unduly prolonged surgical procedure influence the outcome for the patient.

Messages should be conveyed periodically during a long radical surgical procedure to the patient's anxiously waiting family members or significant others to reassure them that their loved one is receiving care from a concerned operating room (OR) team.

ENDOCRINE THERAPY

Tumors arising in organs that are usually under hormonal influence, such as breast and uterus in a female patient and prostate and testes in a male patient, may be stimulated by hormones produced in the endocrine glands. Cellular metabolism is affected by the presence of specific hormone receptors in tumor cells: estrogen and/or progesterone in a female and androgens in a male. Some breast, endometrial, and prostatic cancers depend on these hormones for growth and maintenance. Recurrence or spread of disease may be retarded by therapeutic hormonal manipulation. Endocrine manipulation does not cure, but it can control dissemination of the disease if the tumor progresses beyond the limits of effective surgical resection or radiation therapy. Cancer of the breast or prostate may metastasize to soft tissues or to the brain, lung, liver, and bone.

Hormonal Receptor Site Studies

Identifying hormonal dependence of the primary tumor by receptor site studies is a fairly reliable way of selecting patients who will benefit postoperatively from endocrine manipulation. Following a positive diagnosis of cancer, either by a frozen section biopsy or by pathologic permanent sections, the surgeon will probably request receptor site evaluation of a primary breast, uterine, or prostatic tumor. The tissue specimen removed by surgical resection should *not* be placed in formalin preservative solution because this will alter the receptor cells enough to negate hormonal study.

Endocrine Ablation

Since 1896, surgeons have described positive clinical responses in patients with metastatic breast cancer treated by *endocrine ablation,* the surgical removal of endocrine glands. If the surgeon plans to eliminate endocrine stimulation surgically in a patient with a known hormone-dependent tumor, all sources of the hormone should be ablated.

Bilateral Adrenaloophorectomy

Both adrenal glands and ovaries may be resected to prevent recurrence, control soft tissue metastases, or relieve bone pain from metastatic breast cancer. These may be removed as a one-stage surgical procedure (i.e., bilateral adrenaloophorectomy). If two separate surgical procedures are preferred, bilateral oophorectomy precedes bilateral adrenalectomy, except in menopausal women in whom only the latter surgical procedure may be indicated. (See Chapter 30, p. 622, for discussion of oophorectomy and Chapter 31, p. 647, for discussion of adrenalectomy.)

Bilateral Orchiectomy and Adrenalectomy

Both testes may be removed (i.e., bilateral orchiectomy) to eliminate androgens of testicular origin following prostatectomy for advanced carcinoma of the prostate. Bilateral adrenalectomy may also be indicated.

Hypophysectomy

Enucleation of the pituitary gland (i.e., hypophysectomy) may be indicated to eliminate stimulating hormones produced by the pituitary in patients with recurrent or progressive breast or prostatic cancer.

Hormonal Therapy

Hormones administered orally or intramuscularly can alter cell metabolism by changing the systemic hormonal environment of the body. To be effective, tumor cells must contain receptors. Hormones must bind to these receptors before they can exert an effect on cells.

Androgens

A male sex hormone (i.e., androgen) is given to women with cancer of the breast to inhibit estrogen action following oophorectomy or during the normal postmenopausal life cycle. Preparations of testosterone are most commonly used.

Estrogens

A female sex hormone (i.e., estrogen) is given to both men with prostatic carcinoma and women with breast cancer. Diethylstilbestrol is one of the most common estrogens for both sexes.

Progesterones

Progesterone inhibits proliferation of endometrium and will retard the growth of some endometrial carcinomas. It also is given to retard renal cell and breast cancers.

Antiestrogen Therapy

Patients with medical contraindications to endocrine ablation may receive antiestrogen therapy. An estrogen antagonist deprives an estrogen-dependent tumor of estrogen necessary for its growth. Nafoxidine hydrochloride and tamoxifen citrate (Nolvadex), which are synthetic nonsteroidal drugs, inhibit normal intake of estrogen at estrogen receptor sites. They are taken orally. Tamoxifen may be useful in palliative treatment of advanced breast and ovarian cancer in postmenopausal women.

Corticosteroids

When bilateral adrenalectomy or hypophysectomy is contraindicated, corticosteroids may be administered to suppress estrogen production. Prednisone, cortisone, hydrocortisone, or some other preparation of corticosteroids may be administered as an antiinflammatory agent, along with chemotherapeutic agents given for control of disseminated disease.

PHOTODYNAMIC THERAPY

For photodynamic therapy, also referred to as *photoradiation,* an argon tunable dye laser is used to destroy malignant cells by photochemical reaction. A photosensitive drug, either hematoporphyrin derivative (HpD) from cow's blood (Photofrin) or purified dihematoporphyrin ether, is absorbed by malignant and reticular endothelial cells. The drug is injected intravenously via venipuncture or Hickman catheter 24 to 48 hours before the photodynamic therapy. It is taken up by cells to make them fluorescent and photosensitive. It remains longer in malignant cells than in normal cells before it is excreted from the body. When exposed to light from an argon laser, the tunable rhodamine-B dye laser produces a red beam of approximately 630 nanometers. Other dyes, such as dicyanomethylene, may produce different wavelengths. HpD in cells absorbs the light beam, causing a photochemical reaction. This reaction causes tissue-oxygen molecules to release cytotoxic singlet oxygen and thus destroy tumor cells. The laser can be delivered interstitially, endoscopically, externally, or retrobulbarly, depending on tumor site.

Photodynamic therapy may be used to debulk tumors of the eye, head and neck, breast, esophagus, gastrointestinal tract, bronchus, and bladder. The tunable dye laser may also be used to diagnose tumor cells. The OR should be darkened or have shades to block outside daylight during the laser treatment. After injection of dye and postoperatively, the patient is cautioned to avoid exposure to sunlight or other sources of ultraviolet light. Photosensitivity is the primary side effect of the dye and may last 4 to 6 weeks.

RADIATION THERAPY

Treatment of malignant disease with radiation may be referred to as *radiation therapy, brachytherapy,* or *radiotherapy.* It involves the use of high-voltage irradiation and other radioactive elements to injure or destroy cells. Like surgical resection and photodynamic therapy, radiation is localized therapy applicable for a limited number of specific tumors. Radiation is the emission of electromagnetic waves or atomic particles from the disintegration of nuclei of unstable or radioactive elements. Ionizing radiation is used for therapy.

Ionizing Radiation

Ionization is a physical production of positive and negative ions capable of conducting electricity. Radiation of sufficient energy to disrupt the electronic balance of an atom is *ionizing radiation.* When this takes place in tissue cells or extracellular fluids, the effect can range from minor changes to profound disturbances. Radiation may come from particles of the nuclei of disintegrating atoms or from electromagnetic waves that have no mass. Types of ionizing radiation include the following:

1. *Alpha particles.* Alpha particles are relatively large particles that have a very slight penetrating power. They are stopped by a thin sheet of paper. They have dense ionization but can produce tremendous tissue destruction within a short distance.
2. *Beta particles.* Beta particles, relatively small, are electrical and travel with the speed of light. They have greater penetrating properties than do alpha particles. Their emissions cause tissue necrosis. They produce ionization, which has destructive properties.
3. *Gamma rays and x-rays.* Electromagnetic radiation of short wavelength but high energy, gamma rays and x-rays are capable of completely penetrating the body. They affect tumor tissue more rapidly than normal tissue. Rays are stopped by a thick lead shield. Protons ranging in energy from 30 kilovolts (kV) to 35 million electron volts (eV) are available for treatment of various cancers. Gamma rays are emitted spontaneously from nucleus of the atom of a radioactive element.

Effects of Radiation on Cells

Cancer cells multiply out of normal body control. They are in a state of active, uncontrolled mitosis, the nuclear division of the cytoplasm and nucleus. Radiation affects the metabolic activity of cells. Cells in an active state of mitosis are most susceptible. However, effects of radiation also depend to a large extent on tissue oxygenation. As a tumor grows, the periphery is well oxygenated, but the central portion becomes necrotic and poorly oxygenated. The cells killed by radiation are directly related to both amount of tissue and oxygen within tumor. Therefore the hypoxic effect is a factor in determining therapeutic radiation dose. Gamma rays and x-rays, acting over a period of time, cause a cessation of cell growth and regression of tumor mass. Cells die and are replaced by fibrous tissue.

Sensitivity to radiation varies. Some tumors can be destroyed by a small amount of radiation; others require a large amount. The sensitivity of the normal cells from which the tumor cells are derived determines the sensitivity of the tumor cells. Cells originating from bone marrow and lymphoid tissue are especially susceptible to radiation. Tumors in bone are resistant.

Dosage of radiation cannot be limited solely to the area to be treated. Danger of injuring normal surrounding tissue is a limiting factor in dosage and selection of the most appropriate type of radiation therapy. A factor in dosage is the ratio of tumor tissue to the surrounding normal tissue. Dosage is computed in rads. A *rad* (roentgen absorbed dose) is the unit used to measure the absorbed dose of radiation. One rad is the amount of radiation required to deposit 100 ergs of energy per gram of tissue. The dosage of irradiation delivered to a specific tissue site is measured by distance from the source and duration of exposure by radiophysics or by instruments such as Geiger counters or scintillation probes. Doses are measured in rads to determine whether dosage is adequate for therapy but not so excessive that it would cause damage to normal tissues.

Radiation energy penetration is calculated from the rate of decay or disintegration, known as half-life. *Half-life* is the time required for half the radioactive element to disintegrate and to lose one half its activity by decay.

Sources of Radiation

Although effects are similar, sources and their application for radiation therapy differ. Some sources are implanted into the body in direct contact with tumor tissue; others are passed through the body to the tumor from an external beam.

Radium

Radium is a radioactive metal. Mme. Marie Curie, a research chemist, and her husband, a physicist, discovered and named it in 1898. Several years earlier, Mme. Curie had been given the task of finding out why pitchblende would record its image on a photographic plate. She and her husband knew that pitchblende emitted more radiation than the known minerals in it justified. It took 6 years of painstaking, difficult work for the Curies to isolate radium as a pure element and learn of its radioactive properties. Their research eventually led to the use of radium in the treatment of malignant tumors.

Metallic radium is unstable in air. Radium chloride or bromide salts emit fluorescence and heat. One gram gives off 134 calories per hour. Alpha and beta particles and gamma rays are products of its disintegration. The half-life of radium is about 1620 years; half the remaining life is lost in another 1620 years, and so on. The final product is lead.

Radon

Radon is a dense radioactive gas liberated as the first by-product from the disintegration of radium. Mme. Curie discovered this gas and first named it "emanation." Radon is collected by an intricate process in radiopaque glass or gold capillary tubing. Seeds for implantation are then cut and sealed. Dosage is computed for the hours of insertion into tissue. It is measured in millicurie-hours. The half-life of radon is 4 days; its total life is about 30 days.

Radionuclides

A radionuclide is an element that has been bombarded in a nuclear reactor with radioactive particles. It shows radioactive disintegration and emits either alpha and beta particles or gamma rays. Those emitting beta particles and gamma rays are used primarily for treating malignant tumors. Therapeutic radionuclides may also be referred to as *radiopharmaceuticals*. Historically they were known as *radioactive isotopes*, or *radioisotopes*, and these terms are still found in the literature. Cesium, cobalt, iodine, iridium, and yttrium are the most commonly used elements for therapy. *Brachytherapy*, internal application with sealed sources of radionuclides, has almost totally supplanted the use of radium and radon. The gamma rays of cesium 137, for example, have greater penetrating power than do those of radium.

Radionuclides are controlled by the Atomic Energy Commission and are released only to individuals trained and licensed to use them. Available in liquid or solid forms, they may be ingested orally, infused intravenously, instilled into a body cavity, injected or implanted into a tumor, or applied to the skin externally. The ionizing radiation emitted has an action on tissue similar to that of radium, but radionuclides differ from radium in the following ways:

1. Half-life is short. Radionuclides disintegrate at varying rates depending on their type. Each element has a specific half-life, but each one is different, varying from a few hours, such as the 6 hours of technetium 99, to the 8 days of iodine 131 or the 5.3 years of cobalt 60.
2. Irradiation does not spread so much into adjoining tissue; therefore a stronger dose can be used in a malignant tumor. Radiation is not absorbed by bone and other normal body tissues.
3. Irradiation can be more easily shielded. The surgeon and other personnel get less radiation exposure in placing or removing radionuclides.

Exposure to radionuclides, like exposure to radium and radon, is always potentially dangerous. Radiation may treat cancer, but it can also cause a malignant neoplasm.

Implantation of Radiation Sources

All radiation sources for implantation are prepared in the desired therapeutic dosages by the nuclear medicine department. Many types of sources are used to deliver maximum radiation to the primary tumor. No single type is ideal for every tumor or anatomic site.

Interstitial Needles

Interstitial needles are hollow sheaths, usually made of platinum or Monel metal. Radium salts or radionuclides are encased in platinum or platinum-iridium short units or cells, which in turn are sealed in the metal sheath of the needle for implantation into tumor tissue. A needle may contain one or several short units or cells of the radiation source, depending on the length of needle to be used. Needles vary in length from 10 to 60 mm, with a diameter of 1 to 2 mm. The choice of length depends on the area involved, as well as dosage. Dosage is measured in milligram hours, which can be converted to rads.

Needles, usually containing cesium 137, are implanted in tumors near the body surface or in tissue accessible enough to permit their use, such as in the vagina, cervix, tongue, mouth, or neck. In selected patients, stereotactic techniques are used to implant needles to irradiate brain tumors. In the OR these needles are inserted at periphery of and within the tumor. One end of the needle is pointed and the other has an eye for a heavy (size 2) suture. Needles are threaded to prevent loss while in use and to aid in removal. After the surgeon inserts the needles, the ends of sutures are tied or taped together and taped to the skin in an adjoining area or secured to buttons. Depending on the anatomic site, a template may be used to position and secure needles. The template consists of two acrylic plates with rubber O rings between them that are held together with screws. The plates have holes for insertion of the interstitial needles. The template remains in place until the needles are removed. Needles are usually left in place for 4 to 7 days, depending on planned dosage to the tumor bed.

Interstitial Seeds

Sealed radionuclide seeds may be implanted permanently or temporarily. Because they have a short half-life, gold seeds are permanently implanted, most commonly into the prostate, lungs, or pancreas. Seeds containing cesium 137, iridium 192, or iodine 125 implanted directly into tumor tissue are removed after the desired exposure. Seeds are useful in body cavities, localized areas, and tumors that are not resectable because they are located near major vessels or the spinal cord. Because they are small, seeds can be placed to fit a curved area without immobilization. However, they may move about if there is much motion.

Seeds are 7 mm or less in length, 0.75 mm in diameter, with a wall 0.3 mm thick. Length depends on desired dosage. Seeds can be inserted with or without an invasive surgical procedure. They may be strung on a strand of suture material or placed in a hollow plastic tube with sealed ends. With a needle attached, the strand or tube is woven or pulled through the tumor. Seeds in a plastic tube may be inserted through a hollow needle like a catheter through a trocar. Empty tubes may be inserted in the OR and afterloaded (i.e., seeds put into the tube at a later time and place). A microprocessor-controlled machine that pulls wire attached to radioactive material through the tube may be used for remote afterloading.

Intracavitary Capsules

A sealed capsule of radium, cesium 137, iodine 125, yttrium 192, or cobalt 60 may be placed into a body cavity or orifice. Usually used to treat tumors in the cervix or endometrium of the uterus, a capsule is inserted via the vagina. The capsule may be a single tube of radioactive pins fixed in a tandem loader or a group of individual capsules, each containing one radioactive pin. These methods are used for treating cancer of the uterine corpus.

In a patient with cervical cancer, an instrument such as an Ernst applicator is employed. A metal or plastic tube with radioactive pins is inserted in the uterus. Metal pins are used in conjunction with hyperthermia (see p. 930). The tube is attached to two vaginal ovoids, each containing a radioactive pin, that are placed in the cul-de-sac around the cervix. This type of application delivers the desired dosage in a pear-shaped volume of tissue, which includes the cervix, corpus, and tissue around the cervix but spares the bladder and rectum from high doses of irradiation.

A blunt intracavitary applicator is used to position the parts. The applicator must be held securely and remain fixed to ensure proper dosage to the tumor without injury to normal surrounding structures. The surgeon may suture the applicator to the cervix for stabilization. Vaginal packing is used. Two different methods of application are employed to insert the radiation source.

Afterloading Techniques Afterloading techniques afford the greatest safety for OR personnel. A "cold," unloaded, hollow plastic or metal applicator, such as the Fletcher afterloader, is inserted into or adjacent to tissues to receive radiation. This is done in the OR. After x-ray verification of correct placement, the radiation source is loaded into the applicator at the patient's bedside.

Preloading Techniques Preloading techniques require insertion of the "hot" radiation capsule in the OR by the surgeon. OR personnel should not be permitted in the room during this procedure. To deliver a uniform dose to the desired area, the surgeon inserts an adjustable device, such as the Ernst applicator, designed to hold the radiation source in proper position in the tissues. The bladder and rectum are held away from the area with packs to avoid undesired radiation. To calculate the dosage the surgeon checks the position of the radiation source on x-ray films of the pelvis to measure distances from critical sites.

NOTE All preparations for insertion are made by nursing team members before they leave the room. (They wait in substerile room during insertion.) Preparations include setting sterile table with vaginal packing, antibiotic cream for packing, radiopaque solutions for x-ray studies, basin of sterile water; placing x-ray cassette on the operating table and notifying radiology technician; obtaining the radiation source; positioning patient; and putting a radiation sheet on patient's chart and card on the stretcher.

Intracavitary Colloidal Suspensions

Sterile radioactive colloidal suspensions of gold or phosphorus are used as palliative therapy to limit growth of metastatic tumors in the pleural or peritoneal cavities. The effect is caused by the emission of beta particles, which penetrate tissue so slightly that radioactivity is limited to the immediate area in which the colloidal suspension is placed. A trocar and cannula are introduced into the pleural or peritoneal cavity. The coloidal suspension is injected through the cannula from a lead-shielded syringe. These instruments must be stored in a remote area until decay of radioactivity is complete. Radioactive colloidal gold 198 is most commonly used;

it has a half-life of 2.7 days. It may also be instilled within the bladder.

Safety Rules for Handling Radiation Sources

The following principles of radiation safety for both personnel and patients apply to handling all types of radioactive materials. The cardinal factors of protection are *distance, time,* and *shielding.*

1. Radiation intensity varies inversely with the square of the distance from it; double distance equals one-quarter intensity, etc. Personnel must stay as far from the source as is feasible.
2. Radiation sources (i.e., needles, seeds, capsules, and suspensions) are prepared by personnel in the nuclear medicine department from behind a lead screen with hands protected by lead-lined gloves, if possible, or special forceps during handling.
3. Radiation sources are transported in a long-handled lead carrier so that they are as close to the floor and as far away from the body of the transporter as possible. The lead carrier should be stored away from personnel and patient traffic areas while it is in the OR suite.
4. Each needle, seed, or capsule is counted by the surgeon with the radiation therapist when radiation sources are delivered to the OR. The number is recorded.
5. Glutaraldehyde solution is poured into the lead carrier to completely submerge the radiation sources. When ready to use, the lead carrier is transported into the OR. Needles, seeds, or capsules are removed from the lead container with sterile, long-handled instruments and *rinsed thoroughly* with sterile water.
6. All radiation sources are handled with special, long, ring-handled forceps from behind a lead protection shield. *Never touch radiation sources with bare hands or gloves.* Radiation sources are never handled with a crushing forceps because the seal of hollow containers can be broken. A groove-tipped forceps, designed for this purpose, is used.
7. Radiation sources are handled as quickly as possible to limit the time personnel are exposed to radiation.
8. Account for all radiation sources before and after use. Report any loss at once to the OR nurse manager. Do not remove anything from the room. Call a radiation therapist or nuclear medicine department technician to bring a Geiger counter to locate a lost radiation source. This instrument has a radiation-sensitive gauge with an indicator that moves and a sound that increases when near radioactive substances.

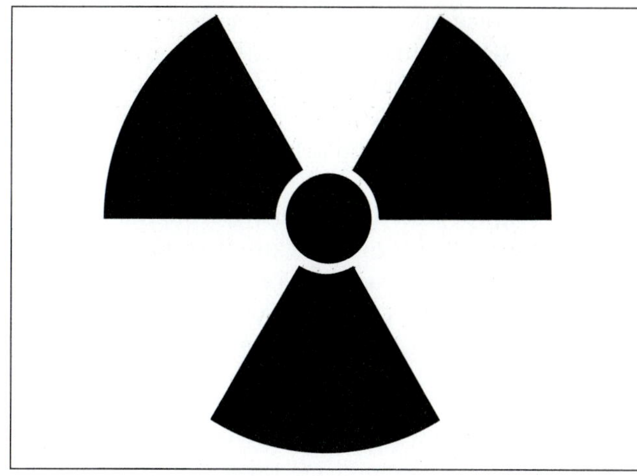

FIGURE 45-1 Universal symbol for radiation. Symbol is dark purple on a solid yellow background.

9. A *radiation documentation* sheet is completed and put in the patient's chart. The surgeon fills in the amount and exact time of insertion and the time the source is to be removed. Each nurse who cares for the patient on the unit signs this sheet in turn just before going off duty, thereby passing responsibility for checking the patient and radiation source to the nurse who relieves. To check needles, sutures attached to each needle are counted.
10. Patient's bed and door of the room are conspicuously labeled with a "radiation in use" card or symbol (Figure 45-1).
11. Radiation source is removed by the surgeon at the exact time indicated so patient will not be overexposed.
12. Be careful—observe rules. Radiation is not seen or felt. See Chapter 10, pp. 144-148, for procedures to monitor and minimize exposure.

External Beam Radiation Therapy

Ionizing radiations of gamma or x-rays generated from machines are used externally to alter tumor cells within the body. This type of radiation therapy is noninvasive.

A maximum dose of radiation is concentrated below the skin on the malignant tumor, with a minimum dose to surrounding tissue. The angle of approach is changed a number of times during treatment to spread amount of radiation to normal tissue over as wide an area as possible. *Orthovoltage,* low-voltage equipment producing 200 to 500 kV, and *megavoltage* equipment, such as cobalt 60 beams and linear accelerators or betatrons, are in use for external beam radiation therapy.

External radiation may be the only therapeutic modality used to cure some cancers. The dosage of radiation that will provide the optimal cure with an acceptable balance of complications is difficult to determine. With the advent of stereotactic techniques and the use of megavoltage equipment, intense rays can deliver cancericidal doses without permanently injuring normal tissue and causing skin irritation. Even so, most oncologists recommend a combination of radiation therapy and surgical resection for many tumors. Radiation therapy may be administered preoperatively and/or postoperatively or intraoperatively. External radiation therapy may also be combined with internal sources such as intracavitary radiation capsules to build up dosage to large tumor areas.

Intraoperative Radiation Therapy

Delivery of a single high dose of radiation directly to an intraabdominal or intrapelvic tumor or tumor bed during a surgical procedure may provide an additional palliative or localized means of control. Normal organs or tissues can be shielded from exposure. Radiation may be used following resection of the bulk of the tumor. An orthovoltage unit may be installed in the OR. The sterile Lucite cone is placed directly over the tumor site. All team members must leave the room during treatment. The room must be lead-lined. In some hospitals the patient is geographically transported from the OR to the radiation therapy department. Following exposure to a megavoltage electron beam, the wound may be closed in the treatment area or the patient may be returned to the OR for further surgery and/or wound closure. The open wound must be covered with a sterile drape during transport, and sterile technique is used for closure.

Stereotactic Radiosurgery

For stereotactic radiosurgery, referred to as the *gamma knife*, highly concentrated doses of gamma rays are directed at an inoperable or deep-seated brain tumor. The localized area is determined by stereotaxis. The neurosurgeon fixes the patient's head within a collimator helmet so that the focusing channels will direct cobalt 60 beams to the tumor. The radiation sources are housed in a large spherical chamber. The helmet fits into the chamber.

CHEMOTHERAPY

In 1854 the first drug used for cancer chemotherapy was synthesized. However, this type of therapy did not attract much attention until after World War II, when reports were published purporting that tumor cells circulate in the venous blood of patients undergoing surgical procedures. Administration of chemotherapeutic agents during and shortly after a surgical procedure, in the hope of destroying these cells, seemed justified in selected patients. Nitrogen mustard was first used in 1942. A cooperative clinical study involving 23 medical centers was begun in 1958 to evaluate the efficacy of triethylenephosphoramide following radical mastectomy. Since then, many researchers have investigated over a quarter of a million compounds in search of systemic antineoplastic substances that would kill tumor cells without excessive toxicity or damage to normal cells.

A variety of chemotherapeutic agents are capable, either alone or in combination, of providing measurable palliative remission or regression of primary and metastatic disease with decrease in size of tumor and no new metastases. In some instances a complete response with disappearance of all clinical evidence of tumor is achieved. The trend is toward earlier and greater use of adjuvant chemotherapy. More than one agent may be administered to enhance the action of another cytotoxic or antigenic substance. Adjuvant therapy is designed to maximize the benefits of each agent in the combination while avoiding overlapping toxicities. The following factors are important in determining the ability of tumor cells to respond to chemotherapy:

1. Size and location of tumor. The smaller the tumor, the easier it will be to reach cells. The mechanism for passage of drugs into the brain differs from that for other body organs.
2. Type of tumor. Cells of solid tumors in the lung, stomach, colon, and breast may be more resistant than cells in the lymphatic system, for example.
3. Combinations of adjunctive and adjuvant therapy. Chemotherapy may be used as an adjunct to all other types of therapy in selected patients. Precise scheduling of dosages is necessary to attain effective results.
4. Specific biochemical requirements of the tumor. Agents are selected according to the appropriateness of their structure and function. More than one agent is usually given.
5. State of cancer cell life cycle. An understanding of this phenomenon is necessary for understanding chemotherapy. Cancer cells go through the same life-cycle phases as do normal cells.

Cell Life Cycle

Deoxyribonucleic acid (DNA) is a double molecule in the cell nucleus that contains its genetic code. DNA is capable of reproducing itself and also of producing ribonucleic acid (RNA), which in turn synthesizes protein. Protein is essential for cellular function. Therefore DNA is vital to cell viability. It regulates the processes of growth, rate of mitosis, differentiation, specialization, and death of cells. Cell division requires assimilation of nutrients in the cell, their incorporation into DNA, synthesis of new DNA, and splitting of DNA to form two new cells. RNA is synthesized in the rest intervals between phases of DNA replication. Duration of the rest interval is related to the proliferative activity of the tissue cells. Malignant tumor cells may proliferate more rapidly than normal cells.

Action of Chemotherapeutic Agents

Antineoplastic cytotoxic agents are destructive to rapidly dividing cells. However, each dose will kill only a fractional portion of the tumor cells present. The action of these agents takes place within the cell, but each agent acts differently to interrupt the cell life cycle. Antineoplastic agents are classified according to their structure and function. Only a few of the many agents in use are mentioned as examples of each classification. Cytotoxic action may be:

1. *Cell-cycle specific.* An agent may affect cell during one or more phases and have no adverse effect during other phases. Some interfere with DNA synthesis; others inhibit mitosis when the cell is most susceptible; still others prolong rest intervals.
   a. *Antimetabolites* affect cells as they enter the DNA synthesis phase, thus interfering with RNA synthesis. This causes death of the cell by inhibiting the DNA cycle. These agents include floxuridine (FUDR), 5-fluorouracil (5-FU), and methotrexate.
   b. *Mitotic inhibitors* prevent cell division in a subphase of mitosis. They may be plant alkaloids such as vinblastine sulfate (Velban), vincristine sulfate (Oncovin), and paclitaxel (Taxol), or enzymes such as L-asparaginase (Elspar).
2. *Cell-cycle nonspecific.* Agents affect the cell throughout the entire life cycle. They have a more prolonged action that is independent of the phases of the life cycle.
   a. *Alkylating agents* denature or inhibit DNA to interfere with mitosis and synthesis, thereby preventing rapid cell growth. Their action is similar to that of radiation therapy. These agents include cyclophosphamide (Cytoxan), melphalan (L-phenylalanine mustard, L-PAM), mechlorethamine hydrochloride (Mustargen), chlorambucil (Leukeran), and cisplatin (Platinol).
   b. *Antibiotics* bind with DNA to block RNA production, thus disrupting cellular metabolism. Those used as antineoplastic agents include dactinomycin, actinomycin D (Cosmegen), bleomycin sulfate (Blenoxane), doxorubicin hydrochloride (Adriamycin), and daunorubicin hydrochloride (Cerubidine).

Indications for Chemotherapy

Patients at risk for or with systemic signs of advanced or disseminated disease, generally indicated by extranodal involvement, may be candidates for chemotherapy preoperatively or postoperatively.

Preoperative Therapy

The objective of preoperative therapy may be to shrink the tumor sufficiently to permit radical surgical resection. Tumor regression with tumor necrosis may occur with or without adjunctive radiation therapy. Agents may eliminate subclinical microscopic metastatic disease.

Postoperative Therapy

Surgical resection followed by regional chemotherapy often can control local disease to keep a tumor in remission. Residual metastatic disease may be treated with systemic chemotherapy to cure the patient or prolong life. Multiple doses may be given over a long period of time (several months to a year or more) to delay recurrence of the tumor.

Administration of Agents

The method of administration depends on how disseminated or localized the tumor cells are and on the agent, or combination of agents, selected. Agents can be instilled locally into a target site by continuous infusion, injected intramuscularly or intrathecally, infused by intravenous push or drip, or ingested orally. A patient with widely disseminated metastatic cells usually receives systemic chemotherapy via the intravenous, intramuscular, or oral route. Agents may be infused regionally for patients whose tumor cannot be removed because of its location (e.g., a primary or metastatic tumor in the liver). The patient may come to the OR for insertion of an indwelling catheter or implantable infusion pump.

Infusion Catheters

An indwelling infusion catheter may be placed percutaneously or directly into a vein or artery or into a body cavity. Continuous or intermittent infusion of the chemotherapeutic agent can be maintained by means of a portable infusion pump attached to the catheter.

Central Venous Catheter Under local anesthesia, a long-term Hickman or other central venous catheter is inserted. The catheter may be used for other purposes (see Chapter 8, p. 111, for discussion of central venous cannulation for hyperalimentation).

Hepatic Artery Catheter Hepatic artery catheterization may be performed to establish regional chemotherapy to metastases in the liver. The catheter may be inserted percutaneously, under local anesthesia, into left axillary artery and threaded into common hepatic artery. This technique eliminates need for laparotomy to cannulate hepatic arteries. However, some patients have variant anatomy that requires a dual catheter delivery system. Vascular reconstruction, ligation, and/or occlusion of an artery may be necessary for local/regional perfusion. Regardless of method of catheterization, an infusion pump is attached to the catheter(s) to deliver the cytotoxic agent to the tumor.

Intraperitoneal Catheter Under local anesthesia, a Tenckhoff catheter is inserted into the peritoneal cavity. Incision in the anterior abdominal wall usually is located just lateral to right or left of rectus abdominis muscle at level of the umbilicus. The anterior rectus sheath is incised to allow a Verres needle to penetrate the peritoneum. Air is injected before catheter is placed in the peritoneal cavity so that the catheter will not kink (i.e., lie straight). A subcutaneous tunnel is made between the initial incision and stab wound to secure the catheter. Intraperitoneal chemotherapy permits delivery of high concentrations of an agent to an ovarian or colorectal tumor without exposing normal tissues systemically. The agent exits the peritoneal cavity via the portal circulation.

Infusion Devices

Devices with reservoirs for the chemotherapeutic agent are implanted into body tissues.

Subcutaneous Infusion Ports Under local anesthesia, a venous access device is implanted subcutaneously for intermittent injections of cytotoxic agent(s). The device consists of a plastic or silicone rubber self-sealing port on a plastic or stainless steel reservoir, depending on the manufacturer. The catheter attached to the reservoir is inserted into a central vein, hepatic artery, peritoneal cavity, or epidural space. A tunnel is created from point where the catheter enters vessel, cavity, or space to a subcutaneous pocket. The pocket is made over a bony prominence or under clavicle to stabilize the port. The reservoir is sutured to underlying fascia. A Huber needle with an angled tip is used to enter the port for heparinizing and infusing agents. Extension tubing may connect the needle to an infusion pump for continuous infusion. Thrombosis and infection are potential complications of long-term venous access devices.

Implantable Infusion Pump With the patient under general anesthesia, an infusion catheter is placed into an artery, vein, body space, or ventricle for localized chemotherapy to liver, head and neck, or brain tumor. The infusion pump device (Infusaid) is implanted in a subcutaneous pocket created in the abdominal wall, beneath the clavicle, or under the scalp. The titanium, stainless steel, and silicone rubber device resembles a hockey puck. The inner reservoir is filled with cytotoxic agent. When the reservoir is collapsed by pressure, the agent is infused into the catheter. The pump must be warmed initially to activate the fluorocarbon propellant in the chamber around the reservoir. It is placed over a bony prominence for support when refilling. The drug is replenished periodically by percutaneous injection. These implanted infusion devices also are used for control of severe systemic conditions, such as diabetes, thromboembolic disease, or pain from a malignancy. Insulin, heparin, or morphine is infused, respectively.

Safe Handling of Agents

Antineoplastic cytotoxic agents have carcinogenic and mutagenic properties, and most can cause local and/or allergic reactions. Personnel must avoid inadvertent direct skin or eye contact, inhalation, and ingestion of these agents during handling. Written precautions and procedures for handling, preparing, administering, and disposing of cytotoxic agents must be followed. Some basic guidelines include:

1. Protect yourself from skin and respiratory contact. Preferably, prepare agents under a vertical laminar flow hood. Whether or not a containment hood is available, wear thick gloves, mask, eye protection, and gown.
2. Wash hands after handling agents and all items that have been in contact with them, including those used for administration.
3. Place all cytotoxic waste in sealed, leakproof bags or containers. Incineration is recommended for all materials used in preparing and administering cytotoxic agents.

Toxic Side Effects

Cytotoxic agents are destructive to rapidly dividing cancer cells, but they also affect rapidly dividing normal cells such as hematopoietic cells of bone marrow, epithelial cells of oral cavity and gastrointestinal tract, and hair follicles. Patients must be informed of the toxic side effects to be expected from the specific agents they are receiving. These can include:

1. *Alopecia.* Loss of hair can occur suddenly or gradually. This can be devastating to the patient's self-image. It is most often caused by the alkylating and plant alkaloid agents and by some antibiotics. Hair grows back after therapy is discontinued.
2. *Bone marrow suppression.* Suppression of bone marrow function is the most hazardous toxic effect from cytotoxic agents. Therapy may have to be discontinued to allow for bone marrow recovery. Suppression increases the patient's susceptibility to:
   a. Leukopenia. White blood cell count is lowered below normal number of leukocytes in the peripheral blood. Leukocytes protect body against invasion of microorganisms. The patient with leukopenia is therefore highly vulnerable to spread of infection from one part of body to another or to acquiring a nosocomial infection from the environment.
   b. Thrombocytopenia. The number of platelets in the blood decreases below normal with variable consequences. Spontaneous hemorrhage into the skin,

sclera, joints, or brain may occur. Normal blood clotting time can be prolonged. The patient may require platelet transfusion.

3. *Gastrointestinal disturbances.* Anorexia, nausea, vomiting, and/or diarrhea are common complaints. Usually these subside within a few hours or days after each dose is administered.
4. *Neurotoxicity.* Symptoms of neurotoxicity to the plant alkaloids usually begin with constipation. Toxicity can progress to impaired sensation, ataxia, and an unsteady gait. The effects are cumulative during the course of therapy but reversible when therapy is discontinued.
5. *Stomatitis.* Ulcerative lesions in the mouth and oropharynx are often early signs of severe toxicity from antimetabolite and antibiotic agents. These can be very painful and may lead to secondary infection.
6. *Vein hyperpigmentation.* A dark discoloration of a vein may occur over the length of the arm during prolonged infusion of some agents. A vesicular rash around the injection site may develop from use of some other agents. Although unsightly, these effects are not uncomfortable for the patient.
7. *Respiratory insufficiency.* Alveolitis, interstitial fibrosis, or other symptoms of respiratory insufficiency may include dyspnea, cough, crackles (rales), and fever. As a result of bone marrow suppression and/or an altered immune system, respiratory infection can disseminate rapidly.
8. *Nephrotoxicity.* Agents excreted exclusively in urine, such as methotrexate and cisplatin, may be toxic to renal function. Adequate hydration before administration is necessary to ensure urinary creatinine clearance. Other agents may cause hematuria.

IMMUNOTHERAPY

Ancient Chinese and Arabic writings describe stimulation of the body's immune system to combat infectious diseases. Immunization against smallpox was practiced in Turkey long before Edward Jenner (1749-1823) developed a vaccine in England in the late eighteenth century. The concept developed by Jenner, Pasteur, Salk, and Sabin, to mention a few historic names, of using vaccinations and immunizations to prevent or treat infectious diseases forms the basis of modern immunotherapy.

Immunotherapy utilizes agents that stimulate or activate the body's own host defense immune system to combat disease. This is the same immune system that normally wards off microorganisms that cause infection. Cancer may become clinically apparent only when the immune system ceases to function properly. Immune response may be defective or become compromised as the disease progresses. Immunosuppression can stimulate tumor growth and prolong wound healing. If the patient can be helped to regain partial or complete immunocompetence, the immune system can be utilized against the "foreignness" of tumor cells.

Attempts to treat cancer by immunization date back to 1895. However, it was not until 1957 that antigens specific for tumors were conclusively demonstrated in animals. Although intensive research has been conducted since that time, applications of immunotherapy as a therapeutic modality remain selective and adjunctive. *Active nonspecific immunotherapy,* thought to be promising in the 1960s, stimulated antibody and lymphocyte production by injecting vaccines of bacille Calmette-Guérin (BCG, a bovine tubercle bacillus), methanol-extracted residue of BCG (MER), and *Corynebacterium parvum* (gram-positive anaerobic bacillus). Further research led to the development in the 1980s of monoclonal antibodies for identifying tumor-associated antigens and the selective use of active specific immunotherapy and biologic response modifiers.

Types and Agents

When the immune system detects antigens, such as tumor cells, it evokes an immune response to destroy them. This may be a *humoral response* of antibodies occurring in blood and tissue fluid outside the cells or a *cell-mediated immunity* taking place within or on the surface of cells. A cell-mediated reaction binds an antigen with an antigen receptor on the surface of T lymphocytes. T lymphocytes differentiate into antigen-specific "killer" cells, "suppressor" cells, "helper" cells, "memory" cells, and lymphokine-producing killer cells. Tumor-specific cytotoxic T cells can be generated from lymphocytes of a tumor-bearing host or from syngeneic lymphocytes. The objective of immunotherapy is to augment, direct, and restore the body's immune functions.

Active Specific Immunotherapy

Active tumor-specific cytotoxic T lymphocytes (CTLs) are obtained from lymphocytes in a tumor mass removed as from kidney or spleen or by resection of metastatic lymph nodes or melanoma. A vaccine is produced from the CTLs. The vaccine of specific tumor antigen stimulates the immune response by making antibodies that attack live cancer cells. Vaccine also can be produced from peripheral blood lymphocytes used to generate CTLs for *specific adoptive cellular immunotherapy.* A series of small doses of these vaccines are administered intradermally.

Biologic Response Modifiers

Agents that have the potential to alter the patient's own reaction to tumor cells (i.e., biologic response modifiers) may be used as single agents or in conjunction with other therapy. *Lymphokines* enhance the body's immune response. Lymphokines are soluble protein molecules produced by sensitized T-helper lymphocytes in contact with specific antigens.

Interleukin-2 Interleukin-2 (IL-2), found in the body in small amounts, helps stimulate and regulate cellular immunity. It also stimulates T lymphocytes to multiply and become activated. Lymphocytes activated with IL-2, known as lymphokine-activated killer (LAK) cells, preferentially lyse malignant cells. By a recombinant process of DNA fusion, an optimal immunomodulating dose of IL-2 with LAK cells is produced. By leukopheresis, the patient's lymphocytes are collected by a blood cell separator. The IL-2 is extracted and fused with cells of *Escherichia coli,* which produce large quantities of IL-2 when they reproduce. This IL-2 is incubated to generate LAK cells before it is prepared for reinfusion into the patient. The LAK cells seem to be tumor-specific when reinfused in combination with recombinant IL-2.

Interferon Interferon, a glycoprotein, directly interacts with T lymphocytes to stimulate production of killer cells. It also directly inhibits growth and division of tumor cells and stimulates antigens. Interferon can be produced from human donor blood, tissue culture, or a recombinant DNA process. Therapy supplements the body's natural supply of interferon.

Monoclonal Antibodies Monoclonal antibodies (MoAbs) can be produced by hybridoma to react with specific antigens. Tumor cells are fused with antibody-producing cells (B lymphocytes) from the spleen of an immunized mouse. The cells that survive, called *hybridomas,* are cloned for the production of monoclonal antibodies. MoAbs are used for radioimmunoimaging to locate both primary and metastatic tumors. They may be given therapeutically for immunoconjugate therapy to target tumor cells.

Active Nonspecific Immunotherapy

Levamisole is a putative immunostimulant given to stimulate host defense. It may be administered alone or with a chemotherapeutic agent such as 5-FU as adjuvant therapy for colorectal cancer.

Advantages of Immunotherapy

Immunotherapeutic agents have a relatively weak killing capacity but no limitation on the kinds of cells that they can destroy. Although highly specific, they can destroy small numbers of tumor cells but are not effective against large numbers. They can regress or eradicate a small tumor mass or eliminate cells resistant to chemotherapy. Combining these agents may accomplish what neither can do alone, either with or without surgical resection—delay recurrence and prolong survival. An immunotherapeutic agent:

1. Attacks only cancer cells
2. Does not damage normal cells
3. Can be continued for long periods with fewer hazardous side effects than chemotherapy

Hyperthermia

Hyperthermia at temperatures of 105.8° to 113° F (41° to 45° C) has a regressive tumoricidal effect with necrosis proportional to thermal dose. Thermal energy inhibits DNA synthesis. Increasing the temperature of tumor cells sensitizes them to the effects of radiation therapy or chemotherapy. Therefore hyperthermia is used as an adjunct to these therapeutic modalities for some tumors. Because drug action is greater at higher temperatures, perfusate is warmed before regional infusion of cytotoxic agents. An extremity also is warmed externally during regional perfusion. Systemic total-body hyperthermia may be applied externally by placing the patient on a hyperthermia blanket or mattress. Systemic hyperthermia can also be produced with extracorporeal circulation via a shunt placed in the thigh.

For localized palliative management of some solid tumors, a surface or interstitial hyperthermia device applies microwave energy. The temperature is measured by probes in target and surrounding normal tissue and controlled by computer adjustment of power. When tissue absorbs microwave radiation, energy converts into heat that dissipates by blood perfusion. Solid tumors with less blood perfusion dissipate heat slowly and hence retain heat longer than normal surrounding tissue.

Hyperalimentation

Cancer can cause weight loss and lead to malnutrition if sufficient nutrients are not supplied to meet the protein demands of the body and the tumor. Tumor cells extract nutrients at a rapid rate at the expense of body mass. Malnutrition depresses established cell-mediated immunity to infection and immunologic reactivity to the tumor. The only hope of cure or palliation of cancer in a malnourished patient may be a treatment that itself produces malnutrition. Healing may be delayed following operative resection in poorly nourished tissues of patients who have some degree of malabsorption of nutrients. This can deter resumption of oral intake after head and neck or gastrointestinal operations. Radiation therapy, chemotherapy, and immunotherapy can cause loss of appetite and/or nausea and often produce vomiting or diarrhea. Adequate nutrition can be maintained before and during treatment with total parenteral nutrition (TPN, see hyperalimentation in Chapter 8, pp. 111-112). Any patient who cannot be nutritionally maintained by other means is a candidate for TPN.

Patients are usually started on hyperalimentation before oncologic therapy and supported postoperatively or throughout other therapy. If the tumor responds to therapy, appetite returns, weight gain is maintained, and immunocompetent cells return as a defense mechanism against tumor cells. During this period, patients who manage their TPN at home must be taught to recognize signs and symptoms of hyperglycemia and hypoglycemia, to test blood for sugar, and to manage a volumetric infusion pump.

FUTURE OF ONCOLOGY

As described, many therapeutic modalities are used, and researchers are constantly seeking others, to improve survival rates and quality of life for patients with neoplasms. The complex nature of the disease makes adjuvant therapy and cancer research a multidisciplinary effort. Early diagnosis, while disease is still localized, is crucial for the selection of appropriate curative therapy. In poor-risk patients with extensive tumors and advanced disease, only palliative therapy may be possible.

Oncologists study the cause (epidemiology) of cancer, as well as the diagnosis, treatment, and rehabilitation of cancer patients. Moreover, patients are demanding that their surgeons give attention to reconstruction of body image and rehabilitation to a useful life. Management of cancer patients must, therefore, be accomplished through the efforts of a multidisciplinary team of surgeons in conjunction with pathologists, radiation therapists, pharmacists, immunologists, oncologists, and others. Nurses in all patient care settings must provide, in addition to physical care, psychologic support for cancer patients and their families.

Development of *hospice care* helps terminally ill cancer patients and their families cope with physical, emotional, and spiritual needs. The roots of hospice care can be traced back to the Middle Ages, but the modern team concept of care was influenced by a British physician in the 1960s. Hospice teams of physicians, nurses, social workers, and clergy provide a network of support that makes home care for the dying feasible.

BIBLIOGRAPHY

Auguste L-J, Damp KA: Radical ilioinguinal lymph node dissection, *AORN J* 58(2):294-300, 1993.

Bloom JR: Early detection of cancer, *Cancer* 74(suppl 4):1464-1473, 1994.

Engleking C: New approaches: innovations in cancer prevention, diagnosis, treatment, and support, *Oncol Nurs Forum* 21(1):62-71, 1994.

Hallenbeck P et al: Cytoreductive surgery and intraperitoneal chemotherapy, *AORN J* 56(1):50-72, 1992.

Kitrow C: Photodynamic therapy for bronchial and esophageal tumors, *AORN J* 55(6):1483-1492, 1992.

Larson DA et al: Stereotaxic irradiation of brain tumors, *Cancer* 65(suppl 3):792-799, 1990.

Larson SM et al: Overview of clinical radioimmunodetection of human tumors, *Cancer* 73(suppl 3):832-835, 1994.

Lilley LL, Scott HB: What you need to know about Taxol, *Am J Nurs* 93(12):46-50, 1993.

Meyer C: New drugs: on the oncology front, *Am J Nurs* 93(3):63-64, 1993.

Nag S et al: Comprehensive surgical radiation oncology, *AORN J* 60(1):27-37, 1994.

Roundtree D: The PIC catheter: a different approach, *Am J Nurs* 91(8):22-26, 1991.

Rowley JD et al: The impact of new DNA diagnostic technology on the management of cancer patients: survey of diagnostic techniques, *Arch Pathol Lab Med* 117(11):1104-1109, 1993.

Way L: *Current surgical diagnosis and treatment,* ed 10, Norwalk Conn, 1994, Appleton-Lange.

Wood LS, Gullo SM: IV vesicants: how to avoid extravasation, *Am J Nurs* 93(4):42-46, 1993.

Index

B

D

M

N

P

U

W

X